Medical Language for Modern Health Care

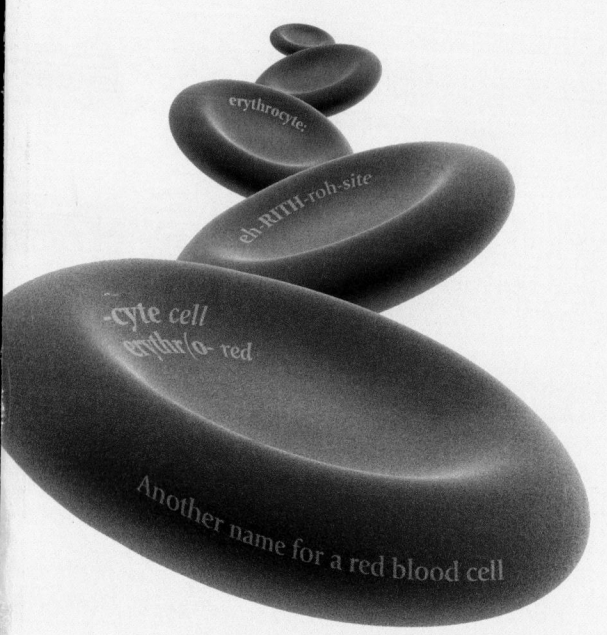

erythrocyte

eh-RITH-roh-site

-cyte cell
erythr/o- red

Another name for a red blood cell

Second Edition

David M. Allan, MA, MD

Karen D. Lockyer, BA, RHIT, CPC

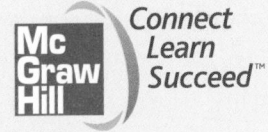

Mc Graw Hill

Connect
Learn
Succeed™

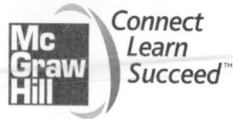

MEDICAL LANGUAGE FOR MODERN HEALTH CARE

Published by McGraw-Hill, a business unit of The McGraw-Hill Companies, Inc., 1221 Avenue of the Americas, New York, NY 10020. Copyright © 2011 by The McGraw-Hill Companies, Inc. All rights reserved. Previous edition © 2008. No part of this publication may be reproduced or distributed in any form or by any means, or stored in a database or retrieval system, without the prior written consent of The McGraw-Hill Companies, Inc., including, but not limited to, in any network or other electronic storage or transmission, or broadcast for distance learning.

Some ancillaries, including electronic and print components, may not be available to customers outside the United States.

 This book is printed on acid-free paper.

1 2 3 4 5 6 7 8 9 0 RJE/RJE 1 0 9 8 7 6 5 4 3 2 1 0

ISBN 978-0-07-337430-7
MHID 0-07-337430-X

Vice president/Editor in chief: *Elizabeth Haefele*
Vice president/Director of marketing: *John E. Biernat*
Publisher: *Kenneth S. Kasee II.*
Senior sponsoring editor: *Debbie Fitzgerald*
Senior developmental editor: *Patricia Hesse*
Marketing manager: *Mary B. Haran*
Lead media producer: *Damian Moshak*
Media development editor: *Marc Mattson*
Director, Editing/Design/Production: *Jess Ann Kosic*
Project manager: *Marlena Pechan*
Senior production supervisor: *Janean A. Utley*
Senior designer: *Srdjan Savanovic*
Lead photo research coordinator: *Carrie K. Burger*
Media project manager: *Cathy L. Tepper*
Outside development house: *Patricia Gillivan, Triple SSS Press Media Development, Inc.*
Cover design: *Srdjan Savanovic*
Typeface: *10.5/12 ITC Giovanni*
Compositor: *Laserwords Private Limited*
Printer: *R. R. Donnelley, Jefferson City, MO*
Cover credit: *© artpartner-images/Gettyimages; Back: blood cells: © Christian Anthony/iStockphoto*

Credits: The credits section for this book begins on page C-1 and is considered an extension of the copyright page.

Library of Congress Cataloging-in-Publication Data

Allan, David, 1942-
 Medical language for modern health care / David M. Allan, Karen D. Lockyer. —2nd ed.
  p. ; cm.
 Includes index.
 ISBN-13: 978-0-07-337430-7 (alk. paper)
 ISBN-10: 0-07-337430-X (alk. paper)
 1. Medicine—Terminology—Programmed instruction. I. Lockyer, Karen. II. Title.
 [DNLM: 1. Medicine. 2. Terminology as Topic. WB 100 A417m 2011]
 R123.A43 2011
 610.1'4—dc22

                                                2009042928

The Internet addresses listed in the text were accurate at the time of publication. The inclusion of a Web site does not indicate an endorsement by the authors or McGraw-Hill, and McGraw-Hill does not guarantee the accuracy of the information presented at these sites.

www.mhhe.com

DAVID ALLAN

David Allan received his medical training at Cambridge University and Guy's Hospital in England. He was Chief Resident in Pediatrics at Bellevue Hospital in New York City before moving to San Diego, California.

Dr. Allan has worked as a family physician in England, a pediatrician in San Diego, and Associate Dean at the University of California, San Diego School of Medicine. He has designed, written, and produced more than 100 award-winning multimedia programs with virtual reality as their conceptual base. Dr. Allan resides happily in San Diego and walks the beach most days.

KAREN LOCKYER

Karen Lockyer holds a degree in Health Information (RHIT), a national coding certification (CPC), and a BA from Rutgers University. She is also a credentialed member of AHIMA (American Health Information Management Association) and AAPC (American Academy of Professional Coders).

Mrs. Lockyer has worked in medical practice administration and the health information management fields for many years. She has taught medical terminology for high school, community college, and workforce development areas at the National Institutes of Health and the federal government's Office of Personnel Management. She has also taught coding and billing for undergraduate and certificate programs at the community college level.

Residing in Southlake, Texas, Karen enjoys the sights and flavors of the Southwest.

BRIEF CONTENTS

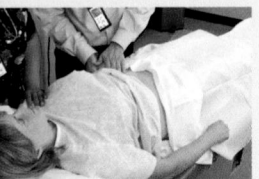
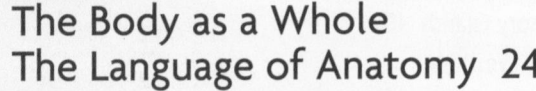
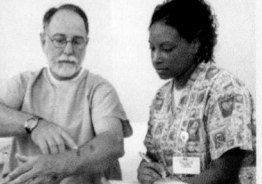

CHAPTER 4 Special Senses of the Eye and Ear
The Languages of Ophthalmology and Otology 98

CHAPTER 5 Musculoskeletal System
The Language of Orthopedics 148

CHAPTER 6 Digestive System
The Language of Gastroenterology 212

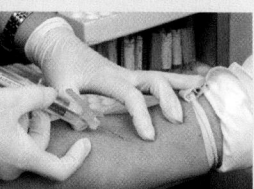
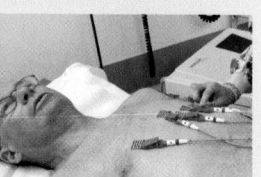

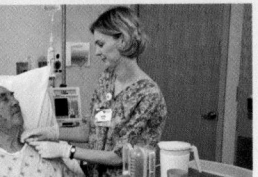
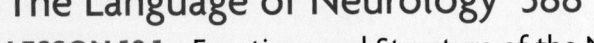

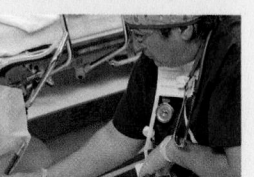
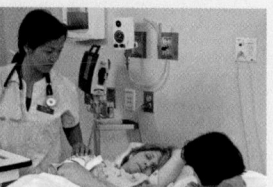

CHAPTER 14

Endocrine System
The Language of Endocrinology 566

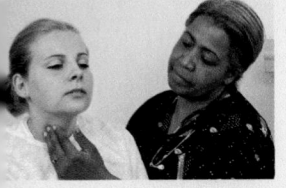

CHAPTER 15

Lymphatic and Immune Systems
The Language of Immunology 606

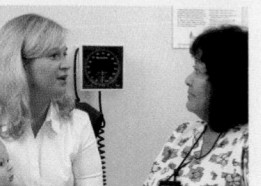

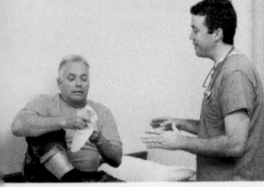

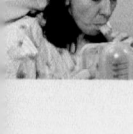

Medical Language for Modern Health Care is designed for you. The development of many medical terminology textbooks and learning programs begins with the question, "What topics should this book or program cover?" This question has been the basis of a host of textbooks available today. There is only one problem: Where do *you*, the student, fit into this question?

To put the focus back on the student, a new question guided the design and writing of *Medical Language for Modern Health Care:*

What medical terminology knowledge and skills do students preparing for careers in modern health care need to be successful?

Time and time again, instructors and students alike have indicated their belief that students learn medical language best when it is connected to real life: real health professionals interacting with real patients in a real medical setting. Just as one of the best ways to learn a foreign language is to be immersed in the language and culture of the country where it is spoken, one of the best ways to learn medical language is to be immersed within a vibrant, authentic, modern health care community.

Medical Language for Modern Health Care helps students learn the terminology and language of modern health care in a way that bridges the gap between the classroom and the clinical setting.

WHAT'S NEW

- Content updated to reflect innovations in health care
- 104 new terms defined in text and analyzed in the Word Analysis and Definition boxes
- New critical thinking exercises added based on the case reports
- Critical thinking exercises related directly to lesson objectives have been added
- New pharmacology Appendix D
- Added exercises to Appendix A
- Updated Appendix B and C
- Updated glossary and index
- **LearnSmart**™ Medical Terminology is a diagnostic study tool that adapts questioning based on an individual's response. A clearly defined learning path is developed for each student and tied to specific learning objectives. **LearnSmart** measures progress and generates student reports for the instructor.
- **McGraw-Hill** *Connect Plus*™ allows students and instructors to access all of their course materials, including the media-rich textbook, in one place. With its unique integrated learning system, *Connect Plus* combines market-leading content, a proven course architecture, and unmatched flexibility to help students apply the principles in the textbook. It contains over 10,000 exercises ranging from spelling, audio definitions, labeling, medical documents, abbreviations, word analysis, and word element definitions.

HOW STUDENTS' NEEDS ARE MET

This book was designed with your needs in mind. You are a student preparing for a career as a health professional. You may already have had a few health care–related courses, or you may just be beginning your studies in the field. While students' backgrounds and interests may differ, you and your classmates share the need to understand medical terminology.

To make sure your needs would be addressed in this book, we asked both students and experienced medical terminology instructors, "What helps students learn medical terminology?" Overwhelmingly, the responses pointed to three common factors:

- Motivation to learn
- Retention of the material
- Opportunities for application and practice

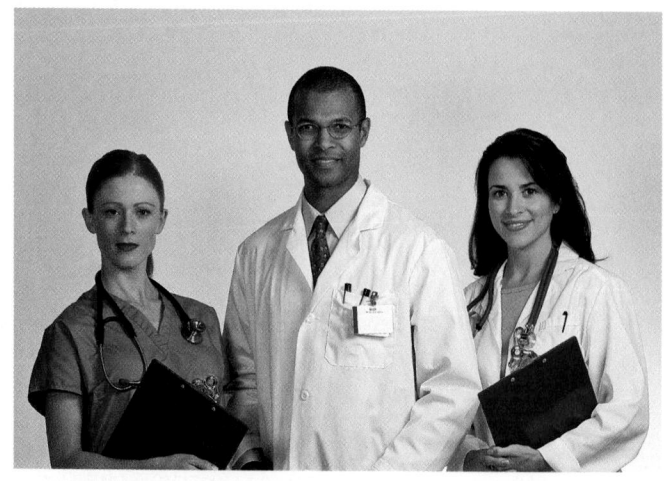

THIS TEXTBOOK INCORPORATES FEATURES DESIGNED TO ADDRESS THESE THREE FACTORS.

Motivation to learn	→	For students to be motivated to learn, what they are learning must be meaningful and relevant. To ensure that the chapters in *Medical Language for Modern Health Care* fit these criteria, the student is asked to step into the role of a health professional in each chapter. Authentic patient cases are used to illustrate how medical language is used on the job.
Retention of the material	→	To learn and remember something new, students must associate it with something they already know or have experienced. As the old saying goes, "Experience is the best teacher." When students encounter new medical terms within the context of a patient case, they are able to remember them more effectively. In addition, each chapter presents medical terms from one body system or medical specialty, which further serves to "tie it all together" to help students retain the knowledge and skills.
Opportunities for application and practice	→	Practice makes perfect. This is especially true for learning medical terminology. This textbook provides many opportunities for students to apply what they are learning. Exercises are included in the lessons, as well as at the end of each chapter. Additional exercises are available on McGraw-Hill *Connect Plus*™.

HOW INSTRUCTORS' NEEDS ARE MET

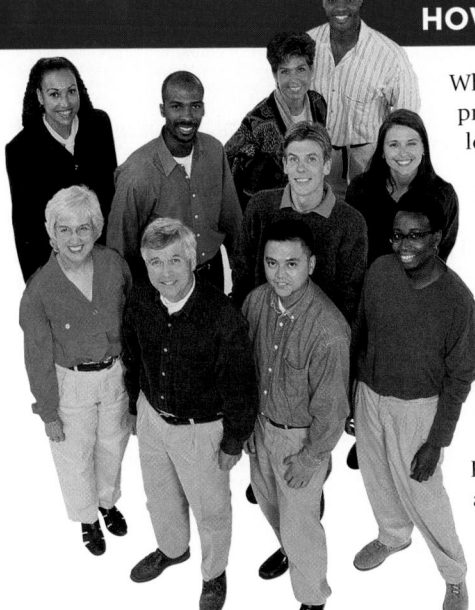

When you use *Medical Language for Modern Health Care*, you will be supported at every point in the program. Each chapter in the book is broken down into lessons, and the Instructor's Manual provides lesson plans and additional materials for each lesson.

Lesson-Based Approach

Each chapter of *Medical Language for Modern Health Care* is divided into lessons covering different aspects of the overall chapter subject. Lessons within a chapter break down into topics. Each topic is designed so that your students will not have to flip back and forth when completing exercises or looking at figures, tables, and boxes. All main concepts and ideas presented in topics begin and end within a two-page "spread." These spreads help learning flow smoothly by ensuring that valuable class and reading time is not wasted on flipping pages.

You Are . . . Your Patient Is . . . Case Reports

Each chapter begins by immediately placing your students in the role of a health professional faced with a situation in which medical communication is necessary. Many different professional health and LPN-level nursing roles are utilized so that your students can "experience" various specialties and positions. The patient cases introduced at the beginning of the chapters are referenced throughout the lessons to further unify the students' experience.

Chapter Outcomes and Lesson Objectives

"I really like the case reports presented in each chapter. This allows the students to immediately use the knowledge they are gaining for a better understanding of the material. Excellent way to introduce students to actively learning instead of passively learning."

Crystal Kitchens, CMT, MA
Richland Community College

The major learning outcomes for each chapter are previewed in the beginning so that you and your students can focus on what they need to know and be able to do by the end of the chapter. Each lesson has outcome-based learning objectives. Accomplishing each lesson's objectives helps ensure that students will be able to achieve the chapter outcomes and, ultimately, the goal of the textbook: They will learn the terminology and language of modern health care.

Word Analysis and Definition (WAD) Boxes

Each lesson contains boxes listing important medical terms and their pronunciation, elements, and definition. Prefixes, suffixes, and roots/combining forms are color-coded. These boxes provide your students with an at-a-glance view of the terms covered. The boxes are excellent for reference as well as for studying and reviewing.

Two-Page Spread and End-of-Chapter Exercises

At the end of each two-page spread are exercises. The spread exercises provide your students with immediate practice using the terms in the spread. These exercises focus on basic understanding and ability to apply the terms. They are an excellent foundation for the end-of-chapter exercises, which are often based on authentic situations, such as interactions with patients and physicians or medical documentation.

The end-of-chapter exercises require your students to understand, accurately apply, and think critically about the medical language they use. Throughout the text, frequent opportunities for application and reinforcement of medical language skills and concepts are provided to help your students build confidence and knowledge. A wide variety of exercises and activities is included to address different medical settings and levels of learning (including knowledge, comprehension, application, analysis, synthesis, and evaluation).

FOR THE INSTRUCTOR:

The **Instructor's Manual** (available online, www.mhhe.com/allanmedlanguage2e) is an invaluable resource for new and experienced medical terminology instructors. All of the components of the *Medical Language for Modern Health Care* textbook program are designed to be coherent and connected in order to create a consistent environment in which students can learn. The Instructor's Manual shows how each component of the textbook program works to support and reinforce the content and strengths of the other components, from art to exercises to content to test bank questions.

The Instructor's Manual contains the following sections:

- **Your Medical Terminology Course—An Introduction to Teaching Medical Terminology**
  The Instructor's Manual contains a helpful introduction to teaching medical terminology, as well as other helpful resources such as:
  - Information about student learning styles and corresponding instructor strategies.
  - Innovative learning activities.
  - Assessment techniques and strategies.
  - Classroom management tips.
  - Techniques for teaching limited-English-proficiency students.

- **Lesson Planning Guide**
  In addition, the Instructor's Manual contains a Lesson Planning Guide with a complete and customizable lesson plan for each of the 76 lessons in the book. Each lesson plan contains a step-by-step 50-minute teaching plan and master copies of handouts. These lessons may be used alone or combined to accommodate different class schedules. The lessons can easily be revised to reflect your preferred topic or sequence or to add or delete topics entirely. Each of the lesson plans is designed to be used with a corresponding PowerPoint® presentation that is available on the Online Learning Center, discussed below.

- **Internet-Based Research Activities**
  The Instructor's Manual also includes Internet-based research activities for each chapter in the book.

The **Online Learning Center, Instructor Resources,** www.mhhe.com/allanmedlanguage2e, contains:

- **Instructor's Manual.** The manual was written by Teleologic Learning Company.

- **McGraw-Hill's EZ-Test Test Generator.** This flexible electronic testing program allows instructors to create tests from book-specific items. It accommodates a wide range of question types, and instructors may add their own questions. Multiple versions of a test can be created, and any test can be exported for use with course management systems such as WebCT, Blackboard, or PageOut. EZ-Test Online is a new service that gives you a place online to easily administer your EZ-Test-created exams and quizzes. The program is available for Windows and Macintosh environments.

- **PowerPoint® Lecture Outlines.** PowerPoint lectures with speaking notes are available for the chapters in the textbook. Each 50-minute lesson plan in the Instructor's Manual Lesson Planning Guide dedicates approximately 20 to 25 minutes to the use of the corresponding ready-made PowerPoint presentations. The PowerPoint presentations, which combine art and lecture notes, are designed to help instructors discuss with students the important points of the lessons. The slides are customizable, allowing instructors to modify lectures to ensure that the needs of their unique students and curricula are met.

- **Image Bank.** The image bank features selected textbook images.

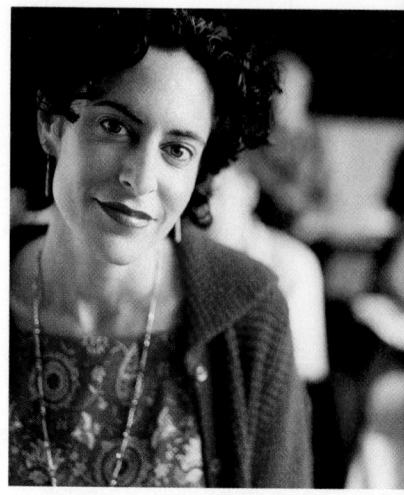

"I love the lesson plans and internet activities provided along with the different teaching techniques and ideas. This is very helpful and saves time. I use a lot of these ideas in my Anatomy course that I teach."

Mindy S. McDonald, CMA
University of Northwestern Ohio

"I have been teaching for 12 years and I have never seen [an Instructor's] Manual as thorough as this manual."

Sherry Jones, COTA/L
Sinclair Community College

COURSE DELIVERY SYSTEMS

With help from our partners, WebCT, Blackboard, TopClass, eCollege, and other course management systems, instructors can take complete control of their course content. These course cartridges also provide online testing and powerful student tracking features.

HOW TO TEACH MEDICAL TERMINOLOGY

The **Online Course for Instructors to Support** *Medical Language for Modern Health Care* is found at the Instructor Resources section of the Online Learning Center, www.mhhe.com/allanmedlanguage2e.

The **How to Teach Medical Terminology online course** provides instructors with the introductory knowledge and resources they need to begin effectively using the *Medical Language for Modern Health Care* textbook and related materials. This course is designed to cover the "basics" of how to effectively teach medical terminology.

How to Teach Medical Terminology allows instructors to choose for themselves which module they wish to take, or they may opt to take a self-assessment survey that will recommend one of the three modules.

- **Module 1** is designed for the inexperienced instructor.
- **Module 2** is designed for the instructor who has previous classroom experience but has never taught medical terminology.
- **Module 3** is designed for the experienced medical terminology instructor who has not previously used a contextualized approach to teaching the subject.

Upon completion of a given module, instructors will take a final assessment designed to demonstrate their understanding and achievement of the learning objectives for that module. Those who score 70% or higher on the final assessment will receive a certificate that can be printed for professional development purposes.

FOR THE STUDENT:

- *Connect Plus+*™ allows students and instructors to access all their course materials, including the media-rich textbook, in one place. With its unique integrated learning system, *Connect Plus+* combines market-leading content, a proven course architecture, and unmatched flexibility to help students apply the principles in the textbook.

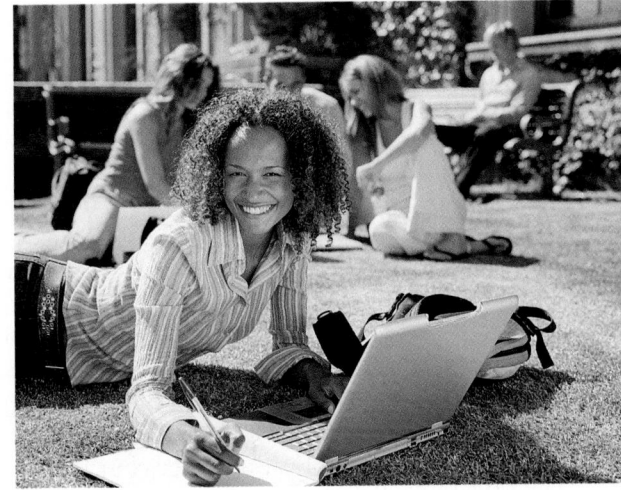

- **LearnSmart**™ Medical Terminology is a diagnostic study tool that adapts questioning based on an individual's response. A clearly defined learning path is developed for each student and tied to specific learning objectives. LearnSmart measures progress and generates student reports for the instructor.

ACKNOWLEDGMENTS

The uniqueness, beauty, and high standards of this book are due to the skills and devotion of a team of people who worked closely and happily together.

We would also like to thank the dedicated staff of Greater Annapolis Medical Group, Annapolis, Maryland, for opening their practice to our photography team.

David Allan

Karen Lockyer

For insightful reviews, criticisms, helpful suggestions, and information, we would like to acknowledge the following:

SECOND EDITION REVIEWERS

Dr. Irfan Akhtar
Career Institute of Health and Technology

Jessica Lynn Alexander, BS, MN
Mississippi University for Women

Suzanne Allen, RMA, RPT
Sanford-Brown Institute

Emil Asdurian, MA
Bramson ORT College

Dr. Joseph H. Balatbat
Sanford-Brown Institute

Nina Beaman, MS, RNC-AWHC, CMA (AAMA)
Bryant & Stratton College

Jean M. Chenu, MS
Genesee Community College

Carolyn Sue Coleman, LPN, AS
National College

Lucinda A. Conley, RHIT
Ozarka College

Mary Alice Conrad, ADN
Delaware Technical and Community College

Lynn M. Egler, RMA, AHI, CPhT
Dorsey Schools

William C. Fiala, BS, MA
University of Akron, Allied Health Department

Nancy Gacke, BA
Southeast Technical Institute

Leslie Harbers, BSN, RMA
National College

Betty Hassler, RN, RMA
National College

Katherine Hawkins, BS, MS
Ivy Tech Community College

Judy Hurtt, MEd
East Central Community College

Carol Lee Jarrell, MLT, AHI
Brown Mackie College

Sherry Jones, COTA/L
Sinclair Community College

Timothy J. Jones, MA
Oklahoma City Community College

Cathy Kelley-Arney, CMA, MLTC, BSHS
National College and National College of Business and Technology

Crystal Kitchens, CMT, MA
Richland Community College

Naomi Kupfer, CMA
Heritage College

LM Liggan, MEd, C-AHI, RMA
Director of Health Care Education, National College

Susan Long, BS
Ogeechee Technician College

Ann M. Lunde, BS, CMT
Waubonsee Community College

Loreen W. MacNichol, CMRS, RMC
Andover College

Allan L. Markezich, PhD
Black Hawk College

Mindy S. McDonald, CMA (AAMA)
University of Northwestern Ohio

Elizabeth L. Miller, CPC CMA

Deborah M. Mullen, CCS-P, CPC, CPC-I
Probill PMCC

Gail P. Orr, BA
National College

Judith L. Paulsen, BA
Vatterott College

Pamela K. Roemershauser, CPC
MedVance Institute

Patricia L. Sell, AAS, BS, MSEd
National College

Shirley J. Shaw, MA
Northland Pioneer College

Gene Simon, RHIA, RMD
Florida Career College

Christine Sproles, RN, BSN, MS
Pensacola Christian College

Susan Stockmaster, MHS
Trident Technical College

Diane Swift, RHIT
State Fair Community College

Kathryn Whitley, RN, MSN, NP-C
Patrick Henry Community College

Cassandra E. Williams, MS, RHIA
Ogeechee Technical College

Kari Williams, BS, DC
Front Range Community College

Marsha L. Wilson, MA, BS, MEd
Clarian Health Sciences Education Center

James R. Woods, MS, RRT, RPFT
Florida Community College

MEDICAL REVIEWERS

Marie Atkinson, MD
Wayne State University School of Medicine
Department of Neurology

Courtney L Barr, MPH, MD
University of Missouri School of Medicine
Department of OB/GYN

Toby C Campbell, MD, MSCI
University of Wisconsin-Madison, Carbone Cancer Center
Department of Hematology/Oncology

Lawrence S. Chan, MD
University of Illinois College of Medicine
Department of Dermatology

Dawn Belt Davis, MD, Ph.D.
University of Wisconsin-Madison
Department of Endocrinology

Julie A. Kovach, MD, FACC, FASE
Wayne State University School of Medicine
Division of Cardiology, Department of Medicine

Noelle K. LoConte, MD
University of Wisconsin-Madison
Dept of Medicine, Section of Hematology/Oncology

Barry Newman, M.D.
PC Tech

Abdul Ghani Sankri-Tarbichi, MD
Wayne State University-School of Medicine

Scott E. Van Valin, MD
Medical College of Wisconsin
Department of Orthopaedic Surgery

Damandeep S. Walia, MD
The University of Kansas Medical Center
Division of Allergy, Clinical Immunology & Rheumatology

Jennifer M. Weiss, MD
University of Wisconsin School of Medicine and Public Health

Fred Arthur Zar, MD
University of Illinois at Chicago
Department of Medicine

Giancarlo F. Zuliani, MD
Wayne State University School of Medicine
Department of Otolaryngology–Head and Neck Surgery

FIRST EDITION REVIEWERS

Anita Dupre Althans, RNC, MSN
Our Lady of Holy Cross College

Summer Aulich, CMA, BS
Ivy Tech State College

Christina L. Baumer, RN, Ph.D., CNOR, CHES
Lancaster General College of Nursing and Health Sciences

Nina Beaman, MS, BA, CMA, RN
Bryant and Stratton College

Paula Bostwick, RN, MSN
Ivy Tech State College—Northeast

Teresa Bruno. BA
EduTek College

Marcella Bucknam, BA
Clarkson College

William, J. Burke, BA
Madison Area Technical College
Blackhawk Area Technical College

Denise Carsillo, RMA, MS
Lincoln College of Technology

Jean M. Chenu, MS, BS
Genesee Community College

Sheila Maxell Cook, MT, LMT
Red Mountain Institute, Inc.

Barbara S. Desch, LVN, CPC, AHI
San Joaquin Valley College
Visalia, CA

Sheryl Daniel, BA, CMT, NMT, BMT
Infinite Healing Massage Therapy

Angela Edwards, RN, BSN
Community Care College

Lynn M. Egler, RMA, AHI, CPhT
Dorsey Schools

Pallavi Eswara, MS
Freelance Science Editor and Writer

Mary Fabink, MSN, M.Ed., RN, CEN
Milligan College

George Fakhoury, MD, DORCP, CMA
Heald College

Penny Fedje, RHIT
North Dakota State College of Science

Melinda J. Fernandez, AA, EMT-P, NR-CMA, NR-RPT, B-Radiologist
Keiser Career College

Kathie Folsom, MS, BSN, RN
Whidbey Island Campus, Skagit ValleyCollege

Mark W. Forquer, BS
Advanced Career Training

Margaret Schell Frazier, CMA, RN, BS
Formerly of Ivy Tech State College—Northeast

Eugenia M. Fulcher, RN, BSN, EdD, CMA
Eastern New Mexico University,

Tracie Fuqua, BS, CMA
Wallace State Community College

Ron Gaines, MS, BS
Cameron University

Mary A. Harmon, BS, CMA, CPC
Med Tech College

Katherine Harper
Pellissippi State Technical Community College

Katherine Hawkins, BS
Ivy Tech Community College of Indiana

Barbara J. Hogg, MLT, RN, BSN
South Arkansas Community College

Janet R. Hunter, MBA, MS, ABD
Northland Pioneer College

Judy Hurtt, M.Ed.
East Central Community College

Frances C. Hutson, MSN, RN
Louisiana Technical College

Sherry Jones, COTA/L
Sinclair Community College

Beverly W. Juett, MS, Ed.S
Midway College

Mike Kennamer, NREMT-P, MPA
Northeast Alabama Community College

Pat King, MA, RHIA
Baker College of Cass City

Crystal Kitchens, MA, CMT
Richland Community College

Judy Kronenberger, RN, CMA, M.Ed
Sinclair Community College

Naomi Kupfer, CMA, CMBS
Heritage College

Wei Li, MD, MSCS
North Georgia Technical College

Patricia B. Lisk, RN, BSN
Augusta Technical College

Martha Luebke, AA, BA, CPC, NIIC
High-Tech Institute

Ann M. Lunde, BS, CMT
Waubonsee Community College

Loreen W. MacNichol, CMRS, RMC
Andover College

Susan Madden, M.Ed, RHIT
Brown College

Alicia Mata, BS, MA
Corinthian Colleges, Inc.

Sister Sheila McGinnis, RN, BSN, CMT
Center for Human Integration

Peggy L. Meli, MS, RHIA, LHRM
Valencia College

Tanya Mercer, BS, RN, RMA
KAPLAN Higher Education Corporation

Maureen E. Russell Messier, CMA, RMA
Brandford Hall Career Intitute

James J. Mizner Jr., BS Pharmacy, MBA
ACT College

Kay A. Nave, CMA, MRT
Hagerstown Business College

Laurence C. Neely, BS, MAE
EPCI College of Technology

Judith L. Neville, BA
Vatterott College

Alice M. Nolan, MBA, RHIA
University of Central Florida

Tammy O'Brien, M.Ed
Augusta Technical College

D.J. Overbey, RN, CCRC
Virginia College at Austin

Murray Paton Pendarvis, Ph.D.
Southern Louisiana University

Roberta Pavy Ramont, RN, EdD
Corinthian Colleges Inc.

Brian David Riffe, BS, CMA, RMA, AHI
National College of Business and Technology

Alan Rosenberg, MS
Allied Schools

Ona Schulz, CMA
Lake Washington Technical College

Janet R. Sesser, BS, RMA, CMA
High-Tech Institute, Inc.

Frances J. Sheehan, Jr., R.Ph., MD
Northern Virginia Community College

Pamela K. Sheffield, CPC
MedVance Institute

Lynn G. Slack, BS, CMA
ICM School of Business and Medical Careers

Karen R. Snipe, CPhT, AS, BA MA
Trident Technical College

John J. Smith, EdD
Director Health Sciences, Corinthian Colleges, Inc.

Robert J. Spears, PA-C
Physician Assistant Program The University of Findlay

Christine Sproles, MS, BSN, RN, CMT
Pensacola Christian College

Cynthia H. Thompson, RN, MA, BS
Davenport University

Megan Treitz
Arapahoe Community College

Marcia Truinfoli, Ph.D.
DNA Goes to School

Valeria D. Truitt, BS, MA
Craven Community College

Ann-Marie Varenna, BS
Sanford Brown Institutue

Mark S. Volpe, MD
Premier Education Group

Bonnie Welniak, RN, MSN
Monroe County Community College

Jay W. Wilborn, M.Ed, MT (ASCP)
National Park Community College

Marsha Lynn Wilson, BS, MS
Clarian Health Sciences Education Center

Nancy H. Wright, RN, BS, CNOR
Virginia College

Review of Case Study Scenarios

Stewart Dadmun, MD
Internist, San Diego, CA

Contextual Approach Promotes Active Learning

Chapters in the textbook are organized by body system in accordance with an overall anatomy and physiology (A&P) approach. Lessons introduce and define terminology through the context of A&P, pathology, and clinical and diagnostic procedures and tests. The organization of the body systems into chapters is based on an "outside to inside" sequence that reflects a physician's differential diagnosis method used during an examination.

To provide students with an authentic context, the medical specialty associated with each body area or system is introduced along with relevant anatomy and physiology. Students actually step into the role of a health professional associated with each specialty. Patient cases and documentation are used to illustrate the real-life application of medical terminology in modern health care: to care for and communicate with patients and to interact with other members of the health care team.

The A&P organizational approach, used in conjunction with an authentic medical setting and patient cases, encourages student motivation and facilitates active, engaged learning.

"Overall, this text has more information (than current text in use) and is divided so that the student has better understanding."

Pamela Sheffield
Roemershauser
MedVance Institute

Innovative Pedagogical Aids Provide a Coherent Learning Program

Each chapter is structured around a consistent and unique framework of pedagogic devices. No matter what the subject matter of a chapter, the structure enables students to develop a consistent learning strategy, making *Medical Language for Modern Health Care* a superior learning tool.

YOU ARE . . . YOUR PATIENT IS

Each chapter opens by placing the student in the role of a health professional related to the specialty and associated body systems and areas covered by the chapter. The student is also introduced to a patient and given information about the patient's case.

LEARNING OUTCOMES

At the same time, **Learning Outcomes** are presented to let students know what they will learn in the chapter. This technique immediately engages students, motivating them to read on to learn how this patient's case (and their role in the patient's care) relates to the medical terminology being introduced in the chapter.

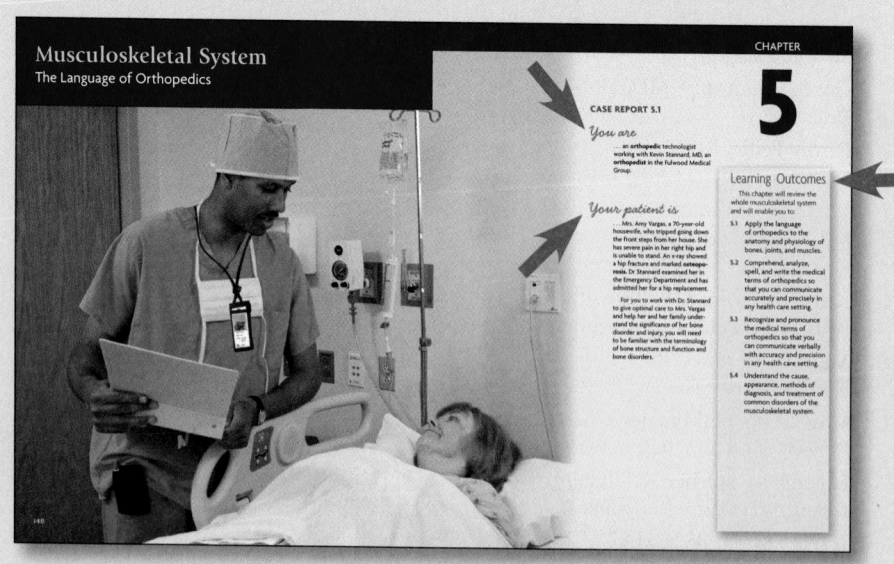

LESSON-BASED ORGANIZATION

"This book is the, as a college instructor, 'Book of my Dreams!'"

Gene Simon
Florida Career College

The chapter content is broken down into chunks, or lessons, to help students digest new information and relate it to previously learned information. Rather than containing many various topics within a chapter, these lessons group the chapter material into logical, streamlined learning units designed to help students achieve the chapter outcomes. Lessons within a chapter build on one another to form a cohesive, coherent experience for the learner.

Each lesson is based on specific **Lesson Objectives** designed to support the students' achievement of the overall chapter outcomes.

Each lesson in a chapter contains an introduction, lesson objectives, lesson topics, Word Analysis and Definition boxes, and lesson exercises. Within each lesson, all topics and information are presented in **self-contained two-page spreads**. This means students no longer have to flip back and forth to see figures on one page that are described on another.

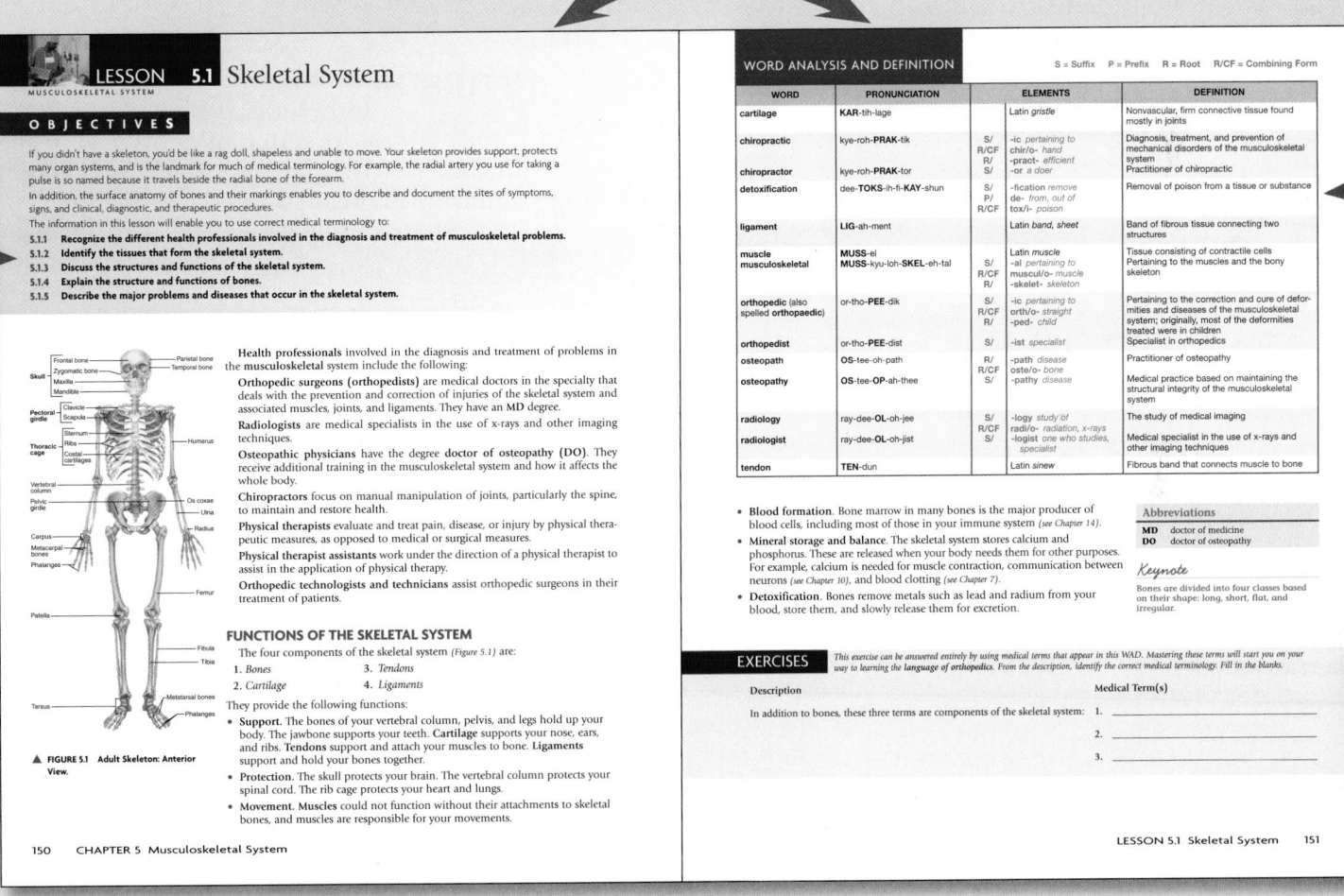

WORD ANALYSIS AND DEFINITION BOXES

The medical terms covered in each lesson are introduced in context, either within a patient case or in the lesson topics. To facilitate easy reference and review, the terms are also listed in boxes as a group. The **Word Analysis and Definition (WAD) boxes** list the term and its pronunciation, elements, and definition in a concise, color-coded, at-a-glance format.

SPREAD AND CHAPTER-END EXERCISES

Each spread within a chapter ends with exercises designed to allow students to check their basic understanding of the terms they just learned. These "checkpoints" can be used by instructors as assignments, in class activities, or by students for self-evaluation.

At the end of each chapter you will find 10 to 15 pages of exercises that ask students to apply what they learned in all lessons of a chapter. These chapter-end exercises reinforce learning and help students go beyond mere memorization to think critically about the medical language they use. In addition to reviewing and recalling the definitions of terms learned in the chapter, students are asked to use medical terms in new and different ways to ensure a thorough understanding.

"These are excellent learning tools for students."

Crystal Kitchens, CMT, MA
Richland Community College

EXERCISES *After you deconstruct the following medical terms into their basic elements, provide a brief definition for each term. Fill in the chart; then fill in the blanks at the end of the exercise. The first one is done for you.*

Medical Term	Prefix	Root/CF	Suffix	Definition of Medical Term
reduction	re	duct	ion	*The restoration of a structure to its normal position*
alignment				
malunion				
hematoma				

Demonstrate your understanding of the terms by finishing this exercise.

1. Use *both* the terms **reduction** and **alignment** in *one sentence.*
   _____
   _____

2. The suffix **oma** means *tumor* as well as *mass.* Briefly explain why a hematoma is not a tumor.
   _____
   _____

3. Explain the difference between a **malunion** and a **nonunion** of a fracture.
   _____
   _____

STUDY HINT BOXES

Study Hint boxes are found throughout the review exercises. They reinforce, and remind students to use, basic study skills.

CHAPTER 5 REVIEW
MUSCULOSKELETAL SYSTEM

T. Choose the correct medical term(s) from the list to complete the sentence. You will not use all the terms.

striation	symphysis	detoxification	intervertebral discs
DMD	orthotic	opposition	pelvis
retinaculum	shoulder girdle	fascicle	acetabulum
popliteal fossa	traction	steroids	fibromyalgia

1. Line or streak across a muscle is called a _____.

2. Transverse, fibrous band on the wrist: _____

3. _____ support and cushion the vertebral column.

4. _____ has no known etiology, no laboratory tests for it, and no known treatment except pain management.

5. Movement that enables the thumb to touch the tips of the other fingers is called _____

6. Cartilaginous joint between two bones: _____

7. Bundle of muscle fibers: _____

8. Dr. Stannard ordered continuous application of weight to the patient's broken leg. He has been placed in _____.

9. _____ cause skeletal muscle to hypertrophy.

10. The hollow at the back of the knee is called the _____.

U. Build your orthopedic terminology by completing the medical terms defined here. After you fill in the element on the line, write the type of element (prefix, root, combining form, suffix) you have used below the line. Fill in the blanks.

1. Removing poison from tissue — de/ _____ / _____

2. Bone disease — osteo/_____

3. Projection above the condyle — _____ /condyle

4. Membrane surrounding a bone — peri/ _____ / _____

5. Region between diaphysis and epiphysis — _____ /physis

6. Bones lacking in calcium — osteo/ _____

7. Inflammation of bone tissue — osteo/ _____ /itis

8. Collection of blood in tissues — _____ /oma

9. Moving toward the midline — _____ /ion

10. Fixation of a joint with surgery — arthro/ _____

V. Knowing the exact number of certain body parts, and their relative positions, will ensure precision in your medical documentation. Match the correct number to the correct term. Use one answer twice.

1. Number of lumbar vertebrae: _____   A. 7

2. Number of bones in the vertebral column: _____   B. 5

3. Number of cervical vertebrae: _____   C. 4

4. Number of components in the skeletal system: _____   D. 12

5. Number of regions in the vertebral column: _____   E. 26

6. Number of thoracic vertebrae: _____

W. Could you explain the difference among these abnormal spinal curvatures to a patient if they ask? _____

lordosis _____

scoliosis _____

kyphosis _____

Which one is the most common defect? _____

Which defect is seen in patients with osteoporosis? _____

> **Study Hint**
> Anything that is referred to as the most powerful, largest, smallest, most common, etc., is probably going to be a test question.

X. Functions of Skeletal Muscles: (Add this to your outline.) Bones and joints would get us nowhere without the muscles to move them. Illustrate how each of these functions is accomplished with skeletal muscles.

Function	How Function Is Effected
Movement	_____
Posture	_____
Body heat	_____
Respiration	_____
Communication	_____

> **Study Hint**
> To help you remember the functions, make up a sentence with each word (mnemonic) starting with the letters M, P, B, R, and C. *Example: Mr. Parker's Body Heat Rose Considerably.*

Y. Employ the *language of orthopedics* to answer the following questions about muscles.

1. What is muscle tone?
   _____
   _____

2. What is muscle contraction?
   _____
   _____

3. What is the difference between muscle atrophy and hypertrophy?
   _____
   _____

VIVID ILLUSTRATIONS AND PHOTOS

Colorful, precise anatomical illustrations and photos lend a realistic view of body structures and correlate to the clinical context of the lessons.

"The illustrations are wonderful. It is one thing to learn the words, but to be able to identify what the word actually 'looks like' is extremely beneficial to the learning process."

Ann M. Lunde, BS, CMT
Waubonesee Community College

BONES, JOINTS, AND MUSCLES OF THE HIP AND THIGH

The **hip joint** is a **ball-and-socket** synovial joint between the head of the femur and the cup-shaped **acetabulum** of the hip bone *(Figure 5.38a)*. A ligament (ligamentum capitis) attached to the head of the femur from the lining of the acetabulum carries blood vessels to the head of the femur to nourish it.

The joint is held in place by a thick joint **capsule** reinforced by strong ligaments that connect the neck of the femur to the rim of the acetabulum *(Figure 5.38b)*.

The **labrum** is the cartilage that forms a rim around the socket of the joint; it cushions the joint and helps keep the head of the femur in place in the socket. Recent improvements in diagnostic techniques have shown that with injury the labrum can tear and cause pain. The tear is diagnosed on MRI and may need surgery to be repaired.

Powerful muscles that support the hip joint and move the thigh have their **origins** on the pelvic girdle and their **insertions** into the femur. Prominent among them are the three **gluteus** muscles, **maximus, medius,** and **minimus** *(Figure 5.38c)*, and the **adductor** muscles that run down the inner thigh.

▲ **FIGURE 5.38 Hip Joint.** (*a*) Right frontal view of a section of hip joint. (*b*) Ligaments of hip joint. (*c*) Muscles of hip and thigh (lateral view).

Disorders and Injuries of the Hip Joint

Hip pointer, usually a football-related injury, is a blow to the rim of the pelvis that leads to bruising of the bone and surrounding tissues.

Osteoarthritis is common in the hip as a result of aging, weight bearing, and repetitive use of the joint. The cartilage on both the acetabulum and the head of the femur degenerates, and eventually there is total loss of the cartilage cushion. The resulting friction between the bones of the head of the femur and the acetabulum leads to pain and loss of mobility.

▲ **FIGURE 5.39 Fracture of Neck of [Femur] in Woman with Osteoporosis.**

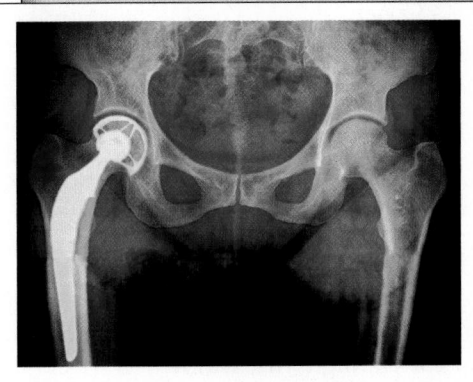

▲ **FIGURE 5.40 Total-Hip Replacement.** Colored x-ray of prosthetic hip.

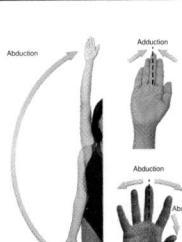
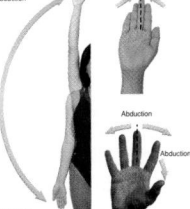
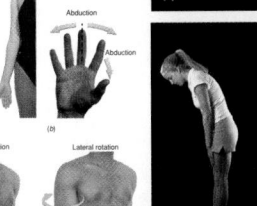
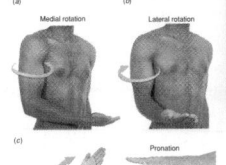
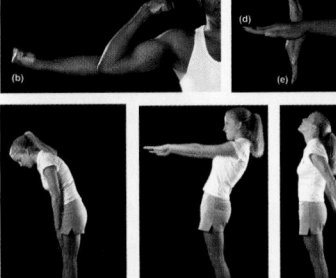
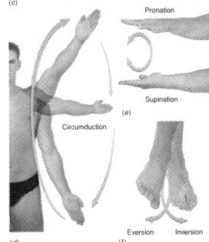

▲ **FIGURE 5.14 Movement of the Limbs.** (*a*) Abduction and adduction of the upper limb. (*b*) Abduction and adduction of the fingers. (*c*) Medial and lateral rotation of the arm. (*d*) Circumduction. (*e*) Pronation and supination of the hand. (*f*) Eversion and inversion of the foot.

▲ **Figure 5.13 Joint Flexion and Extension.** (*a*) Flexion of the elbow. (*b*) Extension of the elbow. (*c*) Extension of the wrist. (*d*) Neutral position of the wrist. (*e*) Flexion of the wrist. (*f*) Flexion of the spine. (*g*) Flexion of the shoulder. (*h*) Extension of the shoulder.

JOINT MOVEMENT

Flexion and Extension of Joints

Flexion (bending) and **extension** (straightening) are shown in the elbow joint *(Figure 5.13a and b)*, in the wrist joint *(Figure 5.13c, d, and e)*, and in the shoulder joint *(Figure 5.13g and h)*.

For most of the rest of the body, flexion is movement of a body part *anterior* to the **coronal plane** *(see Chapter 2)*. Extension is movement *posterior* to the coronal plane. For example, when you bend your trunk forward, that is flexion *(Figure 5.13f)*. When you bend your trunk backward, that is extension *(see Figure 5.13g)*. When you bend your trunk sideways to the right or left, that is called *lateral flexion.*

Abduction and Adduction of Joints

Abduction is movement away from the midline. **Adduction** is movement toward the midline. Abduction of your arm is moving it sideways away from your trunk. Adduction is bringing it back to the side of your trunk *(Figure 5.14a)*. Abduction of your fingers is spreading them apart, away from the middle finger. Adduction is bringing them back together *(Figure 5.14b)*.

Rotation of Joints

Rotation is turning around an axis. Medial rotation of the upper arm bone, the humerus, with the elbow flexed brings the palm of the hand toward the body. Lateral rotation moves the palm away from the body *(Figure 5.14c)*.

Pronation and Supination

When you lie flat on the ground face-down on your belly with your palms touching the ground, you are **prone.** When you lie flat on your back with your spine on the floor and your palms facing up, you are **supine.**

TABLES

Meaningful tables aid in summarizing concepts and lesson topics.

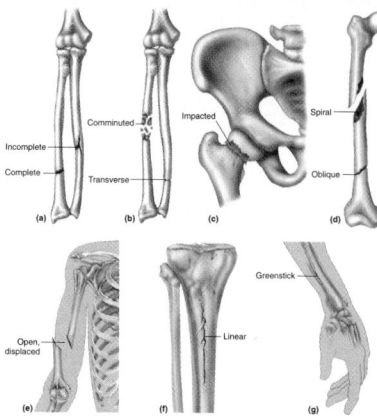

▲ FIGURE 5.9   Bone Fractures.

TABLE 5.1 Classification of Bone Fractures

Name	Description	Reference
Closed	A bone is broken, but the skin is not broken.	Figure 5.9g
Open	A fragment of the fractured bone breaks the skin, or a wound extends to the site of the fracture.	Figure 5.9e
Displaced	The fractured bone parts are out of alignment.	Figure 5.9e
Complete	A bone is broken into at least two fragments.	Figure 5.9a
Incomplete	The fracture does not extend completely across the bone; it can be **hairline** (as in a stress fracture in the foot when there is no separation of the two fragments).	Figure 5.9a
Comminuted	The bone breaks into several pieces, usually two major pieces and several smaller fragments.	Figure 5.9b
Transverse	The fracture is at a right angle to the long axis of the bone.	Figure 5.9b
Impacted	One bone fragment is driven into the other, with resulting shortening of a limb.	Figure 5.9c
Spiral	Fracture spirals a round the long axis of the bone.	Figure 5.9d
Oblique	Diagonal fracture runs across the long axis of the bone.	Figure 5.9d
Linear	Fracture runs parallel to the long axis of the bone.	Figure 5.9f
Greenstick (closed)	This is a partial fracture: one side breaks, the other bends.	Figure 5.9g
Pathologic	Fracture occurs in an area of bone weakened by disease (such as cancer).	—
Compression	Fracture occurs in a vertebra from trauma or pathology leading to the vertebra being crushed.	—

KEYNOTES AND ABBREVIATIONS

Keynotes and Abbreviations offer students additional information correlating to the lesson.

BONE GROWTH AND STRUCTURE

Keynote

Minerals are deposited in bone when the supply is ample and released when they are needed elsewhere.

Factors that affect bone growth include:

1. **Genes.** Genes determine the size and shape of bones and the ultimate adult height.
2. **Nutrition.** Calcium and phosphorus are needed to develop good bone density.
3. **Exercise.** Exercise increases bone density and total bone mass.
4. **Mineral deposition.** Calcium and phosphate are taken from plasma and deposited in bone.
5. **Mineral resorption.** Calcium and phosphate are released from bone back into the plasma when they are needed elsewhere. For example, calcium is needed for muscle contraction, communication between neurons, and blood clotting. Phosphate is a component of DNA and RNA.
6. **Vitamins.** Vitamin A activates osteoblasts; vitamin C is essential for collagen synthesis; vitamin D stimulates absorption, transport, and deposition of calcium and phosphate into bones *(see Chapter 21)*.
7. **Hormones.** For example, growth hormone stimulates the epiphyseal plate to calcify, and estrogen and testosterone accelerate bone growth after puberty and maintain bone density *(see Chapter 13)*.

Structure of Bones

Long bones are the most common type of bone in the body *(Figure 5.2)*.

The shaft of a long bone is called the **diaphysis.** Each end of the bone is called the **epiphysis** and is expanded to provide extra surface area for the attachment of ligaments and tendons.

Sandwiched between the diaphysis and epiphysis is a thin area called the **metaphysis.** Thin layers of cartilage cells in the **epiphyseal plate** enable the diaphysis (bone shaft) to grow in length. When growth stops, compact bone grows into the epiphyseal plate and forms the **epiphyseal line.**

A tough connective tissue sheath called **periosteum** covers the outer surface of all bones and is attached to the compact or **cortical** bone by tough collagen fibers. The periosteum protects the bone and anchors blood vessels and nerves to the surface of the bone.

The hollow cylinder inside the diaphysis is called the **medullary cavity.** It contains bone **marrow** and is lined by a thin membrane called the **endosteum.** The marrow is a fatty tissue that contains blood cells in different stages of development *(see Chapter 7)*.

The endosteum and periosteum contain **osteoblasts,** cells that produce the matrix of new bone tissue. This process is called **osteogenesis.** Bone **matrix** consists of cells, collagen fibers, a gel that supports and suspends the fibers, and calcium phosphate crystals that give bone its hardness.

When osteoblasts are incorporated into the new bone, they become **osteocytes.** These cells, which maintain the matrix, reside in small spaces in the matrix called **lacunae.**

Osteoclasts are produced by the bone marrow. They dissolve calcium, phosphorus, and the organic components of the bone matrix. There is a continual balancing act going on as osteoclasts remove matrix and osteoblasts produce matrix. If osteoclasts outperform the osteoblasts, then **osteoporosis** occurs, as with Mrs. Vargas in the Case Report.

All bones are well supplied with blood *(Figure 5.3)*. The blood vessels travel through the bone in a system of small **haversian (central) canals.** Because of its good blood supply, bone heals well.

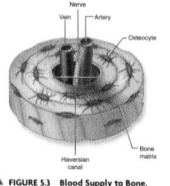

▲ FIGURE 5.2   Femur: Long Bone of the Thigh.

(a) Anterior view   (b) Interior view

▲ FIGURE 5.3   Blood Supply to Bone.

Case Report 5.1 (continued)

On questioning, Mrs. Vargas demonstrated many of the risk factors for osteoporosis, including a family history, lack of exercise, cigarette smoking, inadequate diet, postmenopause, and increasing age.

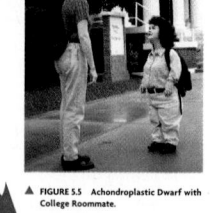

Normal bone   Osteoporotic bone

LM 5×

▲ FIGURE 5.4   Normal Bone and Osteoporotic Bone.

▲ FIGURE 5.5   Achondroplastic Dwarf with College Roommate.

Abbreviations

BMD	bone mineral density
DEXA	dual energy x-ray absorptiometry
FDA	U.S. Food and Drug Administration
IU	international unit(s)

DISEASES OF BONE

Osteoporosis results from a loss of bone density *(Figure 5.4)* when the rate of bone **resorption** exceeds the rate of bone **formation.** It is more common in women than in men, and its incidence increases with age. Ten million people in the United States already have osteoporosis, and 18 million more have low bone density (**osteopenia**) and are at risk for developing osteoporosis.

In women, production of the hormone estrogen decreases after menopause, and its protection against osteoclast activity is lost. This leads to fragile, brittle bones. In men, reduction in testosterone has a similar but less marked effect.

Women at risk for osteoporosis should have bone mineral density (**BMD**) screening using a dual-energy x-ray absorptiometry (**DEXA**) scan. Men and women over age 50 should take 1200 mg of calcium daily and 400 to 600 international units (**IU**) of vitamin D or expose the body to the sun for 15 minutes daily. Chapter 22 covers nutritional needs.

There are several U.S. Food and Drug Administration (**FDA**)–approved medications available for the treatment of osteoporosis. Most inhibit osteoclast activity.

Osteomyelitis is an inflammation of an area of bone due to bacterial infection, usually with a staphylococcus. Untreated tuberculosis can spread from its original infection in the lungs to bones via the bloodstream to produce tuberculous osteomyelitis.

Osteomalacia, known as **rickets** in children, is a disease caused by vitamin D deficiency. When bones lack calcium, they become soft and flexible. They are not strong enough to bear weight and become bowed. Osteomalacia occurs in some developing nations and occasionally in this country when children drink soft drinks instead of milk fortified with vitamin D.

Achondroplasia occurs when the long bones stop growing in childhood but the bones of the axial skeleton are not affected *(Figure 5.5)*. This leads to short-stature individuals who are about 4 feet tall. Intelligence and life span are normal. It is caused by a spontaneous gene mutation that then becomes a dominant gene for succeeding generations.

Osteogenic sarcoma is the most common malignant bone tumor. Peak incidence is between 10 and 15 years of age, and the tumor often occurs around the knee joint.

Osteogenesis imperfecta is a rare genetic disorder, producing very brittle bones that are easily fractured, often **in utero** (while inside the uterus).

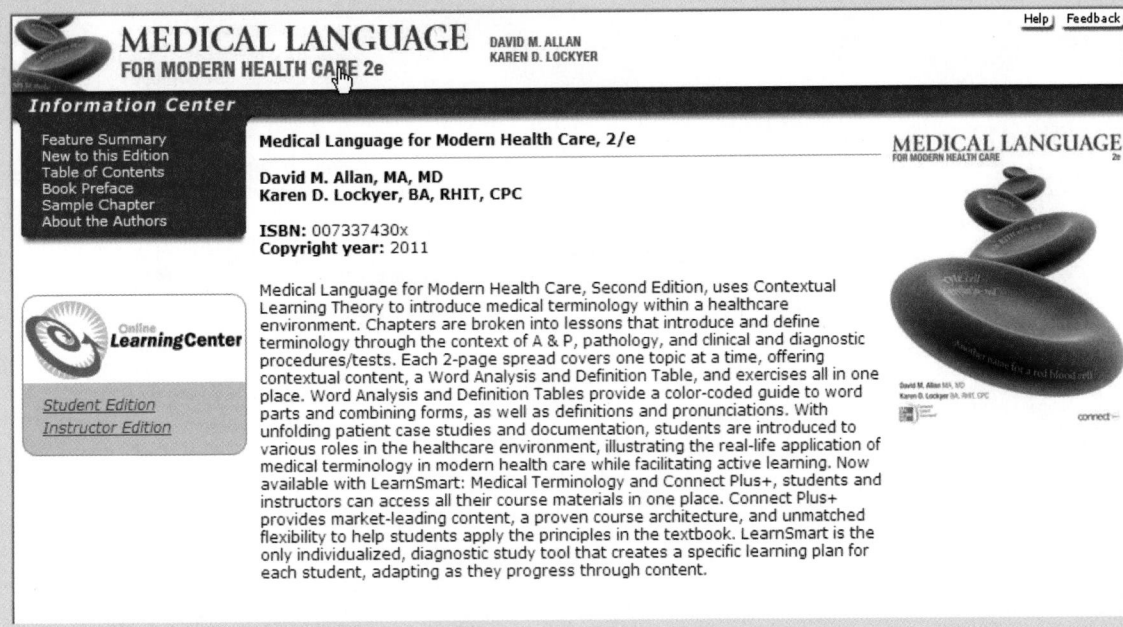

McGraw-Hill **Connect Plus+**™

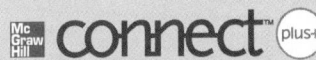

Connect Plus+™ allows students and instructors to access all their **course materials, including the media-rich textbook, in one place.** With its unique integrated learning system, *Connect Plus+* combines market-leading content, a proven course architecture, and unmatched flexibility to help students apply the principles in the textbook.

McGraw-Hill LearnSmart: Medical Terminology

McGraw-Hill *LearnSmart* is a diagnostic learning system that determines the level of student knowledge and then feeds the student appropriate content. Students learn faster and study more efficiently.

As a student works within the system, LearnSmart develops a personal learning path adapted to what the student has learned and retained. LearnSmart is also able to recommend additional study resources to help the student master topics.

In addition to being an innovative, outstanding study tool, LearnSmart provides comprehensive reports for instructors. Results are generated by individual, by topic, and by learning objective. This can provide direction for the instructors during class time or during office hours with individual students. LearnSmart is SCORM compliant so student data can be easily imported into any Learning Management System.

Students and instructors will be able to access LearnSmart anywhere via a Web browser. And for students on the go, it will also be available through any iPhone or iPod Touch.

Learning Medical Language

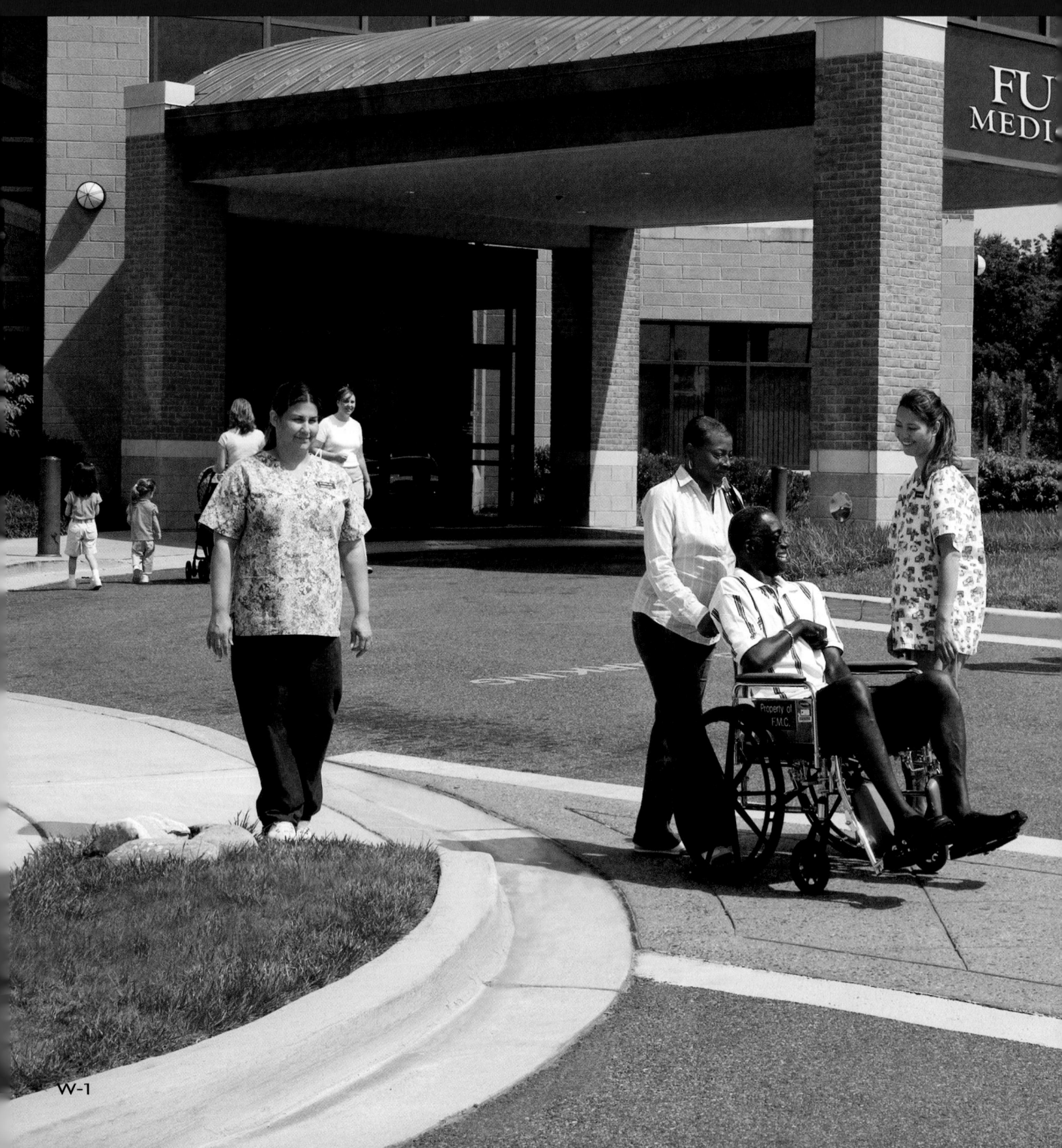

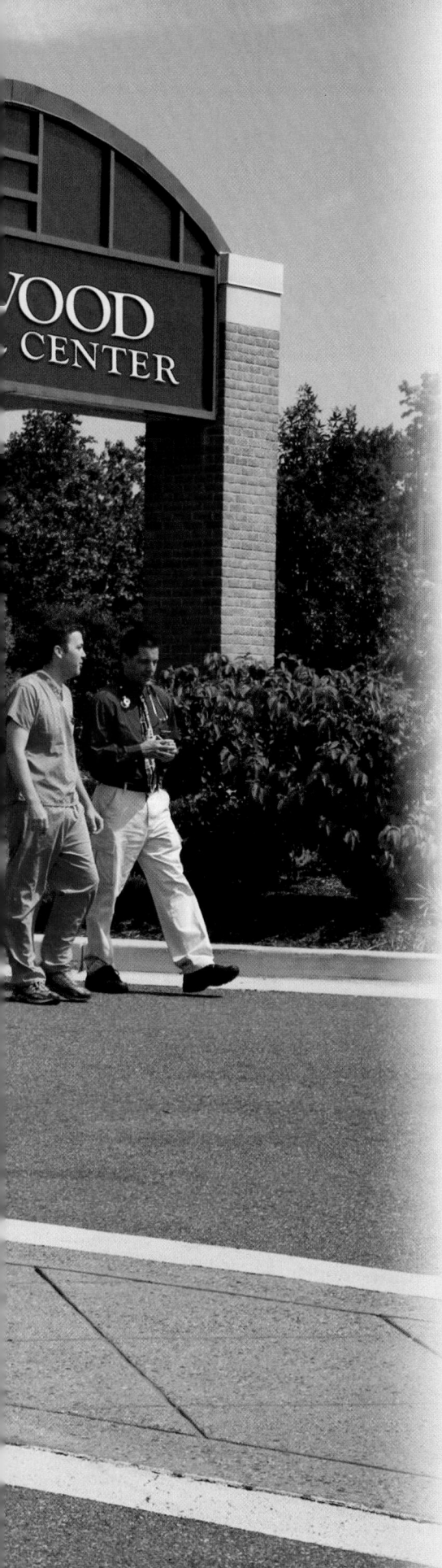

Welcome

You are

. . . a student preparing for a career as a health professional. As part of your training program, you must complete a supervised **externship.** You have just arrived at Fulwood Medical Center for your first day as an **extern.** You are glad to have this opportunity: Fulwood is a busy center with highly skilled, compassionate staff members. Between attending classes at night, working during the day, and raising two children, you have a full schedule. However, the knowledge and skills you are learning in your studies, and at Fulwood, will prepare you for a successful future.

Learning Outcomes

Your journey through this book, and your externship at Fulwood Medical Center, begin with getting to know the surroundings in which you will experience medical language. In order to get the most out of your experience, you need to:

W.1 Understand the role of various members of the health care team so that you can progress through the medical specialties covered in this book.

W.2 Become familiar with the realistic health care context used in this book to help you learn medical terminology.

W.3 Comprehend the value of learning medical terminology in a realistic setting.

W.4 Recognize the importance of effective study and organizational strategies to becoming a lifelong learner.

W.5 Develop effective study habits.

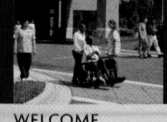
WELCOME

LESSON W.1 | Orientation to Fulwood Medical Center

OBJECTIVES

The information in this lesson will enable you to:

W.1.1 Identify members of the health care team.

W.1.2 Recognize the distinguishing features of Fulwood Medical Center and its role in your study of medical terminology.

W.1.3 Explain the importance of learning medical terminology in a realistic setting.

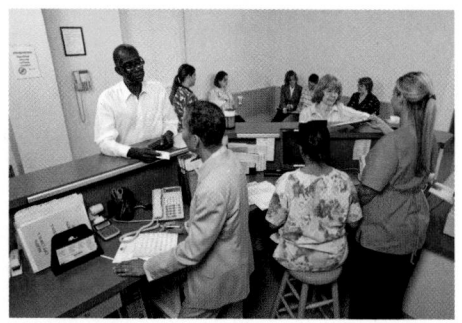

▲ **FIGURE W.1** A Busy Medical Practice at Fulwood Medical Center.

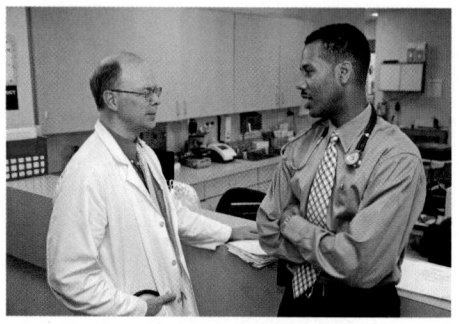

▲ **FIGURE W.2** The primary care physician refers patients to specialists when necessary.

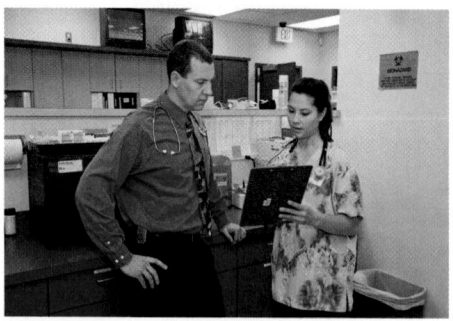

▲ **FIGURE W.3** Physicians and medical assistants provide direct care to patients.

THE HEALTH CARE TEAM

Fulwood Medical Center is a realistic health care setting *(Figure W.1)* that allows you to experience the use of medical language. Each chapter in this book focuses on the medical terminology used in a specific medical specialty and the body systems related to that specialty. A variety of health professionals make up the teams caring for patients in each medical specialty.

As a **health professional**, you are part of a team of medical and other professionals who provide health care services designed to improve the health and well-being of their patients.

The team leader is a medical doctor, or physician, who can be an **MD** (doctor of medicine) or a **DO** (doctor of osteopathy). Most **managed care systems** require the patient to have a **primary care physician** *(Figure W.2)*. This physician can be a **family practitioner, internist,** or **pediatrician** (for children) and is responsible for the continuing overall care of the patient. In managed care, the primary care physician acts as the "gatekeeper" for the patient to enter the system, supervising all care the patient receives.

If needed medical care is beyond the expertise of the primary care physician, the patient is referred to a medical specialist whose expertise is based on a specific body system or even a part of a body system. For example, a **cardiologist** has expertise in diseases of the heart and vascular system, whereas a **dermatologist** specializes in diseases of the skin and an **orthopedist** in problems with the musculoskeletal system. A **gastroenterologist** is an expert in diseases of the whole digestive system, whereas a **colorectal surgeon** specializes only in diseases of the lower gastrointestinal tract.

Other health professionals work under the supervision of the physician and provide direct care to the patient *(Figure W.3)*. These can include a **physician assistant, nurse practitioner, medical assistant,** and, in specialty areas, different therapists, technologists, and technicians with expertise in the use of specific therapeutic and diagnostic tools.

Still other health professionals on the team provide indirect patient care *(Figure W.4)*. These include **administrative medical assistants, transcriptionists, health information technicians, medical insurance billers,** and **coders,** all of whom are essential to providing high-quality patient care.

As you study the language of each medical specialty at Fulwood Medical Center, you will also meet the members of each specialty's health care team and learn more about their roles in caring for the patient.

FIGURE W.4 Administrative medical assistants are among the health professionals who provide indirect care to patients. ▶

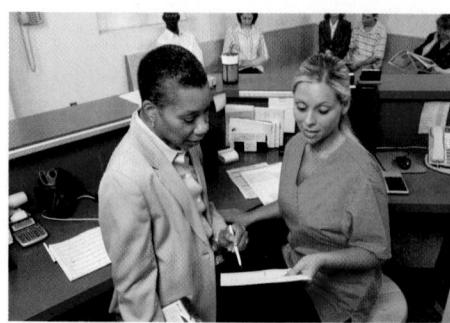

ACTIVELY EXPERIENCING MEDICAL LANGUAGE

Medical terms were created to provide health care professionals a way to communicate with each other and document the care they provide. To provide effective patient care, all health care professionals must be fluent in medical language. One misused or misspelled medical term on a patient record can cause errors that can result in injury or death to patients, incorrect coding or billing of medical claims, and possible fraud charges.

When medical terms are separated from their intended context, as they are in other medical terminology textbooks, it is easy to lose sight of how important it is to use them accurately and precisely. Learning medical terminology in the context of the medical setting reinforces the importance of correct usage and precision in communication.

During your externship at Fulwood Medical Center, you will *experience* medical language. Just as in a real medical center, you will encounter and apply medical terminology in a variety of ways. Actively experiencing medical language will help ensure that you are truly learning, and not simply memorizing, the medical terms in each chapter. Memorizing a term allows you to use it in the same situation (e.g., repeating a definition) but doesn't help you apply it in new situations. Whether you are reading chart notes in a patient's medical record or a description of the treatment prescribed by a physician, you will see medical terms being used for the purpose they were intended.

The Health Care Center

In the lobby, the supervisor of Externship Programs welcomes you and tells you about Fulwood Medical Center. You learn that Fulwood consists of this medical office building and the attached 250-bed hospital. The office building houses physicians practicing primary care, the major medical specialties, and some complementary medicine therapies—in all, nearly 100 physicians in 25 specialty areas. The hospital and the medical offices share pharmacy, laboratory, radiology, physical therapy, health education, and cafeteria facilities, but they have separate main entrances. A directory on the wall near the hospital lobby lists all the departments and doctors and their locations *(Figure W.5)*.

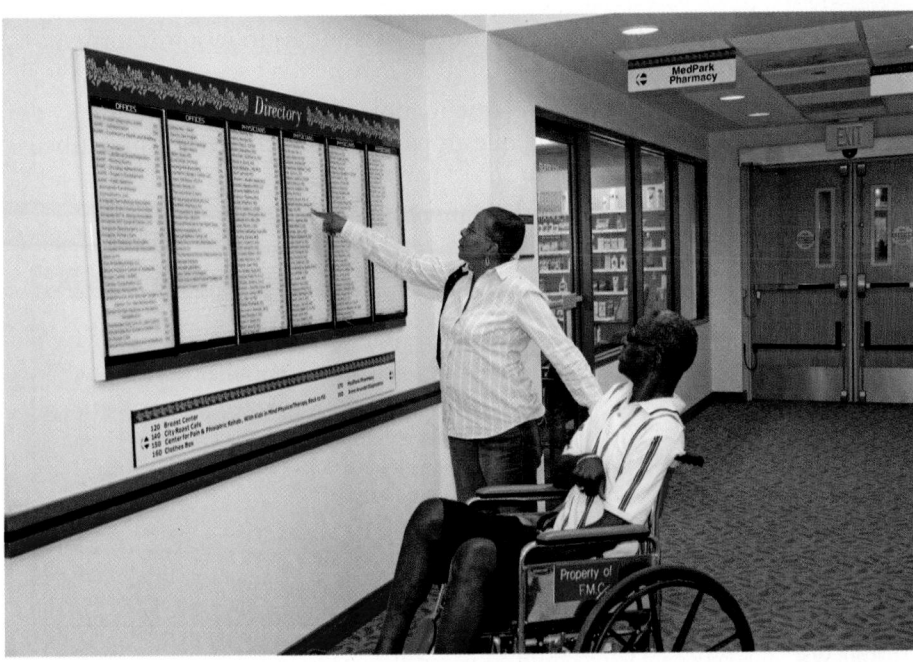

FIGURE W.5 The office directory can help orient visitors within the medical office complex.

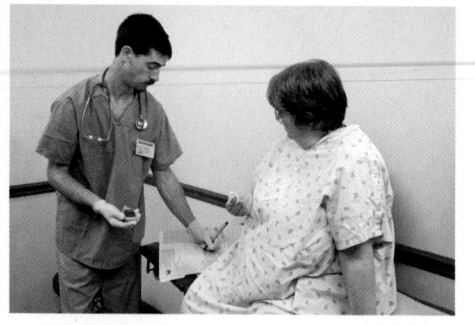

▲ **FIGURE W.6** The CMA interviews the patient to learn more about her condition.

This book goes beyond simply presenting and defining new medical terms. Fulwood Medical Center, with its wide range of patient cases, health professionals, and realistic medical environment, allows you to encounter and discover terms the way they are used in real life: in the different medical settings. Experiencing medical language in this context bridges the gap between what you learn in the classroom and what really happens in the clinical setting.

As you progress through this book,

- You will encounter, and be asked to interact with, patients and health care professionals.
- You will analyze medical records and documentation.
- You will be introduced to diagnostic and therapeutic methods and the pathophysiology of disease.
- You will be able to see how all of these activities depend on effective communication, accurate comprehension, and precise use of medical language.

Below are just a few of the ways you will use medical language on your first day at Fulwood.

Listening and Speaking

You will:

- Listen to patients describing their medical history and explaining their symptoms (*Figure W.6*). A sample conversation between Luis Guitterez, a Certified Medical Assistant (CMA), and Mrs. Jones, a patient, follows:

> **Luis Guitterez, CMA:** "Mrs. Jones, I'm Luis, an assistant to Dr. Lee. The receptionist noticed that you were looking pale and sweaty and notified Dr. Lee."
>
> **Mrs. Jones:** "In the rush to get here this morning, Luis, I didn't have time to eat breakfast. I'm not feeling so well right now . . . I'm diabetic, you know."
>
> **Luis Guitterez, CMA:** "Dr. Lee has asked me to test your blood sugar. As a diabetic, you've done this many times yourself, I'm sure."

- Listen to and carry out physicians' instructions and information concerning patient care.
- Speak to physicians and other health care professionals to report information and ask questions.
- Talk with patients in the course of patient encounters and phone calls, giving instructions and answering questions about the physician's prescribed treatment plans.
- Document your interaction with the patient.

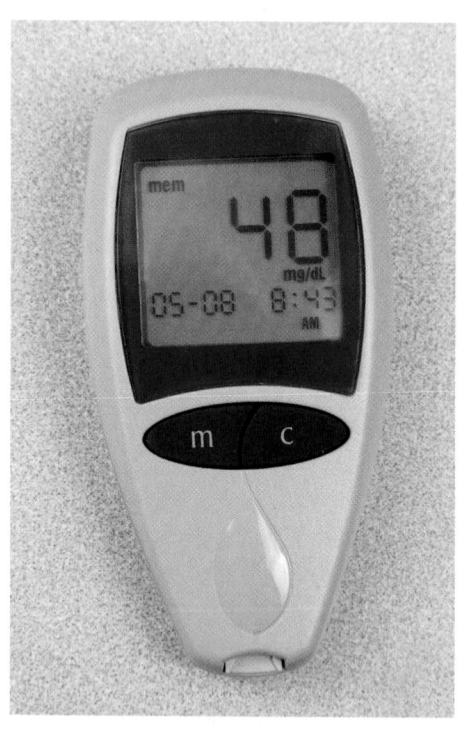

▲ **FIGURE W.7** One of your responsibilities may be to read the results of diagnostic tests, such as this blood sugar reading.

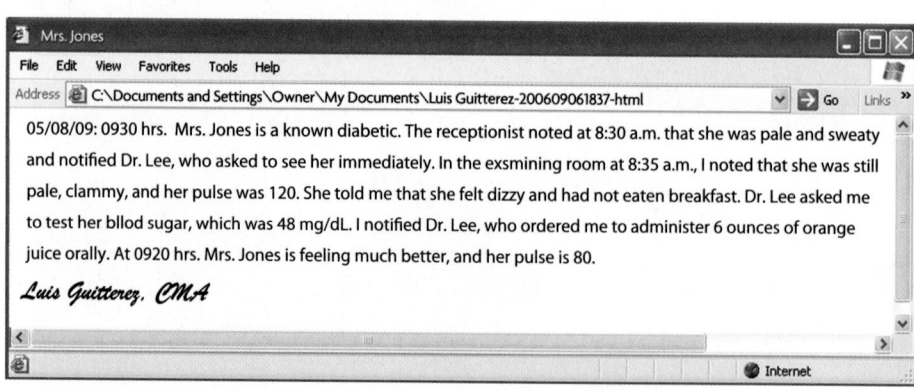

05/08/09: 0930 hrs. Mrs. Jones is a known diabetic. The receptionist noted at 8:30 a.m. that she was pale and sweaty and notified Dr. Lee, who asked to see her immediately. In the exsmining room at 8:35 a.m., I noted that she was still pale, clammy, and her pulse was 120. She told me that she felt dizzy and had not eaten breakfast. Dr. Lee asked me to test her bllod sugar, which was 48 mg/dL. I notified Dr. Lee, who ordered me to administer 6 ounces of orange juice orally. At 0920 hrs. Mrs. Jones is feeling much better, and her pulse is 80.

Luis Guitterez, CMA

▲ **FIGURE W.8** It is important to proofread documentation to ensure its accuracy.

Reading

You will:

- Read physicians' comments and treatment plans in patient medical records and case reports.
- Read the results of physical examinations, procedures, and laboratory and diagnostic tests *(Figure W.7)*.

Writing

You will:

- Document actions taken by yourself and other members of the health care team *(Figure W.8)*.
- Proofread medical documentation to ensure its accuracy.

Thinking Critically

You will:

- Evaluate medical documentation for accuracy *(Figure W.9)*.
- Translate technical medical communication into words patients can understand.
- Analyze unfamiliar medical terms using the strategies presented in this book.

Learning from Patient Cases

You will encounter realistic patient cases throughout this book. These cases ask you to step into the role of a health care professional *(You are …)* and focus on a real patient with real health care needs *(Your patient is …)*.

Taking full advantage of the patient cases in this book allows you to:

- Experience various health care careers.
- Examine the roles you may fill to provide care for patients.
- See the types of documentation needed in these situations.
- Become acquainted with medical terminology in real-life settings.

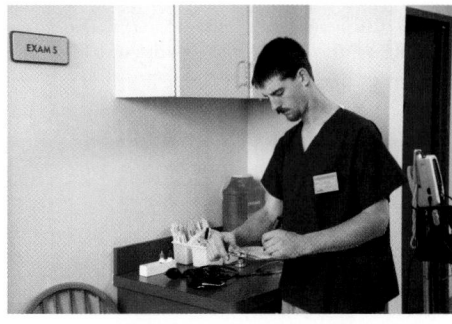

▲ **FIGURE W.9** Your knowledge of medical terminology will help you understand your patients' medical records.

Applying What You Learn

Throughout each chapter, you will be asked to apply and practice what you are learning. These application opportunities are designed to give you practice using medical terms in a variety of ways and for a variety of purposes. Specifically, the exercises will require you to perform tasks you would perform on the job, such as *listening and speaking, reading, writing,* and *thinking critically.* They are designed to help you move beyond simple memorization and become fluent in the language of modern health care.

EXERCISES

Each encounter with medical language improves your ability to (a) understand the medical terms you hear, (b) speak accurately and precisely using medical terms, (c) write accurately and precisely using the appropriate medical terms, (d) read and understand medical terms, and (e) think critically about the medical terms you experience. These five skills are very important for all health care professionals. It is important to be able to identify experiences that build your knowledge and skill with medical language. Write the letter of the skill or skills being used in each blank below. More than one skill may be needed for each activity.

Skills:
- **a.** Understand spoken medical terms.
- **b.** Speak accurately and precisely with medical terms.
- **c.** Read and understand medical terms.
- **d.** Write accurately and precisely with medical terms.
- **e.** Think critically about medical language.
- **f.** Translate medical terms into nonmedical language.

_____ 1. Answering a patient's questions about the physician's diagnosis and instructions.

_____ 2. Taking a phone message when a specialist calls from another facility and has information concerning one of the patients of a physician in your facility.

_____ 3. Proofreading an insurance claim form.

_____ 4. Teaching a patient with special nutritional needs how to modify her diet.

_____ 5. Using the Internet and textbooks to learn more about a family member's disease or condition.

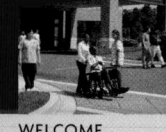

LESSON W.2 Learning Medical Language

WELCOME

The information in this lesson will enable you to:

W.2.1 Recognize the need for a solid understanding of medical terminology.

W.2.2 Justify the need to become a lifelong learner.

W.2.3 Apply organizational and study strategies to help you succeed.

FIGURE W.10 Electronic Report of a Patient's Condition. ▶

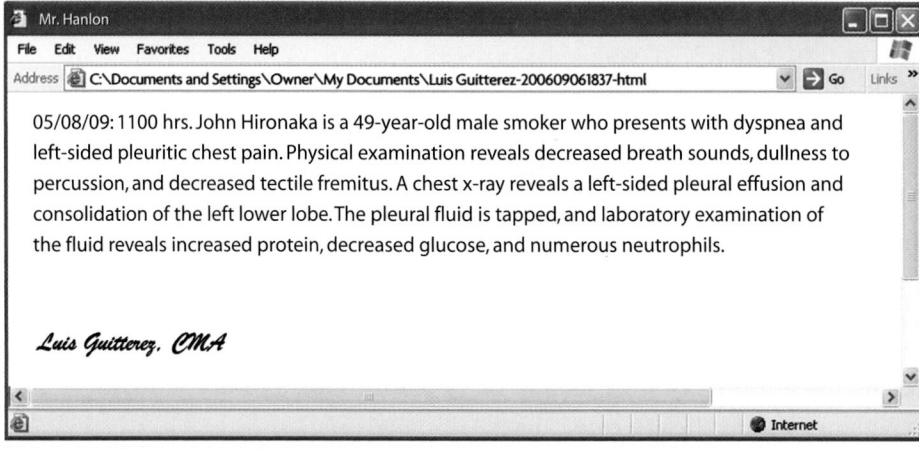

05/08/09: 1100 hrs. John Hironaka is a 49-year-old male smoker who presents with dyspnea and left-sided pleuritic chest pain. Physical examination reveals decreased breath sounds, dullness to percussion, and decreased tectile fremitus. A chest x-ray reveals a left-sided pleural effusion and consolidation of the left lower lobe. The pleural fluid is tapped, and laboratory examination of the fluid reveals increased protein, decreased glucose, and numerous neutrophils.

Luis Guitterez, CMA

WHY YOU SHOULD LEARN MEDICAL TERMINOLOGY

Medical terminology is not just another subject for which you memorize the facts and then forget them when you move on to the next course. Medical language will be used throughout your studies, as well as every day on your job. Nothing you hear or read in your studies or in a health care setting will make sense without an understanding of medical terminology. Once you learn the medical language, however, the world of health care is open to you to explore—and understand.

Even beyond your career goals, everyone is a patient at one time or another. You may also accompany an elderly parent, friend, or child to a doctor or emergency room. Knowing medical terminology makes it easier for you to communicate with physicians and use the Internet to research health information—and ultimately to become a proactive medical consumer.

Figure W.10 shows an electronic report of a patient's condition: something you have to understand as a health professional. Terms like **dyspnea, pleuritic, effusion,** and **neutrophils** are used every day in medical language.

Health care professionals use specific terms to describe and talk about objects and situations they encounter each day. Like every language, medical terminology is changing as new knowledge is discovered. For example, in genetics, today's terminology was unheard of a decade ago. Medical terms become outdated as new knowledge explodes. **Consumption** is now known as **tuberculosis, grippe** as **influenza,** and **whooping cough** as **pertussis.**

Modern medical terminology is an artificial language constructed over centuries by using words and elements from Greek and Latin origins as its building blocks. Some 15,000 or more words are formed from 1200 Greek and Latin roots. It serves as an international language, enabling medical scientists from different countries and in different medical fields to communicate with a common understanding.

In your world as a health care professional, medical terminology enables you to communicate with your team leader, with the other health care professionals on your team, and with other professionals in different disciplines outside your team. Understanding medical terminology also enables you to translate the medical terms into language your patients can understand, improving the quality of their care and demonstrating your professionalism.

In short, if you can't speak the language, you can't join the club *(Figure W.11).*

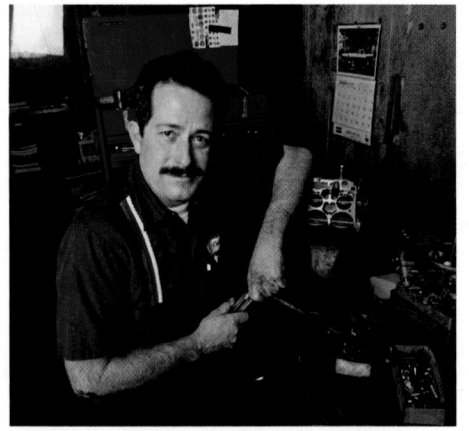

▲ **FIGURE W.11** Every profession has its own language. You may have difficulty understanding your auto mechanic when he tells you that the expansion valve, evaporator core, and orifice tubes in your air-conditioning system need to be replaced.

Lifelong Learning

No matter where you are in your life's journey—an infant trying to walk, a child beginning school, an adolescent working in your first job, a parent changing a diaper, an adult watching television, a grandparent playing with your grandchild—every day provides numerous opportunities for learning. If you actively absorb each piece of learning as it becomes available, you form a foundation on which you can build your continually increasing body of knowledge and experience (*Figure W.12*).

Your current training in medical terminology is necessary for you to be able to continue your education in health care, but it is important to realize that school is just one of the many places where you acquire knowledge. Each time you solve a problem in life, such as working through an argument with a friend or helping your child perform better in school, the knowledge you gain is *your own* answer to *your own* problem. This type of knowledge—discovered through experience—is genuine, real, and trustworthy for you. It is not like what you learned in school, which was determined by some distant authority. Your medical terminology instructor isn't likely to ask a test question on how to unclog your sink. Instead, this type of learning is driven by your needs and goals. The authentic knowledge you gain from solving your own problems, whether by yourself or with the help of other people or resources, motivates you to acquire still more knowledge and helps you grow as a person and as a professional.

When you are working as a health care professional, your ongoing education is an integral and inseparable part of your work activities. Additional classroom training will be needed to keep your skills and professional knowledge up to date. You will also continue to learn on your own through experience. As a health care professional, every time you interact with a patient, read a report, or talk with your team leader or peers, you are given another opportunity to learn.

Everything you do in life results in learning. Your own experience and judgment become your most valuable resources to make your life vivid, strong, creative, and, ultimately, what *you* want it to be. Take advantage of these resources, and use them to maximize your professional and personal success.

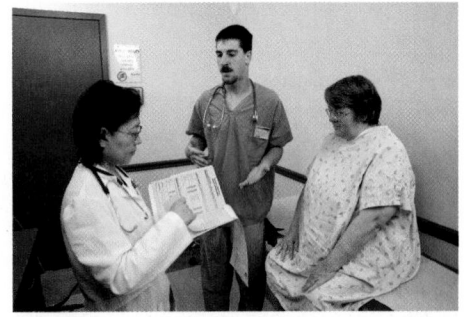

▲ **FIGURE W.12** Learning doesn't stop when you leave the classroom; every time you interact with other health care professionals and patients, you have the opportunity to learn something.

Keynote

As novelist Lillian Smith once said, ***"When you stop learning, stop listening, stop looking and asking questions, always new questions, then it is time to die."***

EXERCISES   *Reflect on the idea of "lifelong learning" and how you can make it work for you to enrich your life's experience. Think about one instance in your life when something you learned (by yourself, from another person, from research, etc.) became the foundation upon which you built further learning and information. Some examples are how to paint a room, clean a fish, use a computer, and cook a meal. Briefly describe that here.*

_____

_____

_____

Now describe why you need to be committed to learning from everyday experiences on the job, and explain how that can help you in your career.

_____

_____

_____

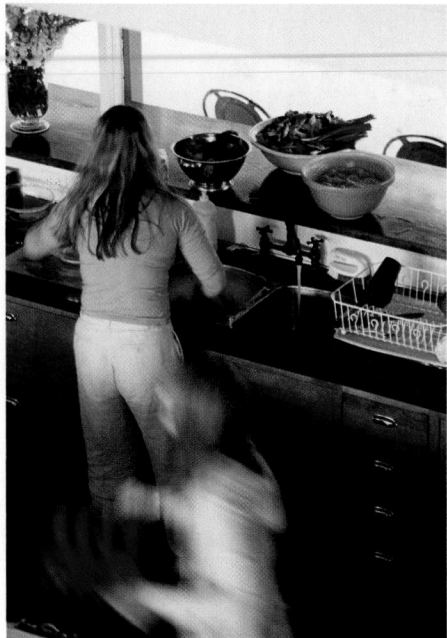

▲ **An Evening at Home.**

STUDY STRATEGIES

- Recognize the stresses you are under.
- Determine what you can change because the situation, people, and events are making excessive demands on you.
- Prioritize mentally and handle each task in the order of importance.

In this case, eat a healthy meal with your kids, enjoy putting them to bed, pay the bills, and then take some deep breaths to relax (or meditate) for 10 minutes. When you feel more relaxed, settle down to review the text, and then go to bed at a reasonable hour. Picking up around the house will have to wait since studying and sleeping are a higher priority. Sound too easy? What other choices do you have to be able to study in an effective way?

- Find ways to give yourself a break from stressful situations.

If you know you have a test every Thursday night, ask your spouse, mother, sister, or friend or someone in your support group to come and put the kids to bed Wednesday night while you go to that person's house or to the library and study. A support group of family and friends is essential to your success, so look for ways to surround yourself with people you can trust and rely on.

This lesson contains strategies you can use to get focused. It will help you learn how to manage your time and your studies to succeed—but this lesson can't do it alone. You are what you put into your studies. You have a lot of time and money invested in your education. Don't waste it now by putting in only half of the effort this class requires. Succeeding in this class, and in life, requires the following:

- Committing with your time and perseverance
- Knowing and motivating yourself
- Getting organized
- Scheduling and managing your time
- Being an active learner

The rest of this lesson will help you learn how to be effective in these areas so that, as you encounter new learning situations during your externship at Fulwood, you will be prepared to handle them.

Committing with Your Time and Perseverance

Understanding—and mastering—what you learn in the classroom and during your externship at Fulwood Medical Center will take time, as well as patience. Nothing worthwhile comes easily. Be committed to your studies, and you will reap the benefits in the long run.

Consider this: Your training in health care is building the foundation for your future career. Sloppy and hurried craftsmanship now will lead only to difficulties later.

Keynote

A few years of committed study time now is nothing compared to the lifetime that awaits you.

Knowing and Motivating Yourself

What type of learner are you? When are you most productive? Know yourself and your limits, and work within them *(Figure W.13)*. Know how to motivate yourself to give your all to your studies and achieve your goals. You are the one who benefits most from your success. If you lack self-motivation and drive, you are the first person who suffers.

Know yourself. Just as there are many types of learners, there is no right or wrong way of learning. Into which category do you fall?

Visual learner. You respond best to "seeing" processes and information. Take advantage of the strengths of your learning style by doing the following:

- Focus on text illustrations and charts, as well as course handouts.
- Check to see if there are animations on the course or text website to help you.
- Consider drawing diagrams in your notes to illustrate concepts.
- Use the contextual and labeling exercises at McGraw-Hill CONNECT.

Auditory learner. You work best by listening to processes and information. Take advantage of the strengths of your learning style by doing the following:

- Listen carefully to—and possibly tape record (with instructor permission)—the lecture.
- Talk information through with a study partner.
- Listen to audio pronunciations of terms at McGraw-Hill CONNECT.

Tactile/kinesthetic learner. You learn best by working "hands on." Take advantage of the strengths of your learning style by doing the following:

- Apply what you have learned in a role-play or realistic scenario.
- Think of ways to apply your critical thinking skills in application-based ways.
- The course text website and McGraw-Hill CONNECT will also help you.

In addition to these suggestions, here are a few helpful hints for students of all learning styles:

- Ask questions to make sure you understand what you hear, read, and do.
- Rephrase what you have heard in lecture and read in the text as you talk with your peers.
- Study with a partner to help you stay committed and double-check your understanding of concepts.

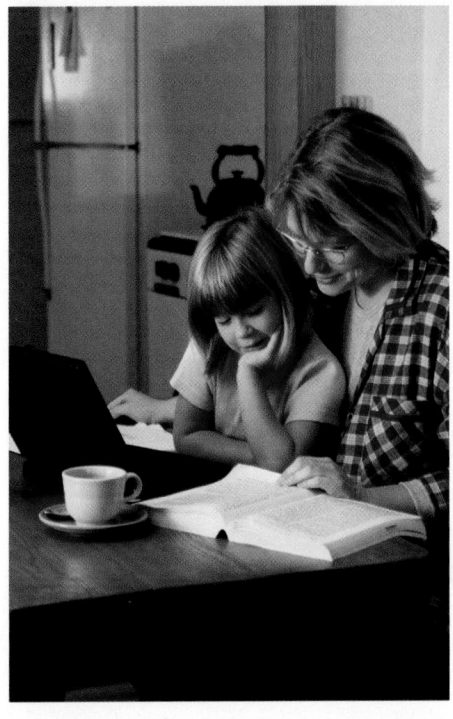

▲ **FIGURE W.13** Identify your own personal preferences for learning, and seek out the resources that will best help you with your studies. Recognize your weaknesses, and try to compensate for or work to improve them.

EXERCISES *Take time to assess your learning style, and use that to aid your study and classroom habits. Identify the type of learner you are, and briefly describe which of the strengths in that style work best for you.*

I am a _____ learner.

This works best for me:

_____

_____

_____

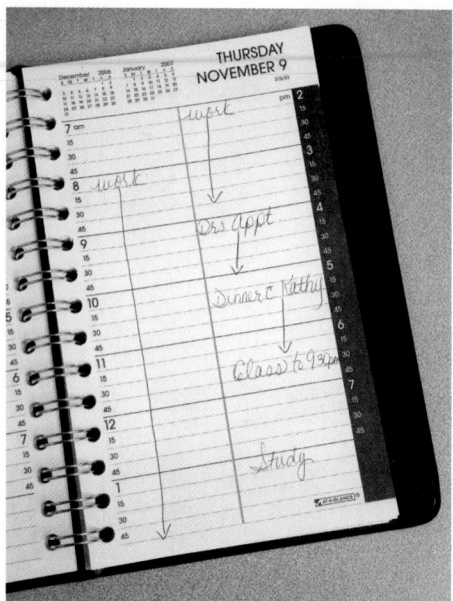

FIGURE W.14 Use a daily planner to organize school, work, family, and leisure time.

STUDY STRATEGIES (continued)

Getting Organized

It seems the more organized you are, the easier things come. This will definitely be the case as you proceed through this class and your externship at Fulwood. Take time now to look around and analyze your life and your study habits. Get organized now, and you'll find you have a little more time—and a lot less stress.

Find a calendar system that works for you. The best kind is one that you can take with you everywhere. To be truly organized, you should integrate all aspects of your life into this one calendar—school, work, family, and leisure *(Figure W.14)*. Some people also find it helpful to have an additional monthly calendar posted in a convenient place (e.g., on the refrigerator) for "at a glance" dates and to have a visual of what is to come. If you do this, be sure you are consistently synchronizing both calendars so that you do not miss anything. (More tips for organizing your calendar can be found in the Scheduling and Managing Your Time section below.) Some sample entries follow:

Thursday

- Work from 8:00 a.m. to 3:30 p.m.
- Doctor's appointment from 4:00 to 4:45
- Dinner from 5:15 to 6:15
- Class from 6:30 to 9:30
- Study from 10:00 to 10:30

Keep everything for your course or courses in one place—and at your fingertips. A three-ring binder works well because it allows you to add or organize handouts and notes from class in any order you prefer. Incorporating your own custom tabs helps you flip instantly to the material you need.

Find your space. Find a place that helps you be organized and focused. If it is a desk or table at home, keep it clean. Clutter adds confusion and stress, and it wastes time. If there are small children in your home, be sure your study materials are kept out of reach. If your "space" is at the library or a relative's house, keep a backpack or bag fully stocked with your text, binder or notes, pens, highlighters, sticky notes, phone numbers of study partners, and anything else you might need.

Scheduling and Managing Your Time

There is never enough time in the week to get everything done. This makes managing your time one of the most difficult tasks to successfully master.

Valuable time can easily be lost. Here are just a few ways time slips away unnoticed:

- **Procrastination**—putting off tasks simply because you don't feel in the mood to do them right away.
- **Distraction**—getting sidetracked by the endless variety of other things that seem easier (or more fun) to do.
- **Underestimating the value of small bits of time**—thinking it isn't worth doing any work because you have something else to do, or someplace else to be, in 20 minutes or so.

Just as you make choices about where to spend your money and how to get the best value for your dollar, you do the same with your time. In order to get the most out of your externship at Fulwood Medical Center and out of your life in general, you have to spend your time wisely. Unlike money, however, time passes whether or not it is what you want. You may be able to save money for future use; but, unfortunately, you can't store away time to use later. However, you *can* plan how you will spend your time in a way that maximizes the quality and the quantity of things you can get done in a day, week, month, or year. If you're like most people, you may not have a good idea of how your time is actually being used.

EXERCISES

Write out all of your activities for a typical week. On average, how many hours each week do you spend sleeping, grooming, eating, working, running errands, attending class, attending your children's activities, and watching TV. Add all of the hours up. There are 168 hours in the week. How many hours do you have left for studying? A sample budget is shown below.

Activity	Number of Hours per Day	Number of Days per Week	Number of Hours per Week
Sleeping	7	7	49
Grooming	1	7	7
Meals: preparation, eating, cleanup	2	7	14
Cleaning, laundry	1	3	3
Commuting to and from school	1	5	5
In class	4	5	20
Doing errands	1	3	3
Family time	3	7	21
Church, workout, hobbies			5
Job			30
Friends, going out, TV, entertainment			6
TOTAL			163
TOTAL HOURS IN A WEEK			168
Hours remaining for study			5

• *Are 5 hours enough for study?*

• *When are they available?*

• *What can you do to increase them?*

Study hours should be spent in a setting that allows you to concentrate on your work and not be distracted. Turn off your cell phone and TV. The biggest question to ask yourself is, "Am I investing my time wisely?" If not, how can you budget your time differently so that more time is spent on higher-priority activities?

STUDY STRATEGIES (continued)

Ten Steps to a Study Schedule That Works   Making a study schedule you will actually follow means knowing yourself and your limits. Implement the following tips to develop a schedule that works for you. Or, if success in the class is not important to you, skip to the next section containing strategies for self-sabotage.

1. **Study when you are most productive.** When are you most productive? Are you a night owl or an early bird? Plan to study when you are most alert and can have uninterrupted segments of time. This could include a quick 5-minute review before class or a 1-hour problem-solving study session with a friend.

2. **Create a set study time for yourself daily.** Having a set schedule for yourself means making a commitment to studying. Write your study time on your calendar, and do not schedule other activities during this time.

3. **Schedule study time using shorter, focused blocks with small breaks.** Studying a little each day rather than cramming the night before a test is a much more effective use of your time. Doing this helps you learn the material and store it in your long-term memory, not just memorize it and forget it after the test. Also, you will be less fatigued and less likely to procrastinate.

4. **Plan time for family, leisure, friends, exercise, and sleep.** Studying should be your main focus, but you need to balance your time—and your life.

5. **Log your projects and homework deadlines.** Record all due dates, tests, and projects in your personal calendar so that you know what is coming. If you have a large project, break the assignment down into smaller targets. Set a goal for the first draft, second draft, and final copy, and record each of these deadlines in your calendar.

6. **Try to complete tasks ahead of schedule.** This will give you a chance to carefully review your work before you hand it in. You'll feel less stressed in the end.

7. **Prioritize.** In your calendar or planner, highlight or number key projects. Do them first; then cross them off when they are completed. Give yourself a pat on the back for getting them done.

8. **Review and reprioritize daily.** Check your scheduled activities each day, and adjust them if priorities have changed.

9. **Resist distractions.** Don't let unscheduled activities take you away from designated study time. The Internet is a notorious time-waster. It is easy to lose hours surfing the Web or instant messaging. It's just as easy to let a 5-minute phone call with a friend turn into a 3-hour conversation. Stick to your schedule.

10. **Multitask when possible.** You may find a lot of extra time you didn't think you had. Review material or deconstruct medical terms in your head while walking to class, doing laundry, or during "mental down time." (**Note:** Mental down time does *not* mean in the middle of lecture.)

How to Sabotage Yourself

If you are determined to **fail,** just follow these simple instructions:

1. Skip class, or, if you do attend, arrive fashionably late.
2. Don't bother studying if you have to be someplace in 20 minutes; that's not enough time to get anything done.
3. Big test coming up? Beat the stress by relaxing with friends, going out for a few beers, or hanging out in an Internet chat room. Be sure to complain to your chat room friends about how there is no way you can pass the test tomorrow.
4. Don't ask questions in class. You are probably the only one who doesn't know the answer, and everyone else will think you are stupid.
5. Don't visit the instructor in his or her office; instructors don't want to be bothered.
6. Be sure to pull an all-nighter before the exam; you don't have time to sleep.
7. The time to begin studying for an exam is the day before the test. Four hours ought to be plenty.
8. When reading the book, yellow highlight most of it. If it's not important, it wouldn't be in the book; and, if it is important, you need to highlight it.
9. Don't take notes in lecture. You can't get it all down anyway, and it would be better just to sit back and listen.
10. Stop reading this book now. Do not continue to the next page to find out how to be an active learner and increase your chances of success in the course.

EXERCISES *Be honest with yourself and self-assess. Are you guilty of any of the tendencies described above? If so, determine to change at least one bad habit before this course begins.*

The habit I would most like to change is:

_____

_____

_____

I recognize that if I change this habit, the **benefit** to me will be:

_____

_____

_____

Remember: Your instructor puts time and effort into preparing this class and marking tests. You need to devote your time and energy to the class as well.

STUDY STRATEGIES (continued)

Being an Active Learner

As you will find out in your externship at Fulwood Medical Center, true learning is active. You can't sit back and let someone else pour knowledge into your head. You need to authentically assume the various health care professional roles you'll play at Fulwood and work to get as much from them as you can. Simply attending your Medical Terminology class is another valuable thing you can do to help yourself. However, it doesn't end there. Here are more ways you can be an active learner and get the most out of your studies.

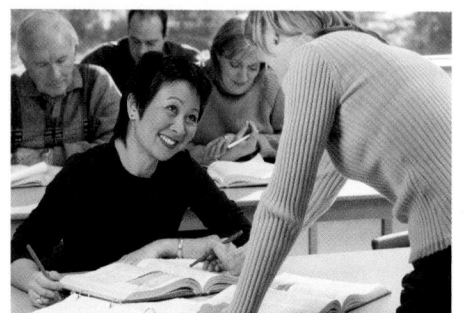

▲ **FIGURE W.15** Being a good listener is important to success.

Getting the Most Out of Lectures

1. **Prepare.** You'll be amazed at how much easier it is to understand the material when you have previewed the chapter before going to class. If you find it difficult to carve out the time, simply arrive at class 5 to 15 minutes earlier than usual and skim the chapter before the lecture begins. This will at least give you an overview of what may be discussed.

2. **Be a good listener.** Most people think they are good listeners, but few really are *(Figure W.15)*. Are you?
   - You can't listen if you are talking or text messaging or looking at your cell phone.
   - You can't listen if you are daydreaming or dozing.
   - Listening and comprehending are two different things. If you don't understand something the instructor is saying, ask a question or jot a note and visit the instructor after class. Don't feel intimidated: You probably aren't the only person who "doesn't get it."

3. **Take good notes.** Here are some tips for successful note-taking:
   - Use a standard-size notebook or, better yet, a three-ring binder with loose-leaf notepaper. The binder will allow you to organize and integrate your notes and handouts.
   - Use a standard black or blue ink pen to take your initial notes. You can annotate later using a pencil, which can be erased if necessary.
   - Start a new page with each lecture or note-taking session.
   - Label each page of your notes with the date and a heading.
   - Focus on the main points, and try to use an outline format to take notes. This will help you capture key ideas and organize subpoints.
   - Review and edit your notes shortly after class—at least within 24 hours—to make sure they make sense. You may also want to compare your notes with those of a study partner later to make sure neither of you has missed anything.

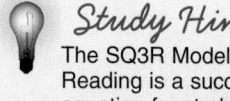

Study Hint

The SQ3R Model for Reading is a successful equation for studying.

Survey what you are going to read.

Question what you are going to learn after the preview.

Read—Read the assignment.

Recite—Stop every once in a while, look up from the book, and put what you've just read into your own words.

Review—After you've finished, review the main points.

Getting the Most Out of Reading

1. **Concentrate on what you are reading.** Survey the titles, outcomes, objectives, and headings in each chapter, and look at the visuals to identify what the chapter is all about.

2. **Use the SQ3R method** (see Study Hint) to help you read actively.

3. **Take notes on key ideas** in the reading.

4. **Write down any questions** you have.

5. **Discuss what you have read** with your study partner.

Performing Well on Tests

1. **Always read the directions.** If you are unsure, ask. Find out if there is a penalty for guessing. If there is not, try to answer every question on the test even if you have to guess at some.

2. **Before you begin, scan the entire test** so that you know how long it is and what types of activities it contains.

3. **Answer the easy questions or sections first** so that you get as much of the exam finished as possible if difficult questions slow you down.
   - When answering multiple-choice questions, eliminate each incorrect option until you are left with the answer that seems most correct to you.
   - When answering matching questions, match all items you know first; then do your best with the ones that remain.
   - When answering essay questions, reword the question as a statement to be sure you have answered it. Give enough examples and explanation to support your points.

4. **Once you have finished the test, use any extra time to check that you have answered all questions.** If you still have time after checking for completion, reread the questions and recheck your answers.

Studying with a Partner or Group

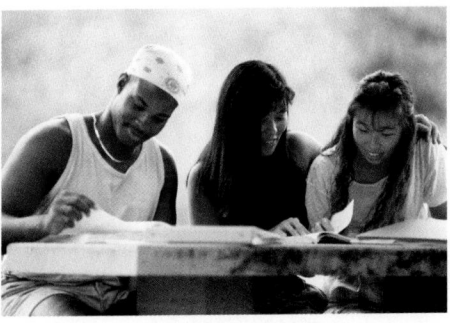

▲ **FIGURE W.16** Studying with a partner can help you succeed, and it can be fun.

1. **Get a study partner.** Schedule set study dates. Talk through the concepts, compare notes, and quiz each other *(Figure W.16)*. Studying with a partner can be fun. Think of it this way: You are multitasking, layering study time and social time. Just be sure the social time doesn't squeeze out the study time.

2. **Don't take advantage of your study partner.** If you can't make a study date or attend a class, let your partner know. You won't have a study partner—or a friend—much longer if it isn't a mutually beneficial arrangement.

3. **Establish a study group.** Choose a few students in the class, including your study partner, with whom to study on a regular basis. Having a group in addition to a study partner ensures that you will still be able to study with others if your partner has to miss a session.

EXERCISES

Budgeting your time is key to being able to take care of your priorities. Follow these steps with the list of tasks you need to get done:

1. Rank each of the tasks in the table in order of its priority (e.g., 1 is the highest priority, 2 is next highest, and so on).

2. On a separate sheet of paper, plan a weekly schedule that will help you accomplish these tasks. Include all seven days of the week, and block off the days in hourly increments.

3. Keep in mind that while some activities have set times, others can be flexible. Also consider that activities like studying and household tasks will need to be done for a period of time *every day*, not just once a week.

   (**Note:** *There is no one "correct" answer to this exercise; however, it is beneficial to see how other students in the class chose to budget their time. Be creative but realistic. Don't forget to budget for travel time between tasks if needed.*)

Weekly Tasks

Studying for Medical Terminology _____	Errands (groceries, etc.) _____	Leisure time _____
Sleep _____	Family time _____	Household chores _____
Medical Terminology class (Tuesday and Thursday 6:30–9:30 p.m.) _____	Work (8:00–3:30 daily) _____	Meals, including preparation & cleanup _____
Church and/or hobbies _____	Exercise _____	Grooming _____

Armed with an understanding of what it takes to be successful, you are now ready to move through this textbook as if engaged in an externship at Fulwood Medical Center.

Anatomy of Word Building
The Language of Health Care

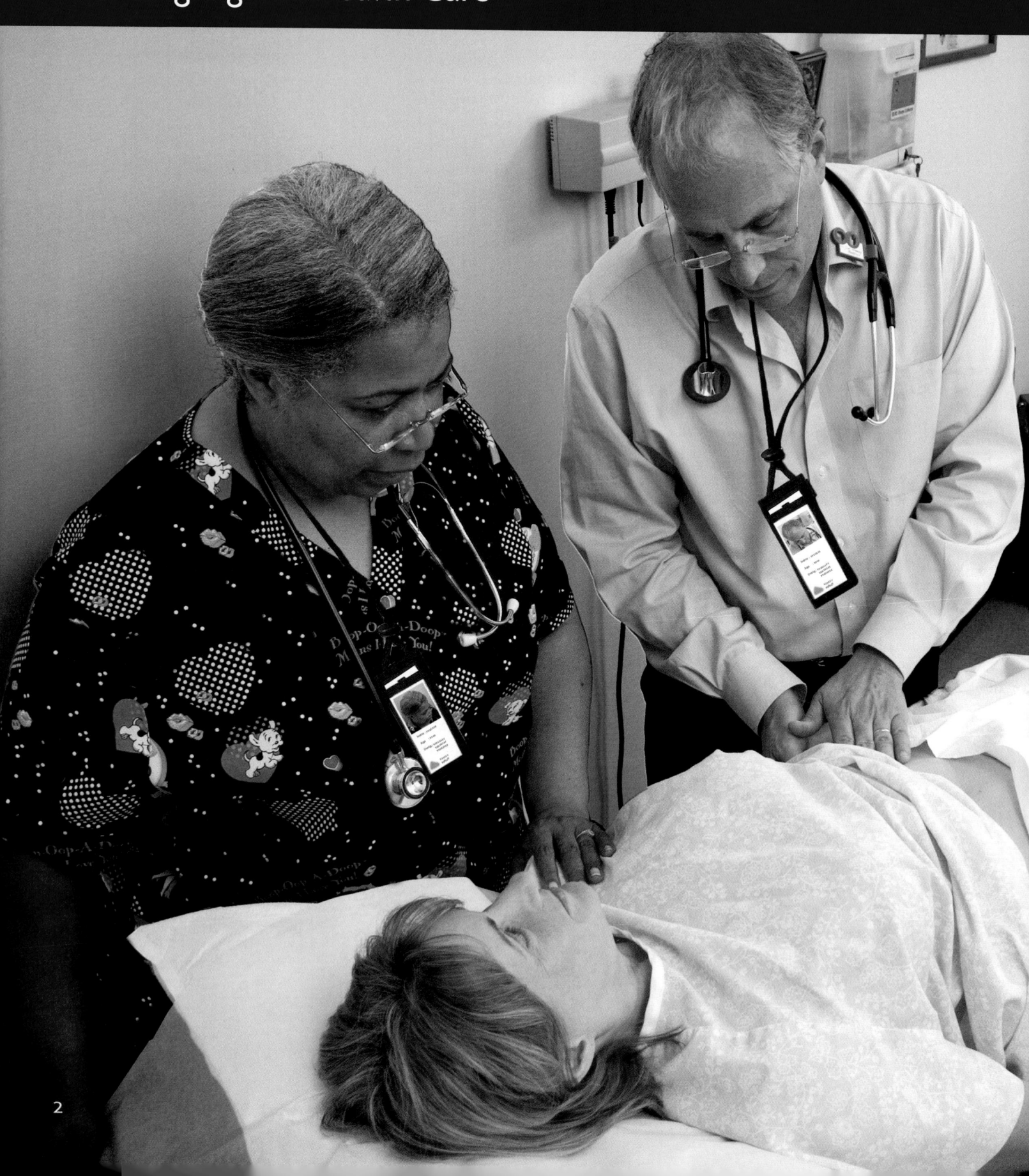

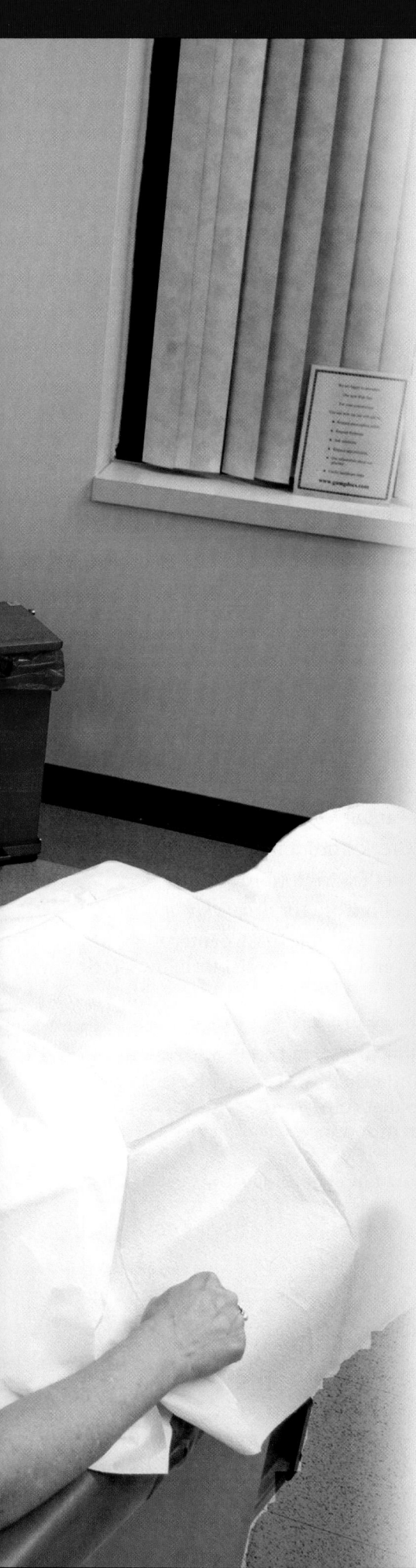

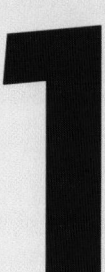
CASE REPORT 1.1

You are

. . . a medical assistant working for
Russell Gordon, MD, a primary care
physician at Fulwood Medical Center.

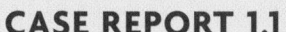

Your patient is

. . . Mrs. Connie Bishop, a 55-year-old
woman who presents with a swelling
in her lower abdomen and shortness
of breath. She has no gynecologic or
gastroenterologic symptoms. Her previous medical history shows recurrent
dermatitis of her hands since a teenager and an arthroscopy for a knee
injury at age 40. Physical examination
reveals a circular mass 6 inches in
diameter in the left lower quadrant of
her abdomen. There is no abnormality in her respiratory or cardiovascular
system.

   Your role is to maintain her medical
record and document her care, assist
Dr. Gordon during his examinations,
explain the examination and treatment
procedures to Mrs. Bishop, and facilitate her referral for specialist care.

Learning Outcomes

   Review the various case reports
shown in this chapter. Pay close
attention to the terms and language
contained in them. You will see that
medicine has its own language. This
language provides all the health
professionals involved in the care of
a patient with the ability to communicate with each other by using
medical terms with precise meanings. This chapter is designed to give
you tools that will enable you to:

1.1 Understand the logic of the
language of medicine and
relate it to your practice as
a health care professional.

1.2 Construct medical terms
using prefixes, roots,
combining forms, and suffixes.

1.3 Use roots, combining forms,
prefixes, and suffixes so that
you can analyze, deconstruct,
and determine the meaning
of medical terms.

1.4 Comprehend, spell, and write
medical terms so that you
communicate and document
accurately and precisely in
any health care setting.

1.5 Recognize and pronounce
medical terms so that you
communicate verbally with
accuracy and precision in
any health care setting.

1.6 Explain the meaning of
medical terms to people
with no medical training.

OBJECTIVES

The technical language of medicine has not arisen at random but has been developed logically from Latin and Greek roots. The first steps to take to understand the logic of the language are to:

1.1.1 Select the root of each medical term.

1.1.2 Identify the meanings of the roots of commonly used medical terms.

1.1.3 Define the terms *combining vowel* and *combining form.*

1.1.4 Construct combining forms for commonly used medical terms.

1.1.5 Identify the combining vowel and combining form of commonly used medical terms.

THE ELEMENTS OF A MEDICAL TERM ARE:

- prefix—the beginning of some words
- root—the foundation of the word that provides its meaning
- combining vowel—vowel that joins a root to another root or to a suffix
- combining form—combination of a root and a combining vowel
- suffix—the ending of some words

ROOTS:

- the constant, unchanging foundation of a medical term
- usually of Greek or Latin origin
- nearly all medical terms have one or more roots

COMBINING VOWEL:

- has no meaning of its own
- joins a root to another root
- joins a root to a suffix
- makes a word easier to pronounce
- "o" is the most common combining vowel, followed by "a"

UNDERSTANDING MEDICAL TERMINOLOGY

To understand and be comfortable with the technical language of medicine is an important key to your successful career as a health professional. Your ability to use the language to communicate verbally and in writing is essential for patient safety, high-quality patient care, interaction with other health care professionals, and your own self-esteem as a health care professional.

Your confidence in using medical terms will increase as you understand the logic of how these terms are built from their individual parts, or **elements.** In addition, understanding the logic will enable you to analyze or "deconstruct" a word, break it down into its elements or its "anatomy," and construct the pieces into a whole to understand its meaning.

The core element of any term is its root. You can use the following information about "roots" to help you understand Mrs. Bishop's Case Report.

Nearly every medical term has at least one root, the element that bears the core meaning of the word. Ninety percent of all roots arise from Greek and Latin words, and many of them have been in use for over 2000 years. For example:

Gynecologic uses the Greek root gynec-, meaning *female.*

Dermatitis has the root dermat- from the Greek word for *skin.*

Arthroscopy has the root arthr- derived from the Greek word for *joint.*

Respiratory uses the root respir- from the Latin word for *to breathe.*

Many words contain more than one root. For example, **gastroenterology** has the root gastr- from the Greek word for *stomach* and the root enter- from the Greek word for *intestine.*

Combining Vowels

You build medical terms on the foundation of a root. Adding a combining vowel onto the end of a root joins that root to other word elements. This vowel has no meaning of its own. It is the vehicle that joins word elements to create medical terms. It also makes the word easier to pronounce. Creating medical terms is like assembling pieces of a jigsaw puzzle.

The vowel "o" is a combining vowel, as shown in gynecologist:

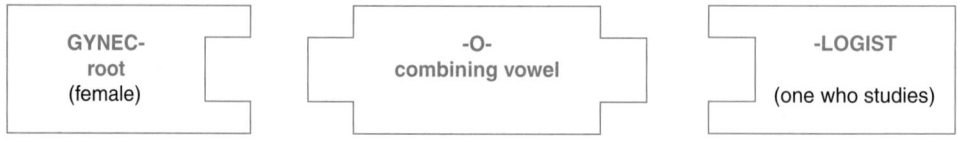

| GYNEC-
root
(female) | -O-
combining vowel | -LOGIST

(one who studies) |

The vowel "a" is a combining vowel, as shown in respiratory:

| RESPIR-
root
(breathing) | -A-
combining vowel | -TORY

(relating to) |

"O" is the most common combining vowel. The vowels "a," "i," and "u" are used less frequently.

Some words have more than one combining vowel. Gastroenterology has two "o" combining vowels attached to different roots.

A combining vowel can be used to link two roots even when the second root begins with a vowel, as shown in gastroenterology:

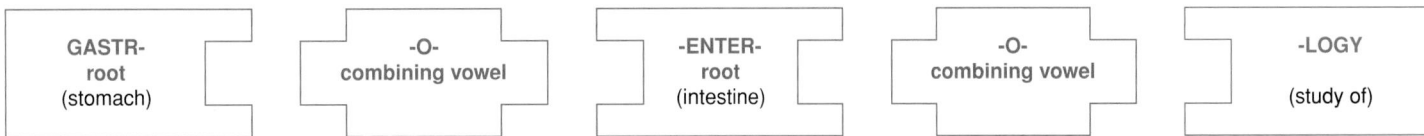

Combining Forms

A root with a combining vowel added to it is called a combining form. For example, the root abd- + the vowel "o," or abd/o-, meaning *belly*, is the combining form for the word **abd/o-men**, or **abdomen**.

Examples of combining forms are:

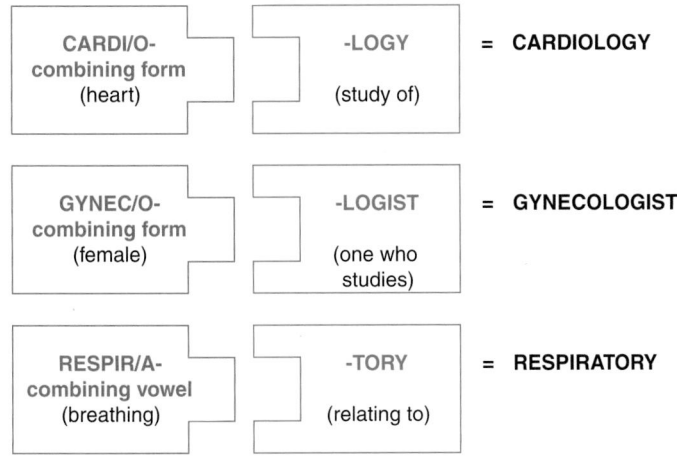

CARDI/O- combining form (heart)	-LOGY (study of) = **CARDIOLOGY**
GYNEC/O- combining form (female)	-LOGIST (one who studies) = **GYNECOLOGIST**
RESPIR/A- combining vowel (breathing)	-TORY (relating to) = **RESPIRATORY**

> **COMBINING FORMS:**
> - combine a root and a combining vowel
> - can be attached to another root or combining form
> - can precede a suffix

An example of a word with two combining forms is **gastroenterology**, the elements of which can be pieced together like this:

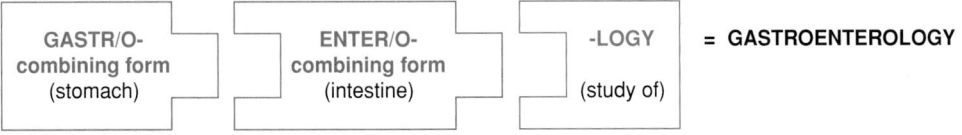

GASTR/O- combining form (stomach)   ENTER/O- combining form (intestine)   -LOGY (study of)   = **GASTROENTEROLOGY**

Keynote

Throughout the book, in word analysis tables, for a **combining form** the root will always be separated from the **combining vowel** by a /.

EXERCISES   *The jigsaw pieces are your visual aid to understanding the logic of how elements form medical terms. Number the puzzle pieces with each statement that pertains to that part of the puzzle. Each puzzle piece will have several numbers. Fill in the blanks.*

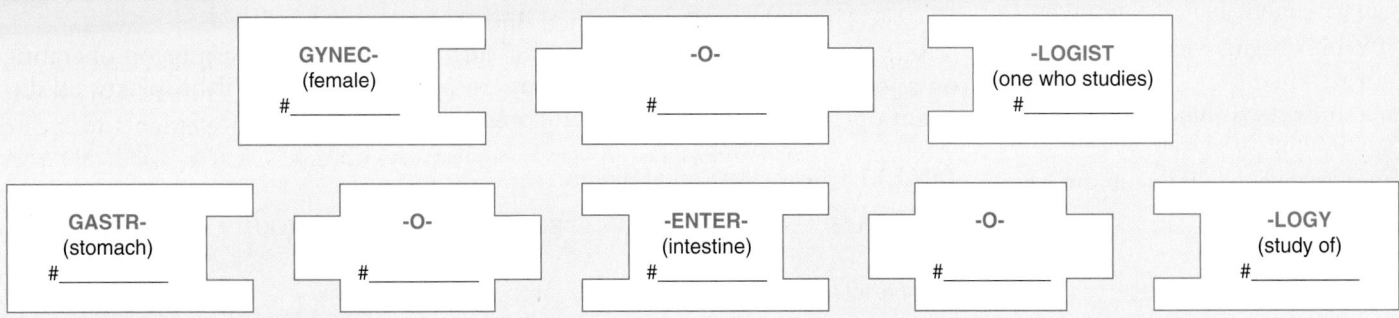

GYNEC- (female) #_____   -O- #_____   -LOGIST (one who studies) #_____

GASTR- (stomach) #_____   -O- #_____   -ENTER- (intestine) #_____   -O- #_____   -LOGY (study of) #_____

Place the numbers of the following statements into the correct puzzle piece.

1. This piece is a root.
2. This piece is a combining vowel.
3. This piece is the end of the term, or the suffix.
4. This piece needs to be in every term.
5. This piece attaches to a root.
6. This piece comes before a suffix.
7. This piece has no meaning of its own.
8. This piece is usually of Greek or Latin origin.

A root + combining vowel = _____ ; examples in these puzzles are the elements _____

OBJECTIVES

Adding a different **suffix** to the end of the same **root** enables you to build a whole new set of words, all with different meanings. Adding a different **prefix** in front of the root also helps to build more medical terms. This lesson will increase your medical word building power by enabling you to:

1.2.1 **Define the term _suffix_.**
1.2.2 **Identify the suffixes of commonly used medical terms and their meanings.**
1.2.3 **Define the term _prefix_.**
1.2.4 **Identify the prefixes of commonly used medical terms and their meanings.**
1.2.5 **Link word elements together to construct medical terms.**
1.2.6 **Dissect word elements to deconstruct medical terms.**

Keynote

A **suffix** is added to the end of a root or combining form to give it a new meaning.

SUFFIX:

- a group of letters
- positioned at the end of a medical term
- attaches to the end of a root or combining form
- can have more than one meaning
- if a suffix begins with a consonant, add a combining vowel to the root
- if a suffix starts with a vowel, no combining vowel is needed
- an occasional medical term can have two suffixes

SUFFIXES AND PREFIXES

Suffixes

You add a suffix onto the end of a word to modify the core of the root and give it a new meaning.

For example, in the medical specialty of cardiology, a cardiologist will often diagnose a cardiopathy.

Another example of the use of suffixes is in the medical specialty of dermatology, when a dermatologist will often diagnose a dermatitis *(Table 1.1)*.

TABLE 1.1 Use of Suffixes

Complete Word	Combining Form	Suffix	Meaning of Suffix	Meaning of Word
dermatitis	dermat- (root)	-itis	*inflammation*	*inflammation of the skin*
dermatologist	dermat/o-	-logist	*one who studies*	*one who studies the skin*
dermatology	dermat/o-	-logy	*study of*	*study of the skin*

In dermatitis, the suffix -itis starts with a vowel so there is no need for a combining vowel, and the suffix is attached directly to the root.

In a different example of the use of suffixes, an orthopedic surgeon operating on a joint can perform an arthroscopy, an arthrodesis, or an arthroplasty, all different operations with different outcomes as shown in *Table 1.2*.

TABLE 1.2 Different Meanings of Suffixes

Complete Word	Combining Form	Suffix	Meaning of Suffix	Meaning of Word
arthroscopy	arthr/o-	-scopy	*visual examination*	*visual examination of a joint*
arthrodesis	arthr/o-	-desis	*fixation*	*fixation of a joint*
arthroplasty	arthr/o-	-plasty	*surgical repair*	*repair of a joint*

You always need a combining vowel before a suffix that begins with a consonant (e.g., dermatology, arthroplasty).

Prefixes

To continue expanding terms derived from the core root of a medical term, you can place a **prefix** at the beginning of the **root**. **Prefixes** are added directly to the **root** or **combining form** and do not require a combining vowel.

For example, you can add the different prefixes peri- and endo- to the same root, cardi-, to produce the different words pericardium and endocardium, which have very different meanings, as shown in *Table 1.3*.

Note that -um is a suffix meaning *structure*.

PREFIX:
- one letter or a group of letters
- precedes a root to give it a different meaning
- can have more than one meaning
- never requires a combining vowel
- an occasional medical term can have two prefixes

TABLE 1.3 Use of Prefixes

Complete Word	Prefix	Meaning of Prefix	Meaning of Word
pericardium	peri-	*around*	structure around the heart
endocardium	endo-	*inside*	structure inside the heart

Similarly, epigastric, hypogastric, and endogastric all have the same root, gastr-, but because of the different prefixes, epi-, hypo-, and endo-, have very different meanings, as shown in *Table 1.4*. Note that -ic is a suffix meaning *pertaining to*.

TABLE 1.4 Different Meanings of Prefixes

Complete Word	Prefix	Meaning of Prefix	Meaning of Word
epigastric	epi-	*above*	pertaining to above the stomach
hypogastric	hypo-	*below*	pertaining to below the stomach
endogastric	endo-	*inside*	pertaining to inside the stomach

EXERCISES

Building onto the elements of roots, combining vowels, and combining forms are the prefixes and suffixes of medical terminology. Prefixes and suffixes are additional word elements that give further meaning to a root or combining form. Develop your knowledge of more word elements with the following exercise. Circle the correct answer, and then rewrite any false statement(s) correctly on the lines below.

1. In a medical term, the suffix will always appear at the end.   T   F

2. Every medical term has to have a prefix.   T   F

3. In the terms **arthroscopy** and **arthrodesis**, the combining form is the same, but the suffix is different.   T   F

4. In the term **endocarditis**, the prefix means *above*.   T   F

5. If a suffix begins with a consonant, you will need a combining vowel before it.   T   F

6. A prefix will always come at the beginning of the term.   T   F

Corrected statements:

_____

_____

_____

_____

_____

In your career as a health professional, the correct, precise pronunciation of medical terms is an essential part of your daily life and of your self-esteem. It is also critical for patient safety and high-quality patient care. The information in this lesson will enable you to:

1.3.1 **Connect the singular and plural components of medical terms.**

1.3.2 **Employ the system for describing pronunciation used in the textbook.**

1.3.3 **Verbalize the pronunciation of medical terms written in the textbook by utilizing the audio glossary found in McGraw-Hill CONNECT as the reference and standard for pronunciation. Your instructor will direct you to McGraw-Hill CONNECT.**

PLURALS AND PRONUNCIATIONS

Plurals

When you change a medical term from singular to plural, it is not as simple as adding an "s," as you often can in the English language. Unfortunately, in medical terms, the end of the word changes in ways that were logical in Latin and Greek but have to be learned by memory in English. This is shown in *Table 1.5.*

TABLE 1.5 Singular and Plural Forms

Singular Ending	Plural Ending	Examples	Singular Ending	Plural Ending	Examples
-a		axilla	-on		ganglion
	-ae	axillae		-a	ganglia
-ax		thorax	-um		septum
	-aces	thoraces		-a	septa
-en		lumen	-us		viscus
	-ina	lumina		-era	viscera
-ex		cortex	-us		villus
	-ices	cortices		-i	villi
-is		diagnosis	-us		corpus
	-es	diagnoses		-ora	corpora
-is		epididymis	-x		phalanx
	-ides	epididymides		-ges	phalanges
-ix		appendix	-y		ovary
	-ices	appendices		-ies	ovaries
-ma		carcinoma	-yx		calyx
	-mata	carcinomata		-ices	calices

Adapted from *Anatomy and Physiology,* 3rd ed., by Kenneth S. Saladin. Copyright © 2004 The McGraw-Hill Companies, Inc. Reprinted with permission.

Pronunciations

In your role as a health professional, pronouncing medical terms correctly and precisely is not only about understanding a conversation when you talk to your peers or your physician. It is also a matter of ensuring patient safety and providing high-quality patient care. One "small error" in writing *ileum* as *ilium*, for example, changes the meaning entirely from a segment of the small intestine to a bone in the pelvis. In most regions, both *ilium* and *ileum* are pronounced **ILL**-ee-um, which is confusing.

Correct pronunciation is essential so that the other health professionals with whom you are working can understand what you are saying. Throughout this textbook, the pronunciation of each medical term will be written out phonetically using modern English language forms. The part(s) of the word to which you give the strongest, or primary, emphasis is written in bold, uppercase letters.

For example, the term **gastroenterology** will be phonetically written **GAS**-troh-en-ter-**OL**-oh-gee, whereas the term **gastritis**, inflammation of the stomach, will be written as gas-**TRY**-tis. **Hemorrhage** will be written as **HEM**-oh-raj, whereas the term **hemostasis,** the stopping of bleeding, will be written he-moh-**STAY**-sis.

The only way you can learn how to pronounce medical terms is to say them repeatedly and have your pronunciation checked against a standard.

The audio glossary that can be found in McGraw-Hill CONNECT is an integral part of your learning program. The new medical terms listed can be easily accessed and listened to so you can perfect your pronunciation.

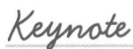

Keynote

Correct pronunciation and spelling enable you to enter the world of health care.

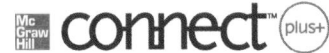

Keynote

Check your pronunciation with the standard in the audio glossary in McGraw-Hill CONNECT. Your instructor will direct you to CONNECT.

EXERCISES

Forming plurals of medical terms can be less difficult if you follow the rules and apply them correctly. The rules are given to you in the following chart—practice changing the medical terms from singular to plural. Fill in the chart.

Singular	Plural	Singular Term	Plural Term	Singular	Plural	Singular Term	Plural Term
-a	-ae	axilla		-on	-a	ganglion	
-ax	-aces	thorax		-um	-a	septum	
-en	-ina	lumen		-us **	-era	viscus	
-ex	-ices	cortex		-us **	-i	villus	
-is *	-es	diagnosis		-us **	-ora	corpus	
-is *	-ides	epididymis		-x	-ges	phalanx	
-ix	-ices	appendix		-y	-ies	ovary	
-ma	-mata	carcinoma		-yx	-ices	calyx	

Note: In the case of the rules with an asterisk (*), both singular terms can end in -is. You have to know on a case-by-case basis which singular terms change to -es and which ones change to -ides.
** The same applies to the singular terms ending in -us—some will form plurals with -era, -i, or -ora.

OBJECTIVES

When you see a medical term you do not understand, the first step you can take to analyze, decipher, or deconstruct the term is to break it down into its component elements or parts. In this lesson you will learn to:

1.4.1 Break down or deconstruct a medical term into its word elements.

1.4.2 Use the word elements to analyze and identify the medical term.

CASE REPORT 1.2

You are

. . . an emergency medical technician (**EMT**) employed in the Emergency Department at Fulwood Medical Center.

Your patient is

. . . Barbara Rotelli, a 17-year-old woman, who presents with **pyrexia** and shaking chills. On her medical record, you read that her physical examination reveals splinter **hemorrhages** under her fingernails and a heart **murmur**. There is blood in her urine. She had **dental** surgery four days ago. A provisional **diagnosis** is made of acute **endocarditis**. You are to prepare her for admission to intensive care.

TO ANALYZE, BREAK DOWN, OR DECONSTRUCT MEDICAL TERMS:

- recognize any suffix at the end of the word and define its meaning
- recognize any prefix at the beginning of the word and define its meaning
- recognize the root and define its meaning
- assemble these meanings together to define the word

Abbreviation

EMT	emergency medical technician

WORD ANALYSIS, DEFINITION, AND PRONUNCIATION

For words you need to define, first identify the suffix.

For example, in the term **endocarditis**, the suffix at the end of the word is **-itis**, which you have learned means *inflammation*.

That leaves **endocard-**. You have learned that **card-** is a root meaning *heart*. So now you have *inflammation of the heart*.

$$Card + itis = \textbf{inflammation of the heart}$$

That leaves **endo-**, which you have learned is a prefix meaning *inside*. So now you can assemble the pieces together to form the word meaning *inflammation of the inside of the heart*:

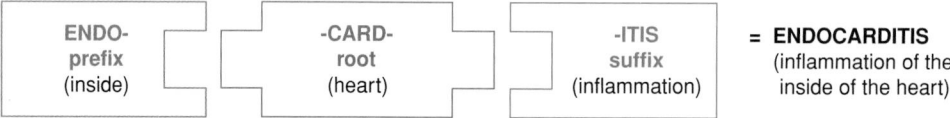

| ENDO-
prefix
(inside) | -CARD-
root
(heart) | -ITIS
suffix
(inflammation) | = **ENDOCARDITIS**
(inflammation of the
inside of the heart) |

You also have learned that the suffix **-um** means *a structure*. So the **endocardium** would be the structure that lines the inside of the heart.

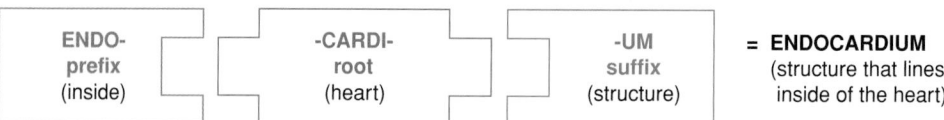

| ENDO-
prefix
(inside) | -CARDI-
root
(heart) | -UM
suffix
(structure) | = **ENDOCARDIUM**
(structure that lines
inside of the heart) |

Therefore, you can understand that **endocarditis** is used to mean that the endocardium lining the heart has become inflamed or infected. Both **card-** and **cardi-** are roots meaning *heart*.

Another example is the word **hemorrhage**, used in Case Report 1.2. The suffix **-rrhage** following the combining vowel "o" is borrowed from the Greek word meaning *to flow profusely*. The root **hem-** is from the Greek word for *blood*. The elements of the medical term **hemorrhage** are assembled together and used to mean *a profuse flow of blood*.

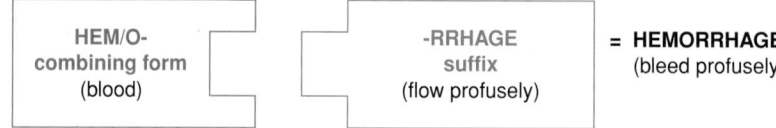

| HEM/O-
combining form
(blood) | -RRHAGE
suffix
(flow profusely) | = **HEMORRHAGE**
(bleed profusely) |

In this book, when the medical terms are broken down into their elements, a hyphen is used to isolate each major element and to identify its position in the whole word.

When a combining form is used, the combining vowel is separated from the root by a slash (/).

One of the key design concepts of this book is that all the textual and visual information you need for any given topic will be on the two-page spread open in front of you. As part of this, in the top right-hand quarter of the two-page spread will be a box designed to give you the elements, definition, and pronunciation of every new medical term that appears in the two pages you are reviewing. For example, the box will look like the following, which refers to the medical terms used on these two pages.

WORD ANALYSIS AND DEFINITION

S = Suffix   P = Prefix   R = Root   R/CF = Combining Form

WORD	PRONUNCIATION		ELEMENTS	DEFINITION
dental	**DEN**-tal	S/ R/	-al *pertaining to* dent- *tooth*	Pertaining to the teeth
dentist dentistry (**Note:** This word has two suffixes and one root.)	**DEN**-tist **DEN**-tis-tree	S/ S/ S/ R/	-ist *specialist* -ry *occupation* -ist- *specialist* dent- *tooth*	Legally qualified specialist in dentistry Evaluation, diagnosis, prevention, and treatment of conditions of the oral cavity and associated structures
diagnosis (noun)	die-ag-**NO**-sis	P/ R/	dia- *complete* -gnosis *knowledge of an abnormal condition*	The determination of the cause of a disease
diagnoses (pl) diagnostic (adj) (**Note:** The "is" in *gnosis* is deleted to allow the word to flow.)	die-ag-**NO**-sees die-ag-**NOS**-tik	S/	-tic *pertaining to*	Pertaining to or establishing a diagnosis
diagnose (verb)	die-ag-**NOSE**	R/	-gnose *recognize an abnormal condition*	To make a diagnosis
endocarditis	**EN**-doh-kar-**DIE**-tis	S/ P/ R/	-itis *inflammation* endo- *within, inner* -card- *heart*	Inflammation of the lining of the heart
endocardium	**EN**-doh-kar-**DEE**-um	S/ R/	-um *structure* cardi- *heart*	The inside lining of the heart
hemorrhage	**HEM**-oh-raj	S/ R/CF	-rrhage *to flow profusely* hem/o- *blood*	To bleed profusely
murmur	**MUR**-mur		Latin *murmur*	Abnormal sound heard on auscultation of the heart or blood vessels
pyrexia	pie-**REK**-see-ah	S/ R/	-ia *condition* pyrex- *fever, heat*	An abnormally high body temperature or fever

Many of the exercises at the end of each spread are based on information found in the Word Analysis and Definition (WAD) box or in the spread.

EXERCISES

To analyze a medical term, simply break the elements down (deconstruct them) into their basic forms. To construct a new term, take the appropriate elements, put them in the correct position in the term, and build your term. **Note:** *Remember that not every term will have all elements present at the same time.*

1. **To deconstruct:** Take the medical term **endocarditis** and break it down into elements. _____ / _____ / _____

P   R/CF   S

The prefix _____ means _____ .

The root _____ means _____ .

The suffix _____ means _____ .

The term **endocarditis** means _____ .

2. **To construct:** Take the following elements and construct a new term with them. _____ / _____ / _____

P   R/CF   S

The element "**um**" means _____ . What type of word element is this? _____

The element "**endo**" means _____ . What type of word element is this? _____

The element "**cardi**" means _____ . What type of word element is this? _____

This term is _____ and means_____ .

OBJECTIVES

This year in the United States, more than 400,000 people will die because of drug reactions and medical errors. Many of these deaths are due to inaccurate or imprecise written or verbal communications between the different members of the health care team. You can avoid making errors in your own communications, and this lesson will help you do that by enabling you to:

1.5.1 **Communicate with precision both verbally and in writing.**

1.5.2 **Utilize word analysis to help ensure the precise use of words.**

You are

... a radiology technician (RT) working in the Radiology Department of Fulwood Medical Center.

Your patient is

... Mrs. Matilda Morones, a 38-year-old woman who presents with sudden onset of severe, colicky right-flank pain and pain in her urethra as she passes urine.

CASE REPORT 1.3

Physical examination has revealed a woman in severe distress with marked tenderness in the right costovertebral angle and in the right lower quadrant of her abdomen. Microscopy of her urine showed numerous red blood cells. The stat abdominal x-ray you have taken reveals a radiopaque stone in the right ureter. She has now become faint and hypotensive.

How are you going to communicate Mrs. Morones' condition as you ask for help and then document her condition and your response?

PRECISION IN COMMUNICATION

In Case Report 1.3, if **hypotension** (low blood pressure) were confused with **hypertension** (high blood pressure), incorrect treatments could be prescribed.

If the patient's **ureter** (the tube from the kidney to the bladder) were confused with the **urethra** (the tube from the bladder to the outside), the consequences could be disastrous.

Here are several other examples of medical terms that can be confused:

The **trapezius** is a back muscle, whereas the **trapezium** is a bone in the wrist.

The **malleus** is a small bone in the middle ear. The **malleolus** is a bony protuberance of your ankle.

Neurology is the study of diseases of the nervous system. **Urology** is the study of diseases of the kidney and bladder and the male reproductive system.

Being a health professional requires the utmost attention to detail and precision, both in written documentation and in verbal communication. A patient's life could be in your hands. In addition, the medical record in which you document a patient's care and your actions is a legal document. It can be used in court as evidence in professional medical liability cases. Any incorrect spelling can reflect badly on the whole health care team.

USE OF WORD ANALYSIS

In Case Report 1.3, **ureter** (you-RET-er) and **urethra** (you-REE-thra) are both simple words with no prefix, combining vowel, or suffix. They are derived from the Greek word for *urine*. They are similar words but have very different anatomical locations *(Chapter 11)*.

Keynote

Communicate verbally and in writing with attention to detail, accuracy, and precision.

Keynote

When you understand the individual word elements that make up a medical term, you are better able to understand clearly the medical terms you are using.

To deconstruct the word **hypotension** (high-po-**TEN**-shun) you start with the suffix -ion, which means *a condition*. Next, the prefix hypo- means *below* or *less than normal*. The root tens- is from the Latin word for *pressure*. So you can place the pieces together to form a word meaning *condition of below-normal pressure*, or low blood pressure.

HYPO- prefix (below, deficient)	-TENS- root (pressure)	-ION suffix (condition)	**= HYPOTENSION** (condition of low blood pressure)

In **hypertension** (high-per-**TEN**-shun), the prefix hyper- means *excessive*. So, when you assemble the pieces together, you have a *condition of excessive pressure*, or high blood pressure.

HYPER- prefix (excessive)	-TENS- root (pressure)	-ION suffix (condition)	**= HYPERTENSION** (condition of high blood pressure)

Your ability to identify the different prefixes of hypo- and hyper- helps to ensure precision in your written and verbal communications.

In the term **costovertebral** (koss-toh-ver-**TEE**-bral), you start with the suffix -al, which means *pertaining to*. Then, separated by the combining vowel "o" are two roots, cost- and vertebr-. The combining form cost/o- is from the Latin word for *a rib*. Vertebr- is from the Latin word for *backbone or spine*. So you have *pertaining to the rib and the spine*.

COST/O- combining form (rib)	-VERTEBR- root (spine)	-AL suffix (pertaining to)	**= COSTOVERTEBRAL** (pertaining to the rib and spine)

The **costovertebral angle** is the angle pertaining to or between the 12th rib and the spine. This angle is a surface anatomy marking for the kidney.

EXERCISES

Precision in Communication: *Verbal and written communication must always be precise and accurate for patient safety and legal requirements. Develop your eyes' and ears' ability to distinguish correct pronunciations, word choice, and spelling to ensure documentation and communication accuracy. Fill in the following blanks:*

1. If the doctor tells you a patient's blood pressure readings were elevated, does the patient have hypertension or hypotension?

   _____

2. If the patient has a problem with his malleolus, would you send him to see an orthopedist (bone specialist) or an ENT (ear, nose and throat) specialist?

   _____

3. If a patient fell off a ladder and injured his back, would it most likely be his trapezius or his trapezium that was hurt?

   _____

4. Does a patient with a kidney infection need to see a urologist or a neurologist?

   _____

5. What is the difference in anatomical location of the ureter and the urethra?

   The ureter is _____ .

   The urethra is _____ .

6. Do you remember what is unusual about the elements of the words **ureter** and **urethra?**

   They have no _____ .

ANATOMY OF WORD BUILDING

CHALLENGE YOUR KNOWLEDGE

A. **Understanding word elements is the key to medical terminology.** Assess your knowledge of word elements by completing the following exercise. Read statements 1 through 15. Each statement applies to a specific word element–root (R), combining vowel (CV), combining form (CF), prefix (P), or suffix (S). Write the number of the statement beside the element to which it applies. The first one is done for you. Every word element in the following list will have more than one correct answer on the line beside it.

Suffix: #_____

Prefix: #_____

Root: #_____

Combining vowel: #_____

Combining form: #___*1*_____

1. Combination of a root and a combining vowel.
2. Different types of surgical procedures can be noted with this element.
3. Usually "o" and "a," but occasionally "i" and "u."
4. "Ic" and "um" are this type of element.
5. Core meaning of the term.
6. In the term **gastroenterology**, which element is present twice?
7. "Endo" is this type of element.
8. Some terms can have more than one.
9. Used to link two roots even when the second root begins with a vowel.
10. In the terms **cardiology, cardiopathy,** and **cardiologist,** which element does not change?
11. "**Abd/o**" is this type of element.
12. Every medical term has at least one.
13. Although opposites, "**hyper**" and "**hypo**" are both this same type of element.
14. Most derive from Greek and Latin words.
15. Can link two roots.

B. **True or False:** Circle the correct answer. On the lines below, rewrite any false answer *correctly*.

1. A term never has more than one root.   T   F

2. Some terms will have no combining vowel.   T   F

3. Modification may be necessary to make a word easier to pronounce.   T   F

4. A vowel must always be present in a combining form.   T   F

Corrected statements:

_____

_____

_____

_____

_____

C. **Root = core meaning of the term and the foundation on which the term is built.** Find the root in each of the following terms, and define it.

Term	Root	Meaning of Root
cardiology	_____	_____
gynecologic	_____	_____
dermatitis	_____	_____
arthroscopy	_____	_____

D. **Root + combining vowel = combining form.** Determine the correct combining form (CF) in the following list of medical terms. Finding the root(s) first will put you on the right track. Fill in the blanks.

Term	Root(s)	Combining Vowel	Combining Form
cardiology	_____	_____	_____
gynecologic	_____	_____	_____
dermatology	_____	_____	_____
arthroscopy	_____	_____	_____

E. **A prefix appears at the beginning of the term, but not every term will have a prefix.** Keeping the same prefix but changing the root and other elements will produce new terms. First, underline the prefix in every term. Then use your knowledge of the meaning of prefixes to fill in the blanks.

1. An **endoscope** is an instrument for looking _____ the body.

   An **endotracheal** tube is inserted _____ the trachea.

2. The **pericardium** is the structure _____ the heart.

   The **perirectal** area is the tissue _____ the rectum.

3. **Epigastric** is the area _____ the stomach.

   Epidermal is the layer of skin _____ the dermal layer.

4. **Hypotension** is _____ blood pressure.

   Hypothyroidism is a condition that occurs when the level of thyroid hormone in your blood is _____ .

5. **Hypertension** is _____ blood pressure.

   Hyperglycemia is _____ sugar content in the blood.

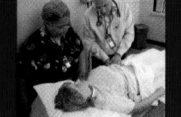

F. **A suffix appears at the end of the term.** Its purpose is to modify the core of the root or combining form and give it new meaning. Your knowledge of suffixes will help you complete this exercise. Circle the correct choice, and finish filling in the blanks. *A hint for the suffix is bolded in each statement.*

1. A **disease** of the heart is cardi/o _____ .

   -logy   -pathy   -plasty

2. Surgical **examination** of a joint is an arthr/o _____ .

   -plasty   -desis   -scopy

3. A **specialist** in the study of skin is a dermat/o _____ .

   -itis   -logy   -logist

4. Visual **examination** of a joint is an arthr/o _____ .

   -plasty   -scopy   -desis

5. A **structure** around the heart is the pericardi _____ .

   -osis   -itis   -um

6. An **inflammation** of the stomach is gastr _____ .

   -logy   -plasty   -itis

7. The **study of** the skin is called dermat/o _____ .

   -pathy   -tosis   -logy

G. **The suffix in this exercise remains the same, but changing the root will change the specialist.** You are looking for a position as a medical assistant. The following practices have advertised on the County Medical Society's job hotline. What are their specialties? (Use your dictionary or glossary if needed.)

Type of Physician   **Medical Specialty**

urologist   _____

gynecologist   _____

gastroenterologist   _____

hematologist   _____

cardiologist   _____

dermatologist   _____

H. **Recognizing word elements will help you "dissect," or deconstruct, a term.** The following terms have an element set in bold. Identify the type of element, and give a brief definition of its meaning.

Term   **Prefix, Root, CF, Suffix**   **Meaning of Element**

arthro**plasty**   _____   _____

endocarditis   _____   _____

hemo**rrhage**   _____   _____

hypotension   _____   _____

hypergastric   _____   _____

I. **To help you master plurals, practice changing singular endings to plural and plural endings to singular in the following exercise.** If you are given a singular word, change it to plural. If you are given a plural word, change it back to singular. The first one is done for you. Fill in the chart; then pick any two terms (singular or plural) and write a sentence for each term on the lines below.

Word	Singular	Plural
carcinomata	*carcinoma*	
ovary		
ganglia		
lumen		
villi		
cortices		
calyx		
epididymis		
axilla		
viscus		
appendices		
corpora		
septum		
diagnosis		
thorax		

1. _____

2. _____

J. **Word elements are the building blocks of medical terminology.** Being able to define word elements will help you use them correctly. Identify the element by placing a check mark (✓) in the correct column; then define the meaning of the element. In the last column, give an example of a medical term containing that element. Fill in the chart.

Element	Prefix	Root/CF	Suffix	Meaning of Element	Medical Term
cardi		✓		*heart*	*endocardium*
entero					
dermat					
logy					
gastro					
scopy					
itis					
gynec					
logist					

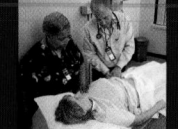

K. Using the elements from the list in Exercise J, answer the following questions:

1. Who is the specialist in the stomach and intestines? _____

2. What is study of the heart called? _____

3. What is inflammation of the skin called? _____

4. What specialist would you see for an inflammation of the skin? _____

5. What is inserting a tube into the stomach for a visual examination called? _____

L. **Spelling is most important in medical terminology.** For example, **ilium** and **ileum** may be similar in appearance and sound, but the difference of one letter makes each a different body part. Choose the correct spelling for the following terms. Fill in the blanks.

1. A Pap smear is part of a _____ exam.

             gynecologik   gyneckologic   gynecologic

2. After a difficult delivery, the patient started to _____ .

             hemorage   hemmorhage   hemorrhage

3. Inflammation of the heart is _____ .

             carditus   carditis   cardiitis

4. A muscle in the back is the _____ .

             trapeze   trapezium   trapezius

5. A bony protuberance in your ankle is the _____ .

             maleus   malius   malleolus

M. **Speak and spell with precision in medical communication.** All terms in the Word Analysis and Definition boxes are spelled phonetically to make them easier for you to learn to pronounce. Be sure you can speak them correctly as well as spell them correctly! Practice, practice, practice. Circle the best answer; then fill in the blanks.

1. The correct pronunciation for an inflammation of the heart is:

    a. EN-do-kar-di-tis

    b. en-DO-kard-itis

    c. EN-doh-kar-DIE-tis

    The correct spelling of this term is _____ .

2. An abnormally high body temperature is:

    a. pie-REK-see-ah

    b. PIE-rek-seeah

    c. pie-REK-see-AH

    The correct spelling of this term is _____ .

3. Profuse bleeding is termed a:

   a. HEM-oh-raj

   b. hem-**OH**-raj

   c. HEM-oh-**RAJ**

Study Hint
Remember to start with the suffix and work back in the term.

   The correct spelling of this term is _____ .

N. **Constructing terms is taking the building blocks of elements and correctly arranging them to form the term you need.** Employ your knowledge of prefixes, roots, combining forms, and suffixes to construct the term required. Fill in the chart.

Meaning	Prefix	Root/Roots	Combining Form	Suffix	Term
Inflammation of the stomach and intestines	_____	_____	_____	_____	_____
Pertaining to the rib and spine	_____	_____	_____	_____	_____
Inflammation of a joint	_____	_____	_____	_____	_____
Visual examination of the stomach	_____	_____	_____	_____	_____
Blood bursting forth	_____	_____	_____	_____	_____
Pertaining to on top of the skin	_____	_____	_____	_____	_____
One who studies the heart	_____	_____	_____	_____	_____
Visual examination within the body	_____	_____	_____	_____	_____

O. **Analyze the following medical terms on the basis of your knowledge of elements.** Put a slash (/) between each element of the terms listed below; then write the definition of each term.

   1. enteric: _____

   2. abdominopelvic: _____

   3. arthroplasty: _____

   4. gastric: _____

   5. costovertebral: _____

P. **The following three elements have something in common.** Fill in the blanks.

Study Hint
Learning elements in groups will help you remember them.

   "**Epi**" means_____ .

   "**Hypo**" means_____ .

   "**Endo**" means_____ .

   1. These are all (circle one):   prefixes   roots   combining forms   suffixes

   2. They can be grouped by (circle one):   color   size   location

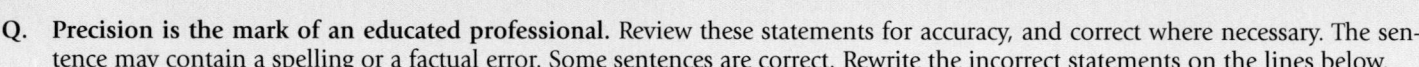

Q. **Precision is the mark of an educated professional.** Review these statements for accuracy, and correct where necessary. The sentence may contain a spelling or a factual error. Some sentences are correct. Rewrite the incorrect statements on the lines below.

1. Patient has a bad case of the hives. I referred her to a neurologist.
2. Discharge diagnosis: resolving cardiitis and cardiopathy.
3. Because of a possible bowel obstruction, I have asked a gastroenterologist to see the patient.
4. Patient is suffering from a topical dermatitis.
5. Due to prolonged hemmorrhaging, the patient needed a blood transfusion.
6. Patient will be scheduled for gastrodesis of her knee on Monday.

Corrected statements:

_____

_____

_____

_____

_____

R. **Terminology Challenge:** Fill in the blanks.

1. Which two prefixes in this chapter are opposites, and what do they mean?

_____ means _____ , and _____ means _____ .

2. Name two suffixes in this chapter that mean *pertaining to.* _____ and _____

3. List two medical specialties that were mentioned in this chapter. _____ and _____

4. What is the medical term for stopping bleeding? _____ *(Watch your spelling!)*

S. **Analyze your word choice to be precise.** Errors in medical documentation are a threat to patient safety and a legal liability. Circle the correct answer.

1. A visual **examination** of the stomach is a:

    gastroscopy   gastropexy   gastrodesis   gastroplasty

2. An **abdominoplasty** would be a surgical:

    fusion   fixation   repair   examination

3. **Endogastric** would be:

    above the stomach   below the stomach   within the stomach   outside the stomach

4. **Arthropathy** would be a disease of:

    skin   joints   arteries   blood vessels

5. If you have a painful **skin** rash, what type of specialist do you need?

    cardiologist   urologist   neurologist   dermatologist

6. The root **respir-** means:

    to walk   to hear   to breathe   to feel

7. If **rhino** means *nose,* what is a surgical repair of a broken nose called?

  rhinodesis   rhinoscopy   rhinoplasty   rhinopexy

8. Which condition would likely affect your heart?

  arthritis   gastritis   dermatitis   carditis

9. Which of these conditions would a neurologist treat?

  migraine   endocarditis   urinary infection   arthritis

Example:

The prefix **hypo-** means _____ ; it can also mean _____ .

1. In hypogastric, hypo- means _____ .

2. In hypotension, hypo- means _____ .

T. **Case Report Questions:** This Case Report is taken from the beginning of Chapter 1. You should feel more comfortable with the medical terminology now. Read the report again, and you will be able to answer the questions. Fill in the blanks.

> **Study Hint**
> Many elements have more than one meaning. You must know both of them because that will make a difference in the use of the medical term.

CASE REPORT 1.1

You are

. . . a medical assistant employed by Russell Gordon, MD, a primary care physician at Fulwood Medical Center.

Your patient is

. . . Mrs. Connie Bishop, a 55-year-old woman who presents with a swelling in her lower abdomen and shortness of breath. She has no gynecologic or gastroenterologic symptoms. Her previous medical history shows recurrent dermatitis of her hands since a teenager and an arthroscopy for a knee injury at age 40. Physical examination reveals a circular mass 6 inches in diameter in the left lower quadrant of her abdomen. There is no abnormality in her respiratory or cardiovascular system.

Your role is to maintain her medical record and document her care, assist Dr. Gordon during his examinations, explain the examination and treatment procedures to Mrs. Bishop, and facilitate her referral for specialist care.

1. What type of skin problem has Mrs. Bishop had since she was a teenager? _____

2. She "has no gynecologic or gastroenterologic symptoms."

   Define **gynecologic.** _____

   Define **gastroenterologic.** _____

3. Her knee injury required what type of procedure? _____

   Describe this procedure. _____

4. She shows "no abnormality in her respiratory or cardiovascular system." Explain this in layman's terms.

   _____

5. What symptoms does Mrs. Bishop have that brought her to Dr. Gordon? _____

   _____

Congratulations! You are on your way to learning medical terminology.

CHAPTER SUMMARY EXERCISE

1. *Listen to the pronunciation of the medical terms as given by your instructor.*
2. *Circle the correct spelling of the medical term.*
3. *Match the correctly spelled terms to the brief descriptions below.*
4. *Write a sentence for each of the 10 terms that appear in this exercise.*

A. SPELLING COMPREHENSION: *Circle the correct spelling of the term.*

1. abdomin	abdumin	abdomen	addumen	adumen
2. cardilogist	cardelogist	cardiologist	cardeologist	cardiollogist
3. respiratory	rispiratory	risperatory	resspiratory	resperatory
4. hemorrhege	hemorrage	hemmorrhage	hemmorage	hemorrhage
5. gastroenterology	gastricenterology	gastrioenterology	gastrology	gastraenterology
6. arthroedisis	artredesis	arthredessis	arthrodesis	arthridisis
7. cardeopathy	cardeeopathy	cardeopathie	cardiopathy	cardiopethy
8. arthriscopy	arthroscopy	artroscopy	arterioscopy	arterioscopie
9. hemostassis	hemostasis	hemmostassis	hematsasis	hemastasis
10. gyneckologic	gynecologic	gynicologic	gynickologic	gynekologic

B. MATCH THE NUMBER OF THE CORRECT TERM IN PART A WITH THE BRIEF DESCRIPTION OF THE TERM BELOW.

a. Stomach and intestines _____

b. Visual examination of a joint _____

c. Stopping bleeding _____

d. Specialist in treating heart problems _____

e. Latin word for *belly* _____

f. Lungs _____

g. Surgical fixation of a joint _____

h. Root means *female* _____

i. To bleed profusely _____

j. Disease of the heart _____

C. USING YOUR KNOWLEDGE OF TERMS 1–10 IN PART A AND THEIR CORRECT SPELLING, WRITE A BRIEF SENTENCE FOR EACH OF THE TERMS AS IT MIGHT APPEAR IN PATIENT DOCUMENTATION.

1. _____

2. _____

3. _____

4. _____

5. _____

6. _____

7. _____

8. _____

9. _____

10. _____

D. YOUR INSTRUCTOR WILL DIRECT YOU TO MCGRAW-HILL CONNECT. OPEN THE AUDIO GLOSSARY AND PRACTICE YOUR PRONUNCIATION OF THE TERMS IN PART A OF THIS EXERCISE.

E. MEET A LESSON OBJECTIVE AND LIST EACH OF THE BUILDING BLOCKS OF A MEDICAL TERM. DESCRIBE THEIR USUAL POSITION IN THE TERM, AND GIVE AN EXAMPLE OF EACH TYPE OF ELEMENT. THEN ANSWER QUESTION #4.

1. Building blocks of a medical term are:

_____   _____   _____   _____   _____

2. Usual position in the term:

_____ usually appears _____

_____ usually appears _____

_____ usually appears _____

_____ usually appears _____

_____ usually appears _____

3. Give an example of each type of element, and its meaning:

Element: _____   Meaning: _____

Element: _____   Meaning: _____

Element: _____   Meaning: _____

Element: _____   Meaning: _____

Element: _____   Meaning: _____

4. To analyze a medical term, where do you start? _____

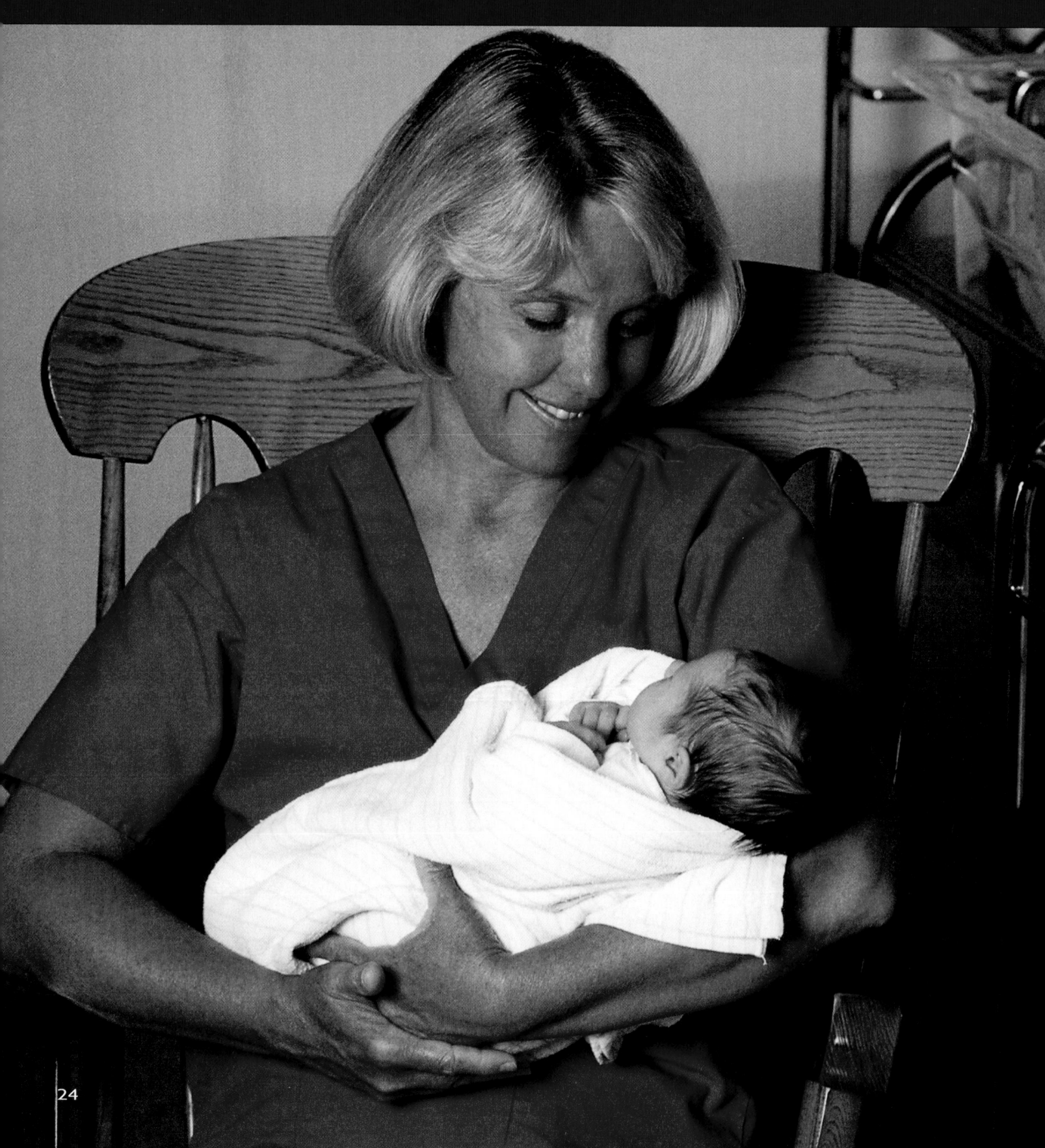

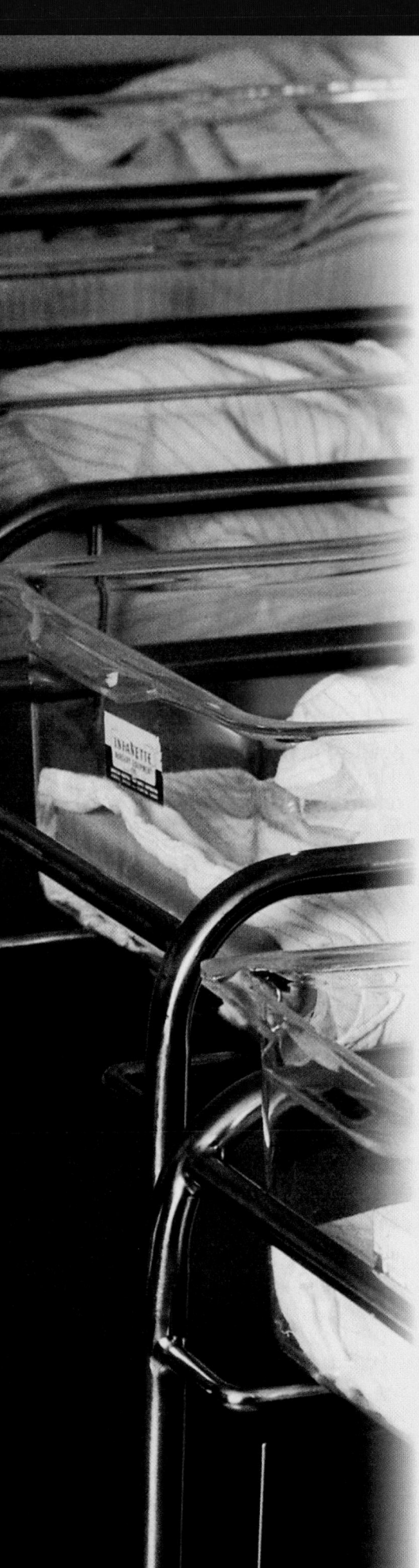

CASE REPORT 2.1

You are

...a certified medical assistant (CMA) employed as an in vitro fertilization coordinator in the Assisted Reproduction Clinic at Fulwood Medical Center.

Your patient is

...Mrs. Mary Arnold, a 35-year-old woman who was unable to conceive. **In vitro fertilization (IVF)** was recommended. After hormone therapy, several healthy and mature eggs were recovered from her ovary. The eggs were combined with her husband's sperm in a laboratory dish where fertilization occurred to form a single cell, called a **zygote**. The cells were allowed to divide for 5 days to become **blastocysts**, and then four cells were implanted in her uterus.

Your role is to guide, counsel, and support Mrs. Arnold and her husband through the decision, implementation, and follow-up for the IVF process.

Learning Outcomes

Each of us begins as a zygote and becomes a whole person. Effective medical treatment recognizes that each organ, tissue, and cell in your body functions in harmony with and affects every other organ, tissue, and cell. Your whole body also includes your thoughts, emotions, and perceptions that affect your health, disease, and recovery. This concept of treating the body as a whole is called **holistic** and requires you to be able to:

2.1 Apply correct medical terms to the anatomy and physiology of the body as a whole.

2.2 Integrate individual body systems into the organization and function of the body as a whole.

2.3 Comprehend, spell, and write medical terms pertaining to the body as a whole so that you communicate and document accurately and precisely in any health care setting.

2.4 Recognize and pronounce medical terms pertaining to the body as a whole so that you communicate verbally with accuracy and precision in any health care setting.

Organization of the Body

OBJECTIVES

All the elements of your body interact with each other to enable your body to be in constant change as it reacts to the environment and to the nourishment you give it.

To understand the structure and function of your body, you need to be able to use correct medical terminology to:

2.1.1 **Identify the structure and functions of the components of a cell.**
2.1.2 **List the four primary groups of tissue, and describe their functions.**
2.1.3 **Identify a major organ, and list the smaller organs contained within it.**
2.1.4 **Name the medical terms associated with cells, tissues, and organs.**

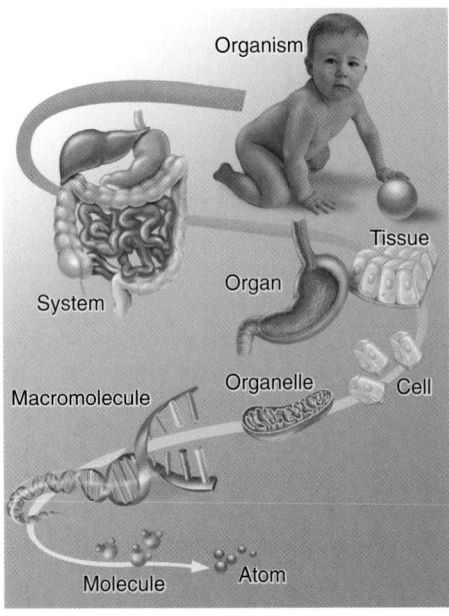

Abbreviation	
IVF	in vitro fertilization

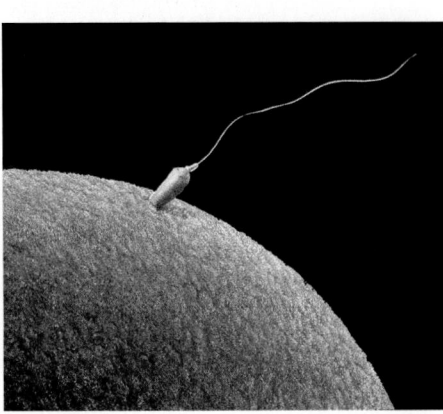

▲ **FIGURE 2.2** **Fertilization of Egg by Single Sperm.**

COMPOSITION OF THE BODY

- The whole body or organism is composed of **organ** systems.
  - Organ systems are composed of organs.
    - Organs are composed of **tissues**.
      - Tissues are composed of cells.
        - Cells are composed in part of **organelles**.
          - Organelles are composed of **molecules**.
            - Molecules are composed of **atoms**.

THE CELL

This single fertilized cell, the **zygote,** is the result of the **fertilization** of an egg **(oocyte)** by a sperm and is the origin of every cell in your body *(Figures 2.1 and 2.2).* The oocyte divides and multiplies into millions of cells that are the basic unit of every tissue and organ. The structure and all of the functions of your tissues and organs are due to their cells. The **cell** is the basic unit of life. **Cytology** is the study of this cell structure and function. Your understanding of the cell will form the basis for your knowledge of the anatomy and physiology of every tissue and organ.

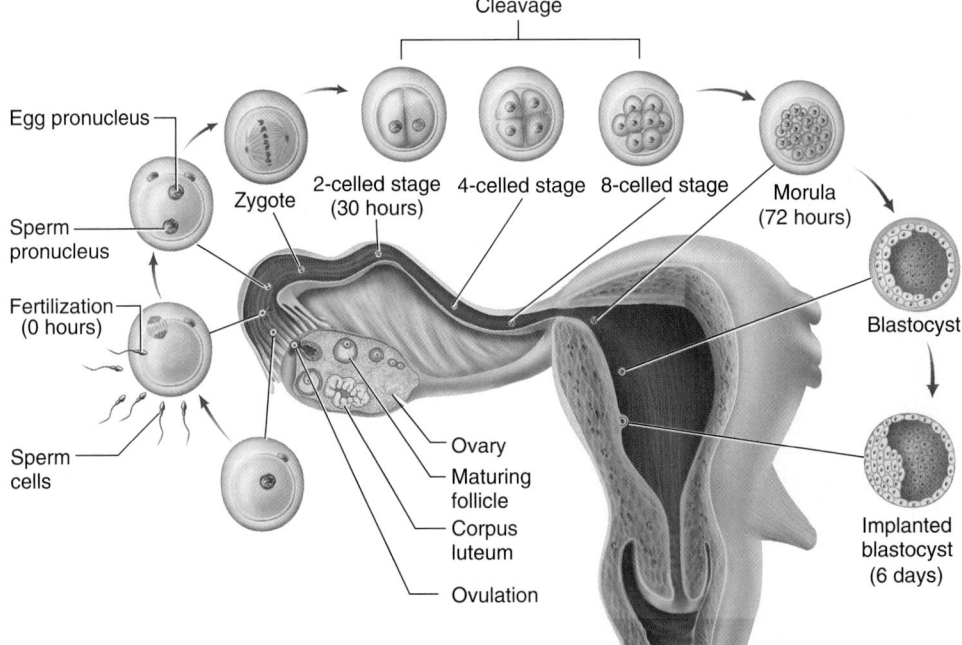

▲ **FIGURE 2.1** **Beginning of Life.**

WORD ANALYSIS AND DEFINITION

WORD	PRONUNCIATION		ELEMENTS	DEFINITION
atom	**AT**-om		Greek *indivisible*	A small unit of matter
blastocyst	**BLAS**-toe-sist	R/CF R/	blast/o *immature cell* -cyst *cyst, sac, bladder*	First 2 weeks of the developing embryo
cell	SELL		Latin *a storeroom*	The smallest unit capable of independent existence
cellular (adj)	**SELL**-you-lar	S/ R/	-ar *pertaining to* cellul- *small cell*	Pertaining to a cell
cytology	**SIGH**-tol-oh-gee	S/ R/CF	-logy *study of* cyt/o- *cell*	Study of the cell
fertilization	FER-til-eye-**ZAY**-shun	S/	-ation *process*	Union of a male sperm and a female egg
fertilize (verb)	**FER**-til-ize	R/	fertiliz- *to bear*	
holistic	ho-**LIS**-tik	S/ R/	-ic *pertaining to* holist- *whole*	Pertaining to the care of the whole person in physical, mental, emotional, and spiritual dimensions
molecule	**MOLL**-eh-kyul	S/	-ule *small*	Very small particle consisting of two or more atoms held tightly together
molecular (adj)	mo-**LEK**-you-lar	R/	molec- *mass*	
oocyte	**OH**-oh-site	S/ R/CF	-cyte *cell* o/o- *egg*	Female egg cell
organ	**OR**-gan		Latin *instrument, tool*	Structure with specific functions in a body system
organelle	**OR**-gah-nell	S/ R/	-elle *small* organ- *organ*	Part of a cell having a specialized function(s)
tissue	**TISH**-you		Latin *to weave*	Collection of similar cells
vitro	**VEE**-troh		Latin *glass*	
in vitro fertilization (IVF)	IN **VEE**-troh FER-til-eye-**ZAY**-shun			Process of combining a sperm and egg in a laboratory dish and placing resulting embryos inside a uterus
zygote	**ZYE**-goat		Greek *yolked*	Cell resulting from the union of the sperm and egg

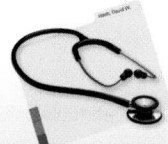

Case Report 2.1 (continued)

Mrs. Arnold achieved pregnancy and delivered a healthy girl at term.

EXERCISES

As you begin your study of medical language, it is important to realize the logic of how terms are formed. Elements are building blocks. You may not see a root in the same position in every term. Not every term requires a prefix and/or a suffix. Build your terms after first reviewing the Word Analysis and Definition (WAD) box. Fill in the blanks.

1. First 2 weeks of the developing embryo   blast/o _____

   R/CF   S

   This term does not have a prefix, and the combining form is at the beginning of the word.

2. Pertaining to a cell   cellul/ _____

   R/CF   S

   This term does not start with a prefix; it starts with a root and ends with a suffix.

3. Study of the cell   cyt/o _____ ;

   R/CF   S

   This term begins with a combining form, which is a root plus a combining vowel. The term ends with a suffix.

   The five elements used to build medical terms are _____, _____, _____, _____, and _____.

> **Study Hint**
> Notice the position of the root in questions 1 and 2. A root can appear at the end of a term or at the beginning of a term, as well as in the middle of a term (its usual place).

STRUCTURE AND FUNCTIONS OF CELLS

As the zygote divides, every cell derived from it becomes a small, complex factory that carries out these basic functions of life:

- *Manufacture* of proteins and lipids
- *Production* and use of energy
- *Communication* with other cells
- *Replication* of deoxyribonucleic acid (**DNA**)
- *Reproduction*

All your cells contain a fluid called **cytoplasm** (**intracellular** fluid) surrounded by a **cell membrane** *(Figure 2.3)*. A single cell may have 10 billion protein molecules inside it.

The cell membrane is made of proteins and lipids and allows water, oxygen, glucose, **electrolytes, steroids,** and alcohol to pass through it. On the outside of the cell membrane are receptors that bind to chemical messengers, such as **hormones** sent by other cells. These are the chemical signals by which your cells communicate with each other. The cytoplasm is a clear, gelatinous substance crowded with different organelles. **Organelles** are small structures that carry out special **metabolic** tasks, the chemical processes that occur in the cell. Examples of organelles are:

- Nucleus
- Endoplasmic reticulum
- Golgi complex or apparatus
- **Mitochondria**

- Nucleolus
- Ribosomes
- Lysosomes

These are defined and their functions detailed in the succeeding pages.

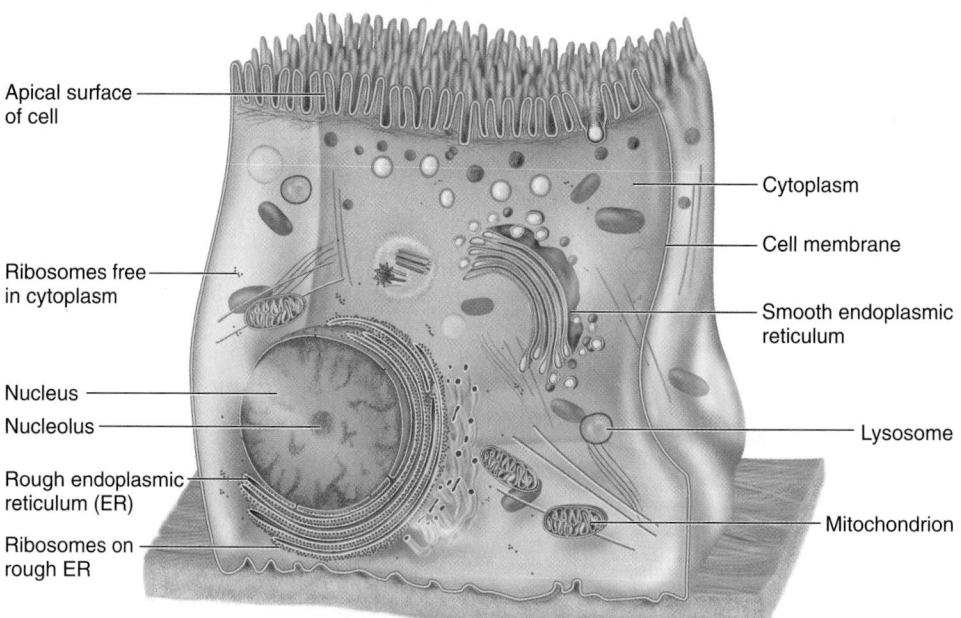

▲ **FIGURE 2.3   Structure of a Representative Cell.**

WORD	PRONUNCIATION		ELEMENTS	DEFINITION
cytoplasm	**SIGH**-toe-plazm	S/ R/CF	-plasm *something formed* cyt/o- *cell*	Clear, gelatinous substance that forms the substance of a cell except for the nucleus
deoxyribonucleic acid (DNA)	dee-**OCK**-see-**RYE**-boh-noo-**KLEE**-ik **ASS**-id		**deoxyribose** *sugar* **nucleic acid** *protein*	Source of hereditary characteristics found in chromosomes
electrolyte	ee-**LEK**-troh-lite	S/ R/CF	-lyte *soluble* electr/o- *electric*	Substance that, when dissolved in a suitable medium, forms electrically charged particles
hormone hormonal (adj)	**HOR**-mohn hor-**MOHN**-al		Greek *set in motion*	Chemical formed in one tissue or organ and carried by the blood to stimulate or inhibit a function of another tissue or organ
intracellular	in-trah-**SELL**-you-lar	S/ P/ R/	-ar *pertaining to* intra- *within* -cellul- *small cell*	Within the cell
membrane membranous (adj)	**MEM**-brain **MEM**-brah-nus		Latin *parchment*	Thin layer of tissue covering a structure or cavity
metabolism metabolic (adj)	meh-**TAB**-oh-lizm met-ah-**BOL**-ik	S/ R/ S/	-ism *condition* metabol- *change* -ic *pertaining to*	The constantly changing physical and chemical processes occurring in the cell Pertaining to metabolism
mitochondrion mitochondria (pl)	my-toe-**KON**-dree-on my-toe-**KON**-dree-ah	S/ R/CF R/CF	-ion *action, condition* mit/o- *thread* chondr/o- *cartilage, rib, granule*	Organelle that generates, stores, and releases energy for cell activities
organelle	**OR**-gah-nell	S/ R/	-elle *small* organ- *organ*	Part of a cell having a specialized function(s)
steroid steroidal (adj)	**STER**-oyd **STER**-oy-dal	S/ R/	-oid *resemble* ster- *solid*	Large family of chemical substances found in many drugs, hormones, and body components

EXERCISES

Continue building your knowledge of elements. Fill in the blanks.

1. Within the cell   _____/cellul/_____

   Add the elements that will complete this medical term. Write under the line the element(s) you have used (P = prefix, R = root, CF = combining form, S = suffix).

2. Substance of a cell except for the nucleus   _____/ _____/plasm

   Add the elements that will complete this medical term. Write under the line the element(s) you have used (P, R, CF, S).

   What makes the difference between a root and a combining form? _____

3. Chemical substance found in drugs   _____/ _____ /oid

   Add the elements that will complete this medical term. Write under the line the element(s) you have used (P, R, CF, S).

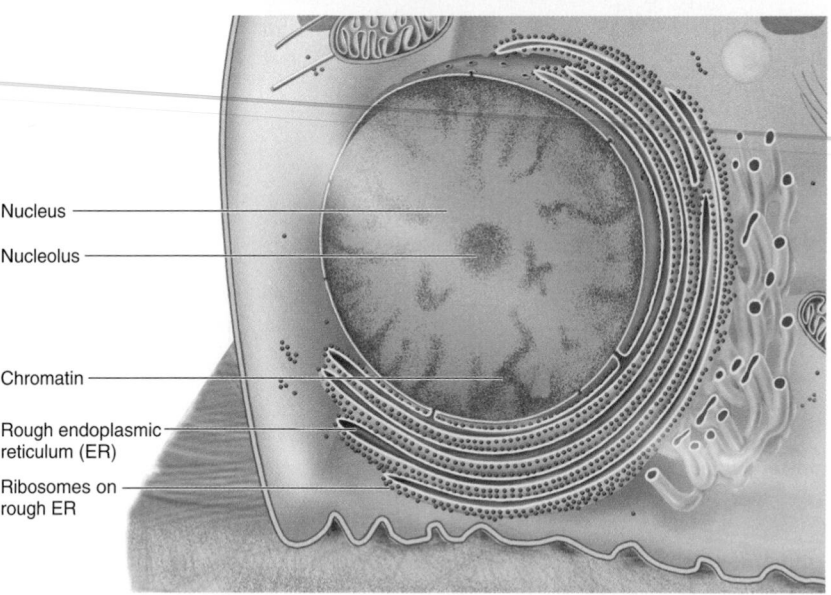

Nucleus

Nucleolus

Chromatin

Rough endoplasmic reticulum (ER)

Ribosomes on rough ER

▲ **FIGURE 2.4   The Nucleus.**

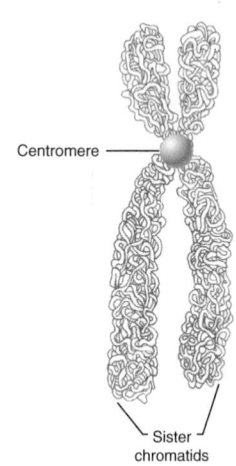

Centromere

Sister chromatids

▲ **FIGURE 2.5**
Chromosome Structure.

STRUCTURE AND FUNCTIONS OF CELLS (continued)

Organelles

The **nucleus** is the largest organelle *(Figure 2.4)*. It directs all the activities of the cell. Most of your cells have one nucleus; red blood cells have none, and some liver cells and muscle cells contain many nuclei. The nucleus is surrounded by its own membrane, which has small openings called pores. Every minute, hundreds of molecules pass through the pores. These molecules include the raw materials for the DNA and RNA synthesis that is ongoing inside the nucleus. (The functions of DNA and RNA are covered in *Chapter 21*.)

Forty-six molecules of DNA and their associated **proteins** are packed into each nucleus as thin strands called **chromatin.** When cells divide, the chromatin condenses to form 46 more densely coiled bodies called **chromosomes** *(Figure 2.5)*. Each chromosome consists of two **chromatids** joined at a pinched spot called the **centromere.** When the cell divides, the two chromatids separate, and each becomes a chromosome in the new cell.

Each nucleus contains a **nucleolus,** a small dense body composed of RNA and protein. It manufactures ribosomes that migrate through the nuclear membrane pores into the cytoplasm.

Ribosomes are organelles involved in the manufacture of protein from simple materials. This process is called **anabolism.**

The **endoplasmic reticulum** is an organelle that manufactures steroids, cholesterol and other lipids, and proteins. It also detoxifies alcohol and other drugs.

The **Golgi complex** (apparatus) synthesizes **carbohydrates** and packages proteins with carbohydrates to form **glycoproteins.**

Lysosomes are organelles that are the garbage disposal units of the cell. They digest and dispose of worn-out organelles as part of the process of cell death. They also digest foreign particles and bacteria.

Mitochondria are the powerhouses of the cells. They extract energy by breaking down compounds such as glucose and fat. This process is called **catabolism.** The energy is used to do the work of the cell; for example, to make a muscle contract.

WORD	PRONUNCIATION		ELEMENTS	DEFINITION
anabolism	an-**AB**-oh-lizm	S/ R/	-ism *condition* anabol- *build up*	The buildup of complex substances in the cell from simpler ones as a part of metabolism
carbohydrate	kar-boh-**HIGH**-drate	S/ R/CF R/	-ate *composed of, pertaining to* carb/o- *carbon* -hydr- *water*	Group of organic food compounds that includes sugars, starch, glycogen, and cellulose
catabolism	kah-**TAB**-oh-lizm	S/ R/	-ism *condition* catabol- *break down*	Breakdown of complex substances into simpler ones as a part of metabolism
centromere	**SEN**-troh-mere	R/CF R/	centr/o- *central* -mere *part*	Junction that holds the two chromatids together to form a chromosome
chromatid	**KROH**-ma-tid	S/ R/	-id *having a particular quality* chromat- *color*	One of the two strands of a chromosome
chromatin	**KROH**-ma-tin	S/ R/	-in *substance, chemical compound* chromat- *color*	Substance composed of DNA that forms chromosomes during cell division
chromosome	**KROH**-moh-sohm	S/ R/CF	-some *body* chrom/o- *color*	Body in the nucleus that contains DNA and genes
endoplasmic reticulum	**EN**-doh-**PLAZ**-mik reh-**TIC**-you-lum	S/ P/ R/ S/ R/	-ic *pertaining to* endo- *inside* -plasm- *to form* -um *structure* reticul- *network*	Structure inside a cell that synthesizes steroids, detoxifies drugs, and manufactures cell membranes
glycoprotein	**GLYE**-koh-**PRO**-teen	R/CF R/	glyc/o- *sugar* -protein *protein*	Combination of carbohydrate and protein
Golgi complex	**GOAL**-jee **KOM**-pleks	 R/	Camillo Golgi, Italian physician, 1843–1926 complex *woven together*	Organelle involved in synthesis of carbohydrates and glycoproteins
lysosome	**LIE**-soh-sohm	S/ R/CF	-some *body* lys/o- *decompose*	Enzyme that digests foreign material and worn out cell components
nucleus nuclear (adj)	**NYU**-klee-us **NYU**-klee-ar	S/ R/	-us *pertaining to* nucle- *nucleus*	Functional center of a cell or structure
nucleolus	nyu-**KLEE**-oh-lus	S/ R/CF	-lus *small* nucle/o- *nucleus*	Small mass within the nucleus
protein	**PRO**-teen	S/ R/CF	-in *substance, chemical compound* prot/e- *first*	Class of food substances based on amino acids
ribosome	**RYE**-bo-sohm	S/ R/CF	-some *body* rib/o- *like a rib*	Structure in the cell that assembles amino acids into protein

EXERCISES

Continue analyzing the logic of medical language. Add the element that will complete this medical term. Write under the line the element you have used (P, R, CF, S). Fill in the blanks.

1. Combination of carbohydrate + protein   _____/protein

   What is unusual about this term? _____

2. Pertaining to something formed inside (the cell)   endo/_____/ _____

   This word contains the main building-block elements for a medical term.

3. Find a term in the WAD that contains an element that means water. _____

CASE REPORT 2.2

Using arthroscopy, the orthopedic surgeon removed his torn **anterior cruci-ate ligament (ACL)** and replaced it with a **graft** from his patellar ligament. The torn **medial collateral ligament** was sutured together. The tear in his medial **meniscus** was repaired. Rehabilitation focused on strengthening the **muscles** around his knee joint and regaining joint mobility.

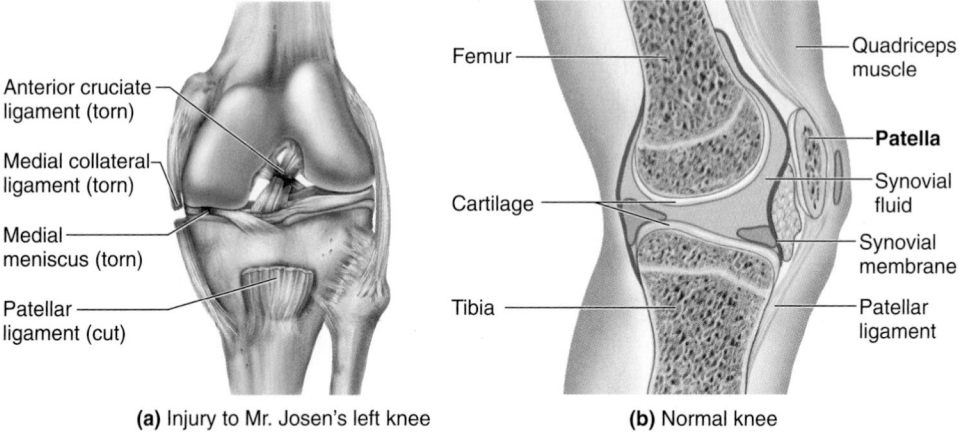

Anterior cruciate ligament (torn)

Medial collateral ligament (torn)

Medial meniscus (torn)

Patellar ligament (cut)

Femur

Quadriceps muscle

Patella

Synovial fluid

Cartilage

Synovial membrane

Tibia

Patellar ligament

(a) Injury to Mr. Josen's left knee

(b) Normal knee

▲ **FIGURE 2.6   Knee Anatomy.**

TISSUES

The knee contains examples of all the different major groups of tissue and will be used in this lesson to illustrate the relation of structure to function in the different tissues. To understand the condition of the 22-year-old in Case Report 2.2, you need a knowledge of tissue structure and function. Ultimately, this is important for your understanding of the anatomy and physiology of organs, organ systems, and the whole body.

Tissues hold your body together. The many tissues of your body have different structures for specialized functions. The different tissues are made of similar cells with unique materials around them that are manufactured by the cells. **Histology** is the study of the structure and function of tissues. The four primary tissue groups are outlined in *Table 2.1*.

TABLE 2.1 The Four Primary Tissue Groups

Type	Function	Location
Connective	Bind, support, protect, fill spaces, store fat	Widely distributed throughout the body; for example, in blood, bone, cartilage, and fat
Epithelial	Protect, **secrete**, absorb, **excrete**	Cover body surface, cover and line internal organs, compose glands
Muscle	Movement	Attached to bones, in the walls of hollow internal organs, in the heart
Nervous	Transmit impulses for **coordination**, sensory reception, motor actions	Brain, spinal cord, nerves

Adapted from *Hole's Human Anatomy and Physiology*, 10th ed., by Shier, Butler, and Lewis. Copyright © 2004 The McGraw-Hill Companies, Inc. Reprinted with permission.

WORD	PRONUNCIATION	ELEMENTS		DEFINITION
anterior (opposite of posterior)	an-**TER**-ee-or	S/ R/	-ior *pertaining to* anter- *before, front part*	Front surface of body; situated in front
collateral	koh-**LAT**-er-al	S/ P/ R/	-al *pertaining to* co- *together* -later- *side*	Situated at the side; having an accessory function
coordinate	ko-**OR**-din-ate	S/	-ate *composed of, pertaining to*	To bring together different structures into a harmonious function
coordination (noun)	ko-**OR**-di-**NAY**-shun	P/ R/CF	co- *together* -ordin- *arrange*	
cruciate	**KRU**-she-ate		Latin *cross*	Shaped like a cross
epithelium	ep-ih-**THEE**-lee-um	S/ P/ R/CF	-um *structure* epi- *upon* -thel/i- *nipple*	Tissue that covers surfaces or lines cavities
epithelial (adj)	ep-ih-**THEE**-lee-al	S/	-al *pertaining to*	
excrete **excretion** (noun)	eks-**KREET** eks-**KREE**-shun		Latin *separate*	To pass waste products of metabolism out of the body Removal of waste products of metabolism out of the body
graft	GRAFT		French *transplant*	Transplantation of living tissue
histology **histologist**	his-**TOL**-oh-jee his-**TOL**-oh-jist	S/ R/CF S/	-logy *study of* hist/o- *tissue* -logist *one who studies*	Structure and function of cells, tissues, and organs
ligament	**LIG**-ah-ment		Latin *band*	Band of fibrous tissue connecting two structures
medial (opposite of lateral)	**ME**-dee-al		Latin *middle*	Nearer to the middle of the body
meniscus **menisci** (pl)	meh-**NISS**-kuss meh-**NISS**-key		Greek *crescent*	Disc of connective tissue cartilage between the bones of a joint; for example, in the knee joint
muscle	**MUSS**-el		Latin *muscle*	A tissue consisting of contractile cells
patella	pah-**TELL**-ah		Latin *small plate*	Thin, circular bone in front of the knee joint that is embedded in the patellar tendon. Also called the kneecap
secrete **secretion** (noun)	se-**KREET** se-**KREE**-shun		Latin *release*	To produce a chemical substance in a cell and release it from the cell

EXERCISES

Change the elements; change the word. *Find a set of terms in the WAD for which changing a single element will change the meaning of the term. Fill in the blanks.*

1. _____/ _____/ _____ means _____ .
   　　P　　　　　　R/CF　　　　　　S

   _____/ _____/ _____ means_____ .
   　　P　　　　　　R/CF　　　　　　S

The element that changed was the _____.

Examples of opposite terms are given in the WAD. Write the terms and their opposites below.

2. _____ is the opposite of _____ .

3. _____ is the opposite of _____ .

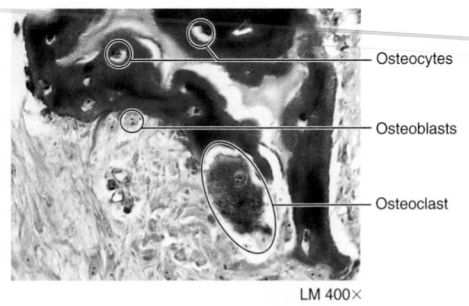

Osteocytes

Osteoblasts

Osteoclast

LM 400×

▲ **FIGURE 2.7** **Bone Tissue.**

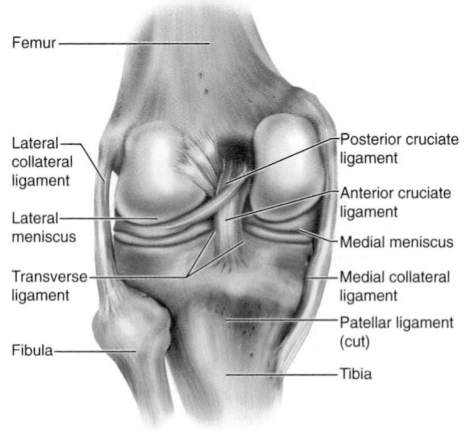

Femur

Lateral collateral ligament

Lateral meniscus

Transverse ligament

Fibula

Posterior cruciate ligament

Anterior cruciate ligament

Medial meniscus

Medial collateral ligament

Patellar ligament (cut)

Tibia

Anterior view

▲ **FIGURE 2.8** **Ligaments of the Knee Joint.**

CONNECTIVE TISSUES IN THE KNEE JOINT

- **Bones** of the knee joint are the femur, tibia, and patella. Bone is the hardest connective tissue due to the presence of calcium mineral salts, mostly calcium phosphate. Bone **matrix** is deposited by bone cells, **osteoblasts,** in concentric patterns around a central canal containing a blood vessel *(Figure 2.7)*. As a result, every osteoblast is close to a supply of **nutrients** from the blood. This enables bones to heal after being fractured. **Osteocytes** are former osteoblasts that maintain the bone matrix. **Osteoclasts** dissolve the bone matrix to release calcium and phosphate into the blood when they are needed elsewhere. Bones as a whole are covered with a thick fibrous tissue called the **periosteum.**

- **Cartilage** has a flexible, rubbery matrix that allows it, as a meniscus, to function as a shock absorber, and as a gliding surface at **articulations** where two bones meet to form a joint. Cartilage has very few blood vessels and heals poorly or not at all. When it is injured or torn, surgical repair is usually necessary. Sometimes (for example, in osteoarthritis) it cannot be repaired. Cartilage also forms the shape of your ear, the tip of your nose, and your larynx.

- **Ligaments** are strips or bands of fibrous connective tissue *(Figure 2.8)*. Cells called **fibroblasts** form a gelatinous (jellylike) matrix and closely packed, parallel **collagen** fibers. These fibers provide the strength the ligament needs. The knee joint has a complex array of 11 ligaments that hold it together, prevent it from rotating when we stand upright, and help prevent dislocations. Their blood supply is poor, so they do not heal well without surgery.

- **Tendons** are thick, strong ligaments that attach muscles to bone.

- The **joint capsule** of the knee joint is attached to the tibia and femur, encloses the joint cavity, and is made of thin, collagen fibrous connective tissue. It is strengthened by fibers that extend over it from the ligaments and muscles surrounding the knee joint. These features are common to most joints.

- The inner surface of many joint capsules is lined with **synovial membrane,** which secretes **synovial fluid.** This fluid is a slippery lubricant retained in the joint cavity by the capsule. It has a texture similar to raw egg white. It makes joint movement almost friction-free and distributes nutrients to the cartilage on the joint surfaces of bone.

- **Muscle tissue** stabilizes the knee joint. Extensions of the tendons of the *quadriceps femoris,* the large muscle in front of the thigh, and of the *semimembranosus muscle* on the rear of the thigh, are major stabilizers. The muscles themselves respectively extend and flex the joint. The structure and functions of these and other skeletal muscles are described in *Chapter 5.*

- **Nervous tissue** extensively supplies all the knee structures, which is why a knee injury is excruciatingly painful. The structure and functions of nervous tissue are described in *Chapter 10.*

WORD	PRONUNCIATION		ELEMENTS	DEFINITION
articulate articulation (noun)	ar-**TIK**-you-late ar-tik-you-**LAY**-shun		Latin *jointed*	To form a joint so as to allow movement Joint formed to allow movement
capsule capsular (adj)	**KAP**-syul **KAP**-syu-lar	S/ R/	-ule *little* caps- *box*	Fibrous tissue layer surrounding a joint or some other structure
cartilage	**KAR**-tih-lage		Latin *gristle*	Nonvascular firm, connective tissue found mostly in joints
collagen	**KOL**-ah-jen	S/ R/CF	-gen *produce, form* coll/a- *glue*	Major protein of connective tissue, cartilage, and bone
fibroblast	**FIE**-bro-blast	S/ R/CF	-blast *germ cell* fibr/o- *fiber*	Cell that forms collagen fibers
matrix	**MAY**-triks		Latin "mater" *mother*	Substance that surrounds cells, is manufactured by the cells, and holds them together
nutrient	**NYU**-tree-ent	S/ R/	-ent *end result* nutri- *nourish*	A substance in food required for normal physiologic function
osteoblast	**OS**-tee-oh-blast	S/ R/CF	-blast *germ cell* oste/o- *bone*	Bone-forming cell
osteoclast osteocyte	**OS**-tee-oh-klast **OS**-tee-oh-site	S/ S/	-clast *break* -cyte *cell*	Bone-removing cell Bone-maintaining cell
periosteum	**PER**-ee-**OSS**-tee-um	S/ P/ R/	-um *tissue* peri- *around* -oste- *bone*	Fibrous membrane covering a bone
synovial (adj)	si-**NOH**-vee-al	S/ P/ R/CF	-al *pertaining to* syn- *together* -ov/i- *egg*	Pertaining to synovial fluid and synovial membrane
tendon	**TEN**-dun		Latin *sinew*	Fibrous band that connects muscle to bone

EXERCISES

Understanding elements is the key to a large medical vocabulary. Work with the following exercise to increase your knowledge of the medical language. Fill in the blanks.

osteoblast   osteoclast   osteocyte

1. These terms all refer to (circle one):   cartilage   bone   collagen   *Be careful!*

   With the element: _____ .

2. Underline the element that changes in every term.

   The element that changes is the (circle one):   P   R   CF   S

3. Osteo**blast** means _____ .

   Osteo**clast** means _____ .

   Osteo**cyte** means _____ .

4. The difference between a **fibroblast** and an **osteoblast** is:

   _____

   _____

5. In question 4, this element has changed: _____; and this element has remained the same: _____ .

CASE REPORT 2.3

Fulwood Medical Center

An 84-year-old man with advanced **Parkinson disease** was having difficulty breathing because his stooped **posture** was compressing his lungs and his loss of muscle control made respiration more difficult. A bout of influenza increased his breathing difficulty, and a **tracheostomy** tube was inserted to help him breathe. He then became unable to swallow, and a feeding tube was inserted. Because of **hypertrophy** of his prostate, he developed a **urinary** tract infection. This led to **septicemia.** The bloodborne infection attacked his kidneys, heart, and lungs, leading to failure of these organs and their organ systems and, ultimately, death.

As described in the Case Report, when organs and organ systems do not function in an **integrated** way, a person can die.

An **organ** is a structure composed of several tissues that work together to carry out specific functions. For example, the skin is an organ that has different tissues in it such as epithelial cells, hair, nails, and glands.

An **organ system** is a group of organs with a specific collective function, such as digestion, circulation, or respiration. For example, the nose, pharynx, larynx, trachea, and bronchi work together to achieve the total function of respiration.

Organ Systems

The body has 11 organ systems, shown in *Table 2.2*. Muscular and skeletal can be considered one organ system, the musculoskeletal system.

All your organ systems work together to ensure that your body's internal environment remains relatively constant. This process is called **homeostasis.** For example, your digestive, respiratory, and circulatory organ systems work together so that (a) every cell in your body receives adequate nutrients and oxygen and (b) waste products from the breakdown of these nutrients during cell metabolism are removed. Your cells can then function normally. Disease affecting an organ or organ system disrupts this game plan of homeostasis.

Keynote

Homeostasis is the coordinated response of all the organs to maintain the internal physiologic stability of an organism.

TABLE 2.2 Organ Systems

Organ System	Major Organs	Major Functions
Integumentary	Skin, hair, nails, sweat glands, sebaceous glands	Protect tissues, regulate body temperature, support sensory receptors
Skeletal	Bones, ligaments, cartilages, tendons	Provide framework, protect soft tissues, provide attachments for muscles, produce blood cells, store inorganic salts
Muscular	Muscles	Cause movements, maintain posture, produce body heat
Nervous	Brain, spinal cord, nerves, sense organs	Detect changes, receive and interpret sensory information, stimulate muscles and glands
Endocrine	Glands that secrete hormones: pituitary, thyroid, parathyroid, adrenal, pancreas, ovaries, testes, pineal, thymus	Control metabolic activities of organs and structures
Cardiovascular	Heart, blood vessels	Move blood and transport substances throughout body
Lymphatic	Lymph vessels and nodes, thymus, spleen	Return tissue fluid to the blood, carry certain absorbed food molecules, defend body against infection
Digestive	Mouth, tongue, teeth, salivary glands, pharynx, esophagus, stomach, liver, gallbladder, pancreas, small and large intestines	Receive, break down, and absorb food, eliminate unabsorbed material
Respiratory	Nasal cavity, pharynx, larynx, trachea, bronchi, lungs	Intake and output air, exchange gases between air and blood
Urinary	Kidneys, ureters, urinary bladder, urethra	Remove wastes from blood, maintain water and electrolyte balance, store and transport urine
Reproductive	*Male:* scrotum, testes, epididymides, vas deferens, seminal vesicles, prostate, bulbourethral glands, urethra, penis	Produce and maintain sperm cells, transfer sperm cells into female reproductive tract, secrete male hormones
	Female: ovaries, uterine (fallopian) tubes, uterus, vagina, vulva	Produce and maintain egg cells, receive sperm cells, support development of an embryo, function in birth process, secrete female hormones

Adapted from *Hole's Human Anatomy and Physiology,* 10th ed., by Shier, Butler, and Lewis. Copyright © 2004 The McGraw-Hill Companies, Inc. Reprinted with permission.

WORD	PRONUNCIATION	ELEMENTS		DEFINITION
homeostasis (**Note:** Hemostasis is very different.)	ho-mee-oh-**STAY**-sis	S/ R/CF	-stasis *stand still, control* home/o- *the same*	Stability or equilibrium of a system or the body's internal environment
hypertrophy	high-**PER**-troh-fee	P/ R/	hyper- *excessive* -trophy *development*	Increase in size, but not in number, of an individual tissue element
integrate	**IN**-teh-grate	S/	-ate *composed of, pertaining to*	To bring together into a complete and harmonious whole
integration (noun)	**IN**-teh-**GRAY**-shun	R/	integr- *whole*	
organ	**OR**-gan		Greek *instrument*	Structure with specific functions in a body system
Parkinson disease	**PAR**-kin-son diz-**EEZ**		James Parkinson, British physician, 1755–1824	Disease of muscular rigidity, tremors, and a masklike facial expression
posture	**POSS**-chur		Latin *placement*	The carriage of the body as a whole and the position of the limbs
septicemia	sep-tih-**SEE**-mee-ah	S/ R/	-emia *blood condition* septic- *infected*	Microorganisms circulating in, and infecting, the blood (blood poisoning)
tracheostomy	tray-kee-**OST**-oh-me	S/ R/CF	-stomy *new opening* trache/o- *windpipe*	Incision into the windpipe, usually so that a tube can be inserted to assist breathing
urinary	**YUR**-in-ary	S/ R/	-ary *pertaining to* urin- *urine*	Pertaining to urine

Organs

Go to *Table 2.2*, and see that each organ system contains several organs. An organ is composed of two or more tissue types that perform a particular function. Each organ has well-defined anatomical boundaries separating it from adjacent structures. The different organs in an organ system are usually interconnected. For example, in the urinary organ system, the organs are the kidneys, ureters, bladder, and urethra, and they are all connected *(Figure 2.9)*.

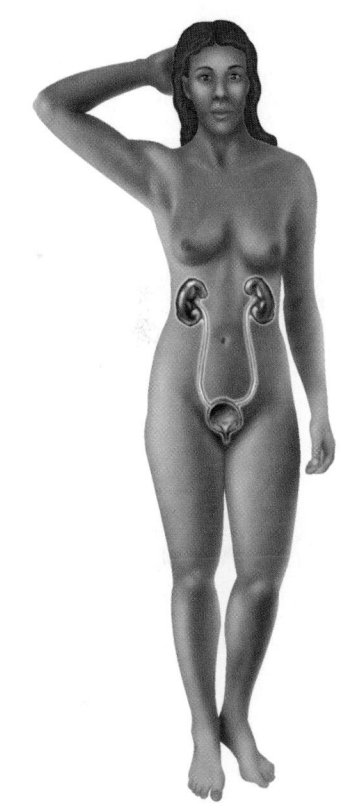

▲ **FIGURE 2.9   Urinary System.**

EXERCISES

Use your knowledge of the building blocks of terms, and **deconstruct** *the following terms into their basic elements. This will give you a better picture of how the words were formed. Fill in the blanks.*

Medical Term	Prefix	Root and/or Combining Form	Suffix	Meaning of Term
homeostasis				
hypertrophy				
septicemia				
tracheostomy				
urinary				

Anatomical Positions, Planes, and Directions

Terms have been developed over the past several thousand years to enable you to describe clearly where different anatomical structures and lesions are in relation to each other. To communicate effectively with other health professionals, it is critical that you are able to use the terminology to describe these positions and relative positions. To do this, you need to be able to use correct medical terminology to:

2.2.1 Define the fundamental anatomical position on which all descriptions of anatomical locations are based.

2.2.2 Describe the different anatomical planes and directions.

2.2.3 Locate the body cavities.

2.2.4 Identify the four abdominal quadrants and three regions.

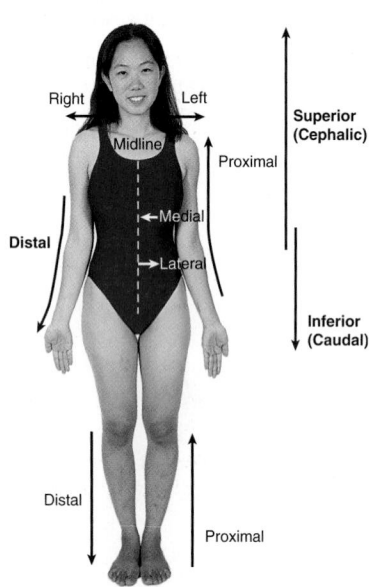

▲ **FIGURE 2.10 Anatomical Position with Directional Terms.**

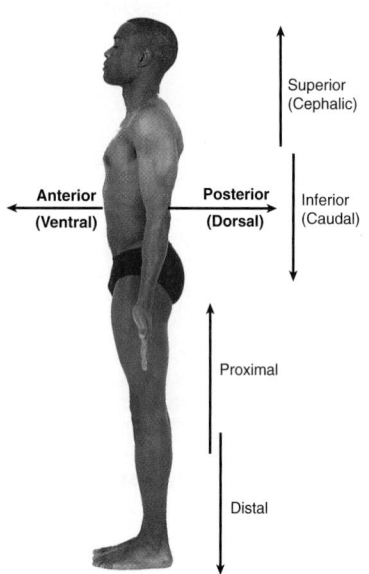

▲ **FIGURE 2.11 Directional Terms.**

ANATOMICAL POSITION

When all **anatomical** descriptions are used, it is assumed that the body is in the anatomical position. The body is standing erect with feet flat on the floor, face and eyes facing forward, and arms at the sides with the palms facing forward *(Figure 2.10)*.

When your palms face forward, the forearm is **supine.** When you lie down flat on your back, you are supine. When your palms face backward, the forearm is **prone.** When you lie down flat on your belly, you are prone.

DIRECTIONAL TERMS

Directional terms describe the position of one structure or part of the body relative to another. These directional terms are shown in *Figures 2.10 and 2.11*.

ANATOMICAL PLANES

Different views of the body are based on imaginary "slices" producing flat surfaces that pass through the body *(Figure 2.12)*. The three major anatomical planes are:

- **Transverse** or **horizontal**—a plane passing across the body parallel to the floor and perpendicular to the body's long axis. It divides the body into an upper (**superior**) portion and a lower (**inferior**) portion.
- **Sagittal**—a vertical plane that divides the body into right and left portions.
- **Frontal** or **coronal**—a vertical plane that divides the body into front (**anterior**) and back (**posterior**) portions.

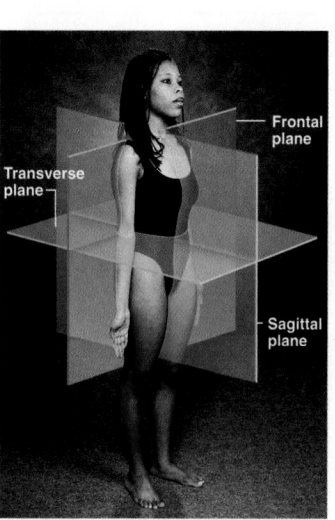

▲ **Figure 2.12 Anatomical Planes.**

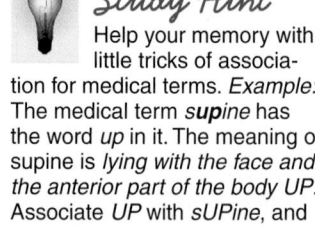

Study Hint

Help your memory with little tricks of association for medical terms. *Example:* The medical term *sup*ine has the word *up* in it. The meaning of supine is *lying with the face and the anterior part of the body UP*. Associate *UP* with s*UP*ine, and you will have no trouble remembering its definition.

Then associate the opposite term, and you will know the meaning of *prone* as well.

WORD ANALYSIS AND DEFINITION

WORD	PRONUNCIATION	ELEMENTS		DEFINITION
anatomy	ah-**NAT**-oh-mee	S/	**-tomy** *process of separating*	Study of the structures of the human body
anatomical (adj)	an-ah-**TOM**-ik-al	R/ S/	**ana-** *apart from* **-ical** *pertaining to*	Pertaining to anatomy
anterior (opposite of posterior)	an-**TER**-ee-or	S/ R/	**-ior** *pertaining to* **anter-** *coming before*	Front surface of body; situated in front
caudal (opposite of cephalic)	**KAW**-dal	S/ R/	**-al** *pertaining to* **caud-** *tail*	Pertaining to or nearer to the tail
cephalic (opposite of caudal)	se-**FAL**-ik	S/ R/	**-ic** *pertaining to* **cephal-** *head*	Pertaining to or nearer to the head
coronal (equivalent to frontal)	**KOR**-oh-nal	S/ R/	**-al** *pertaining to* **coron-** *crown*	Pertaining to the vertical plane dividing the body into anterior and posterior portions
distal (opposite of proximal)	**DISS**-tal	S/ R/	**-al** *pertaining to* **dist-** *away from the center*	Situated away from the center of the body
dorsal (equivalent to posterior)	**DOR**-sal	S/ R/	**-al** *pertaining to* **dors-** *back*	Pertaining to the back or situated behind
frontal (equivalent to coronal)	**FRON**-tal	S/ R/	**-al** *pertaining to* **front-** *front*	Pertaining to the vertical plane dividing the body into anterior and posterior portions
inferior (opposite of superior)	in-**FEE**-ree-or	S/ R/	**-ior** *pertaining to* **infer-** *below*	Situated below
posterior (opposite of anterior)	pos-**TER**-ee-or	S/ R/	**-ior** *pertaining to* **poster-** *coming behind*	Pertaining to the back surface of the body; situated behind
prone (opposite of supine)	PRONE		Latin *bending forward*	Lying face-down, flat on your belly
proximal (opposite of distal)	**PROK**-sih-mal	S/ R/	**-al** *pertaining to* **proxim-** *nearest*	Situated nearest the center of the body
sagittal	**SAJ**-ih-tal	S/ R/	**-al** *pertaining to* **sagitt-** *arrow*	Pertaining to the vertical plane through the body, dividing it into right and left portions
superior (opposite of inferior)	soo-**PEE**-ree-or	S/ R/	**-ior** *pertaining to* **super-** *above*	Situated above
supine (opposite of prone)	soo-**PINE**		Latin *bend backward*	Lying face-up, flat on your spine
transverse	trans-**VERS**		Latin *crosswise*	Pertaining to the horizontal plane dividing the body into upper and lower portions
ventral (equivalent to anterior)	**VEN**-tral	S/ R/	**-al** *pertaining to* **ventr-** *belly*	Pertaining to the belly or situated nearer the surface of the belly

EXERCISES

Each of the following terms from this WAD has one element in bold. You need to identify what type of element it is and define its meaning. Then answer the questions. Fill in the blanks.

1. poster**ior**   Type of element: _____   Meaning: _____

2. **caud**al   Type of element: _____   Meaning: _____

3. **cephal**ic   Type of element: _____   Meaning: _____

4. dis**tal**   Type of element: _____   Meaning: _____

5. **infer**ior   Type of element: _____   Meaning: _____

6. The three elements with the same meaning are _____, _____, and _____.

7. They all mean _____.

> **Study Hint**
> Terms will be easier to remember if you study them in *pairs of opposites*.

BODY CAVITIES

FIGURE 2.13   Body Cavities. ▶

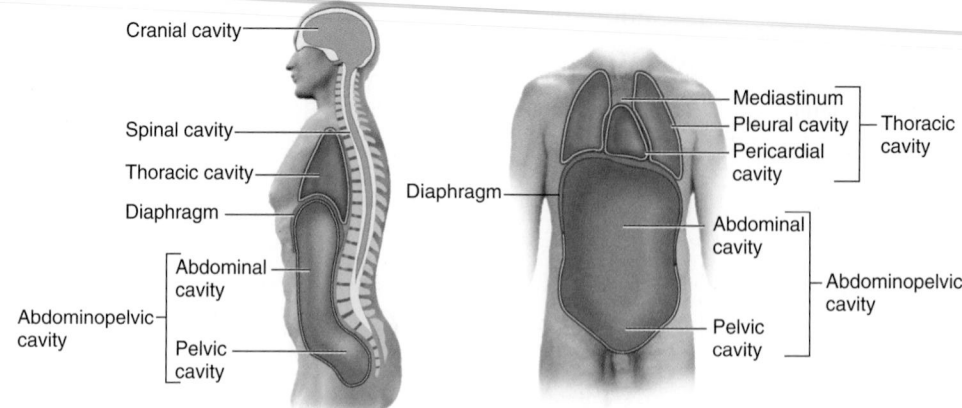

The body contains many **cavities.** Some, like the nasal cavity, open to the outside. Five cavities do not open to the outside and are shown in *Figure 2.13*.

- **Cranial cavity**—contains the brain within the skull.
- **Thoracic cavity**—contains the heart, lungs, thymus gland, trachea, and esophagus, as well as numerous blood vessels and nerves.
- **Abdominal cavity**—is separated from the thoracic cavity by the **diaphragm** and contains the stomach, intestines, liver, spleen, pancreas, and kidneys.
- **Pelvic cavity**—is surrounded by the pelvic bones and contains the urinary bladder, part of the large intestine, the rectum, the anus, and the internal reproductive organs.
- **Spinal cavity**—contains the spinal cord.

The abdominal cavity and pelvic cavity are collectively referred to as the **abdominopelvic cavity.**

Abbreviations

LLQ	left lower quadrant
LUQ	left upper quadrant
RLQ	right lower quadrant
RUQ	right upper quadrant

ABDOMINAL QUADRANTS

One way of referring to the locations of abdominal structures and to the site of abdominal pain and other abnormalities is to divide the abdominal region into **quadrants,** as shown in *Figure 2.14a*. The locations are **right upper quadrant**

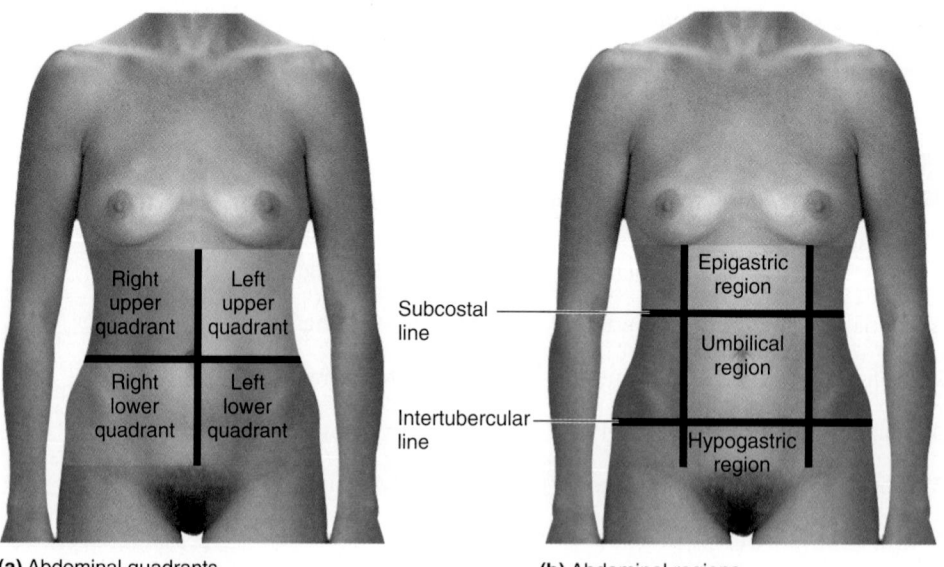

(a) Abdominal quadrants

(b) Abdominal regions

▲ **FIGURE 2.14   Regional Anatomy.**

WORD	PRONUNCIATION	ELEMENTS		DEFINITION
abdomen abdominal (adj)	AB-doh-men ab-DOM-in-al	S/ R/	Latin *abdomen* -al *pertaining to* abdomin- *abdomen*	Part of the trunk between the thorax and pelvis Pertaining to the abdomen
abdominopelvic	ab-DOM-ih-no-PEL-vik	S/ R/CF R/	-ic *pertaining to* abdomin/o- *abdomen* -pelv- *pelvis*	Pertaining to the abdomen and pelvis
cavity cavities (pl)	KAV-ih-tee KAV-ih-tees		Latin *hollow place*	Hollow space or body compartment
diaphragm	DIE-ah-fram		Greek *diaphragm, fence*	The musculomembranous partition separating the abdominal and thoracic cavities
epigastric epigastrium (noun)	ep-ih-GAS-trik ep-ih-GAS-tree-um	S/ P/ R/CF S/	-ic *pertaining to* epi- *above* -gastr/i- *stomach* -um *structure*	Pertaining to the abdominal region above the stomach Abdominal region above the stomach
hypogastric	high-poh-GAS-trik	S/ P/ R/	-ic *pertaining to* hypo- *below* -gastr- *stomach*	Abdominal region below the stomach
quadrant	KWAD-rant		Latin *one quarter*	One-quarter of a circle
umbilical umbilicus (noun)	um-BIL-ih-kal um-BIL-ih-kuss	S/ R/	-al *pertaining to* umbilic- *belly button (navel)*	Pertaining to the umbilicus or the center of the abdomen

(RUQ), left upper quadrant (LUQ), right lower quadrant (RLQ), and **left lower quadrant (LLQ)**.

   In addition, there are three regions in the middle of the abdomen as shown in *Figure 2.14b*. The upper **epigastric region**, the central **umbilical region**, and the lower **hypogastric region**.

EXERCISES

Take a closer look at the breakdown of medical terms. The medical term is given to you. Break it down into elements with a slash (/). Below each element, write the meaning of the element. See how the combination of elements will give you the meaning of the entire term. The first one is done for you. Fill in the blanks.

1. epigastrium

           <u> *epi* </u> / <u> *gastr/i* </u> / <u>   *um*   </u>
            above   *stomach*   *structure*

Study Hint
Remember to start with the suffix and work back to the front of the word.

   Meaning of **epigastrium**:   *abdominal region above the stomach*

2. epigastric

          _____ / _____ / _____

   Meaning of **epigastric**: _____

3. hypogastric

          _____ / _____ / _____

   Meaning of **hypogastric**: _____

4. umbilical

          _____ / _____ / _____

   Meaning of **umbilical**: _____

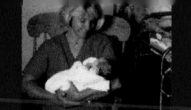
THE BODY AS A WHOLE

CHALLENGE YOUR KNOWLEDGE

A. **Word Elements:** These elements are grouped together to make them easier for you to review. Insert the correct name for the type of element (P, R, CF, S) in the heading of the first column for that group, give the meaning of each element, and **construct** a term using each element.

> **Study Hint**
> Notice that there are several elements with the same meanings.

Element Group =	Meaning of Element	Example of Medical Term Using That Element
endo		
epi		
co		
hyper		
hypo		
intra		
syn		

The elements in the table above are all (P, R, CF, S) _____ .

Element Group =	Meaning of Element	Example of Medical Term Using That Element
blasto		
fibro		
histo		
homeo		
mito		
osteo		
theli		
tracheo		
chromo		
ovi		

The elements in the table above are all (P, R, CF, S) _____ .

Element Group =	Meaning of Element	Example of Medical Term Using That Element
al		
ar		
ary		
ation		
elle		
emia		
oid		
ic		
logy		
stomy		
ule		
um		

The elements in the table above are all (P, R, CF, S) _____ .

B. **Apply your knowledge of the body as a whole with the following exercise.** Fill in the blanks to build the composition of the whole body *from the lowest to the highest order* of the anatomical hierarchy. Two of the blanks have been filled in to help you start the chart.

Atoms		
_____ *Atoms* _____	build	_____ *molecules* _____ .
_____	build	_____ .
_____	build	_____ .
_____	build	_____ .
_____	build	_____ .
_____	build	_____ .
_____	build	_____ .

A small unit of matter is the _____ .

THE BODY AS A WHOLE

C. Abbreviations: Pick any three of these abbreviations, define their meanings, and use each one in a sentence.

IVF   ACL   LLQ   LUQ   RLQ   RUQ

1. _____ means _____ .

   Sentence:

   _____

   _____

   _____

2. _____ means _____ .

   Sentence:

   _____

   _____

   _____

3. _____ means _____ .

   Sentence:

   _____

   _____

   _____

D. Cell Labeling: Read the definitions of the cell components below. In the figure below, write in the name of each component and the number of the definition that describes it.

1. Name means *small nucleus*
2. Manufactures protein
3. Clear, jellylike substance that contains organelles
4. Manufactures cholesterol
5. Cleans up cellular debris
6. Encases the cytoplasm and nucleus
7. Responsible for catabolism
8. Directs activities of the cell

E. **Functions of the Cell:** The basic functions of life are all carried on by each and every cell. Fill in the blanks to name all the functions.

1. _____

2. _____

3. _____

4. _____

5. _____

F. **Organs, Organelles, and Tissue Types:** Through attention and effort, you will learn to recognize the correct spelling of medical terms. Review the pairs of medical terms in the first chart below, and circle the correctly spelled word in each pair. Then insert the correct spelling of each term in the first column of the second chart, and place a check (✓) in the appropriate column to show whether it is an organ, organelle, or tissue type.

1. Circle the correct spelling.

ribosome	galbladder	nevus	mitocondria	conective	nucleolus
ribosomme	gallbladder	nerrvous	mitochondria	connective	nucliolus
muscle	nuceus	lysosones	pancreas	epithelial	reticculum
mussel	nucleus	lysosomes	panncreas	epithellial	reticulum

2. Enter the correctly spelled terms in the first column; then finish filling in the chart by indicating whether the term is an organ, organelle, or tissue type.

Term	Organ	Organelle	Tissue Type

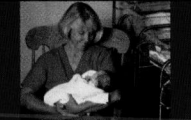

THE BODY AS A WHOLE

G. If you understand the terms in this chapter, you can describe correctly the difference between cytology and histology.

The difference is:

_____

_____

_____

_____

_____

H. **Knowing the meaning of word elements will help you to deconstruct the following terms to explain the differences in their meaning.** First, divide the word into its elements with slashes (/). Circle the suffix, and then fill in the table.

Term	Meaning of Root(s)/CF	Meaning of Suffix	Meaning of Term
homeostasis			
anabolism			
catabolism			
metabolism			
nucleus			
nucleolus			
ribosome			
lysosome			

I. **Terminology Challenge:** Pick what you think are the three most difficult words to spell in this chapter. Write them, pronounce them, and define them here:

1. _____ means _____ .

2. _____ means _____ .

3. _____ means _____ .

Have you checked your spelling? Can you spell them without looking at the book? You will probably see them again on a test.

J. **Organs and Body Systems:** Knowledge of the body's systems will help you master medical terminology. Assign the following organs to an organ system, and describe one major function of that system.

Organ	Organ System	System Function
blood vessels		
cartilage		
epididymis		
fallopian tubes		
hair		
larynx		
liver		
muscles		
spinal cord		
spleen		
sweat glands		
teeth		
thymus		
thyroid gland		

K. **Apply this knowledge of organ systems to answer the following questions.** Circle your choice, but remember to rewrite any false information *correctly* on the blanks at the end of the exercise.

  1. Organs make basic functions happen in an organ system.   T   F

  2. Glands that secrete hormones are in the endocrine system.   T   F

  3. There are 13 different body systems.   T   F

  4. An organ system will have more than one organ.   T   F

  5. Organ systems that are not functioning correctly can disrupt homeostasis.   T   F

Rewrite any false statement(s) with correct information.

_____

_____

_____

_____

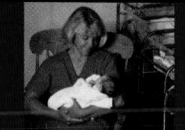
THE BODY AS A WHOLE

L. Build medical terms using your knowledge of elements and their proper position in a medical term. Fill in the blanks.

1. Small mass   molec/ _____

2. Pertaining to below the stomach   _____ / _____ /ic

3. Instrument for viewing a joint   _____ /scope

4. Pertaining to urine   urin/ _____

5. A change of condition   _____ /ism

6. Small organ   organ/ _____

7. Small nucleus   nucleo/ _____

8. Enzyme that digests foreign material   lyso/ _____

Note: *More than one element can have the same meaning. List the elements in this exercise that have the same meaning.*

_____ all mean _____ .

_____ all mean _____ .

M. Anatomical Positions and Planes: You must know anatomical positions to prepare a patient for any type of procedure or surgery. Anatomical planes can help define radiologic studies. Using this knowledge, complete the following.

1. The surgeon needs his patient in the _____ position to remove a lesion on his back.

2. To prepare for a knee arthroscopy, the patient will be in the _____ position.

3. The body is standing erect with feet flat on the floor, face and eyes facing forward, and arms at the sides with the palms facing forward; this is the _____ position.

4. A plane that divides the body into an upper, or superior, portion and a lower, or inferior, portion is called a _____ plane.

5. A frontal plane can also be called a _____ plane.

N. Directional Terms: Along with knowing planes, body cavities, and quadrants, you must know body directional terms in order to be able to document and communicate accurately.

> **Study Hint**
> Learn these terms
> in pairs of opposites.
> The acronym "PADS" will help
> you remember the pairs.

Proximal and distal: Proximal means_____ ; distal means _____ .

Anterior and posterior: Anterior means _____ ; posterior means _____ .

Dorsal and ventral: Dorsal means _____ ; ventral means _____ .

Superior and inferior: Superior means _____ ; inferior means _____ .

O. Demonstrate your knowledge of directional terms and abbreviations by circling the correct choice.

1. The epigastric region is (above/below) the stomach. Therefore, it is (superior/inferior) to the stomach.

2. The umbilical region is so named because it is in the (center/back) of the abdomen and (inferior/superior) to the epigastric region.

3. The hypogastric region is between the (RUQ/LUQ) and the (RLQ/LLQ).

4. In the abbreviation LLQ, the first "L" means (lower/left).

5. The nose is (superior/inferior) to the chin.

6. The spine is (anterior/posterior) to the heart.

7. The umbilicus is (dorsal/ventral) to the spine.

8. The toes are (distal/proximal) to the knee.

P. **Recall and Review:** How well do you remember these word elements from the previous chapter? Try to answer without first looking back to check. Fill in the chart.

Element	Type of Element (P, R, R/CF, S)	Meaning of Element
gynec		
um		
entero		
pathy		
endo		

Q. **Body Cavities:** The organ is given to you. Challenge yourself to place the organ in the correct body cavity, and then place the organ in the correct body system. Fill in the chart.

Organ	Body Cavity	Body System
brain		
gallbladder		
heart		
kidneys		
lungs		
pituitary		
ribs		
spleen		
uterus		

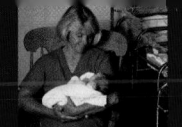

CHAPTER 2 REVIEW

THE BODY AS A WHOLE

R. Classroom Discussion: Pick one topic, and prepare a five-sentence brief summary of your thoughts on the topic. The questions given are only an example of what you might choose to discuss. Turn your preparation notes in to the instructor.

1. Explain the holistic approach to medical treatment. What does this encompass? Do only certain physicians believe in this method? How does one locate this type of physician?

2. Why is homeostasis important to a normally functioning body? What exactly is homeostasis? How is it disrupted? How is it restored?

S. Latin and Greek Terms: There is no easy way to remember these—you just have to know them so that you can relate to their meanings. Match the terms in 1–10 to the meanings in A–J. Fill in the blanks.

_____ 1. atom	_____ 6. matrix	A. A storeroom	F. Small particle
_____ 2. graft	_____ 7. cruciate	B. Cross	G. Mother
_____ 3. hormone	_____ 8. membrane	C. Yolked	H. To set in motion
_____ 4. ligament	_____ 9. meniscus	D. Crescent	I. Transplant
_____ 5. cell	_____ 10. zygote	E. Band	J. Parchment

T. Knowledge of anatomical locations on the body will make your communications with other health professionals precise. Challenge yourself with the following questions. Circle *T* (true) or *F* (false); then rewrite the false answers correctly below.

1. Standing erect with feet flat on the floor, face and eyes facing forward, and arms at the side with palms facing forward is the anatomical position.   T   F

2. A transverse plane is a horizontal plane.   T   F

3. Frontal and sagittal planes are both vertical planes.   T   F

4. Inferior is situated above another part of the body.   T   F

5. Dorsal means the same as **anterior.**   T   F

6. The abdominal cavity contains the urinary bladder.   T   F

7. The thoracic cavity is superior to the pelvic cavity, and the pelvic cavity is inferior to the abdominal cavity.   T   F

8. The diaphragm divides the pelvic cavity and the abdominal cavity.   T   F

9. In RUQ, "Q" means quadrant.   T   F

10. The RUQ and the LUQ can be divided by a sagittal plane.   T   F

Corrected statements:

_____

_____

_____

_____

U. Multiple choice is the format used for most national certification examinations.

1. The single, fertilized cell is called the:

     a. mitochondria   d. zygote

     b. ribosome   e. blastocyst

     c. organelle

2. The word *membrane* means:

   a. small organ

   b. fluid inside a cell

   c. thin layer of tissue

   d. chemical substance

   e. molecule with electrical charge

3. Patella is the medical term for:

   a. ankle

   b. muscle

   c. kneecap

   d. ligament

   e. meniscus

4. Which of the following functions as a shock absorber?

   a. cartilage

   b. muscle

   c. tendon

   d. ligament

   e. blood vessel

5. The prefix endo- means:

   a. outside

   b. within

   c. around

   d. behind

   e. across

6. The study of the function of tissues is called:

   a. cytology

   b. cardiology

   c. dermatology

   d. histology

   e. gastroenterology

7. Two bones that have formed a joint are called:

   a. graft

   b. articulation

   c. homeostasis

   d. metabolism

   e. cartilage

8. How many quadrants are in the body?

   a. one

   b. two

   c. three

   d. four

   e. five

9. Hypogastric refers to a:

   a. body region

   b. directional term

   c. body quadrant

   d. a and b

   e. a and c

THE BODY AS A WHOLE

V. Short Answer and/or Class Discussion: Building up to larger components in the body, expand your knowledge of cells and tissues to organs and organ systems. Write a short answer to each question, and be prepared to discuss your answers with the instructor and class.

1. Define an **organ**.

   _____

   _____

2. What is the difference between an organ and an organ system?

   _____

   _____

   _____

3. It is difficult to imagine skin as an "organ" because it is not a compact size like a liver or heart. Based on the above answers, why, then, is skin an organ?

   _____

   _____

   _____

4. Which body system has skin as a major organ?

   _____

   _____

5. There can be smaller organs within a large organ. Name the smaller organs within the skin and some of their functions.

   _____

   _____

   _____

   _____

6. List all the organ systems in the body.

   _____

   _____

   _____

   _____

   _____

   _____

   _____

W. Now that you have had some practice with the new medical terms, you are ready to read again the following Case Report from earlier in this chapter. Underline all the medical terms, and then answer all the questions. Fill in the blanks.

CASE REPORT 2.2

You are

...a physical therapy assistant employed by the Rehabilitation Unit in Fulwood Medical Center.

Your patient is

...Richard Josen, a 22-year-old man who injured tissues in his left knee playing football. Using arthroscopy, the orthopedic surgeon removed his torn anterior cruciate ligament (ACL) and replaced it with a graft from his patellar ligament. The torn medial collateral ligament was sutured together. The tear in his medial meniscus was repaired. Rehabilitation focused on strengthening the muscles around his knee joint and regaining joint mobility.

1. Define **arthroscopy.** _____

2. What type of specialist will use an **arthroscope?** _____

3. ACL is the abbreviation for _____ .

4. What is a **graft?** _____

5. What does a **meniscus** resemble? _____

6. What is the patella also called? _____

7. What is the opposite of medial? _____

8. Define ligament. _____

9. Describe anterior. _____

10. Define collateral. _____

THE BODY AS A WHOLE

CHAPTER SUMMARY EXERCISE

1. *Listen to the pronunciation of the medical terms as given by your instructor.*
2. *Circle the correct spelling of the medical term.*
3. *Match the correctly spelled terms to the brief descriptions below.*
4. *Write a sentence for each of the 10 terms that appear in this exercise.*

A. SPELLING COMPREHENSION: *Circle the correct spelling of the term.*

1. organale   orgenele   organelle   orgenelle   organel

2. sinovial   sinnovial   synoveal   synevial   synovial

3. rybosome   ribosonme   rhibosome   ribosome   rhybosone

4. diaphram   diaphrame   diaphragm   deaphragm   diafragm

5. traciostomy   trackeostomy   trachiostomy   treckeostomy   tracheostomy

6. nucklii   nucleei   nuclei   neuclei   nucklie

7. zygoat   zigote   zygote   zigotte   zygoate

8. endockrine   endocrine   endoccrine   endockryne   endocrin

9. meniscus   menniscus   menickus   meniskus   meniscuss

10. historyology   histology   hystology   hestology   historology

B. MATCH THE NUMBER OF THE CORRECT TERM IN PART A WITH THE BRIEF DESCRIPTION OF THE TERM BELOW.

a. Manufacture protein   _____

b. Plural of nucleus   _____

c. Opening for tube to assist in breathing   _____

d. Suffix means *small*   _____

e. Separates two body cavities   _____

f. Gland   _____

g. Study of function of tissues   _____

h. Origin of every cell in body   _____

i. Crescent shaped   _____

j. Lubricant   _____

C. USING YOUR KNOWLEDGE OF TERMS 1–15 IN PART A AND THEIR CORRECT SPELLING, WRITE A BRIEF SENTENCE FOR EACH OF THE TERMS AS IT MIGHT APPEAR IN PATIENT DOCUMENTATION.

1. _____

2. _____

3. _____

4. _____

5. _____

6. _____

7. _____

8. _____

9. _____

10. _____

D. YOUR INSTRUCTOR WILL DIRECT YOU TO MCGRAW-HILL CONNECT. OPEN THE AUDIO GLOSSARY AND PRACTICE YOUR PRONUNCIATION OF THE TERMS IN PART A OF THIS EXERCISE.

E. MEET A LESSON OBJECTIVE AND BEGIN APPLYING MEDICAL TERMINOLOGY TO ANSWER THE FOLLOWING QUESTIONS.

1. List the four primary tissue groups and describe their functions.

   _____

   _____

   _____

   _____

2. Identify a major organ and list the smaller organs contained in it.

   _____

   _____

3. Identify the structure and functions of the components of a cell.

   _____

   _____

   _____

   _____

4. Be able to demonstrate on your own body or on a classroom skeleton the names and locations of the:

   a. body cavities.

   b. abdominal quadrants.

   c. body regions.

5. Describe the fundamental anatomical position.

   _____

   _____

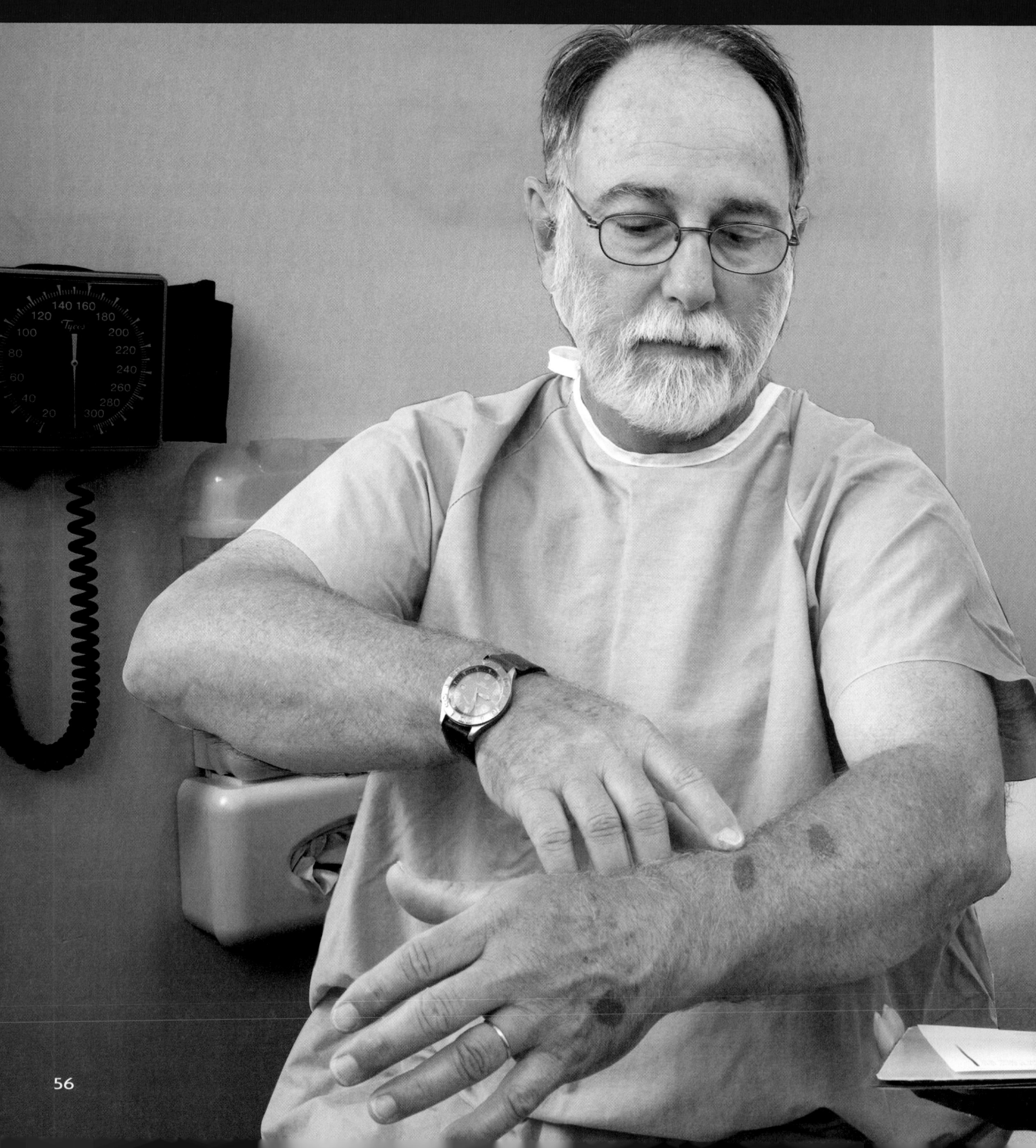

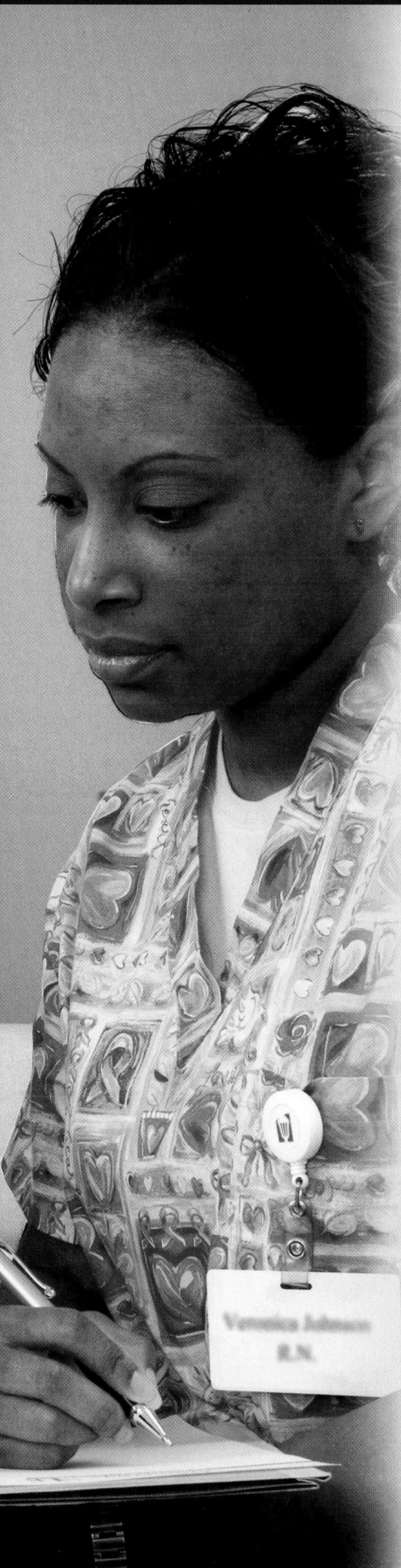

3

CASE REPORT 3.1

You are

... a clinical medical assistant working in the office of dermatologist Dr. Lenore Echols, a member of the Fulwood Medical Group.

Your patient is

... Mr. Rod Andrews, a 60-year-old man, who shows you three skin lesions, two on his left forearm and one on the back of his left hand. On questioning him, you learn that he has been living for the past 10 years in Arizona and has come back home to be near his daughter and young grandchildren. You find no other skin lesions on his body.

Learning Outcomes

In addition to anticipating Dr. Echols' needs for equipment to **biopsy,** diagnose, and treat the **lesions,** you also have to be able to communicate clearly with her in medical terms and to understand her language as she communicates with you and the patient about the **etiology** (cause) and structure of the lesions. You will then need to document the medical history and treatment and communicate clearly with Mr. Andrews about the treatment of his lesions and their **prognosis.**

To perform these tasks, you must be able to:

3.1 Apply the language of dermatology to the anatomy and physiology of the skin and its associated organs.

3.2 Comprehend, analyze, spell, and write the medical terms of dermatology so that you can communicate and document accurately and precisely in any health care setting.

3.3 Recognize and pronounce the medical terms of dermatology so that you can communicate verbally with accuracy and precision in any health care setting.

3.4 Understand the etiology and prognosis of common dermatologic conditions.

Functions and Structure of the Skin

The three lesions on Mr. Andrews' arm and hand developed in the superficial layer of the skin called the **epidermis.** This lesson looks at the structure and functions of the skin and at diseases of the epidermis so that you will be able to:

3.1.1   List the layers of the skin.

3.1.2   Name the tissues in the different layers of the skin.

3.1.3   Identify the functions of the different layers.

3.1.4   Describe certain disorders affecting the superficial layers of the skin, including cancers.

3.1.5   Apply correct medical terminology to the anatomy, physiology, and disorders of the superficial layers of the skin.

Case Report 3.1 (continued)

When Dr. Echols examined Mr. Andrews, she determined clinically that two of his lesions were basal cell **carcinomas** and she treated them with **cryosurgery.** She believed that the third lesion was a **squamous cell** carcinoma, and she performed a **biopsy removal** of that **lesion.** You sent it to the laboratory with a request for **pathological** diagnosis and determination of whether the lesion had been completely removed. This is done by ensuring that a normal skin margin completely surrounds the lesion when it is examined under the **microscope.**

FUNCTIONS AND STRUCTURE OF THE SKIN

The **integumentary organ system** consists of the skin and its associated organs *(Figure 3.1)*. The study and treatment of the integumentary system is called **dermatology.** This organ system receives more medical and personal attention than any other organ system. Your understanding of its structures and functions will be used every day in your professional and personal life.

The skin is the largest organ in your body and accounts for 7% to 8% of your body weight. The skin is the most vulnerable of all your organs because it is continually exposed to chemicals, trauma, infection, radiation, temperature change, humidity variation, and all the pollution of modern life. Your skin is an important part of your own self-image and an important part of total patient care.

Keynote

The skin is the largest and most vulnerable organ in the body.

Keynote

A medical specialist in diseases of the skin is a **dermatologist.**

Keynote

There are four combining forms for skin:
• cutane/o
• derm/a
• dermat/o
• derm/o

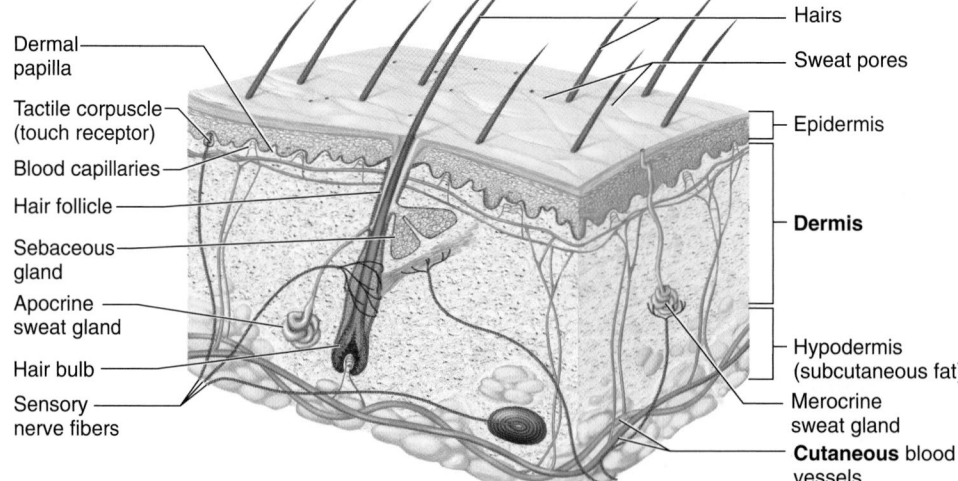

Dermal papilla

Tactile corpuscle (touch receptor)

Blood capillaries

Hair follicle

Sebaceous gland

Apocrine sweat gland

Hair bulb

Sensory nerve fibers

Hairs

Sweat pores

Epidermis

Dermis

Hypodermis (subcutaneous fat)

Merocrine sweat gland

Cutaneous blood vessels

▲ **FIGURE 3.1   Structure of the Skin and Subcutaneous Tissue.**

WORD	PRONUNCIATION	ELEMENTS		DEFINITION
biopsy	**BI**-op-see	S/	-opsy *to view*	Removing tissue from a living person for laboratory examination
biopsy removal (also called **excisional biopsy**)	**BI**-op-see re-**MUV**-al	R/CF	bi/o- *life*	Used for small tumors when complete removal provides tissue for a biopsy and cures the lesion
carcinoma	kar-sih-**NOH**-mah	S/ R/	-oma *tumor, mass* carcin- *cancer*	A malignant and invasive **epithelial** tumor
cryosurgery	cry-oh-**SUR**-jer-ee	S/ R/CF R/	-ery *process of* cry/o- *icy cold* -surg- *operate*	Use of liquid nitrogen or argon gas in a probe to freeze and kill abnormal tissue
cutaneous	kyu-**TAY**-nee-us	S/ R/CF	-ous *pertaining to* cutan/e- *skin*	Pertaining to the skin
dermis dermal (adj)	**DER**-miss **DER**-mal		Greek *skin*	Connective tissue layer of the skin beneath the epidermis
dermatology	der-mah-**TOL**-oh-jee	S/ R/CF	-logy *study of* dermat/o- *skin*	Medical specialty concerned with disorders of the skin
dermatologist	der-mah-**TOL**-oh-jist	S/	-logist *one who studies*	Medical specialist in diseases of the skin
epidermis	ep-ih-**DER**-miss	P/ R/	epi- *upon* -dermis *skin*	Top layer of the skin
epithelium epithelial (adj)	ep-ih-**THEE**-lee-um ep-ih-**THEE**-lee-al	S/ P/ R/CF	-um *tissue* epi- *upon* thel/i- *nipple*	Tissue that covers surfaces or lines cavities
integument	in-**TEG**-you-ment		Latin *a covering*	Organ system that covers the body, the skin being the main organ within the system
integumentary (adj)	in-**TEG**-you-**MEN**-tah-ree	S/ R/	-ary *pertaining to* integument- *covering of the body*	Pertaining to the covering of the body
lesion	**LEE**-zhun		Latin *injury*	Pathological change or injury in a tissue
microscope	**MY**-kroh-skope	P/ R/	micro- *small* -scope *instrument for viewing*	Instrument for viewing something small that cannot be seen in detail by the naked eye
microscopic (adj)	**MY**-kroh-**SKOP**-ik	S/	-ic *pertaining to*	Visible only with the aid of a microscope
pathology pathological (adj)	pa-**THOL**-oh-jee path-oh-**LOJ**-ik-al	S/ R/CF	-logy *study of* path/o- *disease*	Medical specialty dealing with the structural and functional changes of a disease process or the cause, development, and structural changes in disease
prognosis	prog-**NO**-sis	P/ R/	pro- *projecting forward* -gnosis *knowledge*	Forecasting of the probable course of a disease
squamous cell	**SKWAY**-mus SELL		Latin *scaly*	Flat, scalelike epithelial cell

EXERCISES

Review the Word Analysis and Definition (WAD) box before starting this exercise. Build your knowledge of the elements in the language of dermatology. Circle the best answer.

1. The suffix -oma can mean tumor or:

   gland   mass   cancer

2. Circle the term that means *study of*:

   dermatology   dermatologist   dermatitis

3. Cryo- is a combining form that signifies:

   color   temperature   location

4. The term **cutaneous** means *pertaining to*:

   skin   mass   tumor

5. The root in **carcinoma** means:

   surgery   tumor   cancer

6. In the term **microscope,** the prefix signifies:

   size   shape   position

7. The root in **prognosis** means:

   specialist   study of   knowledge

8. The suffix -**opsy** means:

   to view   to cut   to repair

FUNCTIONS OF THE SKIN

Keynote

The skin provides protection, contains sensory organs, and helps control body temperature.

- **Protection.** The skin is physical barrier against injury, chemicals, ultraviolet rays, microbes, and toxins.

- **Water resistance.** You don't swell up every time you take a bath because your skin is water resistant. It also prevents water from leaking out from the body tissues.

- **Temperature regulation.** A network of **capillaries** in the skin opens up or dilates **(vasodilation)** when your body is too hot so that the blood flow increases and the heat from the blood dissipates through your skin. When your body is cold, the capillary network narrows **(vasoconstriction)**, blood flow decreases, and heat is retained in your body *(Chapter 8)*.

- **Vitamin D synthesis.** As little as 15 to 30 minutes of sunlight daily allows your skin cells to initiate the metabolism of vitamin D, which is essential for bone growth and maintenance.

- **Sensation.** Nerve endings that detect touch, pressure, heat, cold, pain, vibration, and tissue injury are particularly numerous on your face, fingers, palms, soles, nipples, and genitals.

- **Excretion and secretion.** Water and small amounts of waste products from cell metabolism are lost through the skin by **excretion** (the process of removal of waste products from the body) and by **secretion** (the process of producing and releasing a substance by a tissue or organ of the body) from your sweat glands.

- **Social functions.** The skin reflects your emotions, blushing when you are self-conscious, going pale when you are frightened, wrinkling when you dislike something.

SKIN AS A BARRIER

The skin is a barrier that is not easily broken. Few infectious organisms can penetrate the skin on their own. Those that do use accidental breaks in the skin or rely on animals such as mosquitoes, fleas, or ticks to puncture the skin to allow access for the infectious organisms. The skin is also a barrier to solar radiation, including ultraviolet (UV) rays.

Blood receives 1% to 2% of its oxygen from diffusion through the skin, and it releases through the skin some carbon dioxide and organic chemicals that attract mosquitoes and other insects to people.

REGIONS OF SKIN SURFACE AREA

The skin's surface area can be divided into regions, each one of which is a fraction or multiple of 9% of the total surface area. This is called the Rule of Nines *(Figure 3.2)*.

The treatment and prognosis for a burn patient depend, in part, on the extent of the body surface that is affected. This is estimated by applying the Rule of Nines to determine the percentage of the skin's surface affected by burns:

- Head and neck are assigned 9% (4½% anterior and 4½% posterior).
- Each arm is 9% (4½% anterior and 4½% posterior).
- Each leg is 18% (9% anterior and 9% posterior).
- The anterior trunk is 18%.
- The posterior trunk is 18%.
- The genitalia are 1%.

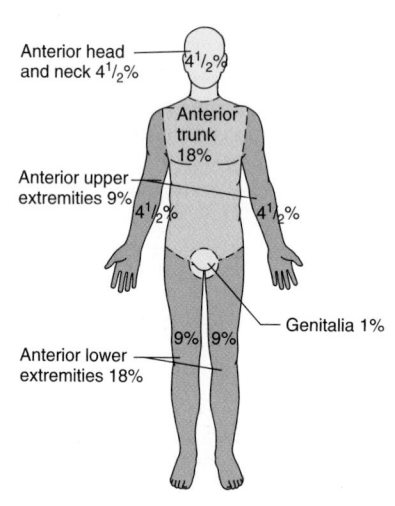

Anterior head and neck 4½%
Anterior trunk 18%
Anterior upper extremities 9%
4½% 4½%
Genitalia 1%
Anterior lower extremities 18%
9% 9%

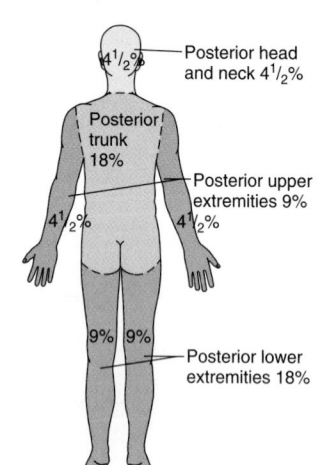

Posterior head and neck 4½%
Posterior trunk 18%
Posterior upper extremities 9%
4½% 4½%
Posterior lower extremities 18%
9% 9%

▲ **FIGURE 3.2 Rule of Nines.**

WORD	PRONUNCIATION	ELEMENTS		DEFINITION
excrete	eks-**KREET**		Latin *remove*	To pass out of the body waste products of metabolism
excretion (noun)	eks-**KREE**-shun			Removal of waste products of metabolism out of the body
function	**FUNK**-shun		Latin *to perform*	The ability of an organ or tissue to perform its special work
protection	pro-**TEK**-shun	S/	-ion *action, condition*	Defense against attack or invasion
protect (verb)		P/	pro- *before*	
		R/	-tect- *to shelter*	
regulation	reg-you-**LAY**-shun	S/	-ation *process*	Control of the way in which a process progresses
	REG-you-late	R/	regul- *to rule*	
regulate (verb)		S/	-ate *pertaining to*	To control the way in which a process progresses
resistance	ree-**ZIS**-tants	S/	-ance *state of*	Ability of an organism to withstand the effects of an antagonistic agent
resist (verb)		R/	resist- *to withstand*	
secrete	se-**KREET**		Latin *to separate*	To produce a chemical substance in a cell and release it from the cell
secretion (noun)	se-**KREE**-shun			
sensation	sen-**SAY**-shun	S/	-ation *process*	The conscious feeling of the effects of a stimulation
sense (verb)		R/	sens- *to feel*	
synthesis	**SIN**-the-sis	P/	syn- *together*	The process of building a compound from different elements
synthesize (verb)	**SIN**-the-size	R/	-thesis *to arrange*	

EXERCISES

The following are functions of the skin—assign one to each statement by filling in the blanks.

protection	water resistance	temperature regulation	vitamin D synthesis
sensation	excretion	secretion	social function

1. water and waste products lost through the skin   _____

2. nerve endings detect touch, pressure, heat   _____

3. prevents leakage from body tissues   _____

4. vasoconstriction or vasodilation   _____

5. production of sweat glands   _____

6. works with sunlight to metabolize   _____

7. blushing   _____

8. physical barrier against toxins   _____

Choose any pair of noun-verb medical terms in the WAD above, and use each term in a sentence of medical documentation.

9. Noun: _____

_____

_____

Verb: _____

_____

_____

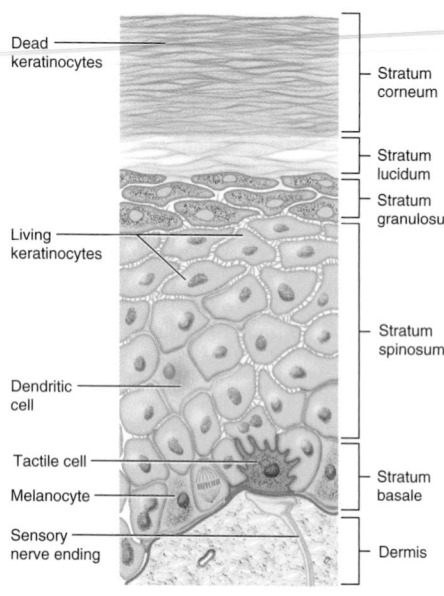

- Dead keratinocytes — Stratum corneum
- Stratum lucidum
- Stratum granulosum
- Living keratinocytes — Stratum spinosum
- Dendritic cell
- Tactile cell — Stratum basale
- Melanocyte
- Sensory nerve ending — Dermis

▲ **FIGURE 3.3** Epidermis.

Keynote

The stratum granulosum waterproofs the skin.

Keynote

The stratum spinosum holds the epidermis together.

STRUCTURE OF THE SKIN: EPIDERMIS

The three lesions that Mr. Andrews had were present in the **epidermis,** the most superficial layer of his skin. This layer:

- **Protects** underlying structures.
- **Withstands** the toxic pollution of modern life.
- **Sheds** its superficial cells and renews them continually throughout life.
- **Provides** a waterproof barrier.

The outer layer of the epidermis, the **stratum corneum** *(Figure 3.3),* is a layer of compact, dead cells packed with **keratin.** These dead cells have no nuclei and are continually shed. **Dandruff** is clumps of these cells stuck together with **sebum,** oil from **sebaceous** glands. Keratin is a tough, scaly protein that is also the basis for hair and nails.

Underneath the stratum corneum on the thick skin of the palms, soles, fingers, and toes is a thin translucent layer of cells, the **stratum lucidum.** These cells are filled with a protein that becomes keratin and are called **keratinocytes.**

In the next layer down, the **stratum granulosum,** these keratinocytes produce a fatty mixture that covers the surface of the cells and waterproofs them. This waterproof barrier not only stops water from getting in and out but also cuts off the supply of nutrients to the keratinocytes above it and they die.

In the next layer, the **stratum spinosum,** the keratinocytes contain nuclei and are firmly attached to each other by numerous spines (hence "spinosum"). This enables the epidermis to be firm and strong.

The **squamous cell carcinoma** *(Figure 3.4)* that Mr. Andrews had on his hand arose from keratinocytes in the stratum spinosum in skin on the back of the hand, face, and ears, areas exposed to sunlight. It responds well to surgical removal but can **metastasize** (spread) to lymph glands if neglected.

The bottom layer of the epidermis, the **stratum basale,** is a single layer of cells that form the keratinocytes. This layer also contains **melanocytes,** which produce the dark pigment **melanin,** and **tactile** (touch) cells attached to sensory nerve fibers. The process in which keratinocytes migrate from this layer to the skin's surface, where they are shed as dead cells, takes about a month.

Mr. Andrews' **basal cell carcinoma** *(Figure 3.5)* began in the cells of the stratum basale and invaded the dermis and epidermis. It is the most common skin cancer and is also the least dangerous because it does not metastasize.

Malignant melanoma *(Figure 3.6)* is the least common skin cancer but is the most deadly. It arises from the melanocytes in the stratum basale. It metastasizes quickly and is fatal if neglected.

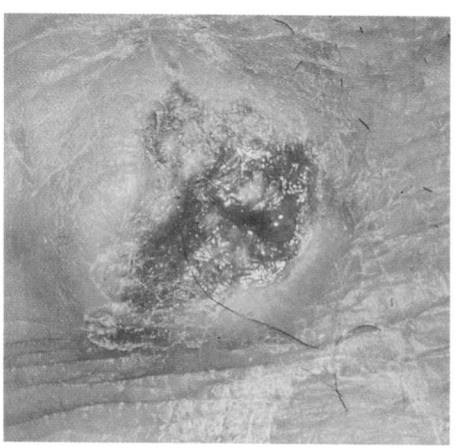

▲ **FIGURE 3.4** Squamous Cell Carcinoma.

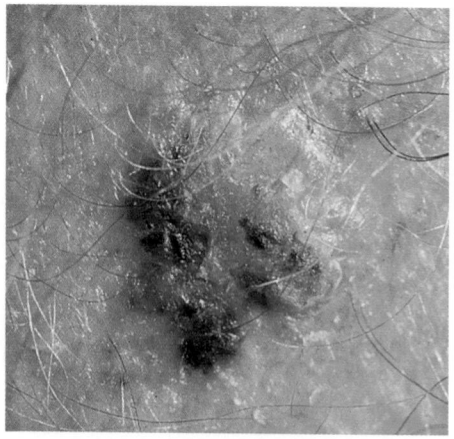

▲ **FIGURE 3.5** Basal Cell Carcinoma.

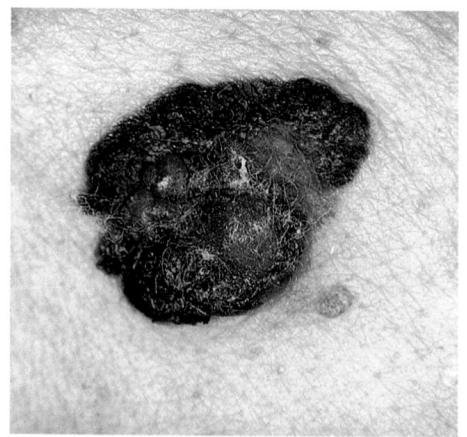

▲ **FIGURE 3.6** Malignant Melanoma.

WORD	PRONUNCIATION	ELEMENTS		DEFINITION
keratin	**KER**-ah-tin		Greek *keratin*	Protein found in the dead outer layer of skin and in nails and hair
keratinocyte	ke-**RAT**-in-oh-site	S/ R/CF	-cyte *cell* keratin/o- *keratin*	Cell producing a tough, horny protein (keratin) in the process of differentiating into the dead cells of the stratum corneum
macule macular (adj)	**MAK**-yul **MAK**-yu-lar		Latin *spot*	Small, flat spot or patch on the skin
malignant	mah-**LIG**-nant	S/ R/	-ant *forming* malign- *harmful*	Tumor that invades surrounding tissues and metastasizes to distant organs
melanin melanocyte	**MEL**-ah-nin **MEL**-ann-oh-cyte	S/ R/CF	Greek *black* -cyte *cell* melan/o- *melanin*	Black pigment found in skin, hair, retina Cell that synthesizes (produces) melanin
melanoma	**MEL**-ah-**NO**-mah	S/	-oma *tumor, mass*	Malignant neoplasm formed from cells that produce melanin
metastasis (noun)	meh-**TAS**-tah-sis	P/ R/	meta- *beyond, subsequent to* -stasis *stagnate, stay in one place*	Spread of a disease from one part of the body to another
metastasize (verb) metastatic (adj)	meh-**TAS**-tah-size meh-tah-**STAT**-ik	S/ S/ R/	-ize *affect in a specific way* -ic *pertaining to* -stat- *stationary*	To spread to distant parts. Pertaining to the character of cells that can metastasize.
sebaceous glands sebum	se-**BAY**-shus GLANZ **SEE**-bum	S/ R/CF	-ous *pertaining to* sebac/e- *wax*	Glands in the dermis that open into hair follicles and secrete an oily fluid called sebum Waxy secretion of the sebaceous glands
stratum basale	**STRAH**-tum ba-**SAL**-eh	S/ R/ R/	-um *tissue* strat- *layer* basal/e *deepest part*	Deepest layer of the epidermis, from which the other cells originate and migrate
tactile	**TAK**-tile		Latin *to touch*	Relating to touch

Case Report 3.1 (continued)

Dr. Echols learned that Mr. Andrews had driven extensively in Arizona while wearing a short-sleeved shirt. His left forearm and hand were exposed to sunlight through the untinted car window to his left. This was an important factor in causing his skin cancers, all of which responded to treatment.

EXERCISES

Apply the correct rule for plurals in question 2, and form the plural of the term **stratum**. *Demonstrate that you know the difference in terms by using each form in a sentence.*

1. Singular: *stratum*
   Sentence:

   _____

2. Plural: _____
   Sentence:

   _____

Medical terms that are nouns can also have an adjectival *form, as seen in* **macule** *and* **macular**. *Use the correct form of each term in the following sentences.*

3. The report from pathology diagnosed the lesion as a _____.

4. The _____ tissue was removed in the biopsy.

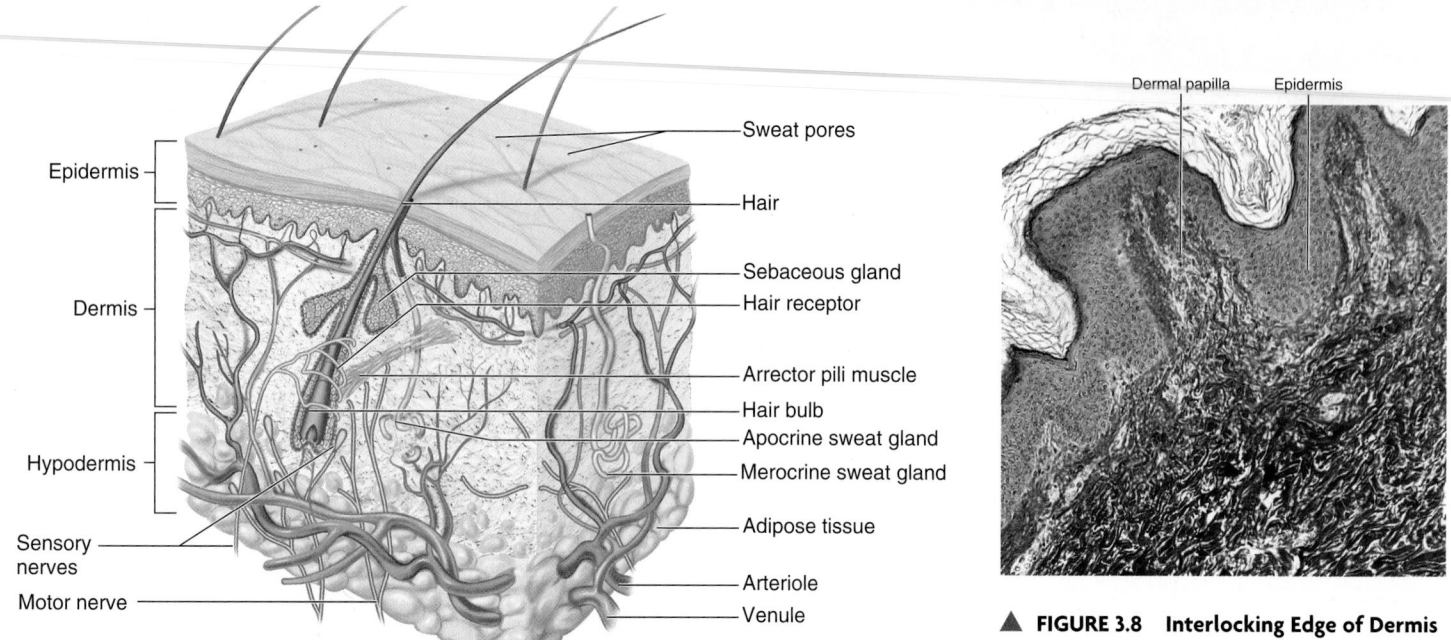

FIGURE 3.7 Dermis and Its Organs.

Labels (left): Epidermis, Dermis, Hypodermis, Sensory nerves, Motor nerve

Labels (right): Sweat pores, Hair, Sebaceous gland, Hair receptor, Arrector pili muscle, Hair bulb, Apocrine sweat gland, Merocrine sweat gland, Adipose tissue, Arteriole, Venule

FIGURE 3.8 Interlocking Edge of Dermis and Epidermis.

Labels: Dermal papilla, Epidermis

STRUCTURE OF THE SKIN: DERMIS

Figure 3.7 shows that the **dermis** is a much thicker connective tissue layer than the epidermis. It consists mostly of **collagen,** with fibers and fibroblasts. It is well supplied with blood vessels and nerves and contains the other **skin organs: sweat glands, sebaceous glands, hair follicles,** and **nail roots.**

The boundary between the dermis and the epidermis is distinct and irregular *(Figure 3.8)*. Upward projections of the dermis, dermal **papillae,** and downward projections of the epidermis, epidermal ridges, interlock to prevent the epidermis from slipping on the dermis. They also produce the ridges and furrows on your skin that are used for fingerprinting.

STRUCTURE OF THE SKIN: HYPODERMIS

This layer beneath the dermis is the site of **subcutaneous** fat (**adipose** tissue). It is also called the **subcutaneous tissue layer.**

CLINICAL APPLICATIONS

Giving Injections

Another important reason why you should be able to identify the layers of the skin is to understand the different sites for giving injections. You will need this information both to keep accurate documentation and, in some states after appropriate training, to be able to give the injections.

The three types of injection are:

- **Intradermal** *(Figure 3.9)*. A short, thin needle is introduced into the dermis between the stratum corneum and the stratum basale. Injected into this site, the medication raises a small **wheal.** This site is used for allergy testing or a **tuberculosis (TB)** test.
- **Subcutaneous (SC).** A longer needle pierces the epidermis and dermis to reach the hypodermis or subcutaneous layer. This site is used for insulin injections.
- **Intramuscular (IM)** *(Figure 3.10)*. A long needle pierces the epidermis, dermis, and subcutaneous layer into the muscles underneath. Some antibiotics can be given by this route.

FIGURE 3.9 Intradermal Injection.

Labels: Medication, Wheal, Epidermis

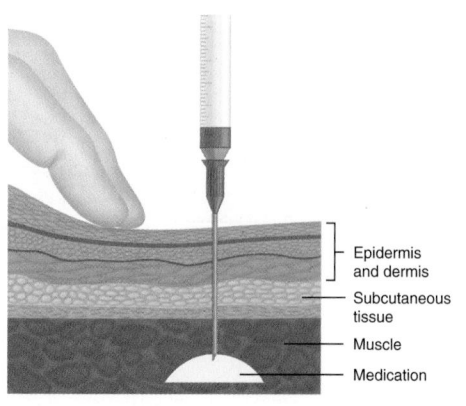

FIGURE 3.10 Intramuscular Injection.

Labels: Epidermis and dermis, Subcutaneous tissue, Muscle, Medication

WORD	PRONUNCIATION	ELEMENTS		DEFINITION
adipose	ADD-i-pose	S/ R/	-ose *condition* adip- *fat*	Containing fat
collagen	KOL-ah-jen	S/ R/	gen *producing* coll/a- *glue*	Major protein of connective tissue, cartilage, and bone
follicle	FOLL-ih-kull		Latin *small sac*	Spherical mass of cells containing a cavity or a small cul-de-sac, such as a hair follicle
hypodermis hypodermic (adj)	high-poh-DER-miss high-poh-DER-mik	P/ R/	hypo- *below* -dermis *skin*	Tissue layer below the dermis
intradermal	in-trah-DER-mal	S/ P/ R/	-al *pertaining to* intra- *within* -derm- *skin*	Within the dermis
intramuscular	in-trah-MUSS-kew-lar	S/ P/ R/	-ar *pertaining to* intra- *within* -muscul- *muscle*	Within the muscle
papilla papillae (pl) papilloma	pah-PILL-ah pah-PILL-ee pap-ih-LOH-mah	 S/ R/CF	Latin *small pimple* -oma *tumor, mass* papill/o- *pimple*	Any small projection Benign projection of epithelial cells
semipermeable membrane	sem-ee-PER-me-ah-bull MEM-brain	S/ P/ R/CF R/	-able *capable of* semi- *half* -perm/e- *pass through* membrane *cover, skin*	A membrane that allows only certain substances to pass through it
subcutaneous (same as hypodermic)	sub-kew-TAY-nee-us	S/ P/ R/CF	-ous *pertaining to* sub- *below* -cutan/e- *skin*	Below the skin
transdermal	trans-DER-mal	S/ P/ R/	-al *pertaining to* trans- *across, through* -derm- *skin*	Going across or through the skin
wheal (also called hives)	WHEEL		Old English *wheal*	Small, itchy swelling of the skin. Wheals raised by an injection do not itch

Transdermal Applications

Some medications can be administered through the skin by an adhesive **transdermal** patch that is applied to the skin. In the patch, a small reservoir contains medication that leaves the reservoir at a known rate through a **semipermeable membrane**. The medication diffuses across the epidermis and enters the blood vessels in the dermis. Medications for motion sickness and cardiac problems, testosterone, birth control hormones, and the chemical nicotine are administered by transdermal patches.

Abbreviations

IM	intramuscular
SC	subcutaneous
TB	tuberculosis

EXERCISES

The following definitions represent medical terms found in this WAD. Find the missing elements and build the terms. Fill in the blanks.

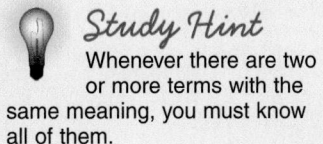

Study Hint
Whenever there are two or more terms with the same meaning, you must know all of them.

1. Going across the skin   trans/_____/ _____

2. Pertaining to wax   sebace/_____

3. Pertaining to within muscle   _____/_____/ar

4. Pertaining to below the skin   _____/dermic

5. Pertaining to below the skin   _____/cutane/_____

LESSON 3.2 Disorders of the Skin

OBJECTIVES

This lesson will enable you to use correct medical terminology to:

3.2.1 **Describe common diseases of the skin.**
3.2.2 **Identify the different types of infections of the skin.**
3.2.3 **Define the types of pharmacologic agents used in the treatment of skin disorders.**
3.2.4 **Describe disorders of the skin.**

CASE REPORT 3.2

Fulwood Medical Center

Mrs. Rose McGinnis, a 72-year-old widow, has been in a nursing home for the past 6 months. She has been unable to get out of bed since surgery to repair a broken hip. She has been depressed and difficult to feed and nurse. Two months ago, she developed decubitus ulcers over her buttocks and left heel. The ulcer over her buttocks became infected with a methicillin-resistant *Staphylococcus aureus* (MRSA). Staphylococcal septicemia ensued, and she died.

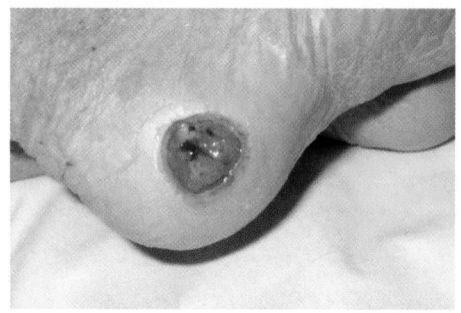

▲ **FIGURE 3.11   Decubitus Ulcer on Heel.**

DISORDERS OF THE SKIN

When a patient lies in one position for a long period, the pressure between the bed and bony body projections, like the lower spine or heel, cuts off the blood supply to the skin and **decubitus (pressure) ulcers** can appear *(Figure 3.11)*. The protective function of the skin is broken, and germs can enter the body.

Other major factors in the breakdown of Rose's skin were that it was thin and dry because of aging. Also, her poor nutritional status had depleted the fatty protective layer in the hypodermis under the skin.

The skin shows the same types of disease as most organs—infections, tumors, malignancies—but, in addition, its protective function makes it the first responder to many irritant and allergenic agents.

CASE REPORT 3.3

Fulwood Medical Center

Ms. Cheryl Fox is a 37-year-old nursing assistant working in a surgical unit in Fulwood Medical Center. Recently her fingers have become red and itchy, with occasional **vesicles.** She has also noticed irritation and swelling of her earlobes and a generalized pruritus. Over the weekends, both the itching and the rash on her hands worsen. A patch test by her dermatologist showed her to be allergic to nickel in rings that she wears on both hands and in her earrings. She wears these on weekends and not during her workdays.

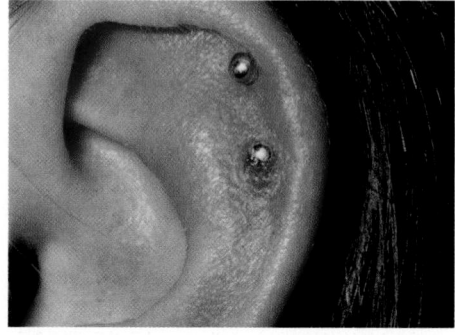

▲ **FIGURE 3.12   Dermatitis of Ear due to Nickel Sensitivity.**

Ms. Fox had a **dermatitis** *(Figure 3.12)*, resulting from direct exposure to an irritating agent. In her case, it was not just a reaction to an irritant. Her form of **atopic (allergic) dermatitis** develops when the body becomes sensitive to an **allergen** such as **latex,** nickel in jewelry, or poison ivy. This whole-body involvement was shown by her systemic symptoms of **pruritus** distant from the local irritant site. She has stopped wearing the rings and earrings.

Eczema is a general term used for inflamed, itchy skin conditions. When the itchy skin is scratched, it becomes **excoriated** and produces the dry, red, scaly patches characteristic of eczema. The atopic dermatitis that Ms. Fox developed to nickel is a common form of eczema.

WORD	PRONUNCIATION	ELEMENTS		DEFINITION
allergen allergenic (adj) allergy allergic (adj)	**AL**-er-jen al-er-**JEN**-ik **AL**-er-jee ah-**LER**-jik	S/ R/	-gen *producing* aller- *allergy*	Substance producing a hypersensitivity (allergic) reaction Hypersensitivity to an allergen
atopy atopic (adj)	**AY**-toh-pee ay-**TOP**-ik		Greek *strangeness*	State of hypersensitivity to an allergen—allergic
decubitus ulcer	de-**KYU**-bit-us **UL**-ser	P/ R/ R/	de- *from* -cubitus *lying down* ulcer *sore*	Sore caused by lying down for long periods of time
dermatitis	der-mah-**TYE**-tis	S/ R/	-itis *inflammation* dermat- *skin*	Inflammation of the skin
eczema eczematous (adj)	**EK**-zeh-mah **EK**-zem-ah-tus	 S/ R/	Greek *to boil or ferment* -tous *pertaining to* eczema- *eczema*	Inflammatory skin disease often with a **serous** discharge
excoriate	eks-**KOR**-ee-ate	S/ P/ R/	-ate *composed of, pertaining to* ex- *away from, out of* -cori- *skin*	To scratch
excoriation (noun)	eks-**KOR**-ee-**AY**-shun	S/	-ation *process*	Scratch marks
latex	**LAY**-tecks		Latin *liquid*	Manufactured from the milky liquid in rubber plants; used for gloves in patient care
mole	MOLE		Latin *spot*	Benign localized area of melanin-producing cells
nevus nevi (pl)	**NEE**-vus **NEE**-vie		Latin *mole, birthmark*	Congenital or acquired lesion of the skin
pruritus pruritic (adj)	proo-**RYE**-tus proo-**RIT**-ik		Latin *to itch*	Itching Itchy
serous	**SEER**-us		Latin *serum*	Thicker and less transparent than water
vesicle	**VES**-ih-kull		Latin *small sac*	Small sac containing liquid; for example, a blister

Sunlight can also be an irritant to the skin, not only by burning it but by leading to cancer when there is excessive exposure, as it did for Mr. Rod Andrews.

Any congenital lesion of the skin, including various types of birthmarks and all **moles**, is referred to as a **nevus**.

Abbreviation

MRSA methicillin-resistant *Staphylococcus aureus*

EXERCISES

Medical terms can have small differences that make them entirely new words. Underline the root of these terms, which stays the same; then focus on how they are different. Insert the correct term in the blanks.

allergen   allergenic   allergy   allergic

1. After many _____ tests, it was determined that she was _____ to mold.

2. There were too many _____ substances in the carpet, and it was removed from the room.

3. Dust mites, peanuts, and pollen are _____.

One of the terms below is a noun (person, place, or thing), and the other term is a verb (action). Identify the noun and verb; then use each term in a sentence.

4. Excor<u>iate</u>   Noun or verb: _____

5. Sentence: _____

6. Excor<u>iation</u>   Noun or verb: _____

7. Sentence: _____

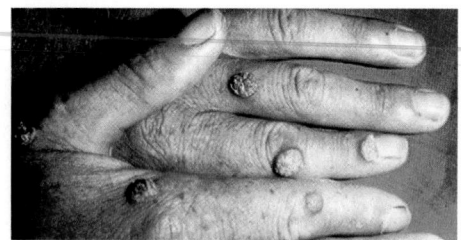

▲ **FIGURE 3.13   Warts of Hands.**

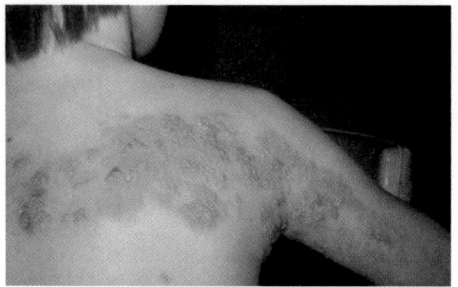

▲ **FIGURE 3.14   Shingles.**

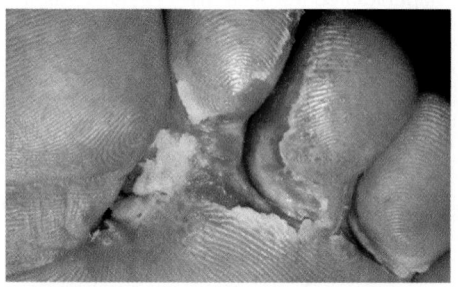

▲ **FIGURE 3.15   Tinea Pedis between Toes.**

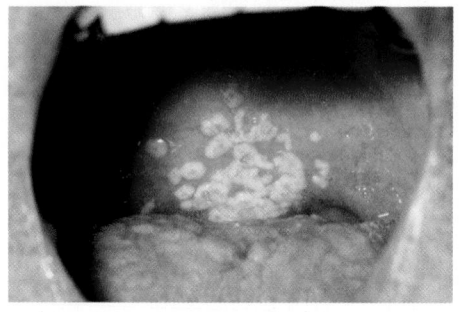

▲ **FIGURE 3.16   Oral Thrush.**

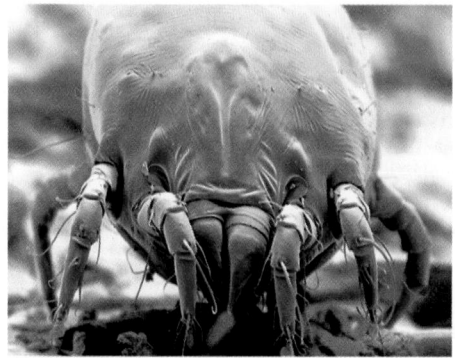

▲ **FIGURE 3.17   House Dust Mite.**

INFECTIONS OF THE SKIN

The skin is also susceptible to the many different types of infections. The following descriptions are examples.

Viral Infections

Warts (verrucas) are caused by the human papillomavirus invading the epidermis and causing the outer epidermal cells to produce a roughened projection from the skin surface *(Figure 3.13)*. Human papillomavirus is discussed extensively in *Chapter 13*.

Varicella-zoster virus causes **chickenpox** in unvaccinated people, forming macules, papules, and vesicles. The virus can then remain dormant in the peripheral nerves for decades before erupting as the painful vesicles of **herpes zoster (shingles)** *(Figure 3.14)*.

Fungal Infections

Tinea is a general term for a group of related skin infections caused by different species of fungi. The fungi live on and are strictly confined to the nonliving stratum corneum and its derivatives, hair and nails, where keratin provides their food. The different types of tinea take their name from the location of the infection.

Tinea pedis, athlete's foot, causes itching, redness, and peeling of the foot, particularly between the toes *(Figure 3.15)*. **Tinea capitis** describes infection of the scalp (ringworm); **tinea corporis** is the name for infections of the body. **Tinea cruris** ("jock itch") is the name for infections of the groin. The fungus spreads from animals, from the soil, and by direct contact with infected individuals. **Tinea versicolor** is characterized by brown and white patches on the trunk.

A yeastlike fungus, *Candida,* can produce recurrent infections of the skin, nails, and mucous membranes. The first sign can be a recurrent diaper rash or thrush in infants. Older children can show recurrent or persistent lesions on the scalp. In adults, chronic **candidiasis** can affect the mouth (**thrush**) *(Figure 3.16)* and vagina, as well as the skin. It can also be associated with diseases of the immune system *(see Chapter 14)*.

Parasitic Infestations

A **parasite** is an organism that lives in contact with and feeds off another organism (host). This process is called an **infestation.** It is different from an **infection.**

Lice are small, wingless, blood-sucking parasites that produce the disease **pediculosis** by attaching their eggs (nits) to hair and clothing *(Table 3.1)*.

"Itch mites" (**scabies**) produce an intense, itching rash, often in the genital area, waist, breast, and armpits. The mites live and lay eggs under the skin.

The skin normally sheds its cells. These tiny specks form some of the dust on our furniture, floors, and carpets. The house dust mite *(Figure 3.17)* thrives on the keratin of these cells and lives well on carpets, upholstery, pillows, and mattresses. Many people are allergic to the inhaled feces of these parasites.

Bacterial Infections

Staphylococcus aureus (commonly called "staph") is the most common bacterium to invade the skin and is the cause of pimples, boils, **carbuncles,** and **impetigo.** It can infect hair follicles and the surrounding tissues to produce **furuncles** and carbuncles. Staph can cause a **cellulitis** of the epidermis and dermis.

Necrotizing fasciitis is caused when some strains of staph and strep produce enzymes that are very toxic and digest the connective tissues and spread into muscle layers.

TABLE 3.1 Pediculosis

Louse (lice, pl)	Attachment of Eggs	Disease
Pediculus capitis	Hair of scalp	Pediculosis capitis
Phthirus pubis (crab-shaped)	Pubic hair	Pediculosis cruris (crabs)
Pediculus humanus	Clothing, body hair	Pediculosis corporis

Word	Pronunciation		Elements	Definition
Candida	**KAN**-did-ah		Latin *dazzling white*	A yeastlike fungus
candidiasis thrush	can-dih-**DIE**-ah-sis THRUSH	S/ R/	-iasis *condition, state of* candid- *Candida*	Infection with the yeastlike fungus *Candida* Infection with *Candida albicans*
carbuncle	**KAR**-bunk-ul		Latin *carbuncle*	Infection of many furuncles in a small area, often on the back of the neck
cellulitis	sell-you-**LIE**-tis	S/ R/	-itis *inflammation* cellul- *small cell*	Infection of subcutaneous connective tissue
furuncle	**FU**-rung-kel		Latin *a boil*	An infected hair follicle that spreads into the tissues around the follicle
herpes zoster (also called **shingles**)	**HER**-pees **ZOS**-ter		**herpes** *to creep or spread* **zoster** *belt, girdle*	Painful eruption of vesicles that follows a dermatome or nerve root on one side of the body
impetigo	im-peh-**TIE**-go		Latin *scabby eruption*	Infection of the skin producing thick, yellow crusts
infection	in-**FEK**-shun	S/ R/	-ion *process* infect- *tainted, internal invasion*	Invasion of the body by disease-producing microorganisms
infestation	in-fes-**TAY**-shun	S/ R/	-ation *process* infest- *invade*	Act of being invaded on the skin by a troublesome other species, such as a parasite
louse lice (pl)	LOWSE LICE		Old English *louse*	Parasitic insect
necrotizing fasciitis	neh-kroh-**TIZE**-ing fash-eh-**EYE**-tis	S/ R/CF S/ S/ R/CF	-ing *quality of* necr/o- *death* -tiz- *pertaining to* -itis *inflammation* fasc/i – *fascia*	Inflammation of fascia, producing death of the tissue
parasite	**PAR**-ah-site		Greek *guest*	An organism that attaches itself to, lives on or in, and derives its nutrition from another species
pediculosis	peh-dick-you-**LOH**-sis	S/ R/	-osis *condition* pedicul- *louse*	An infestation with lice
scabies	**SKAY**-bees		Latin *to scratch*	Skin disease produced by mites
tinea	**TIN**-ee-ah		Latin *worm*	General term for a group of related skin infections caused by different species of fungi
verruca	ver-**ROO**-cah		Latin *wart*	Wart caused by a virus

EXERCISES

Make the WADs work for you. As you read each WAD, notice any elements that may have the same meaning; highlight them, or keep a separate list in the back of your book. This WAD contains two pairs of elements that each have the same meaning. Find the elements, and define them.

A. _____ and _____ both mean _____.

B. _____ and _____ both mean _____.

C. *Match the correct Latin or Greek term to its medical meaning. Circle the best answer.*

1. impetigo: carbuncle   boil   scabby eruption

2. verruca: ulcer   furuncle   wart

3. vesicle: carbuncle   blister   boil

4. scabies: to bleed   to cut   to scratch

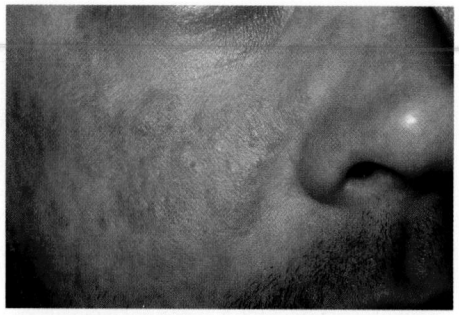

▲ FIGURE 3.18 Systemic Lupus Erythematosus.

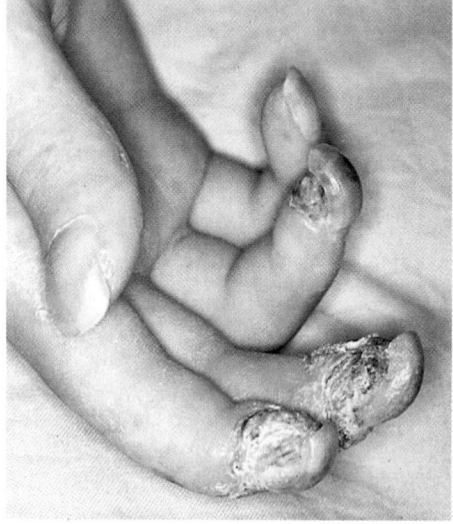

▲ FIGURE 3.19 Scleroderma.

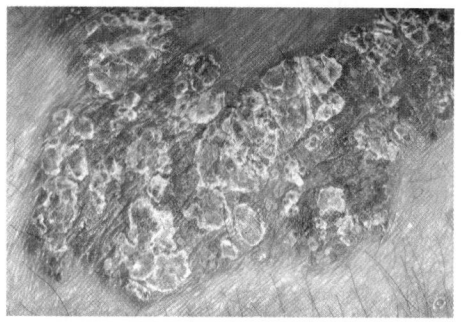

▲ FIGURE 3.20 Psoriasis.

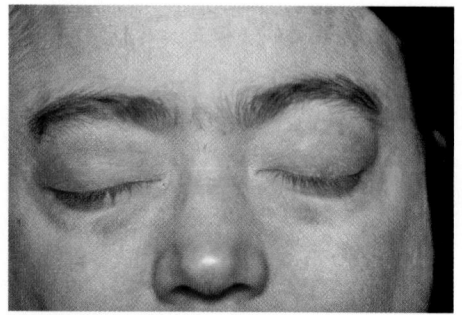

▲ FIGURE 3.21 Periorbital Rash of Dermatomyositis.

DISEASES OF THE SKIN

Collagen Diseases

Collagen, a fibrous protein, accounts for 30% of total body protein. Therefore, collagen diseases can have a dramatic effect all over the body. Collagen diseases, **autoimmune** or otherwise, attack collagen or other components of connective tissue.

Systemic lupus erythematosus (SLE), an autoimmune disease, occurs most commonly in women and produces characteristic skin lesions. A butterfly-shaped, red rash on both cheeks joined across the bridge of the nose is commonly seen *(Figure 3.18)*. It is associated with fever, fatigue, joint pains, and multiple internal organ involvement.

Rosacea produces a similar facial rash to that of SLE, and the underlying capillaries become enlarged and show through the skin. It is thought to be worsened by alcohol and spicy food. Its etiology is unknown. It has no **systemic** complications.

Scleroderma is a chronic, persistent autoimmune disease, occurring more often in women and characterized by hardening and shrinking of the skin that makes it feel leathery *(Figure 3.19)*. Joints show swelling, pain, and stiffness. Internal organs such as the heart, lungs, kidneys, and digestive tract can be involved in a similar process. The etiology is unknown, and there is no effective treatment.

Other Skin Diseases

Psoriasis *(Figure 3.20)* is marked by itchy, flaky, red patches of skin of various sizes covered with white or silvery scales. It appears most commonly on the scalp, elbows, and knees. Its cause is unknown.

Vitiligo produces pale, irregular patches of skin. It is thought to have an autoimmune etiology.

Skin Manifestations of Internal Disease

Signs of the presence of cancer inside the body are often shown by skin lesions, even before the cancer has produced **symptoms** or been diagnosed.

Dermatomyositis *(Figure 3.21)* is often associated with ovarian cancer, which can appear within 4 to 5 years after the skin disease is diagnosed.

Pharmacology

No matter what the cause of skin lesions, a wide range of **topical pharmacologic agents** of different types can be used in their treatment, either to relieve symptoms or to cure the disease.

- **Antipruritics**—topical lotions, ointments, creams, or sprays that relieve itching. **Corticosteroids** such as hydrocortisone are most frequently used.

- **Antibacterials**—topical agents that eliminate the bacteria that cause epidermal infections. The antibiotic neomycin is frequently used in ointments for this purpose.

- **Antifungals**—topical agents that eliminate or inhibit the growth of fungi. Lamisil is used as a cream, gel, or spray.

- **Parasiticides**—topical agents that kill parasites living on the skin. Lindane 1% is in a lotion or shampoo used to kill lice.

- **Keratolytics**—topical agents that peel the stratum corneum away from the other epidermal layers. Salicylic acid is used for this purpose.

- **Anesthetics**—topical agents that relieve pain or itching on the skin's surface. Benzocaine is used for this purpose.

- **Retinoids**—derivatives of **retinoic acid** that are used in the treatment of acne.

WORD	PRONUNCIATION	ELEMENTS		DEFINITION
anesthetic **anesthesia** (noun)	an-es-**THET**-ic an-es-**THEE**-zee-ah	S/ P/ R/	**-ic** *pertaining to* **an-** *without* **-esthet-** *sensation*	Substance that takes away feeling and pain Complete loss of sensation

antipruritic
  pruritus (noun)
  pruritic (adj)
	AN-tee-pru-**RIT**-ik
	proo-**RYE**-tus
	proo-**RIT**-ik
		S/
		P/
		R/
			-ic *pertaining to*
			anti- *against*
			-prurit- *itch*
				Medication against itching
				Itching
				Itchy

corticosteroid	**KOR**-tih-koh-**STEHR**-oyd	S/ R/CF R/	**-oid** *resembling* **cortic/o-** *cortisone* **ster-** *steroid*	A hormone produced by the adrenal cortex
dermatomyositis	**DER**-mah-toe-**MY**-oh-site-is	S/ R/CF R/	**-itis** *inflammation* **dermat/o-** *skin* **-myos-** *muscle*	Inflammation of the skin and muscles
pharmacology **pharmacologic** (adj) **pharmacist** **pharmacy**	far-mah-**KOLL**-oh-jee far-mah-ko-**LOJ**-ik **FAR**-mah-sist **FAR**-mah-see	S/ R/CF S/	**-logy** *study of* **pharmac/o-** *drug* **-ist** *specialist*	Science of the preparation, uses, and effects of drugs Person licensed by the state to prepare and dispense drugs Facility licensed to prepare and dispense drugs
psoriasis	so-**RYE**-ah-sis		Greek *the itch*	Rash characterized by reddish, silver-scaled patches
retinoid	**RET**-ih-noyd		Derived from retinoic acid	A class of keratolytic agents
rosacea	roh-**ZAY**-she-ah		Latin *rosy*	Persistent erythematous rash of the central face
scleroderma	sklair-oh-**DERM**-ah	S/ R/CF	**-derma** *skin* **scler/o-** *hard*	Thickening and hardening of the skin due to new collagen formation
sign (objective) **symptom** (subjective)	SINE **SIMP**-tum		Latin *mark* Greek *sign*	Physical evidence of a disease process Departure from normal health experienced by the patient
symptomatic (adj)	simp-toe-**MAT**-ik	S/ R/	**-ic** *pertaining to* **symptomat-** *symptoms*	Pertaining to the symptoms of a disease
systemic lupus **erythematosus**	sis-**TEM**-ik **LOO**-pus er-ih-**THEE**-mah-toe-sus	S/ R/ S/ R/	**-ic** *pertaining to* **system-** *body system* **lupus** *wolf* **-osus** *condition* **erythemat-** *redness*	Inflammatory connective tissue disease affecting the whole body
topical	**TOP**-ih-kal	S/ R/	**-al** *pertaining to* **topic-** *local*	Medication applied to the skin to obtain a local effect
vitiligo	vit-ill-**EYE**-go		Latin *skin blemish*	Nonpigmented white patches on otherwise normal skin

EXERCISES

Building medical terms and taking them apart force you to focus on the elements they contain. Understanding elements is the key to increasing your medical vocabulary. Deconstruct the following terms to increase your knowledge of their elements. Fill in the chart.

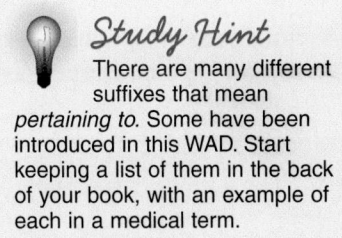

Study Hint

There are many different suffixes that mean *pertaining to*. Some have been introduced in this WAD. Start keeping a list of them in the back of your book, with an example of each in a medical term.

Medical Term	Meaning of Prefix	Meaning of Root/Combining Form	Meaning of Suffix
anesthetic			
antipruritic			
corticosteroid			
pharmacology			
scleroderma			

LESSON 3.3 Accessory Skin Organs

OBJECTIVES

Hair follicles and their associated sebaceous glands, sweat glands, and nails are organs located in your skin. They each have specific anatomical and physiologic characteristics. You must understand their roles in the different functions of the skin and in diseases that affect the skin. This lesson will enable you to use correct medical terminology to:

3.3.1 Name the associated skin organs.
3.3.2 Link the structures of the different organs to their functions.
3.3.3 Describe certain disorders affecting the associated skin organs.
3.3.4 Explain the etiology of certain disorders affecting the associated skin organs.
3.3.5 Identify the anatomy, physiology, and disorders of the associated skin organs.

You are

...a medical assistant working with Lenore Echols, MD, a dermatologist in Fulwood Medical Center.

Your patient is

...Wayne Winter, an 18-year-old man, who has been accepted to college in the fall.

CASE REPORT 3.4

He has had acne since the age of 15 and has tried numerous over-the-counter products. Retinoic acid has also been unsuccessful. He has numerous **comedones, papules, pustules,** and scars on his face and forehead with severe **cystic** lesions and scars on his back. His social life is nonexistent, and he is teased by his peers. He wishes to change all this before he gets to college.

Your role is to document his care and explain to him how to use the medications Dr. Echols prescribes, what their effects will be, and his prognosis.

HAIR FOLLICLES AND SEBACEOUS GLANDS

Each hair follicle has a **sebaceous gland** opening into it *(Figure 3.22)*. The gland secretes into the follicle a mixture of oily, acidic **sebum** and broken-down cells from the base of the gland.

Around puberty, **androgens** are thought to trigger excessive production of sebum from the glands, which then brings excessive numbers of broken-down cells toward the skin surface. This blocks the follicle, forming a **comedo** (whitehead or blackhead). Comedones can stay closed, leading to **papules,** or can **rupture,** allowing bacteria to get in and produce **pustules.** These are the classic signs of **acne,** which is said to affect, in different degrees, about 85% of people between 12 and 25 years *(Figure 3.23)*.

A different skin problem involving the sebaceous glands is **seborrheic dermatitis.** The glands are thought to be inflamed and to produce a different sebum. The skin around the face and scalp is reddened and covered with yellow, greasy scales. In infants, this condition is called cradle cap. Seborrheic dermatitis of the scalp produces **dandruff.**

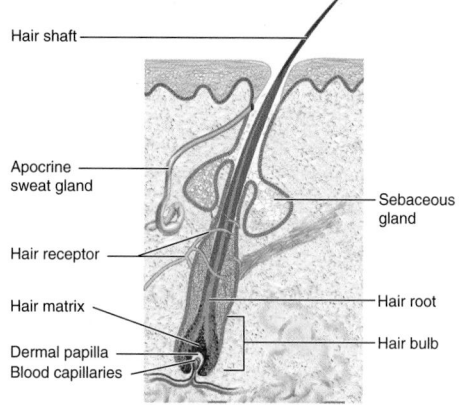

Hair shaft
Apocrine sweat gland
Hair receptor
Hair matrix
Dermal papilla
Blood capillaries
Sebaceous gland
Hair root
Hair bulb

▲ **FIGURE 3.22** **Hair Follicle and Sebaceous Gland.**

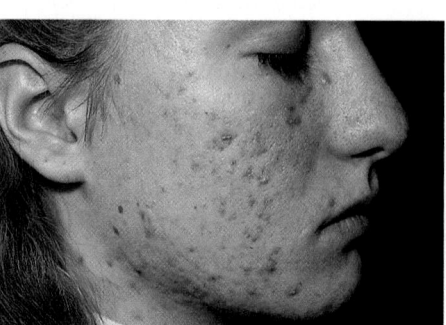

▲ **FIGURE 3.23** **Acne.**

WORD ANALYSIS AND DEFINITION

S = Suffix   P = Prefix   R = Root   R/CF = Combining Form

WORD	PRONUNCIATION	ELEMENTS		DEFINITION
acne	**AK**-nee		Greek *point*	Inflammatory disease of sebaceous glands and hair follicles
androgen	**AN**-droh-jen	S/ R/CF	-gen *to produce* andr/o- *male*	Hormone that promotes masculine characteristics
comedo comedones (pl)	**KOM**-ee-doh		Latin *eat up*	A whitehead or blackhead caused by too much sebum and too many keratin cells blocking the hair follicle
cyst cystic (adj)	SIST **SIS**-tik		Greek *sac, bladder*	An abnormal, fluid-containing sac Relating to a cyst
dandruff	**DAN**-druff		Old English *scurf*	Seborrheic scales from the scalp
papule	**PAP**-yul		Latin *pimple*	Small, circumscribed elevation on the skin
pustule	**PUS**-tyul		Latin *pustule*	Small protuberance on the skin that contains pus
rupture	**RUP**-tyur		Latin *break*	Break or tear of any organ or body part
sebum	**SEE**-bum		Latin *wax*	Waxy secretion of the sebaceous glands
seborrhea seborrheic (adj)	seb-oh-**REE**-ah seb-oh-**REE**-ik	S/ R/CF	-rrhea *flow* seb/o- *sebum*	Excessive amount of sebum

EXERCISES

Match the Greek or Latin term to its medical meaning.

_____ 1. sebum   A. Point

_____ 2. cyst   B. Containing pus

_____ 3. pustule   C. Whitehead, blackhead

_____ 4. acne   D. Wax

_____ 5. comedo   E. Sac, bladder

_____ 6. dandruff   F. Hormone that promotes masculine characteristics

_____ 7. rupture   G. Excessive amount of sebum

_____ 8. androgen   H. Break or tear of any organ or part

_____ 9. papule   I. Seborrheic scales from the scalp

_____ 10. seborrhea   J. Small, circumscribed elevation of the skin

Study Hint
An easy way to remember the meaning of the word **pustule** is as a small protuberance on the skin that contains **pus.**

Study Hint
Make an extra effort to learn the correct spelling of the terms sebo**rrh**ea and seb-o**rrh**eic. The "rrh" combination occurs in other medical terms as well—diar**rh**ea, hemor**rh**age, menor**rh**agia, hernior**rh**aphy, etc. Be alert to this combination of letters in terms. You can be sure these terms will appear on a test.

Read Case Report 3.4 on the opposite page, and circle the best answer for each statement. Rewrite any false statements correctly on the lines below.

1. A *pustule* is filled with pus.   T   F

2. *Acne* is a degenerative disease of the skin.   T   F

3. A *cystic lesion* is filled with hard, packed cells.   T   F

4. An "over-the-counter" product is available without a prescription.   T   F

5. A *comedo* can be either a whitehead or a blackhead.   T   F

Corrections:

_____

_____

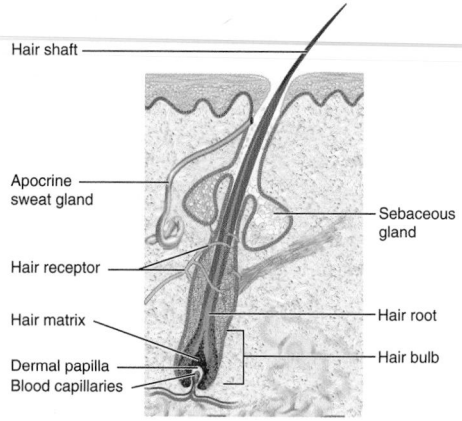

Hair shaft

Apocrine sweat gland

Hair receptor

Hair matrix

Dermal papilla
Blood capillaries

Sebaceous gland

Hair root

Hair bulb

▲ **FIGURE 3.24   Hair Follicle.**

Hair

Each hair, no matter where it is on your body or scalp, originates from epidermal cells at the base (matrix) of a hair follicle. As these cells divide and grow, they push older cells upward away from the source of nutrition in the hair papilla *(Figure 3.24)*. The cells become keratinized and die. They rest for a while; and when a new hair is formed, the old, dead hair is pushed out and drops off.

In cross-section, each hair has three layers *(Figure 3.25a)*. Its core, the **medulla,** is composed of loosely arranged cells containing a flexible keratin. The **cortex** is composed of densely packed cells with a harder keratin that gives hair its stiffness. These cells also contain pigment. The outer **cuticle** is a single layer of scaly, dead keratin cells.

Straight hair is round in cross-section *(Figure 3.25a and b)*. Curly hair is oval *(Figure 3.25c and d)*. Two pigments derived from **melanin (eumelanin** and **pheomelanin)** give hair its natural color. Black and dark brown hair has a lot of a dark form of the pigment eumelanin in the cells of the cortex *(Figure 3.25b)*. Blonde hair has little of this dark pigment but a moderate amount of the lighter form of pheomelanin *(Figure 3.25a)*. Red hair has a lot of the lighter pigment *(Figure 3.25c)*. White or gray hair has no pigment *(Figure 3.25d)*.

A problem with the scalp hair follicle occurs in men when a combination of genetic influence and excess testosterone produces "top of the head" baldness. In most people, aging causes **alopecia,** thinning of the hair and baldness as the follicles shrink and produce thin, wispy hairs.

Scalp hair is thick enough to retain heat. Body hair has no specific function in our present evolution because, in most people, it is too thin to retain heat. Beard, pubic, and **axillary** (armpit) hair reflect sexual maturity. Stronger hairs guard the nostrils and ears to prevent foreign particles from entering. Similarly, eyelashes protect the eyes, and eyebrows help keep perspiration from running into the eyes.

Melanin is in the black skin melanocytes of dark-skinned people and is the pigment generated by sunbathing and tanning. The absence of melanin produces **albinism.**

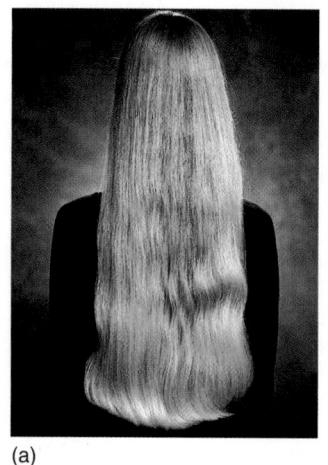
(a)

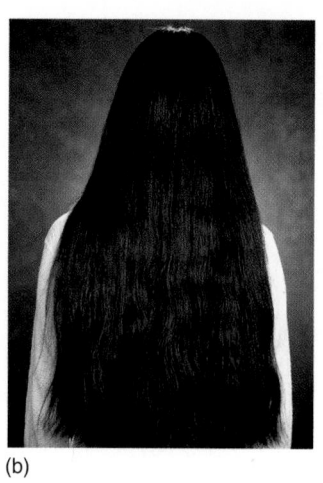
(b)

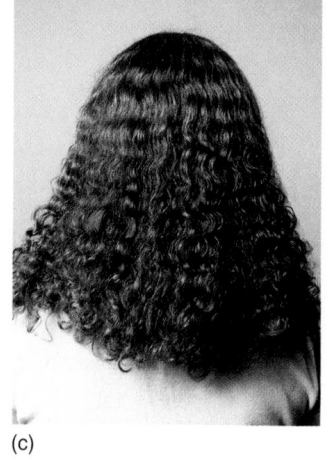
(c)

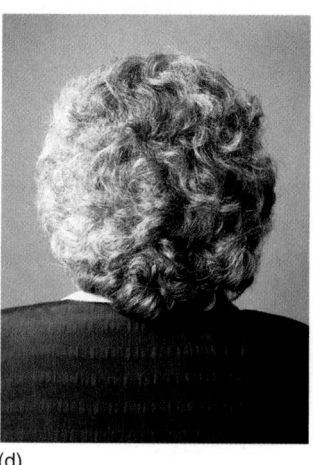
(d)

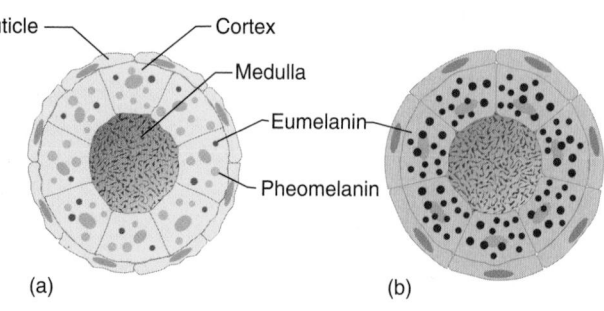

Cuticle — Cortex
— Medulla
— Eumelanin
— Pheomelanin

(a)   (b)

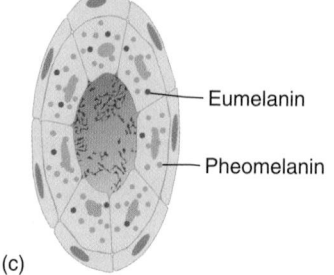

— Eumelanin
— Pheomelanin

(c)

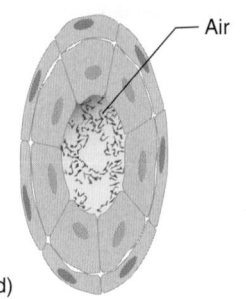

— Air

(d)

▲ **FIGURE 3.25   Basis of Hair Color and Texture.**

WORD	PRONUNCIATION		ELEMENTS	DEFINITION
albinism albino	**AL**-bih-nizm al-**BY**-no	S/ R/	**-ism** *condition* **albin-** *white*	Genetic disorder with lack of melanin Person with albinism
alopecia	al-oh-**PEE**-shah		Greek *mange*	Partial or complete loss of hair, naturally or from medication
axilla axillae (pl) axillary (adj)	**AK**-sill-ah **AK**-sill-ee **AK**-sill-air-ee		Greek *region under a bird's wing*	Medical name for the armpit
cortex cortical (adj) cortices (pl)	**KOR**-teks **KOR**-tih-kal **KOR**-tih-sees		Latin *outer covering*	Outer portion of an organ, such as bone. Gray covering of cerebral hemispheres
cuticle	**KEW**-tih-cul		Diminutive of **cutis** *skin*	Nonliving epidermis at the base of the fingernails and toenails, and the outer layer of hair
medulla medullary (adj)	meh-**DULL**-ah meh-**DULL**-eh-ree		French *middle*	Central portion of a structure surrounded by cortex
melanin eumelanin pheomelanin	**MEL**-ah-nin **YOU**-mel-ah-nin **FEE**-oh-mel-ah-nin	 P/ P/	Greek *black* **eu-** *good, normal* **pheo-** *gray*	Black pigment found in skin, hair, retina The dark form of the pigment melanin The lighter form of melanin

EXERCISES

A good review of the WAD will aid you in answering the following questions about the **language of dermatology**. *Fill in the blanks.*

1. The root _____ denotes the color _____.

2. The medical term for **armpit** is _____.

3. The plural form of **cortex** is _____.

4. The central portion of a structure is the _____, which means _____.

5. The outer portion of an organ is the _____.

6. The medical term for baldness is _____.

7. **Alopecia** can result from natural causes or from _____.

The following nouns all have an adjectival form. Fill in the blanks.

8. Noun: axilla   Adjective: _____

9. Noun: cortex   Adjective: _____

10. Noun: medulla   Adjective: _____

11. Use any one of these adjectives in a sentence.

_____

_____

_____

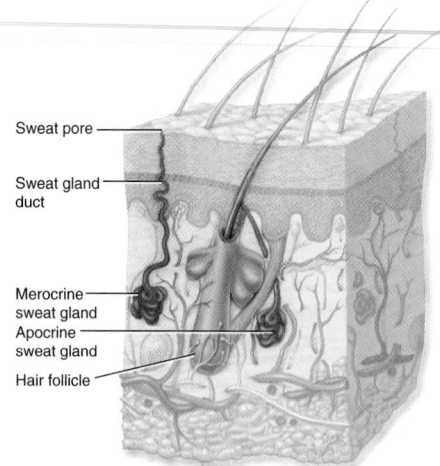

▲ FIGURE 3.26   Sweat Glands.

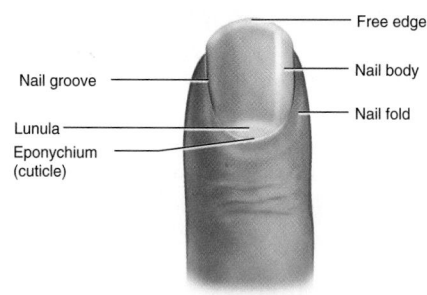

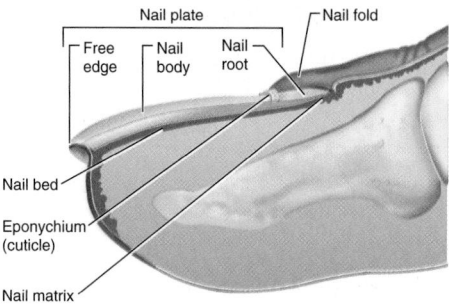

▲ FIGURE 3.27   Anatomy of a Fingernail.

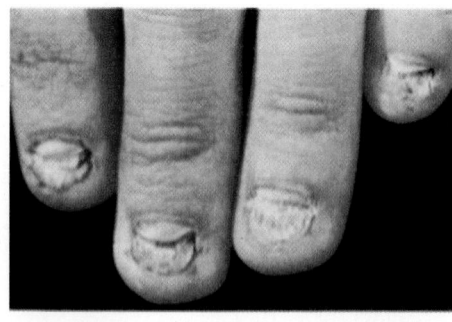

▲ FIGURE 3.28   Onychomycosis (Fungal Infection).

Sweat Glands

You have 3 million to 4 million **merocrine (eccrine)** sweat glands *(Figure 3.26)* scattered all over your skin, with higher concentrations on your palms, soles, and forehead.

Their main function is to produce the watery perspiration (sweat) that cools your body. Your sweat is 99% water; the rest is made up of electrolytes such as sodium chloride, which gives the sweat its salty taste. Some waste products of cell metabolism are also secreted.

In the dermis the sweat gland is a coiled tube lined with epithelial cells that secrete the sweat. Around the tube, muscle cells contract to squeeze the sweat up the tube directly to the surface of the skin.

In your armpits (**axillae**), around your nipples, in your groin, and around your anus, **apocrine** sweat glands produce a thick, cloudy secretion that interacts with normal skin bacteria to produce a distinct, noticeable smell. The ducts of these glands lead directly into hair follicles *(see Figure 3.26)*. They respond to sexual stimulation and stress and secrete chemicals called **pheromones**, which have an effect on the sexual behavior of other people.

Ceruminous glands are found in the external ear canal, where their secretions combine with sebum and dead epidermal cells to form earwax. This wax waterproofs the external ear canal and kills bacteria.

Sweat gland functions are severely affected in a group of diseases termed "ectodermal dysplasia," manifested in the reduction or absence of sweat. They can be involved in the infections that engulf the nearby hair follicles and sebaceous glands.

Mammary glands, a type of modified sweat gland, serve a distinct purpose in reproduction and are therefore discussed in *Chapter 12* under the female reproductive system.

Nails

Nails are formed from the stratum corneum of the epidermis. They consist of closely packed, thin, dead cells that are filled with parallel fibers of hard keratin.

Fingernails grow about 1 millimeter (mm) per week. New cells are added by cell division in the nail **matrix,** which is protected by the nail fold of skin and the cuticle at the base of the nail *(Figure 3.27)*. The nail rests on the nail bed, which consists of the living layers of the epidermis, the strata basale, spinosum, and granulosum.

Diseases of Nails   Fifty percent of all nail disorders are caused by fungal infections and are labeled **onychomycosis** *(Figure 3.28)*. They begin in nails constantly exposed to moisture and warmth; for example, in warm shoes when associated with poor foot hygiene, in the hands of a restaurant dishwasher, under artificial fingernails, and in pedicure bowls if they are not sanitized. The fungus grows under the nail and leads to brittle cracked nails that separate from the underlying nail bed.

Paronychia *(Figure 3.29)* is a bacterial infection, usually staphylococcal, of the base of the nail. The nail fold and cuticle become swollen, red, and painful, and pus forms under the nail and can escape at the side of the nail.

The big-toe nail can grow into the skin at the side of the nail, particularly if pressured by tight, narrow shoes. Infection can then get underneath this ingrown toenail.

The nails can reflect systemic illness. In anemia, the nail bed is pale, and the nails can become spoon-shaped. In conditions producing chronic **hypoxia**, the fingers, toes, and nails become clubbed. **Malnutrition** or severe illness can produce horizontal white lines in the nails.

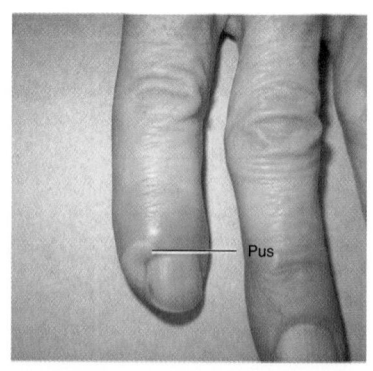

▲ FIGURE 3.29   Paronychia, with Pus at the Corner of the Nail Bed.

WORD	PRONUNCIATION		ELEMENTS	DEFINITION
apocrine	AP-oh-krin	P/ R/	apo- *different from* -crine *secrete*	Apocrine sweat glands open into the hair follicle
cerumen ceruminous (adj)	seh-ROO-men seh-ROO-mih-nus		Latin *wax*	Waxy secretion of the ceruminous glands of the external ear
eccrine	EK-rin		Greek *to secrete*	Coiled sweat gland that occurs in skin all over the body
hypoxia	high-POCK-see-ah	S/ P/ R/	-ia *condition* hyp- *below* -ox- *oxygen*	Decrease below normal levels of oxygen in tissues, gases, or blood
hypoxic (adj)	high-POCK-sik	S/	-ic *pertaining to*	Deficient in oxygen
malnutrition	mal-nyu-TRISH-un	S/ P/ R/	-ion *process* mal- *bad, inadequate* -nutrit- *nourishment*	Inadequate nutrition from poor diet or inadequate absorption of nutrients
matrix	MAY-triks		Latin *womb*	Substance that surrounds cells, is manufactured by the cells, and holds them together
merocrine	MARE-oh-krin	P/ R/	mero- *partial* -crine *secrete*	Another name for eccrine
onychomycosis	oh-ni-koh-my-KOH-sis	S/ R/CF R/	-osis *condition* onych/o- *nail* -myc- *fungus*	Condition of a fungus infection in a nail
paronychia	par-oh-NICK-ee-ah	S/ P/ R/	-ia *condition* para- *alongside* onych- *nail* (**Note:** The vowel "a" at the end of para- is dropped to make the composite word flow more easily.)	Infection alongside the nail
pheromone	FER-oh-moan	P/ R/	pher- *carrying* -omone *excite, stimulate*	Substance that carries and generates a physical attraction for other people

EXERCISES

Work on understanding the meanings of the elements. Deconstruct the medical terms into their elements, and show that you know their meanings. Fill in the blanks.

Medical Term	Prefix	Meaning of Prefix	Root/CF	Meaning of Root/CF	Suffix	Meaning of Suffix
pheromone						
apocrine						
hypoxia						
merocrine						
onychomycosis						
paronychia						

Answer the following questions about the medical terms in this WAD.

A plural form of a term that relates to cells has been intentionally left out of the Word Analysis and Definition box shown above. Find the term, form its plural, and write the rule that applies to that ending.

1. Singular term: _____ Plural term: _____

2. Rule: _____. *Note:* Go back and write the plural form in the Word Analysis and Definition box under the singular term.

LESSON 3.4 Burns and Injuries to the Skin

OBJECTIVES

You have learned that a major role of the skin is protection of your internal organs. In the previous lessons, you have seen the effects of infectious agents on the skin. In this lesson, you will learn the effects of direct injury to the skin, and you will be able to use correct medical terminology to:

3.4.1 **Distinguish the four types of burns.**
3.4.2 **Describe the inflammatory process of the skin when it is injured.**
3.4.3 **Explain the process of healing and repair of the skin.**
3.4.4 **Describe wounds, burns, and the process of healing and repair.**

You are

. . . a burn technologist employed in the Burn Unit at Fulwood Medical Center.

Your patient is

. . . Mr. Steven Hapgood, a 52-year-old man, admitted to the Fulwood Burn Unit with severe burns over his face, chest, and abdomen.

CASE REPORT 3.5

After an evening of drinking, Mr. Hapgood was smoking in bed and fell asleep. His next-door neighbors in the apartment building smelled smoke and called 911. In the Burn Unit, his initial treatment included large volumes of intravenous fluids to prevent **shock.**

Your role will be to participate in Mr. Hapgood's care as a member of the Burn Unit team and to document the care and his response to it.

Keynote

Sunburn causes a first-degree burn.

Scalds can cause second-degree burns.

House fires with prolonged flame contact can cause third-degree burns.

High-voltage electrical injury can cause fourth-degree burns.

Keynote

The prognosis for a burn patient depends on the degree of the burn and on the surface area affected (see page 60).

▼ **FIGURE 3.30**

BURNS

Burns are the leading cause of accidental death. The immediate threats to life are from fluid loss, infection, and the systemic effects of burned dead tissue.

Burns are classified according to the depth of tissue involved *(Figure 3.30)*:

- **First-degree (superficial) burns** involve only the epidermis and produce inflammation with redness, pain, and slight **edema.** Healing occurs in 3 to 5 days without scarring.
- **Second-degree (partial-thickness) burns** involve the epidermis and dermis but leave some of the dermis intact. They produce redness, blisters, and more severe pain. Healing occurs in 2 to 3 weeks with minimal scarring.
- **Third-degree (full-thickness) burns** involve the epidermis, dermis, and subcutaneous tissues, which are often completely destroyed. Healing takes a long time and involves using skin grafts.
- **Fourth-degree burns** destroy all layers of the skin and involve tendons, muscles, and sometimes bones.

Burn injury to the lungs through damage from heat or smoke inhalation is responsible for 60% or more of fatalities from burns.

In partial-thickness burns, **regeneration** of the skin can occur from remaining cells in the stratum basale, from residual hair follicles and sweat glands, and from

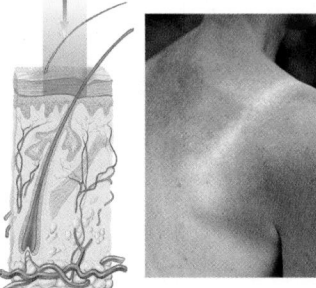

(a) First degree (superficial)

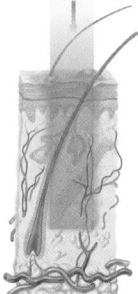

(b) Second degree (partial thickness)

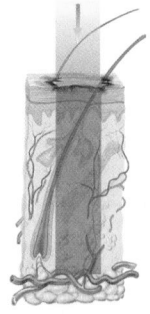

(c) Third degree (full thickness)

WORD ANALYSIS AND DEFINITION

S = Suffix   P = Prefix   R = Root   R/CF = Combining Form

WORD	PRONUNCIATION	ELEMENTS		DEFINITION
allograft	**AL**-oh-graft	P/	allo- *other*	Skin graft from another person or cadaver
		R/	-graft *transplant*	
homograft	**HOH**-moh-graft	P/	homo- *same, alike*	
autograft	**AWE**-toe-graft	P/	auto- *self*	A graft using tissue taken from the individual who is receiving the graft
		R/	-graft *transplant*	
debridement	day-**BREED**-mon	S/	-ment *resulting state*	The removal of injured or necrotic tissue
		P/	de- *take away*	
		R/	-bride- *rubbish*	
edema	ee-**DEE**-mah		Greek *swelling*	Excessive collection of fluid in cells and tissues
edematous (adj)	ee-**DEM**-ah-tus			Marked by edema
eschar	**ESS**-kar		Greek *scab of a burn*	The burned, dead tissue lying on top of third-degree burns
regenerate	ree-**JEN**-eh-rate	S/	-ate *composed of, pertaining to*	Reconstitution of a lost part
regeneration (noun)	ree-**JEN**-eh-**RAY**-shun	P/	re- *again*	
		R/	-gener- *produce*	
shock	SHOCK		German *to clash*	Sudden physical or mental collapse or circulatory collapse
xenograft	**ZEN**-oh-graft	P/	xeno- *foreign*	A graft from another species
		R/	-graft *transplant*	
heterograft	**HET**-er-oh-graft	P/	hetero- *different*	

Case-Report 3.5 *(continued)*

Mr. Hapgood's burns were mostly third-degree. The protective ability of the skin to prevent water loss had been removed, as had the skin barrier against infection. The burned, dead tissue forms an **eschar** that can have toxic effects on the digestive, respiratory, and cardiovascular systems. The eschar was surgically removed by **debridement**.

the edges of the burned area. In full-thickness burns there is no dermal tissue left for regeneration, and skin grafts are needed. The ideal graft is an **autograft** taken from another location on the patient. It is not rejected by the immune system. Mr. Hapgood had autografts taken from his unburned legs and back.

If the patient's burns are too extensive, **allografts** from another person are needed. These are provided by skin banks and taken from deceased people (cadaver). A **homograft** is another name for an allograft. A **xenograft,** or **heterograft,** is a graft from another species; for example, pigs.

Artificial skin is being developed commercially and can stimulate the growth of connective tissues from the patient's underlying tissue.

Keynote

In third- and fourth-degree burns, there is no dermal tissue left for regeneration, and skin grafts are necessary.

Study Hint

Pay special attention to the graft prefixes.

EXERCISES

*Continue your work with elements from the **language of dermatology**. Match the element in 1–12 to its correct meaning in A–L. Fill in the blanks.*

_____ 1. homo-

_____ 2. -bride-

_____ 3. -ate

_____ 4. allo-

_____ 5. -ment

_____ 6. xeno-

_____ 7. -gener-

_____ 8. -graft

_____ 9. auto-

_____ 10. de-

_____ 11. re-

_____ 12. hetero-

A. again

B. foreign

C. produce

D. same, like

E. different

F. other

G. composed of, pertaining to

H. resulting state

I. rubbish

J. transplant

K. self

L. take away

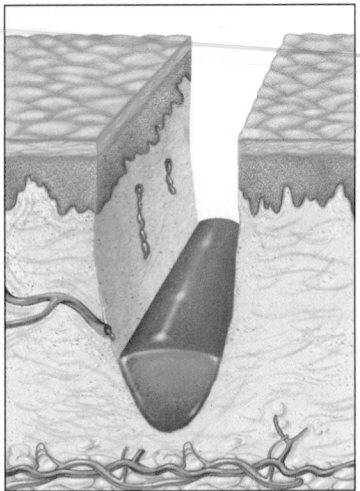

(a) Bleeding into the wound

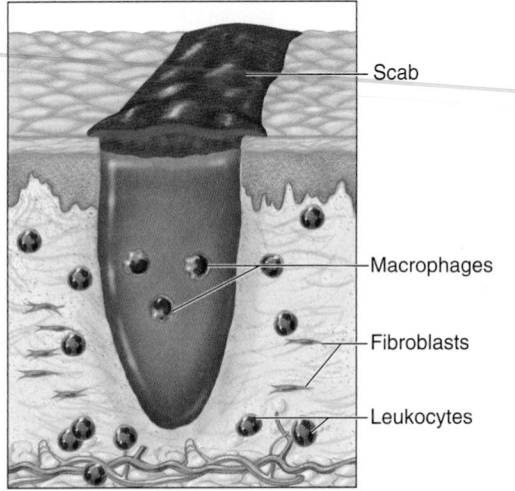

Scab

Macrophages

Fibroblasts

Leukocytes

(b) Scab formation and macrophage activity

▲ FIGURE 3.31   Wound Healing.

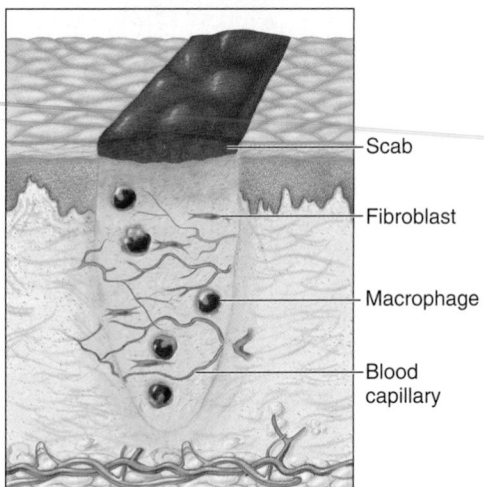

Scab

Fibroblast

Macrophage

Blood capillary

▲ FIGURE 3.32   Formation of Granulation Tissue.

Keynote

A scab seals and protects a wound.

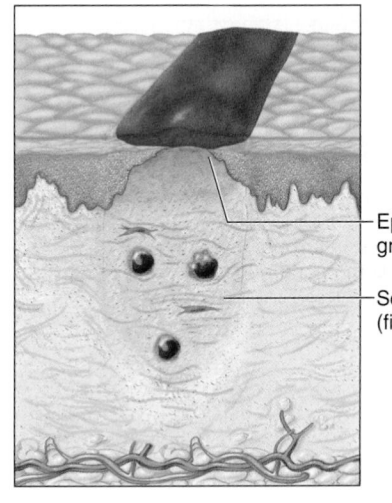

Epidermal growth

Scar tissue (fibrosis)

▲ FIGURE 3.33   Scar Formation.

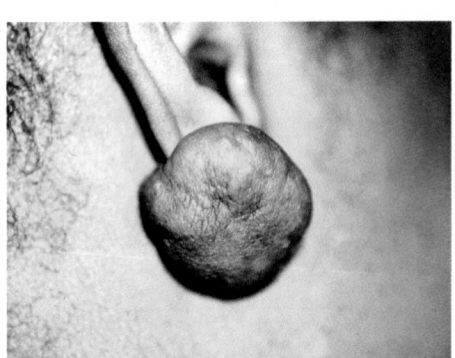

▲ FIGURE 3.34   A Keloid of the Earlobe.
This scar resulted from piercing the ear for earrings.

WOUNDS AND TISSUE REPAIR

If you cut yourself with paper and produce a shallow **laceration** primarily in the epidermis, the epithelial cells along its edges will divide rapidly and fill in the gap. An adhesive bandage helps the process by pulling the edges together.

If you cut yourself more deeply, extending the **wound** into the dermis or hypodermis, or if a surgeon makes an **incision,** then blood vessels in the dermis break and blood escapes into the wound *(Figure 3.31a)*.

This escaped blood forms a **clot** in the wound. The clot consists of the protein **(fibrin)** together with **platelets,** blood cells, and dried tissue fluids trapped in the fibers. **Macrophages** come into the wound with the escaped blood. They digest and clean up the tissue debris. The surface of the clot dries and hardens in the air to form a **scab.** The scab seals and protects the wound from becoming infected *(Figure 3.31b)*.

The clot begins to be invaded by new capillaries from the surrounding dermis. Three or four days after the injury, fibroblasts migrate into the wound and form new collagen fibers that pull the wound together. This soft tissue in the wound is called **granulation tissue** and in unsutured wounds takes a couple of weeks to completely form *(Figure 3.32)*.

As healing continues, surface epithelial cells from the edges of the wound migrate into the area underneath the scab. As this new epithelium thickens, the scab loosens and falls off. Inside the wound, new collagen fibers formed by the fibroblasts form a **scar** to replace the granulation tissue *(Figure 3.33)*. In unsutured wounds, this takes up to a month to complete.

Suturing brings together the edges of the wound to enhance tissue healing. It also reduces the risk of infection and the amount of scarring. A liquid skin adhesive can sometimes be used in place of sutures. Some sutures eventually dissolve, avoiding the need for suture removal. The scar formation and remodeling process may go on for more than a year.

In some people, there is excessive fibrosis and scar tissue formation, producing raised, irregular, lumpy, shiny scars called **keloids** *(Figure 3.34)*. They can extend beyond the edges of the original wound and often return if they are surgically removed. They are most common on the upper body and earlobes.

Surgery on the skin is now being performed using light beams called **lasers.** These beams of light can be focused precisely to vaporize specific lesions on the superficial layers of the skin. The beam removes lesions and creates a fresh surface over which new skin can grow. Healing takes 10 to 15 days and goes through the process described above, with clotting and scabbing.

A superficial scraping of the skin, a mucous membrane, or the cornea *(see Chapter 4)* is called an **abrasion.**

S = Suffix   P = Prefix   R = Root   R/CF = Combining Form

WORD	PRONUNCIATION		ELEMENTS	DEFINITION
abrasion	ah-**BRAY**-shun		Latin *to scrape*	Area of skin or mucous membrane that has been scraped off
clot	KLOT		German *to block*	The mass of fibrin and cells that is produced in a wound
fibrin	**FIE**-brin		Latin *fiber*	Stringy protein fiber that is a component of a blood clot
fibrous (adj)	**FIE**-brus			Tissue containing fibroblasts and fibers
granulation	gran-you-**LAY**-shun	S/ R/	-ation *process* granul- *small grain*	New fibrous tissue formed during wound healing
incision	in-**SIZH**-un	S/ R/	-ion *action, condition* incis- *cut into*	A cut or surgical wound
keloid	**KEY**-loyd		Greek *stain*	Raised, irregular, lumpy, shiny scar due to excess collagen fiber production during healing of a wound
laceration	lass-eh-**RAY**-shun	S/ R/	-ation *process* lacer- *to tear*	A tear of the skin
laser	**LAY**-zer		acronym for *l*ight *a*mplification by *s*timulated *e*mission of *r*adiation	Intense, narrow beam of monochromatic light
macrophage	**MAK**-roh-fayj	P/ R/CF	macro- *large* -phag/e *to eat*	Large white blood cell that removes bacteria, foreign particles, and dead cells
platelet (also called thrombocyte)	**PLAYT**-let		Greek *small plate*	Cell fragment involved in clotting process
scab	SKAB		Old English *crust*	Crust that forms over a wound or sore during healing
scar	SKAR		Greek *scab*	Fibrotic seam that forms when a wound heals
suture	**SOO**-chur		Latin *seam*	Stitch to hold the edges of a wound together
wound	WOOND		Old English *wound*	Any injury that interrupts the continuity of skin or a mucous membrane

EXERCISES

Review the WAD before starting this exercise—the elements and definitions will help you work out the answers. Put on your thinking cap. Fill in the blanks.

1. Reorder these terms into the order of their occurrence.

   scab   scar   clot   wound

   _____

2. How are a *keloid* and a *scar* different?

   _____

3. What is the soft tissue in the wound-healing process called?

   _____

4 What's the relationship between a *clot* and a *scab*?

   _____

5. What is another name for a stitch used to close a wound?

   _____

Congratulations! You have mastered these terms.

INTEGUMENTARY SYSTEM

CHALLENGE YOUR KNOWLEDGE

A. Apply your knowledge of the language of dermatology to the following Case Report from this chapter. Read the report out loud for pronunciation practice. Underline the medical terms, and be sure you understand them. Answer the questions.

CASE REPORT 3.3

Ms. Cheryl Fox is a 37-year-old nursing assistant working in a surgical unit in Fulwood Medical Center. Recently her fingers have become red and itchy, with occasional vesicles. She has also noticed irritation and swelling of her earlobes and a generalized pruritus. Over the weekends, both the itching and the rash on her hands worsen. A patch test by her dermatologist showed her to be allergic to nickel in rings that she wears on both hands and in her earrings. She wears these on weekends and not during her workdays.

1. What diagnostic test did Ms. Fox have to determine the cause of her condition?

   _____

2. List Ms. Fox's symptoms.

   _____

   _____

3. What part of her body was *edematous?*

   _____

4. **Pruritus** is a medical term for _____ .

5. Describe a vesicle. _____

6. What is the *allergen* that Ms. Fox is allergic to? _____

7. A likely diagnosis for Ms. Fox would be (circle one):

       melanoma   dermatitis   vitiligo   candidiasis

B. Identify the following group of elements. Define each element, and use each in a medical term. Complete the analysis by giving the meaning of each medical term. Fill in the chart below.

Element	Meaning of Element	Medical Term	Meaning of Medical Term
an			
anti			
apo			
bi			
cryo			
de			
epi			

Element	Meaning of Element	Medical Term	Meaning of Medical Term
hypo			
intra			
macro			
melan			
para			
peri			
pro			
re			
semi			
sub			
trans			

This entire group in the chart above is what type of element? _____

C. **To have a better understanding of the integumentary system, you must know the** layers of skin and its tissue components, as well as its functions. Fill in the following blanks.

Name the three layers of skin, the type of tissue found in each layer, and the function of each layer of skin.

1. Skin layer: _____

    Tissue(s): _____

    Function(s): _____

2. Skin layer: _____

    Tissue(s): _____

    Function(s): _____

3. Skin layer: _____

    Tissue(s): _____

    Function(s): _____

INTEGUMENTARY SYSTEM

D. **Plurals:** Form the plurals for the following terms.

1. papilla   Plural: _____

2. matrix   Plural: _____

3. cortex   Plural: _____

4. axilla   Plural: _____

E. **Translate to layman's terms.** Expressing yourself verbally is something you will have to do every day on the job. Your patient is asking about the following procedures. In the space given, briefly define each procedure in terms the patient will understand.

1. Cryosurgery:

    _____

    _____

2. Biopsy removal:

    _____

    _____

3. Debridement:

    _____

    _____

F. **The terms in each of the following groups of medical terms have something in common.** Use your knowledge of the *language of dermatology* to determine what links them together. The first one is done for you. Fill in the blanks.

1. epidermis, dermis, and hypodermis   *All are layers of skin.*_____

2. melanoma, malignancy, metastasis _____

3. bee stings, peanuts, cats, pollen _____

4. intradermal, subcutaneous, intramuscular _____

5. merocrine, apocrine, ceruminous _____

6. mole, papule, macule _____

7. parasite, pediculosis, lice _____

8. scleroderma, rosacea, SLE _____

9. paronychia, onychomycosis, matrix _____

10. eschar, debridement, xenograft _____

G. **Diagnoses:** Determining the root(s) of the following diagnoses will help you understand the meaning of the medical term. First, determine the root/combining form(s), then give the meaning of the root/combining form(s), and then provide a brief description of the meaning of the term. Fill in the chart below.

Diagnosis	Root/CF(s)	Meaning of Root/CF	Meaning of Term
candidiasis			
carcinoma			
decubitus ulcer			
dermatitis			
dermatomyositis			
hypoxia			
onychomycosis			
paronychia			
pediculosis			
scleroderma			

H. **Also Known As:** Some medical terms may be known by a more common term. You need to know both. Fill in the blanks with the alternate terms.

1. pressure ulcer = _____

2. cradle cap = _____

3. shingles = _____

4. staph = _____

5. armpit = _____

6. baldness = _____

7. wax = _____

8. whitehead or blackhead = _____

9. athlete's foot = _____

10. hives = _____

11. lice eggs = _____

12. ringworm = _____

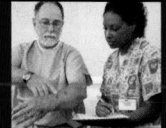

INTEGUMENTARY SYSTEM

I. **Medical vocabulary is filled with terms taken directly from Greek and Latin.** The medical term is given to you—write the definition beside it.

1. dermis _____

2. integument _____

3. mole _____

4. squamous _____

5. collagen _____

6. follicle _____

7. vesicle _____

8. edema _____

9. nevus _____

10. boil _____

J. **Recall and Review:** How well do you remember these word elements from the previous chapter? Try to answer without first looking back to check. Fill in the blanks.

Element	Type of Element (P, R, CF, S)	Meaning of Element
ism	_____	_____
elle	_____	_____
chromat	_____	_____
endo	_____	_____
cyte	_____	_____

K. **Label Exercise:** Identify the integumentary term in phrases 1–6, and write the terms on the correct lines A–F in the illustration.

1. Open into hair follicles

2. Also called subcutaneous tissue layer

3. Top layer of the skin

4. Concentrated on palms, soles of feet, and forehead

5. Layer of skin below epidermis

6. Secrete chemicals called pheromones

B. _____

A. _____

D. _____

E. _____

F. _____

C. _____

L. **The following chart of elements is not complete.** In some cases you are given the element to begin with; in some cases you are given the term that you end with. Work with your integumentary system vocabulary to fill in the missing blanks. There should be an answer in every space of every column.

Element	Type of Element	Meaning of Element	Medical Term Using This Element
adip		*fat or suet*	
	prefix		antigen
oma	suffix		
ment			debridement
	prefix	*icy cold*	
		two/twice	
	suffix	*structure*	
	suffix		androgen
sclero			
		broken	
ox			hypoxia
ation	suffix		
		cell	
		cause	
melan		*becoming black*	

M. **Make a connection from a medical term to an English word.** Fill in the chart below.

Fungal infections that cause human disease are named tinea. Which three body areas host this fungus?

Body Area	Medical Term Is	Correlate to an English Word
1.		pedal
2.		capital/capitol
3.		corporal

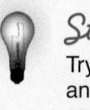

Study Hint
Try to match the term to an English word with the same sense or meaning.

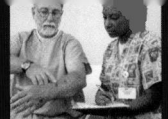

INTEGUMENTARY SYSTEM

N. **Burn treatment is a highly specialized area of care.** Assess what you have learned about burns in Chapter 3. Fill in the blanks.

1. Burns are the leading cause of _____ .

2. A superficial burn is _____ -degree.

3. Burns are classified according to _____ .

4. What degree burns require skin grafts? _____

5. Burn injury can involve other body systems. Name one. _____

6. The immediate threats to life are from _____ , _____ , and _____ .

7. Name three occupations that risk burn injury on the job. _____ , _____ ,

   and _____

8. Name the five different types of skin grafts and where they come from.

   _____ comes from _____ .

   _____ comes from _____ .

   _____ comes from _____ .

   _____ comes from _____ .

   _____ comes from _____ .

O. **Discussion:** Explain this sentence: "Skin is the largest and most vulnerable organ in the body."

   In your discussion of this with your classmates, you must answer these questions:

1. What does *vulnerable* mean? (Look it up in an online dictionary.)

   _____

   _____

2. Why is skin vulnerable?

   _____

   _____

3. What makes skin an organ?

   _____

   _____

P. **Build your medical language of dermatology.** Complete the medical terms by filling in the blanks. The first one is done for you.

1. Study of disorders of the skin   dermato/*logy*

2. To scratch the skin   ex/_____/ate

3. Sore caused by lying in bed   de/_____

4. Infestation with lice   _____/osis

5. Takes away feeling and pain   an/_____/_____

6. Medication against itching   _____/_____ic

7. Infection alongside a nail   _____/_____ia

8. Deficient in oxygen   _____/oxia

9. Forecasting probable course of disease   pro/_____

Q. **Patient Education: In Your Own Words**

Philip was involved in a motor vehicle accident (MVA) and was burned over 60% of his body when his car caught fire. The plastic surgeon has just told Philip he will need extensive grafting to repair his third-degree burns. Pain and nervousness kept Philip from entirely understanding what the surgeon told him. He is asking you for more explanation.

You need to explain to the patient:

1. What an autograft is, and where it will come from.

_____

_____

_____

2. How this procedure will help his skin regenerate.

_____

_____

_____

R. **Use your knowledge of the *language of dermatology* to make the connection with the following medical terms.** Match the medical terms in the left column with the descriptions in the right column.

_____ 1. pruritus   A. Can infiltrate or metastasize

_____ 2. edema   B. Body as a whole

_____ 3. malignancy   C. Instrument for viewing

_____ 4. systemic   D. Swelling

_____ 5. ringworm   E. Infection of the scalp

_____ 6. scope   F. To itch

INTEGUMENTARY SYSTEM

S. **The previous exercises should help you apply your knowledge of the integumentary system and correctly answer the following questions.** Circle the answer.

1. Use of liquid nitrogen to freeze or kill abnormal tissue is called:

   a. biopsy

   b. patch test

   c. cryosurgery

   d. hypodermic injection

   e. infestation

2. A laceration that is *superficial* is not very:

   a. swollen

   b. edematous

   c. deep

   d. purulent

   e. infected

3. Keratinized stratified squamous epithelium is:

   a. stratum spinosum

   b. dandruff

   c. hair follicle

   d. sweat

   e. dermatitis

4. An ointment, cream, or spray prescribed to relieve itching is called:

   a. antifungal

   b. keratolytic

   c. antipruritic

   d. retinoid

   e. antibacterial

5. Subcutaneous fat is another name for:

   a. epidermis

   b. hypodermis

   c. dermis

   d. adipose tissue

   e. follicles

6. This gives hair its stiffness:

   a. the medulla

   b. the follicle

   c. the cortex

   d. the cuticle

   e. the matrix

7. Wounds heal by forming _____ tissue.

   a. connective

   b. muscle

   c. smooth

   d. granulation

   e. purulent

8. Relating to the sense of touch:

   a. strata

   b. tactile

   c. papillae

   d. atopy

   e. excoriation

9. A raised, lumpy, shiny scar due to excess collagen production during wound healing is a:

   a. scab

   b. keloid

   c. matrix

   d. cortex

   e. clot

10. MRSA refers to:

   a. a diagnostic test

   b. a procedure

   c. a blood test

   d. a staph infection

   e. a film study

INTEGUMENTARY SYSTEM

T. Terminology Challenge: Many medical terms can appear in several different forms—a noun (person, place, thing), a verb (action), or an adjective (description). Use the following medical terms to complete the sentences. Note at the end of the sentence whether you have used the noun, verb, or adjectival form of the term. Fill in the blanks.

metastasis   metastasize   metastatic

1. The surgeon predicted that the lesion would _____ to the liver.

   Form used: _____

2. The _____ lesion received radiation therapy, while the primary lesion was surgically removed.

   Form used: _____

3. The pathology report confirmed that there was no _____ of the lesion.

   Form used: _____

Apply your rule for plural endings, and make the plural form of the noun of this medical term. _____

The rule is _____ .

4. Some terms can function as a noun and a verb. "To suture" means to stitch the edges of a wound together (verb). "A suture" is the material used to make the stitch itself (noun). Sutures come in various sizes and materials. Demonstrate your understanding of both terms by creating a sentence of patient documentation for each term.

   Sentence (verb)

   _____

   _____

   Sentence (noun)

   _____

   _____

U. Skin diseases can affect any and all parts of the body. Some skin diseases are an early manifestation of a more serious internal problem. Match the symptom or association in the left column with the correct medical term in the right column. You have more answer choices than you need.

_____ 1. Cause unknown; silvery scales

_____ 2. Butterfly rash

_____ 3. Associated with ovarian cancer

_____ 4. Enlarged capillaries show through skin

_____ 5. Pale patches of skin

_____ 6. Shrinking of skin; hardening

A. pemphigus vulgaris

B. vitiligo

C. rosacea

D. psoriasis

E. seborrheic lesions

F. scleroderma

G. SLE

H. herpes zoster

I. dermatomyositis

V. **Fine-Tune Your Knowledge.** Being able to explain something to someone else means *you* understand it. Explain to your classmates the differences in the terms shown below.

1. What is the difference between an **infestation** and an **infection**? Using correct medical terms, give an example of each.

   _____

   _____

   _____

   _____

2. What is the difference between a **viral** and a **bacterial** infection? Using correct medical terms, give an example of each.

   _____

   _____

   _____

   _____

3. What is the difference between **vasoconstriction** and **vasodilation**? What is the purpose of each?

   _____

   _____

   _____

   _____

W. **Abbreviations appear in written documentation and must be used correctly.** Rewrite the following sentences with the correct abbreviation(s) in the appropriate place.

1. This patient is suffering from septicemia and tuberculosis.

   _____

2. Is this an intramuscular or subcutaneous injection?

   _____

3. Rheumatoid arthritis and systemic lupus erythematosus are classified as autoimmune diseases.

   _____

   _____

INTEGUMENTARY SYSTEM

X. **Continue applying your knowledge of the *language of dermatology* to the integumentary system.** Circle the best choice.

1. A congenital lesion of the skin, including birthmarks and moles, is called a:

   a. macule

   b. papule

   c. vesicle

   d. nevus

   e. melanoma

2. Another name for a pressure ulcer is:

   a. eczema

   b. excoriation

   c. decubitus

   d. edematous

   e. serous

3. Strep enzymes digest connective tissue and spread into muscle layers in:

   a. lesions

   b. atopic dermatitis

   c. cellulitis

   d. ulcers

   e. necrotizing fasciitis

4. The medical term for shingles is:

   a. erysipelas

   b. herpes zoster

   c. impetigo

   d. candidiasis

   e. pediculosis

5. Kaposi sarcoma is associated with:

   a. SC

   b. HIV

   c. SLE

   d. TB

   e. MRSA

Y. **Medical terms that are nouns can also have an adjectival form that must be used in some cases.** Test your knowledge of the correct form of the term to use in the following sentences. Circle the best choice.

1. This puncture wound has completely penetrated the (dermis/dermal).

2. This puncture wound has completely penetrated the (dermis/dermal) layer of skin.

3. Please take this specimen to the (pathological/pathology) department.

4. The (pathology/pathological) diagnosis has not been determined yet.

5. The (anesthesia/anesthetic) properties of the aloe lotion reduced the pain in the sunburn.

Z. **The skin is the largest organ in the body.** Build your knowledge of Chapter 3 terminology with the following exercise. Deconstruct the following medical terms into their word elements. Fill in the chart for each term, and then answer the questions.

Medical Term	Prefix	Root/Combining Form	Suffix	Meaning of Medical Term
biopsy				
carcinoma				
corneum				
cryosurgery				
dermatologist				
epidermis				
integumentary				
keratinocyte				
metastasis				
microscope				
pathological				
prognosis				

1. List the terms that are procedures: _____

2. Write the term for a specialist: _____

3. Name the body system: _____

4. Identify the instrument a pathologist uses:_____

5. Name the top layer of the skin: _____

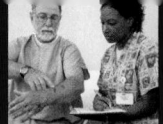

CHAPTER 3 REVIEW

INTEGUMENTARY SYSTEM

CHAPTER SUMMARY EXERCISE

1. *Listen to the pronunciation of the medical terms as given by your instructor.*
2. *Circle the correct spelling of the medical term.*
3. *Match the correctly spelled terms to the brief descriptions below.*
4. *Write a sentence for each of the 10 terms that appear in this exercise.*

A. SPELLING COMPREHENSION: CIRCLE THE CORRECT SPELLING OF THE TERM.

1. ideology	etiology	eteology	iteology	etelogy
2. eczema	eksema	ecczemia	ecczema	ekzema
3. furruncle	furunckle	ferunkle	faruncle	furuncle
4. squamous	squamus	squuamus	sguamus	squamis
5. skleroderma	skeloderma	scleroderma	sccleroderma	sclerroderma
6. wheel	weal	wheil	weel	wheal
7. decubbitus	dicubitus	dekcubitus	decubeitus	decubitus
8. veruca	verruca	veruka	verruka	verukka
9. psoriasis	psoresis	soriasis	soriasus	psorriasus
10. sebacceus	sebaceous	sebbacus	sibacious	sibaceous

B. MATCH THE NUMBER OF THE CORRECT TERM IN PART A WITH THE BRIEF DESCRIPTION OF THE TERM BELOW.

a. Wart _____

b. Means *to itch* _____

c. Hardening and shrinking of the skin _____

d. Secretes a greasy substance called sebum _____

e. From lying down too long _____

f. Inflammatory skin disease with serous discharge _____

g. Layer of scaly cells _____

h. Begins as an infected hair follicle _____

i. Cause is unknown _____

j. Small, itchy swelling of the skin _____

C. USING YOUR KNOWLEDGE OF TERMS 1–10 IN PART A AND THEIR CORRECT SPELLING, WRITE A BRIEF SENTENCE FOR EACH OF THE TERMS AS IT MIGHT APPEAR IN PATIENT DOCUMENTATION.

1. _____

2. _____

3. _____

4. _____

5. _____

6. _____

7. _____

8. _____

9. _____

10. _____

D. YOUR INSTRUCTOR WILL DIRECT YOU TO MCGRAW-HILL CONNECT. OPEN THE AUDIO GLOSSARY AND PRACTICE YOUR PRONUNCIATION OF THE TERMS IN PART A OF THIS EXERCISE.

McGraw Hill **connect**™ (plus+)

E. AFTER READING CASE REPORT 3.5, ANSWER THE FOLLOWING QUESTIONS. *BE PREPARED TO DISCUSS YOUR ANSWERS IN CLASS.*

CASE REPORT 3.5

You are

. . . a burn technologist employed in the Burn Unit at Fulwood Medical Center.

Your patient is

. . . Mr. Steven Hapgood, a 52-year-old man, admitted to the Fulwood Burn Unit with severe burns over his face, chest, and abdomen. After an evening of drinking, Mr. Hapgood was smoking in bed and fell asleep. His next-door neighbors in the apartment building smelled smoke and called 911. In the Burn Unit, his initial treatment included large volumes of intravenous fluids to prevent **shock**.

Your role will be to participate in Mr. Hapgood's care as a member of the Burn Unit team and to document the care and his response to it.

Mr. Hapgood's burns were mostly third-degree. The protective ability of the skin to prevent water loss had been removed, as had the skin barrier against infection. The burned, dead tissue forms an **eschar** that can have toxic effects on the digestive, respiratory, and cardiovascular systems. The eschar was surgically removed by **debridement.**

1. Where are Mr. Hapgood's burns located? _____

2. Because of the extent of his burns, Mr. Hapgood has lost a large volume of body fluids. This could lead to what potentially life-threatening condition? _____

3. How are the fluids replaced? _____

4. Third-degree burns are also known as _____ and involve which layers of skin? _____

5. What two functions of skin have been eliminated due to Mr. Hapgood's large burn area? _____

_____

6. _____ is the medical term for the burned, dead tissue lying on top of third-degree burns, and _____

is the surgical procedure that removes this dead tissue.

7. This burned, dead tissue can have toxic effects on which other body systems? _____

8. Why are burn patients in a special unit and not in rooms with other patients with various diseases and conditions?

_____

9. What other surgical procedure is necessary to promote the growth of new skin for Mr. Hapgood? _____

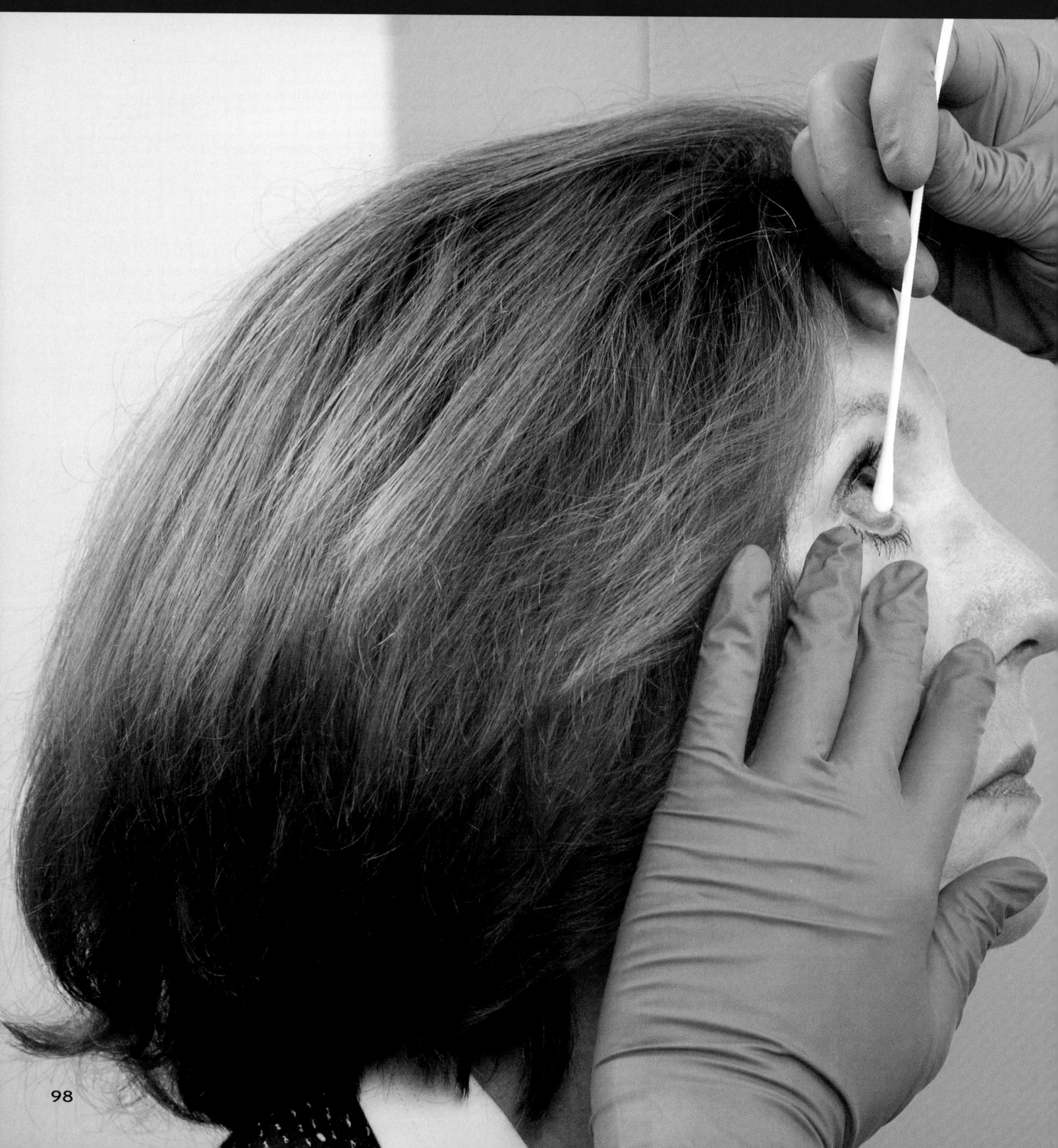

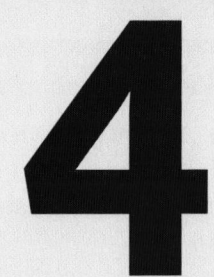
THE EYE AND SEEING

CASE REPORT 4.1

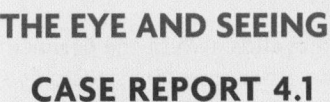

You are

. . . an **ophthalmic** technician **(OT)** working in the office of **ophthalmologist** Angela Chun, MD, a member of the Fulwood Medical Group.

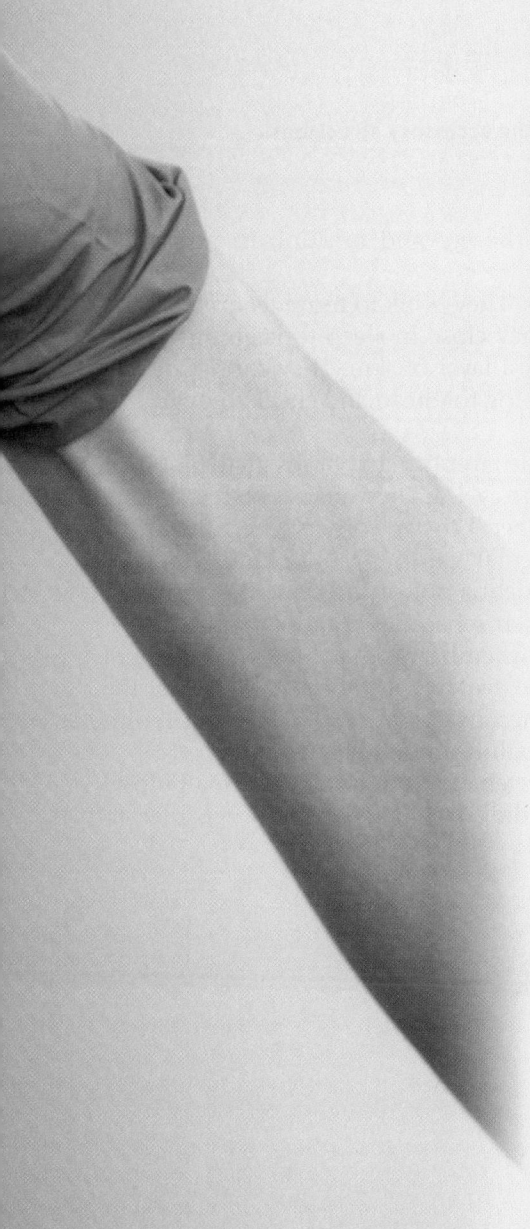

Your patient is

. . . Mrs. Jenny Hughes, a 30-year-old computer software consultant, who walked into the office with painful, red, swollen eyelids and a sticky, **purulent** discharge from both eyes. The administrative medical assistant did not hold her in the reception area, but brought her directly in to you.

Mrs. Hughes complains of headache and photophobia, and her eyelids were stuck together when she woke up this morning. She tells you that, a couple of days earlier, she had gone into a small business office to install software at 10 workstations. One of the employees was absent with **"pink eye."** She wants to know if she could have contracted the disease from that employee's keyboard and how to prevent her husband and two children from getting it.

You have in your hand a clipboard, pen attached, with the office Notice of Privacy Practices and sign-in sheet for her to sign. How do you proceed?

Learning Outcomes

In order to make correct decisions in situations like this, to communicate with Dr. Chun about the patient, to participate in patient education, and to document the patient's care, you need to be able to:

4.1 Apply the language of **ophthalmology** to the anatomy and physiology of the eye and its accessory structures.

4.2 Comprehend, analyze, spell, and write the medical terms of ophthalmology so that you communicate and document accurately and precisely in any health care setting.

4.3 Recognize and pronounce the medical terms of ophthalmology so that you communicate verbally with accuracy and precision in any health care setting.

4.4 Describe the cause, appearance, diagnosis, and treatment of common disorders of the eye and its accessory structures.

NOTE: The sense of smell is discussed as an integral part of the respiratory system (Chapter 9), the sense of taste as an integral part of the digestive system (Chapter 6), and the sense of touch as an integral part of the nervous system (Chapter 10).

LESSON 4.1 Accessory Structures of the Eye

OBJECTIVES

Mrs. Jenny Hughes's **"pink eye"** involved her **conjunctiva** and **eyelids,** two of the **periorbital** accessory structures of the eye, located around the **orbit** and in front of the **eyeball.** The other accessory structures are the **eyebrows and eyelashes** and the **lacrimal (tear) apparatus** (Figure 4.2). All these structures support and protect the exposed front surface of the eye (Figure 4.1).

An understanding of the terminology, anatomy, and physiology of these accessory structures is an essential step to acquire an understanding of how they function to maintain the integrity of the eye.

The information in this lesson will enable you to:

4.1.1 Link the structure of the accessory structures of the eye to the appropriate function.

4.1.2 Explain the roles of the accessory structures in protecting the eye.

4.1.3 Describe some common abnormalities and disorders of the accessory structures.

4.1.4 Apply the correct medical terminology to the anatomy, physiology, and disorders of the accessory structures.

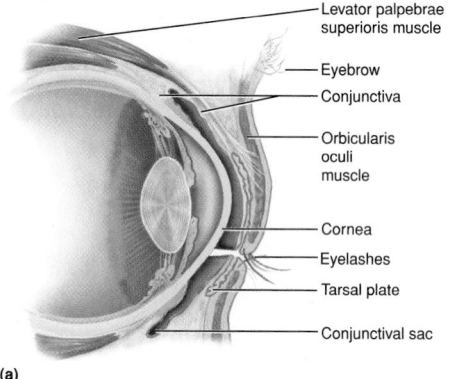

(a)

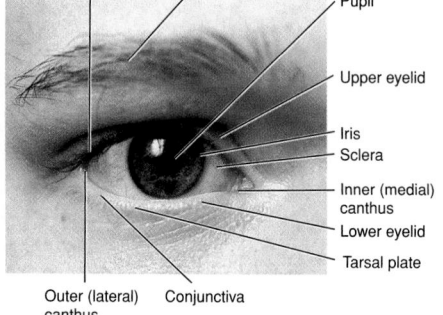

(b)

▲ **FIGURE 4.1 The Eye.** (a) Accessory structures (with eyelid closed). (b) External anatomy.

Abbreviation	
OT	ophthalmic technician

Eyebrows keep sweat from running into the eye and function in nonverbal communication.

Eyelids protect the eye from foreign objects. They blink to move tears across the surface of the eye and sweep debris away. They close in sleep to keep out visual stimuli. They are covered in the body's thinnest layer of skin. They consist mostly of muscle that fans out from each eyelid onto the forehead and cheek to open and close the eyelids.

In the eyelids, a flat, fibrous connective tissue layer (**tarsus**) holds 20 to 25 **tarsal glands,** whose ducts open along the edge of the eyelid. These glands secrete an oily fluid that keeps the eyelids from sticking together. The two corners where the upper and lower eyelids meet are called **canthi** (singular, **canthus**) *(Figure 4.1b).*

Eyelashes are strong hairs that help keep debris out of the eyes. They arise on the edge of the lids from hair follicles with their sebaceous glands.

The **conjunctiva** is a transparent **mucous membrane** that lines the inside of both eyelids and covers all of the front of the eye except the central portion, the **cornea** *(see Figure 4.1a).* In the conjunctiva, numerous goblet cells secrete a thin film of **mucin** that prevents the surface of the eyeball from dehydrating.

The conjunctiva is freely movable over the eyeball. It has numerous small blood vessels and is richly supplied with nerve endings that make it very sensitive to pain.

The **lacrimal apparatus** *(Figure 4.2)* consists of four structures. The **lacrimal (tear) gland,** located in the upper, lateral corner of the orbit, secretes tears. Short **lacrimal ducts** carry the tears to the surface of the conjunctiva. After washing across the conjunctiva, the tears leave the eye at the medial corner of the eye by draining into the **lacrimal sac.** They then flow through the **nasolacrimal duct** into the nose, from where they are swallowed.

The functions of tears are to:

* *Clean and lubricate* the surface of the eye.

* *Deliver* nutrients and oxygen to the conjunctiva.

* *Prevent infection* through a bactericidal enzyme called **lysozyme.**

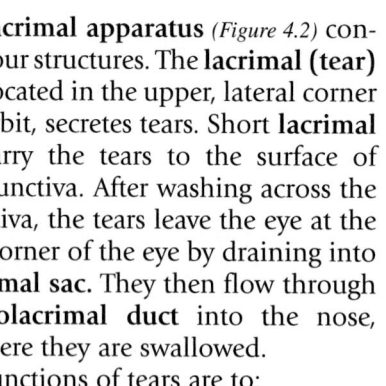

▲ **FIGURE 4.2 Lacrimal Apparatus.**

WORD ANALYSIS AND DEFINITION

S = Suffix   P = Prefix   R = Root   R/CF = Combining Form

WORD	PRONUNCIATION	ELEMENTS		DEFINITION
canthus **canthi (pl)**	**KAN**-thus **KAN**-thi		Greek *corner of the eye*	Corner of the eye where upper and lower lids meet
conjunctiva **conjunctivitis** **conjunctival (adj)**	kon-junk-**TIE**-vah kon-junk-tih-**VI**-tis kon-junk-**TIE**-val	S/ R/ S/	*inner lining of eyelids* Latin -itis *inflammation* conjunctiv- *conjunctiva* -al *pertaining to*	Inner lining of the eyelids Inflammation of the conjunctiva
cornea **corneal (adj)**	**KOR**-nee-ah **KOR**-nee-al		Latin *web, tunic*	The central, transparent part of the outer coat of the eye covering the iris and pupil
lacrimal **nasolacrimal duct**	**LAK**-rim-al **NAY**-zoh-**LAK**-rim-al DUKT	S/ R/ R/CF R/	-al *pertaining to* lacrim- *tears* nas/o- *nose* duct *to lead*	Pertaining to tears Passage from the lacrimal sac to the nose
lysozyme	**LIE**-soh-zime	R/ R/CF	-zyme *enzyme* lys/o- *decomposition*	Enzyme that dissolves the cell walls of bacteria
ophthalmology	off-thal-**MALL**-oh-jee	S/ R/CF	-logy *study of* ophthalm/o- *eye*	Medical specialty that diagnoses and treats diseases of the eye
ophthalmologist	off-thal-**MALL**-oh-jist	S/	-logist *one who studies, specialist*	Medical specialist in ophthalmology
ophthalmic (adj)	off-**THAL**-mik	S/	-ic *pertaining to*	Pertaining to the eye
orbit **orbital (adj)**	**OR**-bit **OR**-bit-al		Latin *circle*	The bony socket that holds the eyeball
periorbital	per-ee-**OR**-bit-al	S/ P/ R/	-al *pertaining to* peri- *around* -orbit- *orbit*	Pertaining to tissues around the orbit
pink eye	PINK EYE		lay term for conjunctivitis	Conjunctivitis
purulent	**PURE**-you-lent	S/ R/	-ulent *abounding in* pur- *pus*	Showing or containing a lot of pus
tarsus (**Note:** *Tarsus* also is used to refer to the seven bones in the instep of the foot.) **tarsal (adj)**	**TAR**-sus **TAR**-sal		Greek *flat*	The flat fibrous plate that gives shape to the outer edges of the eyelids

EXERCISES

Your work with elements is important to build your medical vocabulary. Many of the prefixes and suffixes you see in this chapter you will meet in later chapters and use to build your knowledge of additional medical terms. Fill in the chart.

Medical Term	Prefix	Meaning of Prefix	Root(s)/CF	Meaning of Root(s)/CF	Suffix	Meaning of Suffix
purulent						
conjunctivitis						
lysozyme						
periorbital						
ophthalmology						
nasolacrimal						
ophthalmologist						

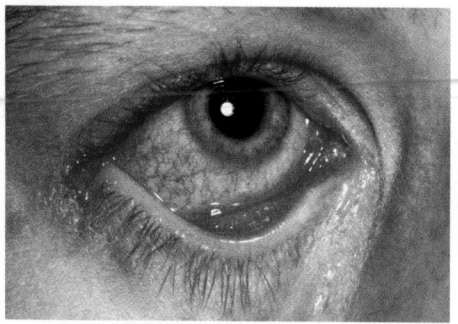

▲ FIGURE 4.3 Conjunctivitis.

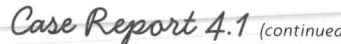

Case Report 4.1 (continued)

Mrs. Jenny Hughes's "pink eye" is called acute **contagious** conjunctivitis *(Figure 4.3)*. It responds well to **antibiotic** eyedrops. Her hands were **contaminated** from the keyboard of the employee who had left work and gone home with "pink eye." Mrs. Hughes transmitted the infection to her eyes by touching or rubbing.

Your documentation of Mrs. Hughes's office visit could read:

Progress Note 04/10/09

Mrs. Jenny Hughes was brought directly into the clinical area at 1030 hrs with what appeared to be conjunctivitis, "pink eye." Both eyelids were red and swollen with a purulent discharge. She complained of headache and **photophobia.** Dr. Chun prescribed Neosporin eyedrops, three drops q.4.h. A swab was sent to the laboratory. I instructed and watched Mrs. Hughes wash her hands and use an alcohol-based hand gel. I then had her sign in and sign our Notice of Privacy Practices. I instructed her in the use of the drops and emphasized home care and hand care measures to prevent the infection from spreading to her family. She was given a return appointment in 1 week and told to call the office if the drops did not help. Daphne Butras, OT. 1055 hrs.

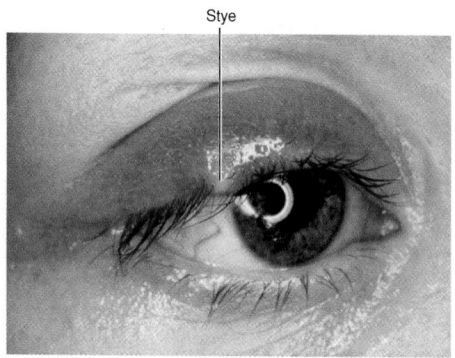

Stye

▲ FIGURE 4.4 **Stye Showing Pus-Filled Cyst.**

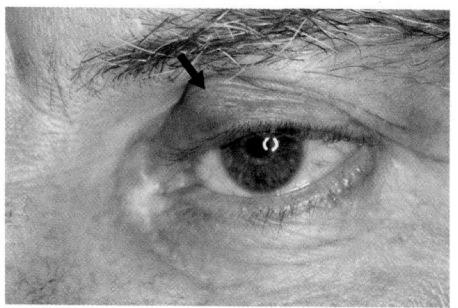

▲ FIGURE 4.5 **Chalazion in Upper Eyelid.**

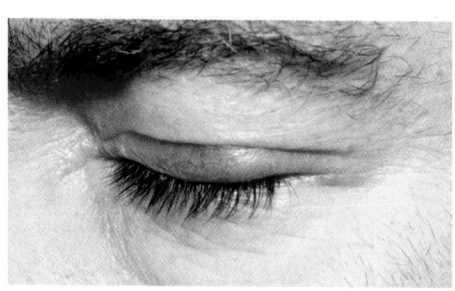

▲ FIGURE 4.6 **Blepharitis.**

DISORDERS OF THE ACCESSORY GLANDS

Conjunctivitis *(Figure 4.3)*, inflammation of the conjunctiva, is more commonly viral than bacterial and can also be caused by irritants such as chlorine, soaps, fumes, and smoke.

Eyelid edema, generalized swelling of the eyelids, is often produced by an allergic reaction *(see Chapter 15)* due to cosmetics, pollen in the air, or stings and bites from insects.

A **stye,** or **hordeolum,** is an infection of an eyelash follicle producing an abscess *(Figure 4.4)*, with localized pain, swelling, redness, and pus formation at the edge of the eyelid.

A **chalazion** is a small, painless, localized, whitish swelling inside the lid when a tarsal gland becomes blocked *(Figure 4.5)*. It can disappear spontaneously or require surgical removal.

Blepharitis occurs when multiple eyelash follicles and tarsal glands become infected. The margin of the eyelid shows persistent redness and crusting and may become ulcerated *(Figure 4.6)*. The infection is usually staphylococcal *(see Chapter 20)*. It is treated with antibiotic ointments.

Dacryostenosis is blockage of the drainage of tears, usually due to narrowing of the nasolacrimal ducts.

Dacryocystitis is an infection of the lacrimal sac, with swelling and pus at the medial corner of the eye.

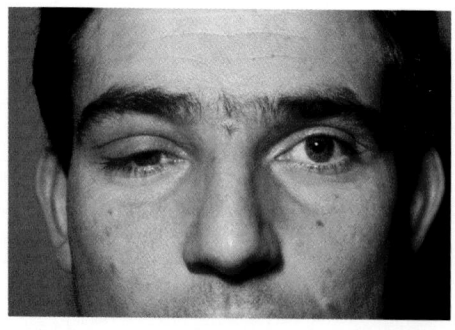

▲ FIGURE 4.7 **Ptosis of Right Eyelid.**

Ptosis occurs when the upper eyelid is constantly drooped over the eye due to **paresis** (partial paralysis) of the muscle that raises the upper lid *(Figure 4.7)*. It can be associated with diabetes, myasthenia gravis, brain tumor, and muscular dystrophy, all of which are described in subsequent chapters. The term **blepharoptosis** is used for sagging of the eyelids due to excess skin. The plastic surgery procedure of **blepharoplasty** is used for the repair of the eyelid.

WORD	PRONUNCIATION	ELEMENTS		DEFINITION
antibiotic	**AN**-tih-bye-**OT**-ik	S/ P/ R/	-tic *pertaining to* anti- *against* -bio- *life*	A substance that has the capacity to destroy bacteria and other microorganisms
blepharitis	blef-ah-**RYE**-tis	S/ R/	-itis *inflammation, infection* blephar- *eyelid*	Inflammation of the eyelid
blepharoptosis	**BLEF**-ah-**ROP**-toe-sis	S/ R/CF	-ptosis *drooping* blephar/o- *eyelid*	Drooping of the upper eyelid
blepharoplasty	**BLEF**-ah-ro-plas-tee	S/	-plasty *surgical repair*	Surgical repair of the eyelid
chalazion	kah-**LAY**-zee-on		Greek *lump*	Cyst on the outer edge of an eyelid
contagious	kon-**TAY**-jus		Latin *touch closely*	Able to be transmitted, as infections transmitted from person to person or from person to air or surface to person
contaminate	kon-**TAM**-in-ate	S/	-ate *composed of, pertaining to*	To cause the presence of an infectious agent to be on any surface
contamination (noun)	**KON**-tam-ih-**NAY**-shun	P/ R/	con- *together* -tamin- *touch*	Presence of an infectious agent on a surface or in substances
dacryocystitis	**DAK**-re-oh-sis-**TIE**-tis	S/ R/CF R/	-itis *inflammation, infection* dacry/o- *tears* -cyst- *sac*	Inflammation of the lacrimal sac
dacryostenosis	**DAK**-re-oh-ste-**NO**-sis	S/ R/	-osis *condition* -sten- *narrowing*	Narrowing of the nasolacrimal duct
hordeolum (also called stye)	hor-**DEE**-oh-lum		Latin *stye in the eye*	Abscess in an eyelash follicle
paresis	par-**EE**-sis		Greek *paralysis*	Partial paralysis
photophobia photophobic (adj)	foh-toe-**FOH**-bee-ah foh-toe-**FOH**-bik	S/ R/CF	-phobia *fear* phot/o- *light*	Fear of the light because it hurts the eyes
ptosis (**Note:** When a word begins with two consonants, the first is silent.)	**TOE**-sis		Greek *drooping*	Sinking down of an eyelid or an organ

EXERCISES

Disorders: *The accessory structures of the eye have their own disorders. The patient conditions are described in the left column; match the condition with the correct medical term (right column) from this lesson. Fill in the blanks.*

_____ 1. Allergic reaction to pollen

_____ 2. Upper eyelid droops over eye

_____ 3. Infection of the lacrimal sac

_____ 4. Produced by a blocked tarsal gland

_____ 5. Blockage of the drainage of tears

_____ 6. Eyelid is red, crusted, and ulcerated

_____ 7. Pus at the edge of the eyelid

A. chalazion

B. hordeolum

C. dacryostenosis

D. blepharitis

E. eyelid edema

F. dacryocystitis

G. ptosis

You are

... an ophthalmic technician working with Angela Chun, MD, an ophthalmologist at Fulwood Medical Center.

Your patient is

... Sam Hughes, a 2½-year-old boy, who has been referred by his pediatrician to Dr. Chun.

CASE REPORT 4.2

His mother, Mrs. Jenny Hughes, states that she has noticed for the past couple of months that his right eye has turned in. The only visual difficulty she has noticed is that he sometimes misses a Cheerio when he tries to grab it. Otherwise, he is healthy.

You are responsible for documenting Sam's diagnostic and therapeutic procedures and explaining the significance of these to his mother.

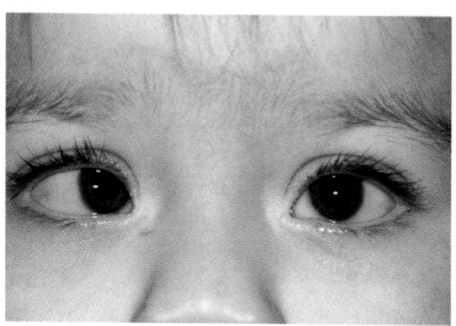

▲ **FIGURE 4.9 Strabismus with Right Eye Turned Inward.**

EXTRINSIC MUSCLES OF THE EYE

Humans, with their two eyes working closely together, have developed very good three-dimensional perception (**stereopsis**) and hand-eye coordination. Stereopsis depends on an accurate alignment of the two eyes.

This alignment is held in place by the coordination of six **extrinsic eye muscles** in each eye that are attached to the inner wall of the orbit and to the outer surface of the eyeball *(Figure 4.8)*. These muscles move the eye in all directions.

When there is muscle imbalance in one eye, as in Sam's case, the alignment breaks down, and the resulting condition is called **strabismus** *(Figure 4.9)*, also known in lay terms as "squinting" or "cross-eyed."

Esotropia is the eye turned in toward the nose. In **congenital** or infantile **esotropia**, both eyes look in toward the nose—the right eye looks to the left, and the left eye looks to the right *(Figure 4.10)*. These children require surgical intervention.

Accommodative esotropia is an inward eye turn, usually noticed around 2 years of age in 1% to 2% of children. In Sam's case, he had an accommodative esotropia in one eye. He will probably respond to treatment using glasses and perhaps a patch over the stronger eye to encourage use of the weaker eye.

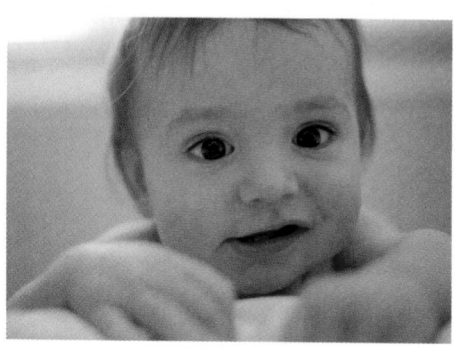

▲ **FIGURE 4.10 Infant with Congenital Bilateral Esotropia.**

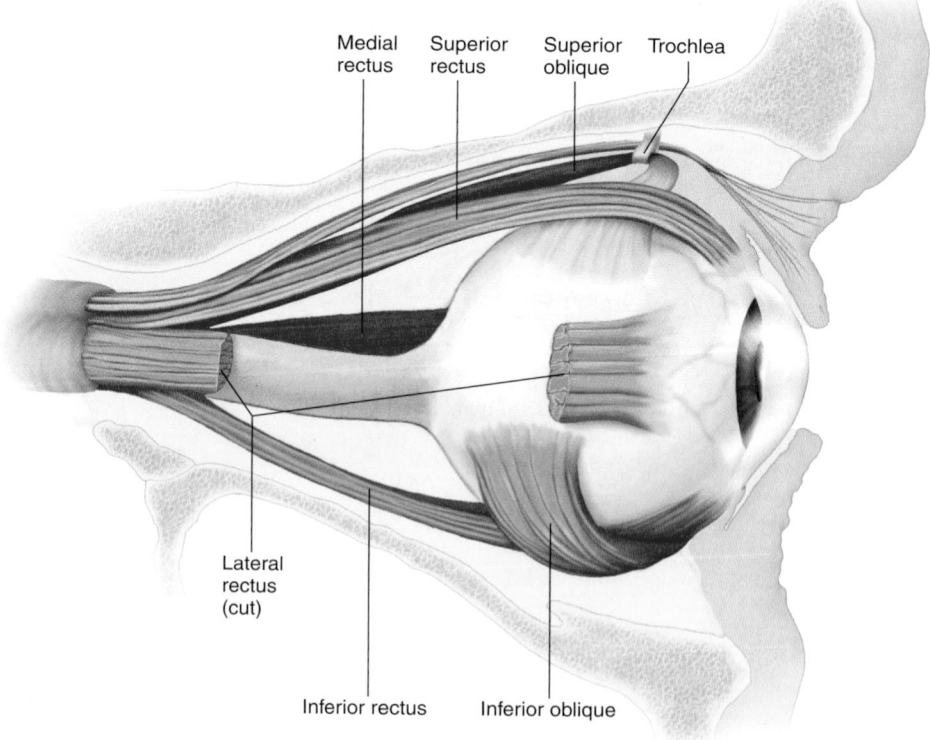

▲ **FIGURE 4.8 Extrinsic Muscles of the Right Eye: Lateral View.**

WORD	PRONUNCIATION	ELEMENTS		DEFINITION
accommodation accommodate (verb)	ah-kom-oh-**DAY**-shun ah-**KOM**-oh-date	S/ P/ R/	-ion *action* ac- *toward* -commodat- *adjust*	The act of adjusting something to make it fit the needs; in the case of the eye, the lens adjusts itself
amblyopia	am-blee-**OH**-pee-ah	P/ R/	ambly- *dull* -opia *sight*	Failure or incomplete development of the pathways of vision to the brain
atropine	**AT**-ro-peen		Greek *belladonna*	Pharmacologic agent used to dilate pupils
congenital	kon-**JEN**-ih-tal	S/ P/ R/	-al *pertaining to* con- *together, with* -genit- *bring forth*	Present at birth, either inherited or due to an event during gestation up to the moment of birth
esotropia	es-oh-**TROH**-pee-ah	S/ P/ R/	-ia *condition* eso- *inward* -trop- *turn*	A turning of the eye inward toward the nose
exotropia	ek-soh-**TROH**-pee-ah	S/ P/ R/	-ia *condition* exo- *outward* -trop- *turn*	A turning of the eye outward away from the nose
extrinsic intrinsic	eks-**TRIN**-sik in-**TRIN**-sik		Latin *on the outer side* Latin *on the inner side*	Extrinsic eye muscles are located on the outside of the eye, as opposed to intrinsic muscles, which are located inside the eye
ocular	**OCK**-you-lar	S/ R/	-ar *pertaining to* ocul- *eye*	Pertaining to the eye
optometrist	op-**TOM**-eh-trist	R/CF S/	opt/o- *vision* -metrist *skilled in measurement*	Someone who is skilled in the measurement of vision but cannot treat eye diseases or prescribe medication
stereopsis	ster-ee-**OP**-sis	S/ R/	-opsis *vision* stere- *three-dimensional*	Three-dimensional vision
strabismus	strah-**BIZ**-mus	S/ R/	-ismus *take action* strab- *squint*	A turning of an eye away from its normal position

Exotropia, an outward turning of one eye, is noticed around 2 to 4 years of age. It will often respond to vision therapy, which includes eye exercises and glasses, from an **optometrist.** Eye muscle surgery may be necessary to establish good **ocular** alignment.

Strabismus is not the same as **amblyopia,** or "lazy eye," which occurs in children when vision in one eye has not developed as well as in the other. It occurs because the eye and the brain are not cooperating for the one eye. Treatment involves getting the child to develop the vision in the weaker eye. This can be done by putting a patch over the stronger eye full-time or part-time or using **atropine** eyedrops to blur the vision in the stronger eye.

Keynote

Amblyopia is the failure or incomplete development of the pathways of vision to the brain.

EXERCISES

Notice in this exercise that not every medical term needs a prefix and/or a suffix; however, every medical term does contain one or more roots and/or combining forms. **Deconstruct** *the following medical terms into their elements. Fill in the chart.*

Medical Term	Prefix	Root(s)/Combining Form	Suffix
strabismus			
exotropia			
accommodation			
optometrist			
esotropia			
amblyopia			
stereopsis			

LESSON 4.2 The Eyeball and Seeing

OBJECTIVES

The eyeball is a fluid-filled globe about 1 inch in diameter. Knowledge of its terminology, structure, and function enables you to understand how we see and what major problems and disorders of the eyeball can arise.

In this lesson, the information will enable you to:

4.2.1 Identify the principal components of the eyeball.

4.2.2 Explain the role of the cornea and the problems that can occur in that structure.

4.2.3 Describe the structure and functions of the lens and its associated structures.

4.2.4 Link the different components of the retina to their functions.

4.2.5 Discuss common disorders of the eyeball and its components.

4.2.6 Apply correct medical terminology to the anatomy, physiology, and disorders of the eyeball.

THE EYEBALL (GLOBE)

The functions of the eyeball are to:

- *Adjust* continuously the amount of light it lets in to reach the retina.
- *Focus* continuously on near and distant objects.
- *Produce images* continuously of those objects and instantly transmit them to the brain.

The front of the eyeball (except for the cornea) is covered by the conjunctiva, a thin layer of tissue that covers the inside of the eyelids and curves over the eyeball to meet the **sclera,** the tough, white outer layer of the eye.

The center of the front of the eye is a transparent, dome-shaped membrane called the **cornea.** The cornea has no blood supply and obtains its nutrients from tears and from fluid in the **anterior chamber** behind it.

When light rays strike the eye, they pass through the cornea. Because of its domed curvature, those rays striking the edge of the cornea are bent toward its center. The light rays then go through the **pupil,** the black opening in the center of the colored area (the **iris**) in the front of the eye.

The pupil controls the amount of light entering the eye. When you are in a dark place, the pupil opens (dilates) to allow more light to enter. When you are in bright light, the pupil closes (constricts) to admit less light. The **sphincter pupillae muscle** *(Figure 4.11)* opens and closes the pupil.

After passing through the pupil, the light rays pass through the transparent **lens.** The ciliary muscle of the **ciliary body** makes the lens thicker and thinner, enabling it to bend the light rays and focus them on the **retina** at the back of the eye. This process of changing focus is called **accommodation.** The process of bending the light rays by the cornea and lens is called **refraction.**

Keynote

The cornea protects the eye and, by changing shape, provides about 60% of the eye's focusing power.

The pupil controls the amount of light entering the eye.

The lens changes its shape to focus rays of light onto the retina.

FIGURE 4.11 Anatomy of the Eyeball. ▼

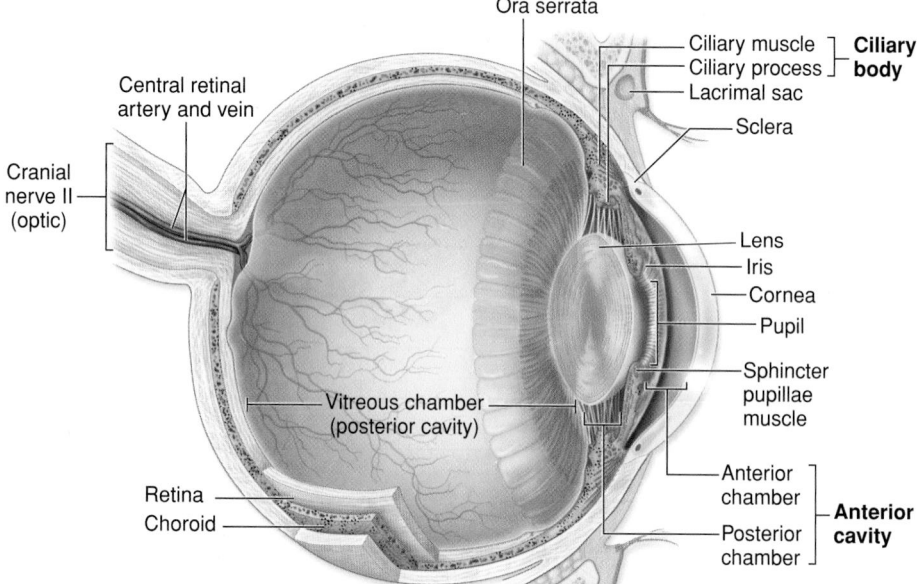

Ora serrata

Central retinal artery and vein

Cranial nerve II (optic)

Ciliary muscle ⎤ **Ciliary**
Ciliary process ⎦ **body**
Lacrimal sac

Sclera

Lens
Iris
Cornea
Pupil

Sphincter pupillae muscle

Vitreous chamber (posterior cavity)

Retina
Choroid

Anterior chamber ⎤ **Anterior**
Posterior chamber ⎦ **cavity**

WORD	PRONUNCIATION	ELEMENTS			DEFINITION
ciliary body	**SILL**-ee-ary **BOD**-ee	S R/ R/	-ary *pertaining to* cili- *eyelid* body *mass*		Muscles that make the eye lens thicker and thinner
iris	**EYE**-ris		Greek *diaphragm of the eye*		Colored portion of the eye with the pupil in its center
lens	LENZ		Latin *lentil shape*		Transparent refractive structure behind the iris
presbyopia	prez-bee-**OH**-pee-ah	R/ R/	-opia *sight* presby- *old man*		Difficulty in nearsighted vision occurring in middle and old age
pupil pupillae (pl) pupillary (adj)	**PYU**-pill pyu-**PILL**-ee **PYU**-pill-**AH**-ree		Latin *pupil*		The opening in the center of the iris that allows light to reach the lens
refract (verb) refraction (noun)	ree-**FRACT** ree-**FRAK**-shun		Latin *break up*		Make a change in direction of, or bend, a ray of light
retina retinal (adj)	**RET**-ih-nah **RET**-ih-nal		Latin *net*		Light-sensitive innermost layer of eyeball
sclera scleral (adj)	**SKLAIR**-ah **SKLAIR**-al	S/ R/	-al *pertaining to* scler- *hard, white of eye*		Fibrous outer covering of the eyeball and the white of the eye
scleritis	sklair-**RI**-tis	S/	-itis *inflammation*		Inflammation of the sclera
sphincter	**SFINK**-ter		Greek *band*		Band of muscle that encircles an opening; when it contracts, the opening squeezes closed

The lens has no supply of blood vessels or nerves. With increasing age, the lens loses its elasticity. When you reach your forties, your eyes may have difficulty focusing on near objects, and the telephone directory can become unreadable without spectacles, a condition called **presbyopia**.

Medical shorthand for a quick normal eye examination can be **PERRLA**, which means *p*upils *e*qual, *r*ound, *r*eactive to *l*ight and *a*ccommodation.

Keynote

Both the cornea and the lens refract light rays. Neither has a blood supply, which compromises healing from injury or disease.

EXERCISES

Components of the Eyeball: *Enhance your knowledge of the components of the eyeball and their functions. This will help you to understand the vision process. Match the phrase in the left column with the appropriate medical term in the right column.*

_____ 1. Colored portion of the eye

_____ 2. Change direction of a ray of light

_____ 3. Opening in the iris

_____ 4. Band of muscle that encircles an opening

_____ 5. Transparent, refractive structure

_____ 6. Difficulty in nearsighted vision

_____ 7. Innermost layer of eyeball

_____ 8. White of the eye

_____ 9. Operate the lens

_____ 10. Normal eye examination

A. lens

B. retina

C. sphincter

D. pupil

E. ciliary body

F. PERRLA

G. refract

H. iris

I. presbyopia

J. sclera

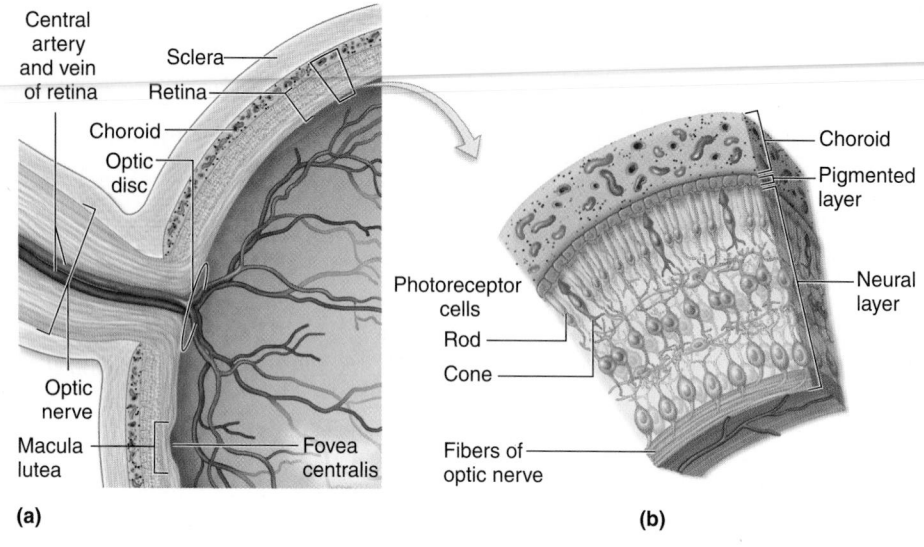

(a)

(b)

▲ **FIGURE 4.12** **Structure of the Retina.**

Keynote

Rods of the retina perceive only dim light and not color. Cones of the retina perceive bright light and color.

Rods and cones are called photoreceptor cells.

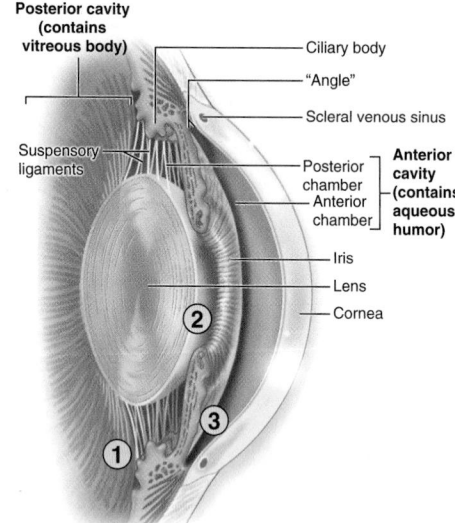

▲ **FIGURE 4.13** **Circulation of Aqueous Humor.**

The Retina

The final destination of the light rays is the **retina**, the thin lining at the back of your eye *(Figure 4.12a)*. It's an area the size of a small postage stamp that has 10 layers of cells. The retina has 130 million **rods** *(Figure 4.12b)*, which perceive only light, not color, and function mostly when the light is dim. There are 6.5 million **cones** *(see Figure 4.12b)*, which are activated by light and color and have precise **visual acuity.** Different cones respond to red, blue, and green light. Your perception of color is based on the intensity of different mixtures of colors from the three types of cones.

Some people have a hereditary lack of response by one or more of the three types of cones and show **color blindness.** The most common form is red-green color blindness, in which these colors and related shades cannot be distinguished from each other.

Rods and cones are called **photoreceptor** cells. The rods and cones convert the energy of the light rays into electrical impulses, and the **optic nerve,** a bundle of more than a million nerve fibers, transmits these impulses to the **visual cortex** at the back of the brain. The area where the optic nerve leaves the retina is called the **optic disc.** Because it has no rods and cones, the optic disc cannot form images and is called the **blind spot.**

Night blindness is the inability to see in poor light. It is a symptom of an underlying problem that can be:

- Uncorrected nearsightedness.
- Cataracts.
- Retinitis pigmentosa.
- Vitamin A deficiency.
- Glaucoma medications (such as pilocarpine) that constrict the pupil.

Just lateral to the optic disc at the back of the retina is a circular, yellowish region called the **macula lutea** *(see Figure 4.12a)*. In the center of the macula is a small pit called the **fovea centralis,** which has 4000 tiny cones and no rods. Each cone has its own nerve fiber, and this makes the fovea the area of sharpest vision. As you read this text, the words are precisely focused on your fovea centralis.

Behind the photoreceptor layer of the retina is a very **vascular** layer called the **choroid.** This layer, together with the iris and **ciliary body,** is called the **uvea.**

Segments of the Eye

The eyeball is divided into two fluid-filled segments separated by the lens and the ciliary muscle. The fluids maintain the shape of the eyeball. In the back, the **posterior cavity** extends from the back of the lens to the retina and contains a transparent jelly called the **vitreous body,** which helps maintain the shape of the eyeball.

In front, the **anterior cavity** extends from the cornea to the lens and is divided into two chambers. The **anterior chamber** extends from the cornea to the iris, and the **posterior chamber** extends from the iris to the lens *(Figure 4.13)*. **Aqueous humor** is produced in the posterior chamber as a filtrate from plasma (step 1). It

WORD ANALYSIS AND DEFINITION

WORD	PRONUNCIATION		ELEMENTS	DEFINITION
aqueous humor	ACHE-we-us HEW-mor	S/ R/CF	-ous *pertaining to* aqu/e- *watery* humor *Greek liquid*	Watery liquid in the anterior and posterior chambers of the eye
choroid	KOR-oid		Greek *membrane*	Region of the retina and uvea
fovea centralis	FOH-vee-ah sen-TRAH-lis		fovea *Latin a pit*	Small pit in the center of the macula that has the highest visual acuity
macula lutea	MAK-you-lah LOO-tee-ah		macula *small spot* lutea *yellow*	Yellowish spot on the back of the retina; contains the fovea centralis
optic optical (adj)	OP-tick OP-tih-kal		Greek *eye*	Pertaining to the eye
photoreceptor	foh-toe-ree-SEP-tor	S/ R/CF R/	-or *that which does something* phot/o- *light* -recept- *receive*	A photoreceptor cell receives light and converts it into electrical impulses
uvea	YOU-vee-ah		vascular layer	Middle coat of eyeball; includes iris, ciliary body, and choroid
uveitis	you-vee-I-tis	S/ R/	-itis *inflammation* uve- *uvea*	Inflammation of the uvea
visual acuity	VIH-zhoo-wal ah-KYU-ih-tee	S/ R/	-al *pertaining to* visu- *sight* acuity *Latin sharpen*	Sharpness and clearness of vision
vitreous humor	VIT-ree-us HEW-mor		Latin *glass*	A gelatinous liquid in the posterior cavity of the eyeball with the appearance of glass

passes through the pupil into the anterior chamber (step 2), where it is continually reabsorbed into a vascular space called the **scleral venous sinus** (step 3) and taken into the venous bloodstream. The aqueous humor also removes waste products and helps maintain the internal chemical environment of the eye.

EXERCISES

The medical terms contained in these two pages will be the answers in the following exercise on the retina and segments of the eye. Review the WAD before you begin the exercise. Circle the best answer.

1. Sharpness and clearness of vision is called:
   a. optical
   b. acuity
   c. vascular
   d. aqueous
   e. choroid

2. The term **photoreceptor** has:
   a. two combining forms and a suffix
   b. a prefix, root, and suffix
   c. a root, a combining form, and a suffix
   d. two roots and a suffix
   e. a suffix and a root

3. The choroid, iris, and ciliary body make up the:
   a. optic disc
   b. blind spot
   c. uvea
   d. visual cortex
   e. optic nerve

4. The gel contained in the posterior cavity is called:
   a. vitreous humor
   b. ciliary body
   c. visual cortex
   d. aqueous humor
   e. macula lutea

5. This helps maintain the shape of the eyeball:
   a. vitreous body
   b. rods
   c. fovea centralis
   d. cones
   e. macula lutea

6. The area of sharpest vision is the:
   a. cornea
   b. rods
   c. macula lutea
   d. fovea centralis
   e. choroid

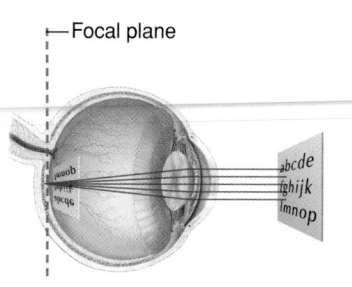

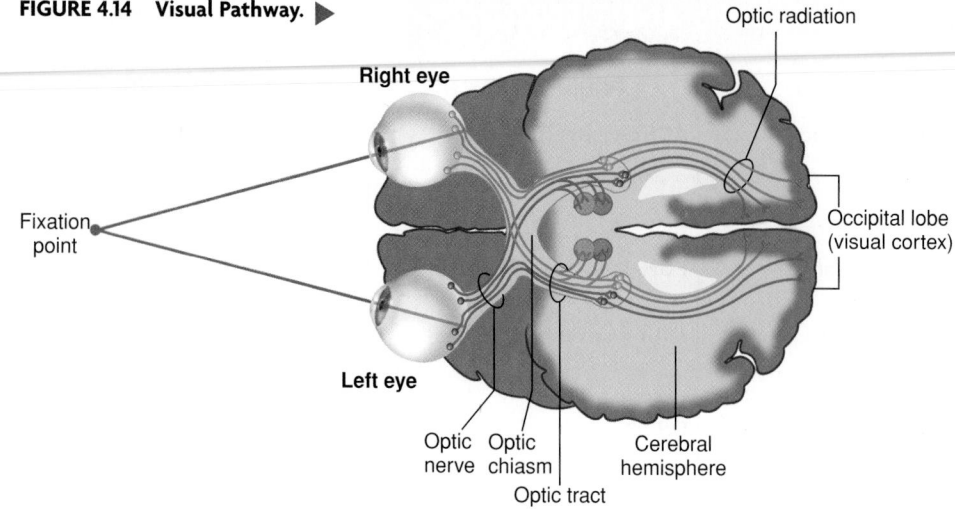

FIGURE 4.14   Visual Pathway. ▶

▲ FIGURE 4.15   Emmetropia, Normal Vision.

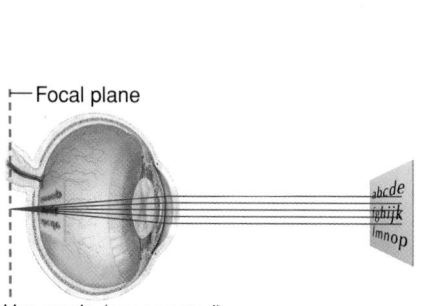

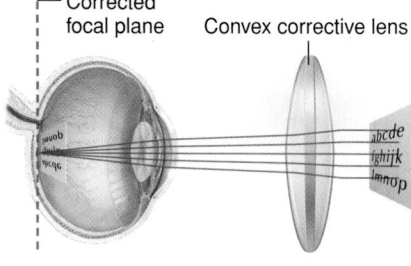

▲ FIGURE 4.16   Hyperopia (Farsightedness).

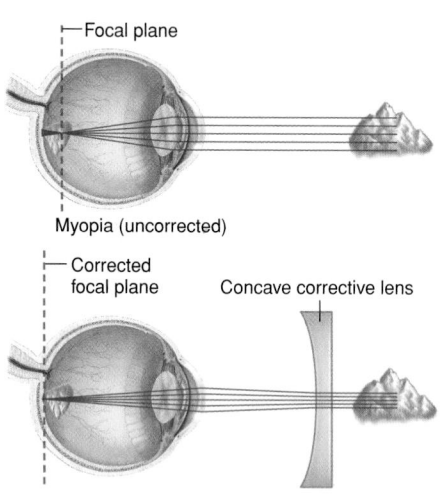

▲ FIGURE 4.17   Myopia (Nearsightedness).

VISUAL PATHWAY

After the optic nerves leave the back of your retina and eyeball, they leave each orbit through the **optic foramen.** They converge into an "X" called the **optic chiasm** *(Figure 4.14).* Here, the fibers from the medial half of each retina cross to the opposite side of the brain.

After leaving the chiasm, the fibers form the **optic tract** and then the **optic radiation** to take the nerve impulses to the **visual cortex** in the **occipital lobes** at the back of your brain. Here the incoming visual stimuli are interpreted.

Refraction

Light is traveling at a speed of 186,000 miles per second when it hits your eye. Light rays that hit the center of your cornea pass straight through, but because of the curvature of the cornea, rays that hit away from center are bent toward the center. The light rays then hit your lens, are bent again, and, in normal vision, the image is focused sharply on your retina *(Figure 4.15).* This normal vision is called **emmetropia.**

Farsighted people are said to have **hyperopia** *(Figure 4.16).* Because the eyeball is shortened, objects close to the eye are focused behind the retina and vision is blurred. Convex lenses are needed to correct the problem.

Nearsighted people are said to have **myopia** *(Figure 4.17).* Because the eyeball is elongated, faraway objects are focused in front of the retina. Vision is blurred. Concave lenses are needed to correct the problem.

In **presbyopia,** when you reach your forties, the lens loses its flexibility, so there is difficulty focusing for near vision. Convex bifocal or transitional lenses are needed for this problem.

In **astigmatism,** unequal curvatures of the cornea cause unequal focusing and blurred images. Cylindrical lenses, which refract light more in one plane than another, are needed to correct this problem.

A surgical procedure, **radial keratotomy,** is used to treat myopia. Radial cuts, like the spokes of a wheel, flatten the cornea and enable it to refract the light rays to focus on the retina.

Laser surgery can also change the shape of the cornea. It can flatten it to correct myopia or alter the outer edges of the cornea to correct hyperopia.

Laser-assisted in situ keratomileusis (LASIK) is being used to treat myopia, hyperopia, and astigmatism. A hinged flap of cornea is reflected (laid back) surgically to expose the midsection of the cornea. A computer-controlled laser, using a cold beam of ultraviolet light, alters the shape of the cornea by vaporizing the tissue.

WORD	PRONUNCIATION		ELEMENTS	DEFINITION
astigmatism	ah-**STIG**-mah-tism	S/ P/ R/	-ism *action* a- *without* -stigmat- *focus*	Inability to focus light rays that enter the eye in different planes
chiasm chiasma (alternative term)	**KYE**-asm **KYE**-az-mah		Greek *cross*	X-shaped crossing of the two optic nerves at the base of the brain
emmetropia	emm-eh-**TROH**-pee-ah	P/ R/	emmetr- *measure* -opia *sight*	Normal refractive condition of the eye
foramen foramina (pl)	fo-**RAY**-men fo-**RAM**-ih-nah		Latin *hole*	An opening through a structure
hyperopia	high-per-**OH**-pee-ah	P/ R/	hyper- *beyond* -opia *sight*	Able to see distant objects but unable to see close objects
in situ	IN **SIGH**-tyu		Latin *in its original place*	In the correct place
keratomileusis	ker-ah-**TOE**-mill-oo-sis	R/ R/CF	-mileusis *lathe* kerat/o- *cornea*	A surgical procedure that involves cutting and shaping the cornea
keratotomy	ker-ah-**TOT**-oh-mee	S/ R/CF	-tomy *surgical incision* kerat/o- *cornea*	Incision in the cornea
myopia (**Note:** An "o" is removed from the elements.)	my-**OH**-pee-ah	P/ R/	myo- *to blink* -opia *sight*	Able to see close objects but unable to see distant objects
presbyopia	prez-bee-**OH**-pee-ah	R/ R/	presby- *old man* -opia *sight*	Difficulty in nearsighted vision occurring in middle and old age
radiation	ray-dee-**AY**-shun	S/ R/	-ation *process* radi- *radius, radiation*	A spreading out, as of anatomical parts
tract	TRAKT		Latin *path*	Bundle of nerve fibers with a common origin and destination

EXERCISES

Create new medical terms by applying different prefixes to the root **opia***. The definition of each term is provided; you construct the medical term. Fill in the blanks.*

Opia means _____.

1. Difficulty in nearsighted vision occurring in middle and old age:

    _____/opia

2. Normal refractive condition of the eye:

    _____/opia

3. Able to see close objects but unable to see distant ones:

    _____/opia

4. Able to see distant objects but unable to see close objects.

    _____/opia

5. *Challenge question:* If **dipl/o** means *double* and *two*, what then is diplopia? _____

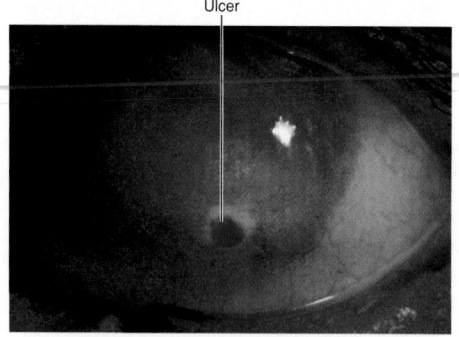

▲ **FIGURE 4.18** Fluorescein-Stained Corneal Ulcer.

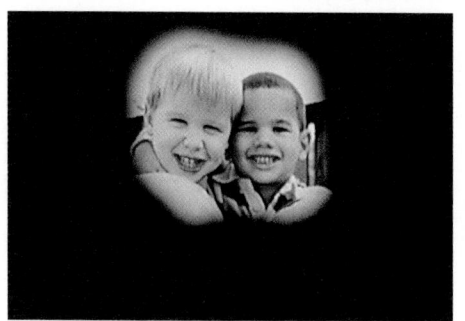

▲ **FIGURE 4.19** Vision with Glaucoma.

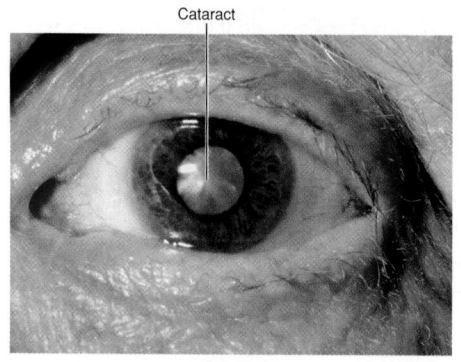

▲ **FIGURE 4.20** Cataract.

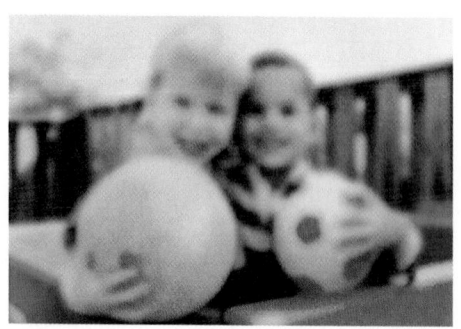

▲ **FIGURE 4.21** Vision with Cataract.

DISORDERS OF THE ANTERIOR EYEBALL

Conjunctivitis is the **infectious,** contagious condition that Mrs. Jenny Hughes had in the opening scenario of this chapter. It can be caused by viruses, many different bacteria, and organisms that cause sexually transmitted diseases (STDs, *Chapter 13*). It is a cause of "bloodshot" eyes.

Allergic conjunctivitis can be part of seasonal **hay fever** or be produced by year-round **allergens** such as animal dander and dust mites *(see Chapter 15)*. **Irritant conjunctivitis** can be caused by air **pollutants** (smoke and fumes) and by chemicals such as chlorine and those found in soaps and cosmetics.

Neonatal conjunctivitis (ophthalmia neonatorum) can be caused by a blocked tear duct in the baby, by the antibiotic eyedrops given routinely at birth, or by sexually transmitted bacteria in an infected mother's birth canal.

Corneal abrasions can be caused by foreign bodies, by direct trauma (such as being poked by a fingernail), or by badly fitting contact lenses. The abrasion can grow into an ulcer. The lesions can be stained with drops of the green dye **fluorescein** to make them more easily visible on examination *(Figure 4.18)*.

Scleritis, inflammation of the sclera (the white outer covering of the eyeball) can affect one or both eyes. It causes dull pain and intense redness and is often associated with rheumatoid arthritis *(see Chapter 5)* and the digestive disorder Crohn disease *(see Chapter 6)*.

Uveitis, inflammation of the iris, ciliary body, and choroid, produces pain, intense photophobia, blurred vision, and constriction of the pupil. There is usually an underlying disease, such as rheumatoid arthritis.

Glaucoma

The circulation of aqueous humor was described earlier in this chapter. If the aqueous humor cannot escape from the eye into the bloodstream, the fluid continues to be produced and pressure builds up inside the eye. The pressure interferes with the blood supply to the retina, causing death of retinal cells. Eventually the optic nerve fibers are damaged. This condition is called **glaucoma** and is a major cause of blindness *(Figure 4.19)*. Treatment is lifelong use of eyedrops to arrest the advance of glaucoma, but lost vision cannot be restored.

Cataracts

A **cataract** is a cloudy or opaque area in the lens *(Figure 4.20)*. It is typically caused by deterioration of the lens due to aging and may be associated with diabetes and with cigarette smoke. It presents with blurring of vision and **photosensitivity** or may be discovered on routine eye examination. It is another major cause of blindness.

The majority of cataracts occur in the center of the lens, but those associated with diabetes can be cortical (around the outside of the lens). Cortical cataracts can cause diminished **peripheral vision** and photosensitivity.

When a cataract interferes with vision *(Figure 4.21)*, the lens needs to be removed and replaced with an artificial **intraocular** lens, which becomes a permanent part of the eye. A surgical technique called **phacoemulsification** uses ultrasonic waves to fragment the cataract, making its removal much easier.

WORD ANALYSIS AND DEFINITION

WORD	PRONUNCIATION		ELEMENTS	DEFINITION
abrasion	ah-**BRAY**-shun		Latin *to scrape off*	Area of skin or mucous membrane that has been scraped off
allergen	**AL**-er-jen	S/ S/ R/	-gen *create* -er- *agent* all- *other, strange*	Substance producing a hypersensitivity (allergic) reaction
allergy allergic (adj)	**AL**-er-jee ah-**LER**-jik	S/ S/	-ergy *process of working* -ic *pertaining to*	Hypersensitivity to an allergen Pertaining to being hypersensitive
cataract	**KAT**-ah-ract		Greek *waterfall*	Complete or partial opacity of the lens
fluorescein	flor-**ESS**-ee-in	P/ R/	fluo- *fluorine* -rescein *resin*	Dye that produces a vivid green color under a blue light to diagnose corneal abrasions and foreign bodies
glaucoma	glau-**KOH**-mah	S/ R/	-oma *mass, tumor* glauc- *lens opacity*	Increased intraocular pressure
infectious	in-**FEK**-shus	S/ R/CF	-ous *pertaining to* infect/i- *internal invasion*	Capable of being transmitted; or caused by infection by a microorganism
intraocular	in-trah-**OCK**-you-lar	S/ P/ R/	-ar *pertaining to* intra- *inside* -ocul- *eye*	Pertaining to the inside of the eye
ophthalmia neonatorum	off-**THAL**-me-ah ne-oh-nay-**TOR**-um	S/ R/ S P/ R/	-ia *condition* ophthalm- *eye* -orum *function of* neo- *new* -nat- *born*	Conjunctivitis of the newborn
neonatal	**NEE**-oh-**NAY**-tal	S/	-al *pertaining to*	Pertaining to the newborn infant
peripheral vision	peh-**RIF**-er-al **VIZH**-un	S/ R/	-al *pertaining to* peripher- *external boundary*	Ability to see objects as they come into the outer edges of the visual field
phacoemulsification	fake-oh-ee-**MUL**-sih-fih-**KAY**-shun	S/ P/ R/	-ation *process* phaco- *lens* -emulsific- *to milk out*	Technique used to fragment the center of the lens into very tiny pieces and suck them out of the eye
photosensitivity photosensitive (adj)	foh-toe-**SEN**-sih-tiv-ih-tee foh-toe-**SEN**-sih-tiv	S/ R/CF R/	-ity *condition* phot/o- *light* -sensitiv- *sensitive*	Condition in which light produces pain in the eye
pollution	poh-**LOO**-shun	S/ R/	-ion *condition* pollut- *to defile*	Condition that is unclean, impure, and a danger to health
pollutant	poh-**LOO**-tant	S/	-ant *pertaining to*	Substance that makes the environment unclean or unpure

EXERCISES

*Review the medical terms in the WAD. Use the **language of ophthalmology** to complete the sentences. You may use a term only one time. Fill in the blanks.*

1. Dust mites and pollen are _____.

2. Scratching your eye with a tree branch produces a(n) _____.

3. _____ produces increased intraocular pressure.

4. Phacoemulsification is a treatment for _____.

5. Sensitivity to light that produces eye pain is _____.

6. Another name for conjunctivitis of the newborn is _____.

7. _____ refers to anything pertaining to the inside of the eye.

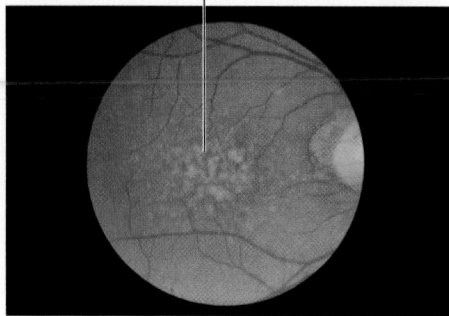

FIGURE 4.22 Ophthalmoscopic View of Macular Degeneration.

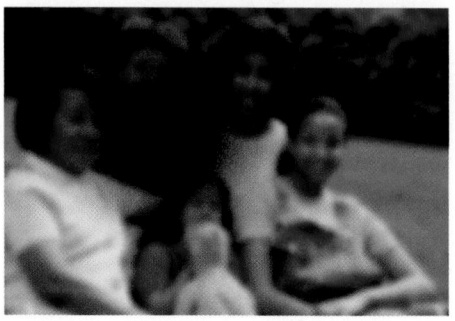

FIGURE 4.23 Vision with Macular Degeneration.

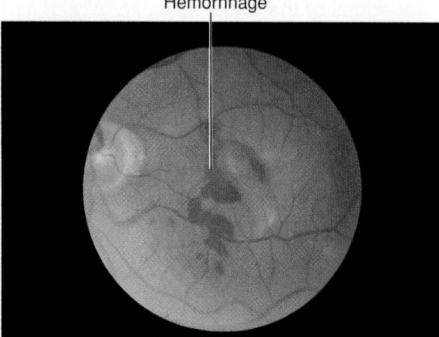

FIGURE 4.24 Ophthalmoscopic View of Diabetic Retinopathy.

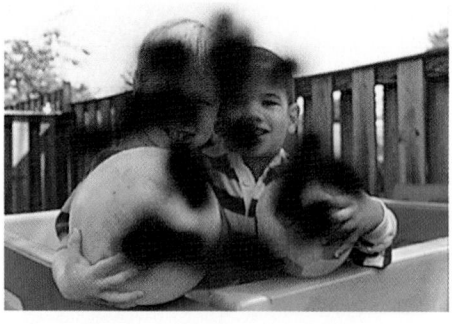

FIGURE 4.25 Vision with Diabetic Retinopathy.

DISEASES OF THE RETINA

Macular Degeneration

Degeneration of the central macula results in loss of visual acuity, with a dark blurry area of vision loss in the center of the visual field *(Figures 4.22 and 4.23)*.

There is photoreceptor cell loss and bleeding, with capillary proliferation and scar formation. The condition can progress to blindness. Most cases occur in people over age 55.

At this time, there is no known cure, but laser **photocoagulation** destroys the abnormal capillaries, thereby slowing the pace of the visual loss.

Retinal Detachment

Separation of the retina from its underlying choroid layer may be partial or complete and produces a retinal tear or hole. The detachment can happen suddenly, without pain. The patient sees a dark shadow invading his peripheral vision. The detachment can be seen on **ophthalmoscopic** examination.

When the retina is detached, photoreceptor cells can die; this condition is a surgical emergency. Treatment of small lesions is by **laser surgery.** The laser creates tiny burns around the tear to "weld" the retina back in place. Another form of treatment, **cryopexy,** freezes the area around the hole to help it reattach to the surrounding retina.

Diabetic Retinopathy

This disease occurs most frequently in diabetics whose blood sugar levels are not controlled. Some 50% of diabetics have **retinopathy.**

In the early stages, **microaneurysms** of the small retinal blood vessels form. There are usually no symptoms. Later, hemorrhages can occur, leading to destruction of the photoreceptor cells (rods and cones) and visual difficulties.

Ophthalmoscopic examination shows the disease *(Figure 4.24)*, and **fluorescein angiography** with pictures taken as the dye passes through the retina reveals more details.

Laser photocoagulation is usually effective in controlling the lesions; but once vision is lost from an area of the retina, it usually does not return *(Figure 4.25)*.

Papilledema

Papilledema is swelling of the optic disc due to increased **intracranial** pressure. It is not a diagnosis; it is a sign of some underlying pathology. It is seen on ophthalmoscopic examination.

Cancer of the Eye

Tumors of the skin of the eyelids include the **squamous cell** and **basal cell carcinomas** and **melanoma** described in *Chapter 3.*

Retinoblastoma is the most common cancer in children and is diagnosed most commonly around 18 months of age. Twenty percent have the cancer in both eyes. The condition can be hereditary.

The first symptom is a white appearance of the pupil **(leukocoria).** With early detection and aggressive treatment based on chemotherapy and laser surgery, 90% of cases are cured.

In adults, the most common cancers are **metastases** to the eye from cancer of the lung in men and the breast in women.

WORD	PRONUNCIATION		ELEMENTS	DEFINITION
angiography	an-jee-**OG**-rah-fee	S/	**-graphy** *process of recording*	Radiography of vessels after injection of contrast material
angiogram	**AN**-jee-oh-gram	R/CF S/	**angi/o-** *blood vessel* **-gram** *a record*	Radiograph obtained after injection of radiopaque contrast material into blood vessels
cryopexy	cry-oh-**PEX**-ee	S/ R/CF	**-pexy** *fixation* **cry/o-** *cold*	Repair of a detached retina by freezing it to surrounding tissue
intracranial	in-trah-**KRAY**-nee-al	S/ P/ R/	**-al** *pertaining to* **intra-** *inside* **-crani-** *skull*	Within the cranium (skull)
laser surgery	**LAY**-zer **SUR**-jer-ee	R/ S/ R/	**laser** *acronym for light amplification by stimulated emission of radiation* **-ery** *process of* **surg-** *operation*	Use of a concentrated, intense narrow beam of electromagnetic radiation for surgery
leukocoria	loo-koh-**KOH**-ree-ah	S/ R/CF R/	**-ia** *condition* **leuk/o-** *white* **cor-** *pupil*	Reflection in pupil of white mass in the eye
metastasis **metastases (pl)**	meh-**TAS**-tah-sis meh-**TAS**-tah-sees	P/ R/	**meta-** *beyond* **-stasis** *stay in one place*	Spread of disease from one part of the body to another
microaneurysm	my-kroh-**AN**-yu-rizm	P/ R/	**micro-** *small* **-aneurysm** *dilation*	Focal dilation of retinal capillaries
ophthalmoscope	off-**THAL**-moh-skope	S/	**-scope** *instrument for viewing*	Instrument for viewing the retina
ophthalmoscopy	**OFF**-thal-**MOS**-koh-pee	S/ R/CF	**-scopy** *to examine, to view* **ophthalm/o-** *eye*	The process of viewing the retina
ophthalmoscopic	**OFF**-thal-**MOS**-koh-pik	S/	**-ic** *pertaining to*	Pertaining to the use of an ophthalmoscope
papilledema	pah-pill-eh-**DEE**-mah	R/ R/	**-edema** *swelling* **papill-** *pimple*	Swelling of the optic disc in the retina
photocoagulation	foh-toe-koh-ag-you-**LAY**-shun	S/ R/CF R/	**-ation** *process* **phot/o-** *light* **-coagul-** *clot*	The use of light (laser beam) to form a clot
retinoblastoma	**RET**-in-oh-blas-**TOE**-mah	S/ R/CF S/	**-oma** *tumor, mass* **retin/o-** *retina* **-blast** *germ cell*	Malignant neoplasm of primitive retinal cells
retinopathy	ret-ih-**NOP**-ah-thee	S/	**-pathy** *disease*	Degenerative disease of the retina

EXERCISES

*Continue your work with elements to help build your knowledge of the **language of ophthalmology**. One element in each of the following medical terms is in bold letters in the left column. Identify the type of element (P, R, CF, S) in the middle column, and then write the meaning of the element in the right column. Fill in the chart.*

Medical Term	Type of Element	Meaning of Element
retino**blast**oma		
meta**stasis**		
intracranial		
cryo**pexy**		
microaneurysm		
ophthalmoscope		
angiography		
photo**coagul**ation		
retino**pathy**		

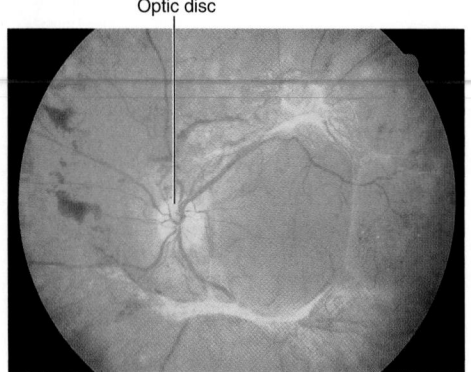

Optic disc

▲ **FIGURE 4.26   Ophthalmoscopic Examination of the Eye.**

Abbreviations	
O.D.	right eye
O.S.	left eye
O.U.	both eyes

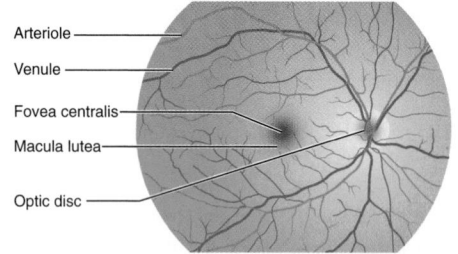

Arteriole
Venule
Fovea centralis
Macula lutea
Optic disc

▲ **FIGURE 4.27   Anatomy of the Fundus.**

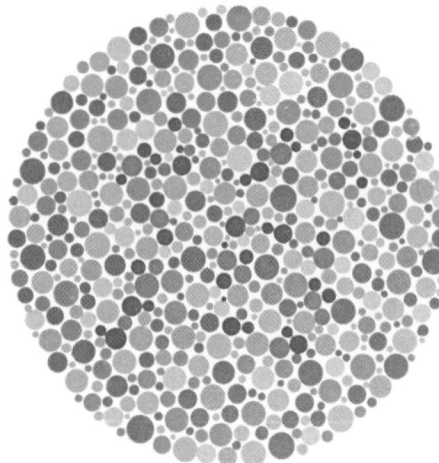

▲ **FIGURE 4.28   Test for Color Blindness.** Reproduced with permission from *Ishihara's Tests for Color Deficiency*, published by Kanehara Trading Inc., Tokyo, Japan. Tests for color deficiency cannot be conducted with this figure. For accurate testing, the original plates should be used.

FIGURE 4.29   Visual Acuity Tests. ▶
(a) Snellen letter chart for distance vision.
(b) Jaeger reading card.

OPHTHALMIC PROCEDURES

As an ophthalmic assistant, you may be trained to perform the following procedures.

Examination of the Retina

When you perform a **fundoscopy** and examine the retina with an **ophthalmoscope**, you can first identify the **optic disc** *(Figure 4.26)*. This is where the optic nerve leaves the back of the eye. The optic disc has no receptor cells and therefore produces a blind spot in the visual field of each eye. In the middle of the disc, a retinal artery enters to supply the **intraocular** structures, and a retinal vein leaves the eye.

Lateral to the optic disc is a yellowish area called the **macula lutea** *(Figure 4.27)*. In the center of the macula is the tiny pit called the **fovea centralis**. This pit is the area of sharpest vision. The arteries and veins of the retina can also be seen and provide clues about vascular diseases *(see Chapter 7)*.

Color Vision

Use illustrations such as those from the **Ishihara color system**. In the example shown in *Figure 4.28*, people with red-green color blindness would not be able to see the number 16 among the colored dots.

Distance Vision

Use the **Snellen letter chart** to test distance vision *(Figure 4.29a)*. The results are recorded as a fraction. For example, when the chart is viewed from 20 feet, line 8 is the smallest line a person with standard vision can read. This is recorded as 20/20. If the patient using her left eye misses two letters on line 8, document it as O.S. 20/20 −2.

Near Vision

Use handheld charts or **Jaeger reading cards** with printed paragraphs of different sizes of print to test near vision *(Figure 4.29b)*.

Visual Fields

Sit 2 feet in front of your patient, who covers one eye. Cover your own opposite eye and bring a pencil into the horizontal and vertical fields. The field is mapped on a visual field grid.

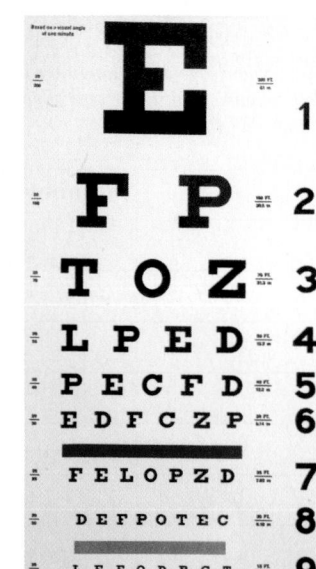

(a)

V = .50 D.

The fourteenth of August was the day fixed upon for the sailing of the brig Pilgrim, on her voyage from Boston round Cape Horn, to the western coast of North America. As she was to get under way early in the afternoon, I made my appearance on board at twelve o'clock in full sea-rig, and with my chest, containing an outfit for a two or three years voyage, which I had undertaken from a determination to cure, if possible, by an entire change of life, and by a long absence from books and study, a weakness of the eyes which had obliged me to give up my pursuits, and which no medical aid seemed likely to cure. The change from the tight dress coat, silk cap and kid gloves of an undergraduate at Cambridge, to the

V = .75 D.

loose duck trousers, checked shirt and tarpaulin hat of a sailor, though somewhat of a transformation, was soon made, and I supposed that I should pass very well for a Jack tar. But it is impossible to deceive the practiced eye in these matters; and while I supposed myself to be looking as salt as Neptune himself, I was, no doubt, known for a landsman by every one on board, as soon as I hove in sight. A sailor has a peculiar cut to his clothes, and a way of wear-

V = 1.   D.

ing them which a green hand can never get. The trousers, tight around the hips, and thence hanging long and loose around the feet, a superabundance of checked shirt, a low-crowned, well-varnished black hat, worn on the back of the head, with half a fathom of black ribbon hanging over the left eye, and a peculiar tie to the black silk neckerchief, with sundry other *details*, are signs the want of which betray the beginner at once.

V = 1.25 D.

Beside the points in my dress which were out of the way, doubtless my complexion and hands would distinguish me from the regular *salt*, who, with a sun-browned cheek, wide step and rolling gait, swings his bronzed and toughened hands athwartships half open, as though just to ready to grasp a rope. "With all my imperfections

V = 1.50 D.

on my head," I joined the crew, and we hauled out into the stream and came to anchor for the night. The next day we were employed in preparation for sea, reeving and studding-sail gear, crossing royal yards, putting on chafing gear, and taking on board our powder. On the

(b)

WORD	PRONUNCIATION		ELEMENTS	DEFINITION
fundus	**FUN**-dus	S/ R/CF S/	Latin *bottom* **-scopy** *to examine* **fund/o-** *fundus* **-ic** *pertaining to*	Part farthest from the opening of a hollow organ
fundoscopy fundoscopic (adj)	fun-**DOS**-koh-pee fun-do-**SKOP**-ik			Examination of the fundus (retina) of the eye
Ishihara color system	ish-ee-**HAR**-ah		Shinobu Ishihara, Japanese ophthalmologist, 1879–1963	Test for color vision defects
Jaeger reading cards	**YA**-ger		Edward Jaeger, Austrian ophthalmologist, 1818–1884	Type in different sizes of print for testing near vision
peripheral vision	peh-**RIF**-er-al **VIZH**-un	S/ R/	**-al** *pertaining to* **peripher-** *external boundary*	Ability to see objects as they come into the outer edges of the visual field
Snellen letter chart	**SNEL**-en		Hermann Snellen, Dutch ophthalmologist, 1834–1908	Test for acuity of distant vision
tonometer	toe-**NOM**-eh-ter	S/ R/CF S/	**-meter** *measure* **ton/o-** *pressure, tension* **-metry** *process of measuring*	Instrument for determining intraocular pressure
tonometry	toe-**NOM**-eh-tree			The measurement of intraocular pressure

Glaucoma

Measure the intraocular pressure with a **tonometer** *(Figure 4.30)*, which determines the eyeball's resistance to indentation or tension.

Administration of Medication

When you are trained as an ophthalmic technician, you will be able to administer eyedrops, creams, and ointments and to irrigate the eye to remove a foreign body.

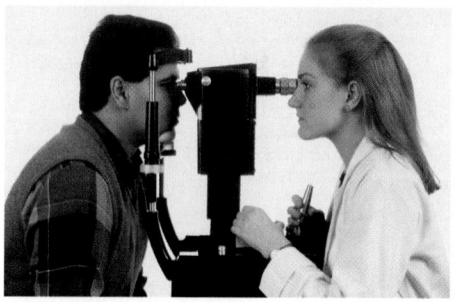

▲ **FIGURE 4.30   Tonometer.**

EXERCISES

The OT in Dr. Chun's office needs to be familiar with all these terms in order to communicate with Dr. Chun and her patients. Show your understanding of the terms by circling the correct answers.

1. Instrument(s) used in an ophthalmologist's office:
   a. tonometer
   b. cystoscope
   c. ophthalmoscope
   d. a and b
   e. a and c

2. Test used to measure color blindness:
   a. Snellen
   b. Jaeger
   c. Ishihara
   d. visual fields
   e. otoscope

3. Peripheral vision measures the outer edge of the:
   a. anterior segment
   b. vitreous body
   c. aqueous humor
   d. posterior segment
   e. visual field

4. A test for near vision is:
   a. Snellen chart
   b. ophthalmoscope
   c. Jaeger cards
   d. Ishihara
   e. visual fields

5. Tonometry measures:
   a. interocular pressure
   b. arterial pressure
   c. venous pressure
   d. intraocular pressure
   e. capillary pressure

6. The part farthest from the opening of a hollow organ:
   a. apex
   b. base
   c. fundus
   d. intraocular
   e. peripheral

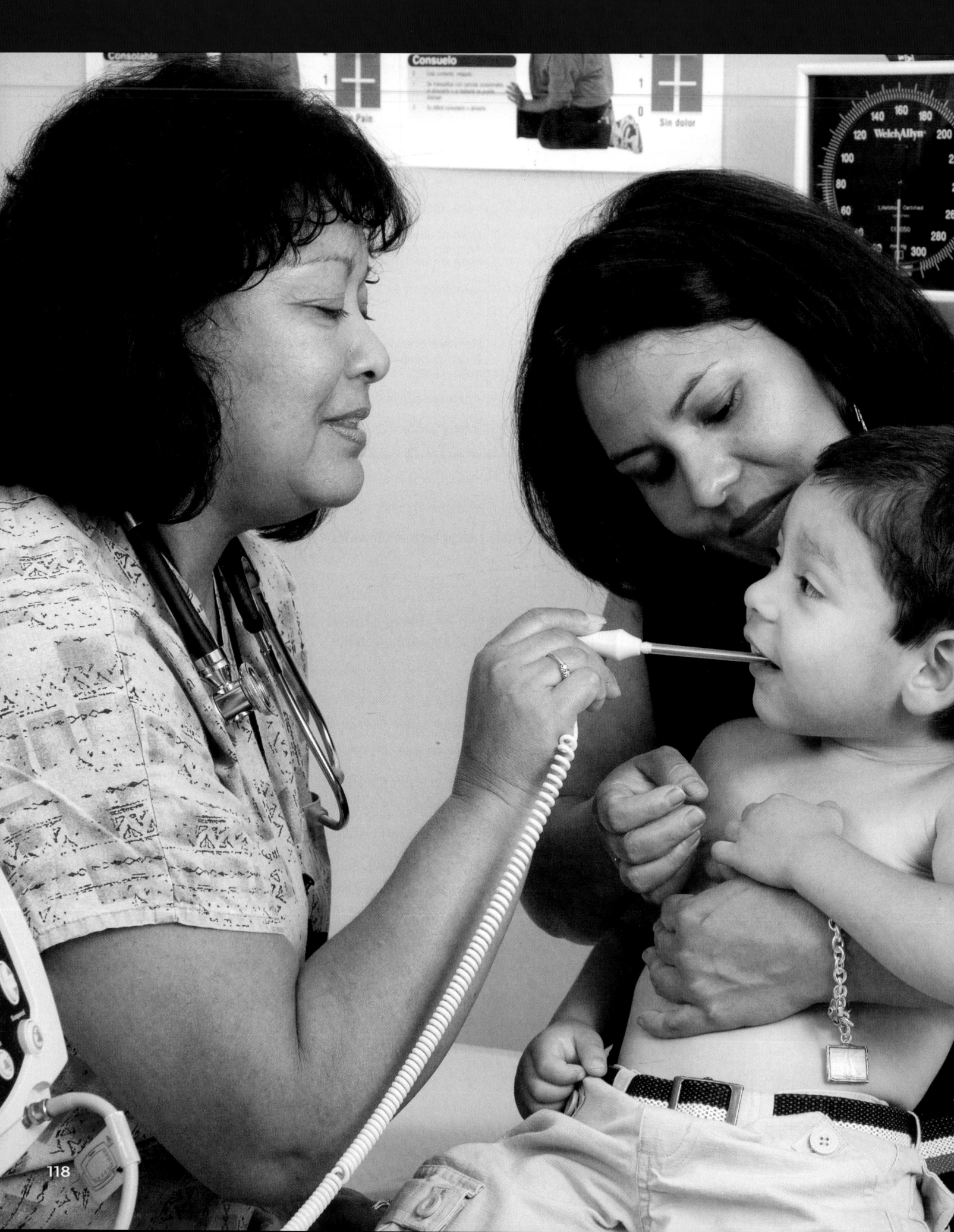

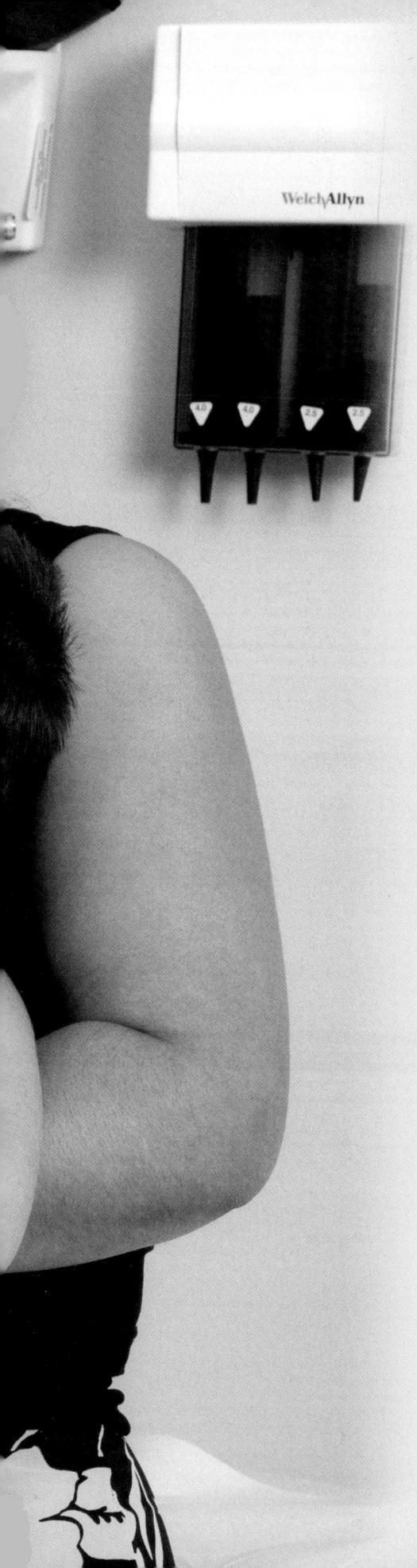

THE EAR AND HEARING

CASE REPORT 4.3

You are

. . . a medical assistant working with **primary care** physician Susan Lee, MD, of the Fulwood Medical Group.

Your patient is

. . . 3-year-old Eddie Cardenas. Mrs. Carmen Cardenas has brought in her son, Eddie. She tells you that he has had a cold for a couple of days. Early this morning he woke up screaming, felt hot, and was tugging his ears. She gave him **acetaminophen** with some orange juice, and he threw up. She also tells you this is the third similar episode in the past year. Since the last time, she is concerned that he is not hearing normally. You see a worried mother and a very unhappy, restless, toddler with a green nasal discharge. His oral temperature taken with an electronic digital thermometer is 102.4°F, pulse 100. You tell her that Dr. Lee will be in to see Eddie as soon as possible.

Learning Outcomes

In order to understand what is going on with Eddie, to communicate with Dr. Lee about him, to respond to the mother's concerns, and to document the office visit, you need to be able to:

4.5 Apply the language of otology to the anatomy and physiology of the ear.

4.6 Comprehend, analyze, spell, and write the medical terms of otology so that you can communicate and document accurately and precisely in any health care setting.

4.7 Recognize and pronounce the medical terms of otology so that you can communicate verbally with accuracy and precision in any health care setting.

4.8 Discuss the cause, appearance, diagnosis, and treatment of common disorders of the ear that lead to hearing loss.

4.9 Describe the cause, appearance, diagnosis, and treatment of common disorders of the ear that lead to difficulty with equilibrium and balance.

OBJECTIVES

To understand your patient's specific problem, you must be able to:

4.3.1 **Describe the structures and functions of the three regions of the ear.**

4.3.2 **Explain how sound waves progress through the ear and are transferred to the brain and recognized as sounds.**

4.3.3 **Identify how common diseases of the ear interfere with the process of hearing.**

4.3.4 **Apply the correct medical terminology to the anatomy, physiology, and disorders of the ear.**

Abbreviations

mg	milligram
p.r.n.	when necessary
q.i.d.	four times each day
q.4.h.	every four hours.

Case Report 4.3 (continued)

Progress Note. 05/10/09

Examination by Dr. Lee showed that Eddie has a **bilateral acute otitis media** with an upper respiratory infection. Dr. Lee is also concerned that Eddie has a **chronic** otitis media with **effusion** that is giving him a hearing loss. She prescribed amoxicillin 250 mg q.i.d. with acetaminophen 160 mg p.r.n. for 10 days, when she will see Eddie again. If, after the acute infection subsides, there remains an effusion with hearing loss, she may need to refer Eddie to an **otologist**. I explained this to Mrs. Cardenas. Luis Guittierez, CMA. 1115 hrs.

The ear has three sections: external, middle, and inner *(Figure 4.31)*.

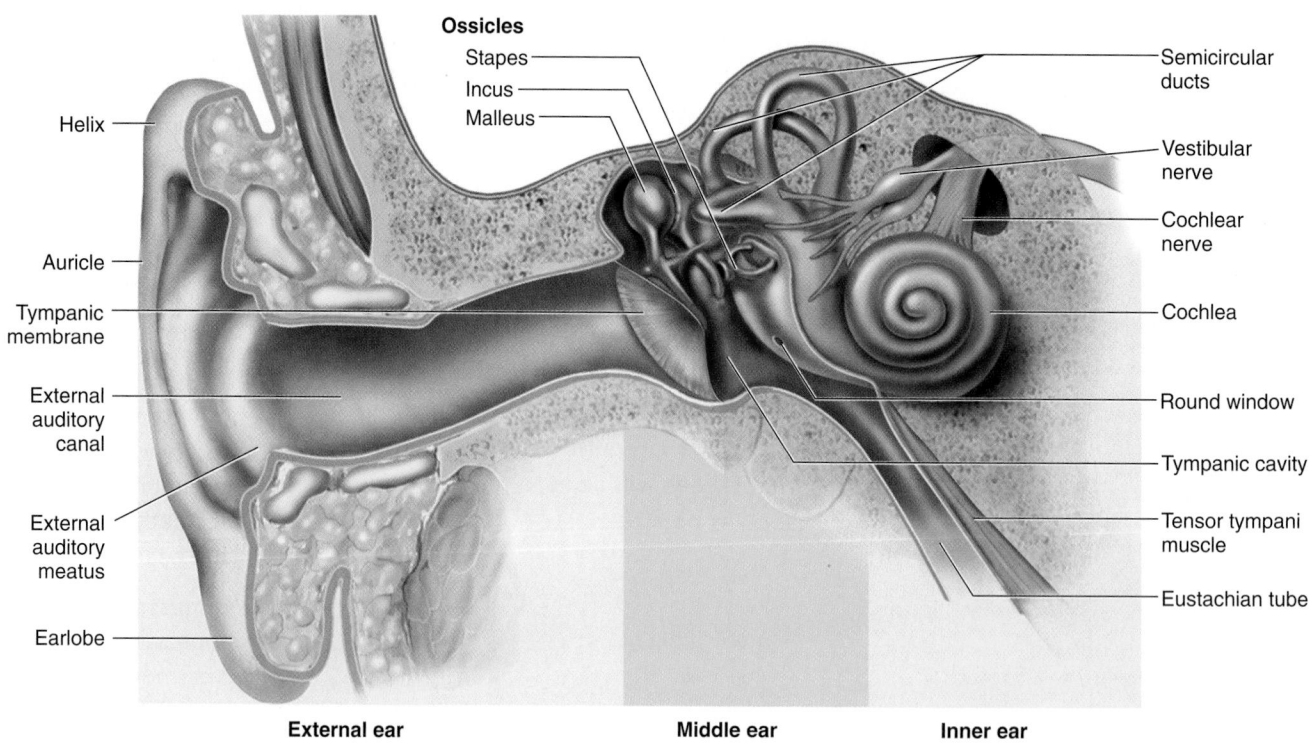

▲ **FIGURE 4.31** **Anatomical Regions of the Ear.**

WORD	PRONUNCIATION	ELEMENTS		DEFINITION
acetaminophen	ah-seat-ah-**MIN**-oh-fen		generic drug name	Medication that is an **analgesic** and an **antipyretic**
acute	ah-**KYUT**		Latin *sharp*	Describes a disease of sudden onset that is usually severe and of short duration
analgesia analgesic	an-al-**JEE**-ze-ah an-al-**JEE**-zic	S/ P/ R/ S/	-ia *condition* an- *without* -alges- *sensation of pain* -ic *pertaining to*	State in which pain is reduced Substance that reduces the response to pain
antipyretic	**AN**-tee-pie-**RET**-ik	S/ P/ R/	-ic *pertaining to* anti- *against* -pyret- *fever*	Agent that reduces fever
bilateral	by-**LAT**-er-al	S/ P/ R/	-al *pertaining to* bi- *two, twice* -later *side*	On two sides; for example, in both ears
chronic	**KRON**-ik		Greek *time*	Describes a persistent, long-term disease
effusion	eh-**FYU**-shun		Latin *pouring out*	Collection of fluid that has escaped from blood vessels into a cavity or tissues
otitis media	oh-**TIE**-tis **ME**-dee-ah	S/ R/ R/	-itis *inflammation* ot- *ear* media *middle*	Inflammation of the middle ear
otologist otology otorhinolaryngologist	oh-**TOL**-oh-jist oh-**TOL**-oh-jee oh-toe-rhino-lah-rin-**GOL**-oh-jist	S/ R/CF S/ R/CF R/CF	-logist *one who studies, specialist* ot/o- *ear* -logy *study of* -rhin/o- *nose* -laryng/o- *larynx*	Medical specialist in diseases of the ear Study of the function and diseases of the ear Ear, nose, and throat medical specialist
primary care	**PRY**-mah-ree KAIR		**primary** Latin *first* **care** Greek *concern*	Comprehensive and preventive health care services that are the first point of care for a patient

EXERCISES

Break these medical terms down into their basic elements. Analyzing each term will help you answer the following questions. Fill in the blanks.

Medical Term	Prefix	Root(s)/CF	Suffix
analgesia			
bilateral			
otitis media			
otologist			
otorhinolaryngologist			

1. A medication that is an analgesic reduces _____.

2. Name another body part that is bilateral. _____

3. What is the difference between an otologist and an otorhinolaryngologist?

_____

4. Where in the ear does otitis media occur? _____

5. Which element is a prefix referring to a number? _____ means _____.

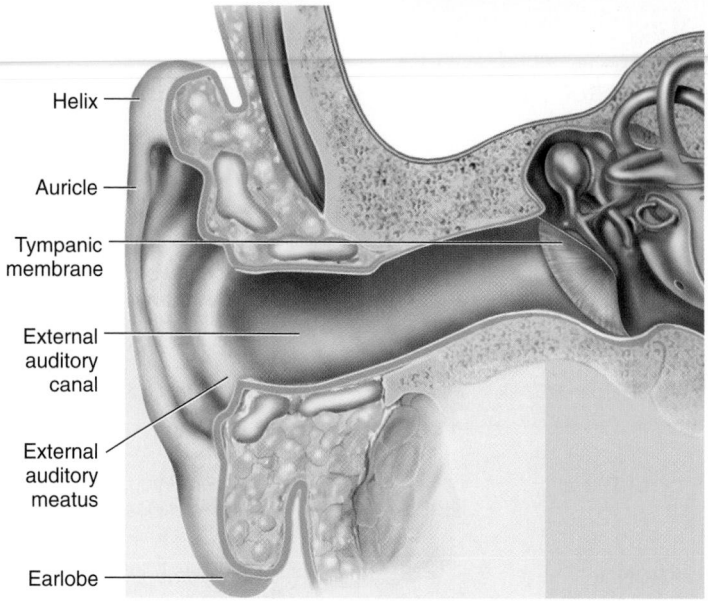

Helix

Auricle

Tympanic
membrane

External
auditory
canal

External
auditory
meatus

Earlobe

▲ FIGURE 4.32   External Ear.

EXTERNAL EAR

The **auricle**, or **pinna**, is a wing-shaped structure that directs sound waves coming through the air into the **external auditory meatus** and **external auditory canal.** This in turn ends at the **tympanic membrane** *(Figure 4.32)*. The external auditory canal not only protects the middle and inner ears but also acts as a resonator to augment the transmission of sound to the middle and inner ears.

The external auditory canal is the only skin-lined cul-de-sac in the body. Its interior is dark, warm, and prone to become moist. These are ideal conditions for bacterial and fungal growth.

The meatus and canal are lined with skin that contains many modified sweat glands called ceruminous glands, which secrete **cerumen.** The cerumen and hairs growing in the meatus help to keep out foreign objects. Cerumen combines with dead skin cells to form **earwax.** Overproduction of cerumen can completely block the external canal, causing hearing loss and preventing examination of the tympanic membrane with an **otoscope.**

If a foreign body, such as a small bead, does get into the canal, or if cerumen becomes **impacted** in the canal, then hearing loss can result.

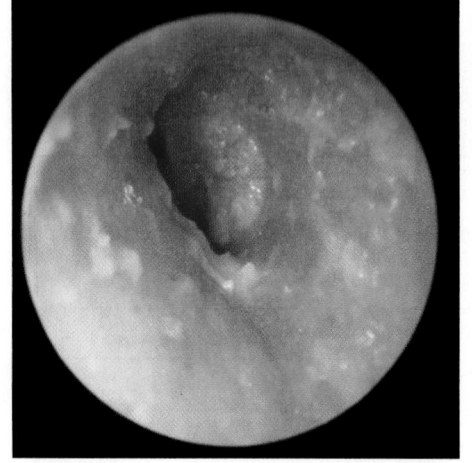

▲ **FIGURE 4.33   Otoscopic View of Otitis Externa with Purulent Exudate.**

DISORDERS OF EXTERNAL EAR

Otitis externa *(Figure 4.33)* is an infection of the lining of the external auditory canal. It produces a painful, red, swollen ear canal, sometimes with purulent drainage. The infection can be bacterial or fungal. Fungal infections are responsible for 10% of otitis externa cases and are called **otomycoses.**

Conditions helping to cause otitis externa include trauma to the canal during attempts to self-clean it; use of unclean earplugs, earphones, or hearing aids; and the presence of other skin diseases, such as seborrhea and psoriasis *(see Chapter 3)*.

Treatment entails thorough cleansing of the canal, acidification with a topical solution of 2% acetic acid in a hydrocortisone solution, and the use of antibiotic drops. Occasionally a wick is needed to enable the topical medications to penetrate down the canal.

Swimmer's ear is a form of otitis externa that comes on after swimming, particularly if the water is polluted.

Excessive earwax can be removed in your physician's office by ear **irrigation** or with a **curette**, a small metal ring at the end of a handle.

WORD ANALYSIS AND DEFINITION

WORD	PRONUNCIATION		ELEMENTS	DEFINITION
auditory	**AW**-dih-tor-ee		Latin *hearing*	Pertaining to the sense or organs of hearing
audiology	aw-dee-**OL**-oh-jee	S/ R/CF	**-logy** *study of* **audi/o-** *hearing*	Study of hearing disorders
audiologist	aw-dee-**OL**-oh-jist	S/	**-logist** *one who studies*	Specialist in evaluation of hearing function
auricle	**AW**-ri-kul		Latin *ear*	The shell-like external ear
cerumen	seh-**ROO**-men		Latin *wax*	Waxy secretion of ceruminous glands of external ear
curette	kyu-**RET**	S/ R/	**-ette** *little* **cur-** *cleanse, cure*	Scoop-shaped instrument for scraping the interior of a cavity or removing new growths
curettage (**Note:** The final "e" of **curette** is dropped because the suffix -age begins with a vowel.)	kyu-reh-**TAHZH**	S/	**-age** *related to*	Scraping the interior of a cavity
impacted	im-**PAK**-ted		Latin *driven in*	Immovably wedged, as with earwax blocking the external canal
irrigation	ih-rih-**GAY**-shun	S/ P/ R/	**-ation** *process* **-ir** *in* **-rig** *water*	Use of water to clean wax out of the external ear canal
meatus	me-**AY**-tus		Latin *go through*	Passage or channel; also used to denote the external opening of a passage
meatal (adj)	me-**AY**-tal			
otomycosis	**OH**-toe-my-**KOH**-sis	S/ R/CF R/CF	**-sis** *abnormal condition* **ot/o-** *ear* **-myc/o-** *fungus*	Fungal infection of the external ear
otoscope	**OH**-toe-skope	S/ R/CF	**-scope** *instrument for viewing* **ot/o-** *ear*	Instrument for examining the ear
otoscopic (adj)	oh-toe-**SKOP**-ik	S/	**-ic** *pertaining to*	Pertaining to examination with an otoscope
otoscopy	oh-**TOS**-koh-pee	S/	**-scopy** *to examine*	Examination of the ear
pinna	**PIN**-ah		Latin *wing*	Another name for auricle
pinnae (pl)	**PIN**-ee			
tympanic	tim-**PAN**-ik	S/ R/	**-ic** *pertaining to* **tympan-** *eardrum, tympanic membrane*	Pertaining to the tympanic membrane or tympanic cavity

EXERCISES

*Every part of the body has its own specialized vocabulary. Test your knowledge of the **language of otology** by matching correct answers. Match the phrase in the left column with the appropriate medical term in the right column.*

_____ 1. External ear fungal infection   A. pinna

_____ 2. External opening of a passage   B. auditory

_____ 3. Instrument for viewing the ear   C. auricle

_____ 4. Procedure for scraping or removing growths   D. tympanic

_____ 5. Shell-like external ear   E. otomycosis

_____ 6. "Driven in"   F. curettage

_____ 7. Another name for auricle   G. meatus

_____ 8. Pertaining to the sense or organs of hearing   H. otoscope

_____ 9. Earwax   I. impacted

_____ 10. Pertaining to the eardrum   J. cerumen

FIGURE 4.34   Middle Ear. ▶

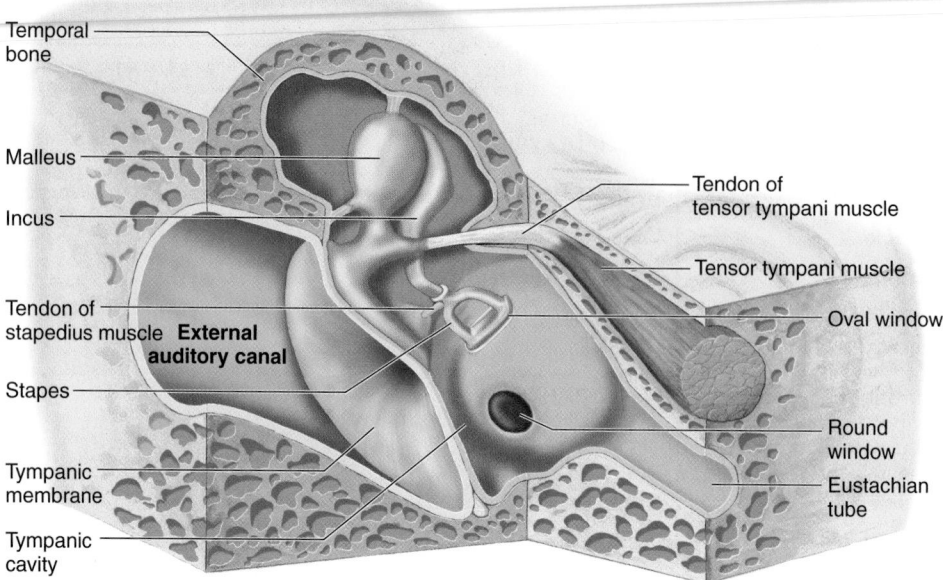

FIGURE 4.34   Middle Ear.

Temporal bone
Malleus
Incus
Tendon of stapedius muscle   **External auditory canal**
Stapes
Tympanic membrane
Tympanic cavity

Tendon of tensor tympani muscle
Tensor tympani muscle
Oval window
Round window
Eustachian tube

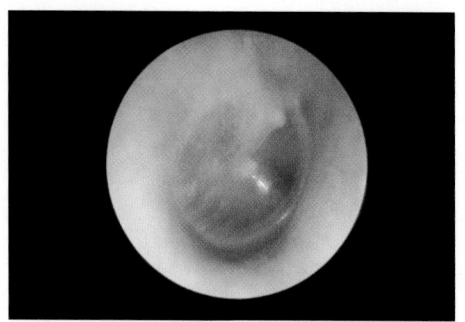

▲ **FIGURE 4.35   Otoscopic View of Normal Tympanic Membrane.**

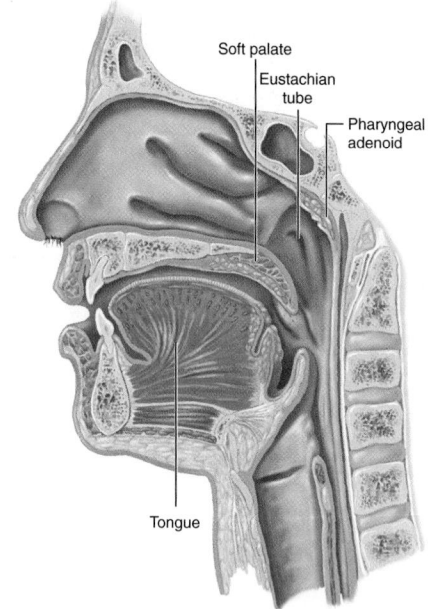

Soft palate
Eustachian tube
Pharyngeal adenoid
Tongue

▲ **FIGURE 4.36   Nasopharynx (Throat).**

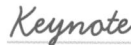
Keynote

The three ossicles amplify sound so that soft sounds can be heard.

MIDDLE EAR

The middle ear has four components: the tympanic membrane, the tympanic cavity, the **eustachian** (auditory) **tube,** and the ossicles *(Figure 4.34).*

1. The **tympanic membrane (eardrum)** is located at the inner end of the external auditory canal. It is suspended in a bony groove, is concave on its outer surface, and vibrates freely as sound waves hit it. It has a good nerve supply and is very sensitive to pain. When examined through the otoscope, it is transparent and reflects light *(Figure 4.35).*

2. The **tympanic cavity** is immediately behind the tympanic membrane. It is filled with air that enters through the eustachian (auditory) tube, and the cavity is continuous with the **mastoid** air cells in the bone behind it. The presence of air in the cavity maintains equal air pressure on both sides of the tympanic membrane, which is essential for normal hearing. The cavity contains the ossicles.

3. The eustachian (auditory) tube *(Figure 4.34)* connects the middle ear with the **nasopharynx** (throat), into which it opens close to the pharyngeal **tonsil (adenoid)** *(Figure 4.36).* In children under 5 years, the tube is not fully developed. It is short and horizontal, and the valvelike flaps in the throat that protect it are not developed. When you are landing in an airplane and moving from a high altitude to a lower one, the air pressure in the external auditory canal increases and pushes the tympanic membrane inward. If your eustachian (auditory) tube is blocked, no air can get into the middle ear to equalize the pressure, and your eardrum is painful. If you can force some air up the eustachian (auditory) tube by chewing or swallowing, then your ear "pops" as the tympanic membrane moves back to its normal position.

4. The three **ossicles**, the **malleus, incus,** and **stapes,** are attached to the wall of the tympanic cavity by tiny ligaments that are covered by a mucous membrane. The malleus is attached to the tympanic membrane and vibrates with the membrane when sound waves hit it. The malleus is also attached to the incus, which also vibrates and passes the vibrations onto the stapes. The stapes is attached to the oval window, an opening that transmits the vibrations to the inner ear. The stapes is the smallest bone in the body.

WORD	PRONUNCIATION		ELEMENTS	DEFINITION
adenoid	**ADD**-eh-noyd	S/ R/	-oid *resembling* aden- *gland*	Single mass of lymphoid tissue in the midline at the back of the throat
eustachian tube (also called **auditory tube**)	you-**STAY**-shun TYUB		Bartolommeo Eustachio, Italian anatomist, 1524–1574	Tube that connects the middle ear to the nasopharynx
incus	**IN**-cuss		Latin *anvil*	Middle one of the three ossicles in the middle ear; shaped like an anvil
malleus	**MAL**-ee-us		Latin *hammer*	Outer (lateral) one of the three ossicles in the middle ear; shaped like a hammer
mastoid	**MASS**-toyd	S/ R/	-oid *resembling* mast- *breast*	Small bony protrusion immediately behind the ear
nasopharynx	**NAY**-zoh-**FAIR**-inks	R/CF R/	nas/o- *nose* -pharynx *throat*	Region of the pharynx at the back of the nose and above the soft palate
ossicle	**OS**-ih-kel	S/ R/CF	-cle *small* oss/i- *bone*	A small bone, particularly relating to the three bones in the middle ear
stapes	**STAY**-peas		Latin *stirrup*	Inner (medial) one of the three ossicles of the middle ear; shaped like a stirrup
tonsil tonsillar (adj)	**TON**-sill **TON**-sih-lar		Latin *tonsil*	Mass of lymphoid tissue on either side of the throat at the back of the tongue

EXERCISES

Answers to the following questions can all be found in the WAD above. Review the terms before you start this exercise. Pay special attention to the spelling. Circle the best choice.

1. In the term **mastoid,** the suffix means:

   condition   resembling   inflammation

2. The element **mast** means:

   throat   breast   ear

3. The **stapes** is:

   gland   ossicle   mastoid

4. The element **pharynx** means:

   throat   nose   gland

5. The term **nasopharynx** is composed of:

   prefix + suffix   root + root   combining form + root

6. This type of tissue is found in an adenoid:

   mucoid   connective   lymphoid

7. The _____ is shaped like a hammer.

   malleus   malleolus   maleus

8. The element **aden** in adenoid is a:

   prefix   root   combining form

9. One of the names for the tube that connects the middle ear to the nasopharynx is the _____ tube.

   eusstachian   eustashian   eustachian

10. The _____ is shaped like an anvil.

    incus   stapes   adenoid

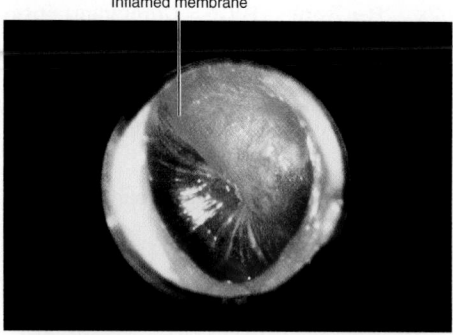

▲ **FIGURE 4.37 Otoscopic View of Otitis Media (Acute), Showing Inflamed Tympanic Membrane.**

Inflamed membrane

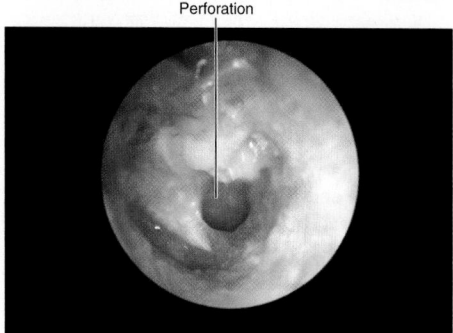

Perforation

▲ **FIGURE 4.38 Otoscopic View of Otitis Media (Chronic) with Perforated Tympanic Membrane.**

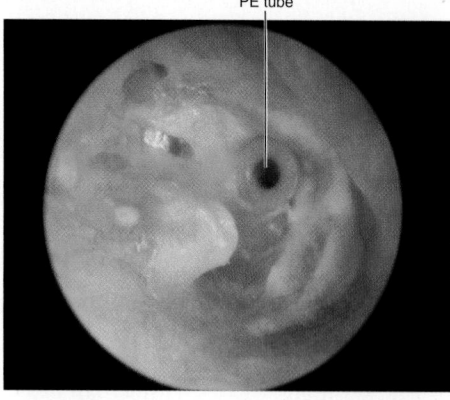

PE tube

▲ **FIGURE 4.39 Pressure-Equalization (PE) Tube in Tympanic Membrane.**

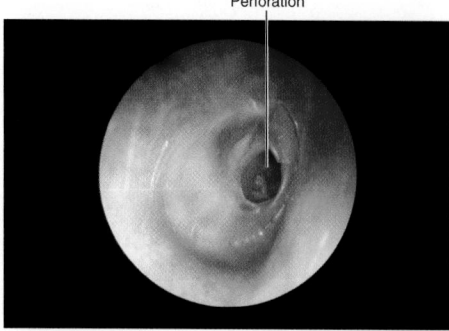

Perforation

▲ **FIGURE 4.40 Perforated Tympanic Membrane.**

Case Report 4.3 (continued)

Eddie Cardenas' ear problems began with his eustachian (auditory) tube. His cold (upper respiratory infection, **URI**, or **coryza**) inflamed the mucous membranes of his throat and auditory tube. Because a young child's auditory tube is short and horizontal, the inflammation spread easily into the middle ear, causing Eddie's acute otitis media (**AOM**). The inflammatory process produced fluid (**effusion**) in the middle ear. His tympanic membrane became painful and inflamed, which you could see through an otoscope *(Figure 4.37).*

DISORDERS OF MIDDLE EAR

Acute otitis media (AOM) is the presence of pus in the middle ear with pain in the ear, fever, and redness of the tympanic membrane. This occurs most often in the first 2 to 4 years of age because:

- Eustachian tubes in children are shorter and more horizontal than in adults, making it easier for bacteria and viruses to find their way into the middle ear from the nasopharynx.
- Adenoids at the back of the nasopharynx near the eustachian tubes can block the opening of the eustachian tubes.
- Children's immune systems are not fully developed until 7 years of age, and they have difficulty fighting infections.

If the infections are viral, they will go away on their own. If bacterial, oral antibiotics may be necessary.

Chronic otitis media occurs when the acute infection subsides but the eustachian tube is still blocked. The **effusion** (fluid) in the middle ear cannot drain out and gradually becomes stickier. This is called **chronic otitis media with effusion (OME)** and produces hearing loss because the sticky fluid prevents the ossicles from vibrating. You can see the fluid through the otoscope *(Figure 4.38).* Dr. Lee was concerned that this had happened to Eddie in his previous ear infection.

If the sticky fluid persists, a **myringotomy** can be performed and a small, hollow plastic tube can be inserted through the tympanic membrane to allow the effusion to drain. The ear tubes have several names: **tympanostomy tubes, pressure-equalization tubes,** or, most commonly, **PE tubes** *(Figure 4.39).* The tube is inserted under general anesthesia as an outpatient surgery. It remains in the ear for 6 to 18 months before it drops out on its own.

A **perforated tympanic membrane** can occur in acute otitis media when pus in the middle ear cannot escape down the eustachian tube. It builds up pressure and perforates the eardrum *(Figure 4.40).* Other causes of perforation include a puncture by a cotton swab, an open-handed slap to the ear, or large pressure changes (as may be induced in scuba diving). Most perforations will heal spontaneously in a month, leaving a small scar.

Cholesteatoma is a complication of chronic otitis media with effusion or of poor eustachian tube function. Chronically inflamed cells in the middle ear multiply and collect into a tumor. They damage the ossicles and can spread to the inner ear. Surgical removal is required.

Otosclerosis is a middle-ear disease that usually affects people between 18 and 35 years of age. It can affect one ear or both and produces a gradual hearing loss for low and soft sounds. Its etiology is unknown. Spongy bone forms around the junction of the oval window and stapes, preventing the stapes from conducting the sound vibrations to the inner ear. The only treatment is to replace the stapes with a metal or plastic **prosthesis.**

WORD	PRONUNCIATION	ELEMENTS		DEFINITION
cholesteatoma	koh-less-tee-ah-**TOE**-mah	S/ R/CF R/	**-oma** *tumor, mass* **chol/e-** *bile* **-steat-** *fat*	Yellow, waxy tumor arising in the middle ear
coryza (also called rhinitis)	ko-**RYE**-zah		Greek *catarrh*	Viral inflammation of the mucous membrane of the nose
effusion	eh-**FYU**-shun		Latin *pouring out*	Collection of fluid that has escaped from blood vessels into a cavity or tissues
myringotomy	mir-in-**GOT**-oh-me	S/ R/CF	**-tomy** *surgical incision* **myring/o-** *tympanic membrane*	Incision in the tympanic membrane
otosclerosis	oh-toe-sklair-**OH**-sis	S/ R/CF R/CF	**-sis** *abnormal condition* **-scler/o-** *hardening* **ot/o-** *ear*	Hardening at the junction of the stapes and oval window that causes loss of hearing
perforated	**PER**-foh-ray-ted		Latin *to bore through*	Punctured with one or more holes
prosthesis	**PROS**-thee-sis		Greek *addition*	Manufactured substitute for a missing part of the body
tympanic	tim-**PAN**-ik	S/ R/	**-ic** *pertaining to* **tympan-** *eardrum, tympanic membrane*	Pertaining to the tympanic membrane or tympanic cavity
tympanostomy	tim-pan-**OS**-toe-me	S/ R/CF	**-stomy** *new opening* **tympan/o-** *eardrum, tympanic membrane*	Surgically created new opening in the tympanic membrane to allow fluid to drain from the middle ear

Abbreviations

AOM acute otitis media
OME otitis media with effusion
PE pressure-equalization tube
URI upper respiratory infection

EXERCISES

Build medical terms. *This is a two-step exercise. Fill in the blanks with the correct element to complete the terms in questions 1–5. Then match the terms in questions 6–9 to their meanings.*

1. Pertaining to the eardrum: _____/ic

2. Hardening at the junction of the stapes and oval window:

    oto/_____/sis

3. Another name for coryza: _____/itis

4. Incision into the tympanic membrane: myringo/_____

5. Yellow, waxy tumor in the middle ear:

    _____/ _____oma

Match the following terms to their meanings.

_____ 6. Manufactured body part   A. coryza

_____ 7. Fluid in a cavity   B. perforated

_____ 8. Common cold   C. prosthesis

_____ 9. Punctured   D. effusion

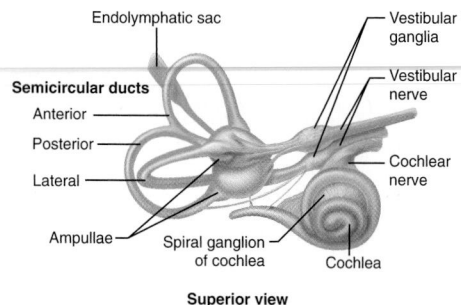

FIGURE 4.41 Inner Ear.

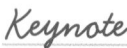

Repeated exposure to loud noise causes hearing loss in young people as well as in older people.

INNER EAR FOR HEARING

The inner ear is a **labyrinth** (*Figure 4.41*) of complex, intricate systems of passages. The passages in the **cochlea,** a part of the labyrinth, contain receptors to translate vibrations into nerve impulses so that the brain can interpret them as different sounds.

The membrane of the oval window separates the middle ear from the vestibule of the inner ear. The stapes (② *in Figure 4.42*) moves the membrane to generate pressure waves in the fluid inside the cochlea ③. The pressure waves cause **vestibular** and **basilar membranes** inside the cochlea to vibrate ④ and sway fine hair cells attached to the basilar membrane ⑤. The hair cells convert this motion into nerve impulses, which travel via the **cochlear nerve** to the brain. The excess pressure waves in the cochlea escape the inner ear via the round window ⑥.

Today, the most common cause of hearing loss is damage to the fine hairs in the cochlea by exposure to repeated loud noise, either related to work (for example, jackhammers, leaf blowers) or to leisure activities (such as amplified music at concerts, personal listening devices, and motorcycles). This is a **sensorineural hearing loss.**

Hearing aids are becoming more sophisticated and smaller, but they do not help people with cochlear damage. **Cochlear implants** are used to bypass the damaged hair cells and directly stimulate cochlear nerve endings.

A **conductive hearing loss** occurs when sound is not conducted efficiently through the external auditory canal to the tympanic membrane and the ossicles. Causes include:

- Middle ear pathology, such as acute otitis media, otitis media with effusion, or a perforated eardrum.
- Impacted cerumen.
- Infected external auditory canal.
- Foreign body in the external canal.

Hearing Test Procedures

Whispered Speech Testing. Ask the patient to cover one ear. Stand 2 feet away from the uncovered ear, whisper words, and ask the patient to repeat them. If the patient cannot repeat them, say the words more loudly. This is a simple screening method.

Weber Test. Strike the tuning fork against your elbow to make a tone, place the tuning fork in the middle of the patient's forehead, and ask whether the tone is louder in one ear or equal on both sides. This determines on which side a hearing loss is located.

Rinne Test. Place the vibrating tuning fork on the mastoid process behind the opening of the ear canal. Then hold it opposite the ear canal. Ask the patient where the tone was louder and/or lasted longer. Normally, sound is heard longer by air conduction at the ear canal than by bone conduction at the mastoid process. The reverse indicates a conductive hearing loss.

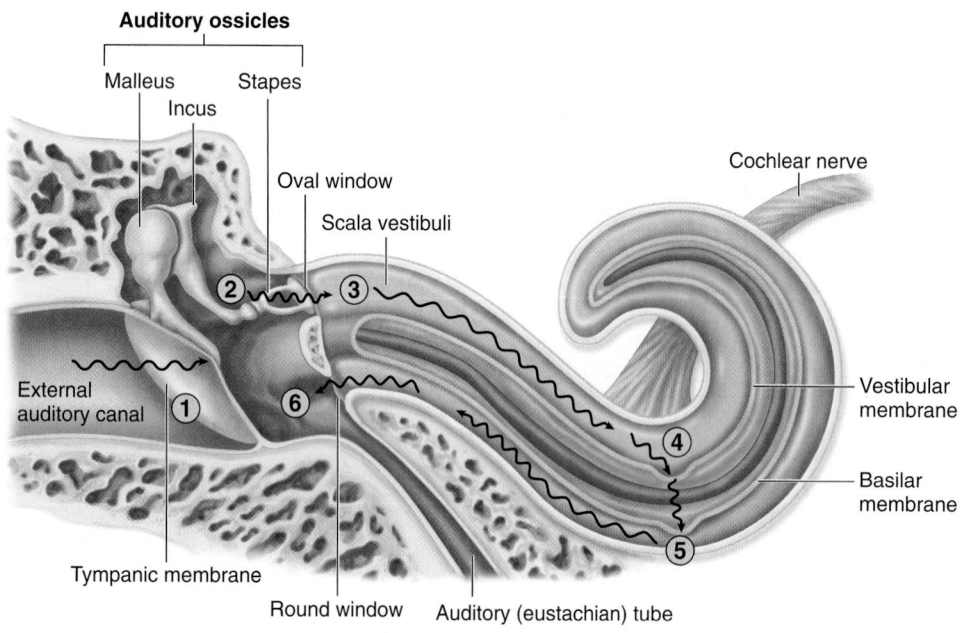

FIGURE 4.42 Hearing Process in the Inner Ear.

WORD	PRONUNCIATION	ELEMENTS		DEFINITION
audiometer	aw-dee-**OM**-ee-ter	S/ R/CF	-meter *measure* audi/o- *hearing*	Instrument to measure hearing
audiometric (adj)	**AW**-dee-oh-**MET**-rik	S/ R/	-ic *pertaining to* metr- *measure*	Pertaining to the measurement of hearing
basilar	**BAS**-ih-lar	S/ R/	-ar *pertaining to* basil- *base, support*	Pertaining to the base of a structure
cochlea cochlear (adj)	**KOK**-lee-ah **KOK**-lee-ar		Latin *snail shell*	An intricate combination of passages; used to describe the part of the inner ear used in hearing
conductive hearing loss	kon-**DUK**-tiv		Latin *to lead*	Hearing loss caused by lesions in the outer ear or middle ear
implant	im-**PLANT**		Latin *to plant*	To insert material into tissues, or the material inserted into tissues
labyrinth labyrinthitis	**LAB**-ih-rinth **LAB**-ih-rin-**THI**-tis	R/ S/	labyrinth- *inner ear* -itis *inflammation*	The inner ear Inflammation of the inner ear
Rinne test	**RIN**-eh TEST		Friedrich Rinne, German otologist, 1819–1868	Test for conductive hearing loss
sensorineural hearing loss	**SEN**-sor-ih-**NYUR**-al	S/ R/CF R/	-al *pertaining to* sensor/i- *sensory* -neur- *nerve*	Hearing loss caused by lesions of the inner ear or the auditory nerve
vestibule vestibular (adj)	**VES**-tih-byul ves-**TIB**-you-lar		Latin *entrance*	Space at the entrance to a canal
Weber test	**VA**-ber TEST		Ernst Weber, German physiologist, 1794–1878	Test for sensorineural hearing loss

Audiometer.   After proper training, use an audiometer to test for hearing loss. The audiometer is an electronic device that generates sounds in different frequencies and intensities and can print out the patient's responses.

When recording the results of hearing testing, **A.D.** is shorthand for the right ear, **A.S.** for the left ear, and **A.U.** for both ears. (*Note:* To avoid confusion with similar abbreviations, the **Joint Commission [JC]** recommends writing out the full terms.)

Abbreviations

A.D.	right ear
A.S.	left ear
A.U.	both ears
JC	Joint Commission

EXERCISES

*Increase your knowledge of the **language of otology** by correctly answering the following questions. Review the WAD; then circle the best answer.*

1. In the term **basilar, basil** is a:

   prefix   root   combining form

2. The entrance to the inner ear is the:

   vestibule   labyrinth   cochlea

3. **Labyrinthitis** is:

   procedure   condition   inflammation

4. The element **neur** means:

   never   nerve   nose

5. An **audiometer** is used to:

   measure   scan   examine

6. An intricate combination of passages in the ear is the:

   cochlea   vestibule   labyrinth

7. The root meaning *hearing* can be found in the word:

   vestibule   audiometric   otology

8. Hearing loss caused by lesions of the inner ear is called _____ hearing loss.

   auditory   basilar   sensorineural

9. The suffix meaning *pertaining to* is found in the term:

   vestibular   labyrinthitis   audiometer

You are

. . . Sonia Ramos, a medical assistant working with Sylvia Thompson, MD, an otolaryngologist at Fulwood Medical Center.

Your patient is

. . . Mr. Ernesto Santiago, a 44-year-old man who was referred to Dr. Thompson by his primary care physician.

CASE REPORT 4.4

Mr. Santiago complains of **recurrent** attacks of nausea and vomiting, a sense of spinning or whirling, and ringing in his ears. The attacks last about 24 hours and are getting more frequent. He has been having trouble hearing quiet speech on his left side.

Your role is to document his investigation, diagnosis, and care and to act as translator between Mr. Santiago and Dr. Thompson.

INNER EAR FOR EQUILIBRIUM AND BALANCE

The **vestibule** and the three **semicircular canals** *(Figure 4.43)* are the organs of balance.

Inside the fluid-filled vestibule are two raised, flat areas (**maculae**) covered with hair cells and a gelatinous material. This gelatinous material contains crystals of calcium and protein called **otoliths**. The position of the head alters the pressure applied to the hair cells by the gelatinous mass. The hair cells respond to horizontal and vertical changes and send impulses to the brain indicating the position to which the head has tilted.

Each of the three fluid-filled semicircular canals has a dilated end called an **ampulla** that contains a mound of hair cells embedded in a gelatinous material that together are called a **crista ampullaris** *(Figure 4.44)*. They detect rotational movements of the head that distort the hair cells and lead to stimulation of connected nerve cells. The nerve impulses travel via the vestibular nerve and go to the brain. From the brain, nerve impulses travel to the muscles to maintain **equilibrium** and balance.

The sensation of spinning or whirling that Mr. Santiago experiences is called **vertigo,** often described by patients as dizziness. The ringing in his ears is called **tinnitus.** Both sensations arise in the inner ear.

Benign paroxysmal positional vertigo (BPPV) is another type of episodic vertigo caused by fragments of the otoliths in the vestibule migrating into the semicircular canals. There they brush against the hair cells, sending conflicting signals to the brain and thereby producing vertigo.

Acute labyrinthitis is an acute viral infection of the labyrinth, producing extreme vertigo, nausea, and vomiting. It usually lasts 1 to 2 weeks.

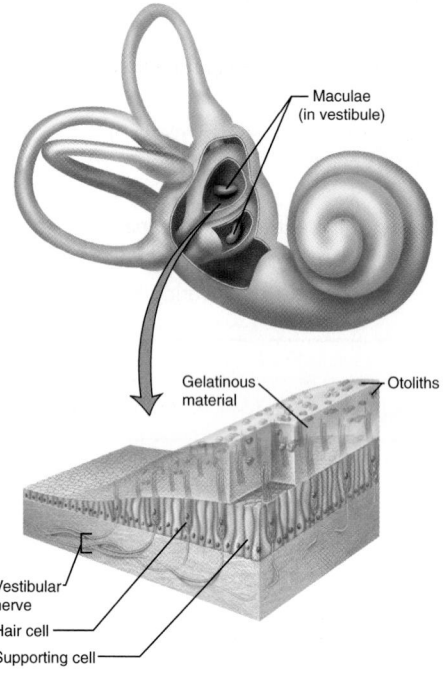

▲ **FIGURE 4.43   Vestibule and Maculae.**

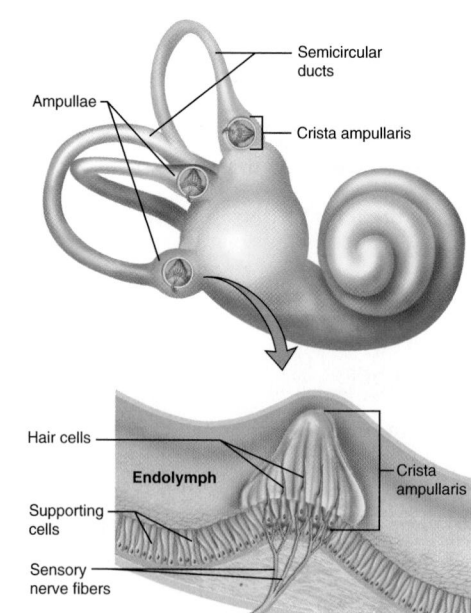

Figure 4.44   **Semicircular Ducts.** ▶

WORD	PRONUNCIATION		ELEMENTS	DEFINITION
ampulla crista ampullaris	am-**PULL**-ah **KRIS**-tah am-**PULL**-air-is	R/ S/ R/	Latin *two-handled bottle* crista *crest* -aris *pertaining to* ampull- *bottle-shaped*	Dilated portion of canal or duct Mound of hair cells and gelatinous material in the ampulla of a semicircular canal
equilibrium	ee-kwi-**LIB**-ree-um	P/ R/	**equi-** *equal* -**librium** *balance*	Being evenly balanced
macula maculae (pl)	**MAK**-you-lah **MAK**-you-lee		Latin *small spot*	Small area of special function; in the ear, a sensory receptor
Ménière disease	men-**YEAR** diz-**EEZ**		Prosper Ménière, French physican, 1799–1862	Disorder of inner ear with cluster of symptoms of acute attacks of tinnitus, vertigo, and hearing loss
otolith	**OH**-toe-lith	S/ R/CF	-lith *stone* ot/o- *ear*	A calcium particle in the vestibule of the inner ear
paroxysmal	par-ock-**SIZ**-mal	S/ R/	-al *pertaining to* -paroxysm- *irritation*	Occurring in sharp, spasmodic episodes
recurrent	ree-**KUR**-ent	S/ P/ R/	-ent *pertaining to* re- *back* curr- *to run*	Symptoms or lesions returning after an intermission
tinnitus	**TIN**-ih-tus		Latin *jingle*	Persistent ringing, whistling, clicking, or booming noise in the ears
vertigo	**VER**-tih-go		Latin *dizziness*	Sensation of spinning or whirling

Case Report 4.4 *(continued)*

The recurrent attacks that Mr. Santiago suffered are called **Ménière disease.** The disease involves the destruction of inner-ear hair cells, but the etiology is unknown, and there is no cure. Dr. Thompson prescribed medication to control his nausea and vomiting.

Abbreviation

BPPV benign paroxysmal positional vertigo

EXERCISES

Challenge your knowledge of the ear by filling in the correct terms for the following definitions. Demonstrate your understanding of the terms by using any one of them correctly in a sentence of your choice. Fill in the blanks.

Definitions	Medical Term
1. Persistent ringing in the ears	_____
2. Sensation of spinning or whirling	_____
3. Occurring in sharp, spasmodic episodes	_____
4. Evenly balanced	_____
5. Dilated portion of a canal or duct	_____
6. Small area of special function	_____
7. Calcium particle in the vestibule	_____
8. Mound of hair cells found in ampulla	_____

Use any one of these terms in a sentence of your choice that is not *a definition.*

_____

_____

SPECIAL SENSES OF THE EYE AND EAR

CHALLENGE YOUR KNOWLEDGE

A. Apply your knowledge of medical terminology to change this paragraph from layman's terms into medical communication. Then practice reading the entire paragraph aloud.

Preoperative Diagnosis: Diabetic _____ (disorder of the retinal blood vessels) with vitreous _____ (sudden discharge of blood), left eye.

Procedure Performed: Laser _____ (clotting together with light) _____ _____ with (surgical removal of vitreous), left eye.

After suitable anesthesia, the patient was prepped and draped in the usual manner. The _____ (inner lining of the eyelid) was well irrigated to remove any debris from the field. A slit _____ (cutting into) was made at four different sites on the _____ (white, outer covering of the eyeball), and the central vitreous cavity was entered. The origin of the bleeding was confined to the _____ _____ (area of sharpest vision). The blood vessels were cauterized with the laser. Fortunately, the _____ _____ (inner lining of the eye) had not become detached, although the vitreous had separated. This was removed in pieces. All operative sites were closed routinely. Ointment, patch, and shield were applied to the affected eye. Patient returned to the postanesthesia care unit for discharge. Patient will be given prescriptions for _____ (medication to destroy bacteria) to be filled when she leaves the hospital. She will follow up with me in the office in 1 week.

B. **Suffixes:** The following terms all have a suffix with a common meaning. Circle the suffix; then identify the common meaning, and define each term.

1. periorbital _____

2. lacrimal _____

3. bactericidal _____

4. intraocular _____

5. neural _____

6. optic _____

7. tarsal _____

8. macular _____

9. retinal _____

10. corneal _____

These suffixes all mean _____ .

C. **Visual Pathway:** In order to better understand the visual pathway, trace its route by putting the following terms in the correct order.

visual cortex   optic chiasm   optic radiation   optic tract   optic foramen   cerebral hemisphere

1. _____

2. _____

3. _____

4. _____

5. _____

6. _____

D. Diagnosis: You are preparing to code the claim forms for various patients seen in the clinic today. The doctor has given each diagnosis in general terms on the charge slip. Not every term in the *ICD-9-CM Index* is cross-referenced, so you must know the medical term to find the code. Write the correct medical term for each general term.

1. Pink eye   _____

2. Sensitivity to light   _____

3. Nearsighted   _____

4. Scratched cornea   _____

5. Inflammation of the iris   _____

6. "Lazy eye"   _____

7. Farsighted   _____

8. Inflamed eyelash and tarsal gland   _____

9. Droopy eyelid   _____

10. Cross-eyed   _____

E. Build medical terms from the following elements. Identify the type of element, its meaning, and a medical term containing that element. The first one is done for you. Fill in the chart.

Element	Prefix	Root/CF	Suffix	Meaning of Element	Example of Medical Term
naso		CF		nose	nasolacrimal
zyme					
ophthalmo					
pur					
bio					
blephar					
cidal					
phobia					
ulcer					
con					
opia					
opto					

F. **Terminology Challenge:** The following medical terms are associated with either an eye specialist or an ear specialist. Check (✓) the appropriate specialist for the term.

Term	Otologist	Ophthalmologist	Term	Otologist	Ophthalmalogist
uveitis			papilledema		
otolith			canthus		
vertigo			audiologist		

G. **Word Elements:** Learning word elements is your most valuable tool for increasing your medical vocabulary. Use your knowledge of word elements to answer the following questions. Circle the correct answer.

1. The root for **tear** is:

   a. blephar

   b. tamin

   c. commodat

   d. strab

   e. lacrim

2. The root of this word means *letting go* and is used to indicate partial paralysis:

   a. parietal

   b. periorbital

   c. paresis

   d. ptosis

   e. presbyopia

3. On the basis of its suffix, you can tell that a **keratotomy** is:

   a. body part

   b. procedure

   c. diagnosis

   d. medication

   e. infection

4. The prefix in **microaneurysm** tells you that this aneurysm is:

   a. large

   b. black

   c. small

   d. painful

   e. red

5. In the term **amblyopia, opia** means:

   a. sound

   b. light

   c. sight

   d. movement

   e. pain

6. **In situ** is a Latin phrase that means: *(Be precise!)*

   a. in this place

   b. in another place

   c. in its original place

   d. in the place

   e. in place of

7. In the terms **retinoblastoma** and **retinopathy,** the combining form tells you that both these terms concern the:

   a. cornea

   b. iris

   c. lens

   d. vitreous body

   e. retina

8. **Angiography** is a radiography of:

   a. organ

   b. bone

   c. blood vessel

   d. muscle

   e. gland

9. In the term **antibiotic, anti** is a prefix that means:

   a. within

   b. outside

   c. on top of

   d. against

   e. around

H. Patient Education: Your patient is confused by some medical terms the doctor has used. Explain to her in simple language the difference between:

1. *hyperopia* and *myopia* _____

_____

_____

2. *dacryocystitis* and *dacryostenosis* _____

_____

_____

I. Prefixes: Use your knowledge of prefixes to deconstruct the terms below; then write the definition of the term. The first one is done for you.

Term	Prefix	Meaning of Prefix	Definition of Term
periorbital	*peri*	*around*	*pertaining to around the orbit*
esotropia	_____	_____	_____
astigmatism	_____	_____	_____
contaminate	_____	_____	_____
accommodation	_____	_____	_____
exotropia	_____	_____	_____
bilateral	_____	_____	_____
analgesic	_____	_____	_____
intraocular	_____	_____	_____

J. Master your documentation—it is a legal record. Circle the most appropriate choice, and insert the correct abbreviation where indicated on the line.

1. Patient complains of sticky eyelids with (purulent/perulent) discharge, both eyes (_____[abbreviation])
   Diagnosis: (scleritis/conjunctivitis)

2. (Refraction/Accommodation) reveals patient's vision now 20/40 in the right eye, with correction.

3. The (diagnosis/prognosis) for Mr. Baker is continued decreasing vision in his right eye (_____[abbreviation]) if his diabetes remains uncontrolled and his (retinopathy/retinoblastoma) worsens.

4. (Opthalmoscopic/Ophthalmoscopic) examination of the left eye (_____[abbreviation]) reveals (microaneurisms/microaneurysms) forming. (Fluoreseen/Fluorescein) angiography is ordered for more details.

K. Discussion Question: Prepare a brief discussion that will address the following questions about Case Report 4.1:

Why was Mrs. Jenny Hughes asked to wash her hands before signing the sign-in sheet?

If she hadn't washed her hands, what could possibly happen?

What sanitary precautions must you take when you work with patients?

What types of precautions could Mrs. Hughes use at home to keep her contagious disease from spreading to the rest of her family?

L. Deconstruct the following medical terms into their word elements and meanings. This group of terms has something in common. What is it? Fill in the blanks.

Medical Term	Prefix	Root/Combining Form	Suffix	Meaning of Medical Term
phacoemulsification				
photocoagulation				
cryopexy				

This group of terms is similar because _____ .

M. Match the Latin and Greek terms in the left column to their meanings in the right column.

_____ 1. orbit   **A.** Flat

_____ 2. extrinsic   **B.** Drooping

_____ 3. chalazion   **C.** On the outer side

_____ 4. cornea   **D.** Paralysis

_____ 5. cortex   **E.** Lump

_____ 6. ptosis   **F.** Corner of the eye

_____ 7. canthus   **G.** Web

_____ 8. contagious   **H.** Circle

_____ 9. tarsus   **I.** Outer shell

_____ 10. paresis   **J.** Touch closely

Use any two terms from this exercise as they would appear in patient documentation.

11. _____

_____

_____

12. _____

_____

_____

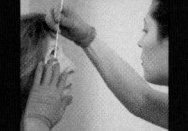
SPECIAL SENSES OF THE EYE AND EAR

N. Patient Documentation. Read the following patient documentation out loud to practice your pronunciation. Certain medical terms are underlined for you. On the lines below, write a definition for each term.

Fulwood Medical Center
3333 Medical Parkway, Fulwood, MI 01234
555-247-6100

Department of: Otology

June 16, 2009

Dear Dr. Lee:

I had the pleasure of seeing your patient Elizabeth Dano in consultation for the first time on June 14, 2009.

This is an 86-year-old woman who comes in with the chief complaint of intermittent <u>vertigo</u>. The patient has known <u>otosclerosis</u> and began having hearing loss in her twenties. Approximately 40 years ago the patient underwent a right <u>stapedectomy</u>, which was not successful. She also states that her hearing continues to get worse each year.

About 3 years ago she began having attacks of dizziness that come on without warning. These lingering feelings of dizziness may last as long as 3 days. Most recently, she had an attack in her doctor's office, which precipitated this consultation.

Her examination in the office today was relatively unremarkable. She specifically had a negative subjective fistula test, so the possibility of this being due to a perilymphatic fistula secondary to the stapedectomy is not very likely. She may indeed have mild <u>*Ménière disease,*</u> which is more common in patients with otosclerosis, but since her attacks are relatively mild, I do not think that any intervention is required at this time. We also know that patients with a known autoimmune disorder such as rheumatoid arthritis can develop immune-mediated inner-ear disease, but this usually is a more insidious and chronic problem, rather than a temporary one. Finally, I think that all things considered, I would not recommend any particular further testing or intervention at this time. I should mention that if her left hearing loss becomes so great that her hearing aid is no longer effective, then we would consider doing a <u>stapedotomy</u> on that ear to once again make her able to use her hearing aid. Obviously, this would be a last-ditch effort, which is not required at this time.

It was a pleasure seeing your patient, and if something new develops, I would be happy to see her in follow-up.

Sincerely,

Albert Aran, M.D.

Definitions: Use your dictionary or glossary for unfamiliar terms. Write the definition for the term on the blank next to it. Then divide terms 2, 3, and 5 into their word elements with slashes.

1. vertigo _____

2. otosclerosis _____

3. stapedectomy _____

4. Ménière disease _____

O. **Patient Documentation:** You must be precise in your use of abbreviations for documentation. Demonstrate your knowledge of abbreviations by filling in the blanks. You are given the medical language—translate it into an abbreviation.

    1. The prescription read: 150 _____ (milligrams) of Cipro, _____ (four times a day).

    2. The patient was diagnosed with _____ (otitis media with effusion) secondary to a _____ (upper respiratory infection).

    3. Since the _____ (acute otitis media) was resolving, the pain medication was used _____ (when necessary).

P. **Build terms from the *language of otology*.** Identify the following elements by checking the appropriate column. Give the meaning of the element; then give an example of a medical term containing that element. The first one is done for you. Fill in the chart.

Element	Prefix	Root/CF	Suffix	Meaning of Element	Medical Term
algesia	____	_____	____	_____	_____
anti	____	_____	____	_____	_____
ette	____	_____	✓	*pain*	*analgesia*
bi	____	_____	____	_____	_____
ot	____	_____	____	_____	_____
rhino	____	_____	____	_____	_____
laryngo	____	_____	____	_____	_____
tympan	____	_____	____	_____	_____
aden	____	_____	____	_____	_____
stomy	____	_____	____	_____	_____
sclero	____	_____	____	_____	_____
audio	____	_____	____	_____	_____

Q. **Teamwork:** You are helping with the orientation of a new medical assistant in the otorhinolaryngologist's office where you work. Can you explain to her the office use for an:

    1. otoscope _____

    _____

    2. audiometer _____

    _____

    3. tonometer _____

    _____

SPECIAL SENSES OF THE EYE AND EAR

R. Apply what you know about the middle ear to choose the answer. Circle the best choice.

1. Which of these is *not* a component of the middle ear?

    a. tympanic membrane

    b. eustachian (auditory) tube

    c. malleus, incus, stapes

    d. nasopharynx

    e. tympanic cavity

2. The eustachian (auditory) tube connects the:

    a. tonsils and nasopharynx

    b. middle ear and nasopharynx

    c. nasopharynx and ossicles

    d. nasopharynx and tympanic membrane

    e. tympanic cavity and tympanic membrane

3. Identify the three ossicles:

    a. pinna, auricle, stapes

    b. eustachian (auditory) tube, mastoid cells, tonsils

    c. nasopharynx, tonsils, middle ear

    d. malleus, incus, stapes

    e. tonsils, stapes, incus

4. What is a complication of chronic otitis media with effusion?

    a. vertigo

    b. acute infection

    c. cholesteatoma

    d. dizziness

    e. nausea

5. Which of these may possibly cause a perforated eardrum?

    a. puncture by a cotton swab

    b. open-handed slap to the ear

    c. scuba diving

    d. pus from acute otitis media

    e. all of the above

S. **Recall and Review:** How well do you remember these word elements from the previous chapter? Try to answer without first looking back to check. Fill in the blanks.

Element	Type of Element (P, R, CF, S)	Meaning of Element
dermato	_____	_____
itis	_____	_____
gnosis	_____	_____
super	_____	_____
um	_____	_____

T. **Terminology Challenge:** *Acute* and *chronic* are two opposite descriptions. Define each term, give an example of an acute condition and a chronic one, and then explain how they are different.

Definition of *acute:* _____

Acute condition: _____

Definition of *chronic:* _____

Chronic condition: _____

How are acute and chronic different?

_____

_____

U. **Schedule Your Patients:** The following doctors and ancillary personnel are seeing patients in the clinic today. Based on the patient's needs, schedule the patient for the correct physician or technician. (In some cases there may be two choices.)

ophthalmologist   optometrist   ophthalmic technician
otologist   otorhinolaryngologist

Patient Needs/Has	Schedule With
refraction	
PE tubes	
phacoemulsification	
instruction in using eyedrops	
cholesteatoma	
patient hit in eye with tree branch	
removal of tonsils and adenoids	
LASIK surgery	
child has bubble gum in nose	
runny nose, stopped-up ears, sore throat	
broken eyeglasses	

SPECIAL SENSES OF THE EYE AND EAR

V. Labeling Exercise: Identify components of the ear. Write the letter of the appropriate description found below the illustration on the numbered line.

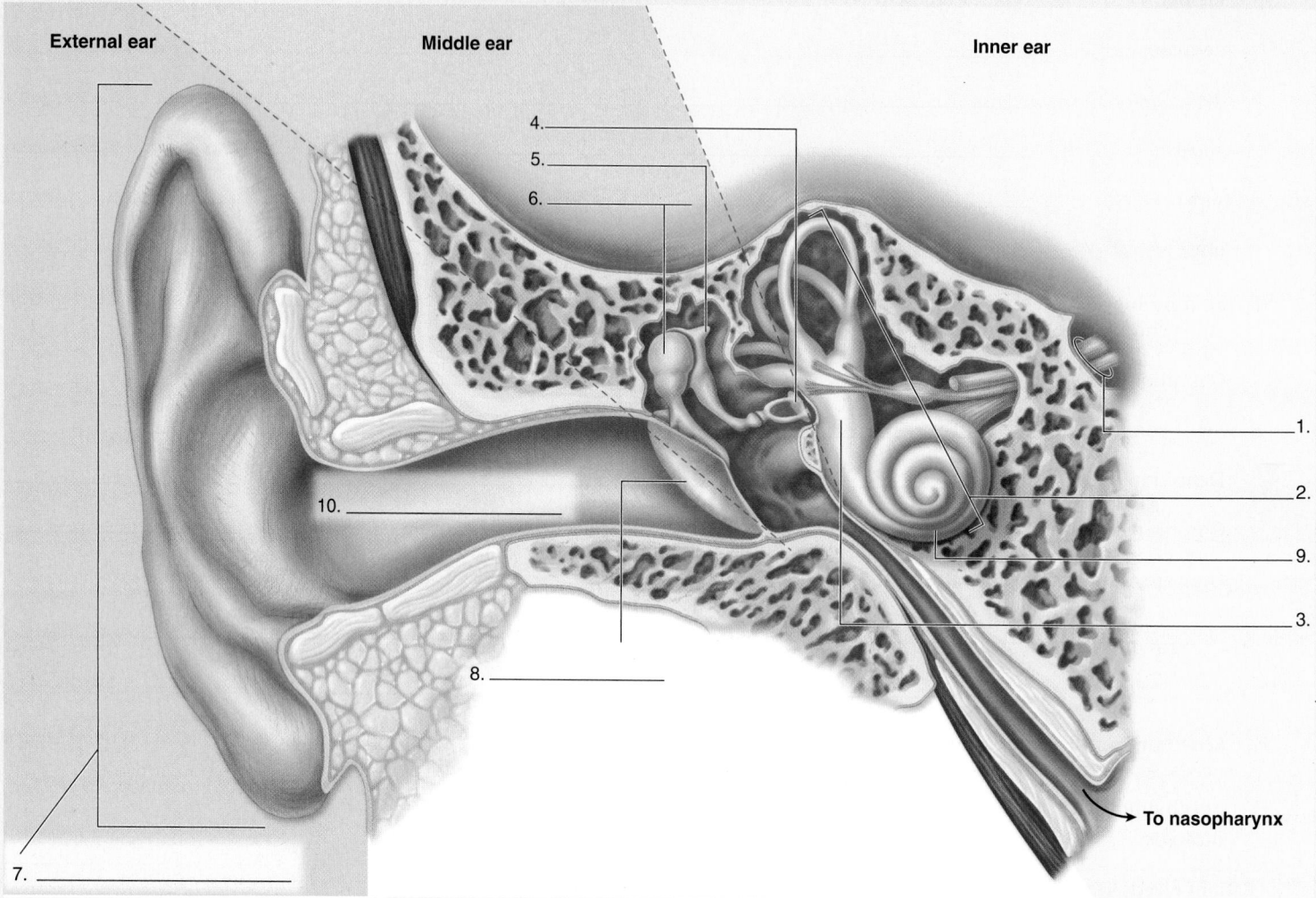

External ear   **Middle ear**   **Inner ear**

4. ____
5. ____
6. ____

1. ____
2. ____
9. ____
3. ____

10. ____

8. ____

7. ____

→ **To nasopharynx**

a. Auditory nerves

b. Inner ear—vestibule and cochlea

c. Eardrum

d. Sound waves travel through here to middle ear

e. Entrance to the inner ear

f. Wing-shaped structure

g. Attached to the oval window

h. "Snail shell" organ of hearing

i. Vibrates with the eardrum when sound waves hit

j. One of three ossicles

W. **Match the Greek and Latin terms in the left column with their meanings in the right column.** Expand your knowledge of the *language of otology.* Fill in the blanks.

_____ 1. chronic

_____ 2. impacted

_____ 3. auricle

_____ 4. vertigo

_____ 5. meatus

_____ 6. effusion

_____ 7. cerumen

_____ 8. pinna

_____ 9. stapes

_____ 10. acute

A. Pouring out

B. Wing

C. Sharp

D. Stirrup

E. Driven in

F. Time

G. Dizziness

H. Ear

I. Wax

J. Go through

X. **Deconstruct the following medical terms.** A portion of the term is in bold—identify that element, and give its meaning. The first one is done for you. Fill in the blanks.

Medical Term	Element	Meaning of Element
otitis	*root*	*ear*
oto**scopy**		
mast**oid**		
cholesteatoma		
myringotomy		
oto**scler**osis		
neural		
equilibrium		
oto**lith**		
paroxysmal		

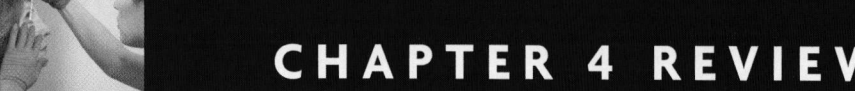

CHAPTER 4 REVIEW

SPECIAL SENSES OF THE EYE AND EAR

Y. Patient Education: Patients will ask you for clarification of certain terms they do not understand or for more explanation of body processes. Be prepared to answer the following questions for your patients.

1. Andrew Baker has severe otosclerosis in his left ear. Dr. Lee has recommended replacement of his stapes with a plastic prosthesis. Explain to Mr. Baker what a prosthesis is, and compare it to other body part replacements he may already have.

Look up **prosthesis** in the glossary. Define **prosthesis.** _____

Name three other types of prostheses that can be inserted into the body. _____

Why can a prosthesis also be considered a "foreign body"?_____

_____

_____

2. Caroline Mason has had many ear problems since she was a child. Frequent infections necessitated PE tubes at a young age. Even after tube removal, she continued to have frequent URIs, tonsillitis, middle-ear infections, impacted cerumen, labyrinthitis, and vertigo later in life.

Can you explain to her the cumulative effect all these previous conditions have had on her hearing loss?

_____

_____

Trace for her the pathway of sound waves through the ear to the brain in order to be recognized as sounds.

_____

_____

_____

_____

How have her previous ear problems interfered with this process?

_____

_____

_____

Is Ms. Mason's condition an acute or chronic condition?

_____

Z. Regions of the Ear: Identify whether the statement references the external, middle, or inner ear by placing a check (✓) in the correct column.

Reference	External Ear	Middle Ear	Inner Ear
swimmer's ear			
otosclerosis			
labyrinthitis			
tympanic membrane			
PE tubes			
otitis externa			
eustachian (auditory) tube			
ossicles			
cochlear implants			

AA. Abbreviations: The following abbreviations are all part of the *language of otology.* Match the abbreviation in the left column with its meaning in the right column.

_____ 1. PE

_____ 2. BPPV

_____ 3. A.S.

_____ 4. p.r.n.

_____ 5. q.i.d.

_____ 6. OME

_____ 7. A.U.

_____ 8. q.4.h.

_____ 9. URI

_____ 10. A.D.

A. Ear infection with fluid collection

B. Both ears

C. Four times each day

D. Right ear

E. Common cold

F. Sensation of spinning or whirling

G. Every 4 hours

H. Pressure-equalization tubes

I. Left ear

J. When necessary

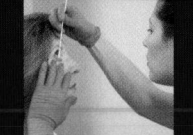
SPECIAL SENSES OF THE EYE AND EAR

CHAPTER SUMMARY EXERCISE

1. *Listen to the pronunciation of the medical terms as given by your instructor.*
2. *Circle the correct spelling of the medical term.*
3. *Match the correctly spelled terms to the brief descriptions below.*
4. *Write a sentence for each of the 10 terms that appear in this exercise.*

A. SPELLING COMPREHENSION: CIRCLE THE CORRECT SPELLING OF THE TERM.

1. chalazion	chelezion	chalezian	chalaziun	chalezium
2. optholmologist	ophtalmologist	optolmologist	ophthalmologist	optalmologist
3. prbyopia	prisbiopia	prisbyopia	pressbiopia	presbyopia
4. blephritis	belpharitis	blepharitis	bleperitis	blephartis
5. strebissmus	strabbismus	strubismis	strabismus	strabithmus
6. amblyopia	ambilopia	amblopia	amblyupia	amblopea
7. petosis	putosis	ptosis	ptysosis	phytosis
8. chiasm	ciasum	ciassum	chesum	chasm
9. antipyrretic	antypiretic	antipyretic	antepiretic	antipieretic
10. yustachian	eustachian	eustacian	eusstacyan	yustachien

B. MATCH THE NUMBER OF THE CORRECT TERM IN PART A WITH THE BRIEF DESCRIPTION OF THE TERM BELOW.

a. Substance that reduces fever   _____

b. Vision not developed equally in both eyes   _____

c. Squinting   _____

d. Cyst on the outer edge of an eyelid   _____

e. Connects middle ear to nasopharynx   _____

f. Nearsighted vision   _____

g. Treats diseases of the eye and prescribes medication   _____

h. Inflammation of the eyelid   _____

i. Two optic nerves cross at the base of the brain   _____

j. Falling or drooping of an eyelid (or organ)   _____

C. USING YOUR KNOWLEDGE OF TERMS 1–10 IN PART A AND THEIR CORRECT SPELLING, WRITE A BRIEF SENTENCE FOR EACH OF THE TERMS AS IT MIGHT APPEAR IN PATIENT DOCUMENTATION.

1. _____

2. _____

3. _____

4. _____

5. _____

6. _____

7. _____

8. _____

9. _____

10. _____

D. YOUR INSTRUCTOR WILL DIRECT YOU TO MCGRAW-HILL CONNECT. OPEN THE AUDIO GLOSSARY AND PRACTICE YOUR PRONUNCIATION OF THE TERMS IN PART A OF THIS EXERCISE.

E. AFTER READING THE PROGRESS NOTE FROM CASE REPORT 4.1, ANSWER THE FOLLOWING QUESTIONS.
BE PREPARED TO DISCUSS YOUR ANSWERS IN CLASS.

Progress Note 04/10/09

Mrs. Jenny Hughes was brought directly into the clinical area at 1030 hrs with what appeared to be conjunctivitis, "pink eye." Both eyelids were red and swollen with a purulent discharge. She complained of headache and **photophobia.** Dr. Chun prescribed Neosporin eyedrops, three drops q.4.h. A swab was sent to the laboratory. I instructed and watched Mrs. Hughes wash her hands and use an alcohol-based hand gel. I then had her sign in and sign our Notice of Privacy Practices. I instructed her in the use of the drops and emphasized home care and hand care measures to prevent the infection from spreading to her family. She was given a return appointment in 1 week and told to call the office if the drops did not help. Daphne Butras, OT. 1055 hrs.

1. Define the term *conjunctivitis.* _____

2. What were the patient's chief complaints? _____

_____

3. Describe Mrs. Hughes's symptoms. _____

_____

4. How often is Mrs. Hughes supposed to use the eyedrops? _____

5. Photophobia is _____ of the light because _____ .

6. If an infection can be spread from person to person, it is considered _____ .

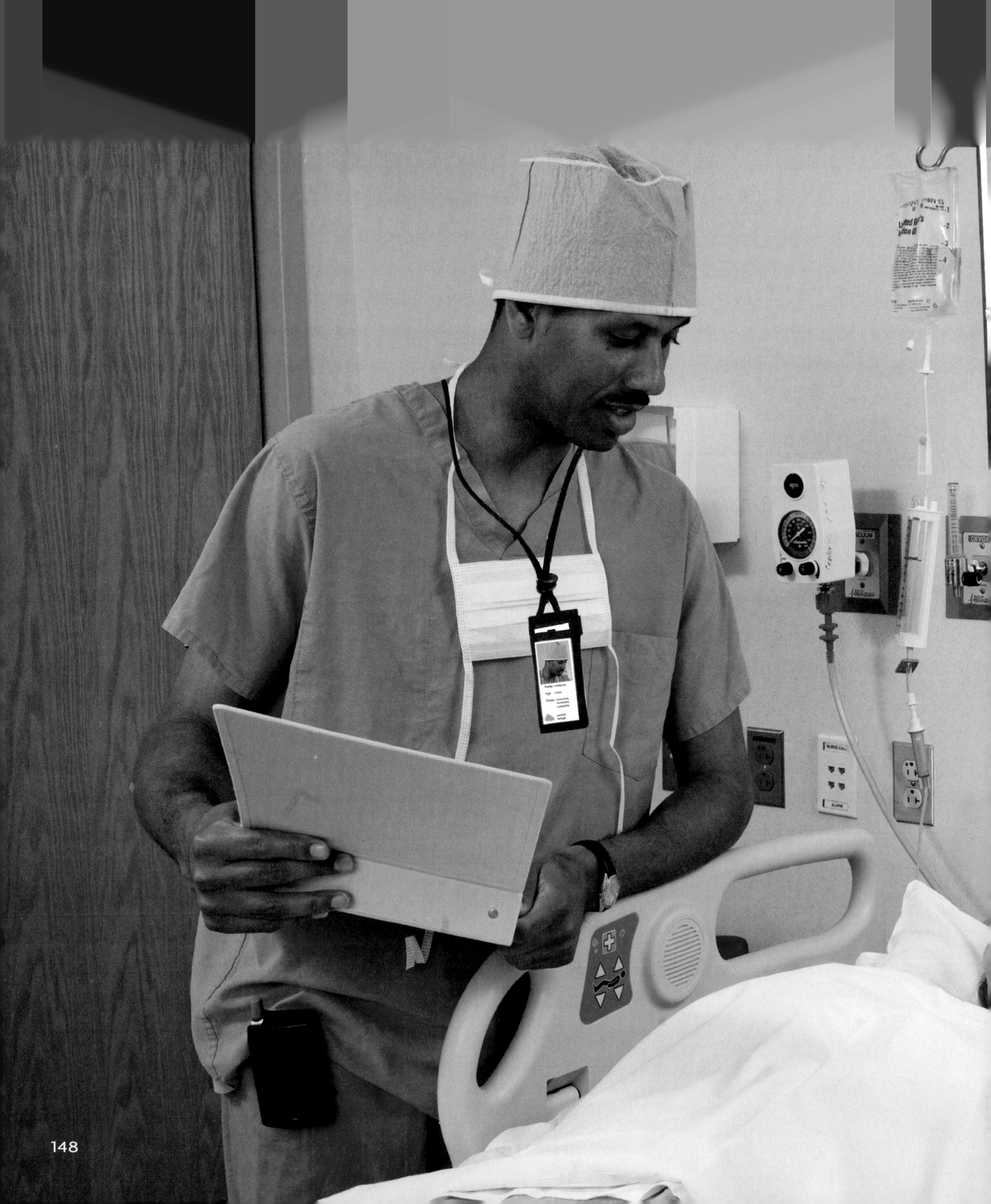

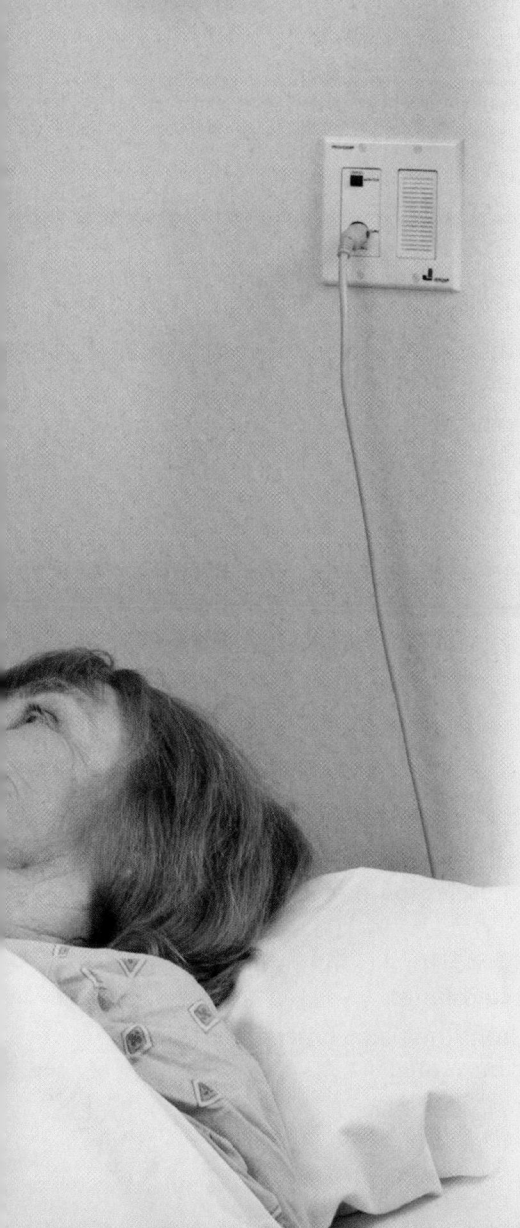

CASE REPORT 5.1

You are

... an **orthopedic** technologist working with Kevin Stannard, MD, an **orthopedist** in the Fulwood Medical Group.

Your patient is

... Mrs. Amy Vargas, a 70-year-old housewife, who tripped going down the front steps from her house. She has severe pain in her right hip and is unable to stand. An x-ray showed a hip fracture and marked **osteoporosis.** Dr Stannard examined her in the Emergency Department and has admitted her for a hip replacement.

For you to work with Dr. Stannard to give optimal care to Mrs. Vargas and help her and her family understand the significance of her bone disorder and injury, you will need to be familiar with the terminology of bone structure and function and bone disorders.

Learning Outcomes

This chapter will review the whole musculoskeletal system and will enable you to:

5.1 Apply the language of orthopedics to the anatomy and physiology of bones, joints, and muscles.

5.2 Comprehend, analyze, spell, and write the medical terms of orthopedics so that you can communicate accurately and precisely in any health care setting.

5.3 Recognize and pronounce the medical terms of orthopedics so that you can communicate verbally with accuracy and precision in any health care setting.

5.4 Understand the cause, appearance, methods of diagnosis, and treatment of common disorders of the musculoskeletal system.

LESSON 5.1 Skeletal System

OBJECTIVES

If you didn't have a skeleton, you'd be like a rag doll, shapeless and unable to move. Your skeleton provides support, protects many organ systems, and is the landmark for much of medical terminology. For example, the radial artery you use for taking a pulse is so named because it travels beside the radial bone of the forearm.

In addition, the surface anatomy of bones and their markings enables you to describe and document the sites of symptoms, signs, and clinical, diagnostic, and therapeutic procedures.

The information in this lesson will enable you to use correct medical terminology to:

5.1.1 Recognize the different health professionals involved in the diagnosis and treatment of musculoskeletal problems.
5.1.2 Identify the tissues that form the skeletal system.
5.1.3 Discuss the structures and functions of the skeletal system.
5.1.4 Explain the structure and functions of bones.
5.1.5 Describe the major problems and diseases that occur in the skeletal system.

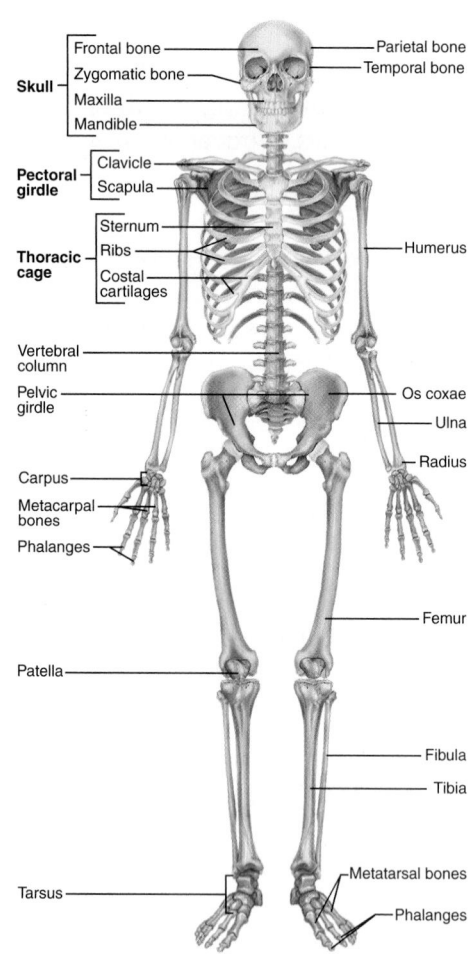

▲ **FIGURE 5.1 Adult Skeleton: Anterior View.**

Health professionals involved in the diagnosis and treatment of problems in the **musculoskeletal** system include the following:

Orthopedic surgeons (orthopedists) are medical doctors in the specialty that deals with the prevention and correction of injuries of the skeletal system and associated muscles, joints, and ligaments. They have an **MD** degree.

Radiologists are medical specialists in the use of x-rays and other imaging techniques.

Osteopathic physicians have the degree **doctor of osteopathy (DO)**. They receive additional training in the musculoskeletal system and how it affects the whole body.

Chiropractors focus on manual manipulation of joints, particularly the spine, to maintain and restore health.

Physical therapists evaluate and treat pain, disease, or injury by physical therapeutic measures, as opposed to medical or surgical measures.

Physical therapist assistants work under the direction of a physical therapist to assist in the application of physical therapy.

Orthopedic technologists and technicians assist orthopedic surgeons in their treatment of patients.

FUNCTIONS OF THE SKELETAL SYSTEM

The four components of the skeletal system *(Figure 5.1)* are:

1. *Bones*   3. *Tendons*
2. *Cartilage*   4. *Ligaments*

They provide the following functions:

- **Support.** The bones of your vertebral column, pelvis, and legs hold up your body. The jawbone supports your teeth. **Cartilage** supports your nose, ears, and ribs. **Tendons** support and attach your muscles to bone. **Ligaments** support and hold your bones together.

- **Protection.** The skull protects your brain. The vertebral column protects your spinal cord. The rib cage protects your heart and lungs.

- **Movement. Muscles** could not function without their attachments to skeletal bones, and muscles are responsible for your movements.

WORD	PRONUNCIATION		ELEMENTS	DEFINITION
cartilage	**KAR**-tih-lage		Latin *gristle*	Nonvascular, firm connective tissue found mostly in joints
chiropractic	kye-roh-**PRAK**-tik	S/ R/CF R/	-ic *pertaining to* chir/o- *hand* -pract- *efficient*	Diagnosis, treatment, and prevention of mechanical disorders of the musculoskeletal system
chiropractor	kye-roh-**PRAK**-tor	S/	-or *a doer*	Practitioner of chiropractic
detoxification	dee-**TOKS**-ih-fi-**KAY**-shun	S/ P/ R/CF	-fication *remove* de- *from, out of* tox/i- *poison*	Removal of poison from a tissue or substance
ligament	**LIG**-ah-ment		Latin *band, sheet*	Band of fibrous tissue connecting two structures
muscle musculoskeletal	**MUSS**-el **MUSS**-kyu-loh-**SKEL**-eh-tal	S/ R/CF R/	Latin *muscle* -al *pertaining to* muscul/o- *muscle* -skelet- *skeleton*	Tissue consisting of contractile cells Pertaining to the muscles and the bony skeleton
orthopedic (also spelled **orthopaedic**)	or-tho-**PEE**-dik	S/ R/CF R/	-ic *pertaining to* orth/o- *straight* -ped- *child*	Pertaining to the correction and cure of deformities and diseases of the musculoskeletal system; originally, most of the deformities treated were in children
orthopedist	or-tho-**PEE**-dist	S/	-ist *specialist*	Specialist in orthopedics
osteopath	**OS**-tee-oh-path	R/ R/CF	-path *disease* oste/o- *bone*	Practitioner of osteopathy
osteopathy	**OS**-tee-**OP**-ah-thee	S/	-pathy *disease*	Medical practice based on maintaining the structural integrity of the musculoskeletal system
radiology	ray-dee-**OL**-oh-jee	S/ R/CF	-logy *study of* radi/o- *radiation, x-rays*	The study of medical imaging
radiologist	ray-dee-**OL**-oh-jist	S/	-logist *one who studies, specialist*	Medical specialist in the use of x-rays and other imaging techniques
tendon	**TEN**-dun		Latin *sinew*	Fibrous band that connects muscle to bone

- **Blood formation.** Bone marrow in many bones is the major producer of blood cells, including most of those in your immune system *(see Chapter 14)*.

- **Mineral storage and balance.** The skeletal system stores calcium and phosphorus. These are released when your body needs them for other purposes. For example, calcium is needed for muscle contraction, communication between neurons *(see Chapter 10)*, and blood clotting *(see Chapter 7)*.

- **Detoxification.** Bones remove metals such as lead and radium from your blood, store them, and slowly release them for excretion.

Abbreviations

MD   doctor of medicine
DO   doctor of osteopathy

Keynote

Bones are divided into four classes based on their shape: long, short, flat, and irregular.

EXERCISES

*This exercise can be answered entirely by using medical terms that appear in this WAD. Mastering these terms will start you on your way to learning the **language of orthopedics**. From the description, identify the correct medical terminology. Fill in the blanks.*

Description | Medical Term(s)

In addition to bones, these three terms are components of the skeletal system:

1. _____

2. _____

3. _____

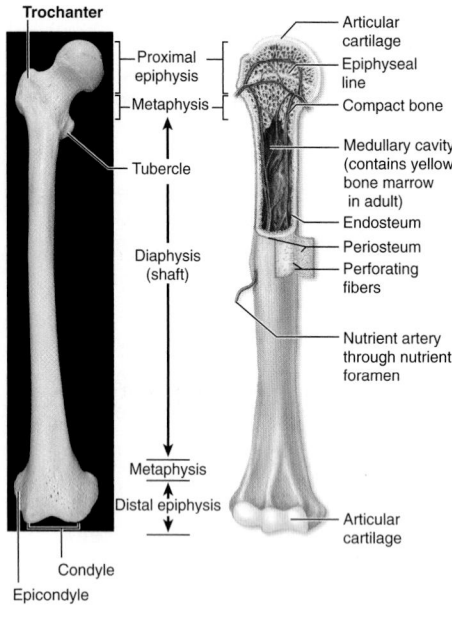

Trochanter
- Proximal epiphysis
- Metaphysis
- Tubercle
- Diaphysis (shaft)
- Metaphysis
- Distal epiphysis
- Condyle
- Epicondyle

- Articular cartilage
- Epiphyseal line
- Compact bone
- Medullary cavity (contains yellow bone marrow in adult)
- Endosteum
- Periosteum
- Perforating fibers
- Nutrient artery through nutrient foramen
- Articular cartilage

(a) Anterior view   (b) Interior view

▲ **FIGURE 5.2   Femur: Long Bone of the Thigh.**

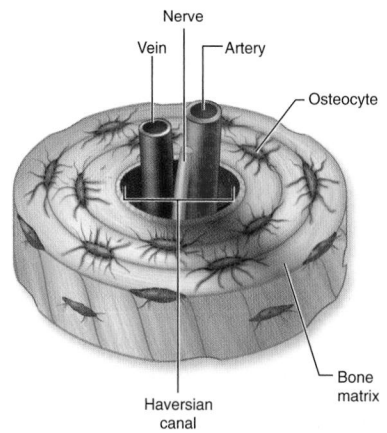

- Nerve
- Vein
- Artery
- Osteocyte
- Haversian canal
- Bone matrix

▲ **FIGURE 5.3   Blood Supply to Bone.**

Factors that affect bone growth include:

1. **Genes.** Genes determine the size and shape of bones and the ultimate adult height.
2. **Nutrition.** Calcium and phosphorus are needed to develop good bone density.
3. **Exercise.** Exercise increases bone density and total bone mass.
4. **Mineral deposition.** Calcium and phosphate are taken from plasma and deposited in bone.
5. **Mineral resorption.** Calcium and phosphate are released from bone back into the plasma when they are needed elsewhere. For example, calcium is needed for muscle contraction, communication between neurons, and blood clotting. Phosphate is a component of DNA and RNA.
6. **Vitamins.** Vitamin A activates osteoblasts; vitamin C is essential for collagen synthesis; vitamin D stimulates absorption, transport, and deposition of calcium and phosphate into bones *(see Chapter 21)*.
7. **Hormones.** For example, growth hormone stimulates the epiphyseal plate to calcify, and estrogen and testosterone accelerate bone growth after puberty and maintain bone density *(see Chapter 13)*.

Structure of Bones

Long bones are the most common type of bone in the body *(Figure 5.2)*.

The shaft of a long bone is called the **diaphysis.** Each end of the bone is called the **epiphysis** and is expanded to provide extra surface area for the attachment of ligaments and tendons.

Sandwiched between the diaphysis and epiphysis is a thin area called the **metaphysis.** Thin layers of cartilage cells in the **epiphyseal plate** enable the diaphysis (bone shaft) to grow in length. When growth stops, compact bone grows into the epiphyseal plate and forms the **epiphyseal line.**

A tough connective tissue sheath called **periosteum** covers the outer surface of all bones and is attached to the compact or **cortical** bone by tough collagen fibers. The periosteum protects the bone and anchors blood vessels and nerves to the surface of the bone.

The hollow cylinder inside the diaphysis is called the **medullary cavity.** It contains bone **marrow** and is lined by a thin membrane called the **endosteum.** The marrow is a fatty tissue that contains blood cells in different stages of development *(see Chapter 7)*.

The endosteum and periosteum contain **osteoblasts,** cells that produce the matrix of new bone tissue. This process is called **osteogenesis.** Bone **matrix** consists of cells, collagen fibers, a gel that supports and suspends the fibers, and calcium phosphate crystals that give bone its hardness.

When osteoblasts are incorporated into the new bone, they become **osteocytes.** These cells, which maintain the matrix, reside in small spaces in the matrix called **lacunae.**

Osteoclasts are produced by the bone marrow. They dissolve calcium, phosphorus, and the organic components of the bone matrix. There is a continual balancing act going on as osteoclasts remove matrix and osteoblasts produce matrix. If osteoclasts outperform the osteoblasts, then **osteoporosis** occurs, as with Mrs. Vargas in the Case Report.

All bones are well supplied with blood *(Figure 5.3)*. The blood vessels travel through the bone in a system of small **haversian (central) canals.** Because of its good blood supply, bone heals well.

S = Suffix   P = Prefix   R = Root   R/CF = Combining Form

WORD	PRONUNCIATION	ELEMENTS		DEFINITION
cortex cortical (adj)	**KOR**-teks **KOR**-tih-cal		Latin *bark*	Outer portion of an organ, such as bone
diaphysis	die-**AF**-ih-sis		Greek *growing between*	The shaft of a long bone
endosteum	en-**DOSS**-tee-um	S/ P/ R/CF	-um *tissue, structure* end- *within* oste/o- *bone*	A membrane of tissue lining the inner (medullary) cavity of a long bone
epiphysis	eh-**PIF**-ih-sis	P/ R/	epi- *upon, above* -physis *growth*	Expanded area at the proximal and distal ends of a long bone that provides increased surface area for attachment of ligaments and tendons
epiphyseal plate	eh-**PIF**-ih-see-al PLATE	S/ R/CF	-al *pertaining to* epiphys/e- *growth*	Layer of cartilage between epiphysis and metaphysis where bone growth occurs
haversian canals (also called **central canals**)	hah-**VER**-shan ka-**NALS**		Clopton Havers, English physician, 1655–1702	Vascular canals in bone
lacuna lacunae (pl)	la-**KOO**-nah la-**KOO**-nee		Latin *a pit, lake*	Small space or cavity within the matrix of bone
marrow	**MAH**-roe		Old English *marrow*	Fatty, blood-forming tissue in the cavities of long bones
matrix	**MAY**-triks		Latin *mother, womb*	Substance that surrounds cells, is manufactured by cells, and holds them together
medulla medullary (adj)	meh-**DULL**-ah **MED**-ul-ah-ree		Latin *marrow*	Central portion of a structure surrounded by cortex
metaphysis	meh-**TAF**-ih-sis	P/ R/	meta- *beyond, after, subsequent to* -physis *growth*	Region between the diaphysis and the epiphysis where bone growth occurs
osteoblast	**OS**-tee-oh-blast	S/ R/CF	-blast *embryo* oste/o- *bone*	Bone-forming cell
osteoclast	**OS**-tee-oh-klast	S/ R/CF	-clast *break down* oste/o- *bone*	Bone-removing cell
osteocyte	**OS**-tee-oh-site	S/ R/CF	-cyte *cell* oste/o- *bone*	Bone-maintaining cell
osteogenesis osteogenic (adj)	**OS**-tee-oh-**JEN**-eh-sis **OS**-tee-oh-**JEN**-ik	S/ R/CF	-genesis *creation* oste/o- *bone*	Creation of new bone
osteoporosis	**OS**-tee-oh-poh-**ROE**-sis	S/ R/CF R/	-osis *condition* oste/o- *bone* -por- *opening*	Condition in which the bones become more porous, brittle, and fragile and are more likely to fracture
periosteum periosteal (adj)	**PER**-ee-**OSS**-tee-um **PER**-ee-**OSS**-tee-al	S/ P/ R/	-um *tissue, structure* peri- *around* oste- *bone*	Strong membrane surrounding a bone
trochanter	troh-**KAN**-ter		Greek *runner*	One of two bony prominences near the head of the femur

EXERCISES

The combining form oste/o- means bone *and is the main element in each of the following terms. You choose the correct suffix to complete the term. Fill in the blanks.*

blast   **cyte**   **genesis**   **clast**   **genic**   **porosis**

The osteo_____ process begins with osteo_____, which produce the matrix of new bone tissue. Osteo_____ has begun. Once these cells incorporate into new bone, they are termed osteo_____. These cells maintain the matrix. Osteo_____ are produced by bone marrow. A delicate balance must be maintained between cells that remove matrix and cells that produce matrix. If more matrix is removed than produced, osteo_____ will result.

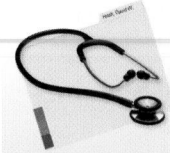

On questioning, Mrs. Vargas demonstrated many of the risk factors for osteoporosis, including a family history, lack of exercise, cigarette smoking, inadequate diet, postmenopause, and increasing age.

Normal bone　　　Osteoporotic bone

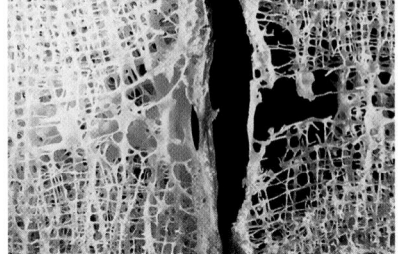

LM 5×

▲ **FIGURE 5.4　Normal Bone and Osteoporotic Bone.**

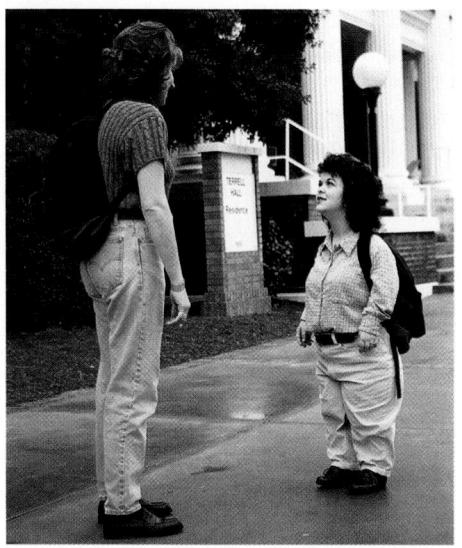

▲ **FIGURE 5.5　Achondroplastic Dwarf with College Roommate.**

Abbreviations

BMD　bone mineral density
DEXA　dual energy x-ray absorptiometry
FDA　U.S. Food and Drug Administration
IU　international unit(s)

DISEASES OF BONE

Osteoporosis results from a loss of bone density *(Figure 5.4)* when the rate of bone **resorption** exceeds the rate of bone **formation.** It is more common in women than in men, and its incidence increases with age. Ten million people in the United States already have osteoporosis, and 18 million more have low bone density (**osteopenia**) and are at risk for developing osteoporosis.

In women, production of the hormone estrogen decreases after menopause, and its protection against osteoclast activity is lost. This leads to fragile, brittle bones. In men, reduction in testosterone has a similar but less marked effect.

Women at risk for osteoporosis should have bone mineral density (**BMD**) screening using a dual-energy x-ray absorptiometry (**DEXA**) scan. Men and women over age 50 should take 1200 mg of calcium daily and 400 to 600 international units (**IU**) of vitamin D or expose the body to the sun for 15 minutes daily. Chapter 22 covers nutritional needs.

There are several U.S. Food and Drug Administration (**FDA**)–approved medications available for the treatment of osteoporosis. Most inhibit osteoclast activity.

Osteomyelitis is an inflammation of an area of bone due to bacterial infection, usually with a staphylococcus. Untreated tuberculosis can spread from its original infection in the lungs to bones via the bloodstream to produce tuberculous osteomyelitis.

Osteomalacia, known as **rickets** in children, is a disease caused by vitamin D deficiency. When bones lack calcium, they become soft and flexible. They are not strong enough to bear weight and become bowed. Osteomalacia occurs in some developing nations and occasionally in this country when children drink soft drinks instead of milk fortified with vitamin D.

Achondroplasia occurs when the long bones stop growing in childhood but the bones of the axial skeleton are not affected *(Figure 5.5)*. This leads to short-stature individuals who are about 4 feet tall. Intelligence and life span are normal. It is caused by a spontaneous gene mutation that then becomes a dominant gene for succeeding generations.

Osteogenic sarcoma is the most common malignant bone tumor. Peak incidence is between 10 and 15 years of age, and the tumor often occurs around the knee joint.

Osteogenesis imperfecta is a rare genetic disorder, producing very brittle bones that are easily fractured, often **in utero** (while inside the uterus).

WORD ANALYSIS AND DEFINITION

WORD	PRONUNCIATION	ELEMENTS		DEFINITION
achondroplasia	a-kon-droh-**PLAY**-ze-ah	S/ P/ R/CF	-plasia *formation* a- *without* -chondr/o- *cartilage*	Condition with abnormal conversion of cartilage into bone, leading to dwarfism
in utero	IN **YOU**-ter-oh		Latin *uterus*	Within the womb; not yet born
osteogenesis imperfecta	**OS**-tee-oh-**JEN**-eh-sis im-per-**FEK**-tah	S/ R/CF R/	-genesis *creation* oste/o- *bone* imperfecta *unfinished*	Inherited condition in which bone formation is incomplete, leading to fragile, easily broken bones
osteomalacia	**OS**-tee-oh-mah-**LAY**-she-ah	S/ R/CF	-malacia *abnormal softness* oste/o- *bone*	Soft, flexible bones lacking in calcium (rickets)
osteomyelitis	**OS**-tee-oh-my-eh-**LIE**-tis	S/ R/CF R/	-itis *inflammation* oste/o- *bone* -myel- *bone marrow*	Inflammation of bone tissue
osteopenia	**OS**-tee-oh-**PEE**-nee-ah	S/ R/CF	-penia *deficient* oste/o- *bone*	Decreased calcification of bone
resorption	ree-**SORP**-shun		Latin *to suck back*	Loss of substance, such as bone
rickets	**RICK**-ets		Old English *to twist*	Disease due to vitamin D deficiency, producing soft, flexible bones
sarcoma	sar-**KOH**-mah	S/ R/	-oma *tumor, mass* sarc- *flesh*	A malignant tumor originating in connective tissue
osteogenic sarcoma	**OS**-tee-oh-**JEN**-ik sar-**KOH**-mah	S/ R/CF	-genic *creation* oste/o- *bone*	Malignant tumor originating in bone-producing cells

EXERCISES

Bone diseases can strike at any age. Refer to the WAD above for the correct terminology to identify each disease. Fill in the blanks.

Identify the disease.

1. Inflammation of an area of bone, usually due to staph infection _____

2. Bone disease in children caused by vitamin D deficiency _____

3. Leads to short stature (height) _____

4. Rare, genetic disorder causing brittle bones _____

5. Decreased calcification of bone _____

6. Most common malignant bone tumor _____

7. Also known as "rickets" in children _____

Questions 8 to 10 relate to the answers in questions 1 to 7 above.

8. "Within the womb, not yet born" is documented as _____.

9. What is the medical term for soft, flexible bones lacking in calcium? _____

10. When bone resorption exceeds bone formation, _____ results.

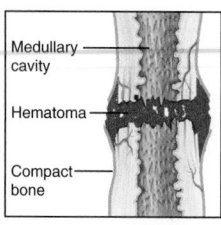

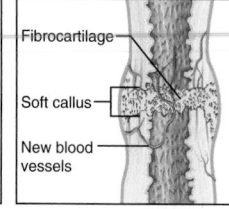

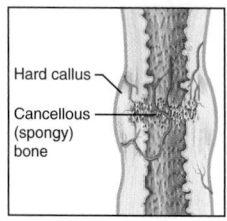

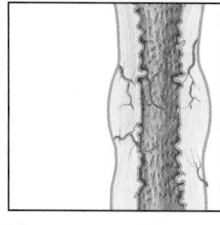

▲ **FIGURE 5.6** **Healing of Bone Fracture.**

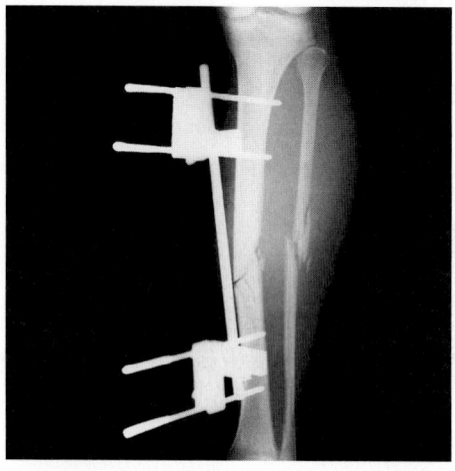

▲ **FIGURE 5.7** **Radiograph of Fractured Limb.** X-Ray of lower-leg fracture set with steel pins and external plate.

Abbreviation	
Fx	fracture

▼ **FIGURE 5.8** **Internal Fixation of Fractures with Screws and Plate.**

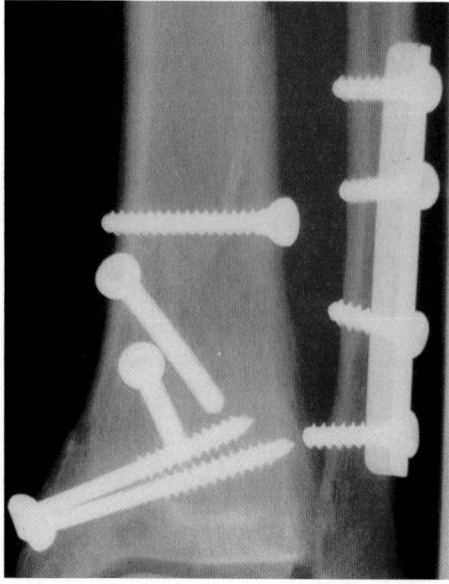

BONE FRACTURES

Healing of Fractures

Step 1: When a bone is fractured, blood vessels bleed into the fracture site, forming a **hematoma** (*Figure 5.6a*).

Step 2: A few days after the fracture (Fx), osteoblasts move into the hematoma and start to produce new bone. This is called a **callus** (*Figure 5.6b*).

Step 3: Osteoblasts produce immature, lacy, **cancellous** (spongy) bone that replaces the callus (*Figure 5.6c*).

Step 4: Osteoblasts continue to produce bone cells. They produce compact bone and fuse the bone segments together (*Figure 5.6d*).

Uncomplicated fractures take 8 to 12 weeks to heal.

Surgical Procedures for Repairing Fractures

The initial goal of fracture treatment is to bring the ends of the bone at the break back opposite each other so that they fit together as they did in the original bone. This is called **alignment.**

External manipulation is used frequently. The bone is pulled from the distal end back into alignment. This process is called **reduction.** Anesthesia may be used.

In external fixation, the alignment is maintained by immobilizing the bone through the use of:

- **Plaster and fiberglass casts**
- **Splints**
- **Traction**—the gentle but continuous application of a pulling force that can align a fracture, reduce muscle spasm, and relieve pain.
- **External fixators**—by which the bone fragments are secured to a strong external steel rod or plate by means of steel pins (*Figure 5.7*).

Internal fixation with materials such as stainless steel and titanium, which are compatible with tissues, enables the patient to return to function quicker and reduces the incidence of **nonunion** and **malunion** (improper healing). The types of internal fixation are:

- **Wires**—used as sutures to "sew" the bone fragments together; this method is often used in the hand.
- **Plates**—extend along both or all fragments of bone and are held in place by screws.
- **Rods**—can be inserted through the medullary cavity of both fragments to align the bones.
- **Screws**—can be used on their own as well as with plates; they are probably the most common form of internal fixation (*Figure 5.8*).
- **Pins**—a long, thick metal pin can be driven down the shaft of a bone from one end.

The types of bone fractures are shown in *Figure 5.9* and described in Table 5.1.

WORD	PRONUNCIATION		ELEMENTS	DEFINITION
alignment	a-**LINE**-ment	S/ P/ R/	**-ment** *resulting state* **a-** (variant of **ad-**) *into* **-lign-** *line*	A state of being in the correct position in relation to other structures
callus (***Note:*** *Callous* is a nonmedical word meaning *insensitive.*)	**KAL**-us		Latin *hard skin*	The mass of fibrous connective tissue that forms at a fracture site and becomes the foundation for the formation of new bone
cancellous	**KAN**-sell-us		Latin *lattice*	Bone that has a spongy or latticelike structure
hematoma	he-mah-**TOH**-mah	S/ R/	**-oma** *tumor, mass* **hemat-** *blood*	Collection of blood that has escaped from the blood vessels into tissue
malunion	mal-**YOU**-nee-un	S/ P/ R/	**-ion** *action, condition, process* **mal-** *bad* **-un-** *one*	Condition in which the two bony ends of a fracture fail to heal together correctly
nonunion	non-**YOU**-nee-un	P/	**non-** *not*	Total failure of healing of a fracture
reduction	ree-**DUCK**-shun	S/ P/ R/	**-ion** *action, condition, process* **re-** *backward* **-duct-** *lead*	The restoration of a structure to its normal position
traction	**TRAK**-shun		Latin *to pull*	A pulling or dragging force

EXERCISES

After you deconstruct the following medical terms into their basic elements, provide a brief definition for each term. Fill in the chart; then fill in the blanks at the end of the exercise. The first one is done for you.

Medical Term	Prefix	Root/CF	Suffix	Definition of Medical Term
reduction	*re*	*duct*	*ion*	*The restoration of a structure to its normal position*
alignment				
malunion				
hematoma				

Demonstrate your understanding of the terms by finishing this exercise.

1. Use *both* the terms **reduction** and **alignment** in *one sentence.*

_____

_____

2. The suffix **oma** means *tumor* as well as *mass.* Briefly explain why a hematoma is not a tumor.

_____

_____

3. Explain the difference between a **malunion** and a **nonunion** of a fracture.

_____

_____

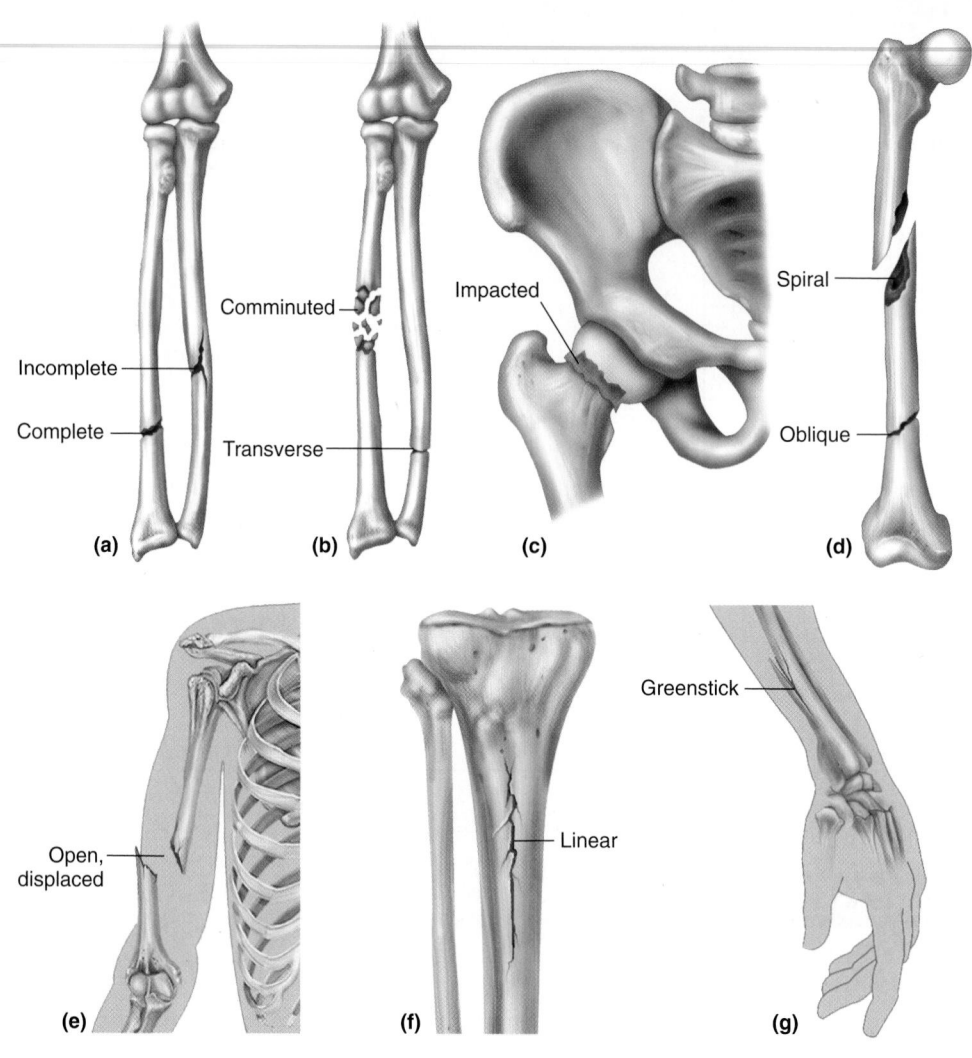

▲ **FIGURE 5.9** **Bone Fractures.**

TABLE 5.1 Classification of Bone Fractures

Name	Description	Reference
Closed	A bone is broken, but the skin is not broken.	Figure 5.9g
Open	A fragment of the fractured bone breaks the skin, or a wound extends to the site of the fracture.	Figure 5.9e
Displaced	The fractured bone parts are out of alignment.	Figure 5.9e
Complete	A bone is broken into at least two fragments.	Figure 5.9a
Incomplete	The fracture does not extend completely across the bone; it can be **hairline** (as in a stress fracture in the foot when there is no separation of the two fragments).	Figure 5.9a
Comminuted	The bone breaks into several pieces, usually two major pieces and several smaller fragments.	Figure 5.9b
Transverse	The fracture is at a right angle to the long axis of the bone.	Figure 5.9b
Impacted	One bone fragment is driven into the other, with resulting shortening of a limb.	Figure 5.9c
Spiral	Fracture spirals a round the long axis of the bone.	Figure 5.9d
Oblique	Diagonal fracture runs across the long axis of the bone.	Figure 5.9d
Linear	Fracture runs parallel to the long axis of the bone.	Figure 5.9f
Greenstick (closed)	This is a partial fracture: one side breaks, the other bends.	Figure 5.9g
Pathologic	Fracture occurs in an area of bone weakened by disease (such as cancer).	—
Compression	Fracture occurs in a vertebra from trauma or pathology leading to the vertebra being crushed.	—

WORD	PRONUNCIATION		ELEMENTS	DEFINITION
closed fracture (opposite of open)	KLOSD **FRAK**-chur	S/ R/	**closed** Latin *hard skin* **-ure** *result of* **fract-** *break*	A bone is broken but the skin over it is intact
comminuted fracture	**KOM**-ih-nyu-ted	S/ R/	**-ed** *pertaining to* **comminut-** *break into small pieces*	A fracture in which the bone is broken into pieces
complete fracture	kom-**PLEET**		Latin *fill up*	A bone is fractured into two separate pieces
compression fracture	kom-**PRESH**-un	S/ R/	**-ion** *condition, action* **compress-** *press together*	Fracture of a vertebra causing loss of height of the vertebra
displaced fracture	dis-**PLAYSD**	P/ R/	**dis-** *apart, away from* **-placed** *in an area*	A fracture in which the fragments are separated and are not in alignment
greenstick fracture	**GREEN**-stik	R/ R/	**green-** *green* **-stick** *branch twig*	A fracture in which one side of the bone is partially broken and the other side is bent. Occurs mostly in children
hairline fracture	**HAIR**-line		Old English *hair* **line** Latin *a mark*	A fracture without separation of the fragments
impacted fracture	im-**PAK**-ted	S/ P/ R/	**-ed** *pertaining to* **im-** *in* **-pact** *driven in*	A fracture in which one bone fragment is driven into the other
incomplete fracture	in-kom-**PLEET**	P/ R/	**in-** *not* **-complete** *fill in*	A fracture that does not extend across the bone, as in a hairline fracture
linear fracture	**LIN**-ee-ar	S/ R/	**-ar** *pertaining to* **line-** *a mark*	A fracture running parallel to the length of the bone
oblique fracture	ob-**LEEK**		Latin *slanting*	A diagonal fracture across the long axis of the bone
open fracture	**OH**-pen		Old English *not enclosed*	The skin over the fracture is broken
pathologic fracture	path-oh-**LOJ**-ik	S/ R/CF R/ S/ R/	**-ic** *pertaining to* **path/o-** *disease* **-log-** *to study* **-ure** *result of* **fract-** *to break*	Fracture occurring at a site already weakened by a disease process, such as cancer
spiral fracture	**SPY**-ral	S/ R/	**-al** *pertaining to* **spir-** *a coil*	A fracture in the shape of a coil
transverse fracture	trans-**VERS**	P/ R/	**trans-** *across* **-verse** *travel*	A fracture perpendicular to the long axis of the bone

EXERCISES

Fractures (Fxs). You are working as the new radiology technician in the Radiology Department at the hospital. You are attempting to identify the types of fractures with the pictures you see on the film. Use the descriptions below to identify the types of fractures. Refer to Table 5.1 on the opposite page.

Fracture Seen on the Film	Type of Fracture
Fx at a right angle to the long axis of the radius	
Femur broken into two clean pieces	
Cancer patient with vertebral Fx	
Broken ankle but no broken skin	
Diagonal Fx across the long axis of the femur	
Fractured hand with bone fragments sticking out	

1. Which one is an open fracture? _____

2. Which one is a closed fracture? _____

OBJECTIVES

Without joints you would be a statue. Joints allow you to move, but movable parts that rub together can wear out. Damage or disease in a joint can make movement very difficult and painful. The structure of any joint, or **articulation,** is directly related to its mobility and function.

To understand, describe, and document your patient's joint problems, you need to be able to use correct medical terminology to:

5.2.1 Classify the different types of joints.

5.2.2 Identify the tissues that form the different joints.

5.2.3 Link structures to functions in the different joints.

5.2.4 Demonstrate an understanding of the major problems and diseases that occur in joints.

You are

. . . an orthopedic technologist working for orthopedic surgeon Kenneth Stannard, MD, at Fulwood Medical Center.

Your patient is

. . . Mr. Hank Johnson, a 63-year-old white male. Mr. Johnson has been active all his life.

CASE REPORT 5.2

In his youth Mr. Johnson played football and baseball. As an adult, he has played racquetball weekly and jogged 3 to 4 miles most mornings on the streets of his neighborhood. For the past year he has had lower-back stiffness and pain, particularly in the mornings. Six months ago, while out hiking, he slid down a mountain on his left side for about 100 feet. He is now having pain in his left groin and thigh, with difficulty walking and climbing stairs.

You are responsible for documenting the doctor's diagnostic procedures and treatment and for making sure that the patient understands the significance of the diagnostic findings and the recommendations for his treatment.

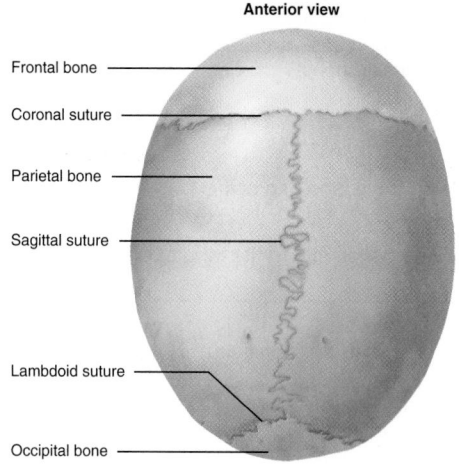

Anterior view

Frontal bone

Coronal suture

Parietal bone

Sagittal suture

Lambdoid suture

Occipital bone

Posterior view

▲ **FIGURE 5.10 Sutures of Skull: Superior View.**

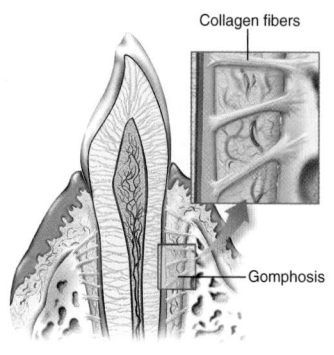

Collagen fibers

Gomphosis

◀ **FIGURE 5.11 Gomphosis between Tooth and Jaw Socket.**

CLASSES OF JOINTS

Joints are classified structurally into three types:

1. **Fibrous** joints are two bones tightly bound together by bands of fibrous tissue with no joint space. They come in three varieties:

   a. **Sutures** occur between the bones of the skull *(Figure 5.10);* the two opposing bones have interlocking processes to add stability to the joint. The **periosteum** on the outer and inner surfaces of the two bones is continuous and holds the joint together.

   b. **Syndesmosis** is a joining of two bones with fibrous ligaments. Their movement is minimal. An example is the joint above the ankle where the tibia and fibula are attached.

   c. **Gomphoses** are pegs that fit into sockets and are held in place by fine collagen fibers. Examples are the joints between teeth and their sockets *(Figure 5.11)*.

2. **Cartilaginous** joints join two bones with cartilage:

   a. **Synchondroses** join two bones with **hyaline** cartilage, which allows little or no movement between them, as between your ribs and costal cartilages.

   b. **Symphyses** join two bones with **fibrocartilage.** An example is the symphysis pubis, where your two pubic bones meet at the front of your pelvis.

WORD	PRONUNCIATION	ELEMENTS		DEFINITION
articulation articulate (verb) articular (adj)	ar-tik-you-**LAY**-shun ar-**TIK**-you-late ar-**TIK**-you-lar	S/ R/	-ation *process* articul- *joint*	A joint
bursa	**BURR**-sah		Latin *purse*	A closed sac containing synovial fluid
fibrocartilage	fie-bro-**KAR**-til-age	R/CF R/CF	fibr/o- *fiber* -cartilag/e *cartilage*	Cartilage containing collagen fibers
gomphosis gomphoses (pl)	gom-**FOE**-sis gom-**FOE**-sees	S/ R/	-osis *condition* gomph- *bolt, nail*	Joint formed by a peg and socket
hyaline	**HIGH**-ah-line		Greek *glass*	Cartilage that looks like frosted glass and contains fine collagen fibers
meniscus menisci (pl)	meh-**NISS**-kuss meh-**NISS**-key		Greek *crescent*	Disc of connective tissue cartilage between the bones of a joint, for example, in the knee joint
suture sutures (pl)	**SOO**-chur		Latin *a seam*	Place where two bones are joined together by a fibrous band continuous with their periosteum, as in the skull
symphysis symphyses (pl)	**SIM**-feh-sis **SIM**-feh-sees		Greek *growing together*	Two bones joined by fibrocartilage
synchondrosis synchondroses (pl)	sin-kon-**DROH**-sis sin-kon-**DROH**-sees	S/ P/ R/	-osis *condition* syn- *together* -chondr- *cartilage*	A rigid articulation (joint) formed by cartilage
syndesmosis syndesmoses (pl)	sin-dez-**MOH**-sis sin-dez-**MOH**-sees	S/ R/	-osis *condition* syndesm- *bind together*	An articulation (joint) formed by ligaments
synovial	si-**NOH**-vee-al	S/ P/ R/CF	-al *pertaining to* syn- *together* -ov/i- *egg*	Pertaining to synovial fluid and synovial membrane

3. **Synovial** joints contain synovial fluid as a lubricant and allow considerable movement *(Figure 5.12)*. Most joints in the legs and arms are synovial joints. The ends of the bones are covered with hyaline **articular** cartilage. In some joints, an additional plate of fibrocartilage is located between the two bones. In the knee, this plate is incomplete and is called a **meniscus**.

A **bursa** is an extension of the synovial joint that forms a cushion between structures that otherwise would rub against each other; for example, in the knee joint between the patellar tendon and the patellar and tibial bones *(Figure 5.12)*.

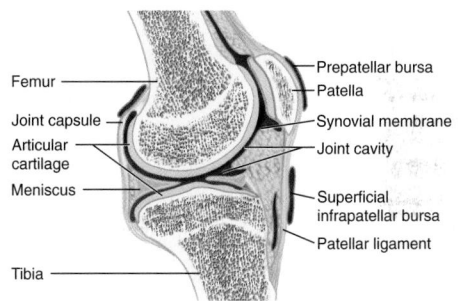

▲ **FIGURE 5.12   Synovial Joint.**

EXERCISES

You must be able to recognize a medical term in its singular and plural forms. In the following chart check (✓) in the appropriate column whether the given term is singular or plural. If you have checked singular, write the plural form of the term in the appropriate column; if you have checked plural, write the singular form of the term in the appropriate column. Fill in the chart; then write the definitions.

Medical Term	Singular	Plural
syndesmoses		
suture		
gomphosis		
menisci		

Define any two of these terms in a sentence.

1. _____

2. _____

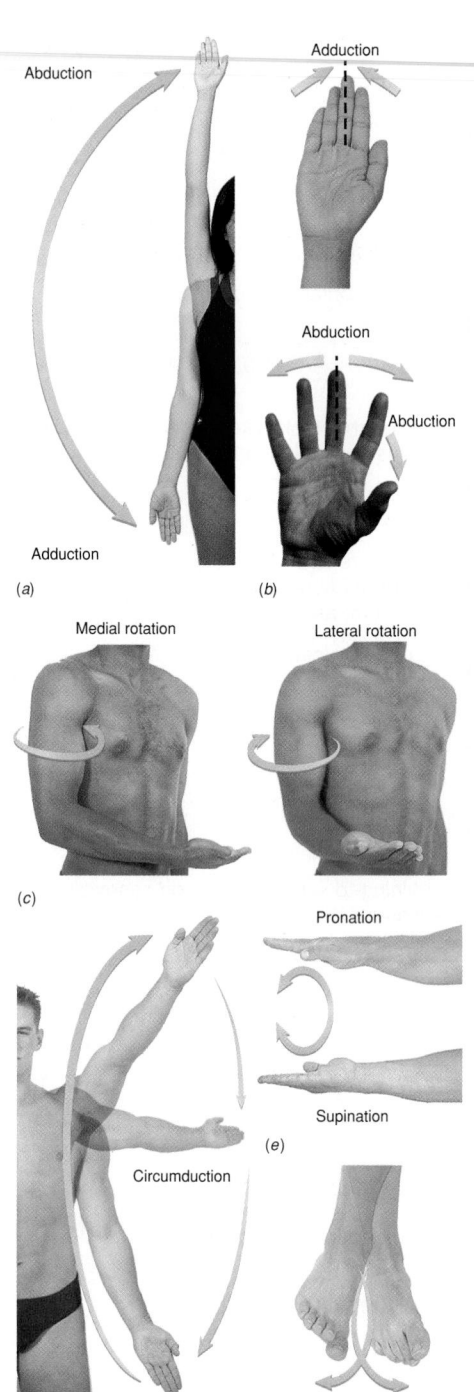

▲ **FIGURE 5.14** **Movement of the Limbs.** (a) Abduction and adduction of the upper limb. (b) Abduction and adduction of the fingers. (c) Medial and lateral rotation of the arm. (d) Circumduction. (e) Pronation and supination of the hand. (f) Eversion and inversion of the foot.

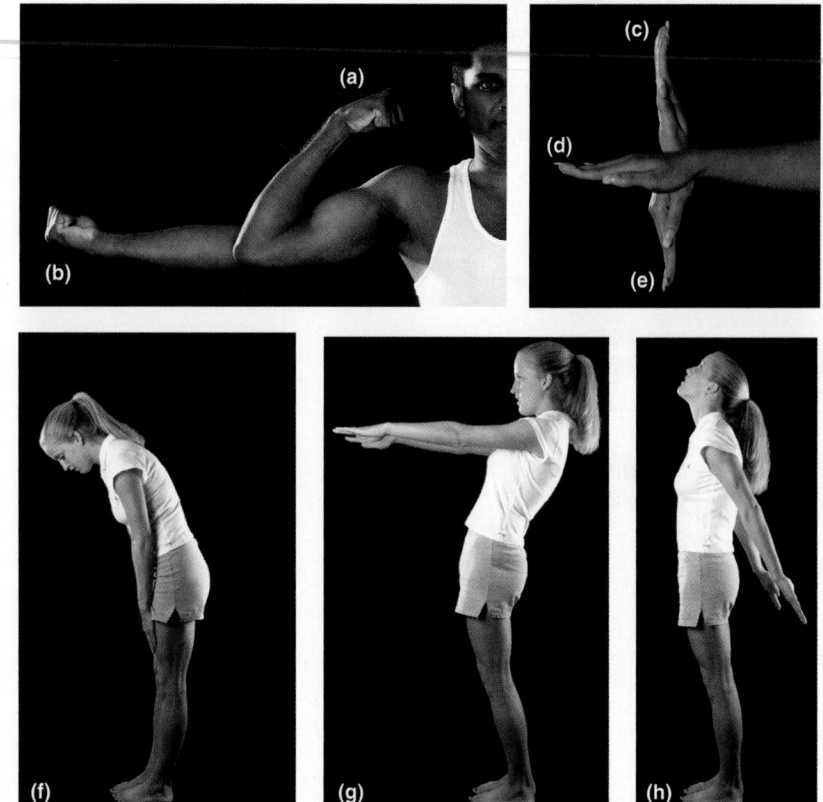

▲ **Figure 5.13** **Joint Flexion and Extension.** (a) Flexion of the elbow. (b) Extension of the elbow. (c) Extension of the wrist. (d) Neutral position of the wrist. (e) Flexion of the wrist. (f) Flexion of the spine. (g) Flexion of the shoulder. (h) Extension of the shoulder.

JOINT MOVEMENT

Flexion and Extension of Joints

Flexion (bending) and **extension** (straightening) are shown in the elbow joint (*Figure 5.13a and b*), in the wrist joint (*Figure 5.13c, d, and e*), and in the shoulder joint (*Figure 5.13g and h*).

For most of the rest of the body, flexion is movement of a body part *anterior* to the **coronal plane** (*see Chapter 2*). Extension is movement *posterior* to the coronal plane. For example, when you bend your trunk forward, that is flexion (*Figure 5.13f*). When you bend your trunk backward, that is extension (*see Figure 5.13g*). When you bend your trunk sideways to the right or left, that is called *lateral flexion*.

Abduction and Adduction of Joints

Abduction is movement away from the midline. **Adduction** is movement toward the midline. Abduction of your arm is moving it sideways away from your trunk. Adduction is bringing it back to the side of your trunk (*Figure 5.14a*). Abduction of your fingers is spreading them apart, away from the middle finger. Adduction is bringing them back together (*Figure 5.14b*).

Rotation of Joints

Rotation is turning around an axis. Medial rotation of the upper arm bone, the humerus, with the elbow flexed brings the palm of the hand toward the body. Lateral rotation moves the palm away from the body (*Figure 5.14c*).

Pronation and Supination

When you lie flat on the ground face-down on your belly with your palms touching the ground, you are **prone.** When you lie flat on your back with your spine on the floor and your palms facing up, you are **supine.**

WORD	PRONUNCIATION	ELEMENTS		DEFINITION
abduction **abduct** (verb)	ab-**DUCK**-shun ab-**DUKT**	S/ P/ R/	**-ion** *process, action* **ab-** *away from* **-duct-** *lead*	Action of moving away from the midline
adduction **adduct** (verb)	ah-**DUCK**-shun ah-**DUCKT**	S/ P/ R/	**-ion** *process, action* **ad-** *toward* **-duct-** *lead*	Action of moving toward the midline
circumduction **circumduct** (verb)	ser-kum-**DUCK**-shun ser-kum-**DUCKT**	S/ P/ R/	**-ion** *process, action* **circum-** *around* **-duct-** *lead*	Movement of an extremity in a circular motion
coronal plane	**KOR**-oh-nal PLAIN	S/ R/	**-al** *pertaining to* **coron-** *crown* **plane** Latin *flat*	Vertical plane dividing the body into anterior and posterior portions
eversion **evert** (verb)	ee-**VER**-shun ee-**VERT**		Latin *overturn*	A turning outward
extension	eks-**TEN**-shun		Latin *stretch out*	Straighten a joint to increase its angle
flexion	**FLEK**-shun		Latin *to bend*	Bend a joint to decrease its angle
inversion **invert** (verb)	in-**VER**-shun in -**VERT**		Latin *to turn about*	A turning inward
prone **pronation** **pronate** (verb)	PRONE pro-**NAY**-shun **PRO**-nate	S/ R/ S/	Latin *prone, lying down* **pronat-** *bend down* **-ion** *process, action*	Lying face-down, flat on your belly Process of lying face-down or of turning a hand or foot with the volar (palm or sole) surface down
supine **supination**	soo-**PINE** soo-pih-**NAY**-shun	S/ R/	Latin *supine, lying face-up* **-ion** *process, action* **supinat-** *bend backward*	Lying face-up, flat on your spine Process of lying face-upward or turning an arm or foot so that the palm or sole is facing up

When you rotate your forearm so that your palm faces the floor, that is **pronation**. When you rotate the forearm so that your palm is facing upward, that is **supination** *(Figure 5.14e)*.

Circumduction of Joints

Circumduction of the shoulder is moving it in a circular movement so that it forms a cone, with the shoulder joint as the apex of the cone *(Figure 5.14d)*.

Inversion and Eversion

When you turn your ankle so that the sole of your foot faces toward the opposite foot, that is supination or **inversion**. When you turn your ankle so that the sole of the foot faces laterally away from the other foot, that is pronation or **eversion** *(Figure 5.14f)*.

> ### Study Hint
> In English, to "abduct" someone is to lead them *away from* (their family) or to kidnap them. Abduction is moving *away from* the midline of the body. Adduction is the *opposite* of abduction.

EXERCISES

Some medical terms can act as both a verb (action) and a noun (person, place or thing). The following pairs of terms are both verbs and nouns. Write the correct form of each term in the blank.

1. circumduct   circumduction

   The baseball pitcher was unable to

   _____ his arm to wind up his pitch.

2. invert   inversion

   A clubfoot would be an _____ of the foot.

3. abduct   abduction

   Moving away from the midline of the body is called

   _____.

4. evert   eversion

   The patient was unable to _____ her ankle due to great pain.

5. adduct   adduction

   The patient was asked to _____ his arms from a horizontal plane toward the center of his chest.

- **Arthrocentesis**—withdrawal of fluid from a joint through a needle. (The suffix -**centesis** means *to puncture*.)

- **Arthrodesis**—fixation or stiffening of a joint by surgery. (The suffix -**desis** means *to fuse together*.)

- **Arthrography**—an x-ray of a joint taken after the injection of a contrast medium into the joint. A contrast medium makes the inside details of the joint visible. (The suffix -**graphy** means *process of recording*.)

- **Arthroplasty**—surgery to restore as far as possible the function of a joint; often involves a total replacement of the joint. (The suffix -**plasty** means *surgical repair*.)

- **Arthroscopy**—the visual examination of the interior of a joint using an **arthroscope**. (The suffix -**scopy** means *to view*.)

Abbreviations

DJD	degenerative joint disease
MCP	metacarpophalangeal
OA	osteoarthritis
PIP	proximal interphalangeal
THR	total-hip replacement
RA	rheumatoid arthritis

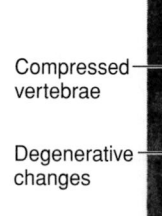

Case Report 5.2 (continued)

By age 65, more than 80% of people have some degree of joint degeneration. Mr. Johnson had always been very physically active, putting a lot of pressure on his weight-bearing joints. At different times in his life he had been overweight, adding to the pressure.

X-rays of his lower back showed **osteoarthritis** of his lower lumbar intervertebral joints and marked osteoarthritis of his left hip joint *(Figure 5.15a and b)*. He received a left total-hip replacement **(THR)** and physiotherapy for his lower back.

DISEASES OF JOINTS

Osteoarthritis (OA) is caused by the breakdown and eventual destruction of cartilage in a joint. It develops as a result of wear and tear and is most common in the weight-bearing joints, the knee, hip, and lower back *(Figure 5.15a)*. Because it is a wear-and-tear disease, it is sometimes called **degenerative joint disease (DJD)**. The degenerative process begins in the articular cartilage, which cracks and frays, eventually exposing the underlying bone.

Rheumatoid arthritis (RA) is a chronic, inflammatory disease that can affect many joints, causing deformity and disability. In *Figure 5.15b*, the hand deformities of RA, swelling of the **metacarpophalangeal (MCP)** and **proximal interphalangeal (PIP)** joints with **ulnar deviation** of the fingers, are shown. The disease process initially causes inflammation of the synovial membrane and then spreads to all other parts of the joint. Rheumatoid arthritis is three times as common in women and often begins in the thirties and forties.

Bursitis is inflammation of a **bursa** that can result from overuse of a joint, repeated trauma, or diseases such as RA.

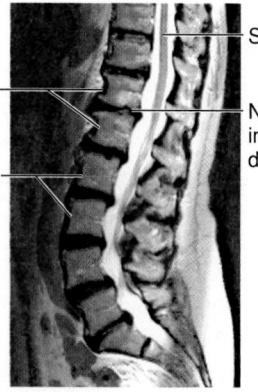

(a) Lumbar vertebrae

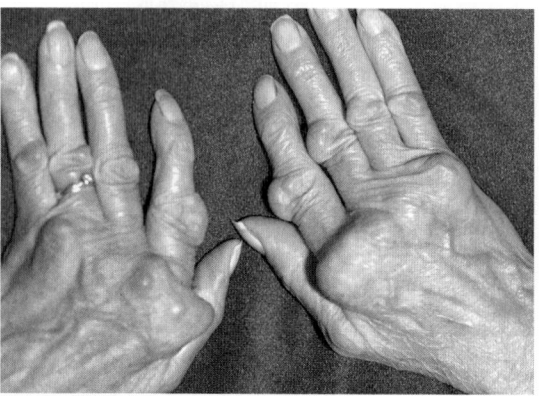

(b)

FIGURE 5.15   Arthritis. (*a*) MRI scan of lumbar vertebrae showing degenerative changes due to osteoarthritis. (*b*) Rheumatoid arthritis of the hands.

WORD ANALYSIS AND DEFINITION

S = Suffix   P = Prefix   R = Root   R/CF = Combining Form

WORD	PRONUNCIATION	ELEMENTS		DEFINITION
arthrocentesis	**AR**-throw-sen-**TEE**-sis	S/ R/	-centesis *to puncture* arthr/o- *joint*	Withdrawal of fluid from a joint through a needle
arthrodesis	ar-**THROW**-dee-sis	S/ R/CF	-desis *bind together* arthr/o- *joint*	Fixation or stiffening of a joint by surgery
arthrography	ar-**THROG**-ra-fee	S/ R/CF	-graphy *process of recording* arthr/o- *joint*	X-ray of a joint taken after the injection of a contrast medium into the joint
arthroplasty	**AR**-throw-plas-tee	S/ R/CF	-plasty *surgical repair* arthr/o- *joint*	Surgery to restore as far as possible the function of a joint
arthroscopy	ar-**THROS**-koh-pee	S/ R/CF	-scopy *to examine, to view* arthr/o- *joint*	Visual examination of the interior of a joint
arthroscope	**AR**-thro-skope	S/	-scope *instrument for viewing*	Endoscope used to examine the interior of a joint
bursa bursitis	**BURR**-sah burr-**SIGH**-tis	S/	Latin *purse* -itis *inflammation*	A closed sac containing synovial fluid Inflammation of a bursa
degenerative	dee-**JEN**-er-a-tiv	S/ R/	-ive *quality of* degenerat- *deteriorate*	Relating to the deterioration of a structure
deviation	de-ve-**A**-shun		Latin *turn from straight path*	A turning aside from a normal course
interphalangeal	**IN**-ter-fay-**LAN**-jee-al	S/ P/ R/CF	-al *pertaining to* inter- *between* -phalang/e- *phalanx*	Pertaining to the joints between two phalanges
metacarpophalangeal	**MET**-ah-**KAR**-poh-fay-**LAN**-jee-al	S/ R/CF P/ R/CF	-al *pertaining to* -phalang/e- *phalanx* meta- *after, beyond* -carp/o- *bones of the wrist*	Pertaining to the joints between the metacarpal bones and phalanges
osteoarthritis	**OS**-tee-oh-ar-**THRI**-tis	S/ R/CF R/	-itis *inflammation* oste/o- *bone* -arthr- *joint*	Chronic inflammatory disease of the joints with pain and loss of function
rheumatoid arthritis (RA)	**RHU**-mah-toyd ar-**THRI**-tis	S/ R/	-oid *resemble* rheumat- *rheumatism*	Disease of connective tissue, with arthritis as a major manifestation
ulna	**UL**-na	R/CF	uln/a *forearm bone*	The medial and larger bone of the forearm
ulnar	**UL**-nar	S/ R/CF	-ar *pertaining to* uln/a- *forearm bone*	Pertaining to the ulna or any of the structures (artery, vein, nerve) named after it

EXERCISES

There are seven terms in this WAD all using the root or combining form arthr/arthro-. For questions 1 through 5, match the description of the procedure for which each patient is scheduled in the left column with the name of the procedure the doctor has ordered in the right column. Then fill in the blanks.

_____ 1. X-ray of a joint after contrast-medium injection

_____ 2. Withdrawal of fluid from the joint with a needle

_____ 3. Surgery to restore or repair joint function

_____ 4. Surgical fixation of the joint

_____ 5. Visual examination of the interior of the joint

A. arthrodesis

B. arthroplasty

C. arthroscopy

D. arthrography

E. arthrocentesis

6. The procedure in question 5 will use an arthro _____.

7. The diagnosis for all these patients could be arthr _____.

OBJECTIVES

In the previous two lessons in this chapter, you have learned how bones of the skeleton support the body and how joints provide mobility. Neither of these functions can occur without muscles to provide both posture and movement. Information in this lesson will enable you to use correct medical terminology to:

5.3.1 **Identify the functions of skeletal muscle and tendons.**

5.3.2 **Describe the structure of skeletal muscle and tendons.**

5.3.3 **Demonstrate an understanding of the major problems and diseases that occur in muscles and tendons.**

You are

...a medical assistant working with Susan Lee, MD, a primary care physician at Fulwood Medical Center.

Your patient is

...Mrs. Mary Carr, a 65-year-old white, retired librarian, who had been in good health until a month ago when she had sudden onset of pain in the muscles of her shoulders and hips.

CASE REPORT 5.3

The pain has become more severe and spread into Mrs. Carr's upper arms, thighs, and lower back. She cannot turn over in bed and cannot get into her car. She has lost 10 pounds in weight and feels constantly tired.

Dr. Lee has diagnosed **polymyalgia rheumatica** and prescribed **prednisone**, 5 mg t.i.d. (three times daily). There has been a marked improvement in her symptoms.

Your role as Dr. Lee's assistant is to ensure that Mrs. Carr understands the use of her medication and to document changes in her symptoms.

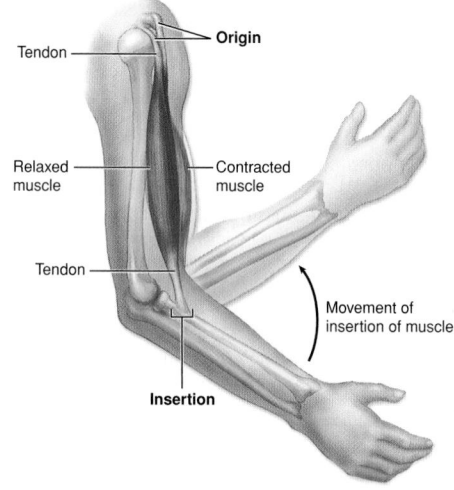

Tendon — Origin

Relaxed muscle — Contracted muscle

Tendon

Movement of insertion of muscle

Insertion

▲ **FIGURE 5.16** **Muscle Contraction.**

Abbreviation

t.i.d. (Latin *ter in die*) three times a day

FUNCTIONS AND STRUCTURE OF SKELETAL MUSCLE

Functions of Skeletal Muscle

Skeletal muscle is attached to one or more bones. It is called **voluntary** because it is under conscious control. Because of their length, muscle cells are usually called muscle **fibers.** Each skeletal muscle consists of bundles of muscle fibers, blood vessels, and nerves, with connective tissue sheets that hold the fibers together and connect the muscle to bone.

Skeletal muscle has the following functions:

1. **Movement.** All skeletal muscles are attached to bones, and when a muscle **contracts** it causes movement of the bones to which it is attached *(Figure 5.16)*. This enables you to walk, run, and work with your hands.

2. **Posture.** The **tone** of skeletal muscles holds you straight when sitting, standing, or moving.

3. **Body heat.** When skeletal muscles contract, heat is produced as a by-product of the energy reaction. This heat is essential to maintain your body temperature.

4. **Respiration.** Skeletal muscles move the chest wall as you breathe.

5. **Communication.** Skeletal muscles enable you to speak, write, type, gesture, and grimace.

Structure of Skeletal Muscle

Skeletal **fibers** are narrow and long, up to 1½ inches (approximately 3.7 cm) in length. Each muscle fiber has a thin layer of connective tissue around it. Bundles of muscle fibers are grouped together into **fascicles** that are also surrounded by a layer of connective tissue. Skeletal muscle fibers contain alternating dark and

WORD	PRONUNCIATION		ELEMENTS	DEFINITION
Duchenne muscular dystrophy	**DOO**-shen **MUSS**-kyu-lar **DISS**-troh-fee	P/ R/	Guillaume Benjamin Duchenne, French neurologist, 1806–1875 **dys-** *bad, difficult* **-trophy** *nourishment*	A condition with symmetrical weakness and wasting of pelvic, shoulder, and proximal limb muscles
fibromyalgia	fie-bro-my-**AL**-jee-ah	S/ R/CF R/	**-algia** *pain* **fibr/o-** *fiber* **-my-** *muscle*	Pain in the muscle fibers
myoglobin	**MY**-oh-**GLOW**-bin	S/ R/CF R/	**-in** *substance* **my/o-** *muscle* **-glob-** *globe*	Protein of muscle that stores and transports oxygen
neurotransmitter (**Note:** *Transmitter* is a word in itself and begins with a prefix.)	**NYUR**-oh-trans-**MIT**-er	S/ R/CF P/ R/	**-er** *agent* **neur/o-** *nerve* **-trans-** *across* **-mitt-** *to send*	Chemical agent that relays messages from one nerve cell to the next
rhabdomyolysis	**RAB**-doh-my-oh-**LIE**-sis	S/ R/CF R/CF	**-lysis** *destruction* **rhabd/o-** *rod shaped* **-my/o-** *muscle*	Destruction of muscle to produce myoglobin
sprain	SPRAIN		root unknown	A wrench or tear in a ligament
strain	STRAIN		Latin *to bind*	Overstretch or tear in a muscle or tendon
tendon **tendinitis** (also spelled **tendonitis**)	**TEN**-dun ten-dih-**NYE**-tis	S/ R/	Latin *sinew* **-itis** *inflammation* **tendin-** *tendon*	Fibrous band that connects muscle to bone Inflammation of a tendon
tenosynovitis	**TEN**-oh-sine-oh-**VIE**-tis	S/ R/CF R/	**-itis** *inflammation* **ten/o-** *tendon* **-synov-** *synovial membrane*	Inflammation of a tendon and its surrounding synovial sheath
thymectomy	thigh-**MEK**-toe-me	S/ R/	**-ectomy** *surgical excision* **thym-** *thymus gland*	Surgical removal of the thymus gland

EXERCISES

The following elements are all contained in the WAD above. Circle the best answer.

1. The suffix **-itis** means: condition   disease   inflammation

2. **Dys** is a: suffix   prefix   root

3. The root **trophy-** means: condition   procedure   nourishment

4. **Fibro** is a: combining form   root   suffix

5. The root **my-** means: tendon   ligament   muscle

6. The suffix **-algia** means: inflammation   pain   swelling

7. **Ectomy** means: fixation   repair   excision

8. **Neuro** means: muscle   nerve   joint

9. **Teno** is a: prefix   root   combining form

LESSON 5.4 Axial Skeleton

OBJECTIVES

To treat patients with spinal injuries and educate them about their problems, you must have a complete knowledge about the structure and functions of their vertebral columns and joints and muscles.

The vertebral column is part of the axial skeleton. In this lesson, information about the axial skeleton, with its joints and the muscles that function in an integrated manner, will enable you to use correct medical terminology to:

5.4.1 Name the regions and bones of the vertebral column.

5.4.2 Describe an intervertebral joint.

5.4.3 Identify the major muscles that hold the vertebral column erect.

5.4.4 Explain the major problems and diseases that affect the vertebral column.

5.4.5 Name the bones of the skull.

5.4.6 Identify the major muscles of mastication and respiration.

You are

. . . a physical therapist assistant working in the Physical Therapy Department of Fulwood Medical Center.

Your patient is

. . . Ms. Nancy Cardenas, a 27-year-old jeweler. Ms. Cardenas was waiting in her car at a traffic light 3 days ago when her car was rear-ended.

CASE REPORT 5.4

She now has severe neck pain radiating down her left arm, with dizziness and headaches. She is unable to go to work. Dr. Stannard has examined her and diagnosed her condition as a **whiplash** injury. A magnetic resonance image (MRI) shows **herniation** of intervertebral discs between C5–C6 and C6–C7. Your role is to implement a regime of physiotherapy, including range-of-motion (ROM) exercises for her neck joints.

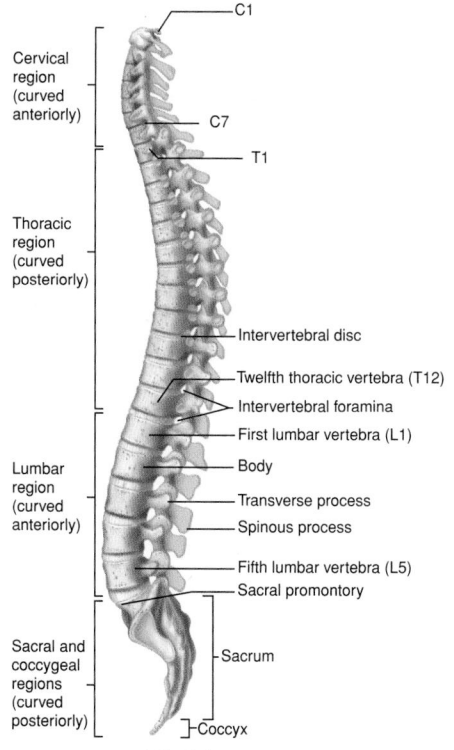

Cervical region (curved anteriorly)

C1

C7

T1

Thoracic region (curved posteriorly)

Intervertebral disc

Twelfth thoracic vertebra (T12)

Intervertebral foramina

First lumbar vertebra (L1)

Lumbar region (curved anteriorly)

Body

Transverse process

Spinous process

Fifth lumbar vertebra (L5)

Sacral promontory

Sacral and coccygeal regions (curved posteriorly)

Sacrum

Coccyx

Lateral view

▲ **FIGURE 5.19 Vertebral Column.**

STRUCTURE OF AXIAL SKELETON

The axial skeleton comprises the:

1. Vertebral column

2. Skull

3. Rib cage

The axial skeleton is the upright axis of the body and protects the brain, spinal cord, heart, and lungs—most of the major centers of our physiology.

The **vertebral column** has 26 bones divided into five regions *(Figure 5.19)*:

1. **Cervical** region, with seven vertebrae, labeled C1 to C7 and curved anteriorly.

2. **Thoracic** region, with 12 vertebrae, labeled T1 to T12 and curved posteriorly.

3. **Lumbar** region, with five vertebrae, labeled L1 to L5 and curved anteriorly.

4. **Sacral** region, with one bone curved posteriorly.

5. **Coccyx** (tailbone), with one bone curved posteriorly.

The **spinal cord** lies protected in the vertebral canal. Spinal nerves leave the spinal cord through the **intervertebral foramina** to travel to other parts of the body.

Intervertebral discs consist of fibrocartilage and inhabit the intervertebral space between the bodies of adjacent vertebrae. They provide additional support and cushioning for the vertebral column. The center of the disc is a gelatinous nucleus pulposus.

WORD	PRONUNCIATION	ELEMENTS		DEFINITION
cervical	**SER**-vih-kal	S/ R/	-al *pertaining to* cervic- *neck*	Pertaining to the neck region
coccyx	**KOK**-sicks		Greek *coccyx*	Small tailbone at the lowest end of the vertebral column
foramen foramina (pl)	fo-**RAY**-men fo-**RAM**-in-ah		Latin *an aperture*	An opening through a structure
herniation herniate (verb)	**HER**-nee-ay-shun **HER**-nee-ate	S/ R/CF	-tion *process, being* herni/a- *rupture*	Protrusion of an anatomical structure from its normal position.
intervertebral	**IN**-ter-**VER**-teh-bral	S/ P/ R/	-al *pertaining to* inter- *between* -vertebr- *vertebra*	The space between two vertebrae
kyphosis kyphotic (adj)	ki-**FOH**-sis ki-**FOT**-ik		French *humpbacked*	A normal posterior curve of the thoracic spine that can be exaggerated in disease
lordosis lordotic (adj)	lore-**DOH**-sis lore-**DOT**-ik		Greek *bend backward*	An exaggerated forward curvature of the lumbar spine
lumbar	**LUM**-bar		Latin *loin*	Region in the back and sides between the ribs and pelvis
sacrum sacral (adj)	**SAY**-crum **SAY**-kral		Latin *sacred*	Segment of the vertebral column that forms part of the pelvis
scoliosis scoliotic (adj)	skoh-lee-**OH**-sis **SKOH**-lee-**OT**-ik		Greek *crooked*	An abnormal lateral curvature of the vertebral column
spine spinal (adj)	SPINE **SPY**-nal		Latin *spine*	Vertebral column, *or* a short projection from a bone
thorax thoracic (adj)	**THO**-racks **THOR**-ass-ik		Greek *breastplate*	The part of the trunk between the abdomen and neck
vertebra vertebrae (pl) vertebral (adj)	**VER**-teh-brah **VER**-teh-bray **VER**-teh-bral		Latin *spinal joint*	One of the bones of the spinal column
whiplash	**WHIP**-lash	R/ R/	whip- *to swing* -lash *end of whip*	Symptoms caused by sudden, uncontrolled extension and flexion of the neck, often in an automobile accident

Abnormal spinal curvatures can result from disease, poor posture, or congenital defects in the vertebrae. The defect that is most common is called **scoliosis,** an abnormal lateral curve in the thoracic region *(Figure 5.20a)*. In older people, particularly with osteoporosis, an exaggerated thoracic curvature is called **kyphosis** *(Figure 5.20b)*. An exaggerated lumbar curve is called **lordosis** *(Figure 5.20c)*.

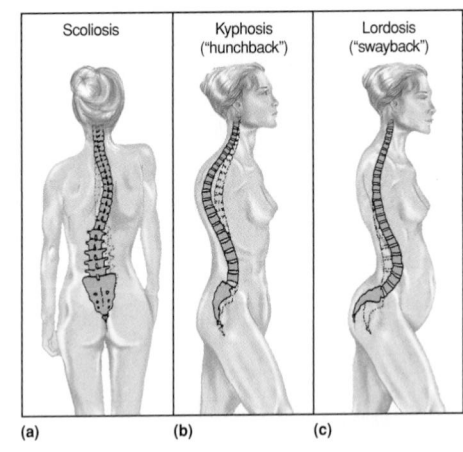

Scoliosis   Kyphosis ("hunchback")   Lordosis ("swayback")

(a)   (b)   (c)

FIGURE 5.20   **Abnormal Spinal Curvatures.** ▶
(a) Scoliosis. (b) Kyphosis. (c) Lordosis.

EXERCISES   *After reading Case Report 5.4 on the opposite page, answer the following questions. Be prepared to discuss your answers in class.*

1. What are Ms. Cardenas' presenting symptoms? _____

2. What medical term means *the space between two vertebrae?* _____

3. What caused the patient's whiplash injury? _____

4. Herniation of a disc means _____ .

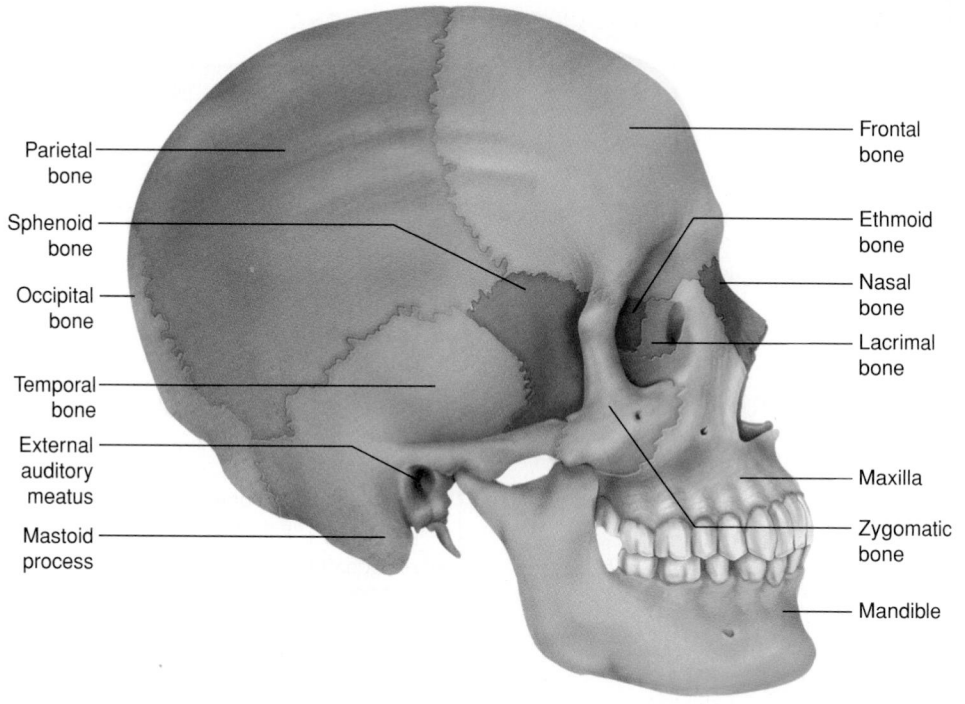

Parietal bone
Sphenoid bone
Occipital bone
Temporal bone
External auditory meatus
Mastoid process
Frontal bone
Ethmoid bone
Nasal bone
Lacrimal bone
Maxilla
Zygomatic bone
Mandible

▲ **FIGURE 5.21   Skull: Right Lateral View.**

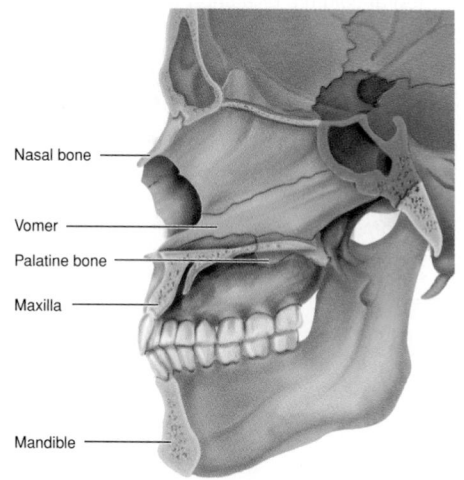

Nasal bone
Vomer
Palatine bone
Maxilla
Mandible

▲ **FIGURE 5.22   Facial Bones.**

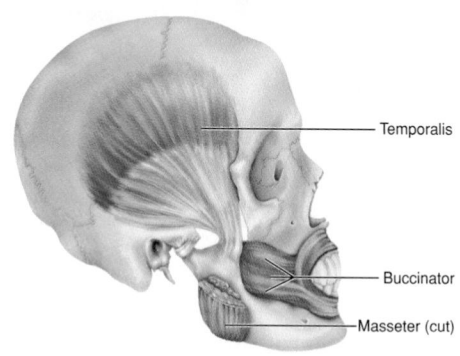

Temporalis
Buccinator
Masseter (cut)

▲ **FIGURE 5.23   Muscles of Chewing.**

THE SKULL

The human skull has 22 bones, 8 of which make up the **cranium,** the upper part of the skull that encloses the **cranial cavity** and protects the brain *(Figure 5.21).* The bones of the cranium are:

1. **Frontal** bone—forms the forehead and the roofs of the orbits and contains a pair of right and left frontal sinuses above the orbits.

2. **Parietal** bones (2)—form the bulging sides and roof of the cranium.

3. **Occipital** bone—forms the back of and part of the base of the cranium.

4. **Temporal** bones (2)—form the sides and part of the base of the cranium.

5. **Sphenoid** bone—forms part of the base of the cranium and the orbits.

6. **Ethmoid** bone—forms parts of the nose and the orbits and is hollow, forming the ethmoid sinuses.

The bones of the cranium are joined together by sutures, joints that appear as seams, covered on the inside and outside by a thin layer of connective tissue.

The lower anterior part of the skull comprises the 14 bones of the facial skeleton *(Figure 5.22; see also Figure 5.21):*

1. **Maxillary** bones (2)—form the upper jaw, hold the upper teeth, and are hollow, forming the maxillary sinuses.

2. **Palatine** bones (2)—are located behind the maxilla.

3. **Zygomatic** bones (2)—form the prominences of the cheeks below the eyes.

4. **Lacrimal** bones (2)—form the medial wall of each eye orbit.

5. **Nasal** bones (2)—form the sides and bridge of the nose.

6. **Vomer** bone—separates the two nasal cavities *(see Figure 5.22).*

7. Inferior nasal **conchae** (2)—fragile bones in the lower nasal cavity.

8. **Mandible**—the lower jawbone, which holds the lower teeth.

The third component of the axial skeleton, the rib cage, is discussed in *Chapter 8.*

Bones, Joints, and Muscles of Mastication

The **temporomandibular joint (TMJ)** connects the condyle of the mandible to a fossa in the temporal bone at the base of the skull. The joint acts like a hinge when you open and close your mouth.

The muscles you use to chew food include:

1. The **masseter,** which raises the jawbone and controls the rate at which you lower it *(Figure 5.23).*

2. The **temporalis,** a fan-shaped muscle that raises the jawbone.

3. The medial **pterygoid,** which closes the jaw and moves it from side to side.

4. The lateral pterygoid, which opens the mouth and moves the jawbone from side to side.

WORD	PRONUNCIATION	ELEMENTS		DEFINITION
concha conchae (pl)	**KON**-kah **KON**-key		Latin *a shell*	Shell-shaped bone on medial wall of nasal cavity
cranium cranial (adj)	**KRAY**-nee-um **KRAY**-nee-al		Greek *skull*	The upper part of the skull that encloses and protects the brain Pertaining to the skull
ethmoid	**ETH**-moyd	S/ R/	-oid *resemble* ethm- *sieve*	Bone that forms the back of the nose and encloses numerous air cells
mandible mandibular (adj)	**MAN**-di-bel man-**DIB**-you-lar	S/ R/	Latin *jaw* -ar *pertaining to* mandibul- *the jaw*	Lower jawbone Pertaining to the mandible
masseter	**MASS**-eh-ter		Greek *to chew*	Muscle that closes the mouth
maxilla maxillary (adj)	mak-**SILL**-ah mak-**SILL**-ary		Latin *jawbone*	Upper jawbone, containing right and left maxillary sinuses
occipital	ock-**SIP**-it-al		Latin *occiput*	The back of the skull
palatine	**PAL**-ah-tine		Latin *palate*	Bone that forms the hard palate and parts of the nose and orbits
parietal	pah-**RYE**-eh-tal	S/ R/	-al *pertaining to* pariet- *wall*	The two bones forming the sidewalls and roof of the cranium
pterygoid	**TER**-ih-goyd	S/ R/	-oid *resemble* pteryg- *wing*	Pterygoid muscles are two wing-shaped muscles that open and close the mouth
sphenoid	**SFEE**-noyd	S/ R/	-oid *resemble* sphen- *wedge*	Wedge-shaped bone at the base of the skull
temporal	**TEM**-por-al	S/ R/	-al *pertaining to* tempor- *temple, side of head*	Bone that forms part of the base and sides of the skull
temporalis muscle	tem-poh-**RAHL**-is **MUSS**-el	S/	-alis *pertaining to*	Muscle attached to temporal bone that opens and closes the jaw
temporomandibular joint (TMJ)	**TEM**-por-oh-man-**DIB**-you-lar JOYNT	S/ R/CF R/	-ar *pertaining to* tempor/o- *temple, side of head* -mandibul- *the jaw*	The joint between the temporal bone and the mandible
vomer	**VOH**-mer		Latin *ploughshare*	Lower nasal septum
zygoma zygomatic (adj)	zye-**GOH**-mah zye-goh-**MAT**-ic		French *yoke*	Bone that forms the prominence of the cheek

Abbreviation

TMJ   temporomandibular joint

EXERCISES

The human skull has 22 bones. Meet a lesson objective by listing the bones of the skull, with a brief description of their location. Fill in the blanks.

These bones make up the cranium (upper skull):

_____   _____

_____   _____

_____   _____

These bones form the lower anterior part of the skull and the facial skeleton:

_____   _____

_____   _____

_____   _____

_____   _____

Appendicular Skeleton, Joints, and Muscles

OBJECTIVES

Attached to the axial skeleton through joints and muscles is the appendicular skeleton, the bones of the upper limbs and the shoulder girdle and those of the lower limbs and the pelvic girdle. These limbs carry out many of the commands issued by your brain in response to changes in your body and in your external environment, particularly in terms of mobility and the manipulation of objects.

An understanding of the terminology, anatomy, and physiology of the bones, joints, and muscles of the limbs and their disorders is a vital part of your overall knowledge of the human body in your work as a health care professional.

Information in this lesson will enable you to use correct medical terminology to:

5.5.1 Describe the structure and functions of the bones, joints, and muscles of the shoulder girdle and upper limbs.

5.5.2 Describe the structure and functions of the bones, joints, and muscles of the pelvic girdle and lower limbs.

5.5.3 Explain the major problems and diseases that affect mobility and other functions of the limbs.

You are

. . . an emergency technician working in the Emergency Department at Fulwood Medical Center.

Your patient is

. . . Mr. Bruce Adams, a 55-year-old construction worker.

CASE REPORT 5.5

Mr. Adams presents with severe pain in his right shoulder that has made him leave work and seek relief. The pain began 3 or 4 months ago; it is worse at the end of the workday and when he has to work with his arm above the shoulder. In the past week, the pain has awakened him from sleep.

A month ago, Mr. Adams reported the symptoms to his employer and was referred to the company physician, who treated him with anti-inflammatory medication and a heating pad. He believes the diagnosis was a shoulder bursitis. He has no previous history of work injuries.

Physical examination shows marked limitation by pain of all passive and active movements of the right shoulder and weakness in all lifting movements.

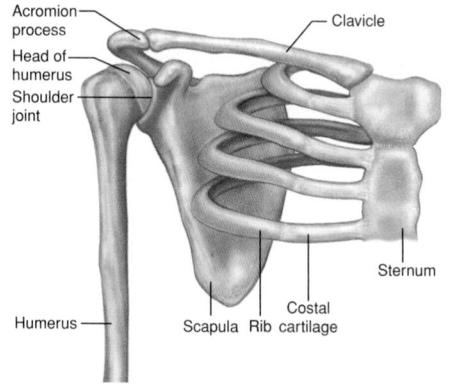

▲ **FIGURE 5.24 Pectoral Girdle.**

Labels: Acromion process, Head of humerus, Shoulder joint, Humerus, Scapula, Rib cartilage, Costal, Clavicle, Sternum

SHOULDER GIRDLE AND UPPER ARM

The **pectoral** (shoulder) **girdle** connects the axial skeleton to the upper limbs and helps with movements of the upper limb.

The bones of the pectoral girdle are the **scapulae** (shoulder blades) and **clavicles** (*Figure 5.24*). The scapula extends over the top of the joint to form a roof called the **acromion**. The acromion is attached to the clavicle at the **acromioclavicular (AC)** joint. This also provides a connection between the axial skeleton, pectoral girdle, and upper arm.

The joint that connects the pectoral girdle to the upper limb is the shoulder joint, located between the scapula and the **humerus** bone of the upper arm (*see Figure 5.24*). This joint is a ball-and-socket joint in which the head of the humerus allows the greatest range of motion of any joint in the body. Because of this, the shoulder joint also is the most unstable joint and is liable to **dislocation.**

Several ligaments hold together the articulating surfaces of the humerus and scapula.

Muscles around the shoulder joint are essential for its stability. Four muscles that originate on the scapula wrap around the joint and fuse to form one large tendon, the **rotator cuff,** which is inserted into the humerus (*Figure 5.25*). This tendon keeps the ball of the humerus tightly in the socket of the scapula and provides the strength that baseball pitchers need. The rotator cuff muscles are:

1. Subscapularis
2. Supraspinatus
3. Infraspinatus
4. Teres minor

Common Disorders of the Shoulder

Rotator cuff tears are the result of the wear and tear of overuse in work situations or in sports actions such as the throwing done by baseball pitchers. The tears

WORD	PRONUNCIATION	ELEMENTS		DEFINITION
acromion acromioclavicular (AC)	ah-**CROW**-mee-on ah-**CROW**-mee-oh- klah-**VICK**-you-lar	S/ R/ S/ R/CF R/	-ion *action* acrom- *extremity* -ar *pertaining to* acromi/o- *acromion* -clavicul- *clavicle*	Lateral end of the scapula, extending over the shoulder joint The joint between the acromion and the clavicle
clavicle clavicular (adj)	**KLAV**-ih-kul klah-**VICK**-you-lar		Latin *collarbone*	Curved bone that forms the anterior part of the pectoral girdle
dislocation	dis-low-**KAY**-shun	S/ P/ R/	-ion *action* dis- *apart* -locat- *a place*	The state of being completely out of joint
humerus	**HYU**-mer-us		Latin *shoulder*	Single bone of the upper arm
pectoral pectoral girdle	**PEK**-tor-al **PEK**-tor-al **GIR**-del	S/ R/	-al *pertaining to* pector- *chest* **girdle** Old English *encircle*	Pertaining to the chest Incomplete bony ring that attaches the upper limb to the axial skeleton
rotator cuff	roh-**TAY**-tor CUFF	S/ R/	-or *a doer* rotat- *rotate* **cuff** Old English *band*	Part of the capsule of the shoulder joint
scapula scapulae (pl) scapular (adj)	**SKAP**-you-lah **SKAP**-you-lee **SKAP**-you-lar	 S/ R/	Latin *shoulder blade* -ar *pertaining to* scapul- *scapula*	Shoulder blade Pertaining to the shoulder blade
subluxation	sub-luck-**SAY**-shun	S/ P/ R/	-ion *action* sub- *under, slightly* -luxat- *dislocate*	An incomplete dislocation in which some contact between the joint surfaces remains

Case Report 5.5 (continued)

When Mr. Adams was evaluated by Dr. Stannard, an x-ray (which looks for bony abnormalities) revealed no shoulder abnormality. An MRI, which shows slices of all tissues, revealed a full-thickness tear of the rotator cuff.

can be partial or complete and usually require surgical repair.

Shoulder separation is a dislocation of the acromioclavicular joint, usually due to a fall on the point of the shoulder.

Shoulder dislocation occurs when the ball of the humerus slips out of the socket of the scapula, usually anteriorly.

Shoulder subluxation occurs when the ball of the humerus slips partially out of position and then moves back in.

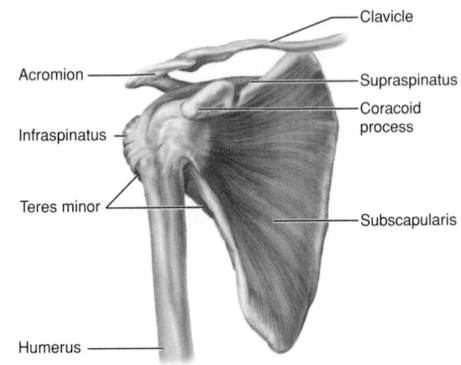

▲ **FIGURE 5.25   Rotator Cuff Muscles.**

EXERCISES   *Use your knowledge of the **language of orthopedics** to complete the following medical terms. The term is defined and partially complete. Add the rest of the elements to complete the term, and write under the line the element(s) you have used. The first one is done for you. Fill in the blanks.*

1. Incomplete dislocation   _____*sub*_____ / _____*luxat*_____ / _____*ion*_____
         P   R   S

2. Joint between acromion and clavicle   _____ / _____ / _____*ar*_____

3. Completely out of joint   _____*dis*_____ / _____ / _____

4. Pertaining to the chest   _____ / _____ / _____*al*_____

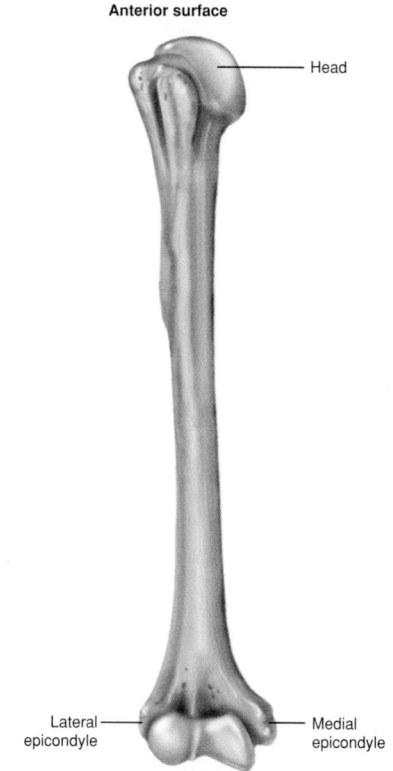

Anterior surface

— Head

Lateral epicondyle — — Medial epicondyle

▲ **FIGURE 5.26** **Humerus.**

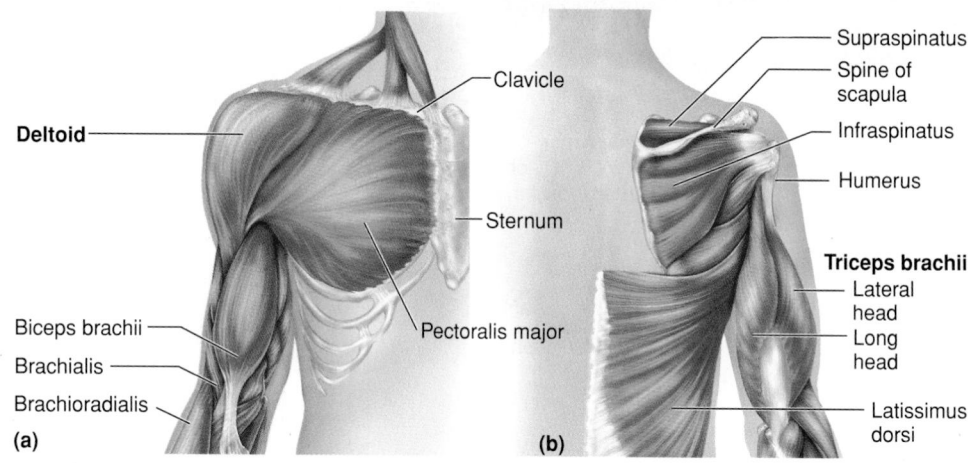

Deltoid ———

— Clavicle

— Sternum

Biceps brachii ———
Brachialis ———
Brachioradialis —
(a)

— Pectoralis major

— Supraspinatus
— Spine of scapula
— Infraspinatus
— Humerus

Triceps brachii
— Lateral head
— Long head

— Latissimus dorsi
(b)

▲ **FIGURE 5.27** **Muscles Joining Arm to Body.** (*a*) Anterior view. (*b*) Posterior view.

UPPER ARM AND ELBOW JOINT

The **humerus** is the long bone of the upper arm (*Figure 5.26*). It extends from the scapula to the elbow joint. Muscles connect it to the pectoral girdle, vertebral column, and ribs. These muscles enable the arm to be freely movable at the shoulder joint. The major anterior muscles are the **deltoid** and **pectoralis major** (*Figure 5.27a*), and among the major posterior muscles is the **latissimus dorsi** (*Figure 5.27b*).

The elbow joint has two **articulations:**

1. A hinge joint between the humerus and **ulna** bone of the forearm, which allows flexion and extension of the elbow.

2. A gliding joint between the humerus and **radius** bone of the forearm, which allows pronation and supination of the forearm and hand.

A joint capsule and ligaments hold the two articulations together.

Muscles that move the elbow joint and forearm have their **origins** on the humerus or pectoral girdle and are **inserted** into the bones of the forearm. On the front of the arm, a group of three muscles (the **biceps brachii, brachialis,** and **brachioradialis**) flexes the forearm at the elbow joint and rotates the forearm and hand laterally (supination) (*Figure 5.28*). On the back of the arm, a single muscle, the **triceps brachii,** extends the elbow joint and forearm (*Figure 5.27b*).

Common Disorders of the Elbow

Tennis elbow is caused by overuse of the elbow joint or poor techniques playing tennis or golf. Tendons of upper-arm and forearm muscles are inserted into the medial and lateral **epicondyles** of the humerus just above the elbow joint (*Figure 5.27*). Small tears in the tendons at their attachments occur with overuse, and eventually enough tears accumulate to cause pain and restrict elbow movement. The pain occurs when straightening the elbow or opening and closing the fingers. Treatment is rest, ice, pain medication, massage, and stretching exercises.

Ligament strains and **bone fractures** due to a heavy fall or a blow to the elbow are also common injuries.

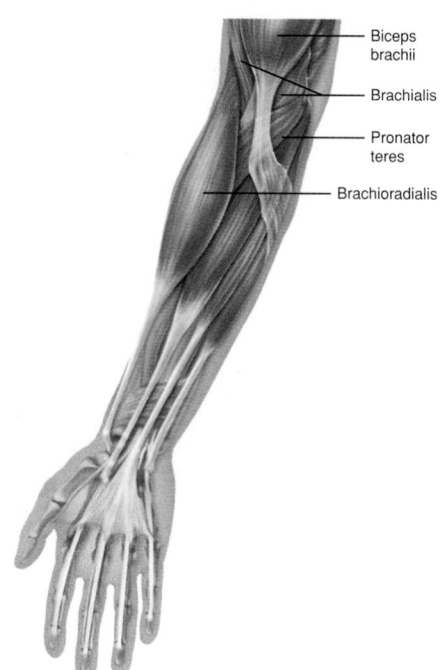

— Biceps brachii
— Brachialis
— Pronator teres
— Brachioradialis

▲ **FIGURE 5.28** **Muscles of Elbow Joint.**

S = Suffix   P = Prefix   R = Root   R/CF = Combining Form

WORD	PRONUNCIATION		ELEMENTS	DEFINITION
biceps brachii	BYE-sepz BRAY-key-eye	P/ R/ R/	bi- *two* -ceps *head* brachii *of the arm*	A muscle of the upper arm that has two heads or points of origin on the scapula
brachialis	BRAY-kee-al-is	S/ R/	-alis *pertaining to* brachi- *arm*	Muscle that lies underneath the biceps and is the strongest flexor of the forearm
brachioradialis	BRAY-kee-oh-RAY-dee-al-is	S/ R/CF R/	-is *belonging to* brachi/o- *arm* -radial- *radius*	Muscle that helps flex the forearm
deltoid	DEL-toyd	S/ R/	-oid *resembling* delt- *Greek letter delta*	Large, fan-shaped muscle connecting the scapula and clavicle to the humerus
epicondyle	ep-ih-KON-dile	P/ R/	epi- *above* -condyle *knuckle*	Projection above the condyle for attachment of a ligament or tendon
insertion	in-SIR-shun	S/ R/	-ion *process* insert- *put together*	The insertion of a muscle is the attachment of a muscle to a more movable part of the skeleton, as distinct from the origin
latissimus dorsi	la-TISS-ih-muss DOOR-sigh	S/ R/ R/	-imus *most* latiss- *wide* dorsi *back*	The widest (broadest) muscle in the back
origin	OR-ih-gin		Latin *source of*	Fixed source of a muscle at its attachment to bone
radius	RAY-dee-us		Latin *spoke of a wheel*	The forearm bone on the thumb side
triceps brachii	TRY-sepz BRAY-key-eye	P/ R/ R/	tri- *three* -ceps *head* brachii *of the arm*	Muscle of the arm that has three heads or points of origin

EXERCISES

There would be no movement without bones and muscles. Reduce the terminology of the following muscles to the basic elements. Fill in the chart; then fill in the blanks with the terms from the chart.

Muscle	Prefix	Root/CF	Suffix
biceps brachii			
brachialis			
brachioradialis			
deltoid			
latissimus dorsi			
triceps brachii			

Using the terms from the chart, write the name of the correct muscle on the line next to its description.

1. Three heads or points of origin _____

2. Strongest flexor of the forearm _____

3. Fan-shaped muscle _____

4. Helps flex the forearm _____

5. Two points of origin on the scapula _____

6. Broadest muscle of the back _____

CASE REPORT 5.6

The office accounting system is computerized, and Ms. Baker works at a keyboard all day, inputting charges and payments. For the past 3 months, she has had constant pain in her right hand, arm, and shoulder. She has numbness and tingling in her fingers and drops things out of her right hand. She is now unable to work.

Dr. Stannard has diagnosed tenosynovitis of the wrist. He has prescribed an anti-inflammatory medication, physiotherapy **(PT)**, and a brace for the wrist. Ms. Baker is to ask for an **ergonomic** keyboard for her computer.

She requires help in filling out her worker's compensation form. (This task is an exercise at the end of the chapter.)

FOREARM AND WRIST

The forearm has two bones, the **radius** on the thumb side and the **ulna** on the little-finger side. They articulate at the wrist joint with the small **carpal** bones. The muscles of the forearm **supinate** and **pronate** the forearm, flex and extend the wrist joint and hand, and move the hand medially and laterally.

Your forearm is bigger near the elbow because the fleshy bellies of the forearm muscles are bulky. Your wrist is much thinner because the muscles have become tendons that pass over the wrist on the way to being inserted into the bones of the fingers. As the tendons pass over the wrist, they are surrounded by sheaths of synovial membrane and held in place on the wrist by a transverse, thick fibrous band called a **retinaculum** *(Figure 5.29)*.

Common Disorders of the Wrist

Ganglion cysts are fluid-filled cysts arising when the synovial tendon sheaths that run over the back of the wrist are irritated or inflamed. They often disappear spontaneously.

Stenosing tenosynovitis is inflammation of the synovial sheaths on the back of the wrist that causes pressure to develop under the retinaculum, producing pain in the wrist. This is what happened to Ms. Baker.

Carpal tunnel syndrome *(Figure 5.29)* develops similarly on the front of the wrist as a result of inflammation and swelling of tendon sheaths arising from overuse of repetitive movements, such as those in computer keyboard operation. The swelling compresses the **median nerve** between the carpal bones and the retinaculum. This causes "pins and needles" or pain and loss of muscle power in the thumb side of the hand. The retinaculum may need to be incised and released (**fasciotomy**).

Colles fracture is a common fracture of the radius just above the wrist joint. It occurs when a person tries to break a fall with an outstretched hand. The distal radius just proximal to the wrist is broken. In some cases, the distal ulnar is also fractured and the wrist joint dislocated. The fracture is diagnosed with an x-ray *(Figure 5.30)*.

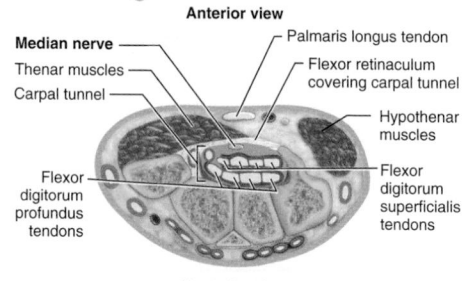

Radius · **Ulna**

Anterior view

Median nerve · Palmaris longus tendon
Thenar muscles · Flexor retinaculum covering carpal tunnel
Carpal tunnel
Hypothenar muscles
Flexor digitorum profundus tendons · Flexor digitorum superficialis tendons

Posterior view

▲ **FIGURE 5.29 Carpal Tunnel: Transverse Section.**

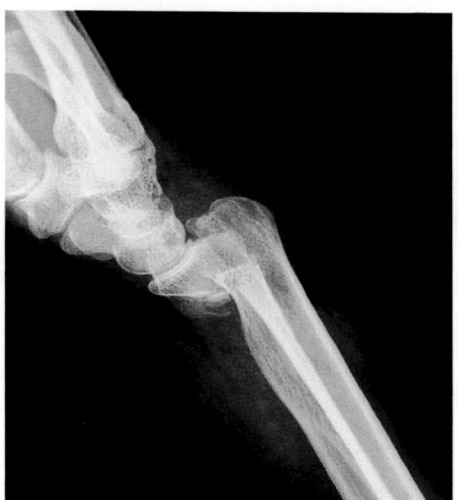

▲ **FIGURE 5.30   X-Ray of Colles Fracture with Radius and Ulna Involved.**

WORD	PRONUNCIATION		ELEMENTS	DEFINITION
carpus carpal (adj)	**KAR**-pus **KAR**-pal	S/ R/	-al *pertaining to* carp- *bones of the wrist*	Collective term for the eight carpal bones of the wrist Pertaining to the wrist
Colles fracture	**KOL**-ez **FRAK**-chur		Abraham Colles, Irish surgeon, 1773–1843	Fracture of the distal radius at the wrist
cyst	SIST		Greek *bladder*	An abnormal, fluid-containing sac
ergonomic	err-go-**NOM**-ick	S/ R/CF R/	-ic *pertaining to* erg/o- *work* -nom- *law*	Describes a workplace tool or equipment designed to prevent worker injury and discomfort
fascia fasciotomy fasciectomy	**FASH**-ee-ah fash-ee-**OT**-oh-me fash-ee-**EK**-toe-me	S/ R/CF S/	Latin *band* -otomy *incision* fasc/i- *fascia* -ectomy *excision*	Sheet of fibrous connective tissue An incision through a band of fascia, usually to relieve pressure on underlying structures Surgical removal of fascia
ganglion ganglionic (adj)	**GANG**-lee-on gang-**LEE**-on-ik		Greek *swelling*	Fluid-containing swelling attached to the synovial sheath of a tendon
pronate	**PRO**-nate		Latin *bend forward*	Rotate the forearm so that the surface of the palm faces posteriorly in the anatomical position
retinaculum	ret-ih-**NACK**-you-lum	S/ R/	-um *structure* retinacul- *hold back*	Fibrous ligament that keeps the tendons in place on the wrist so that they do not "bowstring" when the forearm muscles contract
stenosis	steh-**NOH**-sis		Greek *narrowing*	Narrowing of a passage
supinate	**SOO**-pih-nate		Latin *face up*	Rotate the forearm so that the surface of the palm faces anteriorly in the anatomical position

Abbreviation

PT   physiotherapy

Insert the correct orthopedic terminology from the WAD in the sentences below. You may use a term only one time. Fill in the blanks.

1. Because the patient has _____ tunnel syndrome, she will require a(n) _____ keyboard for her computer at work.

2. The two terms in this WAD that are opposites are _____ and _____.

3. Inflammation of a tendon is tendinitis, but inflammation of a cyst is _____.

4. Constriction produces the narrowing of a passage; _____ will do the same.

5. A fasciectomy is removal of the _____; a cystectomy would be removal of a _____.

6. A _____ is attached to the synovial sheath of a tendon.

7. The _____ is the fibrous ligament that keeps the tendons in place on the wrist.

These questions can be answered from Case Report 5.6 and the text on the opposite page.

8. What type of repetition injury does Ms. Baker have? _____

_____

9. What is the treatment plan for Ms. Baker? _____

_____

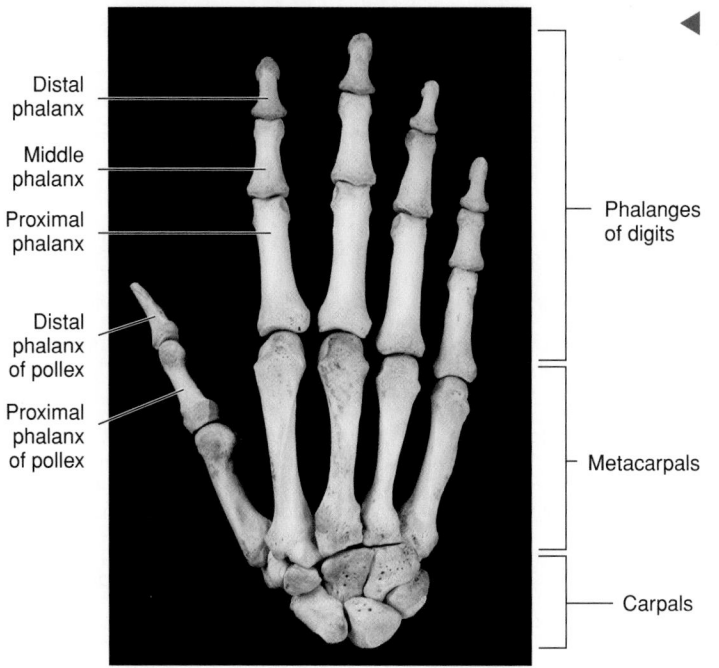

Distal phalanx

Middle phalanx

Proximal phalanx

Distal phalanx of pollex

Proximal phalanx of pollex

Phalanges of digits

Metacarpals

Carpals

(a)

▲ FIGURE 5.31 The Hand. (a) Bones of the hand. (b) Muscles and tendons of the palm of the hand. (c) Muscles and tendons of the dorsum of the hand.

THE HAND

Disorders of and injuries to the hand are among the most common reasons for office and Emergency Department visits and for ambulatory surgical procedures.

The complex structure of the hand *(Figure 5.31)* has evolved in response to the complicated and often very fine movements that modern-day activities require the hand to perform. Examples are making jewelry, repairing a watch, and sewing an artery or nerve back together.

When you look at the **palmar** surface of your hand, at the base of the thumb is a prominent pad of muscles called the **thenar eminence.** A smaller pad of muscles at the base of the little finger is called the **hypothenar eminence** *(Figure 5.32)* The back of the hand is called the **dorsum.**

The five fingers of one hand together have 14 bones called **phalanges.** The thumb has two phalanges. The remaining four fingers have three *(see Figure 5.31a).*

In the palm of the hand, the five bones proximal to the fingers are **metacarpals,** which connect at the wrist to eight small **carpal** bones. These in turn connect the hand to the bones of the forearm *(see Figure 5.31a).*

All these bones require numerous joints with ligaments to connect and stabilize them. The movements of the hand are accomplished by three sets of muscles and tendons:

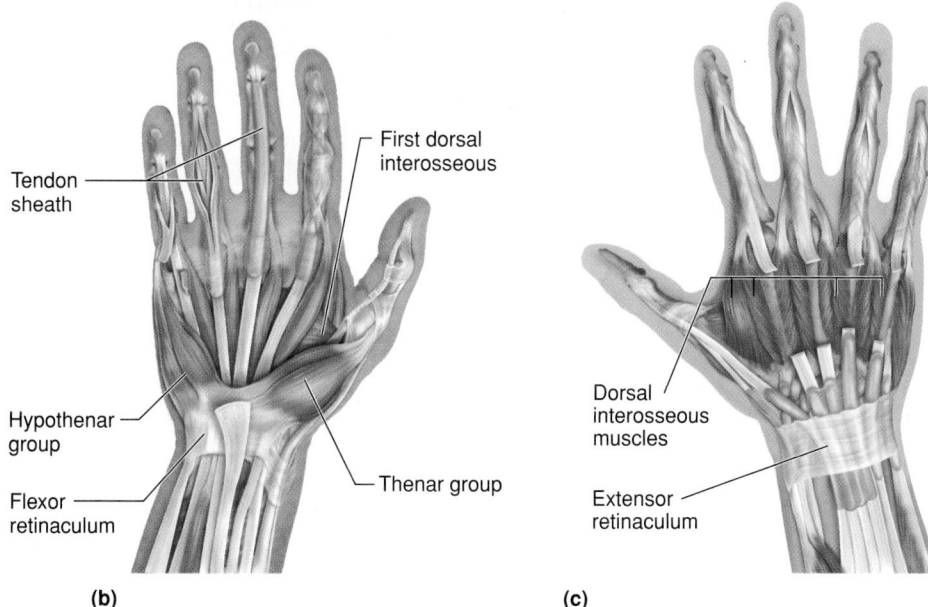

Tendon sheath

First dorsal interosseous

Hypothenar group

Flexor retinaculum

Thenar group

Dorsal interosseous muscles

Extensor retinaculum

(b)

(c)

▼ FIGURE 5.32 Palmar Surface of Hand.

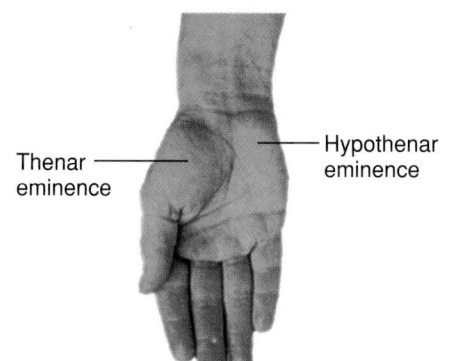

Thenar eminence

Hypothenar eminence

1. The flexor muscles that bend the fingers are located on the front of the forearm and are attached by tendons to the phalanges on the palmar surfaces *(see Figure 5.31b).*

2. The extensor muscles are located on the back of the forearm and are attached by tendons to the dorsal surfaces of the phalanges *(see Figure 5.31c).*

3. Small muscles that originate and insert on the hand are located entirely within the palm and include the **interosseous muscles** between the metacarpals *(see Figure 5.31b and c).* These muscles assist in flexion and extension of the fingers but also adduct and abduct them and enable the thumb to touch the tips of the other fingers, a movement called **opposition.**

WORD	PRONUNCIATION	ELEMENTS		DEFINITION
dorsum dorsal (adj)	**DOR**-sum **DOR**-sal		Latin *back*	Upper, posterior, or back surface Pertaining to the back or situated behind
eminence	**EM**-ih-nens		Latin *stand out*	A higher place or part
hypothenar	high-poh-**THAY**-nar	P/ R/	hypo- *below, smaller* -thenar *palm*	Fleshy eminence at the base of the little finger
interosseous	in-ter-**OSS**-ee-us	S/ P/ R/CF	-ous *pertaining to* inter- *between* -oss/e- *bone*	A structure between bones, such as the muscles between the metacarpals
metacarpal	**MET**-ah-**KAR**-pal	S/ P/ R/	-al *pertaining to* meta- *after* -carp- *bones of the wrist*	The five bones between the carpus and the fingers
opposition	op-oh-**SIH**-shun		Old English *to set against*	The movement of the thumb across the palm of the hand to touch the tips of the other fingers
palm palmar (adj)	PAHLM **PAHL**-mah		Latin *palm*	The flat anterior surface of the hand
phalanx phalanges (pl)	**FAY**-lanks **FAY**-lan-jeez		Greek *line of soldiers*	A bone of a finger or toe
thenar	**THAY**-nar		Greek *palm*	The thenar eminence is the fleshy mass at the base of the thumb

EXERCISES

Because the body has 206 bones, there is an extensive amount of orthopedic vocabulary. Build your knowledge of hand terminology with this exercise. Circle your best choice.

1. The term **dorsum** means: front   back   middle   end

2. The prefix **inter-** means: between   before   behind   beneath

3. The suffix **-ous** means: process   action   full of   pertaining to

4. The prefix **hypo-** means: smaller   larger   twisted   excess

5. The term **metacarpal** refers to: arm   elbow   forearm   hand

6. The suffix **-al** means: pertaining to   one who does   study of   condition

7. The element **osse** refers to: blood   wrist   knuckle   bone

8. Bone of a finger *or* toe is: carpus   fascia   eminence   phalanx

9. The prefix **meta-** means: before   during   after   middle

10. Flesh at the base of the thumb is: thenar   metacarpal   hypothenar   phalanges

11. Higher place or part: emmenince   emminence   eminence   emenince

12. The root **thenar-** means: finger   hand   palm   wrist

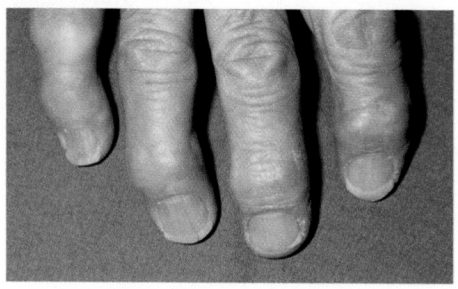

▲ **FIGURE 5.33   Hand with Osteoarthritis.**
Osteoarthritis of hands showing Heberden nodes.

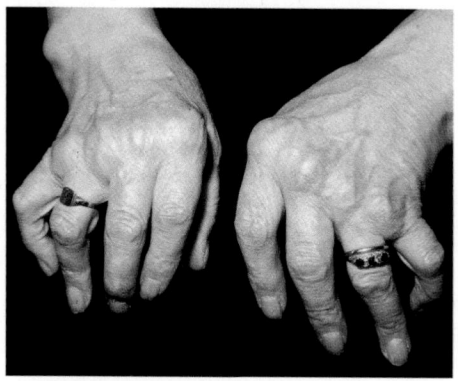

▲ **FIGURE 5.34   Hands with Rheumatoid Arthritis.**

Abbreviations

JRA	juvenile rheumatoid arthritis
RA	rheumatoid arthritis

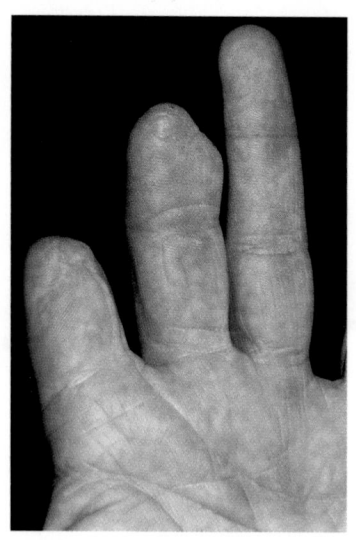

▲ **FIGURE 5.35   Healed Partial Amputation of Two Fingers.**

THE HAND (continued)

Disorders of the Hand

Osteoarthritis in the hand joints occurs from wear and tear, particularly in the joint at the base of the thumb. As a finger joint deteriorates, small bony spurs called **Heberden nodes** form over it *(Figure 5.33)*. William Heberden (1710–1801), a surgeon in Cambridge, England, first described these nodes.

Rheumatoid arthritis (RA), with destruction of joint surfaces, joint capsule, and ligaments, leads to marked **deformity** and joint **instability** *(Figure 5.34)*. It occurs mostly in women, with onset between ages 20 and 50.

The great majority of patients have involvement of the hands where the disease affects the synovial membrane that lines joints and tendons. The abnormal synovial membrane can invade the smooth, gliding joint surfaces and destroy them, or it can invade the surrounding joint capsule and ligaments and cause deformity and joint instability. Lumps known as **rheumatic nodules** form over the small joints of the hand and wrist. The metacarpophalangeal joints can be affected, and this leads to drift of the fingers away from the thumb, called **ulnar deviation.**

Juvenile rheumatoid arthritis (JRA) affects children under the age of 17 with inflammation and stiffness of joints. Many children grow out of it.

Dupuytren contracture is a progressive thickening and contracture of the skin and connective tissues of the palm of the hand.

Injuries of the Hand

Flexor tendon injuries occur as a result of lacerations. Because the flexor tendons lie just beneath the skin on the palmar surfaces of the fingers, they are very **susceptible** to injury even with a shallow laceration. Even after repair, there can be **residual** stiffness and limited motion of the fingers.

Open fractures of hand bones, when the skin is broken and the broken bone penetrates through the break in the skin, can lead to infection of hand tissues.

Partial amputation of a fingertip is a common type of injury, particularly in people who work with sharp tools *(Figure 5.35)*. This type of wound also produces an open phalangeal fracture.

Surgical Procedures of the Hand

Fasciectomy is the surgical removal of the hypertrophied connective tissue to release a contracture.

Tendon reconstruction stitches the two ends of a lacerated tendon back together or inserts a tendon graft.

Arthrodesis is the surgical fixation of a joint to prevent motion. Bone graft, wires, screws, or a plate can be used to stabilize the joint.

Arthroplasty in this setting is the complete replacement of a damaged finger joint with an artificial joint made of silicone rubber.

Reattachment of amputated fingers is performed frequently. The bones are rejoined with plates, wires, or screws. The tendons are reconstructed. Nerves and blood vessels are joined back together using microsurgical instruments.

WORD	PRONUNCIATION	ELEMENTS		DEFINITION
amputation amputate (verb) amputee (noun)	am-pyu-**TAY**-shun **AM**-pyu-tate **AM**-pyu-tee		Latin *cut, prune*	Process of removing a limb, a part of a limb, a breast, or some other projecting part A person with an amputation
contracture	kon-**TRAK**-chur	S/ R/	-ure *process* **contract-** *draw together*	Muscle shortening due to spasm or fibrosis
deformity	de-**FOR**-mih-tee	S/ P/ R/	-ity *condition* **de-** *change of* -form- *form, appearance*	A permanent structural deviation from the normal
Dupuytren	du-pwe-**TRAHN**		Guillaume Dupuytren, French surgeon, 1777–1835	Dupuytren contracture is thickening and shortening of fibrous bands in the palm of the hand
flexor flex	**FLEK**-sor FLEKS		Latin *to bend*	Muscle or tendon that flexes a joint To bend a joint so that the two parts come together
Heberden node	**HEH**-ber-den NOHD		William Heberden, English physician, 1710–1801	Bony lump on the terminal phalanx of the fingers in osteoarthritis
instability	in-stah-**BIL**-ih-tee	S/ P/ R/	-ity *condition* **in-** *not* -stabil- *stand firm*	Abnormal tendency of a joint to partially or fully dislocate
juvenile	**JU**-ven-ile		Latin *youthful*	Between the ages of 2 and 17 years
nodule	**NOD**-yule		Latin *small knot*	Small node or knotlike swelling
residual residue (noun)	re-**ZID**-you-al **REZ**-ih-dyu	S/ R/CF	-al *pertaining to* **resid/u-** *what is left over*	Pertaining to anything left over
rheumatism rheumatic (adj) rheumatoid arthritis	**RU**-mat-izm ru-**MAT**-ik **RHU**-mah-toyd ar-**THRI**-tis	S/ R/ S/ S/	-ism *condition* **rheumat-** *a flow* -ic *pertaining to* -oid *resembling*	Pain in various parts of the musculoskeletal system Disease of connective tissue, with arthritis as a major manifestation
susceptible	suh-**SEP**-tih-bill		Latin *to take up*	Capable of being affected by

EXERCISES   *Demonstrate your knowledge of the difference between these similar terms. Use the correct form of the term in the appropriate place. Fill in the blanks.*

amputation   **amputate**   **amputee**

1. The surgeon has decided to _____ the patient's left leg below the knee. The _____ will be

    performed as soon as possible. Following the surgery, the _____ will be fitted for a new leg prosthesis.

flex   **flexor**

2. The _____ tendons _____ a joint so that the two parts of the joint can come together.

residual   **residue**

3. The _____ in the bottom of the test beaker can be referred to as the _____.

rheumatic   **rheumatoid arthritis**   **rheumatism**

4. _____ is a generic term for _____ pain in various parts of the musculoskeletal system.

    However, _____ is a specific systemic disease affecting many joints.

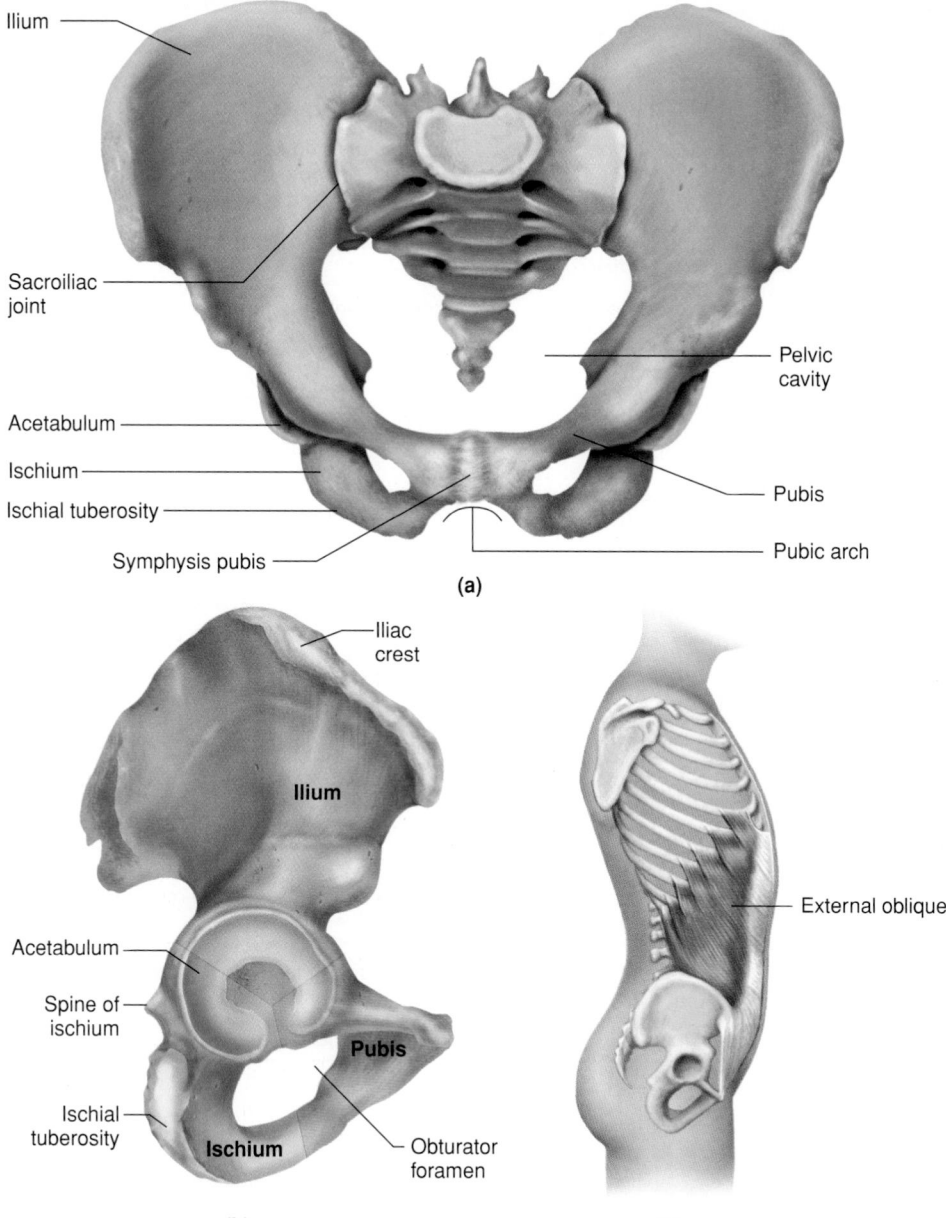

PELVIC GIRDLE

The pelvic girdle *(Figure 5.36)* is the two hip bones that articulate anteriorly with each other at the **symphysis pubis** and posteriorly with the **sacrum** to form the bowl-shaped **pelvis.** The two joints between the **coxae** (hip bones) and the sacrum are the **sacroiliac joints.**

The pelvic girdle has the following functions:

1. Supports the axial skeleton.
2. Transmits the body's weight through to the lower limbs.
3. Provides attachments for the lower limbs.
4. Protects the internal reproductive organs, urinary bladder, and distal end of the large intestine.

Each **os coxa** (hip bone) is a fusion of three bones, the **ilium, ischium,** and **pubis** *(Figure 5.36a).* The fusion takes place in the region of the **acetabulum,** a cup-shaped cavity on the lateral surface of each os coxa that receives the **head** of the **femur** (thigh bone, *Figure 5.36b).*

The lower part of the pelvis is formed by the lower ilium, ischium, and pubic bones that surround a short canal-like cavity. This opening is larger in females than males to allow the infant to pass through during childbirth. The outlet from the cavity is spanned by strong muscular layers through which the rectum, vagina, and urethra pass *(Figure 5.37).*

Muscles anchor the pelvic girdle to the vertebrae and ribs of the axial skeleton. Anteriorly, these are the abdominal muscles that are inserted into the ilium and pubis *(Figure 5.36c).*

▲ **FIGURE 5.36** **Pelvic Girdle.** *(a)* Front view. *(b)* Side view. *(c)* Abdominal muscles supporting the pelvic girdle.

Disorders of the Pelvic Girdle

Sacroiliac joint (SI joint) strain is a common cause of lower-back pain. Unlike most joints, the SI joint is only designed to move ¼ inch (approximately 6 mm) during weight bearing and forward flexion. Its main function is to provide shock absorption for the spine.

During pregnancy, hormones enable connective tissue to relax so that the pelvis can expand enough to allow birth. The stretching in the SI joint ligaments makes it "overmobile" and susceptible to wear-and-tear painful arthritis.

Another cause of pain in the SI joint is trauma, with tearing of the joint ligaments generating too much motion and pain. The pain is felt in the low back, in the buttock, and sometimes in the back and front of the thigh.

A diagnosis of sacroiliac pain can be made by clinical examination, joint x-ray, and CT scan. **Fluoroscopic** injection of local anesthetic into the joint can relieve the pain temporarily. Treatment is usually **stabilization** of the joint with a **brace** and physical therapy to strengthen the low-back muscles. Occasionally, **arthrodesis** of the joint is necessary.

Abbreviation	
SI	sacroiliac

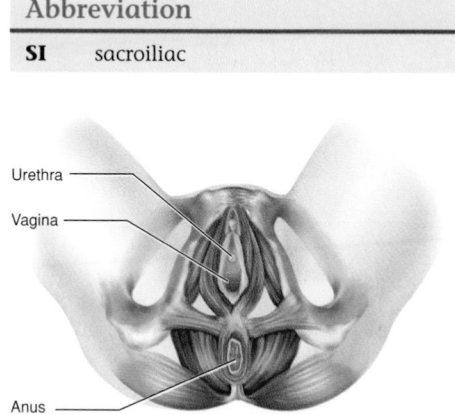

▲ **FIGURE 5.37** **Female Pelvic Outlet.**

WORD	PRONUNCIATION		ELEMENTS	DEFINITION
acetabulum	ass-eh-**TAB**-you-lum		Latin *vinegar cup*	The cup-shaped cavity of the hip bone that receives the head of the femur to form the hip joint
brace	BRACE		Old English *to fasten*	Appliance to support a part of the body in its correct position
coxa coxae (pl)	**COCK**-sah **COCK**-see		Latin *hip bone*	Hip bone
diastasis	die-**ASS**-tah-sis		Greek *separation*	Separation of normally joined parts
femur femoral (adj)	**FEE**-mur **FEM**-oh-ral		Latin *thigh*	The thigh bone
fluoroscopy fluoroscopic (adj)	flor-**OS**-koh-pee flor-oh-**SKOP**-ik	S/ R/CF S/	-scopy *to examine, to view* **fluor/o-** *x-ray beam* -ic *pertaining to*	Examination of structures of the body by x-rays
head	HED		Old English *head*	The rounded extremity of a bone
ilium (**Note:** The ileum is a section of the small intestine [Chapter 6].) ilia (pl)	**ILL**-ee-um **ILL**-ee-ah		Latin *groin*	Large wing-shaped bone at the upper and posterior part of the pelvis
ischium ischial (adj) ischia (pl)	**ISS**-kee-um **ISS**-kee-al **ISS**-kee-ah		Greek *hip*	Lower and posterior part of the hip bone
pelvis pelvic (adj)	**PEL**-vis **PEL**-vic		Latin *basin*	A cup-shaped ring of bone; also a cup-shaped cavity, as in the pelvis of the kidney
pubis pubic (adj)	**PYU**-bis **PYU**-bik	 S/ R/	Latin *pubis* -ic *pertaining to* **pub-** *pubis*	Bony front arch of the pelvis of the hip; also called pubic bone Pertaining to the pubis
sacrum sacral (adj) sacroiliac joint	**SAY**-crum **SAY**-kral say-kroh-**ILL**-ih-ak JOINT	 S/ R/CF R/	Latin *sacred* -ac *pertaining to* **sacr/o-** *sacrum* -ili- *ilium*	Segment of the vertebral column that forms part of the pelvis In the neighborhood of the sacrum The joint between the sacrum and ilium

Diastasis symphysis pubis is another result of the stretching of pelvic ligaments during pregnancy. The softening and stretching of the ligaments of the symphysis pubis stretches the joint between the two pubic bones and leads to pain over the joint and difficulty in walking, climbing stairs, and turning over in bed.

EXERCISES

Match the language of the pelvic girdle to its correct definition. Fill in the blanks.

_____ 1. Receives head of femur

_____ 2. Cup-shaped ring of bones

_____ 3. Posterior part of hip bone

_____ 4. Separation of normally joined parts

_____ 5. Wing-shaped bone, upper part of pelvis

_____ 6. Segment of vertebral column

_____ 7. Thigh bone

A. sacrum

B. ilium

C. diastasis

D. femur

E. pelvis

F. ischium

G. acetabulum

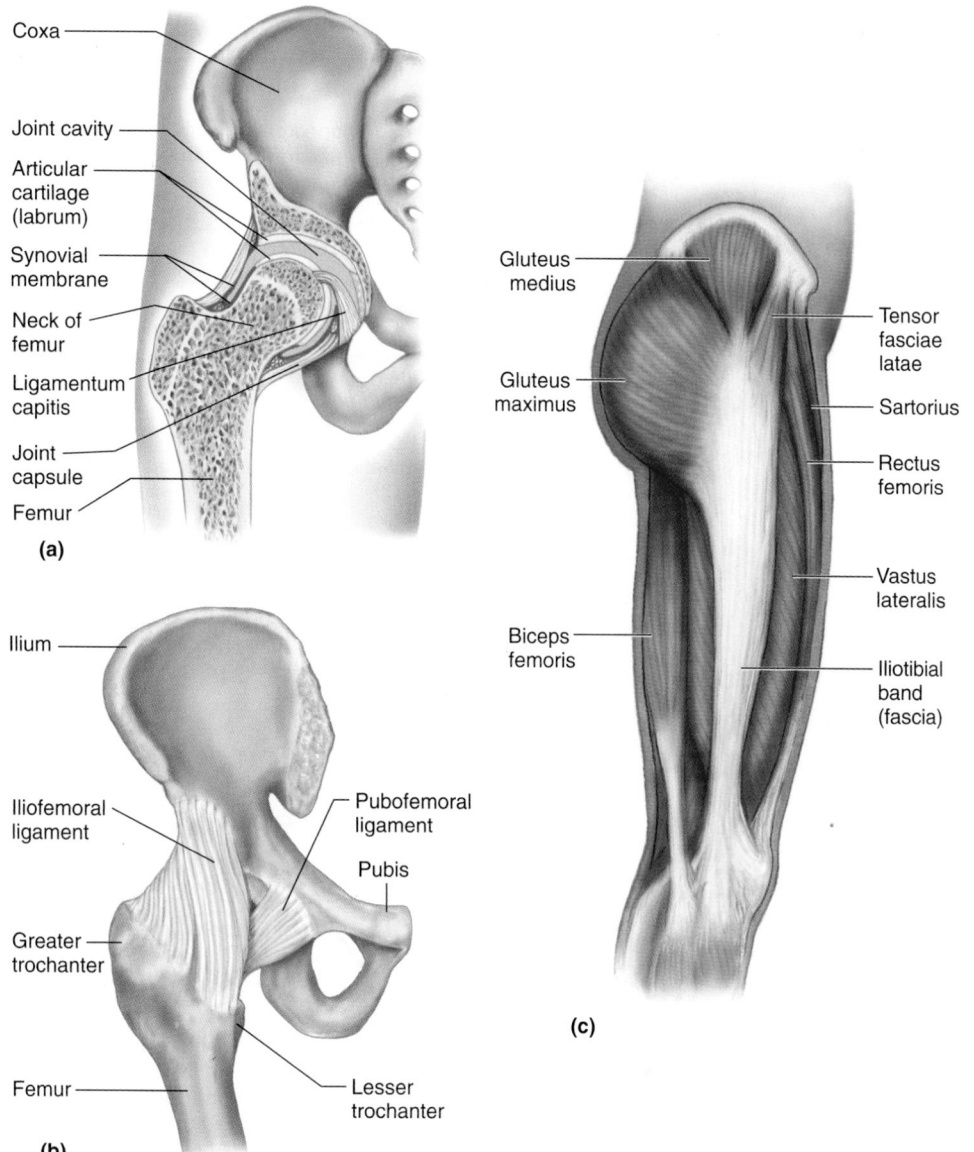

(a)

Coxa
Joint cavity
Articular cartilage (labrum)
Synovial membrane
Neck of femur
Ligamentum capitis
Joint capsule
Femur

(b)

Ilium
Iliofemoral ligament
Greater trochanter
Femur
Pubofemoral ligament
Pubis
Lesser trochanter

(c)

Gluteus medius
Gluteus maximus
Biceps femoris
Tensor fasciae latae
Sartorius
Rectus femoris
Vastus lateralis
Iliotibial band (fascia)

▲ **FIGURE 5.38   Hip Joint.** (*a*) Right frontal view of a section of hip joint. (*b*) Ligaments of hip joint. (*c*) Muscles of hip and thigh (lateral view).

BONES, JOINTS, AND MUSCLES OF THE HIP AND THIGH

The **hip joint** is a **ball-and-socket** synovial joint between the head of the femur and the cup-shaped **acetabulum** of the hip bone (*Figure 5.38a*). A ligament (ligamentum capitis) attached to the head of the femur from the lining of the acetabulum carries blood vessels to the head of the femur to nourish it.

The joint is held in place by a thick joint **capsule** reinforced by strong ligaments that connect the neck of the femur to the rim of the acetabulum (*Figure 5.38b*).

The **labrum** is the cartilage that forms a rim around the socket of the joint; it cushions the joint and helps keep the head of the femur in place in the socket. Recent improvements in diagnostic techniques have shown that with injury the labrum can tear and cause pain. The tear is diagnosed on MRI and may need surgery to be repaired.

Powerful muscles that support the hip joint and move the thigh have their **origins** on the pelvic girdle and their **insertions** into the femur. Prominent among them are the three **gluteus** muscles, **maximus, medius,** and **minimus** (*Figure 5.38c*), and the **adductor** muscles that run down the inner thigh.

Disorders and Injuries of the Hip Joint

Hip pointer, usually a football-related injury, is a blow to the rim of the pelvis that leads to bruising of the bone and surrounding tissues.

Osteoarthritis is common in the hip as a result of aging, weight bearing, and repetitive use of the joint. The cartilage on both the acetabulum and the head of the femur degenerates, and eventually there is total loss of the cartilage cushion. The resulting friction between the bones of the head of the femur and the acetabulum leads to pain and loss of mobility.

Rheumatoid arthritis can also affect the hip, beginning in the synovial membrane and progressing to destroy cartilage and bone.

Avascular necrosis of the femoral head is the necrosis (death) of bone tissue when the blood supply becomes avascular (is cut off), usually as a result of trauma.

Fractures of the neck of the femur occur as a result of falls, most commonly in elderly women with osteoporosis. This is shown in (*Figure 5.39*).

▲ **FIGURE 5.39   Fracture of Neck of Femur in Woman with Osteoporosis.**

WORD	PRONUNCIATION	ELEMENTS		DEFINITION
arthritis	ar-**THRY**-tis	S/ R/	-itis *inflammation* arthr- *joint*	Inflammation of a joint or joints
avascular	a-**VAS**-cue-lar	S/ P/ R/	-ar *pertaining to* a- *without* vascul- *blood vessel*	Without a blood supply
gluteus maximus	**GLU**-tee-us **MAKS**-ih-mus		Greek *buttocks* Latin *the biggest or the greatest*	Refers to a muscle in the buttocks The gluteus maximus muscle is the largest muscle in the body, covering a large part of each buttock
medius	**ME**-dee-us		Latin *middle*	The gluteus medius muscle is partly covered by the gluteus maximus; it originates on the ilium and is inserted into the femur
minimus	**MIN**-ih-mus		Latin *smallest*	The gluteus minimus is the smallest of the gluteal muscles and lies under the gluteus medius
gluteal (adj)	**GLU**-tee-al	S/ R/	-eal *pertaining to* glut- *buttocks*	Pertaining to the buttocks.
labrum	**LAY**-brum		Latin *lip-shaped*	Cartilage that forms a rim around the socket of the hip joint
necrosis necrotic (adj)	neh-**KROH**-sis neh-**KROT**-ik		Greek *death*	Pathologic death of cells or tissue Affected by necrosis
prosthesis	**PROS**-thee-sis		Greek *addition*	Manufactured substitute for a missing part of the body

Surgical Procedures

Arthroplasty, a total replacement of the hip joint with a metal **prosthesis,** is the most common hip surgery today; 150,000 total-hip replacements are performed each year in the United States, mostly for osteoarthritis of the hip joint. The diseased parts of the joint are removed and replaced with artificial parts made of titanium, other metals, and ceramics *(Figure 5.40).*

Arthrocentesis, the aspiration of fluid from the hip joint and replacement of the fluid with a steroid solution, is also performed frequently for osteoarthritis.

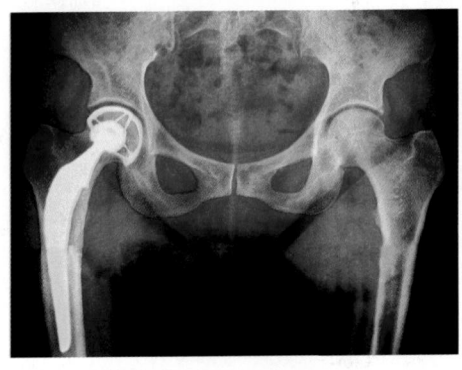

▲ **FIGURE 5.40   Total-Hip Replacement.**
Colored x-ray of prosthetic hip.

EXERCISES

*Continue working with the **language of orthopedics**. Demonstrate your knowledge of the terms by circling the best answer to each question below.*

1. Maximus, medius, and minimus are all:

   bones   muscles   tendons   ligaments   phalanges

2. Gluteus refers to the:

   wrist   hand   buttocks   hip   spine

3. If tissue is dead, it is:

   necrotic   sacral   rheumatic   degenerative   fibrotic

4. Avascular means no:

   living tissue   tendon support   movement   blood supply   inflammation

5. A prosthesis is a(n):

   procedure   cast   diagnostic test   brace   artificial body part

CASE REPORT 5.7

Operative Report.

Gail Griffith, age 17.

Preoperative Diagnosis: Traumatic ACL tear and tear of medial meniscus right knee.

Postoperative Diagnosis: Same.

Procedure Performed: Repair of medial collateral ligament, ACL reconstruction, repair of torn medial meniscus, right knee.

Operative Findings: An avulsed anterior cruciate ligament off the femoral condyle with a tear of the posterior horn of the medial meniscus and tear of medial collateral ligament.

BONES, JOINTS, AND MUSCLES OF THE KNEE AND THIGH

Knee Joint

The knee is a hinged joint formed with four bones:

1. The lower end of the **femur,** shaped like a horseshoe. The two ends of the horseshoe are the medial and lateral femoral **condyles** *(Figure 5.41b).*

2. The flat upper end of the **tibia.**

3. The **patella** (kneecap), a flat triangular bone embedded in the **patellar tendon.** The patella articulates with the femur between its two **condyles** *(Figure 5.41a).*

4. The **fibula,** which forms a separate joint by articulating with the tibia. This is called the **tibiofibular joint** *(see Figure 5.41b).*

Mechanically, the role of the patella is to provide an increase of about 30% in the strength of extension of the knee joint.

Within the knee joint, two crescent-shaped pads of cartilage lie on top of the tibia to articulate with the femoral condyles. They are the **medial** and **lateral menisci.** Their function is to distribute weight more evenly across the joint surface to minimize wear and tear. They play a crucial role in joint stability, lubrication, and transmission of force.

The knee joint has a **fibrous capsule** lined with **synovial membrane** to secrete **synovial fluid,** which provides lubrication for the joint. The joint is held together by **ligaments.** The two ligaments outside the joint are the **medial** and **lateral collateral ligaments.** Two other ligaments are located inside the joint cavity and are called the **anterior cruciate ligament (ACL)** and the **posterior cruciate ligament (PCL).** They cross over each other to form an "X" *(Figure 5.41b).* There are numerous bursae associated with the knee joint *(Figure 5.41a).* Their function is to aid the movement of the patella and the patellar tendon over the bones of the joint.

Thigh Muscles

The thigh muscles move the knee joint and lower leg. The anterior thigh is composed of the large **quadriceps femoris** muscle, which has four heads and is the most powerful muscle in the body. The four muscles converge into the **quadriceps tendon,** which contains the patella, and continue as the patellar tendon to insert into the tibia *(Figure 5.41a).* The quadriceps muscle extends (straightens) the knee joint and, because of the weight of the lower leg, has to be a powerful muscle.

The posterior thigh is composed mostly of the three **hamstring muscles:** the **biceps femoris, semimembranosus,** and **semitendinosus.** They flex (bend) the knee joint and rotate the leg. The hollow at the back of the knee between the hamstring tendons is called the **popliteal fossa.**

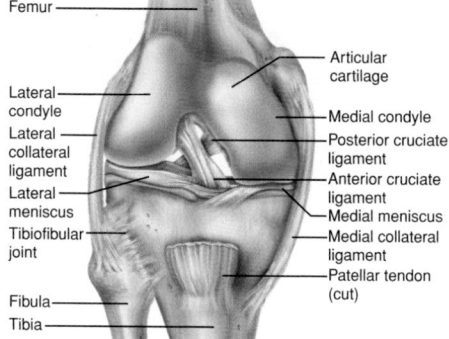

▲ FIGURE 5.41 Knee Joint (*a*) Section of knee joint. (*b*) Right knee joint: anterior view.

Abbreviations	
ACL	anterior cruciate ligament
PCL	posterior cruciate ligament

WORD	PRONUNCIATION	ELEMENTS		DEFINITION
collateral	koh-**LAT**-er-al	S/ P/ R/	-al *pertaining to* co- *together* -later- *side*	Situated at the side, often to bypass an obstruction
condyle	**KON**-dile		Latin *knuckle*	Large, smooth rounded expansion of the end of a bone that forms a joint with another bone
cruciate	**KRU**-she-ate		Latin *cross*	Shaped like a cross
fibula fibular (adj)	**FIB**-you-lah **FIB**-you-lar		Latin *clasp or buckle*	The smaller of the two bones of the lower leg
lateral (opposite of medial)	**LAT**-er-al	S/ R/	-al *pertaining to* later- *side*	Situated at the side of a structure
meniscus menisci (pl)	meh-**NISS**-kuss meh-**NISS**-key		Greek *crescent*	Disc of connective tissue cartilage between the bones of a joint; for example, in the knee joint
patella (kneecap) patellae (pl) patellar (adj)	pah-**TELL**-ah pah-**TELL**-ee pah-**TELL**-ar		Latin *small plate*	Thin, circular bone in front of the knee joint and embedded in the patellar tendon
popliteal fossa	pop-**LIT**-ee-al **FOSS**-ah	S/ R/CF	-al *pertaining to* poplit/e- *ham* **fossa** Latin *ditch*	The hollow at the back of the knee
quadriceps femoris	**KWAD**-rih-seps **FEM**-or-is	P/ R/ S/ R/	quadri- *four* -ceps *head* -is *belonging to* femor- *femur*	An anterior thigh muscle with four heads
tibia tibial (adj)	**TIB**-ee-ah **TIB**-ee-al		Latin *large shinbone*	The larger bone of the lower leg

---

EXERCISES

A medical term must be spelled correctly. Work with a fellow student on this exercise. Cover the WAD while the other student dictates the terms in this WAD to you. Do your best to spell them correctly in the left column. When you are finished, uncover the WAD and check your spelling. If you have made any errors, rewrite the correct spelling in the right column.

Spelling   Corrections

1. _____   _____

2. _____   _____

3. _____   _____

4. _____   _____

5. _____   _____

6. _____   _____

After reading Case Report 5.7 on the opposite page, answer the following questions. Be prepared to discuss your answers in class.

1. The adjective *fibular* means *pertaining to the* _____.

2. Which two terms in the postoperative findings are opposites? _____ and _____

3. If a ligament is described as "collateral," where is it located? _____

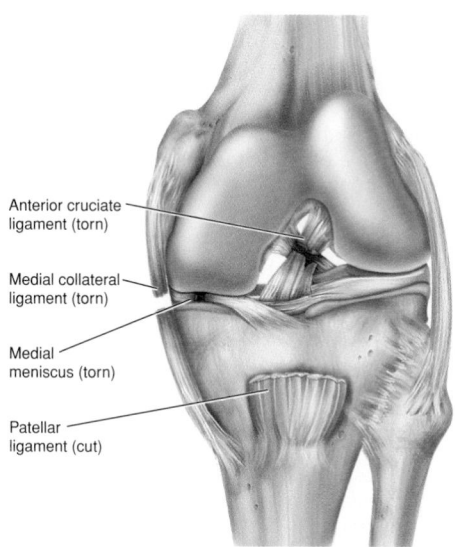

▲ **FIGURE 5.42 Gail Griffith's Knee Injuries.**

Case Report 5.7 (continued)

Gail Griffith, a 17-year-old, landed awkwardly after jumping for a ball during a basketball game. "My knee kinda popped as I landed." She had to be assisted off the court. In the Emergency Room, the knee was swollen and unstable. An MRI showed a complete tear of the medial collateral ligament, a complete tear of the anterior cruciate ligament, and a partial tear (**avulsion**) of the medial meniscus *(Figure 5.42)*. Gail decided to have surgery, even though full recovery would take 6 months to 1 year of rehabilitation.

THE KNEE JOINT

Injuries to the Knee Joint

The **anterior cruciate ligament (ACL)** is the most commonly injured ligament in the knee *(Figure 5.42)*, particularly in female athletes. The injury is often caused by a sudden **hyperflexion** of the knee joint when landing awkwardly on flat ground as in Gail's injury. Because of its poor vascular supply, once torn the ligament does not heal. The knee becomes unstable, risking further joint damage and arthritis. If the ACL has been torn away from its bony insertions, the surgeon will harvest a thin portion of a hamstring or patellar tendon and screw the ends into the tibia and femur. This is a **tendon autograft.** If donated tissue from a tissue bank were used for the graft, it would be called an **allograft.** If tissue from another species is used for a graft, it is called a **xenograft** or a **heterograft.**

Other major ligaments that are commonly injured are the medial and lateral collateral ligaments and the posterior cruciate ligament.

Meniscus injuries result from a twist to the knee. Pain and locking are the result of the torn meniscus flipping in and out of the joint as it moves. Because loss of a meniscus leads to arthritic changes, repair of the meniscus, as in Gail's case, rather than removal is preferred. Removal of a meniscus is a **meniscectomy.**

Patellar problems produce pain that is noticed particularly when descending stairs. The force on the patella when descending stairs is about seven times body weight compared to about two times body weight when ascending stairs.

Chondromalacia patellae (runner's knee) is caused by irritation of the undersurface of the patella.

Patellar subluxation or **dislocation** produces an unstable painful kneecap.

Prepatellar bursitis (housemaid's knee) produces painful swelling over the bursa at the front of the knee and is seen in people who kneel for extended periods of time, such as carpet layers.

Tendinitis of the patellar tendon is produced by overuse during such activities as cycling, running, or dancing. Pain is felt where the tendon is inserted into the tibia. It is treated by RICE.

Rupture of the patellar tendon can occur in the elderly when trying to break a fall or in athletes such as basketball players with their repeated jumping. An MRI can confirm the tear, which may need to be repaired surgically.

Surgical Procedures of the Knee Joint

Arthrocentesis, aspiration of fluid from the knee joint, is used to establish a diagnosis by laboratory examination of the fluid and to drain off infected fluid.

Diagnostic arthroscopy is an exploratory procedure performed using an arthroscope to examine the internal compartments of the knee joint.

Surgical arthroscopy, performed through an arthroscope, can be a **debridement** or removal of torn tissue such as a meniscus or a ligament. It can also be repair of a torn ligament by suturing, tendon autograft, or repair of a torn meniscus.

Arthroplasty involves a total replacement of the knee joint *(Figure 5.43)*, usually because of osteoarthritis of the joint. The lower end of the femur is replaced with a metal shell. The upper end of the tibia is replaced with a metal trough lined with plastic and the back of the patella can be replaced with a plastic button.

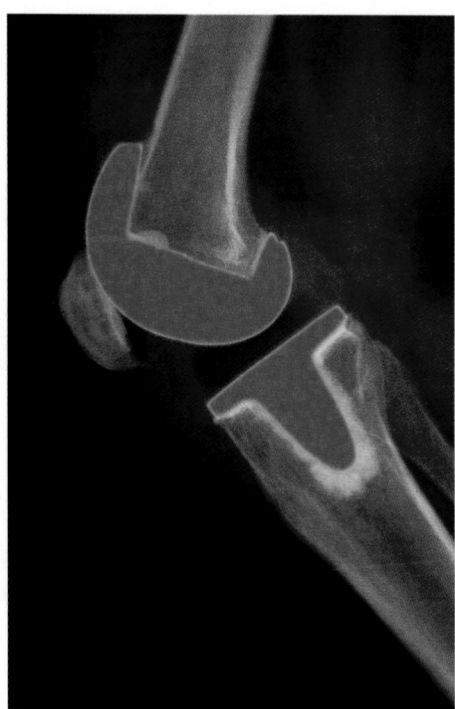

▲ **FIGURE 5.43 Total Knee Replacement.**
Colored x-ray of total knee replacement of left knee.

WORD	PRONUNCIATION	ELEMENTS		DEFINITION
allograft	**AL**-oh-graft	P/ R/	allo- *different* -graft *splice*	Tissue graft from another person or cadaver
autograft	**AWE**-toe-graft	P/ R/	auto- *self, same* -graft *splice*	A graft using tissue taken from the individual who is receiving the graft
avulsion	a-**VUL**-shun		Latin *to tear away*	Forcible separation or tearing away, often of a tendon from bone
chondromalacia	**KON**-dro-mah-**LAY**-she-ah	S/ R/CF	-malacia *abnormal softness* chondr/o- *cartilage*	Softening and degeneration of cartilage
debridement	day-**BREED**-mon	S/ P/ R/	-ment *action* de- *take away* -bride- *rubble*	The removal of injured or necrotic tissue
heterograft (also known as **xenograft**)	**HET**-er-oh-graft	P/ R/	hetero- *different* -graft *splice*	A graft using tissue taken from another species
hyperflexion	high-per-**FLEK**-shun	S/ P/ R/	-ion *action, condition, process* hyper- *excess* -flex- *bend*	Flexion of a limb or part beyond the normal limits
meniscectomy	men-ih-**SEK**-toh-me	S/ R/	-ectomy *excision* menisc- *crescent, meniscus*	Excision (cutting out) of all or part of a meniscus
prepatellar	pree-pah-**TELL**-ar	S/ P/ R/	-ar *pertaining to* pre- *before, in front of* -patell- *patella*	In front of the patella
rupture	**RUP**-tyur		Latin *break*	Break or tear of any organ or body part
tendinitis (also spelled tendonitis)	ten-dih-**NYE**-tis	S/ R/	-itis *inflammation* tendin- *tendon*	Inflammation of a tendon
xenograft (also known as **heterograft**)	**ZEN**-oh-graft	R/CF R/	xen/o- *foreign material* -graft *splice*	A graft from another species

EXERCISES

Recognition of word elements will help you understand the medical term. In each of the following terms, a specific element is in bold. Identify the type of element, and then define that element on the lines provided. Fill in the chart.

Medical Term	Type of Element (P, R, CF, S)	Definition of Element
pre**patell**ar		
tendin**itis**		
hyper**flex**ion		
de**bride**ment		
autograft		
chondromalacia		
menis**cect**omy		
hetero**graft**		
allo**graft**		

BONES, JOINTS, AND MUSCLES OF THE LOWER LEG, ANKLE, AND FOOT

The two bones of the lower leg are the larger and medial **tibia** and the thinner and lateral **fibula.** The lower end of the tibia on its medial border forms a prominent process called the medial **malleolus.** The lower end of the fibula forms the lateral malleolus. You can **palpate** both these prominences at your own ankle.

The muscles of the lower leg move the ankle, foot, and toes. Those on the front of the leg are in a compartment between the tibia and fibula. They **dorsiflex** the foot at the ankle and extend the toes. Those on the lateral side of the leg **evert** the foot.

Those on the back of the leg **plantar flex** the foot at the ankle, flex the toes, and **invert** the foot *(Figure 5.44)*. The **gastrocnemius** muscle forms a large part of the calf. The distal end of it joins with the tendon of the **soleus** muscle to form the **Achilles (calcaneal) tendon,** which is attached to the heel bone (**calcaneus**). The gastrocnemius muscle and the Achilles tendon enable you to "push off" and start running or jumping.

The ankle has two joints:

1. One between the lateral malleolus of the fibula and the talus.

2. One between the medial malleolus of the tibia and the talus.

The **talus** is the most superior of the seven **tarsal** bones of the ankle and proximal foot *(Figure 5.45)*, and its trochlear surface articulates with the tibia. The tarsal bones help the ankle bear the body's weight. Strong ligaments on both sides of the ankle joint hold it together.

Attached to the tarsal bones are the five parallel **metatarsal** bones that form the instep and then fan out to form the ball of the foot, where they bear weight. The toes each have three **phalanges,** except for the big toe, which has only two. This is identical to the thumb and its relation to the hand. The tendons of the leg muscles are inserted into the phalanges.

Disorders and Injuries of the Ankle and Foot

Podiatry is a health care specialty concerned with the diagnosis and treatment of disorders and injuries of the foot.

Bunions occur usually at the base of the big toe and are swellings of the bones that cause the metatarsophalangeal joint to be misaligned and stick out medially. This deformity is called **hallux valgus.**

Strains and sprains are more common in the ankle than in any other joint in the body. A strain is an acute injury resulting from overstretching or overcontraction of a muscle or tendon. A sprain is the result of an abnormal stretch or tear of a ligament. Some severe sprains with tearing of the ligament may require surgical repair.

Pott fracture is a term applied to a variety of fractures in which there is a fracture of the fibula near the ankle, often accompanied by a fracture of the medial malleolus of the tibia *(Figure 5.46)*.

Achilles tendinitis results from a small stretch injury that causes the tendon to become swollen and painful. A larger partial or complete **tear** leads to loss of function with difficulty in walking and no ability to "push off."

Plantar fasciitis is the overstretching or tearing of the dense sheet of fascia that supports the arch of the foot. If the plantar fascia is weak, **pes planus** (flatfoot) can be present.

Ingrown toenails are nails that grow into the skin folds on either side of the toe. They are often infected and painful and may need surgical repair.

Gout is an extremely painful arthritis of the big toe and other joints caused by a buildup of uric acid in the blood, which forms needlelike crystals that accumulate in the joints. Treatment is with allopurinol; some newer drugs are currently being tested.

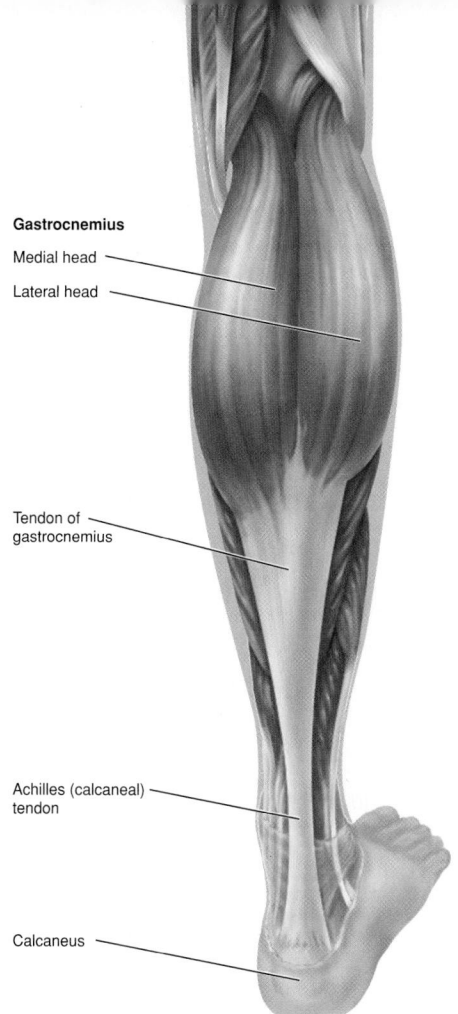

Gastrocnemius
Medial head
Lateral head

Tendon of gastrocnemius

Achilles (calcaneal) tendon

Calcaneus

▲ **FIGURE 5.44 Muscles of Back of Right Lower Leg.**

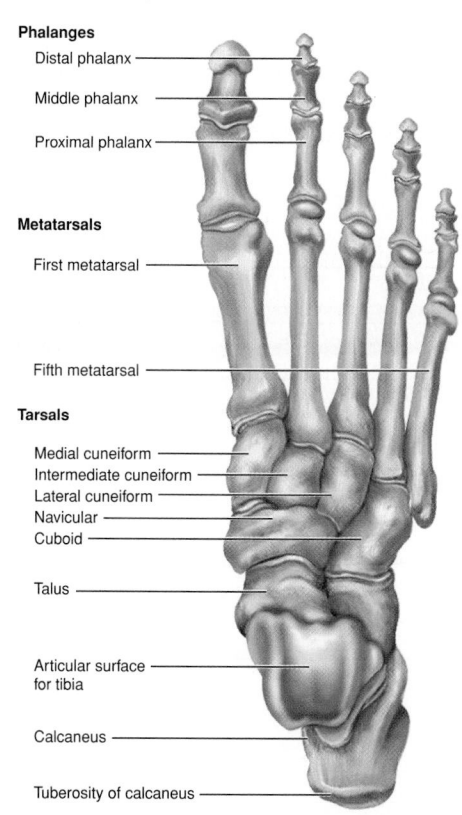

Phalanges
Distal phalanx
Middle phalanx
Proximal phalanx

Metatarsals
First metatarsal

Fifth metatarsal

Tarsals
Medial cuneiform
Intermediate cuneiform
Lateral cuneiform
Navicular
Cuboid

Talus

Articular surface for tibia

Calcaneus

Tuberosity of calcaneus

▲ **FIGURE 5.45 Twenty-six Bones and 33 Joints of Right Foot.**

WORD	PRONUNCIATION	ELEMENTS		DEFINITION
Achilles tendon (also called **calcaneal tendon**)	ah-**KILL**-eeze		a Greek warrior	A tendon formed from gastrocnemius and soleus muscles and inserted into the calcaneus
bunion	**BUN**-yun		French *bump*	A swelling at the base of the big toe
calcaneus **calcaneal** (adj)	kal-**KAY**-knee-us kal-**KAY**-knee-al		Latin *the heel*	Bone of the tarsus that forms the heel
fasciitis (note spelling)	fash-ee-**I**-tis	S/ R/CF	-itis *inflammation* fasc/i- *fascia*	Inflammation of the fascia
gastrocnemius	gas-trok-**NEE**-me-us	S/ R/	-ius *pertaining to* gastrocnem- *calf of leg*	Major muscle in back of the lower leg (the calf)
gout	GOWT		Latin *drop*	Painful arthritis of the big toe and other joints
hallux valgus	**HAL**-uks **VAL**-gus		**hallux** *big toe* **valgus** *turn out*	Deviation of the big toe toward the lateral side of the foot
metatarsus **metatarsal** (adj)	**MET**-ah-**TAR**-sus **MET**-ah-**TAR**-sal	P/ R/ S/	meta- *behind* -tarsus *flat surface* -al *pertaining to*	A collective term referring to the five parallel bones of the foot between the tarsus and the phalanges
pes planus	PES **PLAY**-nuss		**pes** *foot* **planus** *flat surface*	A flat foot with no plantar arch
podiatry **podiatrist**	po-**DIE**-ah-tree po-**DIE**-ah-trist	S/ R/ S/	-iatry *treatment* pod- *foot* -iatrist *practitioner*	Specialty concerned with the diagnosis and treatment of disorders and injuries of the foot Practitioner of podiatry
Pott fracture	POT **FRAK**-chur		Percival Pott, London surgeon, 1714–1788	Fracture of lower end of fibula, often with fracture of tibial malleolus
soleus	**SO**-lee-us		From Latin for "sole of foot"	Large muscle of the calf
talipes	**TAL**-ip-eze	R/ R/	-pes *foot* tali- *ankle bone*	Deformity of the foot involving the talus
talus	**TAY**-luss		Latin *heel bone*	The tarsal bone that articulates with the tibia to form the ankle joint
tarsus **tarsal** (adj)	**TAR**-sus **TAR**-sal		Latin *flat surface*	The collection of seven bones in the foot that form the ankle and instep

EXERCISES

Complete your knowledge of the skeleton by matching the statement in the left column to the appropriate term in the right column.

_____ 1. Forms ankle joint

_____ 2. Flatfoot

_____ 3. Forms ankle and instep

_____ 4. Heel bone

_____ 5. Large muscle of calf

_____ 6. Deviation of big toe

_____ 7. Swelling at base of big toe

_____ 8. Five parallel bones in the foot

_____ 9. Foot deformity involving talus

A. hallux valgus

B. gastrocnemius

C. tarsus

D. talipes

E. pes planus

F. metatarsus

G. talus

H. calcaneus

I. bunion

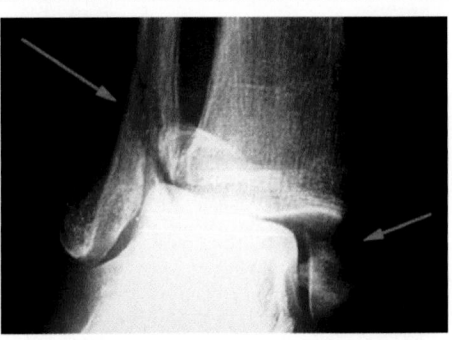

▲ **FIGURE 5.46** Pott Fracture Involving Lower End of Fibula and Medial Malleolus of Tibia.

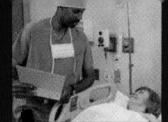
MUSCULOSKELETAL SYSTEM

CHALLENGE YOUR KNOWLEDGE

A. Fill out the disability form for Ms. Lara Baker. Use the information provided in Case Report 5.6, with these additional facts:

1. Ms. Baker must complete her physiotherapy (PT) first, and then return to see Dr. Stannard.

2. Ms. Baker is to remain off work until she has completed PT and returned to see Dr. Stannard in 3 weeks.

3. Dr. Stannard is an MD.

4. Ms. Baker has no other current medical problems.

5. The disability insurance carrier is Empire Insurance Company.

6. On examination, Dr. Stannard has found pain, swelling, numbness, tingling, and reduced grip in Ms. Baker's right hand.

7. The office phone number is on the letterhead, and Dr. Stannard takes calls from 8 to 9 a.m. and again from 3 to 4 p.m., Monday through Friday.

Fulwood Medical Center
3333 Medical Parkway, Fulwood, MI 01234
555-247-6100

Department of Orthopedics
Dr. Stannard 555-247-6100

Doctor's report of occupational injury or illness

Patient name:_____
Patient address:_____
Occupation:_____
Employer:_____
Employer's insurance company:_____
(Please provide insurance claim form to billing manager)_____
Date of onset of illness: (*back date from date seen*)_____
Date seen: (*use current date*)_____
Date last worked: (*use current date*)_____
_____
Patient's description of how injury occurred:_____
Patient's chief complaints:_____
Doctor's findings:_____
Diagnosis:_____
Treatment Plan_____
_____
_____

Any special equipment ordered? No_____Yes_____
If yes, describe equipment: _____
Is there any other current condition that will delay recovery from this injury/illness?
No _____ Yes _____ If yes, describe_____
Is further treatment required? No _____ Yes _____
Followup appointment?   No _____ Yes _____
When _____
Can patient return to work at this time?

YES	NO
No modifications _____	Still in treatment _____
With modification _____	Unable to return to this job _____
Describe restrictions: No lifting _____ No standing _____ No sitting for extended periods of time _____ Other_____	
Full time_____	
Part time only _____	

May we call you concerning this patient? No ——Yes—— Best time:_____
Doctor's name and degree:_____
License number:_____Tax ID#_____
Doctor's signature: (stamped signature not acceptable)

B. **Show your understanding of orthopedic terminology by providing the meaning of the elements for the terms below and then using the term in a sentence.** Slash (/) the terms into elements before you start the exercise.

1. **orthopedic** The combining form is _____ and means _____.
    Sentence:

    _____

    _____

2. **endosteum** The prefix is _____ and means _____.
    Sentence:

    _____

    _____

3. **epiphysis** The root is _____ and means _____.
    Sentence:

    _____

    _____

4. **articulation** The suffix is _____ and means _____.
    Sentence:

    _____

    _____

5. **degenerative** The root is _____ and means _____.
    Sentence:

    _____

    _____

6. **arthrodesis** The suffix is _____ and means _____.
    Sentence:

    _____

    _____

7. **fibromyalgia** The combining form is _____ and means _____.
    Sentence:

    _____

    _____

MUSCULOSKELETAL SYSTEM

C. **The skeleton effects movement and provides support and protection for the entire body.** Help build your knowledge of the skeleton and orthopedic terminology with this minioutline.

The four components of the skeletal system are:

1. _____

2. _____

3. _____

4. _____

These components have the following functions:

1. _____

2. _____

3. _____

4. _____

5. _____

6. _____

Factors that affect bone growth:

1. _____

2. _____

3. _____

4. _____

5. _____

6. _____

7. _____

The most common type of bone in the body is the long bone. Define these terms related to long bones:

1. epiphysis _____

_____

2. diaphysis _____

_____

3. metaphysis _____

_____

4. Covers outer surface of all bones: _____

5. Cartilage cells in the _____ enable the bone shaft to grow in length.

6. The _____ _____ contains the bone marrow and is lined with the membrane

called the _____.

D. **Abbreviations in medical documentation save time for the writer.** You must be sure, however, to interpret them correctly for patient safety. Write the full meaning of each abbreviation on the blank.

1. Eventual treatment for Mrs. Vargas' THR (_____) will involve either an orthopedist or a DO (_____). The PT (_____) department will also provide follow-up care to improve her ROM (_____) and mobility after the surgery. Mrs. Vargas will also take medication to avoid any further DJD (_____).

2. The patient's prescription for pain medication was written for 150 mg (_____) to be taken two times a day. This was not helping her pain so Dr. Stannard increased the frequency to three times a day (_____).

3. BMD (_____) tests and DEXA (_____) scans will determine if osteoporosis is present. If it is, increased IU (_____) of vitamin D may help. There is also FDA-(_____) approved medication available.

4. The patient's MRI (_____) confirmed herniation at her C5–C6 (hint: location _____) vertebral discs.

5. TMJ (_____) syndrome can be diagnosed with an electromyelogram.

Translate sentences 1, 3, and 5 into layman's language for your patient.

6. Sentence 1: _____
   _____
   _____

7. Sentence 3: _____
   _____
   _____

8. Sentence 5:_____
   _____
   _____

MUSCULOSKELETAL SYSTEM

E. **Many professional certification exams are given in multiple-choice format.** Begin deciding on the answer by quickly eliminating the answers you know to be incorrect. Then decide which of the remaining answers is the *best* choice.

1. For an open reduction, internal fixation of a fracture, what surgical hardware could be needed:

   a. wires

   b. rods

   c. plates

   d. screws

   e. any of the above

2. Bone growth occurs at the:

   a. origin

   b. epiphyseal plate

   c. diaphysis

   d. epicondyle

   e. lacuna

3. Inherited condition in which bone formation is incomplete:

   a. osteoarthritis

   b. osteomalacia

   c. osteomyelitis

   d. osteogenesis imperfecta

   e. osteopenia

4. Lubricant for joint movement:

   a. mucin

   b. mucus

   c. mucous

   d. synovial

   e. meniscus

5. Where two bones come together at a joint:

   a. articulation

   b. reduction

   c. mastication

   d. striation

   e. herniation

6. An extension of synovial membrane that forms a cushion to prevent structures from rubbing together:

   a. tendon

   b. periosteum

   c. ligament

   d. bursa

   e. muscle

7. Pulling a bone from the distal end back into alignment:

   a. subluxation

   b. dislocation

   c. reduction

   d. resorption

   e. external fixation

8. The process of lying face-upward, flat on your spine is:

   a. pronation

   b. abduction

   c. adduction

   d. supination

   e. inversion

9. Overstretching or tearing of the dense sheet of tissue that supports the arch of the foot:

   a. pes planus

   b. plantar fasciitis

   c. hallux valgus

   d. Achilles tendinitis

   e. exostosis

10. Joints between the teeth and their sockets are called:

   a. symphyses

   b. gomphoses

   c. sutures

   d. syndesmoses

   e. synchondroses

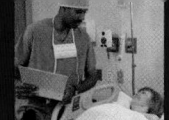
F. Correct spelling and formation of plurals are important in medical documentation. Improve your skill with this exercise. Circle the correct spelling of the singular term, and then form the plural. Use either the singular or the plural form in a sentence.

epiphysis   **epipisis**   **ephysis**   **epyisis**

Plural: _____

Sentence: _____

laccuna   **lacuna**   **lecuna**   **lacunna**

Plural: _____

Sentence: _____

thoraax   **torax**   **thorax**   **thoraxx**

Plural: _____

Sentence: _____

palanx   **phalanx**   **phalynx**   **palanyx**

Plural: _____

Sentence: _____

G. Demonstrate your knowledge of the spinal anatomy by correctly labeling the indicated structures in the following illustration. Place the letter of the appropriate description (below) with the corresponding structure numbered in the figure.

   a. Curved anteriorly, numbers 1 through 7

   b. Also called the "tailbone"

   c. Vertebrae encompassing part of the trunk between the abdomen and the neck

   d. Segment of the vertebral column that forms part of the pelvis

   e. Support and cushion between two vertebrae

   f. L1–L5

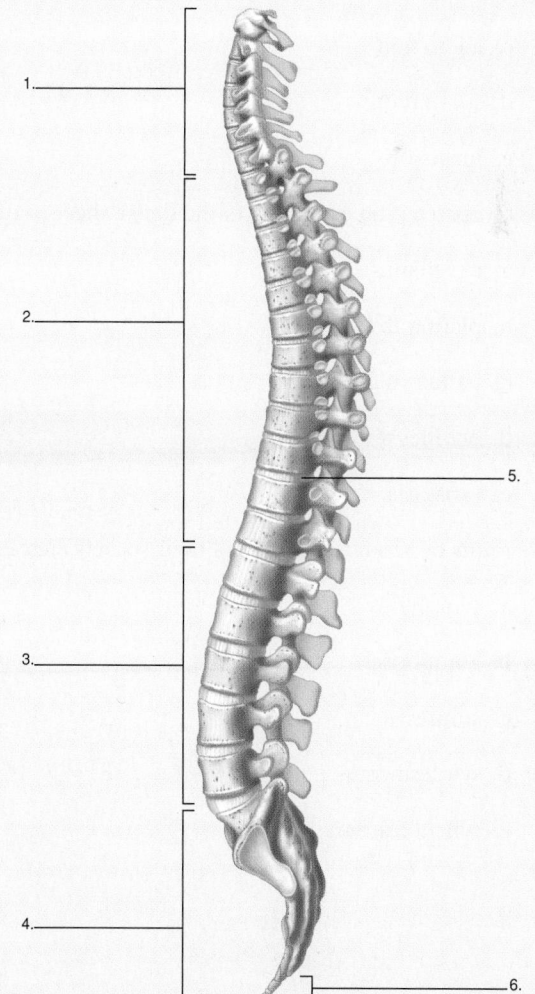

Lateral view

H. **How well do you understand what you read?** Could you explain it to a patient?

First read the paragraph; then translate the medical terms that are written in bold into layman's language for a patient explanation. Use a dictionary or the glossary for terms you don't recognize.

> The two bones of the lower leg are the larger and **medial tibia** and the thinner and **lateral fibula**. The **distal** end of the tibia on its medial border forms a prominent process called the medial **malleolus.** The lower end of the fibula forms the lateral malleolus. You can **palpate** both these **prominences** on your ankle.

1. medial _____

_____

_____

2. tibia _____

_____

_____

3. lateral _____

_____

_____

4. fibula _____

_____

_____

5. distal _____

_____

_____

6. malleolus _____

_____

_____

7. palpate _____

_____

_____

8. prominence _____

_____

_____

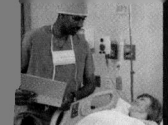

MUSCULOSKELETAL SYSTEM

I. **The following medical terms contain only roots, combining forms, and suffixes.** Identify each element, and then give a brief definition of the medical term. Fill in the chart.

Medical Term	Root(s)/CF(s)	Suffix	Definition of Term
chiropractic			
insertion			
osteoporosis			
hematoma			
pronation			
carpal			

J. **Some medical terms have common layman's terms associated with them.** Write the layman's term for:

femur _____

patella _____

K. **Physical therapists instruct patients in range-of-motion (ROM) exercises to improve mobility.** The exercises are described for you—determine the correct medical term.

abduction   **lateral rotation**   **rotation**   **pronation**   **supination**

inversion   **circumduction**   **medial rotation**   **adduction**   **eversion**

1. Rotating the humerus with the elbow flexed while bringing the palm of the hand toward the

    body is _____.

2. Elbow flexed at 90 degrees, rotate forearm so that palm is facing the floor: _____

3. Sole of the foot faces toward the opposite foot: _____ This is also called _____.

4. Action of moving toward the midline: _____

5. Turning a joint on its axis: _____

6. Sole of the foot faces laterally away from the other foot: _____ or _____

7. Moving the shoulder so that it forms a cone with the shoulder joint as the apex of the cone: _____

8. Spreading fingers apart, away from the middle finger: _____

9. Moving the palm away from the body: _____

10. Lying flat on your back, palms facing up, is _____.

L. **Discussion Question:** Amy Vargas has six different risk factors for osteoporosis. What exactly is a "risk factor"? List each risk factor; then discuss what can or cannot be done to counteract that risk. What steps could Amy have taken to improve her lifestyle and lessen her risk for osteoporosis?

_____

_____

_____

_____

_____

_____

M. **Identify the element by placing a check (✓) in the appropriate column, define the element, and then give an example of a medical term using that element.** Fill in the chart.

	Prefix	Root/CF	Suffix	Meaning of Element	Medical Term Using This Element
ab	_____	_____	_____	_____	_____
algia	_____	_____	_____	_____	_____
circum	_____	_____	_____	_____	_____
duct	_____	_____	_____	_____	_____
dys	_____	_____	_____	_____	_____
hernia	_____	_____	_____	_____	_____
inter	_____	_____	_____	_____	_____
oid	_____	_____	_____	_____	_____
or	_____	_____	_____	_____	_____
osis	_____	_____	_____	_____	_____
syn	_____	_____	_____	_____	_____
trophy	_____	_____	_____	_____	_____

N. **Post the operating room (OR) schedule for the Orthopedic Department.** Convert the description into a medical term for billing the procedure. Fill in the chart.

Description	Medical Term
Insertion right-hip prosthesis	
Removing dead tissue from an open wound of the leg	
Scope examination of left shoulder	
Surgical removal of torn meniscus of left knee	
Withdrawal of fluid from the right knee	
Removal gangrenous right leg	
Surgical removal of hypertrophied connective tissue to release a contracture	

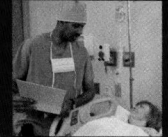
MUSCULOSKELETAL SYSTEM

O. Short Answers: Patients will ask for a layman's explanation of medical terms. If a patient asks, could you explain the difference between the following?

1. Malunion and nonunion of a fracture: _____
_____

2. A muscle strain and a muscle sprain: _____
_____

3. Shoulder separation, dislocation, and subluxation: _____
_____
_____
_____
_____

P. The following prefixes have all appeared in this chapter. The meaning of the prefix is given to you—identify the prefix, and give an example of a medical term that starts with that prefix. Fill in the chart.

Prefix	Meaning of Prefix	Medical Term
	from, out of	
	beyond, making change	
	many	
	without	
	bad	
	backward	
	together	
	away from	
	toward	
	around	

Q. Terminology Challenge: One term in this chapter has alternative spellings—either one is acceptable professionally. Find the term. Fill in the blanks with the alternative spellings and definitions.

One term is an inflammation: _____   _____

Meaning of the term: _____

R. Challenge your knowledge of bones, joints, muscles, tendons, and ligaments by assigning the medical term to the correct category. Place a check (✓) in the appropriate column.

Medical Term	Bone	Joint	Muscle	Tendon	Ligament
ball and socket					
TMJ					
DMD					
gastrocnemius					
rotator cuff					
ACL					
rickets					
dislocation					
compact or cortical					
tenosynovitis					
hinge					
marrow					
acetabulum					
DJD					
Achilles					

S. **Recall and Review:** This exercise on word elements contains some elements from this chapter and the previous chapter. Try to recall the previous elements without turning back in your book. Check the type of element; then write its meaning. Fill in the blanks.

Element	Prefix	Root/CF	Suffix	Meaning of Element
pur	_____	_____	_____	_____
eso	_____	_____	_____	_____
later	_____	_____	_____	_____
ophthalmo	_____	_____	_____	_____
phobia	_____	_____	_____	_____
stereo	_____	_____	_____	_____
strab	_____	_____	_____	_____
teno	_____	_____	_____	_____
um	_____	_____	_____	_____
ure	_____	_____	_____	_____

MUSCULOSKELETAL SYSTEM

T. **Choose the correct medical term(s) from the list to complete the sentence.** You will not use all the terms.

striation	symphysis	detoxification	intervertebral discs
DMD	orthotic	opposition	pelvis
retinaculum	shoulder girdle	fascicle	acetabulum
popliteal fossa	traction	steroids	fibromyalgia

1. Line or streak across a muscle is called a _____.

2. Transverse, fibrous band on the wrist: _____

3. _____ support and cushion the vertebral column.

4. _____ has no known etiology, no laboratory tests for it, and no known treatment except pain management.

5. Movement that enables the thumb to touch the tips of the other fingers is called _____.

6. Cartilaginous joint between two bones: _____

7. Bundle of muscle fibers: _____

8. Dr. Stannard ordered continuous application of weight to the patient's broken leg. He has been placed

   in _____.

9. _____ cause skeletal muscle to hypertrophy.

10. The hollow at the back of the knee is called the _____.

U. **Build your orthopedic terminology by completing the medical terms defined here.** After you fill in the element on the line, write the type of element (prefix, root, combining form, suffix) you have used below the line. Fill in the blanks.

1. Removing poison from tissue   de/ _____ / _____

2. Bone disease   osteo/_____

3. Projection above the condyle   _____ /condyle

4. Membrane surrounding a bone   peri/ _____ / _____

5. Region between diaphysis and epiphysis   _____ /physis

6. Bones lacking in calcium   osteo/ _____

7. Inflammation of bone tissue   osteo/ _____ /itis

8. Collection of blood in tissues   _____ /oma

9. Moving toward the midline   _____ /ion

10. Fixation of a joint with surgery   arthro/ _____

V. Knowing the exact number of certain body parts, and their relative positions, will ensure precision in your medical documentation. Match the correct number to the correct term. Use one answer twice.

1. Number of lumbar vertebrae: _____

2. Number of bones in the vertebral column: _____

3. Number of cervical vertebrae: _____

4. Number of components in the skeletal system: _____

5. Number of regions in the vertebral column: _____

6. Number of thoracic vertebrae: _____

A. 7

B. 5

C. 4

D. 12

E. 26

W. Could you explain the difference among these abnormal spinal curvatures to a patient if they ask?

lordosis _____

scoliosis _____

kyphosis _____

Which one is the most common defect? _____

Which defect is seen in patients with osteoporosis? _____

> **Study Hint**
> Anything that is referred to as the most powerful, largest, smallest, most common, etc., is probably going to be a test question.

X. **Functions of Skeletal Muscles:** (Add this to your outline.) Bones and joints would get us nowhere without the muscles to move them. Illustrate how each of these functions is accomplished with skeletal muscles.

> **Study Hint**
> To help you remember the functions, make up a sentence with each word (mnemonic) starting with the letters M, P, B, R, and C. *Example: Mr. Parker's Body Heat Rose Considerably.*

Function	How Function Is Effected
Movement	_____
Posture	_____
Body heat	_____
Respiration	_____
Communication	_____

Y. Employ the *language of orthopedics* to answer the following questions about muscles.

1. What is muscle tone?

_____

_____

2. What is muscle contraction?

_____

_____

3. What is the difference between muscle atrophy and hypertrophy?

_____

_____

MUSCULOSKELETAL SYSTEM

Z. **The practice needs to hire an additional doctor due to patient volume.** The business manager has asked you to run a computer report that will give you the 10 most frequently billed diagnoses in the orthopedic clinic. You must analyze the report to give the manager the information she needs. The 10 most frequently billed diagnoses are shown below (not in any special order); determine the meaning of the key terms and which body part is affected. The first one is done for you.

Diagnosis	Meaning	Body Part
Osteoarthritis of the patella	*arthritis of the knee*	*knee*
Repair of AC joint		
Herniated discectomy		
Rotator cuff repair		
ACL repair		
Meniscectomy		
THR		
Patellar arthroplasty		
L3–L5 discectomy		

AA. **Demonstrate your knowledge of the upper-body bones and joints by circling the correct answer to these questions.**

1. What is the long bone of the upper arm called?

   radius   ulna   humerus   carpal   scapula

2. What is a likely shoulder injury?

   separation   ACL tear   Colles Fx   ganglion   tenosynovitis

3. What structures hold an articulation together?

   ligaments   tendons   muscles   joint capsule   all of these

4. Incision through a band of fascia is called:

   arthrotomy   fasciectomy   arthrodesis   arthroplasty   fasciotomy

5. What connects the humerus to the pectoral girdle?

   ligaments   tendons   muscles   joints   bones

6. The broadest muscle in the back is the:

   biceps   triceps   brachii   latissimus dorsi   ulna

7. Ganglion cysts are fluid-filled cysts arising from the:

   muscles   joints   synovial tendon sheaths   articulations   bursa

8. Where does a Colles fracture occur?

    arm   leg   shoulder   elbow   wrist

9. Carpal tunnel syndrome develops as a result of inflammation and swelling of:

    bones   ligaments   tendon sheaths   cysts   muscles

10. Four muscles that originate on the scapula, wrap around the joint, and fuse to form one large tendon are called the:

    articulation   rotator cuff   brachialis   scapulae   pectoral

BB. Many medical terms come directly from Greek or Latin. Test your knowledge of these terms with this exercise. Be sure to add a brief definition for the term in the last column. The first one is done for you. Fill in the chart.

Medical Term	Meaning of Greek or Latin	Definition
bursa	*purse*	*closed sac containing synovial fluid*
callus		
cartilage		
condyle		
cortex		
lacuna		
ligament		
matrix		
meniscus		
origin		
rickets		
tendon		

Use any two terms from the above chart in a sentence of patient documentation.

1. _____

   _____

   _____

2. _____

   _____

   _____

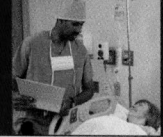

CHAPTER 5 REVIEW

MUSCULOSKELETAL SYSTEM

CHAPTER SUMMARY EXERCISES

1. *Listen to the pronunciation of the medical terms as given by your instructor.*
2. *Circle the correct spelling of the medical term.*
3. *Match the correctly spelled terms to the brief descriptions below.*
4. *Write a sentence for each of the 10 terms that appear in this exercise.*

A. SPELLING COMPREHENSION: CIRCLE THE CORRECT SPELLING OF THE TERM.

1. ephiseal	epiphyseal	epificeal	epyhiseal	epyiseal
2. fastiotomy	fasciotomy	fassiotomy	faseotomy	faciotomy
3. fibromyalgia	febromialgia	fibromialga	febromealga	fibrromialgia
4. peterygoid	pterygoid	terygoid	peterigoid	terigoid
5. interoseus	interossius	interosseous	interosseus	intraosseus
6. syndismosis	syndesmosis	sindesmosis	syndemosis	sindismosis
7. ischium	eschium	eschiom	ischeum	iseum
8. kiposis	kyposis	khyposis	kyphosis	kiphosis
9. coccix	cocyx	coccyx	cockyx	cockix
10. scapulay	scapuae	scalpulay	scappulae	scapulae

B. MATCH THE NUMBER OF THE CORRECT TERM IN PART A WITH THE BRIEF DESCRIPTION OF THE TERM BELOW.

_____ a. Incision and release of retinaculum

_____ b. Tail bone

_____ c. Opens and closes mouth

_____ d. Joint formed by ligaments

_____ e. Lower/posterior part of the hip bone

_____ f. Pain in muscle fibers

_____ g. Compact bone grows in and forms this line

_____ h. Structure between bones

_____ i. Shoulder blades

_____ j. Posterior spinal curve

C. USING YOUR KNOWLEDGE OF TERMS 1–10 IN PART A AND THEIR CORRECT SPELLING, WRITE A BRIEF SENTENCE FOR EACH OF THE TERMS AS IT MIGHT APPEAR IN PATIENT DOCUMENTATION.

1. _____

2. _____

3. _____

4. _____

5. _____

6. _____

7. _____

8. _____

9. _____

10. _____

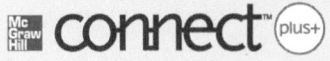

D. YOUR INSTRUCTOR WILL DIRECT YOU TO MCGRAW-HILL CONNECT. OPEN THE AUDIO GLOSSARY AND PRACTICE YOUR PRONUNCIATION OF THE TERMS IN PART A OF THIS EXERCISE.

E. AFTER READING CASE REPORT 5.2, ANSWER THE FOLLOWING QUESTIONS. *BE PREPARED TO DISCUSS YOUR ANSWERS IN CLASS.*

CASE REPORT 5.2

In his youth Mr. Johnson played football and baseball. As an adult, he has played racquetball weekly and jogged 3 to 4 miles most mornings on the streets of his neighborhood. For the past year he has had lower-back stiffness and pain, particularly in the mornings. Six months ago, while out hiking, he slid down a mountain on his left side for about 100 feet. He is now having pain in his left groin and thigh, with difficulty walking and climbing stairs.

By age 65, more than 80% of people have some degree of joint degeneration. Mr. Johnson had always been very physically active, putting a lot of pressure on his weight-bearing joints. At different times in his life he had been overweight, adding to the pressure.

X-rays of his lower back showed **osteoarthritis** of his lower lumbar intervertebral joints and marked osteoarthritis of his left hip joint. He received a left total-hip replacement **(THR)** and physiotherapy for his lower back.

1. Explain to your patient in layman's terms what is meant by "joint degeneration."

_____

_____

2. Describe what is meant by a "weight-bearing" joint and where it is located on the body. _____

3. What physical condition complicated Mr. Johnson's joint problems? _____

_____

4. What is the chronic inflammatory disease of the joints that causes pain and loss of function? _____

5. Where are the "lower lumbar" intervertebral joints located? _____

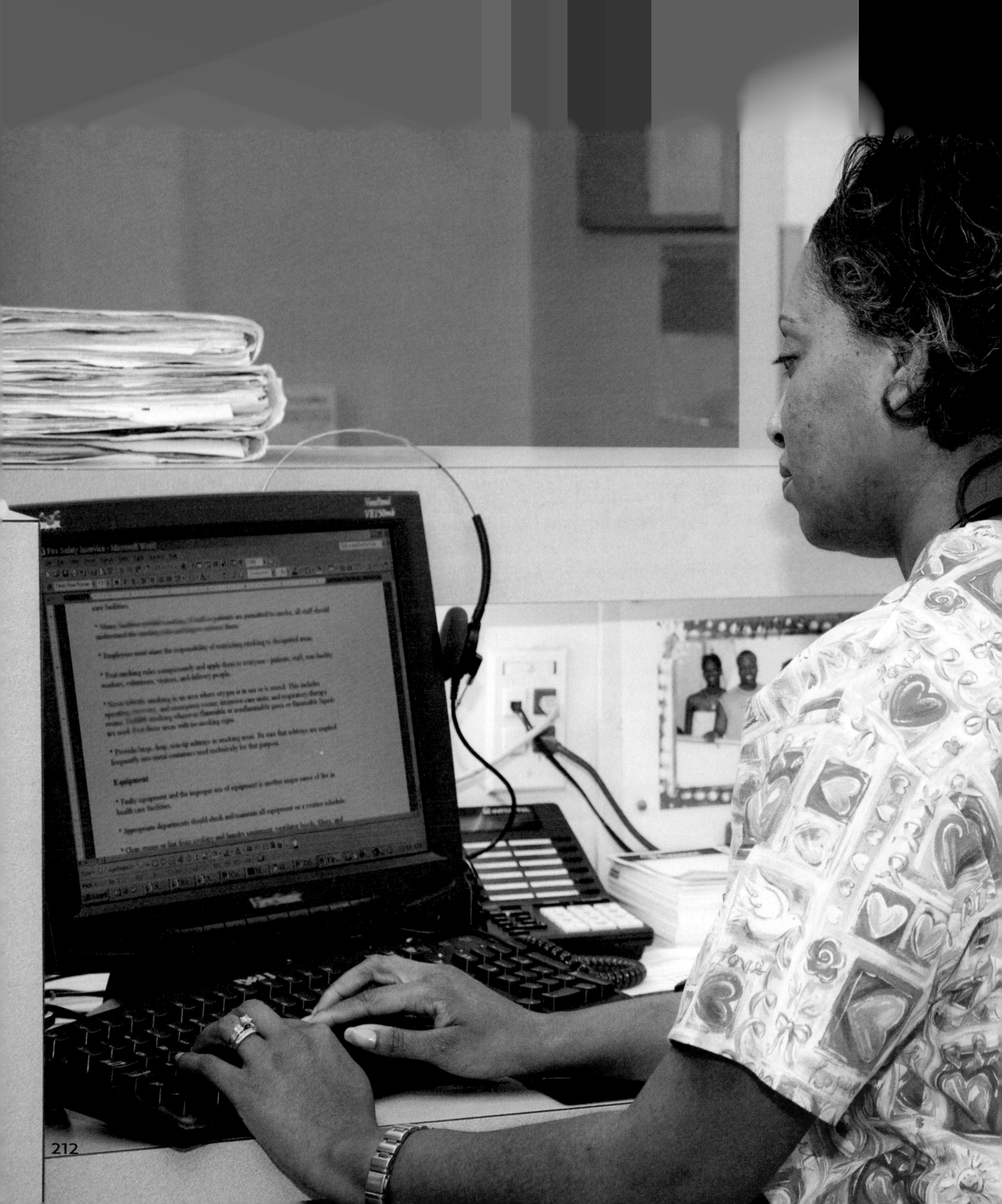

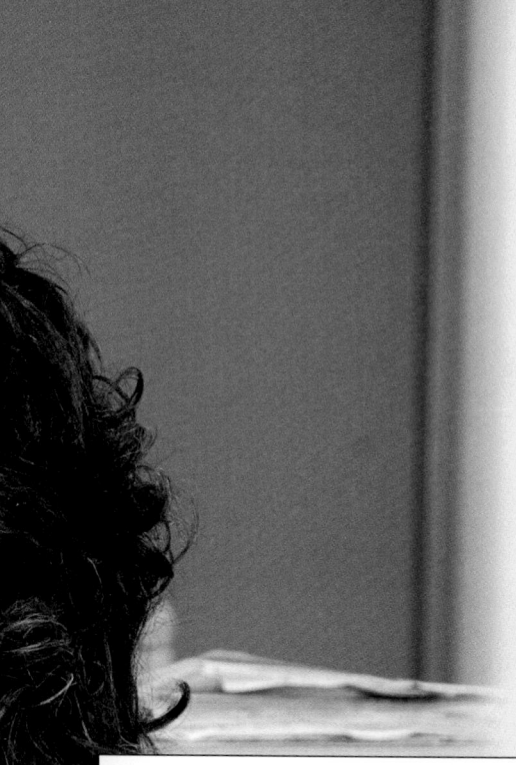

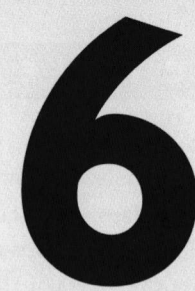
CASE REPORT 6.1

You are

. . . a medical **transcriptionist** at Fulwood Medical Center.

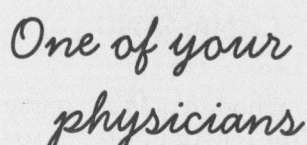

One of your physicians

. . . Dr. Stewart Walsh, has dictated this letter to request authorization for a procedure:

Fulwood Medical Center
3333 Medical Parkway, Fulwood, MI 01234
555-247-6100

Department of: Bariatric Surgery

To: Charles Leavenworth, MD
Medical Director
Lombard Insurance Company

From: Stewart Walsh, MD, FACS
Chief of Surgery
Center for Bariatric Surgery
Fulwood Medical Center

10/06/09

Dear Doctor Leavenworth,

Request for authorization of surgery

Re: Mrs. Martha Jones
Subscriber ID 056437

Mrs. Jones is a 52-year-old former waitress, recently divorced. She is 5 feet 4 inches tall and weighs 275 pounds. She has type 2 diabetes with frequent episodes of hypoglycemia and also ketoacidosis, requiring three different hospitalizations. She now has diabetic retinopathy and peripheral vasculitis. Complicating this is hypertension (185/110), coronary artery disease, and pulmonary edema. Exercise is out of the question because she has marked osteoarthritis of her knees and hips. Mrs. Jones is now housebound, dependent on transportation to our medical center. In spite of monthly meetings with our nutritionist, she has gained 25 pounds in the past 6 months.

At a case conference earlier today, we all recognized that unless we were able to reduce and control her weight, we had no hope of controlling any of her other multiple problems.

Therefore, I am proposing to perform a Roux-en-Y **gastric** bypass using a **laparoscopic** approach. We will need to admit her 2 days prior to surgery to control her blood sugar and cardiovascular problems and anticipate that she will remain in the hospital for 2 days after surgery, barring any complications. My surgical technologist and I have spent time with Mrs. Jones explaining the procedure and its risks, and she is aware and accepting of these. She is also very aware of the necessary follow-up to the procedure and the counseling required for a new lifestyle.

We believe not only that this is an essential procedure medically but that it will reduce in the long term the financial burden of her multiple therapies and improve the quality of the patient's life. Enclosed is supportive documentation of her current history and medical problems.

Your company has designated our hospital as a Center of Excellence for weight-loss surgery, and I look forward to your prompt agreement with this approach for this patient.

Sincerely,

Stewart Walsh, MD, FACS
Chief of Surgery
Fulwood Medical Center

Learning Outcomes

As a medical transcriptionist, you and all health professionals directly and indirectly involved with Mrs. Jones's care need to be able to:

6.1 Apply the language of **gastroenterology** to the anatomy and physiology of the **gastrointestinal** tract, liver, gallbladder, and pancreas.

6.2 Comprehend, analyze, spell, and write the medical terms of gastroenterology so that you can communicate and document accurately and precisely in any health care setting.

6.3 Recognize and pronounce the medical terms of gastroenterology so that you can communicate verbally with accuracy and precision in any health care setting.

6.4 Understand the tests and procedures performed to diagnose and treat gastrointestinal disorders.

In Mrs. Martha Jones's case, the **Roux-en-Y** procedure reduced the size of her available stomach from 2 quarts to 2 ounces. This resulted in her being able to eat less and to absorb less. She had no complications from the **laparoscopic** procedure. In the succeeding 2 months, she lost 15 pounds in weight.

LESSON 6.1 The Digestive System

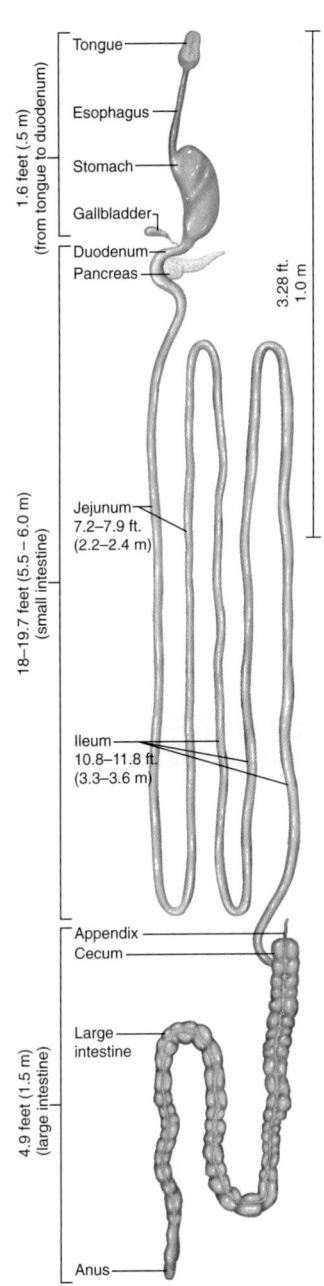

Tongue

Esophagus

Stomach

Gallbladder

Duodenum
Pancreas

1.6 feet (.5 m)
(from tongue to duodenum)

3.28 ft.
1.0 m

Jejunum
7.2–7.9 ft.
(2.2–2.4 m)

18–19.7 feet (5.5 – 6.0 m)
(small intestine)

Ileum
10.8–11.8 ft.
(3.3–3.6 m)

Appendix
Cecum

Large
intestine

4.9 feet (1.5 m)
(large intestine)

Anus

▲ **FIGURE 6.1**
Alimentary Canal.

ALIMENTARY CANAL AND ACCESSORY ORGANS

Every cell in your body requires a constant supply of nourishment. The cells cannot travel, so the nourishment has to be brought to them in a form that can be absorbed across their cell membrane. The foods that you **ingest** cannot be used in their existing form by the cells. The digestive system, through its alimentary canal, breaks down the nutrients in the food into elements that can be transported to the cells via the blood and **lymphatics.** These elements can then be transported across the cell membrane into the cell.

The **digestive system** consists of the **alimentary canal** (digestive tract), which extends from the **mouth** to the **anus,** and **accessory organs** connected to the canal to assist in digestion.

The term **gastrointestinal (GI)** technically refers to the stomach and **intestines** but is often used to mean the whole digestive system. **Gastroenterology** is the study of the digestive system. A **gastroenterologist** is a physician who specializes in the digestive system.

The **alimentary canal** *(Figure 6.1)* includes the:

- Mouth
- Pharynx
- **Esophagus**
- Stomach
- Small intestine
- Large intestine

The **accessory organs** of digestion include the:

- Teeth
- Tongue
- Salivary glands
- Liver
- Gallbladder
- Pancreas

Abbreviation
GI *gastrointestinal*

WORD ANALYSIS AND DEFINITION

S = Suffix   P = Prefix   R = Root   R/CF = Combining Form

WORD	PRONUNCIATION		ELEMENTS	DEFINITION
alimentary	al-ih-**MEN**-tar-ee	S/ R/	-ary *pertaining to* aliment- *nourishment*	Pertaining to the digestive tract
bariatric	bar-ee-**AT**-rik	S/ R/	-atric *treatment* bari- *weight*	Treatment of obesity
digestion	die-**JEST**-shun	S/ R/	-ion *action* digest- *to break down*	Breakdown of food into elements suitable for cell metabolism
digestive (adj)	die-**JEST**-iv	S/	-ive *nature of*	Pertaining to digestion
esophagus	ee-**SOF**-ah-gus		Greek *gullet*	Tube linking the pharynx and the stomach
gastric	**GAS**-trik	S/ R/	-ic *pertaining to* gastr- *stomach*	Pertaining to the stomach
gastroenterology	**GAS**-troh-en-ter-**OL**-oh-gee	S/ R/CF R/CF	-logy *study of* gastr/o- *stomach* -enter/o- *intestine*	Medical specialty of the stomach and intestines
gastroenterologist	**GAS**-troh-en-ter-**OL**-oh-jist	S/	-logist *one who studies*	Medical specialist in gastroenterology
gastrointestinal (GI)	**GAS**-troh-in-**TESS**-tin-al	S/ R/CF R/	-al *pertaining to* gastr/o- *stomach* -intestin- *gut, intestine*	Pertaining to the stomach and intestines
intestine	in-**TES**-tin		Latin *intestine, gut*	The digestive tube from stomach to anus
intestinal (adj)	in-**TES**-tin-al	S/	-al *pertaining to*	
laparoscopy	lap-ah-**ROS**-koh-pee	S/ R/CF	-scopy *to view* lapar/o- *abdomen in general*	Examination of the contents of the abdomen using an endoscope
laparoscope	**LAP**-ah-roh-skope	S/	-scope *instrument for viewing*	Instrument (endoscope) used for viewing the abdominal contents
laparoscopic (adj)	**LAP**-ah-rah-**SKOP**-ik	S/	-ic *pertaining to*	Pertaining to laparoscopy
lymph	LIMF		Latin *spring water*	A clear fluid collected from tissues and transported by vessels to venous circulation
lymphatic (adj)	lim-**FAT**-ik	S/ R/	-atic *pertaining to* lymph- *lymph*	Pertaining to lymph
mouth	MOWTH		Old English *mouth*	External opening of a cavity or canal
Roux-en-Y	**ROO**-on-Y		César Roux, a Swiss surgeon, 1857–1934	Surgical procedure to reduce the size of the stomach
transcript	**TRAN**-skript	P/ R/	trans- *across, through* -script *writing, thing copied*	An exact copy or reproduction
transcription	tran-**SCRIP**-shun	S/	-ion *action, condition*	The action of making a copy of dictated material
transcriptionist	tran-**SCRIP**-shun-ist	S/	-ist *a specialist in*	One who makes the copy of dictated material

EXERCISES

Analyzing the elements can tell you a lot about a medical term. Look closely at the medical terms shown above, and let the elements be your guide. Review the Word Analysis and Definition (WAD) box before you start the exercise. Fill in the blanks.

1. Analyzing the two combining forms shows that the term **gastroenterology** pertains to the _____ and

   the _____.

2. In the term **gastric**, the root _____ has the same meaning as the combining form _____ in the term **gastroenterology**.

3. _____ symptoms pertain to the stomach only. Because Mrs. Jones had stomach and intestinal problems,

   her symptoms can be described as _____. For this condition, she will need a specialist in the study of

   the stomach and intestines, a field known as _____. This type of physician is referred to as

   a _____.

Digestion is both mechanical and chemical.

FUNCTIONS OF THE DIGESTIVE SYSTEM

1. **Ingestion**—the selective intake of food into the mouth. Alternatively, food can be inserted directly into the stomach via a **nasogastric** or stomach tube.

2. **Propulsion**—the mechanical movement of food from the mouth to the anus *(Figure 6.2)*. Normally, this takes 24 to 36 hours. **Mastication** (chewing) breaks down the food into smaller particles so that **digestive enzymes** have a larger surface area with which to interact. **Deglutition,** or swallowing, moves the **bolus** of food from the mouth into the esophagus. **Peristalsis,** or waves of contraction and relaxation, moves material through most of the alimentary canal. **Segmental contractions** in the small intestine move food back and forth to mix it with digestive secretions.

3. **Digestion**—the breakdown of foods into forms that can be transported to and absorbed into cells. This process has two components:

   a. Mechanical digestion breaks larger pieces of food into smaller ones without altering their chemical composition. This process exposes a larger surface area of the food to the action of digestive enzymes.

   b. Chemical digestion breaks down large molecules of food into smaller and simpler chemicals. This process is carried out by digestive enzymes produced by the salivary glands, stomach, small intestine, and pancreas.

   The digestive enzymes have three main groups:
   - **Amylases** that digest carbohydrates
   - **Lipases** that digest fats
   - **Proteases** that digest proteins

4. **Secretion**—the addition throughout the digestive tract of secretions that lubricate, liquefy, and digest the food. Mucus lubricates the food and the lining of the tract. Water liquefies the food to make it easier to digest and absorb. Enzymes break down the food.

5. **Absorption**—the movement of nutrient molecules out of the digestive tract and through the epithelial cells lining the tract into the blood or lymph for transportation to body cells.

6. **Elimination**—the process by which the undigested residue of food is removed from the body.

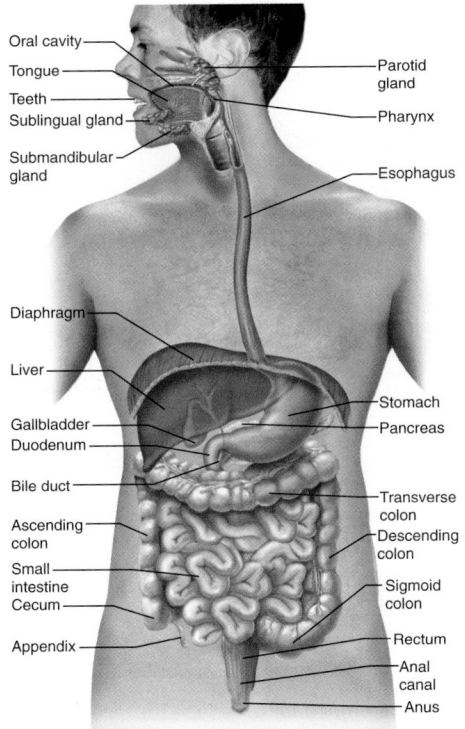

▲ **FIGURE 6.2   The Digestive System.**

Oral cavity
Tongue
Teeth
Sublingual gland
Submandibular gland
Parotid gland
Pharynx
Esophagus
Diaphragm
Liver
Gallbladder
Duodenum
Bile duct
Ascending colon
Small intestine
Cecum
Appendix
Stomach
Pancreas
Transverse colon
Descending colon
Sigmoid colon
Rectum
Anal canal
Anus

WORD	PRONUNCIATION		ELEMENTS	DEFINITION
absorption absorb (verb)	ab-**SORP**-shun ab-**SORB**		Latin *to swallow*	Uptake of nutrients and water by cells in the GI tract
amylase	**AM**-il-aze	S/ R/	-ase *enzyme* amyl- *starch*	One of a group of enzymes that break down starch
bolus	**BOH**-lus		Greek *lump*	Single mass of a substance
deglutition	dee-glue-**TISH**-un	S/ R/	-ion *action* deglutit- *to swallow*	The act of swallowing
elimination	e-lim-ih-**NAY**-shun	S/ R/	-ation *process* elimin- *throw away*	Removal of waste material from the digestive tract
ingestion	in-**JEST**-shun	S/ R/	-ion *action* ingest- *carry in*	Intake of food, either by mouth or through a nasogastric tube
lipase	**LIE**-paze	S/ R/	-ase *enzyme* lip- *fat*	Enzyme that breaks down fat
nasogastric	**NAY**-zoh-**GAS**-trik	S/ R/CF R/	-ic *pertaining to* nas/o- *nose* -gastr- *stomach*	Pertaining to the nose and stomach
peristalsis	per-ih-**STAL**-sis	P/ R/	peri- *around* -stalsis *constrict*	Waves of alternate contraction and relaxation of intestinal wall to move food along the digestive tract
protease	**PRO**-tee-aze	S/ R/CF	-ase *enzyme* prot/e- *protein*	Group of enzymes that break down protein
secrete secretion (noun)	seh-**KREET** seh-**KREE**-shun		Latin *to separate*	To release or give off, as substances produced by cells
segment segmental (adj)	**SEG**-ment **SEG**-ment-al	S/ R/	*Latin to cut* -al *pertaining to* segment- *section*	A section of an organ or structure

EXERCISES

The body process or action has been described for you. Match the definition in the left column to the correct medical term in the right column.

_____ 1. Swallowing

_____ 2. Help lubricate, liquefy, and digest food

_____ 3. Chewing

_____ 4. Removal of waste material

A. mastication

B. elimination

C. deglutition

D. secretion

Build the medical terms by filling in their missing elements.

5. Enzymes that break down protein   _____ /ase

6. The process of throwing away   _____ /ation

7. Enzyme that breaks down fat   lip/ _____

8. Enzyme that breaks down starch   _____ /ase

9. Pertaining to a section of an organ   _____ /al

10. Waves that move food in intestines   peri/ _____

11. On the basis of their suffixes, name the three enzymes in this WAD: _____, _____,

and _____ . All end in _____ .

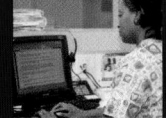

LESSON 6.2 Mouth, Pharynx, and Esophagus

OBJECTIVES

When you pop a piece of chicken and some vegetable into your mouth, you start a cascade of digestive tract events that occur during the following 24 to 36 hours. In this chapter, you will follow a meal of chicken and vegetables as it goes through the digestive tract. In this lesson, you will review the first stages in the cascade while the food is in the mouth and then is swallowed. The information in this lesson will enable you to:

6.2.1 **Identify the structure and functions of the teeth, tongue, and salivary glands.**

6.2.2 **Describe the composition and functions of saliva.**

6.2.3 **Document the process and outcomes of mastication and deglutition.**

6.2.4 **Discuss some common disorders of the mouth, pharynx, and esophagus.**

6.2.5 **Select the correct medical terminology to describe the anatomy, physiology, and disorders of the mouth, pharynx, and esophagus.**

You are

. . . a Certified Medical Assistant working with Susan Lee, MD, a primary care physician at Fulwood Medical Center.

Your patient is

. . . Mrs. Helen Schreiber, a 45-year-old high school principal. Your task is to document her care.

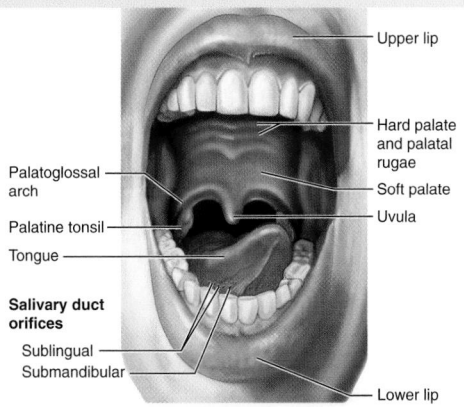

Upper lip

Hard palate and palatal rugae

Soft palate

Uvula

Palatoglossal arch

Palatine tonsil

Tongue

Salivary duct orifices

Sublingual

Submandibular

Lower lip

▲ **FIGURE 6.3** **Mouth (Oral Cavity).**

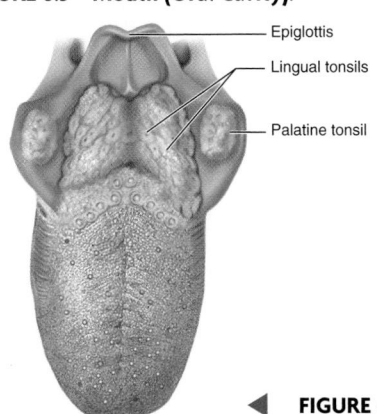

Epiglottis

Lingual tonsils

Palatine tonsil

◀ **FIGURE 6.4**
Tongue.

CASE REPORT 6.2

Documentation.

Mrs. Helen Schreiber, a 45-year-old high school principal, presents with a 6-month history of dry mouth, bleeding gums, and difficulty in chewing and swallowing food.

Questioning by Dr. Susan Lee, her primary care physician, reveals that she also has dry eyes, is having pain in some joints of both hands, and has felt fatigued. Her previous medical history is uneventful. Physical examination shows a dry mouth, mild **gingivitis**, and an **ulcer** on the back of the lower lip. Her salivary glands are not swollen. Her eyes show no **ulceration** or conjunctivitis. The metacarpophalangeal joints of both index fingers are swollen, stiff, and tender. All other systems show no abnormality.

Initial laboratory reports show anemia, decreased **WBC** count, and an elevated **ESR**. Dr. Lee made a provisional diagnosis of **Sjögren syndrome.** The results of blood studies for **SSA** and **SSB** antibodies (Sjögren syndrome antibodies A and B) and rheumatoid factor titers are pending, as are x-rays of her hands.

Mrs. Schreiber was given advice about symptomatic treatment for her dry mouth and will be seen again in 1 week.

Luis Guitterez, **CMA** 06/12/09, 1530 hrs

THE MOUTH AND MASTICATION

The mouth, or **oral** cavity *(Figure 6.3)*, is the entrance to your digestive tract and is the first site of mechanical digestion (through **mastication,** or chewing) and of chemical digestion (through an **enzyme** in saliva).

The cheeks contain the **buccinator** muscles. These muscles hold the chicken and vegetable in place while you chew and your teeth crush and tear them.

The roof of the mouth is called the **palate.** The anterior two-thirds is the bony hard palate. The posterior one-third is the muscular soft palate. The hard palate is covered with folds of epithelium called rugae, which assist the tongue to manipulate food prior to swallowing. The skeletal muscle of the soft palate has a projection called the **uvula** that closes off the nasopharynx during swallowing.

The **tongue** *(Figure 6.4)* moves food around your mouth and helps the cheeks, lips, and gums hold the food in place while you chew it. Small, rough, raised areas on the tongue, called **papillae,** contain some 4000 **taste buds** that react to the chemical nature of the food to give you the different sensations of taste. A taste bud cell lives for 7 to 10 days and is then replaced.

WORD	PRONUNCIATION	ELEMENTS		DEFINITION
buccinator	**BUCK**-sin-a-tor	S/ R/	-ator *agent* buccin- *the cheek*	Buccinator muscle is the muscle in the cheek
enzyme	**EN**-zime	P/ R/	en- *in* -zyme *fermenting, enzyme*	Protein that induces changes in other substances
gingivitis	jin-jih-**VI**-tis	S/ R/	-itis *inflammation* gingiv- *gums*	Inflammation of the gums
masticate	**MAS**-tih-kate	S/	-ate *composed of, pertaining to*	To chew
mastication (noun)	mas-tih-**KAY**-shun	R/	mastic- *chew*	
oral	**OR**-al	S/ R/	-al *pertaining to* or- *mouth*	Pertaining to the mouth
palate	**PAL**-uht		Latin *palate*	Roof of the mouth
papilla papillae (pl)	pah-**PILL**-ah pah-**PILL**-ee		Latin *small pimple*	Any small projection
Sjögren syndrome	**SHOW**-gren **SIN**-drome		Henrik Sjögren, 1899–1986, Swedish ophthalmologist	Autoimmune disease that attacks the glands that produce saliva and tears
taste	TAYST		Latin *to taste*	Sensation from chemicals on the taste buds
tongue	TUNG		Latin *tongue*	Mobile muscle mass in mouth; bears the taste buds
ulcer	**ULL**-cer		Latin *sore*	Erosion of an area of skin or mucosa
ulceration	ull-cer-**A**-shun	S/ R/	-ation *a process* ulcer- *a sore*	Formation of an ulcer
uvula	**YOU**-vyu-lah		Latin *grape*	Fleshy projection of the soft palate

Abbreviations

CMA	Certified Medical Assistant
ESR	erythrocyte sedimentation rate
SSA	Sjögren syndrome antibodies A
SSB	Sjögren syndrome antibodies B
WBC	white blood cell

EXERCISES

After reading Case Report 6.2 on the opposite page, answer the following questions. Be prepared to discuss your answers in class.

1. What are Mrs. Schreiber's presenting symptoms? _____
_____

2. What other complaints does Dr. Lee discover on further questioning of the patient? _____
_____

3. What does Dr. Lee find on physical examination of the patient? _____
_____

4. From Chapter 5 you know the location of the metacarpophalangeal joints. Describe this location (use all the correct terminology).
_____
_____

5. What does "symptomatic treatment" mean? _____
_____

6. What symptoms are specific to the patient's mouth? _____

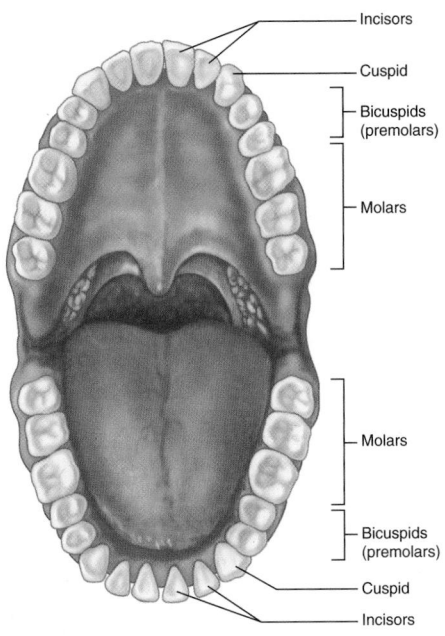

▲ FIGURE 6.5   Adult Teeth.

Labels: Incisors, Cuspid, Bicuspids (premolars), Molars, Molars, Bicuspids (premolars), Cuspid, Incisors

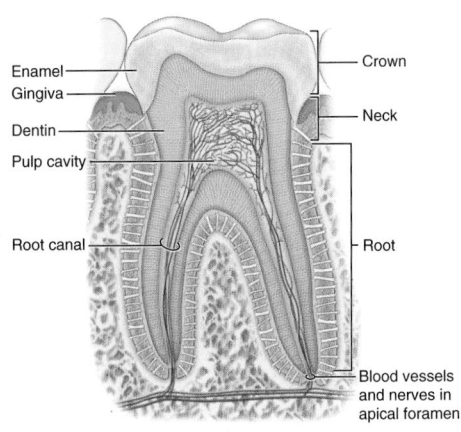

▲ FIGURE 6.6   Anatomy of a Molar.

Labels: Enamel, Gingiva, Dentin, Pulp cavity, Root canal, Crown, Neck, Root, Blood vessels and nerves in apical foramen

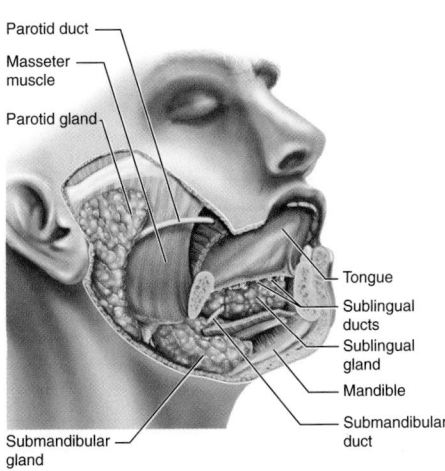

▲ FIGURE 6.7   Salivary Glands.

Labels: Parotid duct, Masseter muscle, Parotid gland, Submandibular gland, Tongue, Sublingual ducts, Sublingual gland, Mandible, Submandibular duct

Adult Teeth

The normal adult has 32 teeth, 16 rooted in the upper jaw (maxilla) and 16 in the lower jaw (mandible). The teeth are the hardest structures in your body, and different teeth *(Figure 6.5)* are designed to handle food in different ways. The eight **incisors** are shaped like a chisel to slice and cut into food. The four **cuspids** have a pointed tip for puncturing and tearing. The eight **bicuspids** and twelve **molars** have flattened surfaces for grinding and crushing food. Your wisdom teeth are molars.

Each tooth has two main parts:

- The **crown,** which projects above the gum and is covered in **enamel,** the hardest substance in the body.
- The **root,** which anchors the tooth to the jaw.

The bulk of the tooth is composed of **dentin,** a substance like bone but harder *(Figure 6.6)*. The dentin surrounds a central **pulp cavity** that contains blood vessels, nerves, and connective tissue. The blood vessels and nerves reach this cavity from the jaw through tubular **root canals.**

Salivary Glands

Salivary glands secrete saliva. The two **parotid** glands, the two **submandibular** glands, the two **sublingual glands** *(Figure 6.7)*, and numerous minor salivary glands scattered in the mucosa of the tongue and cheeks secrete more than a quart of saliva each day.

Saliva is 95% water, and its functions are to:

- Begin starch digestion with the enzyme **amylase.**
- Begin fat digestion through the enzyme **lipase.**
- Prevent the growth of bacteria in the mouth through the enzyme **lysozyme** and the protective **immunoglobulin A (IgA)** *(see Chapter 14).*
- Produce **mucus** to lubricate food to make it easier to swallow.

Case Report 6.2 (continued)

Mrs. Helen Schreiber has Sjögren syndrome, an autoimmune disease *(see Chapter 15)* that affects her salivary glands, stopping production of saliva. This leads to a dry mouth, difficulty in swallowing, and increased bacterial activity in the mouth, causing gingivitis. It is associated with dry eyes and with rheumatoid arthritis, which is beginning in her hands. There is no known cure, and treatment is **symptomatic.**

WORD	PRONUNCIATION		ELEMENTS	DEFINITION
bicuspid (also called **premolar**)	by-**KUSS**-pid	S/ P/ R/	-id *having a particular quality* bi- *two* -cusp- *point*	Having two points; a bicuspid (premolar) tooth has two points
crown	KROWN		Latin *crown*	Part of tooth above the gum
cuspid	**KUSS**-pid	S/ R/	-id *having a particular quality* -cusp- *point*	Tooth with one point
dentin (also spelled dentine)	**DEN**-tin	S/ R/	-in *substance, chemical compound* dent- *tooth*	Dense, ivorylike substance located under the enamel in a tooth
enamel	ee-**NAM**-el		French *enamel*	Hard substance covering a tooth
incisor	in-**SIGH**-zor		Latin *to cut into*	Chisel-shaped tooth
lysozyme	**LIE**-soh-zime	S/ R/CF	-zyme *enzyme* lys/o- *dissolve*	Enzyme that dissolves the cell walls of bacteria
molar	**MO**-lar		Latin *millstone*	One of six teeth in each jaw that grind food
parotid	pah-**ROT**-id	S/ P/ R/	-id *having a particular quality* par- *beside* -ot- *ear*	Parotid gland is the salivary gland beside the ear
pulp	PULP		Latin *flesh*	Dental pulp is the connective tissue in the cavity in the center of the tooth
root	ROOT		Old English *beginning*	Fundamental or beginning part of a structure
saliva salivary (adj)	sa-**LIE**-vah **SAL**-ih-var-ee	S/ R/	Latin *spit* -ary *pertaining to* saliv- *saliva*	Secretion in mouth from salivary glands
sublingual	sub-**LING**-wal	S/ P/ R/	-al *pertaining to* sub- *underneath* -lingu- *tongue*	Underneath the tongue
submandibular	sub-man-**DIB**-you-lar	S/ P/ R/	-ar *pertaining to* sub- *underneath* -mandibul- *the jaw*	Underneath the mandible
symptom	**SIMP**-tum		Greek *sign*	Departure from the normal experienced by a patient
symptomatic	simp-toe-**MAT**-ik	S/ R/	-ic *pertaining to* symptomat- *symptom*	Pertaining to the symptoms of a disease

EXERCISES

Analyze and define the following terms, and determine what makes them similar and what makes them different. Fill in the blanks.

1. submandibular   Definition: _____

2. salivary   Definition: _____

3. sublingual   Definition: _____

4. Now that you have written the definition of each term, it should be obvious what is similar. The similarity is:

_____

5. What makes the terms different? _____

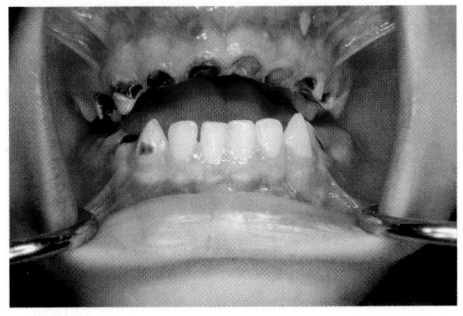

▲ **FIGURE 6.8 Dental Caries.** Child with dental caries.

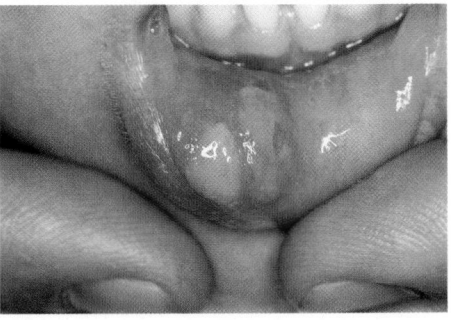

▲ **FIGURE 6.9 Cold Sores.** Ulcer inside lower lip.

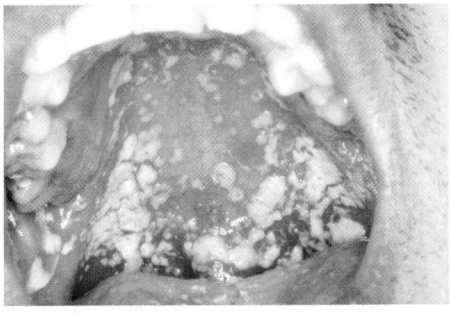

▲ **FIGURE 6.10 Oral Thrush.**

DISORDERS OF THE MOUTH

An accumulation of dental **plaque** (a collection of oral microorganisms and their products) or **dental calculus (tartar)** (calcified deposits at the gingival margin of the teeth) is a precursor to dental disease.

Dental caries, tooth decay and cavity formation, is an erosion of the tooth surface caused by bacteria *(Figure 6.8)*. If untreated, it can lead to an abscess at the root of the tooth. **Gingivitis** is an infection of the gums. **Periodontal disease** occurs when the gums and the jawbone are involved in a disease process. In **periodontitis,** infection causes the gums to pull away from the teeth, forming pockets that become infected. The infection can spread to the underlying bone. Infection of the gums with a purulent discharge is called **pyorrhea.**

The term **stomatitis** is used for any infection of the mouth. The most common infections are:

- **Mouth ulcers,** also called **canker** sores, are erosions of the mucous membrane lining the mouth. The most common type are **aphthous** ulcers, which occur in clusters of small ulcers and last for 3 or 4 days. They are usually related to stress or illness. Ulcers can also be caused by trauma.

- **Cold sores,** also known as fever blisters *(Figure 6.9)*, are recurrent ulcers of the lips, lining of the mouth, and gums due to infection with the virus **herpes simplex type 1 (HSV-1).** Acyclovir is a treatment used, but the ulcers usually clear spontaneously.

- **Thrush** *(Figure 6.10)* is an infection occurring anywhere in the mouth and is caused by the fungus *Candida albicans.* This fungus typically is found in the mouth, but it can multiply out of control as a result of prolonged antibiotic or steroid treatment, cancer chemotherapy, or diabetes. A newborn baby can acquire oral thrush from the mother's vaginal yeast infection during the birth process. Treatment with antifungal agents, such as nystatin or clotrimazole, is usually successful *(see Chapter 19)*.

- **Leukoplakia** is a white plaque seen anywhere in the mouth. It is more common in the elderly, is often associated with smoking or chewing tobacco, and approximately 3% turn into oral cancer. Patients whose immune systems are compromised (for example, with **human immunodeficiency virus [HIV]**) are susceptible to leukoplakia.

- **Oral cancer** *(Figure 6.11)* is mostly a squamous cell carcinoma, occurring often on the lip. Eighty percent of oral cancers are associated with smoking or chewing tobacco. Metastasis occurs to lymph nodes, bone, lung, and liver. The 5-year-survival rate is only 51%.

- **Halitosis** is the medical term for bad breath, which can be found in association with any of the above mouth disorders.

- **Glossodynia** is a painful burning sensation of the tongue. It occurs in postmenopausal women. Its etiology is unknown, and there is no successful treatment.

Abbreviations

HSV-1 herpes simplex virus, type 1
HIV   human immunodeficiency virus

FIGURE 6.11 Oral Cancer. Cancer of the tongue. ▶

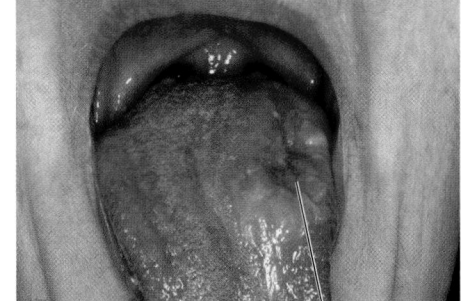

Cancer

WORD	PRONUNCIATION		ELEMENTS	DEFINITION
aphthous ulcer	**AF**-thus **UL**-ser		Greek *ulcer*	Painful small oral ulcer (canker sore)
canker; canker sore (also called **mouth ulcer**)	**KANG**-ker SOAR		Latin *crab*	Nonmedical term for aphthous ulcer
caries	**KARE**-eez		Latin *dry rot*	Bacterial destruction of teeth
gingiva	**JIN**-jih-vah		Latin *gum*	Tissue surrounding teeth and covering the jaw
gingival (adj)	**JIN**-jih-vul	S/ R/	-al *pertaining to* gingiv- *gums*	Pertaining to the gums
gingivitis	jin-jih-**VI**-tis	S/	-itis *inflammation*	Inflammation of the gums
gingivectomy	jin-jih-**VEC**-toe-me	S/	-ectomy *surgical excision*	Surgical removal of diseased gum tissue
glossodynia	gloss-oh-**DIN**-ee-ah	S/ R/CF	-dynia *pain* gloss/o- *tongue*	Painful, burning tongue
halitosis	hal-ih-**TOE**-sis	S/ R/	-osis *condition* halit- *breath*	Bad odor of the breath
leukoplakia	loo-koh-**PLAY**-kee-ah	S/ R/CF R/	-ia *condition* leuk/o- *white* -plak- *plate, plaque*	White patch on oral mucous membrane, often precancerous
periodontal	**PER**-ee-oh-**DON**-tal	S/ P/ R/	-al *pertaining to* peri- *around* -odont- *tooth*	Around a tooth
periodontics	**PER**-ee-oh-**DON**-tiks	S/	-ics *knowledge of*	Branch of dentistry specializing in disorders of tissues around the teeth
periodontist	**PER**-ee-oh-**DON**-tist	S/	-ist *specialist*	Specialist in periodontics
periodontitis	**PER**-ee-oh-don-**TIE**-tis	S/	-itis *inflammation*	Inflammation of tissues around a tooth
plaque	PLAK		French *plate*	Patch of abnormal tissue
pyorrhea	pie-oh-**REE**-ah	S/ R/CF	-rrhea *flow* py/o- *pus*	Purulent discharge
tartar (also called **dental calculus**)	**TAR**-tar		Latin *crust on wine casks*	Calcified deposit at the gingival margin of the teeth
thrush	THRUSH		Root unknown	Infection with *Candida albicans*

EXERCISES

Find the correct suffix to complete the medical terms. Use each suffix only one time. Fill in the blanks; then answer the questions.

1. Inflammation of the gums   gingiv/ _____

2. Specialized branch of dentistry   periodont/ _____

3. Painful, burning tongue   glosso/ _____

4. Around a tooth   periodont/ _____

5. Bad breath   halit/ _____

6. Surgical removal of diseased gums   gingiv/ _____

7. Precancerous white patches   leukoplak/ _____

8. One who specializes in periodontics   periodont/ _____

9. *Aphthous, oral,* and *ulcer* are all terms connected with _____ _____.

10. Dental caries is another name for _____.

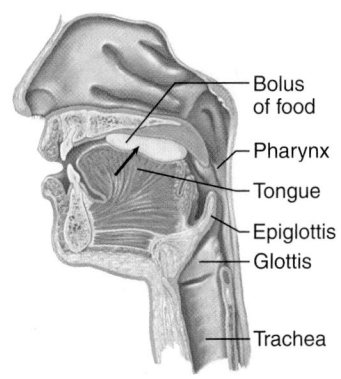

▲ **FIGURE 6.12   Deglutition (Swallowing): Phase One.**

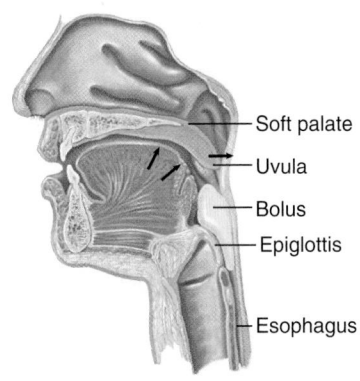

▲ **FIGURE 6.13   Deglutition (Swallowing): Phase Two.**

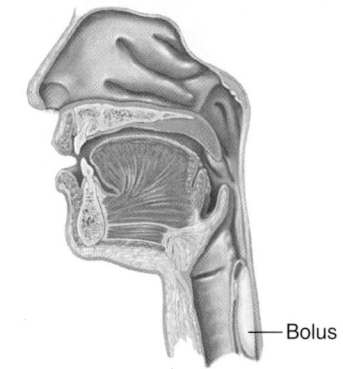

▲ **FIGURE 6.14   Deglutition (Swallowing): Phase Three.**

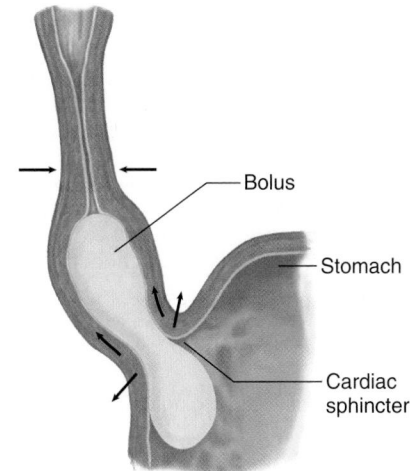

▲ **FIGURE 6.15   Deglutition (Swallowing): Phase Four.**

Abbreviation

GERD gastroesophageal reflux disease

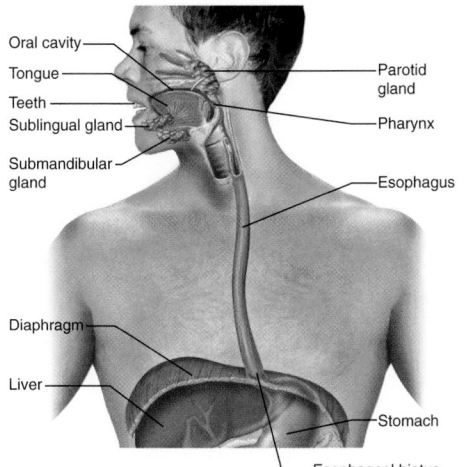

▲ **FIGURE 6.16   Esophagus.**

DEGLUTITION (SWALLOWING)—PHARYNX AND ESOPHAGUS

The pieces of chicken and vegetable that you ingested have now been sliced and ground into small particles by the teeth, partly digested and lubricated by saliva, and rolled into a bolus between the tongue and the hard palate, the bony roof of the mouth *(Figure 6.12)*. The bolus is now ready to be swallowed **(deglutition)**.

- **Phase One.** As you swallow, the bolus of food is pushed backward by your tongue into the **oropharynx**. Once the bolus is in your oropharynx, the tongue pushes up the soft palate and **uvula** to close off the **nasopharynx** at the back of the nose. This prevents food from going up into your nasopharynx and nose *(Figure 6.12)*.

- **Phase Two.** Surrounding the oropharynx are circular muscles called **constrictors**. These muscles contract, forcing the bolus down through the laryngopharynx toward the **esophagus** and pushing the **epiglottis** closed so that food cannot enter the **larynx** and **trachea** *(Figure 6.13)*.

- **Phase Three.** When the bolus reaches the lower end of the **pharynx**, the upper **esophageal sphincter** relaxes and the bolus enters the esophagus, where contractions of the muscles in the wall move the bolus toward the stomach *(Figure 6.14)*.

- **Phase Four.** The esophageal sphincter at the lower end of the esophagus **(cardiac sphincter)** relaxes to allow the bolus to enter the stomach *(Figure 6.15)*.

The **esophagus** *(Figure 6.16)* is a tube 9 to 10 inches long; it pierces the diaphragm at the esophageal **hiatus** to go from the thoracic cavity to the abdominal cavity *(see Chapter 2)*.

Disorders of the Esophagus

Esophagitis is inflammation of the lining of the esophagus that produces a **postprandial** burning chest pain **(heartburn)**, pain on swallowing, and occasional vomiting of blood **(hematemesis)**. The most common cause is **reflux** of the stomach's acid contents into the esophagus, **gastroesophageal reflux disease (GERD)**. **Regurgitation** of stomach contents into the mouth **(water brash)** can occur with resulting hypersalivation.

Hiatal hernia occurs when a portion of the stomach protrudes through the diaphragm alongside the esophagus at the esophageal hiatus. Reflux of acid stomach contents into the esophagus causes an esophagitis. Surgical repair sometimes is necessary and is called a **herniorrhaphy**.

Esophageal varices are **varicose** veins of the esophagus. They are **asymptomatic** until they rupture, causing massive bleeding and hematemesis. They are a complication of cirrhosis of the liver *(Lesson 6.4)*.

Cancer of the esophagus arises from the lining of the tube. Symptoms are difficulty in swallowing **(dysphagia)**, a burning sensation in the chest, and weight loss. Risk factors include cigarettes, alcohol, betel nut chewing, and esophageal reflux. The cancer metastasizes to liver, bone, and lung.

WORD	PRONUNCIATION		ELEMENTS	DEFINITION
deglutition	dee-glue-**TISH**-un		Latin *to swallow*	The act of swallowing
dysphagia	dis-**FAY**-jee-ah	P/ R/	**dys-** *difficult* **-phagia** *swallowing*	Difficulty in swallowing
emesis	**EM**-eh-sis	S/ R/	**-sis** *abnormal condition* **eme-** *to vomit*	Vomit
hematemesis	he-mah-**TEM**-eh-sis	R/	**hemat-** *blood*	Vomiting of red blood
epiglottis	ep-ih-**GLOT**-is	P/ R/	**epi-** *above* **-glottis** *windpipe*	Leaf-shaped plate of cartilage that shuts off larynx during swallowing
esophagus **esophageal (adj)**	ee-**SOF**-ah-gus ee-**SOF**-ah-**JEE**-al	S/ R/	Greek *gullet* **-eal** *pertaining to* **esophag-** *esophagus*	Tube linking the pharynx and stomach
esophagitis	ee-**SOF**-ah-**JI**-tis	S/	**-itis** *inflammation*	Inflammation of the lining of the esophagus
hernia	**HER**-nee-ah		Latin *rupture*	Protrusion of a structure through the tissue that normally contains it
herniorrhaphy	**HER**-nee-**OR**-ah-fee	S/ R/CF	**-rrhaphy** *suture* **herni/o-** *hernia*	Repair of a hernia
herniate (verb)	**HER**-nee-ate	S/	**-ate** *pertaining to*	To protrude
hiatus **hiatal (adj)**	high-**AY**-tus high-**AY**-tal		Latin *an aperture*	An opening through a structure
larynx	**LAIR**-inks		Latin *larynx*	Organ of voice production
nasopharynx	**NAY**-zoh-**FAIR**-inks	R/CF R/	**nas/o-** *nose* **-pharynx** *throat*	Region of the pharynx at the back of the nose and above the soft palate
oropharynx	**OR**-oh-**FAIR**-inks	R/CF R/	**or/o-** *mouth* **-pharynx** *throat*	Region at the back of the mouth between the soft palate and the tip of the epiglottis
pharynx	**FAIR**-inks		Greek *throat*	Air tube from the back of the nose to the larynx
postprandial	post-**PRAN**-dee-al	S/ P/ R/	**-ial** *pertaining to* **post-** *after* **-prand-** *breakfast*	Following a meal
reflux	**REE**-fluks	P/ R/	**re-** *back* **-flux** *flow*	Backward flow
regurgitation	ree-gur-jih-**TAY**-shun	S/ P/ R/	**-ation** *process* **re-** *back* **-gurgit-** *flood*	Expel contents of the stomach into the mouth, short of vomiting
trachea	**TRAY**-kee-ah		Greek *windpipe*	Air tube from the larynx to the bronchi
varix **varices (pl)** **varicose (adj)**	**VAIR**-iks **VAIR**-ih-seez **VAIR**-ih-kos		Latin *dilated vein*	Dilated, tortuous vein Characterized by or affected with varices

---

EXERCISES   *Some of the terms in this chapter are particularly hard to spell and pronounce. Work with the audio glossary at McGraw-Hill CONNECT for pronunciation practice, and remember that spelling is important! Read these sentences aloud after you have circled your choices.*

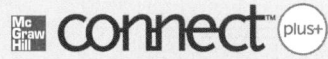

1. (Hyatus/Hiatus) is the Latin word for *opening* and is the opening through the diaphragm for the (esophagis/esophagus).

2. The (eppiglotis/epiglottis) is a leaf-shaped plate of cartilage that acts to cover the opening of the (larynix/larynx) during deglutition.

3. Medication may be ordered (postprandial/postperandial), meaning *taken after meals.*

4. (Hemotemasis/Hematemesis) is the (vomiting/vomitting) of blood.

5. (Esophagitis/Esophogitis) can be caused by reflux disease.

6. (Varricces/Varices) is the plural of (varix/varex) and means *dilated, tortuous vein.* The adjective is (varicose/varricose).

Digestion—Stomach and Small Intestine

The bolus of food that you swallowed has passed down the esophagus. It now enters the stomach, and the process of digestion begins in earnest. The stomach continues the mechanical breakdown of the food particles and begins the chemical digestion of protein and fats. It is in the small intestine that the greatest amount of digestion and absorption occurs. The information in this lesson will enable you to:

6.3.1 Describe the secretions of the stomach and their functions.

6.3.2 Discuss the secretions of the small intestine and their functions.

6.3.3 Explain how food is propelled through the stomach and small intestine.

6.3.4 Detail how the breakdown products of digestion are absorbed from the small intestine.

6.3.5 Use the correct medical terminology to describe the process of digestion in the small intestine.

You are

. . . an **EMT-1** working in the Emergency Department at Fulwood Medical Center.

Your patient is

. . . Mrs. Jan Stark, a 36-year-old pottery maker. Your task is to document her visit.

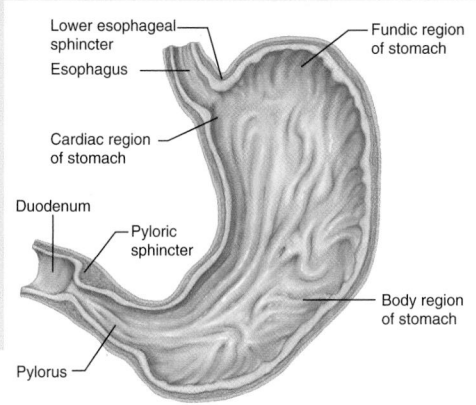

▲ **FIGURE 6.17** Stomach.

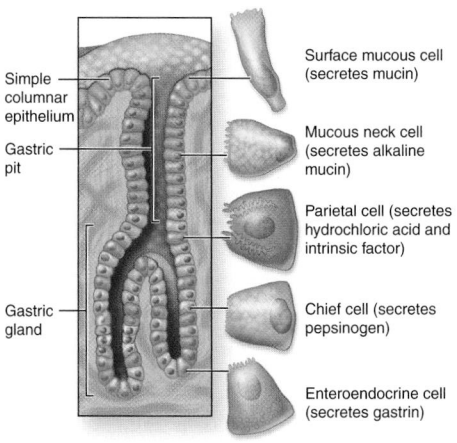

▲ **FIGURE 6.18** Gastric Cells and Their Secretions.

CASE REPORT 6.3

Documentation.

Mrs. Jan Stark, a 36-year-old pottery maker, was admitted to the Emergency Department at 2015 hrs.

She stated the she had passed between 20 and 30 watery, gray stools in the previous 24 hours. She had not passed urine for more than 12 hours. She was markedly **dehydrated** and responded well to infusion of lactated Ringer solution and then D5NS (5% dextrose in normal 0.9% saline).

Questioning revealed that, for the past 10 years, she has had spasmodic episodes of diarrhea and flatulence associated with severe headaches and fatigue. During those episodes her stools were greasy and pale. In the past 3 or 4 months, she has had some difficulties with fine movements as she works on her pottery wheel and has had tingling in her fingers and toes.

Dr. Homer Hilinski, emergency physician, believes her **dehydration** is a result of a **malabsorption syndrome.** An appointment has been made for her to see Dr. Cameron Grabowski, gastroenterologist, tomorrow. She was discharged to her husband's care at midnight. She has been advised to stay on fluids only and to return to the **ER** (Emergency Room) if the diarrhea returns.

Sunil Patel, EMT-1. 06/21/10, 0100 hrs.

DIGESTION: THE STOMACH

The stomach's peristaltic contractions mix different boluses of food together and also push the more liquid contents toward the **pylorus** *(Figure 6.17)*. These contractions and the digestive process work on the boluses of food to produce a mixture of semidigested food called **chyme.**

The cells of the lining of the stomach secrete the following *(Figure 6.18)*:

- **Mucin**—continues to lubricate food and protects the stomach lining.

- **Hydrochloric acid (HCl)**—breaks up the connective tissue of the chicken and the cell walls of the vegetable that you ingested a few seconds ago.

- **Pepsinogen**—hydrochloric acid converts pepsinogen to **pepsin,** an active enzyme that starts to digest the protein in the chicken and vegetable.

- **Intrinsic factor**—is essential for the absorption of vitamin B_{12} in the small intestine *(see Chapter 21)*. Neither chicken nor vegetables contain this factor.

- **Chemical messengers**—stimulate other cells in the gastric mucosa. One of these messengers, **gastrin,** stimulates both the production of HCl and pepsinogen by the stomach cells and the peristaltic contractions of the stomach.

WORD	PRONUNCIATION	ELEMENTS		DEFINITION
chyme	KYME		Greek *juice*	Semifluid, partially digested food passed from the stomach into the duodenum
dehydration	dee-high-**DRAY**-shun	S/ P/ R/	-ation *a process* de- *without* -hydr- *water*	Process of losing body water
duodenum	du-oh-**DEE**-num	S/ R/	-um *structure* duoden- Latin for *twelve*	The first part of the small intestine; approximately 12 finger-breadths (9 to 10 inches) in length
duodenal (adj)	du-oh-**DEE**-nal	S/	-al *pertaining to*	Pertaining to the duodenum
gastrin	**GAS**-trin	S/ R/	-in *substance* gastr- *stomach*	Hormone secreted in the stomach that stimulates secretion of HCl and increases gastric motility
hydrochloric acid (HCl)	high-droh-**KLOR**-ic **ASS**-id	S/ R/CF R/	-ic *pertaining to* hydr/o- *water* -chlor- *green*	HCl is the acid of gastric juice
intrinsic factor	in-**TRIN**-sik **FAK**-tor	S/ R/ R/	-ic *pertaining to* intrins- *on the inside* factor *maker*	Substance that makes the absorption of vitamin B$_{12}$ happen
malabsorption	mal-ab-**SORP**-shun	S/ P/ R/	-ion *action, condition* mal- *bad* -absorpt- *to swallow*	Inadequate gastrointestinal absorption of nutrients
mucus mucous (adj) mucin	**MYU**-kus **MYU**-kus **MYU**-sin		Latin *slime*	Sticky secretion of cells in mucous membranes Relating to mucus or the mucosa Protein element of mucus
pepsin pepsinogen	**PEP**-sin pep-**SIN**-oh-jen	 S/ R/CF	 Greek *to digest* -gen *produce* pepsin/o- *pepsin*	Enzyme produced by the stomach that breaks down protein Converted by HCl in stomach to pepsin
pylorus pyloric (adj)	pie-**LOR**-us pie-**LOR**-ik	S/ R/ S/	-us *pertaining to* pylor- *gate* -ic *pertaining to*	Exit area of the stomach Pertaining to the pylorus

Liquids exit the stomach within 1½ to 2 hours after ingestion. A typical meal like your chicken and vegetable takes 3 to 4 hours to exit. The resulting chyme is held in the pylorus. Peristaltic waves squirt 2 to 3 mL of the chyme at a time through the **pyloric sphincter** into the **duodenum**.

Abbreviations	
ER	emergency room
HCl	hydrochloric acid
EMT-1	emergency medical technician–first responder

EXERCISES

After reading Case Report 6.3 on the opposite page, answer the following questions. Be prepared to discuss your answers in class.

1. What is your body lacking if you are *dehydrated?* _____

2. What is an infusion? _____

3. What are Mrs. Stark's presenting symptoms? _____

_____

4. What symptoms are in Mrs. Stark's past medical history? _____

_____

5. *Malabsorption syndrome* means that Mrs. Stark's body is not absorbing _____ .

DISORDERS OF THE STOMACH

Gastroesophageal reflux disease (GERD) is the regurgitation of stomach contents back into the esophagus, often when a person is lying down at night. The patient experiences burning sensations in the chest and mouth from the acidity of the regurgitation. The acidity can also irritate and ulcerate the lining of the esophagus, causing it to bleed. Scar tissue can form and cause an esophageal **stricture,** with difficulty in swallowing (dysphagia).

Vomiting can result from overdistension or irritation of any part of the digestive tract. A message is sent via the **vagus** nerve to the vomiting center in the brain, which, in turn, stimulates the muscles of the diaphragm and abdominal wall to forcefully contract and expel the stomach contents upward into the esophagus and out the mouth.

Gastritis is an inflammation of the lining of the stomach, producing symptoms of epigastric pain, a feeling of fullness, nausea, and occasional bleeding. Gastritis can be caused by common medications such as aspirin and **NSAIDs** (nonsteroidal anti-inflammatory drugs), by radiotherapy and chemotherapy, and by alcohol and smoking. Treatment is directed at removing the factors causing the gastritis by acid neutralization and suppression of gastric acid (see "Pharmacology of Treating Excess Gastric Acid," below).

Peptic ulcers occur in the stomach and duodenum when the balance between the acid gastric juices and the protection of the mucosal lining breaks down, causing an **erosion** of the lining by the acid *(Figure 6.19)*. Most peptic ulcers are caused by the bacterium *Helicobacter pylori* (*H. pylori*), which produces enzymes that weaken the protective mucus. These ulcers respond to an antibiotic. Use of NSAIDs increases the incidence of peptic ulcers, particularly in the elderly. **Dyspepsia,** epigastric pain with bloating and nausea, is the most common symptom.

Gastric ulcers are peptic ulcers occurring in the stomach. Symptoms are epigastric burning pain after food, nausea, vomiting, and belching. Bleeding can occur from **erosion** of a blood vessel. If untreated, the ulcer can erode through the entire wall, causing a **perforation.**

Gastric cancer can be asymptomatic for a long period and then cause **indigestion, anorexia,** abdominal pain, and weight loss. It affects men twice as often as women. It metastasizes to lymph nodes, liver, peritoneum, chest, and brain. It is usually treated with **resection** and chemotherapy.

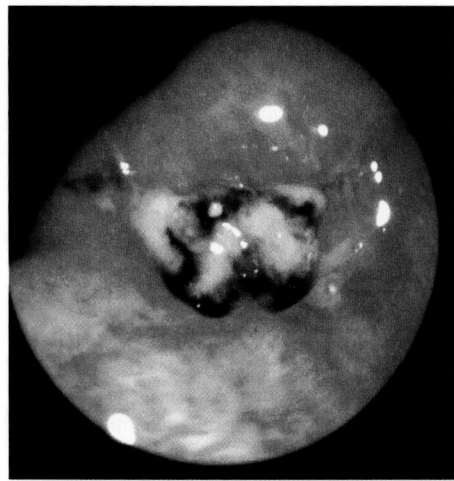

▲ **FIGURE 6.19** **Bleeding Peptic Ulcer.** The yellow floor of the ulcer shows black blood clots. Fresh blood is around the ulcer margin.

Abbreviations

GERD gastroesophageal reflux disease
H₂-blocker histamine-2 receptor antagonist
NSAIDs nonsteroidal anti-inflammatory drugs
PPI proton pump inhibitor

Pharmacology of Treating Excess Gastric Acid

Antacids are taken orally, neutralize gastric acid, and relieve heartburn and acid indigestion. Examples of antacids include:
- Aluminum hydroxide and magnesium hydroxide (Maalox, Mylanta)
- Magnesium hydroxide (Milk of Magnesia)
- Calcium carbonate (Tums, Rolaids)

Histamine-2 receptor antagonists (H₂-blockers) block the production of gastric acid. Examples include:
- Cimetidine (Tagamet)
- Famotidine (Pepcid)
- Ranitidine (Zantac)

Proton pump inhibitors (PPIs) suppress gastric acid secretion by blocking in the lining of the stomach the enzyme system that produces gastric acid. Examples include:
- Omeprazole (Prilosec)
- Lansoprazole (Prevacid)

Sucralfate coats the site of an ulcer and protects it against gastric acid.

Misoprostol diminishes acid production and protects the mucosa. It is used prophylactically in patients taking NSAIDs.

Anti–*H. pylori* therapy is given with two antibiotics (for example, amoxicillin and clarithromycin) with a proton pump inhibitor.

WORD	PRONUNCIATION	ELEMENTS		DEFINITION
anorexia	an-oh-**RECK**-see-ah	S/ P/ R/	-ia *condition* an- *without* -orex- *appetite*	Severe lack of appetite; or an aversion to food
antacid	ant-**ASS**-id	P/ R/	ant- *against* -acid *acid*	Agent that neutralizes acidity
dyspepsia	dis-**PEP**-see-ah	S/ P/ R/	-ia *condition* dys- *difficult, bad* -peps- *digestion*	"Upset stomach," epigastric pain, nausea, and gas
erosion	ee-**ROE**-shun		Latin *to gnaw away*	A shallow ulcer in the lining of a structure
gastritis	gas-**TRY**-tis	S/ R/	-itis *inflammation* gastr- *stomach*	Inflammation of the lining of the stomach
gastroesophageal	**GAS**-troh-ee-sof-ah-**JEE**-al	S/ R/CF R/CF	-al *pertaining to* gastr/o- *stomach* -esophag/e- *esophagus*	Pertaining to the stomach and esophagus
gastroscope	**GAS**-troh-skope	S/ R/CF	-scope *instrument for viewing* gastr/o- *stomach*	Endoscope for examining the inside of the stomach
peptic	**PEP**-tik	S/ R/	-ic *pertaining to* pept- *digest*	Relating to the stomach and duodenum
perforation	per-foh-**RAY**-shun	S/ R/	-ion *action* perforat- *bore through*	Erosion that progresses to become a hole through the wall of a structure
proton pump inhibitor (PPI)	**PRO**-ton PUMP in-**HIB**-ih-tor	R/ R/ S/ R/	proton *first* pump *pump* -or *a doer* inhibit- *repress*	Agent that blocks production of gastric acid
resection resect (verb)	ree-**SEK**-shun	S/ P/ R/	-ion *action, condition* re- *back* -sect- *cut off*	Removal of a specific part of an organ or structure
vagus	**VAY**-gus		Latin *wandering*	Tenth (X) cranial nerve; supplies many different organs throughout the body

EXERCISES

Deconstruct the following medical terms into basic elements. The definitions of the elements will help you understand the meaning of the term. Not every type of element will appear in every term. Fill in the chart.

Medical Term	Meaning of Prefix	Meaning of Root/CF	Meaning of Suffix	Definition of Medical Term
perforation				
peptic				
gastroesophageal				
anorexia				
dyspepsia				
antacid				
gastritis				
gastroscope				

LESSON 6.3 Digestion—Stomach and Small Intestine

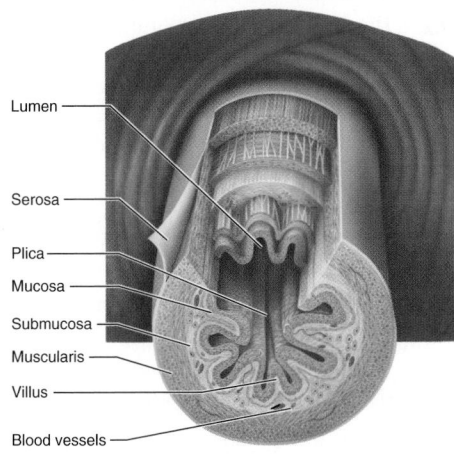

Lumen

Serosa

Plica

Mucosa

Submucosa

Muscularis

Villus

Blood vessels

▲ **FIGURE 6.20   Tissue Layers of Digestive Tract.** An example of the most typical histological structure of the tract.

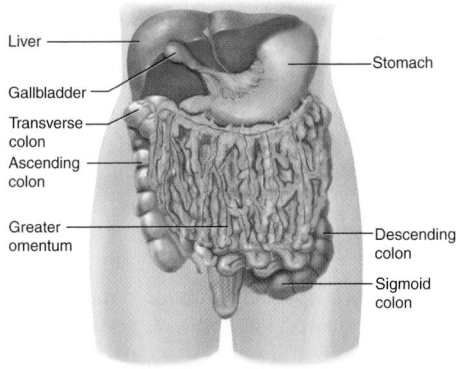

Liver

Gallbladder

Transverse colon

Ascending colon

Greater omentum

Stomach

Descending colon

Sigmoid colon

▲ **FIGURE 6.21   Greater Omentum.**

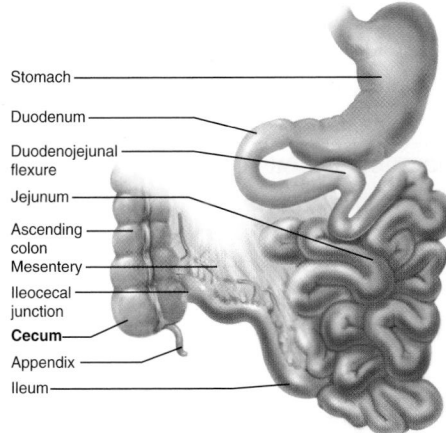

Stomach

Duodenum

Duodenojejunal flexure

Jejunum

Ascending colon

Mesentery

Ileocecal junction

Cecum

Appendix

Ileum

▲ **FIGURE 6.22   Small Intestine.**

SMALL INTESTINE

The small intestine, called "small" because of its diameter, finishes the process of chemical digestion and is responsible for the absorption of most of the nutrients.

Four major layers are present in the wall of the small intestine and in all areas of the digestive tract (*Figure 6.20*):

1. **Mucosa,** or mucous membrane—the layer containing the epithelial cells that line the tract, intestinal glands that secrete the digestive enzymes, and supportive connective tissue. Fingerlike shapes of mucosa called **villi** project into the lumen of the intestine.

2. **Submucosa**—a thick connective tissue layer containing blood vessels, lymphatic vessels, and nerves.

3. **Muscularis**—an inner, circular layer of **smooth muscle** and an outer longitudinal layer of smooth muscle. When the inner circular layer contracts, it decreases the diameter of the tract. When the outer longitudinal layer contracts, it shortens the tract. These two movements create peristalsis and segmental contractions.

4. **Serosa**—an outermost layer of thin connective tissue and a single layer of epithelial cells.

Most of the digestive organs lie within the abdominal cavity (*see Chapter 2*), which is lined by a moist serous membrane called the **peritoneum. Parietal** peritoneum lines the wall of the abdominal cavity. **Visceral** peritoneum (a serosa) covers the external surface of the digestive organs.

The intestines are suspended from the back wall of the abdominal cavity by a **translucent** membrane called the **mesentery,** a continuation of the peritoneum. A fatty portion of the mesentery, called the **greater omentum** (*Figure 6.21*), hangs like an apron in front of all the intestines.

The small intestine (*Figure 6.22*) occupies much of the abdominal cavity, extends from the pylorus of the stomach to the beginning of the large intestine, and has three segments:

1. The **duodenum** is the first 9 to 10 inches of the small intestine. It receives chyme from the stomach, together with pancreatic juices and bile. Here, stomach acid is neutralized, fats are broken up by the bile acids, and pancreatic enzymes take over chemical digestion.

2. The **jejunum** makes up about 40% of the small intestine's length. It is the primary region for chemical digestion and nutrient absorption.

3. The **ileum** makes up about 55% of the small intestine's length. It ends at the **ileocecal** valve, a sphincter that controls entry into the large intestine.

From the duodenum to the middle of the ileum, the lining of the small intestine is thrown into circular folds called **plicae.** Along their surface, the plicae have tiny fingerlike villi. The plicae and villi increase the surface area over which secretions can act on the food and through which nutrients can be absorbed. The folds also act as "speed bumps" to slow down the movement of chyme through the small intestine. The cells at the tip of the villi are shed and renewed every 3 or 4 days.

Digestion in the Small Intestine

After leaving the stomach as chyme, the food spends 3 to 5 hours in the small intestine, from which most of the nutrients are absorbed.

Secretion from the small intestine cells is mostly water, mucus, and enzymes. Peristaltic movements of the small intestine have three functions:

1. Mix chyme with intestinal and pancreatic juices and with bile.

2. Churn chyme to make contact with the mucosa for digestion and absorption.

3. Move the residue toward the large intestine.

WORD	PRONUNCIATION		ELEMENTS	DEFINITION
cecum	**SEE**-kum		Latin *blind*	Blind pouch that is the first part of the large intestine
ileum ileocecal	**ILL**-ee-um **ILL**-ee-oh-**SEE**-cal	S/ R/CF R/	Latin *to roll up* -al *pertaining to* ile/o- *ileum* -cec- *cecum*	Third portion of the small intestine Pertaining to the junction of the ileum and cecum
jejunum jejunal (adj)	je-**JEW**-num je-**JEW**-nal		Latin *empty*	Segment of small intestine between the duodenum and the ileum where most of the nutrients are absorbed
mesentery mesenteric (adj)	**MESS**-en-ter-ree **MESS**-en-ter-ik	P/ R/ S/	mes- *middle* -entery *intestine* -ic *pertaining to*	A double layer of peritoneum enclosing the abdominal viscera
mucosa (another name for **mucous membrane**) mucosal (adj)	myu-**KOH**-sah myu-**KOH**-sal		Latin *mucus*	Lining of a tubular structure Pertaining to the mucosa
muscularis	muss-kyu-**LAR**-is	S/ R/	-aris *pertaining to* muscul- *muscle*	The muscular layer of a hollow organ or tube
omentum omental (adj)	oh-**MEN**-tum oh-**MEN**-tal		Latin *membrane that encloses the bowels*	Membrane that encloses the bowels
pancreas	**PAN**-kree-as		Greek *sweetbread*	Lobulated gland, the head of which is tucked into the curve of the duodenum
peritoneum peritoneal (adj)	per-ih-toe-**NEE**-um per-ih-toe-**NEE**-al		Latin *to stretch over*	Membrane that lines the abdominal cavity
plica plicae (pl)	**PLEE**-cah **PLEE**-key		Latin *fold*	Fold in a mucous membrane
serosa serosal (adj)	seh-**ROH**-sa seh-**ROH**-sal		Latin *serous, watery*	Outermost covering of the alimentary tract
submucosa	sub-mew-**KOH**-sa	P/ R/	sub- *under* -mucosa *lining of a cavity*	Tissue layer underneath the mucosa
villus villi (pl)	**VILL**-us **VILL**-eye		Latin *shaggy hair*	Thin, hairlike projection, particularly of a mucous membrane lining a cavity
viscus (**Note: Viscous** is pronounced the same but means something *sticky*.) viscera (pl) visceral (adj)	**VISS**-kus **VISS**-er-ah **VISS**-er-al		Latin *internal organ* Latin *soft internal organs*	Hollow, walled, internal organ Internal organs, particularly in the abdomen Pertaining to the internal organs

EXERCISES

Greek and Latin terms do not deconstruct into basic elements, so you must know them for what they are. Build your knowledge of these terms by matching the phrase in the left column to the correct medical term in the right column.

1. To roll up _____   A. viscus

2. Membrance that encloses bowels _____   B. peritoneum

3. Watery _____   C. mucosa

4. Shaggy hair _____   D. plica

5. Internal organ _____   E. cecum

6. Fold _____   F. omentum

7. Empty _____   G. ileum

8. To stretch over _____   H. serosa

9. Lining of a tubular structure _____   I. villus

10. Blind _____   J. jejunum

Digestion—Liver, Gallbladder, and Pancreas

The liver and pancreas secrete enzymes that are responsible for most of the digestion that occurs in the small intestine. It is essential to understand the function of these enzymes as they relate to digestion, and you will need to be able to:

6.4.1 **Identify the functions of the liver, gallbladder, bile ducts, and pancreas.**

6.4.2 **Describe the functions of the digestive secretions of the liver and pancreas.**

6.4.3 **Explain common disorders of the liver, gallbladder, bile ducts, and pancreas.**

6.4.4 **Apply the correct medical terminology to describe the anatomy, physiology, and common disorders of the liver, gallbladder, bile ducts, and pancreas.**

You are

. . . a Certified Medical Assistant working with Susan Lee, MD, a primary care physician at Fulwood Medical Center.

Your patient is

. . . Mrs. Sandra Jacobs, a 46-year-old mother of four. Your task is to document her care.

CASE REPORT 6.4

Mrs. Sandra Jacobs, a 46-year-old mother of four, presents in Dr. Susan Lee's primary care clinic with episodes of crampy pain in her right upper quadrant associated with nausea and vomiting. The pain often occurs after eating fast food. She has not noticed fever or jaundice. Physical examination reveals an obese white woman with a positive **Murphy sign.** Her BP (blood pressure) is 170/90, and she has slight pedal edema. A **provisional diagnosis** of **gallstones** has been made. She has been referred for an ultrasound examination, and an appointment has been made to see Dr. Stewart Walsh in the Surgery Department.

I explained to her the etiology of her gallstones and the need for surgical removal of the gallbladder, and I discussed with her a low-fat, 1500-calorie diet sheet.

Luis Guitterez, CMA. 06/12/09, 1430 hrs.

LIVER

The **liver,** the body's largest internal organ, is a complex structure located under the right ribs and below the diaphragm *(Figure 6.23)*.

The liver has multiple functions, including to:

- **Manufacture** and excrete **bile.** Although it contains no digestive enzymes, bile plays key roles in digestion. It neutralizes the acidic chyme so that pancreatic enzymes can function. Bile salts **emulsify** fat. Bile acids are synthesized from **cholesterol,** and bile also contains cholesterol and fat-soluble vitamins.

- **Remove** the pigment **bilirubin** from the bloodstream and excrete it in bile. Bilirubin is produced as a breakdown product of hemoglobin during phagocytosis by macrophages in the spleen and liver. It is dark yellow and is responsible for the brown color of feces and for the yellow color of skin in **jaundice.**

- **Remove** excess glucose (sugar) from the blood and store it as **glycogen** and release glucose when needed by the body.

- **Convert** proteins and fats into glucose, a process called **gluconeogenesis.**

- **Store** fat and the fat-soluble vitamins A, D, E, and K.

- **Manufacture** blood proteins, including those necessary for clotting *(see Chapter 7)*.

- **Remove** toxins from the blood.

A major reason that the liver can perform all these functions is that venous blood is returned from all the intestines to join into the **portal** vein that takes the blood directly to the liver.

The liver cells secrete bile into narrow channels that converge on the underside of the liver to form the common **hepatic duct.**

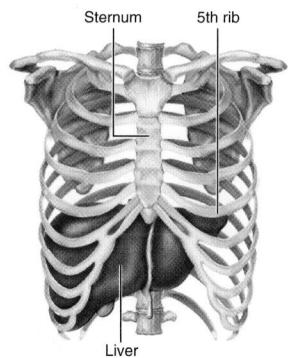

Sternum   5th rib

Liver

▲ **FIGURE 6.23 Location of Liver.**

Keynote

Only the production of bile relates the liver to digestion.

WORD	PRONUNCIATION		ELEMENTS	DEFINITION
bile bile acids biliary (adj)	BILE BILE ASS-ids BILL-ee-air-ee	 S/ R/CF	Latin *bile* -ary *pertaining to* bil/i- *bile*	Fluid secreted by the liver into the duodenum Steroids synthesized from cholesterol Pertaining to bile or the biliary tract
bilirubin	bill-ee-RU-bin	S/ R/CF	-rubin *rust colored* bil/i- *bile*	Bile pigment formed in the liver from hemoglobin
cholesterol	koh-LESS-ter-ol	R/CF S/	chol/e- *bile* -sterol *steroid*	Steroid formed in liver cells; the most abundant steroid in tissues and circulates in the plasma attached to proteins of different densities
emulsify emulsion (noun)	ee-MUL-sih-fye ee-MUL-shun	S/ R/	-ify *to become* emuls- *suspend in a liquid*	Break up into very small droplets to suspend in a solution (emulsion)
gallstone	GAWL-stone	R/ R/	gall- *bile* stone *pebble*	Hard mass of cholesterol, calcium, and bilirubin that can be formed in gallbladder and bile duct
gluconeogenesis	GLU-ko-nee-oh-JEN-eh-sis	S/ R/CF P/	-genesis *creation* gluc/o- *sugar* -neo- *new*	Formation of glucose from noncarbohydrate sources
glycogen	GLYE-koh-gen	S/ R/CF	-gen *produce, create* glyc/o- *sugar*	The body's principal carbohydrate reserve, stored in the liver and skeletal muscle
hepatic hepatitis	hep-AT-ik hep-ah-TIE-tis	S/ R/ S/	-ic *pertaining to* hepat- *liver* -itis *inflammation*	Pertaining to the liver Inflammation of the liver
jaundice	JAWN-dis		French *yellow*	Yellow staining of tissues with bile pigments, including bilirubin
liver	LIV-er		Old English *liver*	Body's largest internal organ located in right upper quadrant of abdomen
Murphy sign	MUR-fee SINE		John B. Murphy, Chicago surgeon, 1857–1916	Tenderness in the right subcostal area on inspiration, associated with acute cholecystitis
portal vein	POR-tal VANE		Latin *gate*	The vein that carries blood from the intestines to the liver
provisional diagnosis (also called preliminary diagnosis)	pro-VISH-un-al die-ag-NO-sis	S/ R/	-al *pertaining to* provision- *provide*	A temporary diagnosis pending further examination or testing

---

EXERCISES

Use this exercise as a quick review of the elements in the WAD. Circle the correct choice.

1. In the term **hepatic**, the root means:

   pancreas   stomach   liver

2. The term **gallstone** is composed of:

   root + CF   root + root   root + suffix

3. The term **biliary** is composed of a:

   prefix + root   root + suffix   CF + suffix

4. To break up into small droplets suspended in a solution is to:

   emulsify   secrete   liquefy

5. In the term **gallstone**, one of the roots means:

   enzyme   acid   bile

6. Which is formed in the liver cells?

   cholesterol   gallstone   insulin

7. In the term **gluconeogenesis**, *neo* means:

   never   new   negative

8. The combining form in the term **glycogen** means:

   sugar   enzyme   bile

DISORDERS OF THE LIVER

Hepatitis is an inflammation of the liver causing jaundice. Viral hepatitis is the most common cause of hepatitis and is related to three major types of virus:

1. **Hepatitis A virus (HAV)** is highly contagious and causes a mild to severe infection. It is transmitted by the **fecal-oral route** through contaminated food. It frequently occurs in schools, camps, and institutions.

2. **Hepatitis B virus (HBV)** is transmitted through contact with blood, semen, vaginal secretions, saliva, or a needle prick and through sharing contaminated needles. Some people become chronic carriers of the virus in their blood.

3. **Hepatitis C virus (HCV)** is transmitted by blood-to-blood contact; it is often asymptomatic. It can be cured in 51% of patients with antiviral treatment, but can progress to chronic hepatitis and cirrhosis.

In addition, **hepatitis D** can occur in association with hepatitis B, making the infection worse. **Hepatitis E** is similar to hepatitis A and occurs mostly in under-developed countries.

Other causes of hepatitis include abuse of alcohol; autoimmune hepatitis; metabolic disorders such as Wilson's disease and diabetes mellitus; other viruses, such as mononucleosis and cytomegalovirus *(see Chapter 20)*; and drugs such as acetaminophen.

Symptoms include nausea, vomiting and loss of appetite, joint pain, and sore muscles. Signs include jaundice, fever, and tenderness in the right upper quadrant of the abdomen.

Chronic hepatitis occurs when the acute hepatitis is not healed after 6 months. It progresses slowly, can last for years, and is difficult to treat.

Cirrhosis of the liver is a chronic, irreversible disease, replacing normal liver cells with hard, fibrous scar tissue *(Figure 6.24)*. It is the seventh leading cause of death in the United States. The most common cause of **cirrhosis** is alcoholism. In cirrhosis, the

Keynote

Vaccines are available to prevent hepatitis A and B.

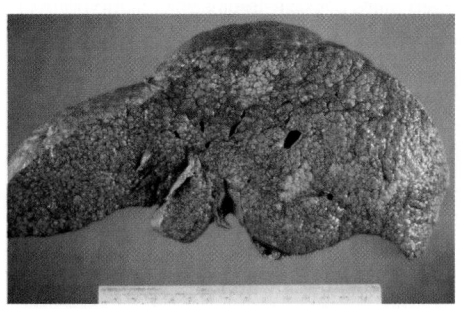

▲ **FIGURE 6.24** **Cirrhosis of Liver.**

Abbreviations

ALP	alkaline phosphatase
ALT	alanine aminotransferase (also known as SGPT)
AST	aspartate aminotransferase (also known as SGOT)
GGT	gamma-glutamyl transpeptidase
HAV	hepatitis A virus
HBV	hepatitis B virus
HCV	hepatitis C virus
LFT	Liver Function Test
PT	prothrombin time
SGOT	serum glutamic oxaloacetic acid transaminase (also known as AST)
SGPT	serum glutamic-pyruvic transaminase (also known as ALT)

Liver Function Tests

Liver Function Tests (LFTs) are a group of tests to show how well your liver is functioning. They are divided into four categories:

1. Measuring liver proteins in blood serum

   • Total proteins, albumin, and globulin (*see Chapter 7*) are low when there is liver damage.

2. Measuring liver enzymes in blood serum

   • Enzymes made in the liver, known as **transaminases**, include **alanine aminotransferase (ALT;** also known as **serum glutamic-pyruvic transaminase,** or SGPT) and **aspartate aminotransferase (AST;** also known as **serum glutamic oxaloacetic acid transaminase,** or SGOT). Elevated levels of these enzymes in the blood indicate liver damage.

   • **Prothrombin** is a protein involved in blood clotting that is made in the liver. Low blood levels resulting from liver disease increase the time it takes blood to clot, and the **prothrombin time (PT)** test is elevated (*see Chapter 7*).

3. Measuring cholestatic liver enzymes in the blood serum

   • **Alkaline phosphatase (ALP)** metabolizes phosphorus and makes energy available for the body. Elevated blood levels are found in liver and biliary tract disorders.

   • **Gamma-glutamyl transpeptidase (GGT)** is elevated in liver disease.

4. Measuring bilirubin in the bloodstream

   • **Bilirubin** is formed in the liver from hemoglobin and secreted into the biliary system. If the liver is damaged, bilirubin can leak out into the bloodstream, producing elevated levels and jaundice.

WORD	PRONUNCIATION		ELEMENTS	DEFINITION
alanine aminotransferase (ALT) aspartate aminotransferase (AST)	**AL**-ah-neen ah-**ME**-no-**TRANS**-fer-aze as-**PAR**-tate ah-me-no-**TRANS**-fer-aze	S/ R/CF R/	**alanine** *an amino acid* -ase *enzyme* amin/o- *nitrogen compound* -transfer- *carry* **aspartate** *an amino acid*	Enzymes that are found in liver cells and leak out into the bloodstream when the cells are damaged, enabling liver damage to be diagnosed
ascites	ah-**SIGH**-teez	S/ R/	-ites *associated with* asc- *belly*	Accumulation of fluid in the abdominal cavity
cholestatic	koh-les-**TAT**-ik	S/ R/ R/CF	-ic *pertaining to* -stat- *standing still* chol/e- *bile*	Stopping the flow of bile
cirrhosis	sir-**ROE**-sis	S/ R/	-osis *condition* cirrh- *yellow*	Extensive fibrotic liver disease
hemangioma	he-**MAN**-jee-oh-mah	S/ R/ R/	-oma *tumor, mass* hem- *blood* -angi- *blood vessel*	Abnormal mass of proliferating blood vessels
hemochromatosis	**HE**-mah-krom-ah-**TOE**-sis	S/ R/ R/CF	-osis *condition* -chromat- *color* hem/o- *blood*	Dangerously high levels of iron in the body with deposition of iron pigments in tissues
phosphatase	**FOS**-fah-tase	S/ R/	-ase *enzyme* phosphat- *phosphorus*	Enzyme that liberates phosphorus
prothrombin	pro-**THROM**-bin	P/ R/	pro- *before* -thrombin *clot*	Protein formed by the liver and converted to thrombin in the blood-clotting mechanism

damage sustained to the liver is irreversible, and there is no known cure. Treatment is symptomatic. When cirrhosis blocks the flow of blood in the portal vein, the back-pressure produces **ascites,** an accumulation of fluid in the abdominal cavity.

Cancer of the liver as a primary cancer typically arises in patients with chronic liver disease, usually from HBV infection. A more common form of liver cancer is secondary deposits of metastases from a primary cancer in colon, lung, breast, or prostate.

Benign liver tumors are often small and symptom-free and include **hepatocellular adenoma** and **hemangioma.**

Hemochromatosis is caused by the absorption of too much iron, which is stored throughout the body mostly in the liver, and can lead to liver failure.

Wilson disease is the retention of too much copper in the liver and can also lead to liver failure.

EXERCISES

Work on recognizing the elements contained in this lesson's WAD. Know the medical terms in which they will appear. Fill in the chart. The first one is done for you.

Element	Meaning of Element	Type of Element (P, R, CF, S)	Medical Term Containing This Element
pro	*before*	*P*	*prothrombin*
osis			
hemo			
asc			
cirrh			
stat			
ase			
thrombin			

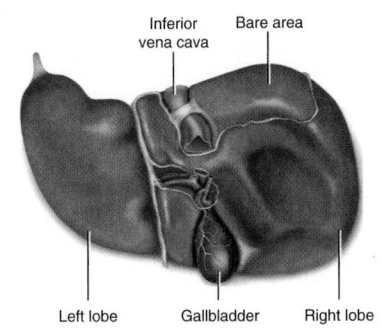

(a)

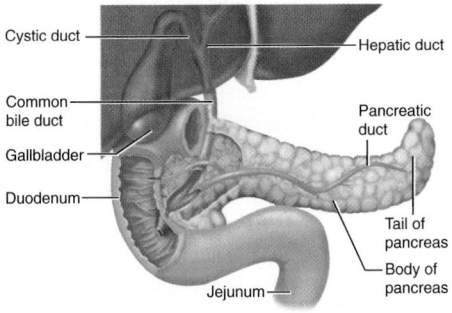

(b)

▲ **FIGURE 6.25** **Gallbladder and Biliary Tract** (a) Underside of liver. (b) Anatomy of gallbladder, pancreas, and biliary tract.

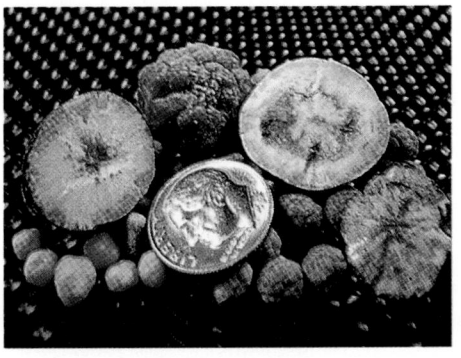

▲ **FIGURE 6.26** **Gallstones.**

Abbreviations

ERCP	endoscopic retrograde cholangio-pancreatography
RBC	red blood cell

GALLBLADDER AND BILIARY TRACT

On the underside of the liver is the **gallbladder** *(Figure 6.25a)*, which stores and concentrates the bile that the liver produces. The **cystic duct** from the gallbladder joins with the **hepatic duct** to form the **common bile duct.** The system of ducts to get the bile from the liver to the duodenum is called the **biliary tract** *(Figure 6.25b)*

When acid and fat arrive in the duodenum, cells in the lining of the duodenum secrete a hormone, **cholecystokinin,** which causes the gallbladder to contract and force bile into the bile duct and, from there, into the duodenum. Cholecystokinin also stimulates the production of pancreatic enzymes.

Disorders of the Gallbladder

Gallstones (cholelithiasis) can form in the gallbladder from excess cholesterol, bile salts, and bile pigment *(Figure 6.26)*. The stones can vary in size and number. Risk factors are **obesity**, high-cholesterol diets, multiple pregnancies, and rapid weight loss. Mrs. Jacobs presented in the Emergency Department with the classic gallstone symptoms of severe waves of right upper quadrant pain (**biliary colic**), nausea, and vomiting. **Cholelithotomy** is the operative removal of one or more gallstones. If small stones become impacted in the common bile duct, this is called **choledocholithiasis.** This can cause biliary colic and jaundice (see below).

Cholecystitis is an acute or chronic inflammation of the gallbladder usually associated with cholelithiasis and obstruction of the cystic duct with a stone. Acute colicky pain in the right upper quadrant with nausea and vomiting are followed by jaundice, dark urine (because bilirubin backs up into the blood and is excreted by the kidneys), and pale-colored stools (because bilirubin cannot get into the duodenum).

Jaundice (icterus) is a symptom of many different diseases in the biliary tract and liver. It is a yellow discoloration of the skin and sclera of the eyes *(see Chapter 3)* caused by deposits of bilirubin just below the outer layers of the skin. Bilirubin is a breakdown product of hemoglobin that occurs as old **red blood cells (RBCs)** are destroyed. Bilirubin is removed from the bloodstream by the liver and excreted in bile.

Jaundice occurs when there is an increased concentration of bilirubin circulating in the bloodstream. There are three categories of disease that cause jaundice:

1. **Obstructive jaundice** is a result of the blockage of bile between the liver and the duodenum, usually due to gallstones in the common bile duct or to a carcinoma of the head of the pancreas impinging on the common duct.

2. **Hemolytic jaundice** results from an accelerated destruction of red blood cells such that the liver cannot remove the excess bilirubin fast enough. This is most often seen in newborn infants with hemolytic jaundice due to blood group incompatibility between mother and infant.

3. **Hepatocellular jaundice** occurs when an infection or poison injures the liver cells, preventing the removal of bilirubin from the blood. This occurs in viral hepatitis.

Procedures for the Biliary System

- **Cholangiography** requires injection of a dye intravenously, followed by x-ray of the biliary system so that the biliary system can be visualized.

- **Cholecystectomy** is surgical removal of the gallbladder through open cholecystectomy or laparoscopic cholecystectomy. A method to remove stones and leave the gallbladder intact involves using **endoscopic retrograde cholangiopancreatography (ERCP)**. An endoscope is passed orally into the duodenum and a guide wire is inserted into the common bile duct so that stones can be identified and removed by a balloon sweep of the duct.

- **Cholelithotomy** is the surgical removal of one or more gallstones from any part of the biliary tract.

WORD ANALYSIS AND DEFINITION

S = Suffix   P = Prefix   R = Root   R/CF = Combining Form

WORD	PRONUNCIATION		ELEMENTS	DEFINITION
cholangiography	KOH-lan-jee-OG-rah-fee	S/ R/ R/CF	-graphy *process of recording* chol- *bile* -angi/o- *blood vessel, lymph vessel*	X-ray of the bile ducts after injection or ingestion of a contrast medium
cholecystectomy	KOH-leh-sis-TECK-toe-me	S/ R/CF R/	-ectomy *surgical excision* chol/e- *bile* -cyst- *bladder*	Surgical removal of the gallbladder
cholecystitis	KOH-leh-sis-TIE-tis	S/ R/CF R/	-itis *inflammation* chol/e- *bile* -cyst- *bladder*	Inflammation of the gallbladder
cholecystokinin	KOH-leh-sis-toe-KIE-nin	S/ R/CF R/CF	-kinin *move in* chol/e- *bile* -cyst/o- *bladder*	Hormone secreted by the lining of the intestine that stimulates secretion of pancreatic enzymes and contraction of the gallbladder
choledocholithiasis	koh-leh-DOH-koh-lih-THIGH-ah-sis	S/ R/CF R/	-iasis *condition* choledoch/o- *common bile duct* -lith- *stone*	Presence of a gallstone(s) in the common bile duct
cholelithiasis	KOH-leh-lih-THIGH-ah-sis	S/ R/CF R/	-iasis *condition* chol/e- *bile* -lith- *stone*	Condition of having bile stones (gallstones)
cholelithotomy	KOH-leh-lih-THOT-oh-me	S/	-otomy *surgical incision*	Surgical removal of a gallstone(s)
gallbladder	GAWL-blad-er	R/	gall- *bile* Old English *bladder*	Receptacle on inferior surface of the liver for storing bile
hemolysis	he-MOL-ih-sis	S/ R/CF	-lysis *destroy* hem/o- *blood*	Destruction of red blood cells so that hemoglobin is liberated
hemolytic (adj)	he-moh-LIT-ik	S/ R/	-tic *pertaining to* -ly- *break down*	Pertaining to the process of destruction of red blood cells
hepatocellular	HEP-ah-toe-SELL-you-lar	S/ R/ R/CF	-ar *pertaining to* -cellul- *small cell* hepat/o- *liver*	Pertaining to liver cells
obesity	oh-BEE-sih-tee		Latin *fat*	Excessive amount of fat in the body

EXERCISES

In this exercise the root or combining form remains the same, but the addition of other elements will construct entirely different medical terms. Use this group of elements, in addition to **chol/e**, *to form the medical terms that are defined. Some elements you will use more than once; some elements you will not use at all. Fill in the blanks.*

The element **chol/e** means _____.

Add these elements to **chol/e** *to form the medical terms defined below:*

lith	lysis	iasis	graphy	ectomy	osis	cyst
angi/o	kinin	nephr/o	cyst/o	hemat/o	tripsy	itis

1. Condition of bile (gall)stones _____

2. Surgical removal of the gallbladder _____

3. Inflammation of the gallbladder _____

4. Using contrast medium to see bile ducts _____

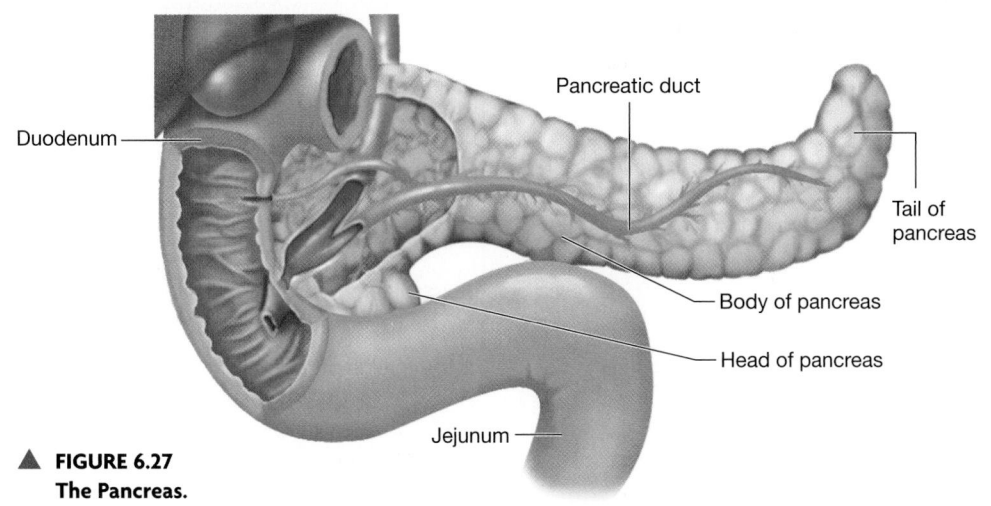

▲ FIGURE 6.27
The Pancreas.

PANCREAS

The pancreas is a spongy gland, the head of which is encircled by the duodenum. Most of the pancreas secretes digestive juices.

The pancreas is called an **exocrine** gland, and the pancreatic digestive juices formed in the **acinar cells** are excreted through the pancreatic duct. The pancreatic duct joins the common bile duct shortly before it opens into the duodenum *(Figure 6.27)*. Pancreatic and bile juices then enter the duodenum.

In the same parts of the pancreas as those in which pancreatic enzymes are produced, pancreatic **islet cells** secrete the hormones insulin and glucagon *(see Chapter 14)*, which go directly into the bloodstream. This part of the pancreas is an **endocrine** gland *(Figure 6.28)*.

Pancreatic juices contain:

1. **Electrolytes,** including the alkaline sodium bicarbonate, that make the pancreatic juice alkaline and help neutralize the acid chyme as it comes from the stomach.

2. **Enzymes:**
   - **Amylase** breaks down the **polysaccharide** starch into **disaccharides** and **monosaccharides.**
   - **Lipase** breaks down **triglyceride** fat molecules into **fatty acids** and **monoglycerides.**
   - **Trypsin, chymotrypsin,** and **carboxypeptidase** split proteins into their amino acids.

Pancreatic secretions are regulated by both the nervous and endocrine systems. While food is being digested in the stomach, nervous impulses stimulate the pancreas to produce its juices. When chyme enters the duodenum, the hormone **secretin,** produced in the duodenal mucosa, stimulates the pancreas to produce large volumes of watery fluid. Another hormone, **cholecystokinin,** is produced in the intestinal mucosa to stimulate production of pancreatic enzymes. Both hormones travel from the intestine via the bloodstream to the pancreas.

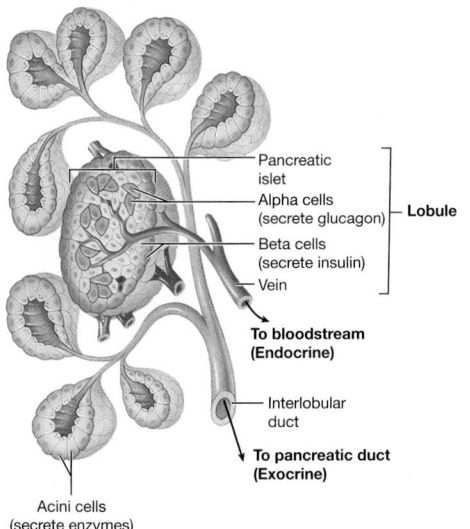

▲ FIGURE 6.28 **Exocrine and Endocrine Aspects of Pancreas.**

Keynote

The prognosis of pancreatic cancer is poor, with only a 15% to 20% 5-year survival rate.

Abbreviation
CF cystic fibrosis

Disorders of the Pancreas

Pancreatitis is inflammation of the pancreas. The acute disease ranges from a mild, self-limiting episode to an acute life-threatening emergency with severe abdominal pain, nausea, vomiting, and a rapid fall in blood pressure. In the **chronic** form, there is a progressive destruction of pancreatic tissue leading to **malabsorption** and diabetes. Factors in the development of pancreatitis are biliary tract disease, gallstones, and alcoholism. The pancreatic enzyme **trypsin** builds up and digests parts of the pancreas, causing the intense pain.

Pancreatic cancer is the fourth leading cause of cancer-related death. It occurs twice as often in males as in females. Incidence peaks in the 40- to 60-year-old range. The cancer can be asymptomatic in its early stages and is difficult to detect. The treatment is surgical resection of the cancer.

Diabetes, in which insulin production is shut down or severely reduced or its effects are resisted by body cells, is discussed in *Chapter 14.*

Cystic fibrosis (CF) is an inherited disease that becomes apparent in infancy or childhood. It affects exocrine glands in multiple body systems, including the respiratory and digestive systems.

WORD	PRONUNCIATION	ELEMENTS		DEFINITION
acinar cells	**ASS**-in-ar SELLS	S/ R/	-ar *pertaining to* acin- *grape*	Enzyme-secreting cells of the pancreas
carboxypeptidase	kar-box-ee-**PEP**-tide-ase	S/ R/ R/	-ase *enzyme* carboxy- *group of organic compounds* -peptid- *digestion*	Enzyme that breaks down protein
disaccharide	die-**SACK**-ah-ride	S/ P/ R/	-ide *having a particular quality* di- *two* -sacchar- *sugar*	A combination of two monosaccharides; for example, table sugar
endocrine gland	**EN**-doh-krin GLAND	P/ R/	endo- *within* -crine *secrete*	A gland that produces an internal or hormonal secretion and secretes it into the bloodstream
exocrine gland	**EK**-soh-krin GLAND	P/ R/	exo- *outward* -crine *secrete*	A gland that secretes outwardly through excretory ducts
fatty acid	**FAT**-ee **ASS**-id		Old English *fat* Latin *sour*	An acid obtained from the hydrolysis of fats
islet cells	I-let SELLS		islet *small island*	Hormone-secreting cells of the pancreas
monoglyceride	mon-oh-**GLISS**-eh-ride	S/ P/ R/	-ide *having a particular quality* mono- *one* -glycer- *glycerol*	A fatty substance with a single fatty acid
diglyceride triglyceride	die-**GLISS**-eh-ride tri-**GLISS**-eh-ride	P/ P/	di- *two* tri- *three*	Substance with two fatty acids Substance with three fatty acids
monosaccharide	**MON**-oh-**SACK**-ah-ride	S/ P/ R/	-ide *having a particular quality* mono- *one* -sacchar- *sugar*	Simplest form of sugar; for example, glucose
polysaccharide	pol-ee-**SACK**-ah-ride	P/	poly- *many*	A combination of many saccharides; for example, starch
pancreas	**PAN**-kree-as		Greek *sweetbread*	Lobulated gland, the head of which is tucked into the curve of the duodenum
pancreatic (adj)	pan-kree-**AT**-ik	S/ R/	-ic *pertaining to* pancreat- *pancreas*	
pancreatitis	**PAN**-kree-ah-**TIE**-tis	S/	-itis *inflammation*	Inflammation of the pancreas
secretin	se-**KREE**-tin	S/ R/	-in *substance, chemical compound* secret- *separate*	Hormone produced by duodenum to stimulate pancreatic juice
trypsin	**TRIP**-sin	S/ R/	-in *substance, chemical compound* tryps- *friction*	Enzyme that breaks down protein
chymotrypsin	kye-moh-**TRIP**-sin	R/CF	chym/o- *chyme*	Trypsin found in chyme

EXERCISES

*Grouping elements of similar meaning or category will help you remember them. This exercise contains only prefixes of number. Fill in the number for the element, **define** the medical terms, and then **define** the English terms with the same elements. Fill in the blanks.*

Prefixes indicating numbers:

1. mono = (number) _____

2. di = _____

3. tri = _____

4. poly = _____

Medical terms:

5. monoglyceride: _____

6. disaccharide: _____

7. triglyceride: _____

8. polysaccharide: _____

English terms:

9. Monorail: _____

10. Divide: _____

11. Triangle: _____

12. Polygon: _____

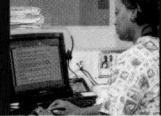

LESSON 6.5 Absorption and Malabsorption

DIGESTIVE SYSTEM

In the previous lessons in this chapter, you have learned the digestive secretions of the different segments of the digestive tract, liver, and pancreas. This information can now be brought together to review the overall process of digestion so that you will be able to:

6.5.1 Explain the chemical digestion and absorption of proteins, carbohydrates, and fats.

6.5.2 Describe disorders of chemical digestion and absorption.

6.5.3 Select the correct medical terminology to describe chemical digestion, absorption, and malabsorption.

Keynote

Proteins are broken down into amino acids.

Minerals are electrolytes.

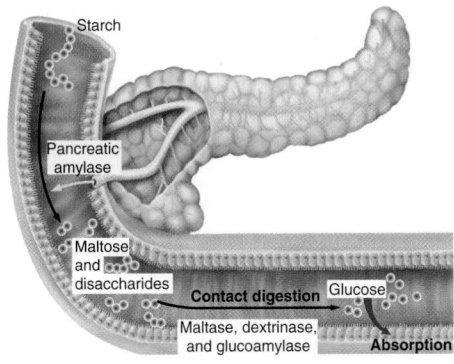

▲ **FIGURE 6.29** **Starch Digestion in the Small Intestine.**

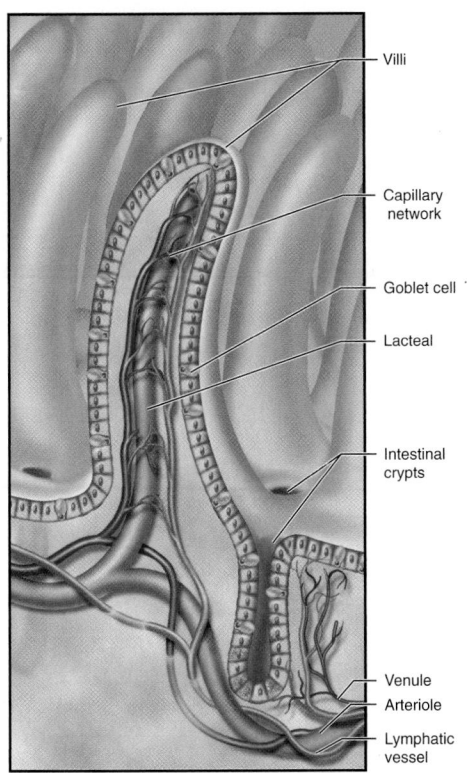

▲ **FIGURE 6.30** **Intestinal Villi.**

CHEMICAL DIGESTION, ABSORPTION, AND TRANSPORT

When the remains of the chicken and vegetable arrive in your duodenum, they have been reduced to very small particles by mastication and gastric peristalsis, and they have been mixed with other boluses of food.

Thus far, 10% of their carbohydrates have been partially digested by salivary amylase, operating mostly in the mouth; 10% to 15% of their protein has been partially digested by **proteases** in the stomach; and 10% of their fats have been digested by the salivary lipase operating in the stomach.

Carbohydrates are ingested in three forms:

1. **Polysaccharides,** such as starches.

2. **Disaccharides,** such as sucrose (table sugar) and lactose (milk sugar).

3. **Monosaccharides,** such as glucose and fructose (found in fruits) and galactose (found in milk).

In the small intestine, polysaccharides are broken down by pancreatic amylase into disaccharides *(Figure 6.29)*. Disaccharides are broken down to monosaccharides by maltase and dextrinase, enzymes secreted by the cells lining the villi of the small intestine.

The monosaccharides are taken up by the lining cells and transferred to the capillaries of the villi. They are then carried by the portal vein to the liver, where the nonglucose sugars are converted to glucose.

Proteins arrive in the duodenum and small intestine only 10% to 20% digested by gastric pepsin. Enzymes attached to the villi of the small intestine, together with the pancreatic enzyme trypsin, break down the remaining proteins to **amino acids.**

The amino acids are taken in by the epithelial cells of the small intestine, released into the capillaries of the villi, and carried away in the hepatic portal circulation. They are transported into cells all over the body, to be used as building blocks for new tissue formation.

Lipids (including fats) enter the duodenum and small intestine as large globules that have to be emulsified by bile salts into smaller droplets so that pancreatic lipase can digest the fats into very small droplets of free fatty acids and monoglycerides. There is enough pancreatic lipase in the duodenum to digest average amounts of fat within 1 or 2 minutes.

The very small droplets are absorbed by the intestinal cells and then taken into the lymphatic system by the **lacteals** inside the villi. The white, fatty lymphatic **chyle** eventually reaches the thoracic duct and is transferred into the left subclavian vein of the bloodstream *(see Chapter 7)*. The chyle is carried by the blood and stored in adipose tissue.

The fat-soluble vitamins (A, D, E, and K; *see Chapter 22*) are absorbed with the lipids.

Water that is ingested is 92% absorbed by the small intestine and taken into the bloodstream through the capillaries in the villi *(Figure 6.30)*. Water-soluble vitamins (C and the B-complex) are absorbed with water with the exception of vitamin B_{12}. This is a large molecule that has to bind with intrinsic factor from the stomach so that cells in the distant ileum can receive it and pass it through to the bloodstream.

Minerals are absorbed along the whole length of the small intestine. Iron and calcium are absorbed according to the body's needs. The other minerals are absorbed regardless of need, and the kidneys excrete the surplus.

S = Suffix   P = Prefix   R = Root   R/CF = Combining Form

WORD	PRONUNCIATION	ELEMENTS		DEFINITION
amino acid	ah-**ME**-no **ASS**-id	R/CF	**amin/o-** *nitrogen compound*	The basic building block of protein
carbohydrate	kar-boh-**HIGH**-drate	S/ R/CF R/	**-ate** *composed of* **carb/o-** *carbon* **-hydr-** *water*	Group of organic food compounds that includes sugars, starch, glycogen, and cellulose
chyle (contrast **chyme,** page 227)	KYLE		Greek *juice*	A milky fluid that results from the digestion and absorption of fats in the small intestine
lacteal	**LAK**-tee-al	S/ R/CF	**-al** *pertaining to* **lact/e-** *milk*	A lymphatic vessel carrying chyle away from the intestine
lipid	**LIP**-id		Greek *fat*	General term for all types of fatty compounds; for example, cholesterol, triglycerides, and fatty acids
mineral	**MIN**-er-al	S/ R/	**-al** *pertaining to* **miner-** *mines*	Inorganic compound usually found in earth's crust
protein	**PRO**-teen		Greek *first, primary*	Class of food substances based on amino acids

EXERCISES

Apply your medical vocabulary to answer the following questions about digestion. Circle the best choice.

1. The suffix that is used to form the names of enzymes is:
   a. -ic
   b. -al
   c. -ase
   d. -ous
   e. -ion

2. A word derived from the Greek for *juice*:
   a. lipid
   b. protein
   c. protease
   d. chyle
   e. lacteal

3. Group of organic food compounds that includes sugars, starch, glycogen, and cellulose:
   a. proteins
   b. fats
   c. lipids
   d. carbohydrates
   e. calories

4. The root **hydr-** means:
   a. blood
   b. juice
   c. water
   d. milk
   e. bile

5. General term for all fatty compounds:
   a. bile
   b. protein
   c. carbohydrate
   d. lipid
   e. protease

6. What is another name for a mineral?
   a. enzyme
   b. electrolyte
   c. lipid
   d. hormone
   e. fatty acid

7. The basic building block of protein is:
   a. carbohydrate
   b. protease
   c. amino acid
   d. lipid
   e. chyle

8. The combining form **lact/e** means:
   a. protein
   b. water
   c. carbon
   d. milk
   e. juice

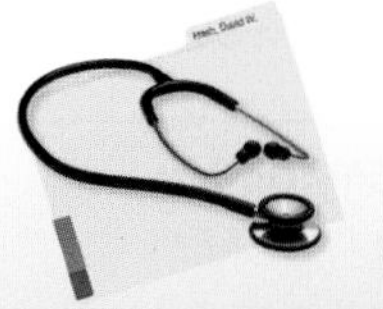

Case Report 6.4 (continued)

Mrs. Jan Stark, who presented in the Emergency Department with dehydration, was found to have **celiac disease,** a sensitivity to the protein **gluten** that is found in wheat, rye, barley, and oats. This disease involves the destruction of epithelial cells of the digestive tract lining, so intestinal enzymes are not being produced and absorption is not taking place.

Her difficulties with fine motor movement were the result of a **neuropathy** caused by vitamin B_{12} deficiency because of the lack of intrinsic factor to enable B_{12} to be absorbed. The diagnosis was made by an intestinal biopsy through oral endoscopy. A diet free of such gluten-containing foods as breads, cereals, cookies, and beer relieved her symptoms.

Disorders of Absorption

Malabsorption syndromes refer to a group of diseases in which intestinal absorption of nutrients is impaired.

Malnutrition can arise from malabsorption or from insufficient food intake as a result of famine, poverty, or loss of appetite due to cancer or terminal illness. Many of the poor and elderly in this country suffer from malnutrition. When the body experiences prolonged deprivation of calories and nutrients, it breaks down its own tissues to meet these needs.

Lactose intolerance occurs when the small intestine is not producing sufficient **lactase** to break down the milk sugar lactose. The result is **diarrhea** and cramps. Lactase can be taken in pill form before eating dairy products, and/or lactose can be avoided by using soy products rather than milk products.

Crohn disease (or **regional enteritis**) is an inflammation of the small intestine (frequently in the ileum) and occasionally also in the large intestine. The symptoms are abdominal pain, diarrhea, fatigue, and weight loss. Malabsorption is common, and children with Crohn disease may have delayed development and stunted growth.

Constipation occurs when fecal movement through the large intestine is slow, causing too much water to be reabsorbed by the large intestine. The feces become hardened. Factors causing constipation are lack of dietary fiber, lack of exercise, and emotional upset.

Gastroenteritis (stomach "flu") is an infection of the stomach and intestine that can be caused by a large variety of bacteria and viruses. It causes vomiting, diarrhea, and fever. An outbreak of gastroenteritis can sometimes be traced to contaminated food or water. The Norwalk virus and rotaviruses are major causes of diarrhea in infants and children.

Dysentery is a severe form of bacterial gastroenteritis with blood and mucus in frequent, watery stools. It can lead to dehydration.

Keynote

In malnutrition, the body breaks down its own tissues to meet its nutritional and metabolic needs.

Milk sugar is lactose. The enzyme lactase breaks down lactose to glucose.

Diarrhea is caused by irritation of the intestinal lining so that feces pass through the intestine too quickly for adequate amounts of water to be reabsorbed.

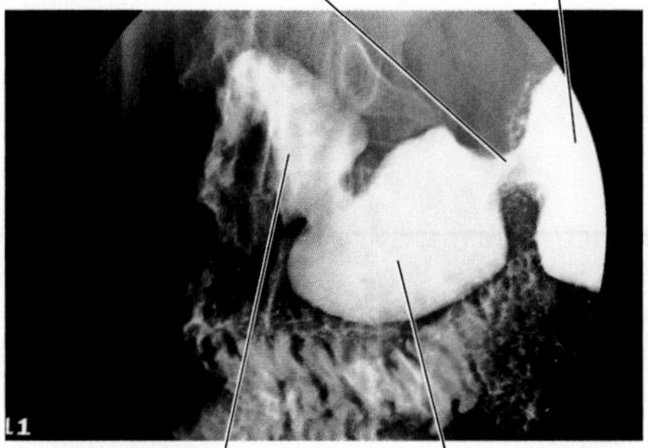

▲ **FIGURE 6.31 Barium Meal.** Barium meal showing pylorus and duodenum.

Diagnostic Procedures for the Upper Digestive Tract

- **Barium swallow.** The patient ingests barium sulfate, a contrast material, to show details of the pharynx and esophagus on x-ray.

- **Barium meal.** This procedure uses barium sulfate to study the distal esophagus, stomach, and duodenum on x-ray (*Figure 6.31*).

- **Enteroscopy.** An oral endoscope is used to visualize and biopsy tumors and ulcers and to control bleeding from the esophagus, stomach, and duodenum. This procedure is also called **esophagogastroduodenoscopy.**

- **Angiography.** This procedure uses dye to highlight blood vessels. It can be used to define the site of bleeding in the intestinal tract.

WORD ANALYSIS AND DEFINITION

S = Suffix   P = Prefix   R = Root   R/CF = Combining Form

WORD	PRONUNCIATION		ELEMENTS	DEFINITION
celiac celiac disease	**SEE**-lee-ack **SEE**-lee-ack diz-**EEZ**	S/ R/ P/ R/	Greek *belly* -ac *pertaining to* celi- *abdomen* dis- *apart* -ease *normal function*	Relating to the abdominal cavity Disease caused by sensitivity to gluten
constipation	kon-stih-**PAY**-shun	S/ R/	-ation *process* constip- *press together*	Hard, infrequent bowel movements
Crohn disease (also called **regional enteritis**)	KRONE diz-**EEZ** **RE**-jun-al en-ter-**I**-tis		Burrill Crohn, New York gastroenterologist, 1884–1993	Inflammatory bowel disease with narrowing and thickening of the terminal small bowel
diarrhea	die-ah-**REE**-ah	P/ R/	dia- *complete, through* -rrhea *flow, discharge*	Abnormally frequent and loose stools
dysentery	**DIS**-en-tare-ee	P/ R/	dys- *bad, difficult* -entery *intestine*	Disease with diarrhea, bowel spasms, fever, and dehydration
enteroscope enteroscopy	**EN**-ter-oh-**SKOPE** en-ter-**OSS**-koh-pee	S/ R/CF S/	-scope *instrument for viewing* enter/o- *intestine* -scopy *to examine, to view*	Slender, tubular instrument with light source and camera to visualize the digestive tract The examination of the lining of the digestive tract
gastroenteritis	**GAS**-troh-en-ter-**I**-tis	S/ R/ R/CF	-itis *inflammation* -enter- *intestine* gastr/o- *stomach*	Inflammation of the stomach and intestines
gluten	**GLU**-ten		Latin *glue*	Insoluble protein found in wheat, barley, and oats
intolerance	in-**TOL**-er-ance		Latin *unable to cope with*	Inability of the small intestine to digest and dispose of a particular dietary constituent
lactose lactase	**LAK**-toes **LAK**-tase	S/ R/	Latin *milk sugar* -ase *enzyme* lact- *milk*	The disaccharide found in cow's milk Enzyme that breaks down lactose to glucose and galactose
neuropathy	nyu-**ROP**-ah-thee	S/ R/CF	-pathy *disease* neur/o- *nerve*	Any disease of the nervous system

EXERCISES

Study the terms and elements in this WAD. Notice that some terms are formed with only a prefix and a root, while others are formed with a root and a suffix. **The only element that needs to be present in every term is a root or combining form.** *The definitions for the terms are given, as well as the element placement in the term. Write the correct term on each blank.*

1. Abnormally frequent and
   loose stools   _____ / _____
                   P   R

2. Any disease of the
   nervous system   _____ / _____
                 R/CF   S

3. Instrument for looking
   in the intestine   _____ / _____
                 R/CF   S

4. Infrequent bowel
   movements   _____ / _____
                   R   S

5. Enzyme that breaks
   down lactose   _____ / _____
                   R   S

6. Relating to the
   abdominal cavity   _____ / _____
                   R   S

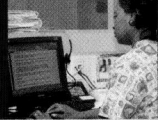

Elimination and the Large Intestine

OBJECTIVES

After the nutrients have been digested and absorbed in the small intestine, the residual materials have to be prepared in the large intestine for elimination from the body. The information in this lesson will enable you to:

6.6.1 Describe the structure of the large intestine.

6.6.2 Explain the functions of the large intestine.

6.6.3 Summarize common disorders of the large intestine.

6.6.4 Select the correct medical terminology to describe the anatomy, physiology, and disorders of the large intestine.

Keynote

A sphincter is a ring of smooth muscle that forms a one-way valve.

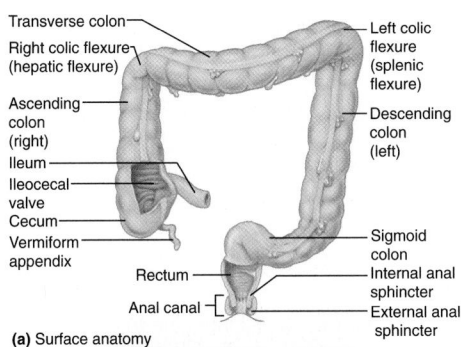

(a) Surface anatomy

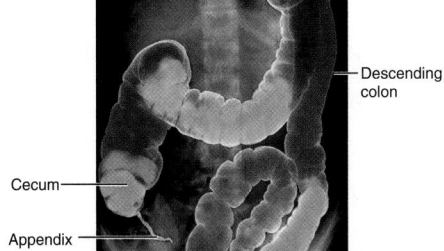

(b) X-ray of large intestine following a barium enema

▲ **FIGURE 6.32   Large Intestine.** *(a)* Surface anatomy. *(b)* Radiograph of large intestine following barium enema.

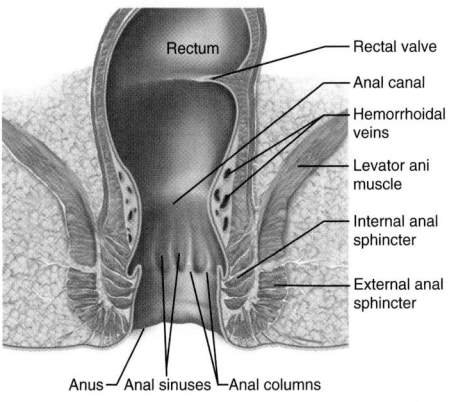

▲ **FIGURE 6.33   Anal Canal.**

STRUCTURE AND FUNCTIONS OF THE LARGE INTESTINE

Structure of the Large Intestine

The **large intestine** is so named because its diameter is much greater than that of the small intestine. It forms a **perimeter** in the abdominal cavity around the central mass of the small intestine *(Figure 6.32a)*.

At the junction between the small and large intestines, a ring of smooth muscle called the **ileocecal sphincter** forms a one-way valve. This allows chyme to pass into the large intestine and prevents the contents of the large intestine from backing up into the ileum.

At the beginning of the large intestine, the **cecum** is a pouch in the lower right quadrant of the abdomen *(Figure 6.32a)*. A narrow tube with a closed end, the **vermiform appendix,** projects downward from the cecum. The function of the appendix is not known.

The **ascending colon** begins at the cecum, extends upward until, just underneath the liver, it makes a sharp left turn at the hepatic **flexure** and becomes the transverse colon. At the left side of the abdomen, near the spleen at the splenic flexure, the transverse colon turns downward to form the descending colon. At the pelvic brim, the **descending** colon makes an S-shaped curve, the **sigmoid** colon, which descends in the pelvis to become the **rectum** and then the **anal canal.**

The rectum has three transverse folds, rectal valves that enable it to retain feces while passing gas (**flatus**). Intestinal gas is 90% nitrogen and oxygen, ingested while breathing and eating, together with methane, hydrogen, sulfites, and carbon dioxide contributed from bacterial fermentation of undigested food. This yields pungent ammonia and foul-smelling hydrogen sulphide to give gas and feces their characteristic odor.

The anal canal is the last 1 to 2 inches of the large intestine, opening to the outside as the **anus.** The mucous membrane is folded into six to eight longitudinal **anal columns.** **Feces,** pressing against the columns causes them to produce more mucus to lubricate the canal during **defecation.** Two sphincter muscles guard the anus *(Figure 6.33)*: an internal sphincter, composed of smooth muscle from the intestinal wall, and an external sphincter, composed of skeletal muscle that you can control voluntarily.

Functions of the Large Intestine

- **Absorption** of water and electrolytes. The large intestine receives more than 1 liter (1.05 quarts) of chyme each day from the small intestine and reabsorbs water and electrolytes to reduce the volume to 100 to 150 mL of feces to be eliminated by defecation.
- **Secretion** of mucus that protects the intestinal wall and holds particles of fecal matter together.
- **Digestion** by the bacteria that inhabit the large intestine of any food remnants that have escaped the digestive enzymes of the small intestine.
- **Peristalsis,** which, in the large intestine, happens only a few times a day to produce mass movements toward the rectum. Often when you ingest food into your stomach, your **gastrocolic reflex** will generate a mass movement of feces.
- **Elimination** of materials that were not digested or absorbed.

WORD	PRONUNCIATION		ELEMENTS	DEFINITION
anus anal (adj)	**A**-nuss **A**-nal		Latin *ring*	Terminal opening of the digestive tract through which feces are discharged
appendix	ah-**PEN**-dicks		Latin *appendage*	Small blind projection from the pouch of the cecum
appendectomy	ah-pen-**DEK**-toe-me	R/ S/	**append-** *appendix* **-ectomy** *surgical excision*	Surgical removal of the appendix
vermiform	**VER**-mih-form		Latin *wormlike*	Worm shaped; used as a descriptor for the appendix
appendicitis	ah-pen-dih-**SIGH**-tis	S/ S/	**-ic** *pertaining to* **-itis** *inflammation*	Inflammation of the appendix
colon	**KOH**-lon		Greek *colon*	The large intestine, extending from the cecum to the rectum
colic	**KOL**-ik	S/ R/	**-ic** *pertaining to* **col-** *colon*	Spasmodic, crampy pains in the abdomen
colitis	koh-**LIE**-tis	S/	**-itis** *inflammation*	Inflammation of the colon
feces	**FEE**-sees		Latin *dregs*	Undigested, waste material discharged from the bowel
fecal (adj)	**FEE**-kal	S/ R/	**-al** *pertaining to* **-fec-** *feces*	Pertaining to feces
defecation defecate (verb)	def-eh-**KAY**-shun **DEF**-eh-kate	S/ P/	**-ation** *process* **de-** *from, out of*	Evacuation of feces from the rectum and anus
flatus flatulence flatulent (adj)	**FLAY**-tus **FLAT**-you-lents **FLAT**-you-lent	S/ R/	Latin *blowing* **-ence** *forming* **flatul-** *excessive gas*	Gas or air expelled through the anus Excessive amount of gas in the stomach and intestines
flexure	**FLECK**-shur		Latin *bend*	A bend in a structure
gastrocolic reflex	gas-troh-**KOL**-ik **RE**-fleks	S/ R/CF R/ R/	**-ic** *pertaining to* **gastr/o-** *stomach* **-col-** *colon* **reflex** *bend back*	Taking food into stomach leads to mass movement of feces in the colon and the desire to defecate
ileocecal sphincter	**ILL**-ee-oh-**SEE**-cal **SFINK**-ter	S/ R/CF R/	**-al** *pertaining to* **ile/o-** *ileum* **-cec-** *cecum* **sphincter** *Greek band*	Band of muscle that encircles the junction of the ileum and cecum
perimeter	peh-**RIM**-eh-ter	P/ R/	**peri-** *around* **-meter** *measure*	An edge or border
rectum rectal (adj)	**RECK**-tum **RECK**-tal	S/ R/	Latin *straight* **-al** *pertaining to* **rect-** *rectum*	Terminal part of the colon from the sigmoid to the anal canal Pertaining to the rectum
sigmoid	**SIG**-moyd	S/ R/	**-oid** *resembling* **sigm-** *Greek letter "S"*	Sigmoid colon is shaped like an "S"

EXERCISES

Attack a medical term with your analytical skills. Break these terms down into their elements to define the word. Fill in the chart.

Medical Term	Meaning of Prefix	Meaning of Root/Combining Form	Meaning of Suffix	Definition
colitis				
defecation				
colic				
ileocecal				

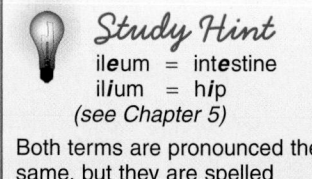

Study Hint

il**e**um = int**e**stine
il**i**um = h**i**p
(see Chapter 5)

Both terms are pronounced the same, but they are spelled differently. Be precise!

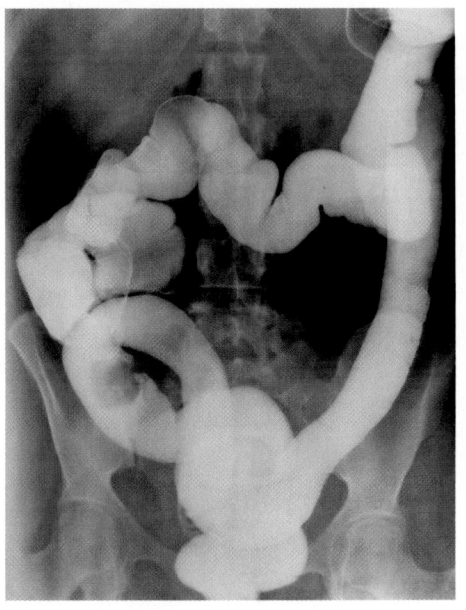

▲ FIGURE 6.34 Barium Enema Showing Diverticulosis.

▲ FIGURE 6.35 Barium Enema Showing Cancer of the Colon (orange area).

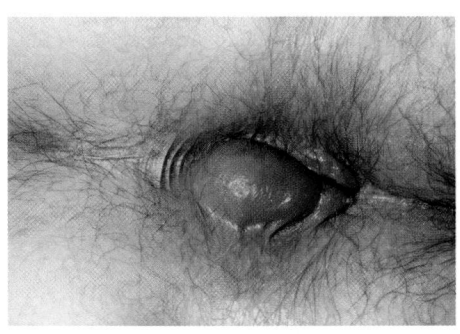

▲ FIGURE 6.36 External Hemorrhoid.
Hemorrhoid protruding from anus.

DISORDERS OF THE LARGE INTESTINE AND ANAL CANAL

Disorders of the Large Intestine

Appendicitis is the most common cause of acute abdominal pain in the right lower quadrant. On palpation, tenderness over the **McBurney point,** one-third the distance from the anterior superior iliac crest to the umbilicus *(see Chapter 5),* suggests appendicitis. If neglected, the inflamed appendix can rupture, leading to **peritonitis.** This is strongly suggested by the presence of **rebound tenderness,** in which a stab of severe pain is produced when the abdominal wall, which has been pressed in slowly, is released rapidly. A surgical appendectomy, usually performed through laparoscopy, is the treatment for appendicitis.

Diverticulosis is the presence of small pouches bulging outward through weak spots in the lining of the large intestine *(Figure 6.34).* They are asymptomatic until the pouches become infected and inflamed, a condition called **diverticulitis.** This condition causes abdominal pain, vomiting, constipation, and fever. Complications, such as perforation and abscess formation, can occur. The most likely cause of diverticular disease (diverticulosis and diverticulitis) is a low-fiber diet.

Ulcerative colitis is an extensive inflammation and ulceration of the lining of the large intestine. It produces bouts of bloody diarrhea, crampy pain, and often weight loss and electrolyte imbalance.

Irritable bowel syndrome (IBS) is an increasingly common large-bowel disorder, presenting with crampy pains, gas, and changes in bowel habits to either constipation or diarrhea. There are no anatomical changes seen in the bowel, and the cause is unknown.

Polyps are masses of tissue arising from the wall of the large intestine that protrude into the bowel **lumen.** They vary in size and shape. Most are benign. Endoscopic biopsy can determine if they are **precancerous** or cancerous.

Colon and **rectal cancers** *(Figure 6.35)* are the second leading cause of cancer deaths after lung cancer. The majority occur in the rectum and sigmoid colon. These cancers spread by:

1. Direct extension through the bowel wall.

2. **Metastasis** to regional lymph nodes.

3. Moving down the lumen of the bowel.

4. Bloodborne **metastases** to liver, lung, bone, and brain.

Obstruction of the large bowel can be caused by cancers, large polyps, or diverticulitis.

Intussusception is a form of obstruction whereby a tumor in the lumen of the bowel, together with its segment of bowel, is telescoped into the immediately distal segment of bowel.

Proctitis is inflammation of the lining of the rectum, often associated with ulcerative colitis, Crohn disease, or radiation therapy. Symptoms are **anorectal** pain, rectal bleeding, and excess mucus in the **stool.**

Disorders of the Anal Canal

Hemorrhoids are dilated veins in the submucosa of the anal canal, often associated with pregnancy, chronic **constipation,** diarrhea, or aging. They protrude into the anal canal (internal hemorrhoid) or bulge out along the edge of the anus (external hemorrhoid, *Figure 6.36*), producing pain and bright red blood from the anus. A **thrombosed** hemorrhoid, in which blood has clotted, is very painful.

Anal fissures are tears in the lining of the anal canal, such as may occur with difficult bowel movements (BMs).

Anal fistulas occur following abscesses in the anal glands. The anal canal has six or seven glands in the posterior canal that secrete mucus to lubricate the canal. If the glands become infected, abscesses form that, when they heal, can form a passage (fistula) between the anal canal and the skin outside the anus.

S = Suffix   P = Prefix   R = Root   R/CF = Combining Form

WORD	PRONUNCIATION		ELEMENTS	DEFINITION
bowel	BOUGH-el		Latin *sausage*	Another name for intestine
diverticulum diverticula (pl) diverticulosis	die-ver-**TICK**-you-lum die-ver-**TICK**-you-lah **DIE**-ver-tick-you-**LOW**-sis	S/ R/ S/	-um *tissue* diverticul- *by-road* -osis *condition*	A pouchlike opening or sac from a tubular structure (e.g., gut) Presence of a number of small pouches in the wall of the large intestine
diverticulitis	**DIE**-ver-tick-you-**LIE**-tis	S/	-itis *inflammation*	Inflammation of the diverticula
fissure	**FISH**-ur		Latin *slit*	Deep furrow or cleft
fistula	**FIS**-tyu-lah		Latin *pipe, tube*	Abnormal passage
hemorrhoid hemorrhoids (pl) hemorrhoidectomy	**HEM**-oh-royd **HEM**-oh-roy-**DEK**-toh-me	S/ R/CF S/	-rrhoid *flow* hem/o- *blood* -ectomy *excision*	Dilated rectal vein producing painful anal swelling Surgical removal of hemorrhoids
intussusception	**IN**-tuss-sus-**SEP**-shun	S/ P/ R/	-ion *action* intus- *within* -suscept- *to take up*	The slipping of one part of bowel inside another to cause obstruction
lumen	**LOO**-men		Latin *light, window*	The interior space of a tubelike structure
McBurney point	mack-**BUR**-nee POYNT		Charles McBurney, New York surgeon, 1845–1913	One-third the distance from anterior superior iliac spine to umbilicus
metastasis metastases (pl)	meh-**TAS**-tah-sis meh-**TAS**-tah-seez	P/ R/	meta- *beyond* -stasis *placement*	Spread of a disease from one part of the body to another
peritoneum	per-ih-toe-**NEE**-um	S/ R/CF	-um *tissue* periton/e- *stretch over*	Membrane that lines the abdominal cavity
peritoneal (adj) peritonitis	**PER**-ih-toe-**NEE**-al **PER**-ih-toe-**NIE**-tis	S/ S/	-al *pertaining to* -itis *inflammation*	Pertaining to the peritoneum Inflammation of the peritoneum
polyp polyposis polypectomy	**POL**-ip pol-ih-**POH**-sis pol-ip-**ECK**-toh-mee	R/ S/ S/	polyp- *polyp* -osis *condition* -ectomy *excision*	Mass of tissue that projects into the lumen of the bowel Presence of several polyps Excision or removal of a polyp
precancerous	pree-**KAN**-sir-us	S/ P/ R/	-ous *pertaining to* pre- *before* -cancer- *cancer*	Lesion from which a cancer can develop
proctitis	prok-**TIE**-tis	S/ R/	-itis *inflammation* proct- *anus and rectum*	Inflammation of the lining of the rectum
ulcerative	**UL**-sir-ah-tiv	S/ R/	-ative *quality of* ulcer- *a sore*	Marked by an ulcer or ulcers

Abbreviations

BM   bowel movement
IBS   irritable bowel syndrome

EXERCISES

This exercise focuses on the suffixes in this WAD. The suffix is your first clue to the meaning of a medical term. Challenge your knowledge of suffixes by filling in the blanks. Some answers you will use twice because more than one suffix can have the same meaning.

_____ 1. -um

_____ 2. -ous

_____ 3. -osis

_____ 4. -ion

_____ 5. -itis

_____ 6. -rrhoid

_____ 7. -ative

_____ 8. -al

_____ 9. -ectomy

A. flow

B. action

C. inflammation

D. tissue

E. pertaining to

F. condition

G. excision

H. quality of

Risk factors that can cause GI bleeding
include alcohol, smoking, and a low-fiber
diet.

GASTROINTESTINAL (GI) BLEEDING

Bleeding can occur anywhere in the gastrointestinal tract from a variety of causes, as described in the preceding sections. The bleeding can be internal and painless. It can present in different ways to provide a clue to the site of bleeding:

- **Hematemesis**—the vomiting of bright red blood, which indicates an upper GI source of ongoing bleeding (esophagus, stomach, duodenum).

- **Vomiting of "coffee grounds"**—occurs when bleeding from an upper GI source has slowed or stopped; red hemoglobin has been converted to brown hematin by gastric acids.

- **Hematochezia**—the passage of bright red bloody stools; usually indicates lower GI bowel bleeding from the sigmoid colon, rectum, or anus.

- **Melena**—the passage of black tarry stools; usually indicates upper GI bleeding. The blood is digested and hemoglobin is oxidized as it passes through the intestine to produce the black color. Melena can continue for several days after a severe hemorrhage.

- **Occult blood**—no bleeding seen in the stool, but a chemical fecal occult blood test (**Hemoccult test**) is positive. The chronic source of the bleeding can be anywhere in the GI tract.

Consuming black licorice, Pepto-Bismol, or blueberries can produce black stools.

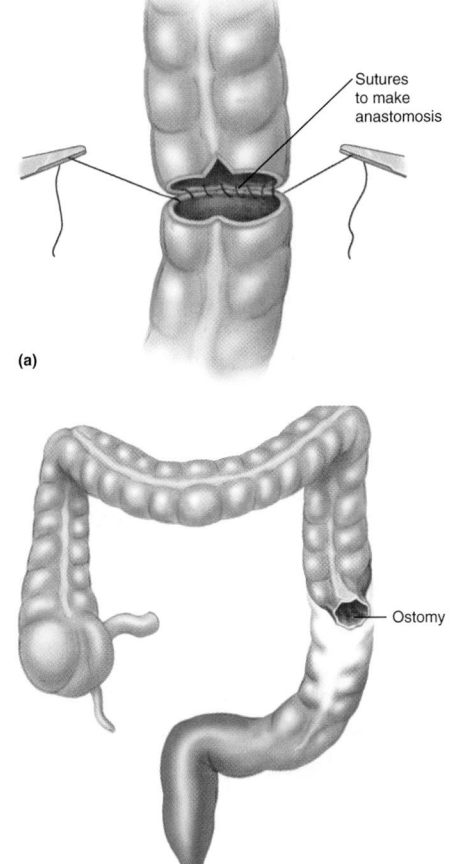

Sutures to make anastomosis

(a)

Ostomy

(b)

▲ **FIGURE 6.37   Intestinal Resections.**
(*a*) Anastomosis. (*b*) Ostomy.

Common Diagnostic and Therapeutic Procedures

- **Fecal occult blood test** (Hemoccult) is used to detect the presence of blood not visible to the naked eye.

- **Nasogastric aspiration and lavage**—the presence of bright red blood indicates active upper GI bleeding; "coffee grounds" indicate the bleeding has slowed or stopped.

- **Upper GI barium x-rays** are less accurate than endoscopy at identifying the bleeding lesion.

- **Barium enema**—a radiographic contrast material is injected into the large intestine as an enema and x-ray films are taken *(see Figures 6.32b, 6.34, and 6.35)*.

- **Endoscopy** enables direct visual examination of the intestine with a flexible tube containing light-transmitting glass fibers or a video transmitter that sends back an enlarged image. **Panendoscopy** examines the esophagus, stomach, and duodenum and provides the highest yield of information to establish the source of upper GI bleeding. Endoscopy can also be used to perform a biopsy, remove polyps (**polypectomy**), and **coagulate** bleeding lesions.

- **Anoscopy** examines the anus and lower rectum with a rigid instrument.

- **Flexible sigmoidoscopy** examines the rectum and sigmoid colon.

- **Flexible colonoscopy** examines the whole length of the colon.

- **Gastroscopy** examines the stomach.

- **Intestinal resections** are used to surgically remove diseased portions of the intestine. The remaining portions of the intestine can be joined together through an **anastomosis** *(Figure 6.37a)*. If there is insufficient bowel remaining, an **ostomy** *(Figure 6.37b)* can be performed, where the end of the bowel opens onto the skin at a **stoma. Ileostomy** and **colostomy** are two common procedures.

- **Digital rectal exam**—the physician palpates the rectum and prostate gland with an index finger.

WORD	PRONUNCIATION		ELEMENTS	DEFINITION
anastomosis anastomoses (pl)	ah-**NAS**-to-**MO**-sis ah-**NAS**-to-**MO**-sez	S/ R/	-osis *condition* **anastom-** *join together*	A surgically made union between two tubular structures
coagulate	koh-**AG**-you-late	S/ R/	-ate *composed of, pertaining to* **coagul-** *clotting*	Form a clot
endoscope	**EN**-doh-skope	P/	endo- *within, inside*	Instrument for examining the inside of a tubular or hollow organ
endoscopic (adj)	**EN**-doh-**SKOP**-ik	S/ S/	-ic *pertaining to* -scope *instrument for viewing*	
endoscopy anoscopy colonoscopy	en-**DOS**-koh-pee **A**-nos-koh-pee koh-lon-**OSS**-koh-pee	S/ R/CF R/CF	-scopy *to examine* **an/o-** *anus* **colon/o-** *colon*	The use of an endoscope Endoscopic examination of the anus Examination of the inside of the colon by endoscopy
gastroscopy ileoscopy panendoscopy (*Note:* two prefixes)	gas-**TROS**-koh-pee ill-ee-**OS**-koh-pee pan-en-**DOS**-koh-pee	R/CF R/CF P/	**gastr/o-** *stomach* **ile/o-** *ileum* **pan-** *all*	Endoscopic examination of the stomach Endoscopic examination of the ileum Examination of the inside of the esophagus, stomach, and upper duodenum using a flexible fiber-optic endoscope
proctoscopy	prok-**TOSS**-koh-pee	R/CF	**proct/o-** *anus and rectum*	Examination of the inside of the anus and the rectum by endoscopy
sigmoidoscopy	sig-moi-**DOS**-koh-pee	R/CF	**sigmoid/o-** *sigmoid colon*	Endoscopic examination of the sigmoid colon
enema	**EN**-eh-mah		Greek *injection*	An injection of fluid into the rectum
hematochezia	he-mat-oh-**KEY**-zee-ah	S/ R/CF	-chezia *pass a stool* **hemat/o-** *blood*	The passage of red, bloody stools
melena	mel-**EN**-ah		Greek *black*	The passage of black, tarry stools
occult Hemoccult test	oh-**KULT** **HEEM**-oh-kult TEST		Latin *to hide*	Not visible on the surface *Hemoccult* (trade name for a fecal occult blood test)
ostomy colostomy ileostomy	**OS**-toe-me ko-**LOSS**-toe-me ill-ee-**OS**-toe-me	S/ R/ R/ R/	-stomy *new opening* **os-** *mouth* **col-** *colon* **ile-** *ileum*	Surgery to create an artificial opening into a tubular structure Artificial opening from the colon to the outside of the body Artificial opening from the ileum to the outside of the body
stoma	**STOW**-mah		Greek *mouth*	Artificial opening

EXERCISES

Scope *and* scopy *are two suffixes you will see attached to many medical terms you will meet in later chapters.* Scope *is the actual instrument used in the procedure. The procedure itself is the* scopy. *Utilize your medical vocabulary to fill in the blanks for this exercise.*

Instrument	Procedure Term	Definition of Procedure
endoscope		
colonoscope		
proctoscope		
anoscope		
gastroscope		
ileoscope		
sigmoidoscope		

Note: Endoscope *is a generic (general) term that means any instrument used to examine the inside of a tubular or hollow organ. The instrument obtains its specific name from the organ it is used to examine. Thus, an instrument used to view a bronchus is a bronchoscope specifically, but it is also an endoscope in general.*

LESSON 6.6 **Elimination and the Large Instestine**   **249**

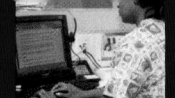

DIGESTIVE SYSTEM

CHALLENGE YOUR KNOWLEDGE

A. **Can you interpret the following colonoscopy report for this patient?** First, read the report out loud. Underline the medical terminology. If you need to, consult a dictionary or your glossary for additional help. Fill in the blanks.

> **Preoperative Diagnosis:** History of (H/O) multiple colonic polyps.
>
> **Postoperative Diagnosis:** Normal colon.
> In the left lateral position, the colonoscope was advanced into the rectum without difficulty. Examination of the rectum was normal. The sigmoid and descending colon revealed extensive diverticular disease but no evidence of colonic polyp disease. The transverse colon was examined to the hepatic flexure. There were no abnormalities of the transverse colon. The ascending colon was examined to the ileocecal valve. This was confirmed by abdominal wall transillumination. There were no abnormalities of the ascending colon. The patient tolerated the procedure well and was discharged from the endoscopy suite in good condition. In view of his age and a clean colonoscopy, I have recommended no further surveillance.

1. Based on the prefixes, what is the difference between the pre- and postoperative diagnoses?

    pre- = _____ post- = _____
    Why are the diagnoses sometimes different?

    _____

2. Describe the left lateral position. _____

3. What instrument was used for this procedure? _____

4. Give another adjective meaning *extensive*. _____

5. Deconstruct **diverticulosis,** and write its meaning. _____

6. Define **polyp.** _____

7. Based on the prefix trans-, in which position does the transverse colon lie? _____

8. Again, using the prefix trans-, what does **transillumination** mean? _____

9. What does a "clean colonoscopy" mean? _____

10. Is it good or bad that the physician is recommending "no further surveillance." Explain your answer.

    _____

B. **While every medical term does not need a prefix, most medical terms will have a suffix, which appears at the end of the term.** Remember that *there can be more than one suffix with the same meaning.* Fill in the chart.

Suffix	Meaning of Suffix	Example of Medical Term Using This Suffix
-al		
-ar		
-ary		
-ase		
-dynia		

Suffix	Meaning of Suffix	Example of Medical Term Using This Suffix
-ectomy		
-ia		
-ics		
-id		
-ist		
-itis		
-osis		
-zyme		

C. **Patient Education—In Your Own Words:** If you had to explain each of the specific functions of the digestive system to a patient, what would you say? Translate the medical terms into language the patient can understand. Fill in the blanks.

1. ingestion: _____

2. propulsion: _____

3. digestion: _____

4. secretion: _____

5. absorption: _____

6. elimination: _____

D. **Using all the terms in part C, trace the process of digestion in a paragraph.** The exercise has been started for you. Underline all the terms in your writing to make sure you have used every one.

The process of digestion begins in the mouth where (go on from here)

_____

_____

_____

_____

_____

_____

DIGESTIVE SYSTEM

E. **Dental assistants, or anyone working in an Oral Surgery Department, need to have a thorough knowledge of the mouth and the mastication process.** Your knowledge of medical terms will help you communicate with the dentist or oral surgeon and the patients. Match the correct answer to the statements below.

_____ 1. Grind and crush food   A. mouth

_____ 2. Projects above the gum/covered with enamel   B. pulp cavity

_____ 3. Cheek muscles   C. root canal

_____ 4. Destroys tooth enamel and dentin   D. caries

_____ 5. Contains blood vessels, nerves, tissue   E. root

_____ 6. Harder than bone   F. gingivitis

_____ 7. Oral cavity   G. papillae

_____ 8. Dental decay   H. crown

_____ 9. Anchors tooth to jaw   I. tartar

_____ 10. Inflammation of the gum   J. buccinator

_____ 11. Nerves reach the tooth through this   K. bicuspids and molars

_____ 12. Contain the taste buds   L. dentin

F. **Be aware of singular and plural terms.** Insert the correct medical terms in the blanks; watch for spelling. You will not use all the terms.

diverticulitis   **diverticulum**   **diverticulosis**   **diverticula**

1. What starts out as a single _____, if left untreated, can lead to many _____.

   The condition of having a number of these small pouches in the wall of the large intestine is known

   as _____. Should these pouches become inflamed, _____ will result.

metastasses   **metastases**   **metastize**   **metastasis**

2. What was originally thought to be a single _____ to the patient's lung was proved to be multiple

   _____ to lung, kidney, and bone.

polypectomy   **polyposis**   **polyp (singular)**

3. The first polyp was found on sigmoidoscopy. A follow-up colonoscopy 6 months later found several more

   (plural) _____ in the large intestine. Diagnosis is _____. Proposed treat-

   ment is _____.

peritoneum   **peritonitis**   **peritoneal**

4. The _____ laceration sliced completely through the _____. Because of an

   infection in the wound, the patient developed _____.

G. Deconstruct and Define: The following medical terms can all designate a diagnosis or a condition. Use your knowledge of basic elements to deconstruct these terms and determine their meanings. First, slash (/) the terms into elements; then fill in the chart.

Medical Term	Prefix	Root/CF	Suffix	Meaning of Medical Term
dysphagia				
esophagitis				
hematemesis				
pyrosis				
reflux				
regurgitation				

H. Abbreviations: Choose the abbreviation that is best described in the statement, and fill it in on the blank provided. On the line below the statement, write out the meaning of the abbreviation you have chosen. There are more answers than questions. The first one is done for you. Fill in the blanks.

GI   SSA   GERD   HAV   ESWL   SGOT   CF   BM

1. Final act of elimination   Abbreviation __*BM*_____

   Meaning: _____*bowel movement*_____

2. Backing up into the esophagus   Abbreviation: _____

   Meaning: _____

3. Digestive system component   Abbreviation: _____

   Meaning: _____

4. Liver disease indicator   Abbreviation: _____

   Meaning: _____

5. Inherited disease that affects exocrine glands   Abbreviation: _____

   Meaning: _____

I. Group Recall: The following colors all have a Latin or Greek term associated with them. Fill in the blanks with the element, and provide a medical term where it is used.

White: _____   Term: _____

Yellow: _____   Term: _____

Rust: _____   Term: _____

DIGESTIVE SYSTEM

J. **Word elements are the keys to unlocking medical terms.** Assess your knowledge of elements with this exercise.

1. Where is the inflammation in **hepatitis**?

   a. the belly

   b. the liver

   c. the pancreas

   d. the mouth

   e. the intestine

2. In the term **submucosa,** the prefix means:

   a. over

   b. under

   c. around

   d. inside

   e. across

3. The color denoted in the term **leukoplakia** is:

   a. green

   b. black

   c. white

   d. yellow

   e. red

4. The element **os** means:

   a. stomach

   b. mouth

   c. eye

   d. liver

   e. ear

5. If the root **cyst** means *bladder,* what is a **cystectomy**?

   a. bladder irrigation

   b. bladder removal

   c. bladder examination

   d. bladder laceration

   e. bladder hemorrhage

6. If a medication is given **postprandial**, you will take it after:

   a. exercise

   b. drinking water

   c. meals

   d. a vitamin

   e. waking up

7. **Gingivitis** has a root that means:

   a. opening

   b. teeth

   c. gum

   d. decay

   e. enzyme

8. A **cholecystectomy** is:

   a. procedure

   b. diagnosis

   c. inflammation

   d. discharge

   e. instrument

9. What is the adjective used to describe a dilated, tortuous vein?

   a. adipose

   b. varicose

   c. edematous

   d. pyloric

   e. segmental

10. On the basis of the suffix, you know that the **peritoneum** will be:

    a. opening

    b. incision

    c. structure

    d. tumor

    e. matrix

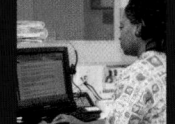

CHAPTER 6 REVIEW

DIGESTIVE SYSTEM

K. **Element:** The following elements are a mixture of the prefixes, roots, combining forms, and suffixes contained in this chapter. In your study of medical terminology, it is important for you to be able to identify the types of elements and their definitions. This will aid you in determining the meaning of the medical term. Fill in the chart.

Identify each element with a check mark (✓) in the proper column. Then provide a meaning for the element. The first one is done for you.

Element	Prefix	Root/CF	Suffix	Meaning of Element
al			✓	*pertaining to*
atric				
bari				
bi				
cusp				
dynia				
glosso				
id				
lingu				
peri				
stalsis				
sub				

Now take any combination of elements from this chart and form a complete medical term. Define the term based on the meaning of the elements given in the chart.

Medical term: _____ / _____ / _____

                                 Prefix   Root/CF   Suffix

Meaning of medical term: _____

L. **Discussion Questions:** Draw on your knowledge of the **language of gastroenterology** to discuss the following questions. Prepare a short answer. Be certain you can define every term you are using.

1. What is the bony roof of the mouth called? _____

   What birth defect is associated with this part of the body? _____

   What large facial bone is connected to this part of the body? (*Hint: See Chapter 5.*) _____

2. Why do teeth have to be the hardest structures in the body?

   _____

   _____

3. Remember what you learned in *Chapter 5* about the role of muscles in the body. What are the buccinator muscles responsible for, and how does that tie in with question 2?

   _____

   _____

M. Recall and Review: The following exercise on word elements contains some elements from this chapter and the previous chapter. Try to recall the previous elements without turning back in your book. Check (✓) the type of element; then write its meaning. Fill in the blanks.

Element	Prefix	Root/CF	Suffix	Meaning of Element
clast	_____	_____	_____	_____
de	_____	_____	_____	_____
hydr	_____	_____	_____	_____
lacte	_____	_____	_____	_____
malacia	_____	_____	_____	_____

N. Patient Education—In Your Own Words: Your knowledge of medical terminology usually must be translated into layman's terms if you are going to explain something the patient can comprehend. Prepare a short answer that will help your patient understand the *difference* between:

1. A *polypectomy* and an *enteroscopy:*

_____

_____

_____

2. *Sublingual* and *subcutaneous* medication (**Hint:** Think back to *Chapter 3*):

_____

_____

_____

O. Deconstruct: No matter how long or how short the medical term, reducing it to elements will provide the meaning. Deconstruct with slashes the following two medical terms into their elemental meanings. Fill in the blanks. Divide and conquer your terms!

esophagogastroduodenoscopy

Prefix	Meaning of Prefix	Root(s)/CF	Meaning of Root(s)/CF	Suffix	Meaning of Suffix

1. The meaning of *esophagogastroduodenoscopy* is:

_____

_____

_____

oral

Prefix	Meaning of Prefix	Root(s)/CF	Meaning of Root(s)/CF	Suffix	Meaning of Suffix

2. The meaning of *oral* is:

_____

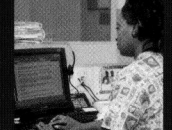

DIGESTIVE SYSTEM

P. As a body system, the digestive system has a lot of different disorders. Can you pair the correct organ with its disease or condition and write a brief definition of the term? Fill in the chart.

Term	Organ	Definition
aphthous ulcers	_____	_____
cholecystitis	_____	_____
choledocholithiasis	_____	_____
cirrhosis	_____	_____
Crohn disease	_____	_____
diverticulitis	_____	_____
dysphagia	_____	_____
GERD	_____	_____
IBS	_____	_____
liver	_____	_____
intussusception	_____	_____
pancreatitis	_____	_____
proctitis	_____	_____

Q. Medical terms that are nouns can also have an adjective form. Each statement has the noun form in parentheses; you must fill in the correct form of the adjective on the blank. Fill in the blanks.

1. The patient's (digestion) _____ symptoms were resolved with the new medication.

2. Due to an obstruction, the (pylorus) _____ sphincter was necrotic.

3. The (lymph) _____ tissues were sent to the pathologist for examination.

4. The patient is suffering from (pancreas) _____ cancer.

5. The (saliva) _____ gland was removed and sent to pathology.

6. Due to infection, the patient's (intestine) _____ surgery has been postponed until next week.

7. (Hemolysis) _____ jaundice results from RBC destruction and excess bilirubin.

8. The patient's (esophagus) _____ varices were bleeding.

9. The (laparoscope) _____ surgery poses less risk to the patient.

10. The (segment) _____ resection of the intestine is scheduled for later today.

R. Supply the missing element(s) that will complete the medical term. Beneath the line, write the type of word element(s) you have used. Some terms may require more than one element. Fill in the blanks. The first one is done for you.

1. Inflammation of the appendix   appendic*itis* _____
                                            Suffix

2. Part of the colon shaped like an "S"   sigm _____

3. Pertaining to the anus

an_____

4. Excessive amount of gas

flatul_____

5. To bend back

_____ flex

6. Inflammation of the colon

col_____

7. Pertaining to the anus and rectum

ano_____ al

8. Evacuation of feces from the rectum and anus

de_____

9. An edge or a border

_____ meter

10. Pertaining to the colon

_____ic

S. **The following medical terms have their origins in Greek and Latin.** Give a definition for each term; then use any three terms in sentences of your choice. Fill in the blanks.

Medical Term	Definition
bolus	
incisor	
uvula	
ulcer	
lymph	
saliva	
canker	
esophagus	
pulp	
caries	
palate	

1. _____

_____

2. _____

_____

3. _____

_____

DIGESTIVE SYSTEM

T. Documentation:

> Mrs. Helen Schreiber, a 45-year-old high school principal, presents with a 6-month history of dry mouth, bleeding gums, and difficulty in chewing and swallowing food. Questioning by Dr. Susan Lee, her primary care physician, reveals that she also has dry eyes, is having pain in some joints of both hands, and has felt fatigued.
>
> Her previous medical history is uneventful. Physical examination shows a dry mouth, mild gingivitis, and an ulcer on the back of the lower lip. Her salivary glands are not swollen. Her eyes show no ulceration or conjunctivitis. The metacarpophalangeal joints of both index fingers are swollen, stiff, and tender. All other systems show no abnormality.
>
> Initial laboratory reports show anemia, decreased WBC count, and an elevated ESR. Dr. Lee made a provisional diagnosis of Sjögren syndrome. The results of blood studies for SSA and SSB antibodies and for rheumatoid factor titers are pending, as are x-rays of her hands. Mrs. Schreiber was given advice about symptomatic treatment for her dry mouth and will be seen again in 1 week.
>
> Luis Guitterez, CMA. 06/12/09, 1530 hrs.

Helen Schreiber's medical record of her visit to Dr. Susan Lee contains terms from this and previous chapters. Reinforce your knowledge of the language of medicine by answering the following questions based on this scenario. Fill in the blanks.

1. List all of Mrs. Schreiber's signs and symptoms.

   _____

   _____

   _____

2. Which symptoms pertain to the digestive system? _____

3. Which other body systems are presenting symptoms? _____

4. Examination of Mrs. Schreiber's eyes revealed no conjunctivitis. What is conjunctivitis?

   _____

U. Terminology Challenge: Dr. Lee made a *provisional* diagnosis for Mrs. Schreiber of Sjögren syndrome. Use your glossary to learn the meaning of the term **provisional diagnosis.** Write your notes here.

_____

_____

_____

V. Precision in Documentation: Get the stone in the right place: **cholelithiasis** or **choledocholithiasis?** Make the correct choice of medical terminology. Fill in the blanks.

1. Patient's films revealed a stone in the common bile duct.

   Diagnosis: _____

2. The presence of a stone in the patient's gallbladder was confirmed by the radiologist.

   Diagnosis: _____

W. **Build your knowledge of the digestive system by correctly answering the following questions.** Circle the best choice.

1. What lines the wall of the abdominal cavity?

    a. omentum

    b. periosteum

    c. viscera

    d. parietal peritoneum

    e. serosa

2. Medical term for the act of swallowing:

    a. micturition

    b. digestion

    c. mastication

    d. deglutition

    e. absorption

3. **Peristalsis** means:

    a. waves of contractions

    b. segment of the intestine

    c. an enzyme

    d. chewing food

    e. ingestion

4. Which of the following is *not* a component of the digestive system?

    a. alimentary canal

    b. digestive tract

    c. salivary glands

    d. pancreas

    e. trachea

5. Mechanical movement of food from the mouth to the anus:

    a. digestion

    b. elimination

    c. propulsion

    d. mastication

    e. ingestion

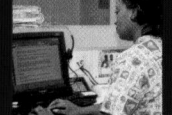

DIGESTIVE SYSTEM

X. **Prefixes make the difference in precision.** Analyze the two pairs of medical terms. Write a brief description of how they differ, based on their prefixes.

1. *emesis* and *hematemesis*

_____

_____

2. *symptomatic* and *asymptomatic*

_____

_____

Y. **Precision in Documentation:** You may someday find yourself doing medical transcription in a hospital or physician's office. Proofread the letter Dr. Walsh has sent to the patient's insurance company, asking for preauthorization for her surgery. Underline or highlight all the errors; then rewrite the correct terms on the lines below the dictation. Then add a brief definition of each term.

> Request for Authorization of Surgery
> Re: Mrs. Martha Jones
> Subscriber ID # 056437
>
> Dear Doctor Leavenworth,
>
> Mrs. Jones is a 52-year-old former waitress, recently divorced. She is 5 feet 4 inches tall and weighs 275 pounds. She has type 2 diabeetes with frequent episodes of hyperglycemia and also ketoacidoses, requiring three different hospitalizations. She now has diabetick retinnopathy and peripheral vascullitis. Complicating this is hypertension (185/110), coronery artery disease, and pulmonary edema. Exercise is out of the question because she has marked osteoarrthritis of her knees and hips. Mrs. Jones is now housebound, dependent on her daughter for transportation to our medical center. In spite of monthly meetings with our nutritionist, she has gained 25 pounds in the past 6 months.

Write the correct form of the misspelled words with a brief definition for each term here.

Corrections	Definitions
_____	_____
_____	_____
_____	_____
_____	_____
_____	_____
_____	_____
_____	_____
_____	_____

Z. Your knowledge of medical terminology will increase if you focus on similarities and differences in medical terms. Fill in the blanks.

  1. One word element makes lactose different from lactase.

     The word element is a _____ .

     Lactose means _____ .

     Lactase means _____ .

  2. One word element makes an enteroscope different from an endoscope.

     The word element is a _____ .

     An enteroscope is _____ .

     An endoscope is _____ .

AA. Check the accuracy of your chart documentation. The following patients have presented to the gastroenterology clinic today. Can you correctly complete their documentation?

  1. Caroline Mason presents today with severe _____ (vomiting of blood), which has been getting

     progressively worse. _____ (looking within by a scope) reveals _____-atous

     (swollen) _____ (pertaining to the esophagus) _____ (dilated veins).

  2. Andrew Baker reported to the Fulwood Emergency Room yesterday with symptoms of _____

     (following a meal) burning chest pain and _____ (vomiting of blood). Dr. Lee admitted him

     to the GI service for further diagnostic tests and possible surgery.

BB. Many medical terms that are nouns also have an adjectival form. Correctly apply these six medical terms to the following sentences. Fill in the blanks.

mucous   **mucin**   **mucus**   **mucosal**   **mucosa**   **submucosa**

  1. The lining of a tubular structure is referred to as the _____.

  2. A sticky film containing mucin is _____.

  3. The term for *pertaining to* the mucosa is _____.

  4. The tissue layer beneath the mucosa is the _____.

  5. _____ is a secretion from the mucosal glands.

  6. _____ means *relating to mucus or the mucosa*.

  7. Which two terms have similar meanings? _____ and _____

  8. Which two terms are pronounced the same but spelled differently? _____

     and _____

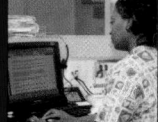
DIGESTIVE SYSTEM

CHAPTER SUMMARY EXERCISE

1. *Listen to the pronunciation of the medical terms as given by your instructor or at McGraw-Hill CONNECT.*
2. *Circle the correct spelling of the medical term.*
3. *Match the correctly spelled terms to the brief descriptions below.*
4. *Write a sentence for each of the 10 terms that appear in this exercise.*

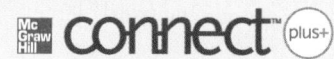

A. SPELLING COMPREHENSION: CIRCLE THE CORRECT SPELLING OF THE TERM.

1. laperoscopie	laparoscopy	leperoscopie	leporoscopy	laporoscopie
2. hematemesis	hemmatemisis	hematimisis	hematemis	hematimisus
3. parrotid	paratid	poratid	parotid	parritid
4. jegjunum	jejuunum	jedgejunum	jeghjunem	jejunum
5. mesentery	mesantery	mesenterie	mesanterie	messantery
6. hematochezia	hemetocizia	hemmatocizia	hemocizia	hematocizia
7. leukoplakkia	leukopakia	leukopiccia	leukoplakia	leukkophakia
8. degluetition	deglutition	deeglutition	degglutation	deglutation
9. varices	varixes	verixces	vericces	varicces
10. aphous	aphtous	appthous	aphthous	affthous

B. MATCH THE NUMBER OF THE CORRECT TERM IN PART A WITH THE BRIEF DESCRIPTION OF THE TERM BELOW.

a. Act of swallowing _____

b. Double layer of peritoneum enclosing viscera _____

c. Small ulcer in the mouth _____

d. Vomiting of blood _____

e. Examining abdomen with an endoscope _____

f. Dilated, tortuous veins _____

g. Most nutrients absorbed here _____

h. White plaque in the mouth _____

i. Red, bloody stools _____

j. Salivary gland beside the ear _____

C. USING YOUR KNOWLEDGE OF TERMS 1–10 IN PART A AND THEIR CORRECT SPELLING, WRITE A BRIEF SENTENCE FOR EACH OF THE TERMS AS IT MIGHT APPEAR IN PATIENT DOCUMENTATION.

1. _____

2. _____

3. _____

4. _____

5. _____

6. _____

7. _____

8. _____

9. _____

10. _____

D. **YOUR INSTRUCTOR WILL DIRECT YOU TO MCGRAW-HILL CONNECT. OPEN THE AUDIO GLOSSARY AND PRACTICE YOUR PRONUNCIATION OF THE TERMS IN PART A OF THIS EXERCISE.**

E. **AFTER READING CASE REPORT 6.4, ANSWER THE FOLLOWING QUESTIONS.** *BE PREPARED TO DISCUSS YOUR ANSWERS IN CLASS.*

CASE REPORT 6.4

You are

. . . a Certified Medical Assistant working with Susan Lee, MD, a primary care physician at Fulwood Medical Center.

Your patient is

. . . Mrs. Sandra Jacobs, a 46-year-old mother of four. Your task is to document her care.

Mrs. Sandra Jacobs, a 46-year-old mother of four, presents in Dr. Susan Lee's primary care clinic with episodes of crampy pain in her right upper quadrant associated with nausea and vomiting. The pain often occurs after eating fast food. She has not noticed fever or jaundice. Physical examination reveals an obese white woman with a positive **Murphy sign.** Her BP (blood pressure) is 170/90, and she has slight pedal edema. A provisional diagnosis of **gallstones** has been made. She has been referred for an ultrasound examination, and an appointment has been made to see Dr. Stewart Walsh in the Surgery Department.

I explained to her the etiology of her gallstones and the need for surgical removal of the stones, and I discussed with her a low-fat, 1500-calorie diet sheet.

Luis Guitterez, CMA. 06/12/09, 1430 hrs.

1. Demonstrate to the class the location of your *right upper quadrant*. _____

2. Define *jaundice*. _____
_____

3. What is a *positive Murphy's sign?* _____
_____

4. What makes a diagnosis *provisional?* _____
_____

5. What are the patient's presenting symptoms? _____
_____

6. What additional diagnostic test is Mrs. Jacobs scheduled for? _____
_____

7. In a dictionary, look up the meaning of the word *etiology*. _____
_____

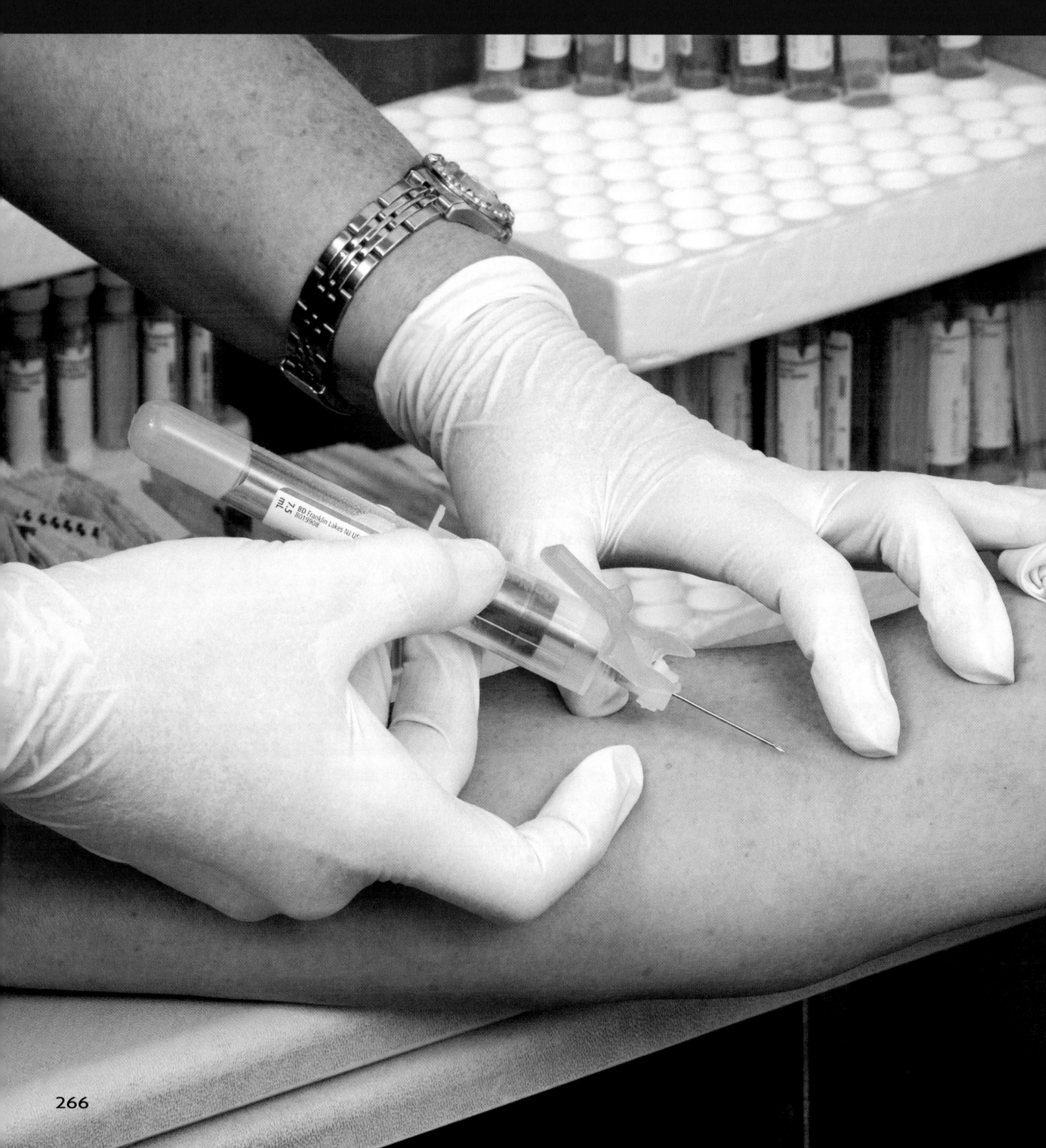

Blood
The Language of Hematology

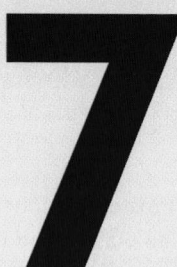
CASE REPORT 7.1

You are

... a medical assistant working with Susan Lee, MD, a primary care physician at Fulwood Medical Center

Your patient is

... Mrs. Luisa Sosin, a 47-year-old woman who presented a week ago with fatigue, lethargy, and muscle weakness. Physical examination revealed **pallor** of her skin, a pulse rate of 90, and a respiratory rate of 20. Dr. Lee referred her for extensive blood work. Dr. Lee also determined that the patient had been taking aspirin and **NSAIDs (nonsteroidal anti-inflammatory drugs)** for the past 6 months for low-back pain.

You are responsible for documenting her investigation and care. She is your next patient, and you are reviewing this laboratory report:

Learning Outcomes

To understand this report, to be able to communicate intelligently with Dr. Lee about the patient, and to document Mrs. Sosin's medical care, you need to have knowledge of the anatomy, physiology, and medical terminology of **hematology.**

This chapter will provide you with information that enables you to:

7.1 Apply the language of hematology to the anatomy and physiology of the blood.

7.2 Comprehend, analyze, spell, and write the medical terms of hematology so that you can communicate and document accurately and precisely in any health care setting.

7.3 Recognize and pronounce the medical terms of hematology so that you can communicate verbally with accuracy and precision in any health care setting.

7.4 Explain the effects of common disorders of the blood on health.

Laboratory Report

Luisa Sosin, ID # 7248412
Blood smear: Red blood cells are **microcytic, hypochromic,** and **poikilocytic.**

Red Blood Cell **Index**	Patient's Result	Reference Range
Hemoglobin Concentration	10.4g/dL	12–16 g/**dL** (grams per deciliter)
Mean **Corpuscular** Volume (**MCV**)	71 fL	86–98 **fL** (femtoliters)
Mean **Corpuscular** Hemoglobin (**MCH**)	21.5 **pg**/cell (picograms per cell)	26–32 g/dL
Mean Corpuscular Hemoglobin Concentration (**MCHC**)	27.5%	32%–36%
Serum Iron	35 μg/100 mL	50–150 μg/100 mL (micrograms per 100 milliliters)
Serum Ferritin	20 μg/100 mL	5–280 μg/100 mL
Total Iron-Binding Capacity (**TIBC**)	500 μg/100 mL	250–410 μg/100 mL

The reference range is the usual range of test values for a healthy population.

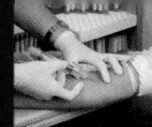

LESSON 7.1 Components of Blood

OBJECTIVES

The information in this lesson relates to the composition, functions, and uses of blood and will enable you to use correct medical terminology to:

7.1.1 **Identify the components of blood.**

7.1.2 **Describe plasma and its functions.**

7.1.3 **Explain the functions of blood.**

Abbreviations

dL   deciliter; one-tenth of a liter

fL   femtoliter; one-quadrillionth of a liter

L   liter

Hct   hematocrit

MCH   mean corpuscular hemoglobin; the average amount of hemoglobin in the average red blood cell

MCHC mean corpuscular hemoglobin concentration; the average concentration of hemoglobin in a given volume of red blood cells

MCV   mean corpuscular volume, the average volume of a red blood cell

μg   microgram; one-millionth of a gram; sometimes written as mcg

NSAID nonsteroidal anti-inflammatory drug

pg   picogram; one-trillionth of a gram

RBC   red blood cell

TIBC   total iron-binding capacity; the amount of iron needed to saturate transferrin, the protein that transports iron in the blood

WBC   white blood cell

COMPONENTS OF BLOOD

Blood is a type of connective tissue and consists of cells contained in a liquid matrix.

Blood volume varies with body size and the amount of adipose tissue. An average-size adult has about 5 L (10 pints) of blood that represents some 8% of body weight.

If a specimen of blood is collected in a tube and centrifuged, the cells of the blood are packed into the bottom of the tube *(Figure 7.1)*. These cells are called the formed elements of blood and consist of 99% red blood cells (**RBCs**), together with white blood cells (**WBCs**) and platelets. The blood sample is normally about 45% formed elements.

The **hematocrit (Hct)** is the percentage of total blood volume composed of red blood cells. The red blood cells can account for 40% to 54% of the total blood volume in normal males and 38% to 47% in females.

Plasma is the remaining 55% of the blood sample. It is a clear, yellowish liquid that is 91% water. Plasma is the fluid noncellular part of blood. Plasma is a **colloid,** a liquid that contains suspended particles, most of which are plasma proteins:

- **Albumin**—makes up 58% of the proteins.
- **Globulin**—makes up 38% of the plasma proteins. Antibodies are globulins *(see Chapter 15).*
- **Fibrinogen**—makes up 4% of the plasma proteins and is part of the mechanism for blood clotting *(see Lesson 7.4).*

Nutrients, waste products, hormones, and **enzymes** are dissolved in plasma for transportation.

When blood is allowed to clot and the solid clot is removed, **serum** is left. Serum is identical to plasma except for the absence of clotting proteins.

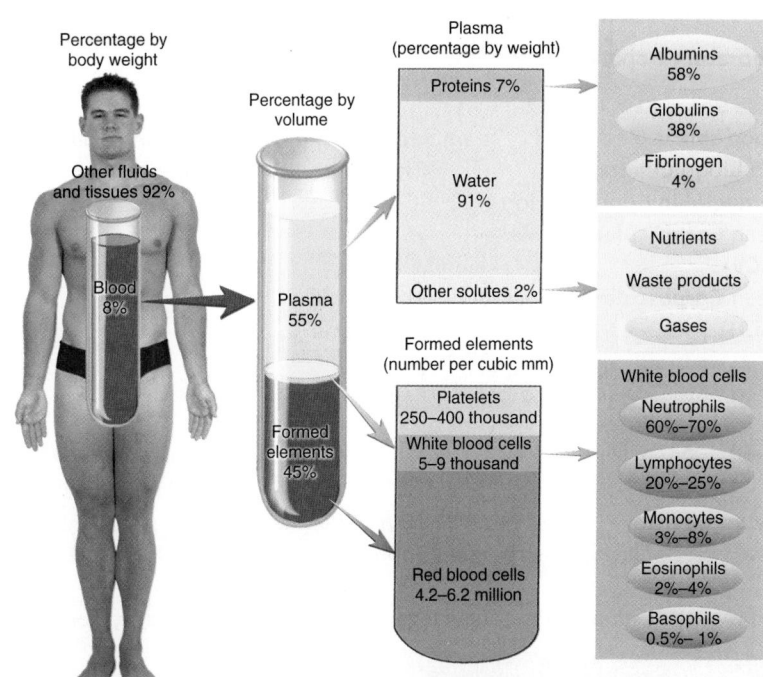

FIGURE 7.1   Components of Blood.

WORD ANALYSIS AND DEFINITION

S = Suffix   P = Prefix   R = Root   R/CF = Combining Form

WORD	PRONUNCIATION		ELEMENTS	DEFINITION
albumin	al-**BYU**-min		Latin *white of an egg*	Simple, soluble protein
colloid	**COLL**-oyd	S/ R/	-oid *appearance of* coll- *glue*	Liquid containing suspended particles
corpuscle corpuscular (adj)	**KOR**-pus-ul kor-**PUS**-kyu-lar	S/ R/	-cle *small* corpus- *body*	A blood cell
ferritin	**FER**-ih-tin	S/ R/	-in *chemical* ferrit- *iron*	Iron-protein complex that regulates iron storage and transport
fibrin	**FIE**-brin		Latin *fiber*	Stringy protein fiber that is a component of a blood clot
fibrinogen	fie-**BRIN**-oh-jen	S/ R/CF	-gen *create, produce* fibrin/o- *fibrin*	Precursor of fibrin in blood-clotting process
globulin	**GLOB**-you-lin		Latin *globule*	Family of blood proteins
hematocrit (Hct)	**HE**-mat-oh-krit	S/ R/CF	-crit *to separate* hemat/o- *blood*	Percentage of red blood cells in the blood
hematology hematologist	he-mah-**TOL**-oh-jee he-mah-**TOL**-oh-jist	S/ S/	-logy *study of* -logist *specialist*	Medical specialty of disorders of the blood Specialist in hematology
hemoglobin	**HE**-moh-**GLOW**-bin	R/ R/CF	-globin *protein* hem/o- *blood*	Red-pigmented protein that is the main component of red blood cells
hypochromic	high-poh-**CROW**-mik	S/ P/ R/	-ic *pertaining to* hypo- *deficient, below* -chrom- *color*	Pale in color, as in RBCs when hemoglobin is deficient
index indices (pl)	**IN**-deks **IN**-dih-seez		Latin *one that points out*	A standard indicator of measurement
microcytic	my-kroh-**SIT**-ik	S/ P/ R/	-ic *pertaining to* micro- *small* -cyt- *cell*	Pertaining to a small cell
pallor	**PAL**-or		Latin *paleness*	Paleness of the skin
plasma	**PLAZ**-mah		Greek *something formed*	Fluid, noncellular component of blood
poikilocytic	**POY**-key-low-**SIT**-ik	S/ P/ R/	-ic *pertaining to* poikilo- *irregular* -cyt- *cell*	Pertaining to an irregular-shaped RBC
serum	**SEER**-um		Latin *whey*	Fluid remaining after removal of cells and fibrin clot

EXERCISES

Know your elements—they will increase your medical vocabulary! This exercise consists of elements taken from this Word Analysis and Definition (WAD) box. Match the element to its correct meaning.

_____ 1. oid   A. small

_____ 2. micro   B. color

_____ 3. cyt   C. deficient, below

_____ 4. crit   D. iron

_____ 5. chrom   E. create, produce

_____ 6. hypo   F. appearance of

_____ 7. gen   G. to separate

_____ 8. ferrit   H. cell

FUNCTIONS OF BLOOD

The functions of the blood are to:

1. **Maintain the body's homeostasis** (*see Chapter 2*).

2. **Maintain body temperature.** Warm blood is transported from the interior of the body to its surface, where heat is released from the blood.

3. **Transport nutrients, vitamins, and minerals** from digestive system and storage areas to organs and cells where they are needed. Examples of nutrients are glucose and amino acids (*see Chapter 6*).

4. **Transport waste products** from cells and organs to the liver and kidneys for detoxification and excretion. Examples are **creatinine, urea,** bilirubin, and lactic acid (*see Chapter 11*).

5. **Transport hormones** from endocrine glands to the target cells. Examples are insulin and thyroxin (*see Chapter 14*).

6. **Transport gases** to and from the lungs and cells. Examples are oxygen and carbon dioxide (*see Chapter 9*).

7. **Protect against foreign substances.** Cells and chemicals in the blood are an important part of the immune system for dealing with microorganisms and toxins (*see Chapter 15*).

8. **Form clots.** This provides protection against blood loss and is the first step in tissue repair and restoration of normal function.

9. **Regulate pH and osmosis.**

Hydrogen ion concentration is measured using a **pH** scale to show the balance between **acid** and **alkaline** in any solution. Pure water is the neutral solution and has a pH of 7.0. Solutions with a pH less than 7.0 are acidic. Solutions with a pH greater than 7.0 are alkaline (or basic). Blood has a pH between 7.35 and 7.45 and must be maintained within that range for life to continue. **Buffer** systems in the blood are used to maintain the correct pH range. Examples of buffer systems are bicarbonate and phosphate.

Osmosis is the passage of water through a selectively permeable membrane, such as a cell membrane, from the "more watery" side to the "less watery" side. All cells exchange water by osmosis, and red blood cells exchange 100 times their own volume across the cell membrane every second.

Viscosity, the resistance of a fluid to flow, is an important element that affects the blood's ability to flow through blood vessels. Whole blood is five times as viscous as water. If the viscosity decreases because red blood cells are deficient (as in **anemia**), this enables blood to flow more easily and puts a strain on the heart because of the increased amount of blood being returned to it in a unit of time.

Keynote

Failure to maintain the normal pH range of the blood between 7.35 and 7.45 can cause paralysis and death.

Abbreviations

CBC   complete blood count
ESR   erythrocyte sedimentation rate
pH   hydrogen ion concentration
RBC   red blood cell count
WBC   white blood cell count

Laboratory Studies for Blood

- **A complete blood count (CBC)** is a combination of:

  1. Red blood cell **(RBC)** count and indices.

  2. White blood cell **(WBC)** count and differential WBC count.

  3. Platelet count.
  In some laboratories a CBC does not include the differential white blood cell count. This may need to be requested separately. White blood cells are addressed in *Lesson 7.3.*

- **Erythrocyte sedimentation rate (ESR)** is a nonspecific measure of inflammation. This test is falling out of use as other more specific tests are developed.

WORD	PRONUNCIATION		ELEMENTS	DEFINITION
acid	**ASS**-id		Latin *sour*	Substance with a pH below 7.0
alkaline (also called basic)	**AL**-kah-line	S/ R/	**-ine** *pertaining to, substance* **alkal-** *base*	Substance with a pH above 7.0
anemia	ah-**NEE**-me-ah	P/ R/	**an-** *without, lacking* **-emia** *blood*	Decreased number of red blood cells
anemic (adj)	ah-**NEE**-mik	S/	**-ic** *pertaining to*	Pertaining to or suffering from anemia
buffer	**BUFF**-er		Latin *cushion*	Substance that resists a change in pH
creatinine	kree-**AT**-ih-neen	S/ R/	**-ine** *pertaining to, substance* **creatin-** *creatine*	Breakdown product of the skeletal muscle protein creatine
erythrocyte	eh-**RITH**-roh-site	S/ R/CF	**-cyte** *cell* **erythr/o-** *red*	Another name for a red blood cell
homeostasis	ho-mee-oh-**STAY**-sis	R/ R/CF	**-stasis** *stay in one place* **home/o-** *the same*	Stability or equilibrium of a system or the body's internal environment
osmosis	oz-**MO**-sis	S/ R/	**-sis** *process* **osmo-** *push*	The passage of water across a cell membrane
sediment	**SED**-ih-ment	S/ R/	Latin *to settle* **-ation** *process* **sediment-** *a settling*	Insoluble material that settles to the bottom of a liquid
sedimentation	**SED**-ih-men-**TAY**-shun			Formation of a sediment
urea	you-**REE**-ah		Greek *urine*	End product of nitrogen metabolism
viscous viscosity	**VISS**-kus vis-**KOS**-ih-tee		Latin *sticky*	Sticky; resistant to flowing The resistance of a fluid to flow

EXERCISES

You will help yourself in this exercise if you first slash (/) the bold medical terms into their elements. Review the WAD before you start to fill in the blanks.

1. In the term **sedimentation,** the suffix means _____.

2. If something is a buffer, it acts as a _____.

3. **Viscous** is a term meaning _____.

4. In the term **erythrocyte,** the suffix means _____.

5. *A state of equilibrium* means something remains _____.

6. The suffix in **homeostasis** means _____.

7. Urea comes from the Greek meaning _____.

8. The opposite of acid is _____.

9. The prefix in **anemia** means _____.

10. In the term **osmosis,** the root means _____.

11. _____ and _____ are two terms in the WAD that relate to blood.

12. _____ settles to the bottom of a liquid.

LESSON 7.2 Red Blood Cells (Erythrocytes)

OBJECTIVES

In your bloodstream at this moment are approximately 25 trillion red blood cells (RBCs). Approximately 2.5 million of them are being destroyed every second. This means that 1% of your red blood cells are destroyed and replaced every day of your life.

It is crucial to understand the reasons for this dynamic process and to be familiar with the critical role that the red blood cells play in maintaining life. This lesson will provide you with the information to use correct medical terminology to:

7.2.1 Link the structure of red blood cells to their functions.

7.2.2 Identify the roles of hemoglobin in maintaining homeostasis.

7.2.3 Describe the life history of red blood cells.

7.2.4 Recognize some common disorders of red blood cells.

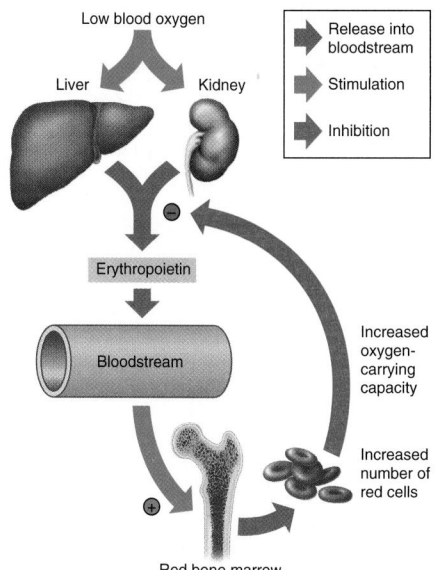

▲ **FIGURE 7.3   Control of RBC Production.**

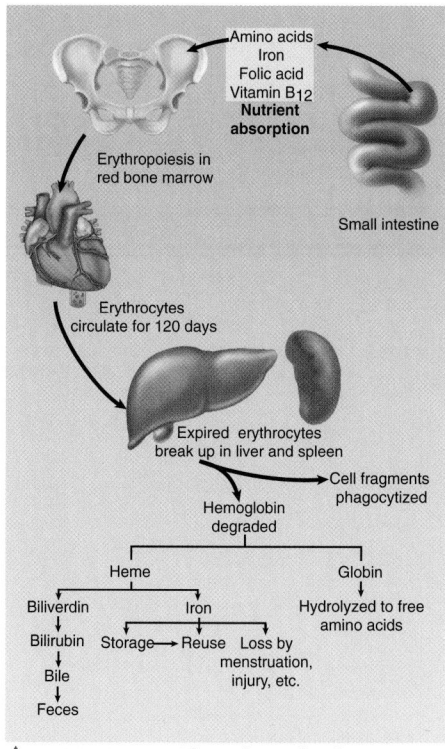

▲ **FIGURE 7.4   Life and Death of RBCs.**

FIGURE 7.2   Red Blood Cells. ▶

Top view
(a)   (b)

STRUCTURE AND FUNCTION OF RED BLOOD CELLS

Structure of Red Blood Cells

The main component of RBCs is **hemoglobin (Hb)**, which gives the cell its red color. Hemoglobin occupies about one-third of the total cell volume and is composed of the iron-containing pigment **heme** bound to a protein called **globin**. The rest of the red blood cell consists of the cell membrane, water, electrolytes, and enzymes. Mature RBCs do not have a nucleus.

Each RBC is a **biconcave** disc with edges that are thicker than the center (*Figure 7.2*). This biconcave shape gives the disc a larger surface area than if it were a sphere. The biconcave surface area enables a more rapid flow of gases into and out of the RBC.

Red blood cells are unable to move themselves and are dependent on the heart and blood vessels to move them around the body.

Function of Red Blood Cells

The functions of the RBCs are to:

1. **Transport oxygen (O_2)** from the lungs to cells all over the body. Oxygen is transported in combination with hemoglobin (**oxyhemoglobin**).
2. **Transport carbon dioxide (CO_2)** from the tissue cells to the lungs for excretion.
3. **Transport nitric oxide (NO)**, a gas produced by cells lining the blood vessels that signals smooth muscle to relax and is also a transmitter of signals between nerve cells.

Life History of Red Blood Cells

Red blood cell formation (**erythropoiesis**) occurs in the spaces in bones filled with red bone marrow. **Hematopoietic stem cells** become nucleated **erythroblasts** and then nonnucleated erythrocytes, which are released into the bloodstream.

A hormone, **erythropoietin**, produced by the kidneys and liver, controls the rate of RBC production (*Figure 7.3*). A lack of oxygen in the body's tissues triggers the release of erythropoietin, which travels in the blood to the red bone marrow to stimulate RBC production.

Red blood cell production is also influenced by the availability of iron, the B vitamins B_{12} and folic acid, and amino acids through absorption from the digestive tract (*Figure 7.4*).

WORD	PRONUNCATION		ELEMENTS	DEFINITION
biconcave	bi-**KON**-cave	P/ R/	bi- *two, double* -concave *arched, hollow*	Having a hollowed surface on both sides of a structure
erythroblast	eh-**RITH**-ro-blast	S/ R/CF	-blast *germ cell* erythr/o- *red*	Precursor to a red blood cell
erythropoiesis	eh-**RITH**-ro-poy-**EE**-sis	S/ R/CF	-poiesis *to make* erythr/o- *red*	The formation of red blood cells
erythropoietin	eh-**RITH**-ro-**POY**-ee-tin	S/ R/CF	-poietin *the maker* erythr/o- *red*	Protein secreted by the kidney that stimulates red blood cell production
hematopoietic	**HE**-mah-toh-poy-**ET**-ick	S/ S/ R/CF	-ic *pertaining to* -poiet- *the making* hemat/o- *blood*	Pertaining to the making of red blood cells
heme	HEEM		Greek *blood*	The iron-based component of hemoglobin that carries oxygen
macrophage	**MAK**-roh-fayj	P/ R/CF	macro- *large* -phag/e *to eat*	Large white blood cell that removes bacteria, foreign particles, and dead cells
oxyhemoglobin	**OCK**-see-he-moh-**GLOW**-bin	R/CF R/CF R/	ox/y- *oxygen* hem/o- *blood* -globin *protein*	Hemoglobin in combination with oxygen

The average life span of an RBC is 120 days, during which time the cell has circulated through the body about 75,000 times. With age, the cells become more fragile, and squeezing through tiny capillaries ruptures them. **Macrophages** in the liver and spleen take up the hemoglobin that is released and break it down into its components heme and globin. The heme is broken down into iron and into a rust-colored pigment called bilirubin *(see Chapter 6.)*

Abbreviations

CO₂	carbon dioxide
Hb	hemoglobin; may also be written as Hgb
NO	nitric oxide
O₂	oxygen

EXERCISES

Some of the medical terms from this WAD are defined for you. One word in the definition is in bold; find the element in the term that has the same meaning. **The first one is done for you.** *Fill in the blanks.*

1. **macrophage:**   Element   _____*macro*_____   =   _____*large*_____

   Definition: **large** white blood cell that removes bacteria and dead cells

2. **erythroblast:**   Element   _____   =   _____

   Definition: **precursor** to red blood cell

3. **biconcave:**   Element   _____   =   _____

   Definition: having a hollowed surface on **both** sides of a structure

4. **erythropoiesis:**   Element   _____   =   _____

   Definition: the **formation** of red blood cells

5. **hemoglobin:**   Element   _____   =   _____

   Definition: red color and oxygen transporter of red **blood** cells

6. **erythropoietin**   Element   _____   =   _____

   Definition: protein that is secreted by kidney and stimulates **red blood cell** production

7. **hematopoietic:**   Element   _____   =   _____

   Definition: **pertaining to** the making of red blood cells

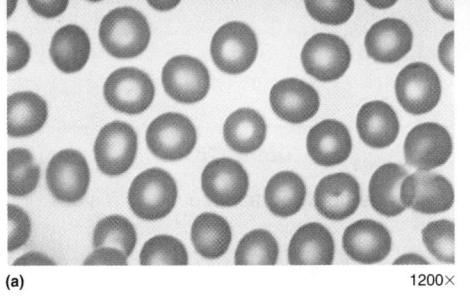

(a)   1200×

▲ **FIGURE 7.5   Red Blood Cells.**
(*a*) Normal RBCs. (*b*) Hypochromic RBCs.

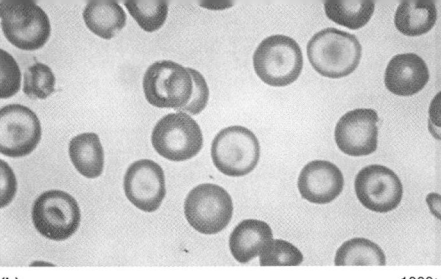

(b)   1000×

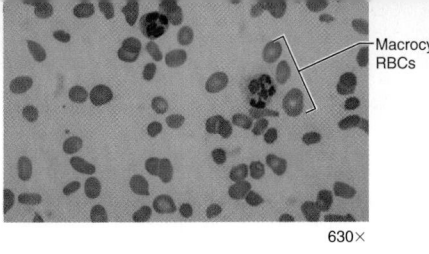

630×

▲ **FIGURE 7.6   Macrocytic Cells in Pernicious Anemia.**

Keynote

Anemia reduces the oxygen-carrying capacity of blood.

Hemolysis liberates hemoglobin from RBCs.

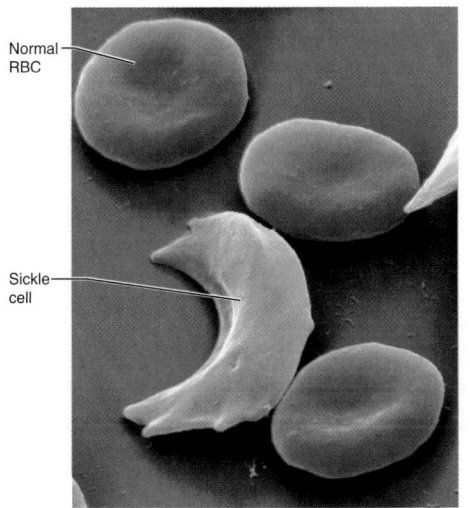

Normal
RBC

Sickle
cell

▲ **FIGURE 7.7   Sickle Cell Anemia.**

DISORDERS OF RED BLOOD CELLS

Anemia is a reduction in the number of RBCs or in the amount of hemoglobin each RBC contains (*Figure 7.5*). Both of these conditions reduce the oxygen-carrying capacity of the blood and produce the symptoms of shortness of breath (**SOB**) and fatigue. They also produce pallor because of the deficiency of the red-colored oxyhemoglobin, the combination of oxygen and hemoglobin.

There are several types of anemia:

- **Iron-deficiency anemia** is the diagnosis for Mrs. Luisa Sosin. In her case, the cause was chronic bleeding from her gastrointestinal tract due to the aspirin and other painkillers she was taking. Her stools were positive for occult blood. Other causes can be heavy menstrual bleeding or a diet deficient in iron.

- **Pernicious anemia (PA)** is due to vitamin B$_{12}$ deficiency. This is caused by a shortage of *intrinsic factor* (*see Chapter 6*), which is normally secreted by cells in the lining of the stomach and binds with vitamin B$_{12}$; this complex is absorbed into the bloodstream. Without vitamin B$_{12}$, hemoglobin cannot be formed. The RBCs decrease in number and in hemoglobin concentration and increase in size (**macrocytic,** *Figure 7.6*).

- **Sickle cell anemia** (also called sickle cell disease) is a genetic disorder found most commonly in African Americans, Africans, and some Mediterranean populations. It results from the production of an abnormal hemoglobin that causes the RBCs to form a rigid sickle cell shape (*Figure 7.7*). The abnormal cells are sticky, clump together (**agglutinate**), and block small capillaries. This causes intense pain in the **hypoxic** tissues (a sickle cell crisis) and can cause stroke and kidney and heart failure.

  There is a minor form of the disease, sickle cell trait, in which symptoms rarely occur and do not progress to the full-blown disease.

- **Hemolytic anemia** is due to excessive destruction of normal and abnormal RBCs. **Hemolysis** can be caused by such toxic substances as snake and spider venoms, mushroom toxins, and drug reactions. Trauma to RBCs by hemodialysis or heart-lung machines can produce a hemolytic anemia.

- **Aplastic anemia** is a condition in which the bone marrow is unable to produce sufficient new cells of all types—red cells, white cells, and platelets. It can be associated with exposure to radiation, benzene, and certain drugs.

- **Hemoglobinopathies,** such as sickle cell disease and **thalassemia,** with their inherited abnormal hemoglobins, also cause hemolysis.

  Hemolysis can also occur through **incompatible** blood transfusions or maternal-fetal incompatibilities (*see Lesson 7.5*). Jaundice is a complication.

- **Polycythemia vera** is an overproduction of RBCs and WBCs due to an unknown cause.

Case Report 7.1 (continued)

Because Mrs. Luisa Sosin was deficient in iron and hemoglobin, her RBCs were small (microcytic) and lacked the red color of oxyhemoglobin (hypochromic; *Figure 7.5*), and some were irregular-shaped (poikilocytic) rather than the normal, round shape. The volume of each cell, mean corpuscular volume (MCV), and the amount of hemoglobin in each cell, mean corpuscular hemoglobin (MCH), were decreased. The amount of iron in her blood (serum iron) and the amount of ferritin in her serum were decreased. Her total iron-binding capacity was raised because the shortage of iron resulted in an increased availability of the protein to which iron is bound in the bloodstream.

WORD	PRONUNCIATION	ELEMENTS		DEFINITION
agglutinate	ah-**GLUE**-tin-ate	S/ P/ R/	-ate *composed of, pertaining to* ag- *to* -glutin- *stick together, glue*	Stick together to form clumps
aplastic anemia	a-**PLAS**-tik ah-**NEE**-me-ah	S/ P/ R/	-tic *pertaining to* a- *without* -plas- *formation*	Condition in which the bone marrow is unable to produce sufficient red cells, white cells, and platelets
hemoglobinopathy	**HE**-mo-**GLOW**-bih-**NOP**-ah-thee	S/ R/CF R/CF	-pathy *disease* hem/o- *blood* -globin/o- *protein*	Disease caused by the presence of an abnormal hemoglobin in the red blood cells
hemolysis hemolytic (adj)	he-**MOL**-ih-sis he-moh-**LIT**-ik	S/ R/CF S/ R/	-lysis *destruction* hem/o- *blood* -ic *pertaining to* -lyt- *destroy*	Destruction of red blood cells so that hemoglobin is liberated Pertaining to the process of destruction of red blood cells
hypoxia hypoxic (**Note:** The surplus "o" is not used.)	high-**POCK**-see-ah high-**POCK**-sik	S/ S/ P/ R/	-ia *condition* -ic *pertaining to* hypo- *deficient* -ox- *oxygen*	Decrease below normal levels of oxygen in tissues, gases, or blood Deficient in oxygen
incompatible	in-kom-**PAT**-ih-bul	S/ P/ R/	-ible *can do* in- *not* -compat- *tolerate*	Substances that interfere with each other physiologically
macrocyte macrocytic (adj)	**MAK**-roh-site mak-roh-**SIT**-ik	P/ R/CF S/	macro- *large* -cyt/e *cell* -ic *pertaining to*	Large red blood cell Pertaining to macrocytes
pernicious anemia (PA)	per-**NISH**-us ah-**NEE**-me-ah	 P/ R/	pernicious Latin *destructive* an- *without, lack of* -emia *blood*	Chronic anemia due to lack of vitamin B$_{12}$
polycythemia vera	**POL**-ee-sigh-**THEE**-me-ah **VEH**-rah	P/ R/ R/	poly- *many, much* -cyth- *cell* -emia *blood* vera Latin *truth*	Chronic disease with bone marrow hyperplasia and increase in number of RBCs and in blood volume
thalassemia	thal-ah-**SEE**-me-ah	S/ R/	-emia *blood condition* thalass- *sea*	Group of inherited blood disorders that produce a hemolytic anemia

EXERCISES

After reading Case Report 7.1 on the opposite page, answer the following questions. Be prepared to discuss your answers in class.

1. If a term means *deficient in*, what element would it start with? (Be specific.) _____

2. What is the opposite of *microcytic?* _____

3. The condition in which the bone marrow is unable to produce sufficient red cells, white cells, and platelets is _____ .

4. *Hypochromic* means _____ .

5. Why is oxyhemoglobin a red color? (*Hint:* Study the elements.)

_____

6. Mrs. Sosin's RBCs showed a decrease in _____ and _____ .

7. _____ and _____ were raised in Mrs. Sosin's blood, and that resulted in _____

_____ .

LESSON 7.3 White Blood Cells (Leukocytes)

OBJECTIVES

The information in this lesson will enable you to use correct medical terminology to:

7.3.1 **Distinguish the different types of white blood cells.**
7.3.2 **Explain the functions of the different types of white blood cells.**
7.3.3 **Describe white blood cell counts and differential white blood cell counts.**
7.3.4 **Describe the effect of common disorders of white blood cells on health.**

You are

. . . a laboratory technician reviewing a peripheral blood smear.

Your patient is

. . . Mrs. Latisha Masters, a 27-year-old student.

CASE REPORT 7.2

Mrs. Masters presented with a 5-day history of fatigue, low-grade fever, and sore throat. Physical examination showed tonsillitis with bilateral, enlarged, tender cervical lymph nodes and an enlarged spleen.

The white blood cell (WBC) count you performed showed 9200 cells per cubic millimeter. The peripheral smear you are looking at is reported as showing the presence of atypical mononuclear cells with abundant cytoplasm.

TYPES OF WHITE BLOOD CELLS

Granulocytes

Keynote

Neutrophils, eosinophils, and basophils are granulocytes.

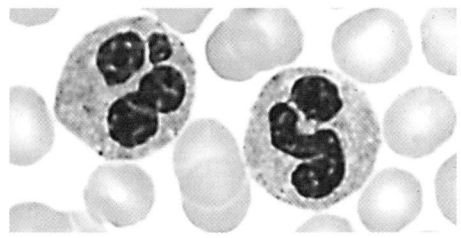

▲ **FIGURE 7.8 Neutrophils Are Granulocytes.**

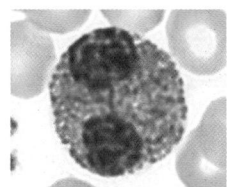

▲ **FIGURE 7.9 Eosinophils Are Granulocytes.**

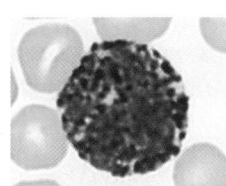

▲ **FIGURE 7.10 Basophils Are Granulocytes.**

FIGURE 7.11 Monocytes Are Agranulocytes. ►

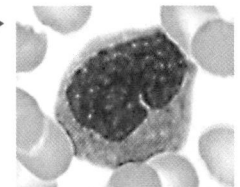

1. **Neutrophils** *(Figure 7.8)* are normally 50% to 70% of the total WBC count. They are also called **polymorphonuclear leukocytes (PMNLs).** These cells phagocytize bacteria, fungi, and some viruses and secrete a group of enzymes called lysozymes, which destroy some bacteria. In bacterial infections, the number and percentage of neutrophils increase dramatically. In **neutropenia,** the number of neutrophils is diminished below normal.

2. **Eosinophils** *(Figure 7.9)* are normally 2% to 4% of the total WBC count. They are mobile cells that leave the bloodstream to enter tissue undergoing an allergic response. In allergic reactions, the number and percentage of eosinophils increase.

3. **Basophils** *(Figure 7.10)* are normally less than 1% of the total WBC count. Basophils migrate to damaged tissues, where they release histamine (which increases blood flow) and **heparin** (which prevents blood clotting).

Because of their granular cytoplasm, the above three types of WBCs are called **granulocytes.** Their granules are the sites for production of enzymes and chemicals.

Agranulocytes

Because monocytes and lymphocytes have no granules in their cytoplasm, they are called **agranulocytes.**

4. **Monocytes** *(Figure 7.11)* are the largest blood cell and are normally 3% to 8% of the total WBC count. Monocytes leave the bloodstream and become macrophages that phagocytize bacteria, dead neutrophils, and dead cells in the tissues.

5. **Lymphocytes** *(Figure 7.12)* are normally 25% to 35% of the total WBC count. They are the smallest type of WBC. Lymphocytes are produced in red bone marrow and migrate through the bloodstream to lymphatic tissues—lymph nodes, tonsils, spleen, and thymus—where they proliferate.

WORD	PRONUNCIATION	ELEMENTS		DEFINITION
agranulocyte	a-**GRAN**-you-lo-site	P/ S/ R/CF	a- *without, not* -cyte *cell* -granul/o- *granule*	A white blood cell without any granules in its cytoplasm
antibody antibodies (pl)	**AN**-tih-body	P/ R/	anti- *against* body- *substance*	Protein produced in response to an antigen
basophil	**BAY**-so-fill	S/ R/CF	-phil *attraction* bas/o- *base*	A basophil's granules attract a basic blue stain in the laboratory
differential	dif-er-**EN**-shal	S/ R/	-ial *pertaining to* different- *not identical*	A differential white blood cell count lists percentages of the different leukocytes in a blood sample
eosinophil	ee-oh-**SIN**-oh-fill	S/ R/CF	-phil *attraction* eosin/o- *dawn*	An eosinophil's granules attract a rosy-red color on staining
granulocyte	**GRAN**-you-loh-site	R/CF R/CF	-cyt/e *cell* granul/o- *small grain*	A white blood cell that contains multiple small granules in its cytoplasm
heparin	**HEP**-ah-rin	S/ R/	-in *chemical* hepar- *liver*	An anticoagulant secreted particularly by liver cells
immunoglobulin	**IM**-you-noh-**GLOB**-you-lin	S/ R/CF R/	-in *chemical* immun/o- *immune response* -globul- *protein*	Specific protein evoked by an antigen. All antibodies are immunoglobulins
leukocyte (alternative spelling leucocyte)	**LOO**-koh-site	R/CF R/CF	-cyt/e *cell* leuk/o- *white*	Another term for a white blood cell
leukocytosis leukopenia	**LOO**-koh-sigh-**TOE**-sis loo-koh-**PEE**-nee-ah	S/ S/	-osis *condition* -penia *deficiency*	An excessive number of white blood cells A deficient number of white blood cells
lymphocyte	**LIM**-foh-site	R/CF R/CF	-cyt/e *cell* lymph/o- *lymph*	Small white blood cell with a large nucleus
monocyte	**MON**-oh-site	P/ R/CF	mono- *single* -cyt/e *cell*	Large white blood cell with a single nucleus
neutrophil neutropenia	**NEW**-troh-fill **NEW**-troh-**PEE**-nee-uh	S/ R/CF S/	-phil *attraction* neutr/o- *neutral* -penia *deficiency*	A neutrophil's granules take up purple stain equally whether the stain is acid or alkaline A deficiency of neutrophils
polymorphonuclear	**POL**-ee-more-foh-**NEW**-klee-ar	S/ P/ R/CF R/	-ar *pertaining to* poly- *many* morph/o- *shape* -nucle- *nucleus*	White blood cell with a multilobed nucleus

There are two main types of lymphocyte:

a. **B cells** that differentiate into plasma cells. These are stimulated by bacteria or toxins to produce **antibodies,** or **immunoglobulins (Igs).**

b. **T cells** that attach directly to foreign antigen bearing cells such as bacteria, which they kill with toxins they secrete.

In a laboratory report, a **differential white blood cell count (DIFF)** lists the percentages of the different leukocytes in a blood sample.

Abbreviations

DIFF	differential white blood cell count
Ig	immunoglobulin
PMNL	polymorphonuclear leukocyte

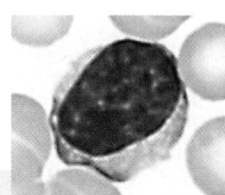

FIGURE 7.12 ▶
Lymphocytes are Agranulocytes.

EXERCISES

Pick the correct suffix to complete the medical term. One element will remain the same in each group of terms. Review the WAD before you start the exercise. Fill in the blanks.

-penia   -cyte   -cytosis

1. An excessive number of white blood cells is _____ .

2. Another term for a white blood cell is _____ .

3. A deficient number of white blood cells is _____ .

Case Report 7.2 (continued)

Latisha Masters' blood smear indicated a diagnosis of infectious **mononucleosis** caused by the **Epstein-Barr virus (EBV)**. This virus infects WBCs. A positive **heterophile reaction (Monospot test)** was present.

Infectious mononucleosis occurs in the 15- to 25-year-old population. Its cause, the Epstein-Barr virus (EBV), is a very common virus, a member of the herpes virus family *(see Chapter 20)*. The EBV is transmitted by exchange of saliva, as in kissing. In patients with symptoms compatible with infectious mononucleosis, a positive Monospot test is diagnostic.

Keynote

Leukocytosis is the presence of too many white blood cells.

Leukopenia is the presence of too few white blood cells.

Pancytopenia is the presence of too few RBCs, WBCs, and platelets.

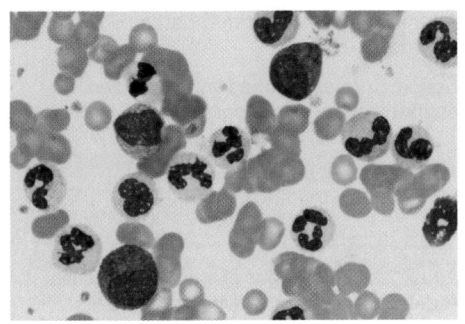

▲ **FIGURE 7.13   Myeloid Leukemia.**

Keynote

Acute lymphoblastic leukemia is the most common leukemia in children.

DISORDERS OF WHITE BLOOD CELLS

Normally a cubic millimeter (**mm³**) of blood contains 5000 to 10,000 white blood cells.

Leukocytosis is defined as a total WBC count exceeding 10,000/mm³. When the majority of the increased cells are neutrophils (polymorphonuclear leukocytes), an acute infection is usually present; for example, appendicitis or bacterial pneumonia.

Allergic reactions increase the number of eosinophils. Typhoid fever, malaria, and tuberculosis increase the number of monocytes. Whooping cough and infectious mononucleosis increase the number of lymphocytes.

Leukemia is cancer of the hematopoietic tissues and produces a high number of leukocytes and their **precursors** in the WBC count. As the **leukemic** cells proliferate, they take over the bone marrow and cause a deficiency of normal RBCs, WBCs, and **platelets**. This makes the patient anemic and vulnerable to infection and bleeding.

Myeloid leukemia is characterized by uncontrolled production of granulocytes and their precursors *(Figure 7.13)*. It can be in an acute or chronic form.

Lymphoid leukemia is characterized by uncontrolled production of lymphocytes. It can be in an acute or chronic form. **Acute lymphoblastic leukemia (ALL)** is the most common form of childhood cancer and is curable with modern treatments, such as chemotherapy and bone marrow and umbilical cord **stem cell** transplants.

Leukopenia results when the WBC count drops below 5000 cells/mm³ of blood. Leukopenia is seen in viral infections such as measles, mumps, chickenpox, poliomyelitis, and AIDS.

Pancytopenia occurs when the erythrocytes (RBCs), leukocytes (WBCs), and thrombocytes (**platelets**) in the circulating blood are all markedly reduced. This can occur with cancer chemotherapy.

Abbreviations

ALL	acute lymphoblastic leukemia
EBV	Epstein-Barr virus
HLA	human leukocyte antigen
mm³	cubic millimeter

Procedures

- **Bone marrow biopsy** or **aspiration** is often performed as part of the diagnostic work-up in patients with aplastic anemia, leukemias, lymphomas, and/or multiple myeloma. The specimen is usually taken from the posterior iliac crest of the pelvis *(see Chapter 5)*.

- **Bone marrow transplant** is the transfer of bone marrow from a healthy, compatible donor to a patient with aplastic anemia, leukemia, lymphoma, multiple myeloma, or other diseases. Compatibility requires having the same type of **human leukocyte antigen (HLA)** in a blood sample.

WORD	PRONUNCIATION	ELEMENTS		DEFINITION
aspiration	**AS**-pih-**RAY**-shun	S/ R/	-ion *process* **aspirat-** *to breathe*	Removal by suction of fluid or gas from a body cavity
heterophile (adj)	**HET**-er-oh-file	S/ R/CF	-phile *attraction* **heter/o-** *different*	Pertaining to antibodies present during a disease but not directed against the causative agent
leukemia leukemic (adj)	loo-**KEE**-mee-ah loo-**KEE**-mick	S/ R/	-emia *blood* **leuk-** *white*	Disease in which the blood is taken over by white blood cells and their precursors
lymphoid	**LIM**-foyd	S/ R/	-oid *resembling* **lymph-** *lymph*	Resembling lymphatic tissue
mononucleosis	**MON**-oh-nyu-klee-**OH**-sis	S/ P/ R/	-osis *condition* **mono-** *single* **-nucle-** *nucleus*	Presence of large numbers of mononuclear leukocytes
Monospot test	**MON**-oh-spot TEST		Trade name	Detects heterophile antibodies in infectious mononucleosis
myeloid	**MY**-eh-loyd	S/ R/	-oid *resembling* **myel-** *bone marrow*	Resembling cells derived from bone marrow
pancytopenia	**PAN**-site-oh-**PEE**-nee-ah	S/ P/ R/CF	-penia *deficiency* **pan-** *all* **-cyt/o-** *cell*	Deficiency of all types of blood cells
platelet (also called **thrombocyte**)	**PLAYT**-let	S/ R/	-let *small* **plate-** *flat*	Cell fragment involved in clotting process
precursor	pree-**KUR**-sir	P/ R/	**pre-** *before, in front of* -cursor *run*	Cell or substance formed earlier in the development of the cell or substance
stem cell	STEM SELL		**stem** Old English *stalk of a plant*	Undifferentiated cell found in a differentiated tissue that can divide to yield the specialized cells in that tissue

EXERCISES

*Test yourself on the **language of hematology** as it appears in the text and Case Report 7.2 on the opposite page.*

1. Use the glossary or an online medical dictionary to define *infectious*.

_____

2. Rewrite this sentence in your own words: "In patients with symptoms compatible with infectious mononucleosis, a positive Monospot test is diagnostic."

_____

_____

_____

3. "Infectious mononucleosis is caused by the EBV, and this infects WBCs." Explain this sentence to your patient in words she can understand.

_____

_____

_____

4. What is cancer of the hematopoietic tissues called? _____

5. What blood disease appears in viral infections such as measles, mumps, chickenpox, and AIDS? _____

6. "As the leukemic cells proliferate, they take over the bone marrow and cause <u>deficiency of normal RBCs, WBCs, and platelets</u>." What one medical word can be substituted for the underlined phrase and mean the same thing? _____

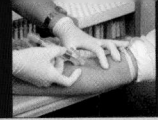

LESSON 7.4 Hemostasis

OBJECTIVES

When you are employed in any clinical area in health care—in an office, in a hospital, or out in the field—at many times in your career, you will be faced with a patient who is bleeding.

Before you can take blood for laboratory examination, you need to have an awareness of the medical terminology for possible diagnoses and the appropriate tests that will be performed. In this lesson, information will be available for you to use correct medical terminology to:

7.4.1 **Identify the functions of platelets.**

7.4.2 **Specify the body's mechanisms for controlling bleeding.**

7.4.3 **Describe the methods of producing blood clots.**

7.4.4 **Explain some disorders of blood clotting.**

You are

... an **emergency medical technician (EMT)** employed in the Fulwood Medical Center Emergency Department.

Your patient is

... Janis Tierney, a 17-year-old high school student.

CASE REPORT 7.3

Ms. Tierney presents with fainting at school. She is pale. Her pulse is 90. Blood pressure is 100/60. She tells you that she is having a menstrual period with excessive bleeding. Her physical examination is otherwise unremarkable. She has a history of easy bruising and recurrent nosebleeds and an episode of severe bleeding after a tooth extraction.

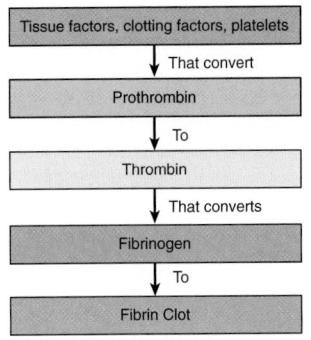

▲ **FIGURE 7.14   Blood Coagulation.**

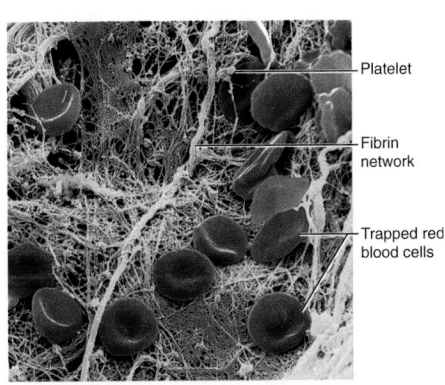

SEM 1400×

▲ **FIGURE 7.15   Blood Clot.**

Hemostasis, the control of bleeding, is a vital issue in maintaining homeostasis, the state of equilibrium of the body. Uncontrolled bleeding can take the body out of balance by decreasing blood volume and lowering blood pressure, leading to death.

Platelets (also called **thrombocytes)** play a key role in hemostasis. They are minute fragments of large bone marrow cells called **megakaryocytes**. They consist of a small amount of granular cytoplasm surrounded by a plasma membrane and have no nucleus. Platelet granules secrete chemicals that are critical to hemostasis:

- **Coagulation factors**—proteins and enzymes—that initiate the process.
- **Vasoconstrictors** that cause constriction in injured blood vessels.
- **Chemicals** that attract neutrophils and monocytes to sites of inflammation.

  Hemostasis is achieved through a three-step mechanism:

1. **Vascular spasm**—an immediate but temporary constriction of the injured blood vessel.
2. **Platelet plug formation**—an accumulation of platelets that bind themselves together and adhere to surrounding tissues. The binding and adhesion of platelets is mediated through **von Willebrand factor (vWF)**, a protein produced by the cells lining blood vessels.
3. **Blood coagulation**—the process beginning with the production of molecules that make **prothrombin** and **thrombin** and finishing with the formation of a blood clot that traps blood cells, platelets, and tissue fluid in a network of fibrin *(Figures 7.14 and 7.15)*.

After a blood clot forms, platelets adhere to strands of fibrin and contract to pull the fibers closer together. As the blood clot shrinks, it pulls the edges of the broken blood vessel together. **Fibroblasts** invade the clot to produce a fibrous connective tissue that seals the blood vessel.

WORD	PRONUNCIATION	ELEMENTS		DEFINITION
anticoagulant	AN-tee-ko-AG-you-lant	S/ P/ R/	-ant *forming* anti- *against* -coagul- *clump*	Substance that prevents clotting
coagulant coagulation	koh-ag-you-LANT koh-ag-you-LAY-shun	S/ S/	-ant *forming* -ation *process*	Substance that induces clotting The process of blood clotting
fibroblast	FIE-bro-blast	S/ R/CF	-blast *immature cell* fibr/o- *fiber*	Cell that forms collagen fibers
hemostasis (*Note:* Homeostasis has a very different meaning.)	he-moh-STAY-sis	S/ R/CF	-stasis *control, stop* hem/o- *blood*	Controlling or stopping bleeding
megakaryocyte	MEG-ah-kair-ee-oh-site	P/ R/CF R/CF	mega- *enormous* -cyt/e *cell* kary/o- *nucleus*	Large cell with large nucleus. Parts of the cytoplasm break off to form platelets
platelet (also called **thrombocyte**)	PLAYT-let	S/ R/	-let *small* plate- *flat*	Cell fragment involved in the clotting process
prothrombin	pro-THROM-bin	P/ R/	pro- *before* -thrombin *clot*	Protein formed by the liver and converted to thrombin in the blood-clotting mechanism
thrombin thrombocyte (also called **platelet**) thrombus thrombosis	THROM-bin THROM-boh-site THROM-bus throm-BOH-sis	R/CF R/CF	Greek *clot* -cyt/e *cell* thromb/o- *clot*	Enzyme that forms fibrin Another name for a platelet A clot attached to a diseased blood vessel or heart lining Formation of a thrombus.

Case Report 7.3 *(continued)*

Janis Tierney, who presented in the ER with heavy menstrual bleeding, has a deficiency of von Willebrand factor (vWF). Her platelets are unable to stick together or adhere to the wall of an injured blood vessel, and a platelet plug cannot form in the lining of her uterus to help end her menstrual flow. Von Willebrand disease (vWD) is the most common hereditary bleeding disorder. It affects at least 1% of the population and both sexes equally.

Abbreviations

EMT emergency medical technician
vWD von Willebrand disease
vWF von Willebrand factor

EXERCISES

After reading Case Report 7.3 on the opposite page and above, answer the following questions. Be prepared to discuss your answers in class.

1. Ms. Tierney is documented as being "pale." What medical term means *pale*? _____

2. In Ms. Tierney's current and past medical history, what symptoms are related to her blood condition?

   a. _____

   b. _____

   c. _____

   d. _____

3. Another medical term meaning *platelets* is _____.

   Another medical term meaning *RBCs* is _____.

   Another medical term meaning *WBCs* is _____.

   Together, this group of terms is considered the _____ of blood.

4. _____ is the most common hereditary bleeding disorder.

5. Hereditary means _____.

A thrombus is a clot. An embolus is a piece of thrombus that breaks off.

Abbreviations

aPTT	activated partial thromboplastin time
DIC	disseminated intravascular coagulation
HUS	hemolytic-uremic syndrome
INR	international normalized ratio
ITP	idiopathic (or immunologic) thrombocytopenic purpura
PT	prothrombin time
tPA	tissue plasminogen activator
TTP	thrombotic thrombocytopenic purpura

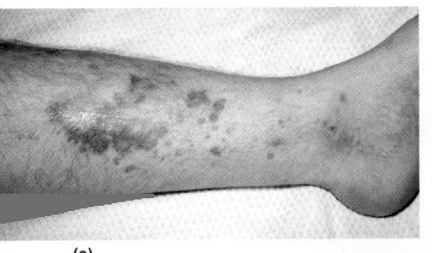
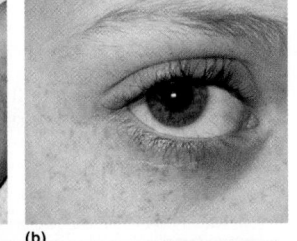

(a)   (b)

FIGURE 7.16 ▲
Subsurface Bleeding.
(a) Purpura.
(b) Petechiae.
(c) Bruises.

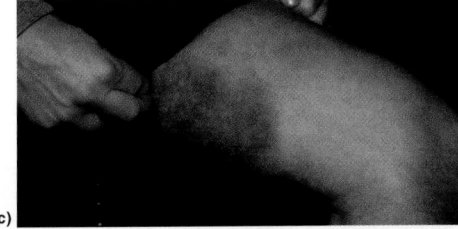

(c)

DISORDERS OF COAGULATION (COAGULOPATHIES)

Hemophilia in its classical form (hemophilia A) is a disease males inherit from their mothers and is due to a deficiency of a coagulation factor, called factor VIII. The disorder causes painful bleeding into skin, joints, and muscles. Concentrated factor VIII is given intravenously to reduce the symptoms.

Von Willebrand disease (vWD) is a deficiency of a specific protein of the factor VIII complex that is different from the part involved in hemophilia.

Disseminated intravascular coagulation (DIC) occurs when the clotting mechanism is activated simultaneously throughout the cardiovascular system. The trigger is usually a severe bacterial infection. Small clots form and obstruct blood flow into tissues and organs, particularly the kidney, leading to renal failure. As the clotting mechanisms are overwhelmed, severe bleeding occurs.

Thrombus formation (**thrombosis**) is a clot that attaches to diseased or damaged areas on the walls of blood vessels or the heart. If part of the thrombus breaks loose and moves through the circulation, it is called an **embolus.**

Thrombocytopenia is a low platelet count (below a 100,000/mm³ of blood). It occurs when bone marrow is destroyed by radiation, chemotherapy, or leukemia. Small capillary hemorrhages called **petechiae** and bruises can be seen in the skin. **Idiopathic (immunologic) thrombocytopenic purpura (ITP)** is an acute self-limiting form of the disease usually seen in children.

Thrombotic thrombocytopenic purpura (TTP) and **hemolytic-uremic syndrome (HUS)** are acute, potentially fatal disorders in which loose strands of fibrin are deposited in numerous small blood vessels. This causes damage to platelets and RBCs, causing thrombocytopenia and hemolytic anemia.

Henoch-Schönlein purpura (anaphylactoid purpura) is a disorder involving purpura, joint pain, and **glomerulonephritis** *(see Chapter 11).* The etiology is unknown. Most cases resolve spontaneously.

Purpura is bleeding into the skin from small arterioles that produces a larger individual lesion than petechiae from capillary bleeding *(Figure 7.16).* **Bruises** (or **hematomas**) are **extravasations** of blood from all types of blood vessels.

Laboratory Tests to Evaluate Blood Coagulation

- **Platelet count** has a normal range of 130,000 to 400,000 platelets/mm³ of blood.

- **Prothrombin time (PT)** is prolonged in deficiencies of some coagulation factors and fibrinogen. It is used to monitor the dose of **warfarin (Coumadin).** It is now reported as an **international normalized ratio (INR)** instead of in seconds.

- **Activated partial thromboplastin time (aPTT)** is prolonged in deficiencies of certain coagulation factors, including factor VIII and fibrinogen. It is used to monitor the dose of heparin.

Pharmacology of Blood Clotting

- **Aspirin** reduces platelet adherence and aggregation. It is used in 81-mg doses to reduce the incidence of heart attacks.

- **Heparin** is a polysaccharide that prevents prothrombin and fibrin formation. It has to be given **parenterally** (not through the digestive tract), and recently a form of heparin that can be given subcutaneously has been approved. Its dose is monitored by activated partial thromboplastin time (aPTT).

- **Hirudin** is a potent anticoagulant, produced by **recombinant DNA technology.** It blocks thrombin formation.

- **Warfarin (Coumadin)** inhibits the synthesis of prothrombin and other coagulation factors, so acts as an anticoagulant. It is given by mouth, and its dose is monitored by prothrombin times, which are reported as an International Normalized Ratio (INR).

- **Streptokinase,** derived from hemolytic streptococci, dissolves the fibrin in blood clots. Given intravenously within 3 to 4 hours of a heart attack, it is often effective in dissolving the clot that has caused the heart attack.

- **Tissue plasminogen activator (tPA)** binds strongly to fibrin and dissolves clots that have caused heart attacks. It is similar in effect and use to streptokinase. Reteplase and urokinase are forms of tPA.

WORD	PRONUNCIATION		ELEMENTS	DEFINITION
coagulopathy coagulopathies (pl)	koh-ag-you-**LOP**-ah-thee	S/ R/CF	-pathy *disease* coagul/o- *clotting*	Disorder of blood clotting
disseminate	dih-**SEM**-in-ate	S/ P/ R/	-ate *composed of, pertaining to* dis- *apart* -semin- *scatter seed*	Widely scattered throughout the body or an organ
embolus	**EM**-boh-lus		Greek *plug, stopper*	Detached piece of thrombus, a mass of bacteria, quantity of air, or foreign body that blocks a blood vessel
extravasate	eks-**TRAV**-ah-sate	S/ P/ R/	-ate *composed of, pertaining to* extra- *out of, outside* -vas- *blood vessel*	To ooze out from a vessel into the tissues
hematoma (also called **bruise**)	he-mah-**TOH**-mah	S/ R/	-oma *mass, tumor* hemat- *blood*	Collection of blood that has escaped from the blood vessels into tissue
hemophilia	he-moh-**FILL**-ee-ah	S/ R/CF	-philia *attraction* hem/o- *blood*	An inherited disease from a deficiency of clotting factor VIII
petechia petechiae (pl)	peh-**TEE**-kee-ah peh-**TEE**-kee-ee		Latin *spot on the skin*	Pinpoint capillary hemorrhagic spot in the skin
purpura	**PUR**-pyu-rah		Greek *purple*	Skin hemorrhages that are red initially and then turn purple
recombinant DNA	ree-**KOM**-bin-ant dee-en-a	S/ P/ R/	-ant *forming* re- *again* -combin- *combine*	DNA (deoxyribonucleic acid) altered by inserting a new sequence of DNA into the chain
streptokinase	strep-toe-**KI**-nase	P/ R/	strepto- *curved* -kinase *enzyme*	An enzyme that dissolves clots
thrombocytopenia	**THROM**-boh-site-oh-**PEE**-nee-ah	S/ R/CF R/CF	-penia *deficiency* thromb/o- *clot* -cyt/o- *cell*	Deficiency of platelets in circulating blood
warfarin	**WAR**-fuh-rin		Named after *Wisconsin Alumni Research Foundation*, which funded its discovery	Anticoagulant; also used as rat poison

EXERCISES

Answers to the following questions can be found on the two-page spread open in front of you. Fill in the blanks. Be prepared to discuss your answers in class.

1. Small, *capillary hemorrhages* are called _____.

2. Bleeding from larger blood vessels called _____ produces *purpura*.

3. What is the difference between an *embolus* and a *thrombus*?

    embolus: _____

    thrombus: _____

4. What is another term for a hematoma? _____

5. Translate the following sentence into language your patient can understand.

    "Aspirin reduces platelet adherence and aggregation. It is used in 81-mg doses to reduce the incidence of myocardial infarction."

    _____

    _____

    _____

6. Deficiency of platelets in circulating blood is called _____.

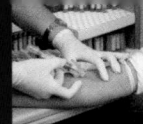
LESSON 7.5 Blood Groups and Transfusions

OBJECTIVES

To make an appropriate decision, it is critical that you are able to use correct medical terminology to:

7.5.1 **List the different blood groups.**
7.5.2 **Explain what determines a person's ABO blood type and how this relates to transfusion compatibility.**
7.5.3 **Describe the effect of an incompatibility between mother and fetus in the Rh blood type.**

You are

...an emergency medical technician—paramedic (EMT-P) working in the Level One Trauma Unit at Fulwood Medical Center.

Your patient is

...Miss Joanne Rodi, an 18-year-old student.

CASE REPORT 7.4

Ms. Rodi has been admitted to the unit from the operating room after surgery for multiple fractures in a car accident. She is receiving a blood transfusion. You document that her temperature has risen to 102°F and her respirations to 24 per minute and she has chills. You take her blood pressure; it has fallen to 90/60. What should you do?

Abbreviations	
EMT-P	emergency medical technician—paramedic
HDN	hemolytic disease of the newborn
Rh	rhesus
RhoGAM	rhesus immune globulin

Keynote

All blood groups are inherited.

Rh factor is an antigen on the surface of a red blood cell.

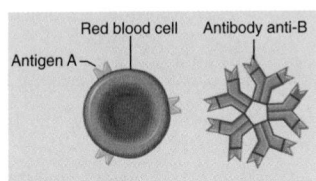

(a) Type A blood

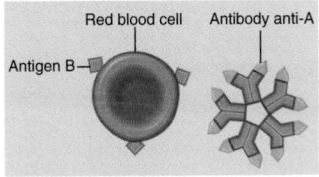

(b) Type B blood

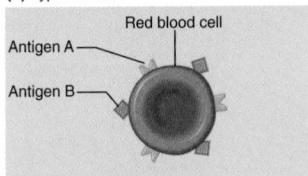

(c) Type AB blood

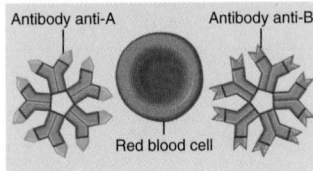

(d) Type O blood

▲ **FIGURE 7.17** **Blood Types.**

RED CELL ANTIGENS

On the surfaces of red blood cells are molecules called antigens. In the plasma, antibodies are present. Each antibody can combine with only a specific antigen. If the plasma antibodies combine with a red cell antigen, bridges are formed that connect the red cells together. This is called **agglutination,** or clumping, of the cells. Hemolysis (rupture) of the cells also occurs.

The antigens on the surfaces of the cells have been categorized into groups, of which two are the most important. These are the ABO and Rh blood groups.

ABO Blood Group

The two major antigens on the cell surface are antigen A and antigen B *(Figure 7.17)*.

A person with only antigen A has *type A* blood.

A person with only antigen B has *type B* blood.

A person with both antigen A and antigen B has *type AB* blood and is a universal recipient who can receive blood from any other type in the ABO system.

A person with neither antigen has *type O* blood and is a universal donor able to give blood to any other person no matter what that person's blood type is.

Figure 7.17 shows the different combinations of antigens and antibodies in the different blood types.

A **transfusion** of blood or packed red blood cells replaces lost red blood cells to restore the blood's oxygen-carrying capacity. In **autologous** donation and transfusion, people donate their own blood ahead of time to be given to them if necessary during a surgical procedure.

Case Report 7.4 (continued)

In Miss Rodi's case, she has type A blood and, by mistake, received blood of type AB, which agglutinated in the presence of her anti-B antibodies. Your immediate response is to stop the transfusion, replace it with a saline **infusion,** call your supervisor, and notify the doctor.

WORD	PRONUNCIATION	ELEMENTS		DEFINITION
agglutination	ah-glue-tih-**NAY**-shun	S/ P/ R/	-ation *process* ag- *to* -glutin- *glue*	Process by which cells or other particles adhere to each other to form clumps
autologous	awe-**TOL**-oh-gus	P/ R/	auto- *self, same* -logous *relation*	Blood transfusion with the same person as donor and recipient
erythroblastosis fetalis	eh-**RITH**-ro-blast-oh-sis fee-**TAH**-lis	S/ R/CF R/ S/ R/ S/	-osis *condition* erythr/o- *red* -blast- *germ cell, immature cell* -is *belonging to* fet- *fetus* -al *pertaining to*	Hemolytic disease of the newborn due to Rh incompatibility
infusion	in-**FYU**-zhun	P/ R/	in- *in* -fusion *to pour*	Introduction intravenously of a substance other than blood
spherocyte spherocytosis	**SFEAR**-oh-site **SFEAR**-oh-site-oh-sis	S/ R/CF S/	-cyte *cell* spher/o- *sphere* -osis *condition*	A spherical cell Presence of spherocytes in blood
transfusion	trans-**FYU**-zhun	P/ R/	trans- *across* -fusion *to pour*	Transfer of blood or a blood component from donor to recipient

Rh Blood Group

If an **Rh** antigen is present on an RBC surface, the blood is said to be Rh-positive (Rh⁺). If there is no Rh antigen on the surface, the blood is Rh-negative (Rh⁻). The presence or absence of Rh antigen is inherited.

If an Rh-negative person receives a transfusion of Rh-positive blood, anti-Rh antibodies will be produced. This can cause RBC agglutination and hemolysis.

If an Rh-negative woman and an Rh-positive man conceive an Rh-positive child *(Figure 7.18a)*, the placenta normally prevents maternal and fetal blood from mixing. However, at birth or during a miscarriage, fetal cells can enter the mother's bloodstream. These Rh-positive cells stimulate the mother's tissues to produce Rh-antibodies *(Figure 7.18b)*.

If the mother becomes pregnant with a second Rh-positive fetus, her Rh-antibodies can cross the placenta and agglutinate and hemolyze the fetal RBCs *(Figure 7.18c)*. This causes hemolytic disease of the newborn (**HDN**, or **erythroblastosis fetalis**).

Hemolytic disease of the newborn due to Rh-incompatibility can be prevented. The Rh-negative mother after giving birth to an Rh-positive child should be given Rh-immune globulin (RhoGAM).

Other causes of hemolytic disease in the newborn include ABO incompatibility, incompatibility in other blood group systems, hereditary **spherocytosis**, and some infections acquired before birth.

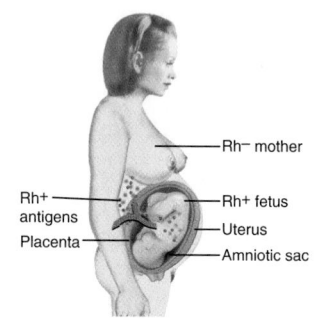

(a) First pregnancy

Rh⁻ mother
Rh+ antigens
Rh+ fetus
Uterus
Placenta
Amniotic sac

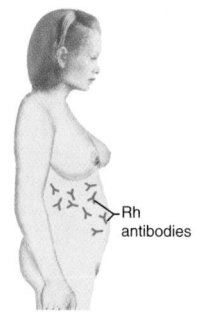

(b) Between pregnancies

Rh antibodies

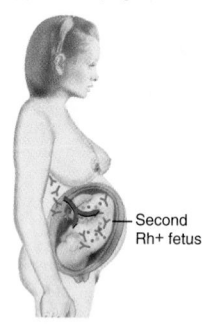

(c) Second pregnancy

Second Rh+ fetus

▲ **FIGURE 7.18   Hemolytic Disease of the Newborn.**

EXERCISES

Review the elements in this WAD before starting this exercise. Match the elements in column 1 with the correct meanings in column 2.

_____   1. logous   A. condition

_____   2. fusion   B. self

_____   3. trans   C. to pour

_____   4. blast   D. across

_____   5. osis   E. relation

_____   6. auto   F. germ cell

BLOOD
CHALLENGE YOUR KNOWLEDGE

A. **Patient Education:** Mrs. Sosin has asked you to interpret the results of her blood work for her. Use your knowledge of blood to explain in your own words her test results.

> Examination of her peripheral smear reveals her RBCs to be microcytic, hypochromic, and poikilocytic. Laboratory examination reveals a hemoglobin concentration of 10.4 g/dL (normal range 12–16 g/dL).

1. Define for the patient:

   RBC: _____

   microcytic: _____

   hypochromic: _____

   poikilocytic: _____

   hemoglobin: _____

2. In your own words, describe to the patient the role of hemoglobin in the blood.

   _____

   _____

   _____

3. Is Mrs. Sosin's hemoglobin concentration within normal limits (WNL)? _____

B. **Recall:** The following elements are grouped according to type. Write the meaning of the element, give a medical term containing that element, and briefly define the medical term. Then identify the group as either prefixes, roots/CFs, or suffixes. Fill in the chart.

Element	Meaning of Element	Medical Term	Meaning of Medical Term
emia			
globin			
in			
ine			
lysis			
oid			
penia			
poiesis			
sis			

This is a group of _____ .

C. **Choose the appropriate abbreviation, or meaning of abbreviation, to fill in the patient documentation.**

1. The patient's _____ (Hct) last week showed normal _____ (RBCs), but the (CBC) _____ showed an abnormal number of _____ (WBCs). Her blood values this week were _____ (WNL).

2. The patient's _____ (MCV) and _____ (MCH) both showed decreased values on his recent blood test.

3. Laboratory work proved Latisha's mononucleosis to be caused by the _____ (EBV).

4. Orders for this patient's preop testing before her surgery will include a _____ (PT) and an _____ (aPTT).

5. Possible admitting diagnoses for this patient include _____ (vWD) or _____ (ALL).

6. This patient was given a drug containing _____ (tPA) in the Emergency Room following his heart attack.

D. **With the possible exception of the appendix, everything in the body has a function.** The functions are listed below. Assign each a letter for the blood component that performs the function.

   A. A function of a red blood cell (RBC)
   B. A function of a white blood cell (WBC)
   C. A function of a platelet
   D. A function of plasma

1. Transport oxygen   _____

2. Help maintain hemostasis   _____

3. Migrate to damaged tissues and release histamine   _____

4. Carry nutrients, hormones, and enzymes to cells   _____

5. Dissolve cellular waste products   _____

6. Secrete lysozymes   _____

7. Transport carbon dioxide   _____

8. Seal off injury and hemorrhage   _____

9. Provide fluid environment to formed elements   _____

10. Transport nitric oxide   _____

BLOOD

E. Medical terminology is a language of small nuances that make a difference.

Determine the difference between the pairs of terms listed below. Underline the element that makes the difference in the term; then provide a brief definition for each term.

1. *transfusion* and *infusion*

   _____

   _____

   _____

2. *hemostasis* and *homeostasis*

   _____

   _____

   _____

3. *pancytopenia* and *thrombocytopenia*

   _____

   _____

   _____

4. In the group of terms in questions 1 through 3, in each pair the _____ (type of element) stays the same.

F. **Build medical terms from the following group of elements.** The definition is given to you; fill in the medical term. You will not use every element, and some you may use twice. Fill in the blanks.

Use a combination of these elements to complete the terms:

ic	micro	auto	osis	hypo	crit
ox	ary	cyte	thrombo	macro	ar

1. Another name for an RBC   erythro _____

2. Pertaining to a small cell   _____cyt_____

3. Blood transfusion with the same person as both donor and recipient   _____logous

4. Large red blood cell   _____cyte

5. Percentage of red blood cells in blood   hemato _____

6. Deficient in oxygen   _____/_____ic

7. Same as a platelet   _____/cyte

8. Formation of a clot   thromb/_____

G. **True or False:** The following statements about blood are either true or false. Circle the correct answer. Rewrite the false statement(s) correctly on the lines below.

1. The formed elements of blood are RBCs, WBCs, platelets, and serum. T F

2. Buffer systems in the blood maintain the correct pH range. T F

3. Serum is identical to plasma except for the absence of clotting proteins. T F

4. Sickle cell anemia is a genetic disorder. T F

5. All cells exchange water by thrombosis. T F

6. Plasma is the fluid, noncellular part of blood. T F

7. The bloodstream is a liquid transport system. T F

8. Whole blood is less viscous than water. T F

9. Monocytes are the largest blood cells. T F

10. Erythropoiesis occurs in bone spaces filled with red bone marrow. T F

Corrections:

_____

_____

_____

_____

_____

_____

_____

_____

_____

H. **Documentation:** Take the patient's own words and translate them into medical language for documentation.

1. "I am always tired, have no energy or 'get up and go,' and my arms and legs ache a lot of the time."

This patient complains of _____

_____ .

Take the doctor's words and translate them into language the patient can understand.

2. "In sickle cell disease, the abnormal cells agglutinate and occlude small capillaries, and this causes the intense pain in the hypoxic tissues. This is the sickle cell crisis."

_____

_____

_____

_____

BLOOD

I. **Multiple Choice:** Use the *language of hematology* to answer the following questions. Remember that in the case of multiple choice, there is only one *best* answer.

1. Blood volume varies with:

   a. your body size

   b. the amount of your adipose tissue

   c. only b

   d. only a

   e. both a and b

2. The percentage of red blood cells in a blood sample is called the:

   a. hemoglobin

   b. hematocrit

   c. hematemesis

   d. hemolysis

   e. hemostasis

3. In the term **hypochromic,** the root means:

   a. blood

   b. center

   c. color

   d. glue

   e. air

4. How many types of WBCs also qualify as granulocytes?

   a. one

   b. two

   c. three

   d. four

   e. five

5. **Myeloid leukemia** is a disorder of:

   a. RBCs

   b. WBCs

   c. platelets

   d. plasma

   e. hemoglobin

6. In the term **erythrocyte,** the combining form means:

   a. yellow

   b. red

   c. white

   d. black

   e. blue

7. **Heparin** is:

   a. antidepressant

   b. antihistamine

   c. antibody

   d. anticoagulant

   e. antibiotic

8. Which of these terms can be connected with blood?

   a. liquid matrix

   b. connective tissue

   c. formed elements

   d. a and c

   e. a, b, and c

9. The largest white blood cell is:

   a. monocyte

   b. macrophage

   c. eosinophil

   d. basophil

   e. neutrophil

10. What is plasma minus its protein fibrinogen?

   a. hemoglobin

   b. antithrombin

   c. plasmin

   d. serum

   e. a formed element

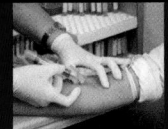
BLOOD

J. **Team Exercise:** Pair with a fellow student or group of students. Choose three medical terms in this chapter that you find the most difficult to remember or understand. Write them, pronounce them, and then use each term in a brief sentence that is a definition. Place a check mark (✓) on the appropriate line once you have practiced the pronunciations. Take turns quizzing the other students on your terms, and see if you can answer their term questions. Track if there is a pattern of certain terms that you all find difficult. *Use this exercise as a study review.*

1. Term:_____   Pronunciation practiced: _____

    Definition:

    _____

    _____

2. Term: _____   Pronunciation practiced: _____

    Definition:

    _____

    _____

3. Term: _____   Pronunciation practiced: _____

    Definition:

    _____

    _____

K. **Medical terms may be similar in appearance.** You need to use your knowledge of prefixes, roots, and suffixes to help determine the difference between similar terms. Using the terms below, correctly insert them into the following paragraph.

erythrocyte   **erythroblast**   **erythroblastosis**   **erythropoiesis**   **erythropoietin**

The immature RBC (_____) undergoes the process of formation (_____) in the red bone marrow.

Too many immature cells result in a condition known as _____. A mature RBC is called an _____.

The hormone _____ controls the rate of RBC production.

L. **Discussion Questions:** Prepare a brief discussion on either topic.
    1. What is the major concern in transfusions? What types of safeguards can be used to prevent a patient getting the wrong blood in a transfusion? Why is it a good thing to know your own blood type?
    2. What is the function of buffer systems in the blood? Give some examples. What is the pH range of blood?

M. **Terminology Challenge:**

erythrocyte   **leukemia**   **purpura**

This group of medical terms has something in common. What is it?_____

N. **Meet the lesson and chapter objectives** by testing your knowledge of the blood and its components. *Use this exercise as a study review before a test.* Fill in the blanks.

1. Name the functions of blood:

   a. _____

   b. _____

   c. _____

   d. _____

   e. _____

   f. _____

   g. _____

   h. _____

   i. _____

2. List the formed elements of blood and give one function for each:

   a. Component: _____ Function: _____

   b. Component: _____ Function: _____

   c. Component: _____ Function: _____

3. Plasma transports:

   a. _____

   b. _____

   c. _____

   d. _____

4. The different types of WBCs are:

   a. _____

   b. _____

   c. _____

   d. _____

   e. _____

5. List the different blood groups:

   a. _____

   b. _____

   c. _____

   d. _____

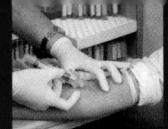

BLOOD

O. **There are many diseases associated with the various components of blood.** Circle the correct choice in the descriptions below; then, on the blanks, write in which blood component is associated with the disease you circled. Use RBC, WBC, and P (for platelet) for blood component notations.

Blood Component

1. Chronic bleeding from the gastrointestinal tract can cause:
   iron-deficiency anemia   pernicious anemia   sickle cell anemia   _____

2. Deficiency of a specific protein of the factor VIII complex:
   thrombus   von Willebrand disease   iron-deficiency anemia   _____

3. Cancer of the hematopoietic tissues is called:
   leukemia   lukemia   lukemmia   _____

4. Disease resulting from vitamin B_{12} deficiency:
   pernicious anemia   hemolytic anemia   polycythemia vera   _____

5. A disease males inherit from their mothers:
   hemmaphilia   hemophilia   hemmophilia   _____

6. Hereditary disease found mostly in people of African descent:
   sickle cell anemia   iron-deficiency anemia   polycythemia vera   _____

7. Numerous small clots form and obstruct blood flow into organs:
   DIC   vWD   tPA   _____

8. Seen in viral infections such as measles and mumps:
   leukopenia   leukocytosis   leukemia   _____

9. Low blood cell count that produces a tendency to bleed:
   thrombocitopenia   thrombocytopenia   thrombocytopennia   _____

10. Destruction of blood cells by toxic substances:
    polycythemia vera   hemolytic anemia   pernicious anemia   _____

P. **Pharmacology of Blood Clotting:** Anyone working with patients must have a knowledge of prescribed drugs and their function. Match the correct drug to its purpose.

_____ 1. Dissolves fibrin in blood clots

_____ 2. Reduces platelet adherence

_____ 3. Prevents prothrombin and fibrin formation

_____ 4. Inhibits formation of prothrombin

_____ 5. Inhibits synthesis of coagulation factors

A. heparin

B. tPA

C. Coumadin

D. streptokinase

E. aspirin

Q. Meet a lesson objective and list the different blood types in the ABO blood group. Be sure to note which type is the "universal donor" and which type is the "universal recipient." *Do you know your own blood type, and that of your spouse or children?*

The two major antigens on the cell surface are antigen A and antigen B.

1. A person with only antigen A has type _____ blood.
2. A person with only antigen B has type _____ blood.
3. A person with *both* antigen A and antigen B has type _____ blood.
4. A person with *neither* antigen A nor antigen B has type _____ blood.

Because the blood type in question 4 has *neither* antigen, it is compatible with any blood type; therefore, it is the universal (donor/recipient) _____.

Because the blood type in question 3 has *both* antigens, it is the universal (donor/recipient) _____.

> **Study Hint**
> The same two letters in the word *donor* will be your hint to the blood type.

R. **Recall and Review:** How well do you remember these word elements from the previous chapter? Try to answer without first looking back to check. Fill in the blanks.

Element	Type of Element (P, R, CF, S)	Meaning of Element
laparo	_____	_____
zyme	_____	_____
gingiv	_____	_____
phagia	_____	_____
hydro	_____	_____

S. **Demonstrate your knowledge of word elements by deconstructing the following medical terms.** Then write the term next to the appropriate statement below.

Term	Prefix	Root/CF	Suffix
leukocytosis			
hypochromic			
vasoconstrictor			
poikilocytic			
precursor			
anemia			
microcytic			
osmosis			
hemoglobin			
pancytopenia			

1. That which comes before something_____

2. Pertaining to a small cell _____

3. Decreased number of red blood cells _____

4. Passage of water across a cell membrane_____

5. Pigmented protein in RBCs_____

6. Excessively high WBC count _____

7. Deficiency of all formed elements in the blood_____

8. Agent that causes narrowing of blood vessels_____

9. Pertaining to an RBC of irregular shape _____

10. Pale in color _____

BLOOD

T. **Test your knowledge of blood, blood groups, and Rh factor by choosing the correct answer to the following questions.** Circle the best answer.

1. A person with both antigen A and antigen B will have:

   a. blood type O

   b. blood type A

   c. blood type B

   d. blood type AB

   e. none of these blood types

2. Where are antibodies synthesized after birth?

   a. in the heart

   b. in the blood

   c. in the arteries

   d. in the plasma

   e. in the veins

3. What normally prevents maternal and fetal blood from mixing during pregnancy?

   a. cell membranes

   b. the peritoneum

   c. the placenta

   d. the amniotic sac

   e. the matrix

4. Blood is said to be Rh-positive if:

   a. the Rh antigen is present on the RBC surface

   b. the Rh antibody is present in the blood type

   c. the Rh antibody is present in the plasma

   d. the Rh antigen is present on the WBCs

   e. the blood type is AB

5. **Agglutination** occurs when:

   a. you have not been vaccinated

   b. you are given the wrong blood type

   c. your antibodies are low

   d. your hematocrit is high

   e. you are Rh-positive

6. The term **transfusion** is used only for:

    a. plasma

    b. whole blood

    c. blood or a blood component

    d. saline solution

    e. intravenous (IV) antibiotics

U. **Word Association:**

The medical term **viscous** means _____. Equate this to something seen in everyday life that has the same consistency.

Example: _____

V. **How well do you understand what you read?** First, read the paragraph aloud to check your pronunciation. Then, read the paragraph again and underline the medical terms. Enter the term in the left column of the chart next to its correct meaning.

When a lab tech takes a blood sample, he spins it in a centrifuge. Formed elements are separated from the colloidal suspension and are packed into the bottom of the tube. The patient's hematocrit can be determined from this test. Whole blood contains all the formed elements. Transfusions can be done with either whole blood or only certain portions of the formed elements—only transfusing RBCs or platelets, for instance. The remaining part (55%) of a blood sample is the plasma, which is mostly water. Plasma provides the fluid transport for the formed elements as well as nutrients, hormones and enzymes for body cells. Waste cell products dissolve in plasma and are excreted through the kidneys and liver.

Term	Meaning
	To dispose of
	Liquid containing particles that do not settle
	Introduction of blood or a blood component into a vein
	Something life sustaining
	Blood clotting cell
	Instrument for separating a blood sample
	Stimulates function of an organ or tissue
	Erythrocyte
	Liquid transport system
	Induces chemical changes in other substances
	Percentage of RBCs in the blood

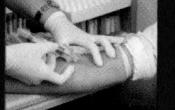

CHAPTER 7 REVIEW

BLOOD

CHAPTER SUMMARY EXERCISE

1. *Listen to the pronunciation of the medical terms as given by your instructor.*
2. *Circle the correct spelling of the medical term.*
3. *Match the correctly spelled terms to the brief descriptions below.*
4. *Write a sentence for each of the 10 terms that appear in this exercise.*

A. SPELLING COMPREHENSION: CIRCLE THE CORRECT SPELLING OF THE TERM.

1. autollogus	autologis	autoligus	autologous	autolagus
2. creatinnine	creatinine	creatynine	creatonin	creatyine
3. erythropoesis	errythropoesis	erythropoisus	erythropuesis	erythropoiesis
4. leukocytusis	leukocytosis	lukocytosis	leukocitosis	lukocitossis
5. feretin	ferrittin	ferriten	ferritin	feriton
6. pitichia	petickia	petechia	petikia	peteckia
7. centrifuje	centerfuge	senterfuge	centrifuge	sentrifuge
8. ossmosis	ossmossis	osmosis	osmoses	osmossus
9. apherises	apheresis	aperisis	aperhisis	apherisus
10. agluetinate	agglutenate	aguentinate	agglutonate	agglutinate

B. MATCH THE NUMBER OF THE CORRECT TERM IN PART A WITH THE BRIEF DESCRIPTION OF THE TERM BELOW.

_____ **a.** Passage of fluid across a cell membrane

_____ **b.** Removing only platelets and returning the rest to the donor

_____ **c.** Regulates iron storage and transport

_____ **d.** Separates particles in a suspension

_____ **e.** Formation of red blood cells

_____ **f.** Donating your own blood for your surgery

_____ **g.** Minute hemorrhage in the skin

_____ **h.** Clump together

_____ **i.** Excessive number of WBCs

_____ **j.** Protein found in skeletal muscle

C. USING YOUR KNOWLEDGE OF TERMS 1–10 IN PART A AND THEIR CORRECT SPELLING, WRITE A BRIEF SENTENCE FOR EACH OF THE TERMS AS IT MIGHT APPEAR IN PATIENT DOCUMENTATION.

1. _____

2. _____

3. _____

4. _____

5. _____

6. _____

7. _____

8. _____

9. _____

10. _____

D. YOUR INSTRUCTOR WILL DIRECT YOU TO MCGRAW-HILL CONNECT. OPEN THE AUDIO GLOSSARY AND PRACTICE YOUR PRONOUNCIATION OF THE TERMS IN PART A OF THIS EXERCISE.

E. AFTER READING CASE REPORT 7.4, ANSWER THE FOLLOWING QUESTIONS. *BE PREPARED TO DISCUSS YOUR ANSWERS IN CLASS.*

CASE REPORT 7.4

You are

. . . an emergency medical technician–paramedic (EMT-P) working in the Level One Trauma Unit at Fulwood Medical Center.

Your patient is

. . . Miss Joanne Rodi, an 18-year-old student, who has been admitted to the unit from the operating room after surgery for multiple fractures in a car accident.

Miss Rodi is receiving a blood transfusion. You document that her temperature has risen to 102°F and her respirations to 24 per minute and she has chills. You take her blood pressure; it has fallen to 90/60. What should you do?

In Miss Rodi's case, she has type A blood and, by mistake, received blood of type AB, which agglutinated in the presence of her anti-B antibodies. Your immediate response is to stop the transfusion, replace it with a saline **infusion,** call your supervisor, and notify the doctor.

1. If a *transfusion* consists of blood or blood components, what does an *infusion* carry?

_____

2. What is meant by the phrase "blood cells *agglutinate*"?

_____

3. Can you think of a study hint that will help you remember what *agglutinate* means? _____

_____

4. What were Miss Rodi's symptoms once the blood started to agglutinate?

_____

_____

5. What specific antigen did Miss Rodi's type A blood react to? _____

6. Define the medical term *incompatible*. _____

7. Write a sentence of documentation in Miss Rodi's case, using the term incompatible. _____

_____

_____

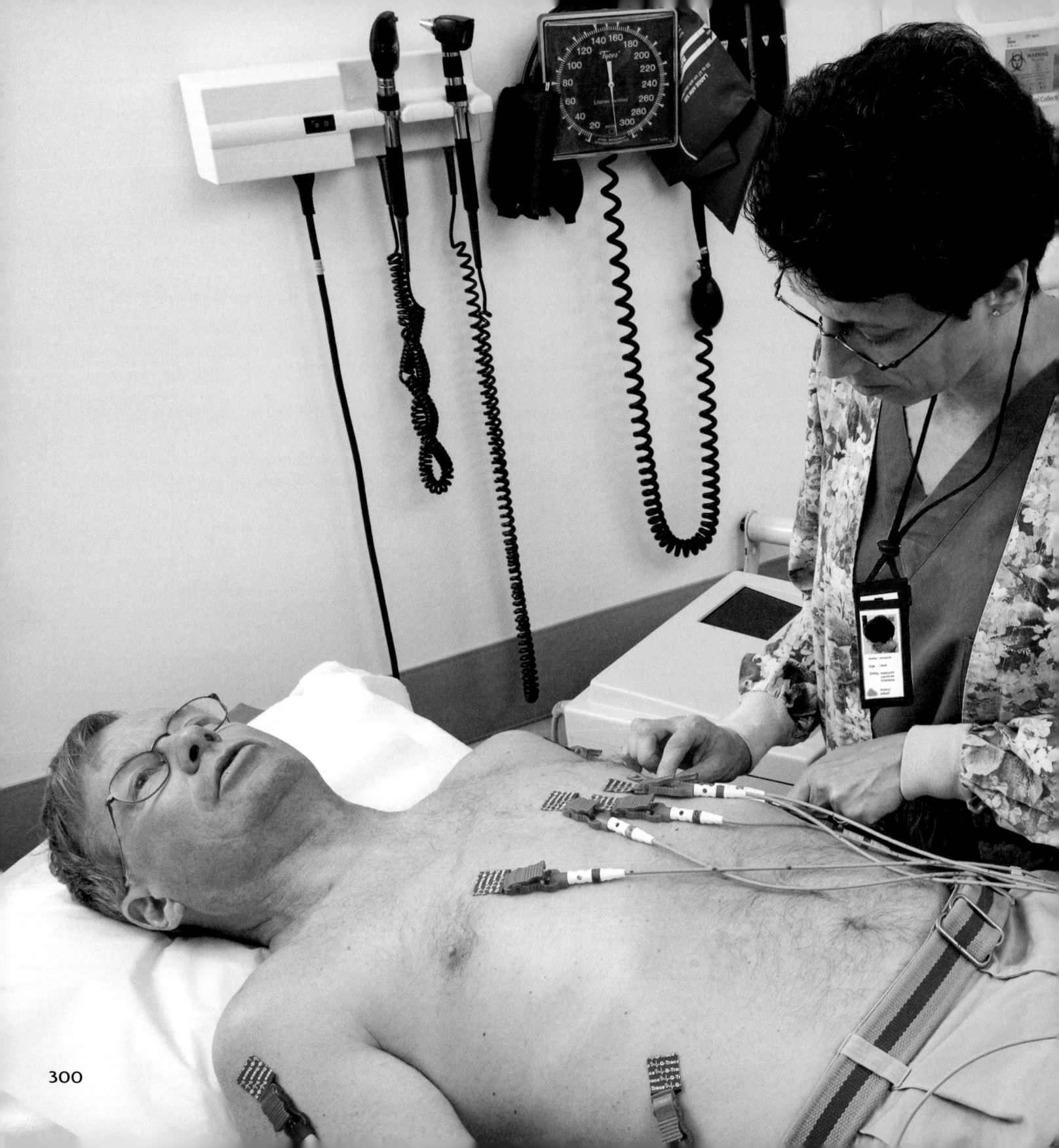

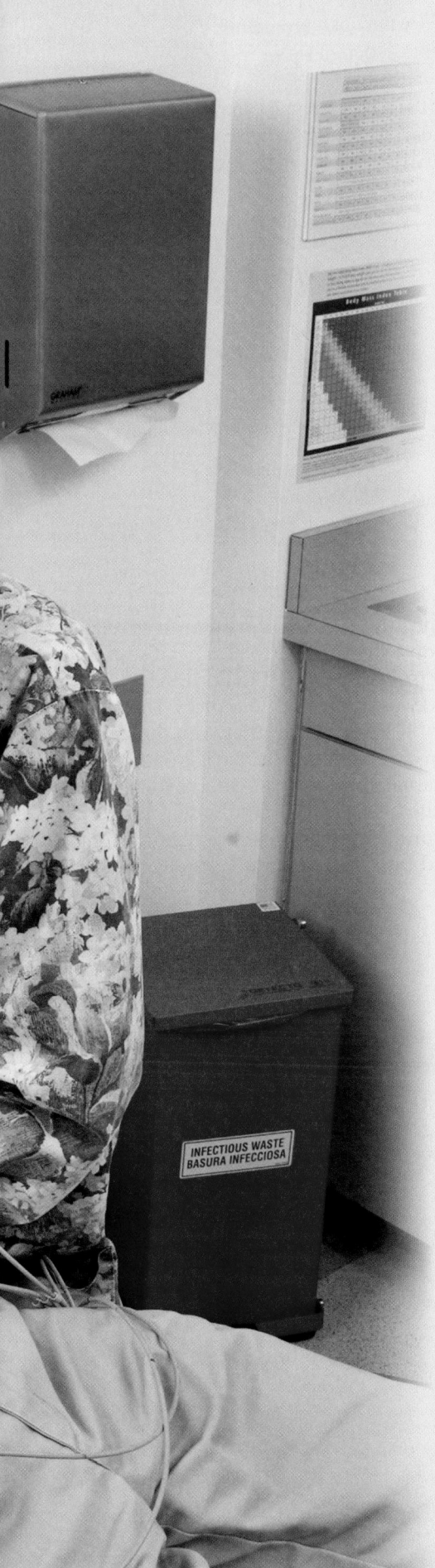

8

CASE REPORT 8.1

You are

. . . a cardiovascular technologist (**CVT**) employed by the **Cardiology** Department at Fulwood Medical Center. You have been called to the Emergency Department **STAT** to take an electrocardiogram (**ECG** or **EKG**).

Your patient is

. . . Mr. Hank Johnson. From his medical records, you see that he is the 64-year-old owner of a printing company.

Eight months previously, he had a left total hip replacement. In the past 3 months, Mr. Johnson has returned to his daily workouts. This morning while riding his exercise bike, he felt tightness in his chest. He kept on cycling and developed pain in the center of his chest radiating down his left arm and up into his jaw. He became **diaphoretic.** His personal trainer called 911.

You perform the ECG, and the automatic report describes abnormalities in the chest leads.

As you remove the electrodes, Mr. Johnson complains that he is feeling faint and short of breath (**SOB**). You are the only person in the room.

Learning Outcomes

To understand the ECG report and to determine what you should do next, you need to have knowledge of the heart's pumping mechanisms, its blood supply, the electrical properties of cardiac muscle, **and the medical terminology to communicate and understand that information.** No matter in which discipline or setting a health professional works, the condition of the patient's heart will always be a factor during diagnosis, treatment, and communication. You need to be able to:

8.1 Apply the language of cardiology to the anatomy and physiology of the **cardiovascular** system.

8.2 Comprehend, analyze, spell, and write the terms of cardiology so that you communicate and document accurately and precisely in any health care setting.

8.3 Recognize and pronounce the medical terms of cardiology so that you communicate and document verbally with accuracy and precision in any health care setting.

8.4 Explain the effects of common disorders of the cardiovascular system on health.

LESSON 8.1 Heart

CARDIOVASCULAR SYSTEM

OBJECTIVES

If you have a healthy heart rate of 60 beats per minute and you live to be 80 years old, your heart will beat (contract and relax) at least 2,522,880,000 times. Your heart pumps approximately 2000 gallons of blood each day. In 80 years of life, it will have pumped a total of 58,400,000 gallons of blood. If your heart is unable to maintain this ability to pump blood for just a few minutes, your life is in danger.

When the heart fails, there is no circulation of blood, tissues are deprived of oxygen and nutrients, and metabolic wastes accumulate. Your cells die.

The information in this lesson will enable you to use correct medical terminology to:

8.1.1 Describe the location of the heart and its relation to other structures.

8.1.2 Discuss the functions of the heart.

8.1.3 Identify the chambers of the heart and the pathway blood takes through them.

8.1.4 Explain the causes of the sounds of the heartbeat heard through a stethoscope.

8.1.5 Specify the blood supply to the heart muscle.

8.1.6 Distinguish between contraction and relaxation during the heart cycle.

8.1.7 Detail the electrical properties of the heart.

ANATOMY OF THE HEART

Location of the Heart

It is important to know the position of the heart so that you can perform effective **cardiopulmonary resuscitation (CPR)**, position a **stethoscope** to hear heart sounds, or position the **electrodes** correctly for an **electrocardiogram (ECG or EKG)**.

The heart is roughly the size of your fist and weighs around 10 ounces. The heart is a blunt cone, pointing down and to the left. It lies obliquely between the lungs, with one-third of its mass behind the **sternum** and two-thirds to the left of the sternum *(Figure 8.1a)*. The **apex** can normally be palpated in the fifth **intercostal** space, between the fifth and sixth ribs. The base of the heart lies behind the sternum and the second intercostal space, between the second and third ribs. The region of the thoracic cavity in which the heart lies is called the **mediastinum**. *(Figure 8.1b)*

Abbreviations	
CPR	cardiopulmonary resuscitation
CVT	cardiovascular technician
ECG	electrocardiogram
EKG	electrocardiogram
SOB	shortness of breath
STAT	immediately

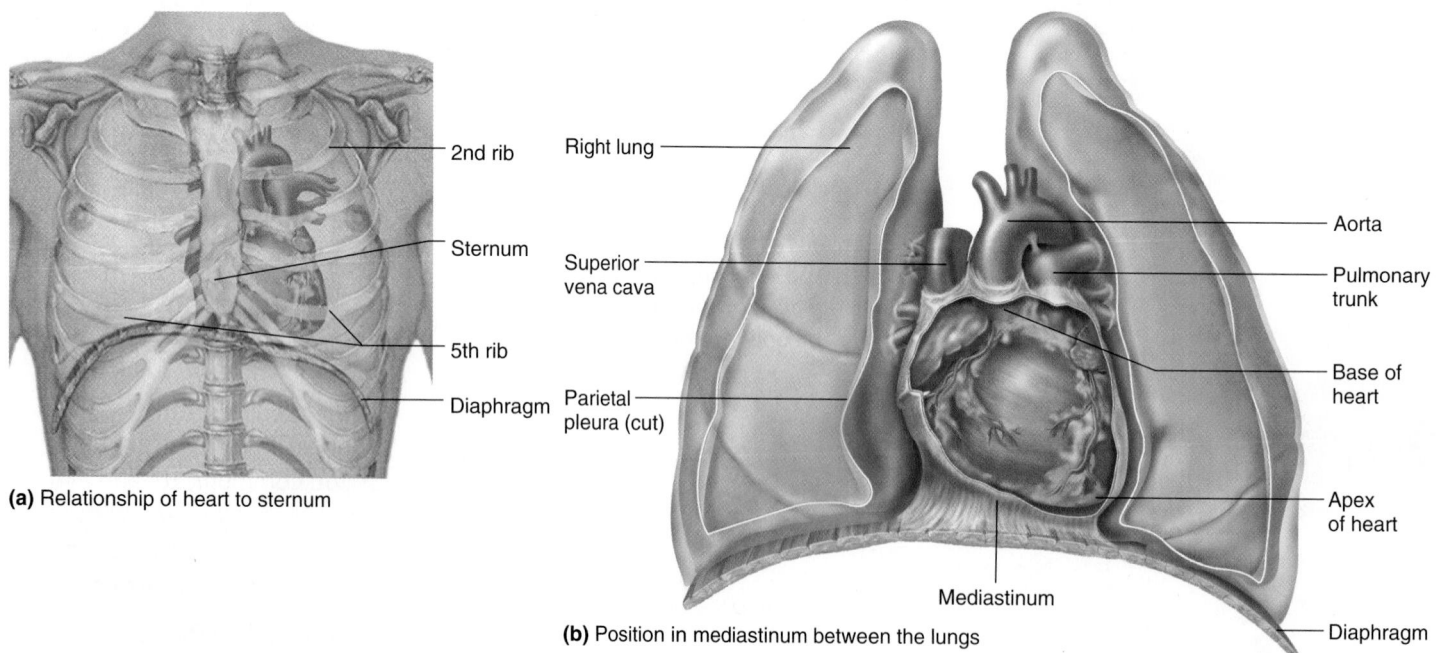

(a) Relationship of heart to sternum

2nd rib — Sternum — 5th rib — Diaphragm

Right lung — Aorta — Superior vena cava — Pulmonary trunk — Parietal pleura (cut) — Base of heart — Apex of heart — Mediastinum — Diaphragm

(b) Position in mediastinum between the lungs

▲ **FIGURE 8.1 Position of Heart in Thoracic Cavity.**

WORD	PRONUNCIATION		ELEMENTS	DEFINITION
apex	**A**-peks		Latin *summit or tip*	Tip or end of cone-shaped structure, such as the heart
cardiac	**KAR**-dee-ak	S/ R/	-ac *pertaining to* cardi- *heart*	Pertaining to the heart
cardiogenic	**KAR**-dee-oh-**JEN**-ik	S/ R/	-ic *pertaining to* -gen *produce, create*	Of cardiac origin
cardiologist	kar-dee-**OL**-oh-jist	R/CF S/	cardi/o- *heart* -logist *specialist*	A medical specialist in diagnosis and treatment of the heart (cardiology)
cardiology	kar-dee-**OL**-oh-jee	S/	-logy *study of*	Medical specialty of diseases of the heart
cardiopulmonary resuscitation	**KAR**-dee-oh-**PUL**-mo-nary ree-sus-ih-**TAY**-shun	S/ R/CF R/ S/ R/	-ary *pertaining to* cardi/o- *heart* -pulmon- *lung* -ation *process* resuscit- *revival from apparent death*	The attempt to restore cardiac and pulmonary function
cardiovascular	**KAR**-dee-oh-**VAS**-kyu-lar	S/ R/CF R/	-ar *pertaining to* cardi/o- *heart* -vascul- *blood vessel*	Pertaining to the heart and blood vessels
diaphoretic (adj)	**DIE**-ah-foh-**RET**-ic	S/ R/	-etic *pertaining to* diaphor- *sweat*	Pertaining to sweat or perspiration
diaphoresis (noun)	**DIE**-ah-foh-**REE**-sis	S/	-esis *abnormal condition*	Sweat or perspiration
electrocardiogram (ECG or EKG)	ee-lek-troh-**KAR**-dee-oh-gram	S/ R/CF R/CF	-gram *a record* electr/o- *electricity* -cardi/o- *heart*	Record of the electrical signals of the heart
electrocardiograph electrocardiography	ee-lek-troh-**KAR**-dee-oh-graf ee-**LEK**-troh-kar-dee-**OG**-rah-fee	S/ S/	-graph *to record* -graphy *process of recording*	Machine that makes the electrocardiogram Interpretation of electrocardiograms
electrode	ee-**LEK**-trode	S/ R/	-ode *way, road* electr- *electricity*	A device for conducting electricity
intercostal	**IN**-ter-**KOS**-tal	S/ P/ R/	-al *pertaining to* inter- *between* -cost- *rib*	The space between two ribs
mediastinum	**ME**-dee-ass-**TIE**-num	S/ P/ R/	-um *structure* media- *middle* -stin- *partition*	Area between the lungs containing the heart, aorta, venae cavae, esophagus, and trachea
sternum	**STIR**-num		Latin *chest*	Long, flat bone forming the center of the anterior wall of the chest
stethoscope	**STETH**-oh-skope	S/ R/CF	-scope *instrument* steth/o- *chest*	Instrument for listening to cardiac and respiratory sounds

EXERCISES

*Build your **language of cardiology** by completing the following documentation. There is only one best answer for each blank.*

1. **cardiology**   **cardiovascular**   **cardiologist**   **cardiac**

   The universal root/combining form in these terms is _____, which means _____.

   The _____ Department sent a specialist to examine the patient in the Emergency Room. The _____

   ordered an angioplasty, which showed three obstructed arteries in the patient's heart, so the _____ surgeon was noti-

   fied immediately to perform _____ surgery.

2. **electrode**   **electrocardiogram**   **electrocardiograph**   **electrocardiography**

   The patient was scheduled for _____ today. The CVT attached the _____ to the patient's chest and

   proceeded to turn on the _____. Unfortunately, a malfunction of the machine prevented him from obtaining the

   _____. This study will have to be rescheduled for the patient.

FUNCTIONS AND STRUCTURE OF THE HEART

Functions of the Heart

1. **Pump blood.** Contractions of the heart generate the pressure to produce movement of blood through the blood vessels.
2. **Route blood.** The heart can be described as two pumps: a pump on the right side of the heart that sends blood through the **pulmonary** circulation of the lungs and back to the pump on the left side, which sends blood through the **systemic** circulation of the body. The valves of the heart ensure this one-way flow of blood.
3. **Regulate blood supply.** The changing metabolic needs of tissues and organs (for example, when you exercise) are met by changes in the rate and force of the heart's contraction.

Structure of the Heart

The heart wall consists of four layers *(Figure 8.2)*:

1. **Endocardium**—a single layer of cells over a thin layer of connective tissue lining the heart.
2. **Myocardium**—cardiac muscle cells that enable the heart to contract.
3. **Epicardium**—an outer single layer of cells overlying a thin layer of connective tissue.
4. **Pericardium**—a connective tissue sac that surrounds and protects the heart. It consists of an inner **visceral** and outer **parietal** layer, between which is the **pericardial** cavity. The cavity contains a **lubricant** fluid that allows the heart to beat with very little friction around it.

Blood Supply to Heart Muscle Because the heart beats continually and strongly, it requires an abundant supply of oxygen and nutrients. To meet this need, the cardiac muscle has its own blood circulation, the **coronary circulation** *(Figure 8.3)*.

Immediately above the aortic valve in the root of the aorta, the right and left **coronary arteries** exit from the aorta and divide into branches to begin the coronary circulation.

After the blood has flowed through the arteries into the capillaries of the myocardium, it drains into veins that flow into the right atrium, where the blood mixes with deoxygenated blood from the body.

If any of the coronary arteries become blocked, the blood supply to a part of the cardiac muscle is cut off (**ischemia**), and those cells supplied by that artery die (undergo **necrosis**) within minutes. This is a **myocardial infarction (MI),** what many call a "heart attack."

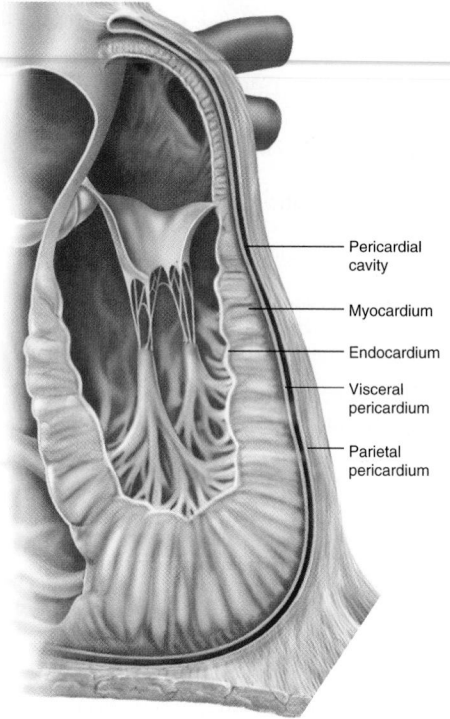

▲ **FIGURE 8.2   Heart Wall.**

Pericardial cavity
Myocardium
Endocardium
Visceral pericardium
Parietal pericardium

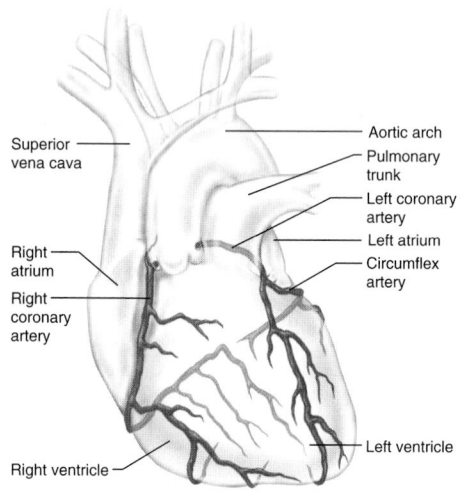

Superior vena cava
Aortic arch
Pulmonary trunk
Left coronary artery
Left atrium
Circumflex artery
Right atrium
Right coronary artery
Left ventricle
Right ventricle

▲ **FIGURE 8.3   Coronary Arterial Circulation.**

Abbreviation	
MI	myocardial infarction ("heart attack")

Case Report 8.1 *(continued)*

Changes on Mr. Johnson's ECG show he was having a myocardial infarction. Cardiac muscle cells have very limited capability to replicate, and the repair of muscle cell death is mainly by **fibrosis.** This limits cardiac function and will contribute to a diminished ability of Mr. Johnson's heart muscle to contract normally after he recovers from the heart attack.

WORD ANALYSIS AND DEFINITION

WORD	PRONUNCIATION	ELEMENTS		DEFINITION
coronary circulation	KOR-oh-nair-ee SER-kyu-LAY-shun	S/ R/	-ary *pertaining to* coron- *crown*	Blood flow through the vessels supplying the heart
endocardium endocardial (adj)	EN-doh-KAR-dee-um EN-doh-KAR-dee-al	S/ P/ R/	-um *structure* endo- *inside* -cardi- *heart*	The inside lining of the heart
epicardium	EP-ih-kar-DEE-um	S/ P/ R/	-um *structure* epi- *upon, above* -cardi- *heart*	The outer layer of the heart wall
fibrosis fibrotic (adj)	fie-BROH-sis fie-BROT-ik	S/ R/CF	-sis *condition* fibr/o- *fiber*	Repair of dead tissue cells by formation of fibrous tissue
infarct infarction	in-FARKT in-FARK-shun	S/ P/ R/	-ion *process* in- *in* -farct- *stuff*	Area of cell death resulting from an infarction Sudden blockage of an artery
ischemia ischemic (adj)	is-KEE-me-ah is-KEE-mik	R/ R/	-emia *blood* isch- *to keep back*	Lack of blood supply to a tissue
lubricant	LOO-bri-cant	S/ R/	-ant *forming* lubric- *make slippery*	Substance for reducing friction
myocardium myocardial (adj)	MY-oh-KAR-dee-um MY-oh-KAR-dee-al	S/ R/CF R/ S/	-um *structure* my/o- *muscle* -cardi- *heart* -al *pertaining to*	All the heart muscle
necrosis necrotic (adj)	neh-KROH-sis neh-KROT-ik	S/ R/ S/ R/CF	-osis *condition* necr- *death* -tic *pertaining to* necr/o- *death*	Pathologic death of tissue or cells Affected by necrosis
parietal	pah-RYE-eh-tal	S/ R/	-al *pertaining to* pariet- *wall*	Pertaining to the outer layer of the pericardium and other body cavities
pericardium pericardial (adj)	per-ih-KAR-dee-um per-ih-KAR-dee-al	S/ P/ R/ S/	-um *structure* peri- *around* -cardi- *heart* -al *pertaining to*	Structure around the heart
pulmonary	PULL-moh-nar-ee	S/ R/	-ary *pertaining to* pulmon- *lung*	Pertaining to the lungs and their blood supply
systemic	sis-TEM-ik	S/ R/	-ic *pertaining to* system- *body as a whole*	Relating to the entire organism
visceral	VISS-er-al	S/ R/	-al *pertaining to* viscer- *an organ*	Pertaining to the internal organs

EXERCISES

Deconstruct the following medical terms into their basic elements by filling in the chart. Knowledge of elements will help increase your medical vocabulary.

Medical Term	Prefix	Root/CF	Suffix	Meaning of Term
myocardium				
infarction				
endocardium				
visceral				
parietal				
ischemia				
pericardium				

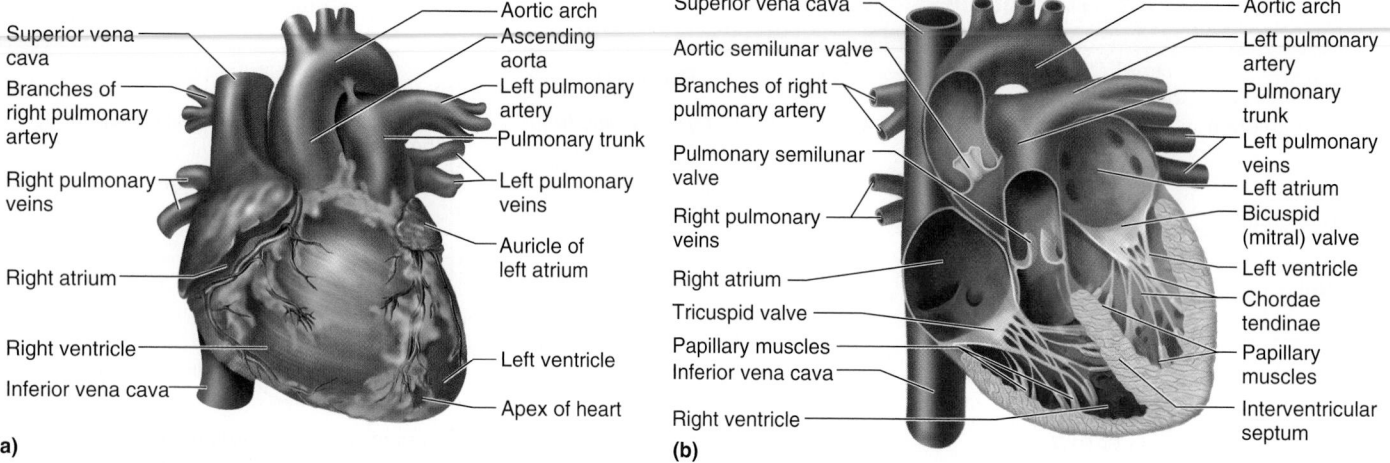

(a)

Superior vena cava
Branches of right pulmonary artery
Right pulmonary veins
Right atrium
Right ventricle
Inferior vena cava

Aortic arch
Ascending aorta
Left pulmonary artery
Pulmonary trunk
Left pulmonary veins
Auricle of left atrium
Left ventricle
Apex of heart

(b)

Superior vena cava
Aortic semilunar valve
Branches of right pulmonary artery
Pulmonary semilunar valve
Right pulmonary veins
Right atrium
Tricuspid valve
Papillary muscles
Inferior vena cava
Right ventricle

Aortic arch
Left pulmonary artery
Pulmonary trunk
Left pulmonary veins
Left atrium
Bicuspid (mitral) valve
Left ventricle
Chordae tendinae
Papillary muscles
Interventricular septum

▲ **FIGURE 8.4 External (a) and Internal (b) Anatomy of the Heart: Frontal View.**

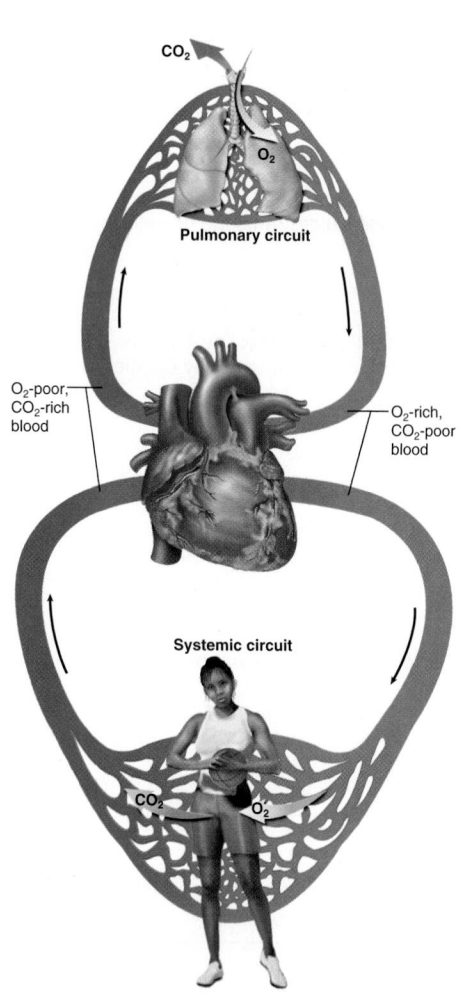

CO₂
O₂
Pulmonary circuit
O₂-poor, CO₂-rich blood
O₂-rich, CO₂-poor blood
Systemic circuit
CO₂
O₂

▲ **FIGURE 8.5 General Schematic of the Cardiovascular Circulation**

Keynote

The pulmonary circulation is the only place in the body where deoxygenated blood is carried in arteries and oxygenated blood is carried in veins.

BLOOD FLOW THROUGH THE HEART

The heart has four chambers *(Figure 8.4b)*:

1. Right **atrium**
2. Right **ventricle**
3. Left atrium
4. Left ventricle

The right and left sides of the heart are separated by the cardiac **septum,** which can be described in two sections:

- The right and left atria are separated by a thin muscle wall called the **interatrial** septum.
- The right and left ventricles are separated by a thicker muscle wall called the **interventricular** septum.
- In addition, the **atrioventricular (AV) septum** is located between and behind the right atrium and left ventricle.

Blood circulates around the body (through the systemic circulation) to unload oxygen and nutrients and pick up carbon dioxide and metabolic waste products. This **deoxygenated** blood returns to the heart via the **superior and inferior venae cavae.** These large veins open into the right atrium. When the right atrium contracts, the blood flows through the **tricuspid valve** into the right ventricle. The tricuspid valve then shuts so that, when the right ventricle contracts, blood cannot flow back into the atrium.

When the right ventricle contracts, the blood is pushed out through the **semilunar pulmonary valve** into the **pulmonary trunk** *(Figure 8.4a and b)* to begin the pulmonary circulation. The pulmonary valve then shuts to prevent blood flowing back into the ventricle. The pulmonary trunk divides into two arteries; the right pulmonary artery goes to the right lung, and the left pulmonary artery goes to the left lung. In the lungs, carbon dioxide is unloaded and oxygen is picked up from the air by the blood. The oxygen-rich blood is returned to the heart by the pulmonary veins *(Figure 8.4a and b)*.

The blood from the pulmonary veins flows into the left atrium. When the atrium contracts, the blood flows through the **mitral** (or **bicuspid**) valve into the left ventricle. The bicuspid valve then shuts so that blood cannot flow back into the left atrium when the ventricle contracts.

When the left ventricle contracts, the oxygenated blood is forced out under pressure through the **aortic** semilunar valve into the **aorta,** to return to circulating round the body in the systemic circulation *(Figure 8.5)*. The aortic valve then shuts so that blood cannot flow back into the left ventricle. The four valves all allow the blood to flow only in one direction.

The bicuspid and tricuspid valves are anchored to the floor of the ventricles by stringlike **chordae tendineae** *(Figure 8.4b)*.

WORD	PRONUNCIATION		ELEMENTS	DEFINITION
aorta **aortic** (adj)	a-**OR**-tuh a-**OR**-tic		Greek *lift up*	Main trunk of the systemic arterial system
atrium **atria** (pl) **atrial** (adj)	**A**-tree-um **A**-tree-ah **A**-tree-al		Latin *entrance*	Chamber where blood enters the heart on both right and left sides
atrioventricular (AV)	**A**-tree-oh-ven-**TRICK**-you-lar	S/ R/CF R/	-ar *pertaining to* atri/o- *entrance, atrium* -ventricul- *ventricle*	Pertaining to both the atrium and the ventricle
bicuspid	by-**KUSS**-pid	S/ P/ R/	-id *having a particular quality* bi- *two* -cusp- *point*	Having two points; a bicuspid heart valve has two flaps
chordae tendineae	**KOR**-dee ten-**DIN**-ee		Latin *cord* Latin *tendon*	Tendinous cords attaching the bicuspid and tricuspid valves to the heart wall
interatrial	**IN**-ter-**AY**-tree-al	S/ P/ R/	-al *pertaining to* inter- *between* -atri- *atrium, entrance*	Between the atria of the heart
interventricular	**IN**-ter-ven-**TRIK**-you-lar	S/ P/ R/	-ar *pertaining to* inter- *between* -ventricul- *ventricle*	Between the ventricles of the heart
mitral	**MY**-tral		Latin *turban*	Shaped like the headdress of a Catholic bishop
semilunar	sem-ee-**LOO**-nar	S/ P/ R/	-ar *pertaining to* semi- *half* -lun- *moon*	Appears like a half moon
septum **septa** (pl)	**SEP**-tum **SEP**-tah		Latin *partition*	A wall dividing two cavities
tricuspid	try-**KUSS**-pid	S/ P/ R/	-id *having a particular quality* tri- *three* -cusp- *point*	Having three points; a tricuspid heart valve has three flaps
vena cava **venae cavae** (pl)	**VEE**-nah **KAY**-vah **VEE**-nee **KAY**-vee	R/CF R/	ven/a *vein* cava *cave*	One of the two largest veins in the body
ventricle	**VEN**-trih-kel		Latin *small belly*	Chamber of the heart or brain

EXERCISES

Plurals of medical terms follow certain established rules. Apply these rules and change the singular forms into plurals. Then write one sentence for either the singular or plural term.

1. Singular: atrium   Plural: _____

   Sentence: _____

2. Singular: septum   Plural: _____

   Sentence: _____

3. Singular: vena cava   Plural: _____

   Sentence: _____

4 Singular: ventricle   Plural: _____

   Sentence: _____

FIGURE 8.6
Ventricular Systole.

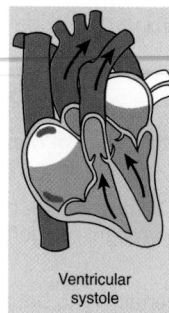

Ventricular systole

THE CARDIAC CYCLE

The action of the four heart chambers is coordinated. When the atria contract (atrial **systole**), the ventricles relax (ventricular **diastole,** or ventricular filling). When the atria relax (atrial diastole), the ventricles contract (ventricular systole) *(Figure 8.6)*. Then the atria and ventricles all relax briefly. This series of events is a complete cardiac cycle, or heartbeat.

The "*lub*-dub, *lub*-dub" sounds heard through the stethoscope are made by the snap of the heart valves as they close.

If there is an abnormality in valve closure, it will produce an added-on, abnormal sound called a **murmur.**

Electrical Properties of the Heart

As the cardiac muscles contract, they generate a small electrical current. Because the muscle cells are coupled together electrically, they stimulate their neighbor cells so that the myocardium of the atria, and that of the ventricles, each acts as a *single* unit.

To keep the heart beating in a rhythm, a **conduction system** is in place. It consists of five components *(Figure 8.7)*:

1. A small region of specialized muscle cells in the right atrium initiates the electrical current and therefore the heartbeat. This area is called the **sinoatrial (SA) node.** It is the **pacemaker** of heart rhythm.

2. Electrical signals from the SA node spread out through the atria and then come back together at the **atrioventricular (AV) node.** This is the electrical gateway to the ventricles, and normally electrical currents cannot get to the ventricles by any other route.

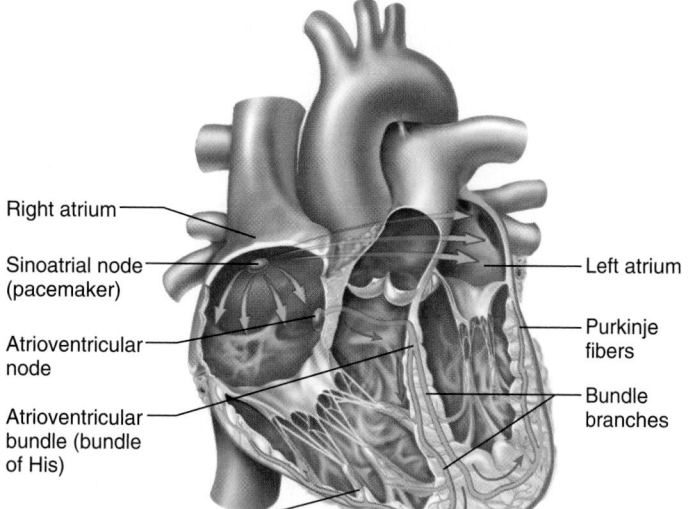

Right atrium

Sinoatrial node (pacemaker)

Atrioventricular node

Atrioventricular bundle (bundle of His)

Purkinje fibers

Left atrium

Purkinje fibers

Bundle branches

▲ **FIGURE 8.7 Cardiac Conduction System.**

Abbreviations	
AV	atrioventricular
SA	sinoatrial

Keynote

The normal rate of heartbeat is 60 to 80 beats per minute. A heart rate slower than 60 is called **bradycardia** *(Figure 8-8)*. A heart rate faster than 100 is called **tachycardia** *(Figure 8.9)*.

Keynote

The normal heartbeat with normal electrical conduction through the heart leading to a ventricular rate of around 60 to 80 beats per minute is called **sinus rhythm.** Any abnormal cardiac rhythm is called an **arrythmia** or a **dysrhythmia.**

3. Electrical signals leave the AV node to reach the ventricles through the atrioventricular bundle, called the **bundle of His.**

4. This AV bundle divides into the right and left **bundle branches,** which supply the two ventricles.

5. From the two bundle branches, **Purkinje fibers** spread through the ventricular myocardium and distribute the electrical stimuli to cause contraction of the ventricular myocardium.

An instrument called an electrocardiograph picks up the electrical changes in the heart muscle and amplifies them to record an electrocardiogram in the form of five waves *(Figure 8.10)*. The waves are labeled P, Q, R, S, and T.

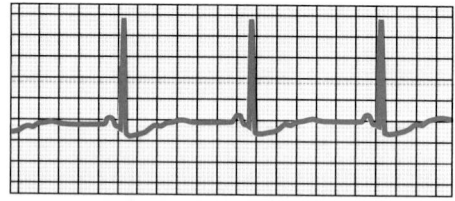

▲ **FIGURE 8.8 Bradycardia.**

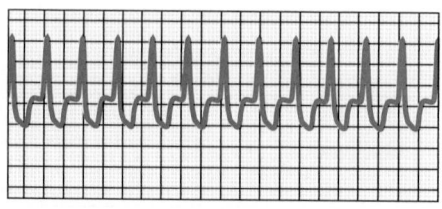

▲ **FIGURE 8.9 Tachycardia.**

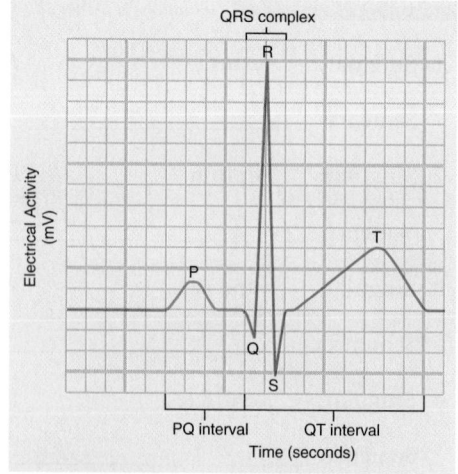

QRS complex

R

Electrical Activity (mV)

P

Q

S

T

PQ interval   QT interval

Time (seconds)

▲ **FIGURE 8.10 Normal Electrocardiogram.**

WORD ANALYSIS AND DEFINITION

WORD	PRONUNCIATION	ELEMENTS		DEFINITION
arrhythmia (note the double "rr")	a-**RITH**-me-ah	S/ P/ R/	-ia *condition* a- *without* -rrhythm- *rhythm*	An abnormal heart rhythm
atrioventricular (AV)	A-tree-oh-ven-**TRICK**-you-lar	S/ R/CF R/	-ar *pertaining to* atri/o- *entrance, atrium* -ventricul- *ventricle*	Pertaining to both the atrium and ventricle
bradycardia	brad-ee-**KAR**-dee-ah	S/ P/ R/	-ia *condition* brady- *slow* -card- *heart*	Slow heart rate (below 60 beats per minute)
bundle of His	**BUN**-del of HISS		Wilhelm His, 1831–1904, Swiss anatomist	Pathway for electrical signals to be transmitted to the ventricles
conduction	kon-**DUCK**-shun	S/ P/ R/	-ion *process* con- *together, with* -duct- *lead*	Process of transmitting energy
diastole diastolic (adj)	die-**AS**-toe-lee die-as-**TOL**-ik		Greek *dilation*	Dilation of heart cavities, during which they fill with blood
dysrhythmia (note the single "r")	dis-**RITH**-me-ah	S/ P/ R/	-ia *condition* dys- *bad, difficult* -rhythm- *rhythm*	An abnormal heart rhythm
murmur	**MUR**-mur		Latin *low voice*	Abnormal heart sound heard on auscultation of the heart or blood vessels
pacemaker	**PACE**-may-ker	S/ R/	-maker *one who makes* pace- *step, pace*	Device that regulates cardiac electrical activity
Purkinje fibers	per-**KIN**-jee fi-**BERS**		Johannes von Purkinje, Bohemian anatomist and physiologist, 1787–1869	Network of nerve fibers in the myocardium
sinoatrial (SA) node	sigh-noh-**AY**-tree-al NODE	S/ R/CF R/	-al *pertaining to* sin/o- *sinus* -atri- *entrance, atrium*	The center of modified cardiac muscle fibers in the wall of the right atrium that acts as the pacemaker for the heart rhythm
sinus rhythm	**SIGH**-nus **RITH**-um		**sinus** *channel, cavity* **rhythm** Greek *to flow*	The normal (optimal) heart rhythm arising from the sinoatrial node
systole systolic (adj)	**SIS**-toe-lee sis-**TOL**-ik		Greek *contraction*	Contraction of the heart muscle
tachycardia	tak-ih-**KAR**-dee-ah	S/ P/ R/	-ia *condition* tachy- *rapid* -card- *heart*	Rapid heart rate (above 100 beats per minute)

EXERCISES

Both of the following terms have similar roots and suffixes, but the prefixes make the difference. Deconstruct each term using slashes; then provide a meaning for each element on the line. Analyze the terms, and explain how they are different.

1. bradycardia: _____ / _____ / _____

                                                P   R   S

Meaning of bradycardia: _____

2. tachycardia: _____ / _____ / _____

                                                P   R   S

Meaning of tachycardia:_____

3. The difference between bradycardia and tachycardia is _____

_____

_____ .

DISORDERS OF THE HEART

Abnormal Heart Rhythms

Arrhythmias are abnormal or irregular heartbeats, and four types are commonly seen:

1. **Premature** beats may originate in either the atrium and the ventricle or both, may occur in individuals of all ages, and may be associated with caffeine and stress.

2. **Atrial fibrillation** occurs when the two atria quiver rather than contract in an organized fashion to pump blood into the ventricle. This causes blood to pool in the atria and sometimes clot. **Paroxysmal atrial tachycardia (PAT)** presents with periods of rapid, regular heartbeats that originate in the atrium. The episodes begin and end abruptly. The heart rate speeds up to 160 to 200 beats per minute.

3. **Ventricular arrhythmias** consist of several types. **Ventricular tachycardia** is a rapid heartbeat arising in the ventricles. **Premature ventricular contractions (PVCs)** occur when extra impulses arise from a ventricle. **Ventricular fibrillation (V-fib)** is characterized by ventricles going out of control, quivering, and beating ineffectively instead of pumping.

4. **Heart block** occurs when interference in cardiac electrical conduction causes the contractions of the atria to fail to coordinate with the contractions of the ventricles.

Palpitations are unpleasant sensations of a rapid or irregular heartbeat that last a few seconds or minutes. They can be brought on by exercise, anxiety, and stimulants like caffeine. Occasionally they can be due to an arrhythmia.

The arrhythmias can be treated with medications, but some patients require mechanical **pacemakers.** These artificial pacemakers consist of a battery, electronic circuits, and computer memory to generate electronic signals. The signals are carried along thin, insulated wires to the heart muscle. The most common need for a pacemaker is a very slow heart rate (bradycardia).

People with life-threatening arrhythmias may need an **implantable cardioverter/defibrillator (ICD),** which senses abnormal rhythms and gives the heart a small electrical shock to return the rhythm to normal.

In emergency situations, external **cardioversion** is performed through **automatic external defibrillators (AEDs)** *(Figure 8.11)* that send an electrical shock to the heart to restore a normal contraction rhythm.

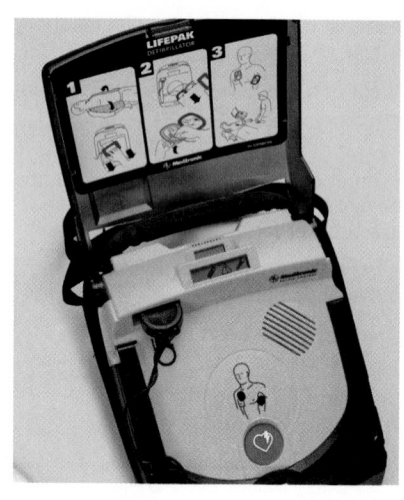

▲ **FIGURE 8.11 Automatic External Defibrillator.**

WORD ANALYSIS AND DEFINITION

WORD	PRONUNCIATION	ELEMENTS		DEFINITION
cardioversion (also called **defibrillation**)	**KAR**-dee-oh-**VER**-shun	S/ R/CF R/	**-ion** *action, process* **cardi/o-** *heart* **-vers-** *turn*	Restoration of a normal heart rhythm by electrical shock
cardioverter	**KAR**-dee-oh-**VER**-ter			Device used to generate electrical shock
defibrillation	dee-fib-rih-**LAY**-shun	S/ P/ R/	**-ation** *process* **de-** *without, away from* **-fibrill-** *small fiber*	Restoration of uncontrolled twitching of cardiac muscle fibers to normal rhythm
defibrillator	dee-fib-rih-**LAY**-tor	S/	**-ator** *instrument*	Instrument for defibrillation
fibrillation	fi-brih-**LAY**-shun	S/ R/	**-ation** *process* **fibrill-** *small fiber*	Uncontrolled quivering or twitching of the heart muscle
implantable	im-**PLAN**-tah-bul	S/ P/ R/	**-able** *capable of* **im-** *in* **-plant-** *insert*	Able to be inserted into tissues
pacemaker	**PACE**-may-ker	S/ R/	**-maker** *one who makes* **pace-** *step, pace*	Device that regulates cardiac electrical activity
palpitation	pal-pih-**TAY**-shun	S/ R/	**-ation** *process* **palpit-** *throb*	Forcible, rapid beat of the heart felt by the patient
paroxysmal	par-ock-**SIZ**-mal	S/ R/	**-al** *pertaining to* **paroxysm-** *irritation*	Occurring in sharp, spasmodic episodes

EXERCISES

The definitions for the medical terms in this Word Analysis and Definition (WAD) box are given to you—break the term down into its basic elements. Notice in particular which terms do not have prefixes or suffixes. Every term must have a root and/or combining form.

1. Forceful, rapid beat of the heart   _____ / _____ / _____
    P   R/CF   S

2. Uncontrolled heart muscle twitching   _____ / _____ / _____
    P   R/CF   S

3. Changes abnormal rhythm to normal   _____ / _____ / _____
    P   R/CF   S

4. Device inserted into body tissues   _____ / _____ / _____
    P   R/CF   S

5. Sharp, spasmodic episodes   _____ / _____ / _____
    P   R/CF   S

6. Device that regulates cardiac electrical activity _____ / _____ / _____
    P   R/CF   S

7. What is another term for cardioversion? _____

8. What are the only terms in the WAD that contain all three elements? _____ and _____

Use one of the terms in a sentence that is not a definition.

9. Sentence: _____

_____

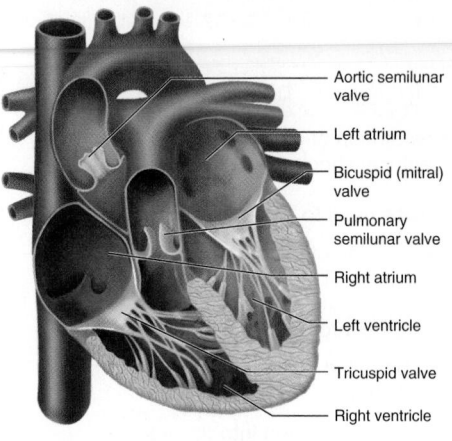

Aortic semilunar valve
Left atrium
Bicuspid (mitral) valve
Pulmonary semilunar valve
Right atrium
Left ventricle
Tricuspid valve
Right ventricle

▲ **FIGURE 8.12   Heart Valves.**

DISORDERS OF THE HEART (continued)

Disorders of the Heart Valves

Heart valves can **malfunction** in two basic ways:

1. **Stenosis** occurs when the valve does not open fully, and its opening is narrowed (constricted). Blood cannot flow freely through the valve and accumulates behind the valve.

2. **Incompetence** or **insufficiency** occurs when the valve cannot close fully, and blood can **regurgitate** (flow back) through the valve to the chamber from which it started.

Mitral valve stenosis can occur following rheumatic fever. Because the blood cannot flow freely through the valve, the left atrium becomes dilated. Eventually, **chronic heart failure** results. (*Figure 8.12* enables you to review the locations of the valves and chambers.)

Mitral valve incompetence occurs when there is leakage back through the valve as the left ventricle contracts. The left atrium becomes dilated. Again, chronic heart failure results.

Mitral valve prolapse occurs when the cusps of the valve bulge back into the left atrium when the left ventricle contracts. This allows blood to flow back into the atrium.

A prolapsed or incompetent mitral valve can often be repaired. If a valve replacement is necessary, there are two types of artificial valves to choose from:

1. **A mechanical (prosthetic) valve.** Various models and designs are made from different metal alloys and plastics.

2. **Tissue valve.** This can come from a pig or cow (occasionally from a human), or a valve can be constructed of tissue from the patient's own pericardium.

Aortic valve stenosis is common in the elderly when the valves become calcified due to **atherosclerosis.** Blood flow into the systemic circuit is diminished, leading to dizziness and fainting. The left ventricle dilates, hypertrophies, and ultimately fails.

Aortic valve incompetence initially produces few symptoms other than a murmur, but eventually the left ventricle fails.

Rheumatic fever is an inflammatory disease. If a sore throat caused by group A beta-hemolytic streptococcus *(see Chapter 20)* is not treated with a complete course of antibiotics, antibodies to the bacteria can develop and attack normal tissue. Multiple joints are inflamed, and an endocarditis can affect the function of the heart valves, particularly the mitral and aortic valves.

Disorders of the Heart Wall

Endocarditis is inflammation of the lining of the heart. It is usually secondary to an infection elsewhere. Intravenous drug users and people with damaged heart valves are at high risk for endocarditis.

Myocarditis is inflammation of the heart muscle. It can be bacterial, viral, or fungal in origin or a complication of other diseases such as influenza.

Pericarditis is inflammation of the covering of the heart. The inflammation causes an exudate (pericardial **effusion**) to be released into the pericardial space. This interferes with the heart's ability to contract and expand normally, and cardiac output falls—a condition called **cardiac tamponade.**

Cardiomyopathy is a weakening of the heart muscle that causes it to pump inadequately. The etiology can be viral, idiopathic (when the cause is unknown), or alcoholic. It causes **cardiomegaly** and heart failure.

WORD	PRONUNCIATION	ELEMENTS		DEFINITION
cardiomegaly	**KAR**-dee-oh-**MEG**-ah-lee	S/ R/CF	-megaly *enlargement* cardi/o- *heart*	Enlargement of the heart
cardiomyopathy	**KAR**-dee-oh-my-**OP**-ah-thee	S/ R/CF R/CF	-pathy *disease* cardi/o- *heart* -my/o- *muscle*	Disease of heart muscle, the myocardium
cor pulmonale	KOR pul-moh-**NAH**-lee	S/ R/ R/	-ale *pertaining to* cor *heart* pulmon- *lung*	Right-sided heart failure arising from chronic lung disease
effusion	eh-**FYU**-shun		Latin *pouring out*	Collection of fluid that has escaped from blood vessels into a cavity or tissues
endocarditis	**EN**-doh-kar-**DIE**-tis	S/ P/ R/	-itis *inflammation* endo- *within* -card- *heart*	Inflammation of the lining of the heart
incompetence	in-**KOM**-peh-tense	S/ P/ R/	-ence *quality of* in- *not* -compet- *strive together*	Failure of valves to close completely
insufficiency	in-suh-**FISH**-en-see	S/ P/ R/CF	-ency *quality of* in- *not* -suffic/i- *enough*	Lack of completeness of function; in the heart, failure of a valve to close properly
malfunction	mal-**FUNK**-shun	S/ P/ R/	-ion *action, condition* mal- *bad, inadequate* -funct- *perform*	Inadequate or abnormal function
myocarditis	**MY**-oh-kar-**DIE**-tis	S/ R/CF R/	-itis *inflammation* my/o- *muscle* -card- *heart*	Inflammation of the heart muscle
pericarditis	**PER**-ih-kar-**DIE**-tis	S/ P/ R/	-itis *inflammation* peri- *around* -card- *heart*	Inflammation of the pericardium, the covering of the heart
prolapse	pro-**LAPS**		Latin *a falling*	The falling or slipping of a body part from its normal position
prosthesis prosthetic (adj)	**PROS**-thee-sis pros-**THET**-ik		Greek *an addition*	A manufactured substitute for a missing or diseased part of the body
regurgitate	ree-**GUR**-jih-tate	S/ P/ R/	-ate *pertaining to* re- *back* -gurgit- *flood*	To flow backward; in this case, through a heart valve
stenosis	steh-**NOH**-sis	S/ R/CF	-sis *abnormal condition* sten/o- *narrow*	Narrowing of a canal or passage, as in the narrowing of a heart valve
tamponade	tam-po-**NAID**	S/ R/	-ade *process* tampon- *plug*	Pathologic compression of an organ such as the heart

EXERCISES

Use your knowledge of the **language of cardiology** to match the description in the left column with the correct medical term in the right column. Fill in the blanks.

_____ 1. Weakening of heart muscle

_____ 2. Inflammation that causes exudates

_____ 3. Cusps of valve bulge back into atrium

_____ 4. Constricted valve opening

_____ 5. Failure of right ventricle to pump properly

_____ 6. Cardiomyopathy can be the cause

_____ 7. Causes valve regurgitation

_____ 8. Inflammatory disease that affects the heart

A. incompetence

B. cardiomegaly

C. cor pulmonale

D. pericarditis

E. rheumatic fever

F. cardiomyopathy

G. prolapse

H. stenosis

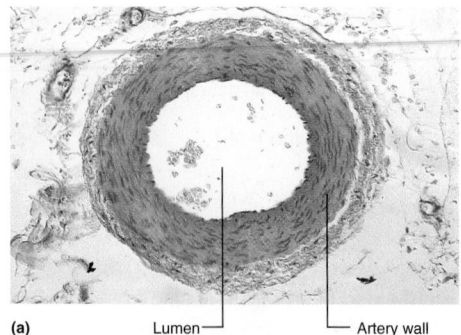

(a) Lumen — Artery wall

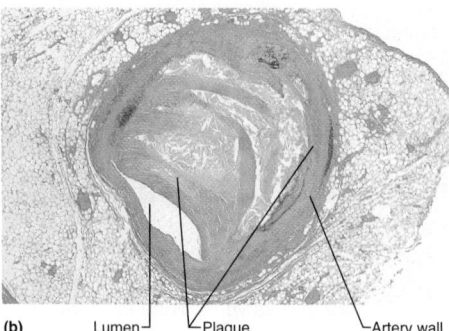

(b) Lumen — Plaque — Artery wall

▲ **FIGURE 8.13   Arterial Structure.**
(*a*) Normal coronary artery. (*b*) Advanced atherosclerosis.

Abbreviations

ASHD arteriosclerotic heart disease
CAD coronary artery disease
MI   myocardial infarction

Keynote

All these risk factors can be reduced by changes in lifestyle.

Keynote

Cardiac arrest is the sudden cessation of cardiac activity resulting from **anoxia**. The ECG shows a flat line, **asystole** (*Figure 8.14*).

DISORDERS OF THE HEART (continued)
Coronary Artery Disease (CAD)

The arteries supplying the myocardium become narrowed by atherosclerotic **plaques,** called **atheroma.** As the atheroma increases, the lumen of the artery becomes more and more narrow (*compare Figure 8.13a and b*). The blood supplied to the cardiac muscle by the artery is reduced. Platelet aggregation can occur on the plaque to form a blood clot (**coronary thrombosis**). Atherosclerosis is the most common form of **arteriosclerosis** (hardening of the arteries) and can lead to **arteriosclerotic heart disease (ASHD).**

Angina pectoris, pain in the chest on exertion, is often the first symptom of reduced oxygen supply to the myocardium. The pain goes away if the exertion is stopped or if a **nitroglycerin** tablet is placed under the tongue (**sublingually**).

Myocardial infarction (MI) is the death of myocardial cells caused by the lack of blood supply (ischemia) when an artery eventually becomes blocked (**occluded**). Sudden, severe, crushing **substernal** or left chest pain is experienced. If the ischemia is not reversed within 4 to 6 hours, the muscle cells die (undergo **necrosis**).

Cardiogenic shock occurs when the heart fails to pump effectively and organs and tissues are **perfused** inadequately. The pulse is weak and rapid, and blood pressure drops. The patient becomes pale, cold, sweaty, and anxious.

The other form of circulatory shock is **hypovolemic shock,** in which there is a loss of blood volume, often from hemorrhage or dehydration.

Risk factors for CAD include:

- Obesity
- Lack of exercise (**sedentary**)
- Tobacco
- Diabetes mellitus
- High blood pressure (**hypertension**)
- Elevated serum cholesterol (*see Chapter 20*)
- Stress

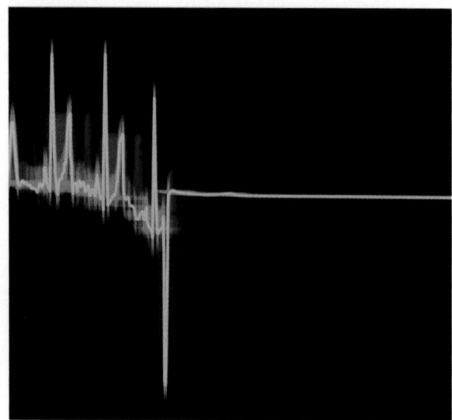

▲ **FIGURE 8.14   Electrocardiogram (ECG) Showing Asystole.**

WORD	PRONUNCIATION		ELEMENTS	DEFINITION
anoxia	an-**OCK**-see-ah	S/ P/ R/	-ia *condition* an- *without* -ox *oxygen*	Without oxygen
anoxic (adj)	an-**OCK**-sik	S/	-ic *pertaining to*	Pertaining to or suffering from a lack of oxygen
arteriosclerosis	ar-**TIER**-ee-oh-skler-**OH**-sis	S/ R/CF R/CF	-sis *abnormal condition* arteri/o- *artery* -scler/o- *hardness*	Hardening of the arteries
arteriosclerotic (adj)	ar-**TIER**-ee-oh-skler-**OT**-ik	S/	-tic *pertaining to*	Pertaining to or suffering from arteriosclerosis
asystole	a-**SIS**-toe-lee	P/ R/CF	a- *without* -systole/e *contraction*	Absence of contractions of the heart
atheroma	ath-er-**ROE**-mah	S/ R/	-oma *tumor* ather- *porridge, gruel*	Lipid deposit in the lining of an artery
atherectomy	ath-er-**EK**-toe-me	S/ R/CF	-ectomy *excision* ather/o- *porridge, gruel*	Surgical removal of the atheroma
atherosclerosis	**ATH**-er-oh-skler-**OH**-sis	S/ R/CF	-sis *abnormal condition* -scler/o- *hardness*	Atheroma in arteries
hypovolemic	**HIGH**-poh-vo-**LEE**-mick	S/ P/ R/	-emic *in the blood* hypo- *below* -vol- *volume*	Having decreased blood volume in the body
occlude (verb) occlusion (noun)	o-**KLUDE** o-**KLU**-zhun		Latin *to close*	To close, plug, or completely obstruct A complete obstruction
perfuse	per-**FYUSE**		Latin *to pour*	To force blood to flow through a lumen or a vascular bed
perfusion (noun)	per-**FYU**-shun	S/ R/	-ion *action, condition* perfus- *to pour*	The act of perfusing
plaque	PLAK		French *a plate*	Patch of abnormal tissue
sedentary	sed-en-**TER**-ee	S/ R/	-ary *pertaining to* sedent- *sitting*	Accustomed to little exercise or movement
sublingual	sub-**LING**-wal	S/ P/ R/	-al *pertaining to* sub- *under* -lingu- *tongue*	Underneath the tongue
substernal	sub-**STER**-nal	S/ P/ R/	-al *pertaining to* sub- *under* -stern- *breastbone*	Under the sternum or breastbone

EXERCISES

Consult this WAD for the best medical terms to complete the following sentences in patient documentation. Fill in the blanks.

1. His _____ (little exercise or movement) lifestyle, coupled with obesity, increases his risk factors for a heart attack.

2. Schedule the patient for a(n) _____ (surgical removal of lipid deposit in artery lining) as soon as possible.

3. _____ (absence of heart contractions) occurred at 2251 hrs, and the patient was pronounced dead.

4. Angioplasty showed a large clot _____ (completely obstructing) her left coronary artery.

5. The bullet entered his left _____ (under the breastbone) area and exited his back.

6. The patient's diagnostic studies show clear evidence of _____ (patch of abnormal tissue) in a coronary heart artery.

7. Cardiogenic shock occurred, and the patient's tissues were not _____ (forcing blood through a vascular bed or lumen) adequately.

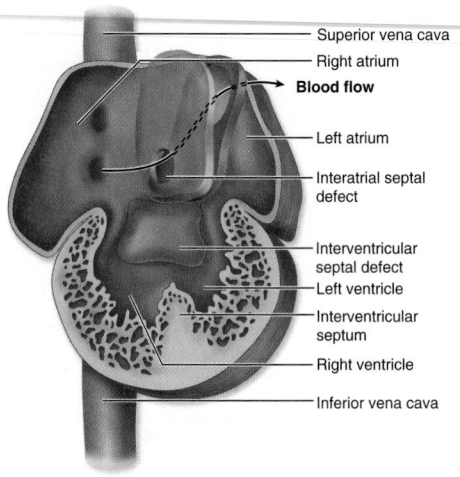

▲ **FIGURE 8.15 Atrial and Ventricular Septal Defects.**

Labels on figure:
Superior vena cava
Right atrium
Blood flow
Left atrium
Interatrial septal defect
Interventricular septal defect
Left ventricle
Interventricular septum
Right ventricle
Inferior vena cava

Keynote

All these risk factors can be reduced by changes in lifestyle.

Hypertension is the major cause of heart failure, stroke, and kidney failure.

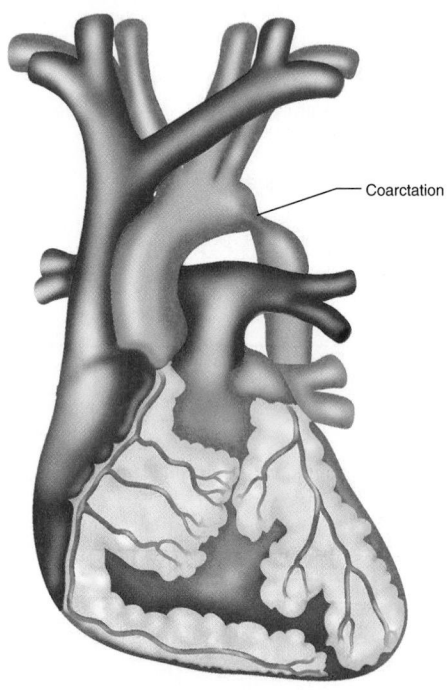

Label on figure: Coarctation

▲ **FIGURE 8.16 Coarctation of Aorta.**

Abbreviations

ASD	atrial septal defect
CHD	congenital heart disease
CHF	congestive heart failure
Hg	mercury
PDA	patent ductus arteriosus
SOB	shortness of breath
TOF	tetralogy of Fallot
VSD	ventricular septal defect

DISORDERS OF THE HEART (continued)

Hypertensive Heart Disease

Hypertension is the most common cardiovascular disorder in this country, affecting more than 20% of the adult population. It results from a prolonged elevated blood pressure throughout the vascular system. The high pressure forces the ventricles to work harder to pump blood. Eventually, the myocardium becomes strained and less efficient. It is the major cause of heart failure, stroke, and kidney failure.

High blood pressure is currently defined as a blood pressure reading at or above 140/90 mm **Hg** (mercury). A normal blood pressure is below 120/80 mm Hg. The first number, or **systolic** reading, reflects the blood pressure when the heart is contracting. The second number, or **diastolic** reading, reflects blood pressure when the heart is relaxed between contractions.

Primary (essential) hypertension is the most common type of hypertension. Its etiology is unknown. Its risk factors are:

- Overweight
- Tobacco
- Stress
- Lack of exercise
- Alcohol

Secondary hypertension results from other diseases such as kidney disease, atherosclerosis, and hyperthyroidism.

Malignant hypertension is a rare, severe, life-threatening form of hypertension in which the blood pressure reading can be greater than 200/120 mm Hg. Aggressive intervention is indicated to reduce the blood pressure.

Prehypertension, with a systolic pressure between 120 and 139 mm Hg and a diastolic pressure between 80 and 90 mm Hg, may indicate an increased risk for cardiovascular disease.

Congestive Heart Failure (CHF)

Congestive heart failure occurs with the inability of the heart to supply enough cardiac output to meet the body's metabolic needs. The patient shows shortness of breath (**SOB**) and **orthopnea.**

The most common conditions leading to CHF are:

- Cardiac ischemia
- Valvular regurgitation
- Cardiomyopathy
- Severe hypertension
- Aortic **stenosis**
- Chronic lung disease

Congenital Heart Disease (CHD)

Congenital heart disease is the result of abnormal development of the heart in the fetus.

Common congenital defects include:

- **Atrial septal defect (ASD).** A hole in the interatrial septum allows blood to **shunt** from the higher-pressure left atrium to the lower-pressure right atrium *(Figure 8.15)*.

- **Ventricular septal defect (VSD).** A hole in the interventricular septum allows blood to shunt from the higher-pressure left ventricle to the lower-pressure right ventricle *(see Figure 8.15)*.

- **Patent ductus arteriosus (PDA).** The ductus arteriosus is a normal blood vessel in the fetus that usually closes within 24 hours of birth. When the artery remains open (patent), blood can shunt from the aorta to the pulmonary artery, and the higher-pressure causes damage to the lungs.

- **Coarctation of the aorta.** This is a narrowing of the aorta shortly after the artery to the left arm branches from the aorta *(Figure 8.16)*. It causes **hypertension** in the arms behind the narrowing and **hypotension** in the lower limbs and organs like the kidney below the narrowing.

- **Tetralogy of Fallot (TOF).** This is a **syndrome** with four congenital heart defects. All these congenital abnormalities can be surgically repaired.

WORD	PRONUNCIATION	ELEMENTS		DEFINITION
coarctation	koh-ark-**TAY**-shun	S/ R/	-ation *process* coarct- *press together*	Constriction stenosis, particularly of the aorta
congenital	kon-**JEN**-ih-tal	S/ P/ R/	-al *pertaining to* con- *together, with* -genit- *bring forth*	Present at birth, either inherited or due to an event during gestation up to the moment of birth
defect	**DEE**-fect		Latin *to lack*	An absence, malformation, or imperfection
hypertension	**HIGH**-per-**TEN**-shun	S/ P/ R/	-ion *action, condition* hyper- *excessive* -tens- *pressure*	Persistent high arterial blood pressure
hypertensive hypotension prehypertension	**HIGH**-per-**TEN**-siv **HIGH**-poh-**TEN**-shun pree-**HIGH**-per-**TEN**-shun	S/ P/ P/	-ive *quality of* hypo- *low, below* pre- *before*	Suffering from hypertension Persistent low arterial blood pressure Precursor to hypertension
orthopnea	or-**THOP**-nee-ah	S/ R/CF	-pnea *breathe* orth/o- *straight*	Difficulty in breathing when lying flat
orthopneic (adj)	or-**THOP**-nee-ik	S/	-ic *pertaining to*	Pertaining to or affected by orthopnea
patent ductus arteriosus	**PAY**-tent **DUK**-tus ar-**TER**-ee-oh-sus	R/ R/ R/	patent *lie open* ductus *leading* arteriosus *like an artery*	An open, direct channel between the aorta and the pulmonary artery
shunt	SHUNT		Middle English *divert*	A bypass or diversion of fluid; in this case, blood
syndrome	**SIN**-drohm	P/ R/	syn- *together* -drome *running*	Combination of signs and symptoms associated with a particular disease process
tetralogy of Fallot (TOF)	teh-**TRAL**-oh-jee OF fah-**LOW**	 P/ S/	Etienne-Louis Fallot, French physician 1850–1911 tetra- *four* -logy *study of*	Set of four congenital heart defects occurring together

---

EXERCISES

Abbreviations need to be used carefully so that you communicate exactly what is necessary. The following sentences contain abbreviations—translate the abbreviations into their correct medical terms. Rewrite the sentences without the abbreviations, and convey the same message. Check your spelling!

1. ASD, TOF, VSD, and PDA are all examples of CHD.

2. CHF occurs with the inability of the heart to supply enough cardiac output to meet the body's metabolic needs.

3. High blood pressure is a reading at or above 140/90 mm Hg.

CARDIOLOGIC TESTS

Blood Tests

Lipid profile helps determine the risk of CAD and comprises:

- Total cholesterol
- **High-density lipoprotein (HDL)** ("good cholesterol")
- **Low-density lipoprotein (LDL)** ("bad cholesterol")
- **Triglycerides**

These are discussed in *Chapter 22*.

B-type natriuretic peptide (BNP), a brain hormone, is used to diagnose and monitor congestive heart failure and to predict the course of end-stage heart failure.

C-reactive protein (CRP), produced by the endothelial cells of arteries, has been identified as a risk factor for atherosclerosis and CAD.

Homocysteine is an amino acid in the blood. Elevated levels are related to a higher risk of CAD, stroke, and peripheral vascular disease.

Creatine kinase (CK) is an enzyme released into the blood by dead myocardial cells in MI.

Troponin I and T are part of a protein complex in muscle that is released into the blood during myocardial injury. Troponin I is found in heart muscle but not in skeletal muscle. Its presence in blood is therefore a highly sensitive indicator of a recent MI. Both CK and Troponin I and T are used to confirm a suspected MI.

Diagnostic Tests

Electrocardiogram (ECG or EKG) is a paper record of the electrical signals of your heart.

Cardiac stress testing is an exercise tolerance test to raise your heart rate and monitor the effect on cardiac function. **Nuclear imaging** of the heart, using an injection of a radioactive substance, can be used with the stress test.

Persantine/thallium exercise testing is used for people unable to engage in physical exercise. It combines nuclear imaging with a drug that increases the demand on the heart.

Echocardiography uses ultrasound waves to study cardiac function. The test is performed by a **sonographer,** who places a **transducer** on the patient's chest.

Transesophageal echocardiography (TEE) involves insertion of a small probe into the esophagus to record the anatomy and function of heart valves.

Holter monitor is a continuous ECG recorded on a tape recorder cassette as you work, play, and rest.

Event monitor is used for patients whose symptoms occur sporadically. A monitor is held over the chest when an event occurs. The data are stored and transmitted by telephone to a monitoring station.

Ambulatory blood pressure monitor provides a record of your blood pressure over a 24-hour period as you go about your daily activities.

Electron beam tomography (EBT) is a scan that identifies calcium deposits in arteries.

Magnetic resonance imaging (MRI) can produce detailed images of the heart and identify sections of cardiac muscle that are not receiving an adequate blood supply.

Cardiac catheterization detects patterns of pressures and blood flows in the heart. A thin tube is guided into the heart under x-ray guidance after being inserted into a vein or artery.

Coronary angiogram uses a contrast dye injected during cardiac catheterization to identify coronary artery blockages.

Abbreviations	
BNP	B-type natriuretic peptide
CK	creatine kinase
CRP	C-reactive protein
EBT	electron beam tomography
HDL	high-density lipoprotein
LDL	low-density lipoprotein
MRI	magnetic resonance imaging
TEE	transesophageal echocardiography

WORD ANALYSIS AND DEFINITION

S = Suffix   P = Prefix   R = Root   R/CF = Combining Form

WORD	PRONUNCIATION	ELEMENTS		DEFINITION
catheter	**KATH**-eh-ter		Greek *to send down*	Hollow tube that allows passage of fluid into or out of a body cavity, organ, or vessel
catheterize (verb)	**KATH**-eh-teh-**RIZE**	S/	**-ize** *action*	To introduce a catheter
		S/	**-er-** *agent*	
		R/	**cathet-** *catheter*	
catheterization (***Note:*** Unusual three suffixes.)	**KATH**-eh-ter-ih-**ZAY**-shun	S/	**-ation** *process*	Introduction of a catheter
creatine kinase	**KREE**-ah-teen **KI**-naze	S/	**-ine** *pertaining to*	Enzyme elevated in plasma following heart muscle damage in myocardial infarction
		R/	**creat-** *flesh*	
		S/	**-ase** *enzyme*	
		R/	**kin-** *motion*	
echocardiography	**EK**-oh-kar-dee-**OG**-rah-fee	S/	**-graphy** *process of recording*	Ultrasound recording of heart function
		R/CF	**ech/o-** *sound wave*	
		R/CF	**-cardi/o-** *heart*	
homocysteine	ho-moh-**SIS**-teen	P/	**homo-** *same*	An amino acid similar to cysteine
		R	**-cysteine** *an amino acid*	
lipoprotein	**LIE**-poh-pro-teen	R/CF	**lip/o-** *fat*	Molecules made of combinations of fat and protein
		R/	**-protein** *protein*	
natriuretic peptide	**NAH**-tree-you-**RET**-ik **PEP**-tide	S/	**-ic** *pertaining to*	Protein that increases the excretion of sodium
		R/CF	**natr/i-** *sodium*	
		R/	**-uret-** *ureter*	
		S/	**-ide** *having a particular quality*	
		R/	**pept-** *amino acid*	
sonograph	**SON**-oh-graf	S/	**-graph** *to record*	Instrument that uses sound waves to create images of structures
		R/CF	**son/o-** *sound*	
sonographer	so-**NOG**-rah-fer	S/	**-grapher** *one who records*	The technician who performs a sonogram
sonogram	**SON**-oh-gram	S/	**-gram** *a record*	Image obtained by using a sonograph
tomography	toe-**MOG**-rah-fee	S/	**-graphy** *process of recording*	Radiographic image of a selected slice of tissue
		R/CF	**tom/o-** *section, cut*	
transducer	trans-**DYU**-sir	P/	**trans-** *across*	Device that converts energy from one form to another
		R/	**-ducer** *to lead*	
triglyceride	tri-**GLISS**-eh-ride	S/	**-ide** *having a particular quality*	Any of a group of fats containing three fatty acids
		P/	**tri-** *three*	
		R/	**-glycer-** *glycerol*	

EXERCISES

Identify the type of element and its meaning in the appropriate column. The first one is done for you. Fill in the blanks.

Element	Meaning of Prefix	Meaning of Root/CF	Meaning of Suffix
ase			*Enzyme*
cardio			
creat			
echo			
graphy			
homo			
ide			

TREATMENT PROCEDURES

The most immediate need in the treatment of MI is to provide perfusion to get blood and oxygen to the affected myocardium. This can be attempted in several ways:

1. **Clot-busting drugs (thrombolysis).** Streptokinase or tissue plasminogen activator (**tPA**) are injected within a few hours of the MI to dissolve the thrombus.

2. **Artery-cleaning angioplasty (percutaneous transluminal coronary angioplasty [PTCA]).** A balloon-tipped catheter is guided to the site of the blockage and inflated to expand the artery from the inside by compressing the plaque against the walls of the artery.

3. **Stent placement.** To reduce the likelihood that the artery will close up again (occlude), a wire mesh tube, or stent, is placed inside the vessel. Some stents (**drug-eluting** stents) are covered with a special medication to help keep the artery open.

4. **Coronary artery bypass surgery (CABG).** Healthy blood vessels harvested from the leg, chest, or arm are used to detour the blood around blocked coronary arteries. This procedure is used mostly for people with extensive disease in several arteries. The procedure is performed using a heart-lung machine that pumps the recipient's blood through the machine to oxygenate it while surgery is performed. More recently, the procedure is being performed "off-pump" with the heart still beating.

5. **Rotational atherectomy.** A high-speed rotational device is used to "sand" away plaque. This procedure has limited acceptance.

Other procedures used in cardiology include:

- **Cardioversion (defibrillation).** An arrhythmia is converted back to a normal rhythm with an electrical shock.
- **Radiofrequency ablation.** A catheter with an electrode in its tip is guided into the heart and used to destroy the cells from which abnormal cardiac rhythms are originating.
- **Heart transplant.** The heart of a recently deceased person (donor) is transplanted to the recipient after the recipient's diseased heart has been removed. The immune characteristics of the donor and recipient have to be a close match *(see Chapter 15).*

Abbreviations

ACE angiotensin-converting enzyme
CABG coronary artery bypass graft
PTCA percutaneous transluminal coronary angioplasty
tPA tissue plasminogen activator

Cardiac Pharmacology

Clinically, six types of cardiac drugs are in use:

1. **Anticoagulants** are drugs that reduce susceptibility to thrombus formation. These include aspirin, warfarin (Coumadin), and heparin.

2. **Chronotropic drugs** alter the heart rate. Epinephrine (adrenaline), norepinephrine, and atropine increase the heart rate. Quinidine, procainamide, lidocaine, and propranolol slow the heart.

3. **Inotropic drugs** alter the contractions of the myocardium. Digitalis and its derivatives, digoxin and digitoxin, increase the strength of contractions of the myocardium, leading to increased cardiac output.

4. **Diuretics** indirectly affect the heart by stimulating urinary fluid loss to lessen the fluid volume with which the heart has to cope. Thiazides are an example. Diuril (chlorthiazide) is a thiazide diuretic. Lasix (furosemide) is a loop diuretic; Aldactone (spironolactone) is a potassium-sparing diuretic.

5. **Antiarrhythmics** change the electrical properties of the myocardial cells to restore normal rate and rhythm. Beta-blockers (**beta-adrenergic-blocking agents**) reduce the rate and strength of myocardial contraction and are used in treating arrhythmias.

6. **Vasodilators** relax smooth muscle in arterioles. For example, nitroglycerin dilates both peripheral and coronary blood vessels. **Calcium channel blockers** have the dual effect of reducing contractility and dilating coronary arteries. **Angiotensin-converting enzyme inhibitors** (**ACE** inhibitors) dilate arteries and veins and can be used to treat hypertension.

WORD	PRONUNCIATION		ELEMENTS	DEFINITION
ablation	ab-**LAY**-shun	S/ R/	-ion *process* **ablat-** *take away*	Removal of a tissue to destroy its function
adrenergic	ad-re-**NER**-jik	S/ R/ R/	-ic *pertaining to* **adren-** *adrenal gland* **-erg-** *work*	Relating to the autonomic nervous system
angioplasty	**AN**-jee-oh-**PLAS**-tee	S/ R/CF	-plasty *formation* **angi/o-** *blood vessel*	Recanalization of a blood vessel by surgery
angiotensin	an-jee-oh-**TEN**-sin	S/	-tensin *tense, taut*	An agent that constricts blood vessels
beta	**BAY**-tah		Greek	Second letter in the Greek alphabet
chronotropic	**KRONE**-oh-**TROH**-pic	S/ R/CF	-tropic *change* **chron/o-** *time*	Affecting the heart rate
diuretic	die-you-**RET**-ik	S/ P/ R/	-ic *pertaining to* **di-** *from dia—throughout* **-uret-** *urine, urination*	Agent that increases urine output
inotropic	**IN**-oh-**TROH**-pic	S/ R/	-tropic *change* **ino-** *sinew*	Affecting the contractility of cardiac muscle
stent	STENT		Charles Stent, English dentist, nineteenth century	Wire mesh tube used to keep arteries open

EXERCISES

Deconstruct the medical terms in this chart to their basic elements. Fill in the blanks.

Medical Term	Prefix	Root/CF	Suffix
angiotensin			
inotropic			
ablation			
diuretic			
adrenergic			
chronotropic			
angioplasty			

Choose any two terms from the table above, and use each in a sentence that is not a definition.

1. _____

   _____

2. _____

   _____

OBJECTIVES

To understand the etiologies and effects of Mrs. Jones's problems (see Case Report 8.2) and communicate with her and Dr. Bannerjee about them, you need to have the medical terminology and knowledge to be able to:

8.2.1 Explain the functions of the peripheral circulation.

8.2.2 Link the structure of the different blood vessels to their functions.

8.2.3 Identify the major arteries and veins in the body.

8.2.4 Explain the dynamics and control of blood flow.

8.2.5 Describe the effects of common disorders of the circulatory system on health.

You are

. . . a medical assistant working for Dr. Lokesh Bannerjee, a cardiologist in Fulwood Medical Center.

Your patient is

. . . Mrs. Martha Jones. You are documenting her medical record after Dr. Bannerjee interviewed, examined, and reported his findings back to Dr. Susan Lee, who referred Mrs. Jones to Dr. Bannerjee.

CASE REPORT 8.2

Documentation.

Fulwood Medical Center
Consultation Request and Report Form

Patient's Name: Jones, MARTHA   Age: 52
To: Dr. LOKESH BANNERJEE   Department: Cardiology
From: Dr. Susan Lee   Department: Primary Care
Patient's Location: FULWOOD MEDICAL CENTER
Type of Consultation Desired:
☐ Consultation Only
☐ Consulation and follow Jointly
☒ Accept in Transfer
Referring Diagnoses: CLAUDICATION, POSSIBLE DVT
Reason for Consultation: severe pain in both legs on walking

Signature: _____   Date: 2/21/10   Time 1105 hrs
Consultation Report: by Lokesh Bannerjee
Chief complaint: Pt. c/o severe pain in both legs on walking about 100 yards or climbing a flight of stairs. Pain is so severe she must stop and wait 5 mins. before she can go on. For the past two weeks she has noticed soreness and hardness along a vein in her left calf.
Past medical history: Known type 2 diabetic with hypertension, CAD, diabetic retinopathy, and OA of her hips and knees. Several episodes of ketoacidosis and one of pulmonary edema. Bariatric surgery performed 8 months prior at 275 lbs.
Medications: metformin, verapamil, propanolol, Mevacor
Allergies: NKA
Physical examination: Ht: 5'2" Wt: 190 lbs. BP: 170/100 sitting. P: 80, regular. Both feet show slight pitting edema and skin is pale, cold, and dry. Small ulcer on lateral margin of each big toe. Varicosities, both legs. Tender cord in superficial vein of left calf. Flexion of left foot produces pain in left calf. Chest clear. Heart sounds unremarkable. No loss of sensation in legs or feet.
Impression: 1. Varicose veins, both legs.
       2. severe claudication, both legs.
       3. probable deep vein thrombosis, left leg
       4. possible peripheral neuropathy
       5. H/o diabetes type 2, CAD, hypertension, retinopathy, OA
Plan: Admit patient to cardiology unit stat for IV heparin and conversion to oral anticoagulant therapy with Coumadin. Doppler studies, venogram, and angiogram have been ordered.

Signature: _____   Date 2/21/10   Time 1250 hrs

ORDER # 267116 ANDRUS CLINI-REC ® PRIMARY CARE CHARTING SYSTEM • © BIBBERO SYSTEMS, INC. • PETALUMA, CA
TO REORDER CALL TOLL FREE: (800) BIBBERO (800-242-9330)   MFG IN U.S.A.

WORD	PRONUNCIATION	ELEMENTS		DEFINITION
angiogram	**AN**-jee-oh-gram	S/ R/CF	**-gram** *a record* **angi/o-** *blood vessel*	Radiograph obtained after injection of radiopaque contrast material into blood vessels
artery	**AR**-ter-ee		Greek *artery*	Thick-walled blood vessel carrying blood away from the heart
circulation	ser-kyu-**LAY**-shun		Latin *to encircle*	Continuous movement of blood through the heart and blood vessels
claudication	klaw-dih-**KAY**-shun	S/ R/	**-ation** *process* **claudic-** *limping*	Intermittent leg pain and limping
diffuse diffusion	dih-**FUSE** dih-**FYU**-zhun		Latin *to pull in different directions*	To disseminate or spread out The means by which small particles move between tissues
Doppler	**DOP**-ler		Johann Doppler, Austrian mathematician and physicist, 1803–1853	Diagnostic instrument that sends an ultra-sonic beam into the body
hemodynamics	**HE**-moh-die-**NAM**-iks	S/ R/CF R/	**-ics** *knowledge of* **hem/o-** *blood* **-dynam-** *power*	The science of the blood flow through the circulation
varix varices (pl) varicose (adj) varicosities	**VAIR**-iks **VAIR**-ih-sees **VAIR**-ih-kos vair-ih-**KOS**-ih-tees	S/ R/	Latin *dilated vein* **-ose** *full of* **varic-** *dilated, tortuous vein*	Dilated, tortuous vein Characterized by varices Collection of varicose veins
vein venogram venous (adj)	VANE **VEE**-noh-gram **VEE**-nuss	S/ R/CF S/	Latin *vein* **-gram** *a record* **ven/o-** *vein* **-ous** *pertaining to*	Blood vessel carrying blood toward heart Radiograph of veins after injection of radiopaque contrast material Pertaining to venous blood or the venous circulation

FUNCTIONS OF THE PERIPHERAL CIRCULATION

The peripheral **circulation** fulfills a number of functions:

1. **Carries blood.** The blood vessels carry oxygenated blood that the heart has pumped to all the tissues of the body and then return the deoxygenated blood to the heart.

2. **Transports.** The peripheral circulation carries oxygen, nutrients, hormones, and enzymes that **diffuse** from the blood into the cells. Waste products and carbon dioxide diffuse back from the cells into the peripheral circulation and are carried to the lungs, liver, and kidney for excretion.

3. **Maintains homeostasis.** The peripheral circulation directs blood flow to tissues to enable them to meet their metabolic needs. This determines the speed of delivery of oxygen and nutrients and the speed of waste removal. The principles of blood flow are called **hemodynamics.**

4. **Regulates blood pressure.** The ability of the **arteries** in the peripheral circulation to expand and contract in coordination with the systole and diastole of the heartbeat maintains a steady flow of blood and blood pressure to the tissues.

EXERCISES

Terms from this WAD can all be correctly inserted into the following paragraph of radiology documentation. Watch your singular and plural forms of terms. Fill in the blanks.

veins	varicosities	varix	vein	varicose	varices	venogram

1. The _____ performed on this patient's left saphenous and popliteal _____ shows the following: One slightly engorged and dilated _____ at the midpoint of the saphenous _____ and several _____ at the terminal end of the popliteal. Diagnosis: _____ veins. These _____ need immediate attention by a vascular surgeon.

2. This can be described as a **hemo**_____ study of the patient's _____.

There are two major circulations, the **pulmonary** and the **systemic.**

Pulmonary Circulation

Deoxygenated blood from the body flows into the right atrium of the heart and then into the right ventricle that pumps it out into the pulmonary trunk *(Figure 8.17)*. This trunk branches into the right pulmonary artery to the right lung and the left pulmonary artery to the left lung. Gas exchange occurs between the air in the lungs and blood *(see Chapter 9)*. Carbon dioxide is removed from the blood and excreted into the air. Oxygen is taken into the blood from the air in the lungs.

The blood exits each lung through two pulmonary veins. All four pulmonary veins take blood into the left atrium of the heart.

Systemic Arterial Circulation

Oxygenated blood enters the left side of the heart from the pulmonary veins. The blood passes through the left atrium into the left ventricle. The ventricle pumps it out into the **aorta,** which takes the blood to all areas of the body. This is the systemic circulation.

The aorta is described in four parts:

1. **Ascending aorta,** which gives rise to the coronary circulation. Right and left coronary arteries branch from it to supply the myocardium.

2. **Aortic arch** *(Figure 8.18)*, which has three main branches:

   a. **Brachiocephalic artery,** a short artery that divides into two arteries:
      i. **Right common carotid artery,** which supplies the right side of the head, brain, and neck.
      ii. **Right subclavian artery,** which supplies the right upper limb.

   b. **Left common carotid artery,** which supplies the left side of the head, brain, and neck. The right and left common carotid arteries divide into two branches:
      i. The **internal carotid** artery, which enters the cranial cavity through a foramen in the base of the skull and supplies the brain.
      ii. The **external carotid** artery, which supplies the neck and face.

   c. **Left subclavian artery,** which supplies the left upper limb.

3. **Thoracic aorta,** which has two major groups of branches:

   a. **Visceral** branches—small **bronchial arteries** that supply the bronchi and bronchioles *(see Chapter 9)*, the esophagus, and the pericardium.

   b. **Parietal** branches—**intercostal arteries** that supply the chest wall and a **phrenic artery** that supplies the diaphragm.

4. **Abdominal aorta,** which has two major groups of branches:

   a. **Visceral branches** that supply the abdominal organs:
      i. **Celiac trunk,** which supplies the stomach, liver, gallbladder, pancreas, and spleen.
      ii. **Superior mesenteric artery,** which supplies the small intestine and part of the large intestine.
      iii. **Inferior mesenteric artery,** which supplies the remainder of the large intestine.
      iv. Paired **renal arteries,** which supply the kidneys and adrenal glands.
      v. Paired **gonadal arteries,** which supply the testes or ovaries.

   b. Four pairs of **lumbar** arteries that supply the abdominal wall.

At the level of the fifth lumbar vertebra (at the top of the pelvis), the aorta divides into the right and left **common iliac arteries.** Visceral branches from these arteries supply the urinary bladder, uterus, and vagina. The common iliac arteries give off an internal iliac artery to supply the pelvis. The common iliac artery becomes the external iliac artery and then the femoral artery as it goes down the thigh and supplies the lower limb. The pulse that can be felt in the back of the knee is the **popliteal artery.**

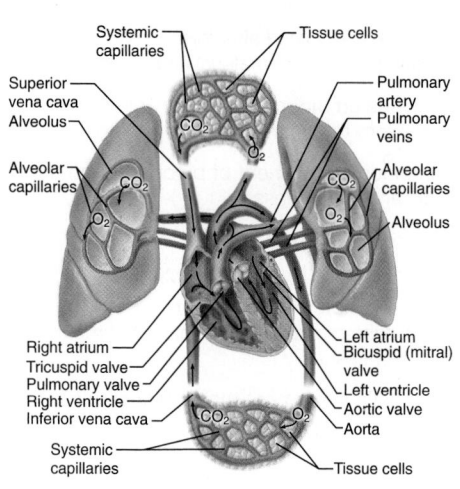

▲ **FIGURE 8.17   Systemic and Pulmonary Circulations.**

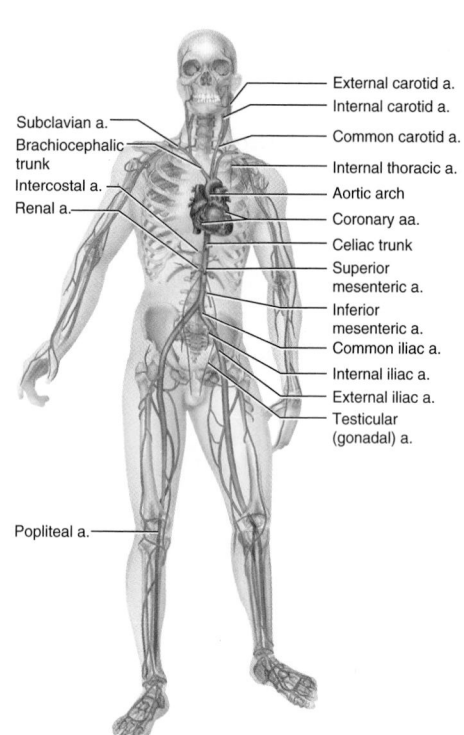

▲ **FIGURE 8.18   The Major Systemic Arteries.** (*a.* = artery; *aa.* = arteries)

WORD	PRONUNCIATION	ELEMENTS		DEFINITION
brachiocephalic	**BRAY**-kee-oh-seh-**FAL**-ik	S/ R/CF R/	-ic *pertaining to* brachi/o- *arm* -cephal- *head*	Pertaining to the head and arm, as an artery supplying blood to both
carotid	kah-**ROT**-id		Greek *carotid arteries*	Main artery of the neck
gonad gonadal (adj)	**GO**-nad go-**NAD**-al		Greek *seed*	Testis or ovary
iliac	**ILL**-ee-ack		Latin *groin, flank*	Pertaining to or near the ilium (pelvic bone)
popliteal	pop-**LIT**-ee-al	S/ R/CF	-al *pertaining to* poplit/e- *back of knee*	Pertaining to the back of the knee
subclavian	sub-**CLAY**-vee-an	S/ P/ R/	-ian *one who does* sub- *under* -clav- *clavicle*	Underneath the clavicle

EXERCISES

Utilize the medical terminology of the circulatory system, and circle the correct answers.

1. The pulse that can be felt at the back of the knee is the:

   aorta   popliteal vein   carotid artery   popliteal artery

2. Blood in the systemic circulation is:

   oxygenated   viscous   deoxygenated   clotted

3. The blood exits each lung through:

   vena cava   pulmonary veins   aorta   pulmonary arteries

4. The _____ arteries supply the chest wall.

   phrenic   visceral   intercostal   mesenteric

5. The *coronary circulation* arises in the:

   thoracic aorta   carotid arteries   ascending aorta   subclavian arteries

6. *Carbon dioxide* is removed from the blood and excreted through:

   dehydration   inspiration   inhalation   expiration

7. The *gonadal* arteries supply the:

   testes   ovaries   kidneys   testes and ovaries

8. *Deoxygenated blood* from the body flows into the:

   right atrium   right ventricle   left atrium   left ventricle

9. This circulation takes blood to all areas of the body:

   coronary   pulmonary   cardiovascular   systemic

10. *Gas exchange* occurs between the air in the lungs and the:

    heart   blood   ventricles   windpipe

11. The *subclavian* artery is located:

    above the heart   below the stomach   above the neck   below the collarbone

12. _____ is a term relating to the abdominal cavity.

    thoracic   iliac   celiac   brachiocephalic

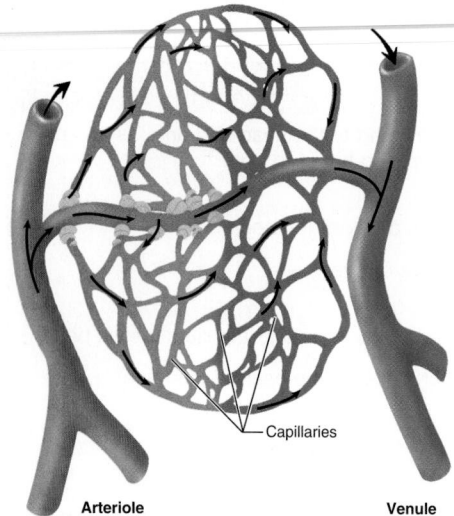

▲ FIGURE 8.19 Capillary Bed.

BLOOD VESSELS IN THE CIRCULATIONS

Arterioles, Capillaries, and Venules

As the arteries branch farther away from the heart and distribute blood to specific organs, they become smaller, muscular vessels called **arterioles.** By contracting and relaxing, these arterioles are the primary controllers by which the body directs the relative amounts of blood that organs and structures receive.

From there, the blood flows into **capillaries** and **capillary beds** *(Figure 8.19).* There are approximately 10 billion capillaries in the body. Each capillary consists of only a single layer of endothelium supported by a thin connective tissue basement membrane. Between the overlapping endothelial cells are thin slits through which larger water-soluble substances can pass. Red blood cells flow through the small capillaries in single file.

From the capillaries, tiny **venules** accept the blood and merge to form **veins.** The veins form reservoirs for blood and at any moment 60% to 70% of the total blood volume is contained in the venules and veins.

The circulatory system exists to serve the capillaries because capillaries are the only place where water and materials are exchanged between the blood and tissue fluids.

Diffusion is the means by which this capillary exchange occurs. Nutrients and oxygen diffuse from a higher concentration in the capillaries to a lower concentration in the **interstitial** fluid around the cells. Waste products diffuse from a higher concentration in the interstitial fluid to a lower concentration in the capillaries.

Systemic Venous Circulation

There are three major types of veins *(Figure 8.20):*

1. **Superficial**—such as those you can see under the skin of your arms and hands.

2. **Deep**—run parallel to arteries and drain the same tissues that the arteries supply.

3. **Venous sinuses**—in the head and heart and have specific functions.

In the lower limb, the superficial veins merge to form the **saphenous vein.** The deep veins form the **femoral vein** *(see Chapter 5).* They join together with veins from the pelvis to form the **common iliac vein.** The right and left common iliac veins form the **inferior vena cava (IVC).**

Veins draining the abdominal organs merge into the **hepatic portal vein** *(see Chapter 6),* which delivers nutrients from the stomach and intestines to the liver. Within the liver, the nutrients are either stored or converted into chemicals that can be used by other cells in the body. The blood leaves the liver in **hepatic veins** that drain into the IVC.

In the upper limb, the superficial veins merge to form the **axillary vein** *(see Chapter 5).* The deep veins alongside the limb arteries empty into the **brachial veins.**

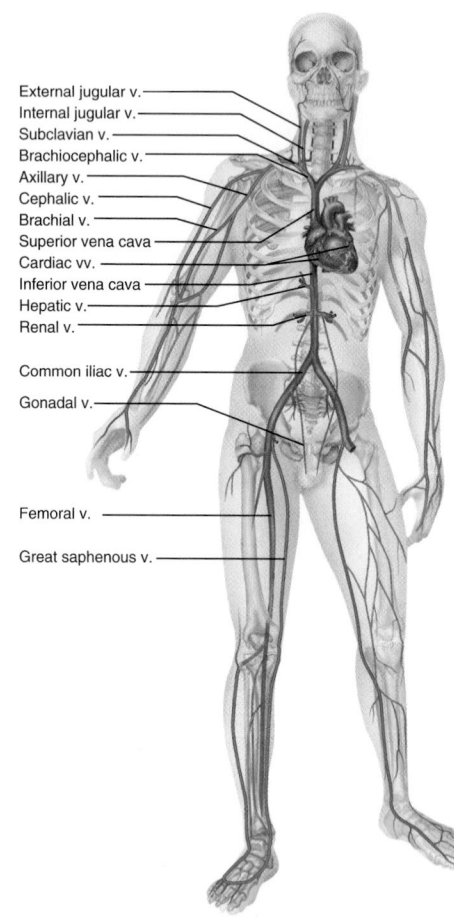

External jugular v.
Internal jugular v.
Subclavian v.
Brachiocephalic v.
Axillary v.
Cephalic v.
Brachial v.
Superior vena cava
Cardiac vv.
Inferior vena cava
Hepatic v.
Renal v.
Common iliac v.
Gonadal v.
Femoral v.
Great saphenous v.

▲ FIGURE 8.20 The Major Systemic Veins.
(*v.* = vein; *vv.* = veins)

Abbreviations	
IVC	inferior vena cava
SVC	superior vena cava

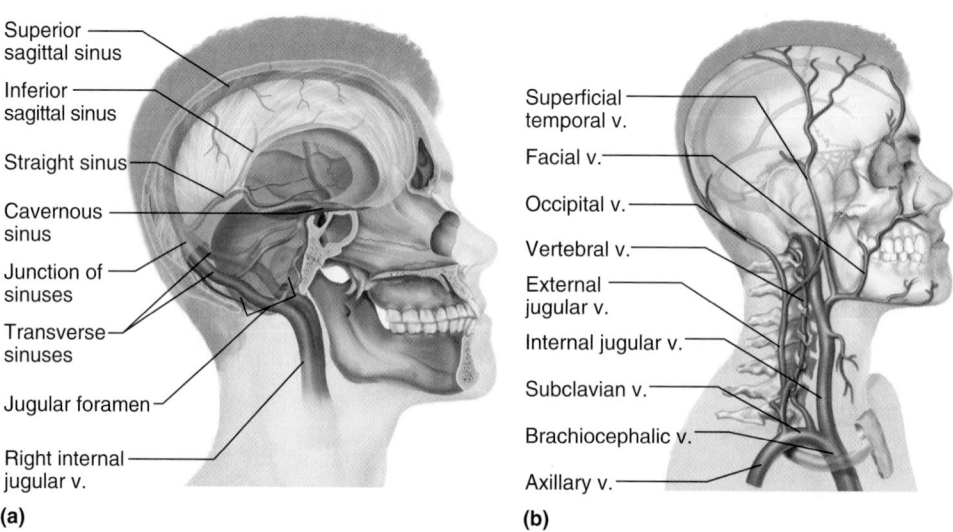

Superior sagittal sinus
Inferior sagittal sinus
Straight sinus
Cavernous sinus
Junction of sinuses
Transverse sinuses
Jugular foramen
Right internal jugular v.

Superficial temporal v.
Facial v.
Occipital v.
Vertebral v.
External jugular v.
Internal jugular v.
Subclavian v.
Brachiocephalic v.
Axillary v.

(a)   (b)

▲ FIGURE 8.21 Cranial Circulation. (*a*) Deep venous drainage of cranial cavity. (*b*) Superficial venous drainage of skull. (*v.* = vein)

WORD	PRONUNCIATION	ELEMENTS		DEFINITION
arteriole	ar-**TER**-ee-ole	S/ R/	Latin *small artery* -ole *small* arteri- *artery*	Small terminal artery leading into the capillary network
axilla	**AK**-sill-ah	S/ R/	Latin *armpit* -ary *pertaining to* axill- *armpit*	Medical name for the armpit
axillary (adj)	**AK**-sil-air-ee			
brachial	**BRAY**-kee-al	S/ R/	-ial *pertaining to* brachi- *arm*	Pertaining to the arm
capillary	**KAP**-ih-lair-ee	S/ R/	-ary *pertaining to* capill- *hairlike structure*	Minute blood vessel betweeen the arterial and venous systems
femoral	**FEM**-oh-ral	S/ R/	-al *pertaining to* femor- *femur*	Pertaining to the femur
interstitial	in-ter-**STISH**-al	S/ R/	-ial *pertaining to* interstit- *spaces within tissues*	Pertaining to spaces between cells in a tissue or organ
jugular	**JUG**-you-lar	S/ R/	-ar *pertaining to* jugul- *throat*	Pertaining to the throat
saphenous	**SAPH**-ih-nus		Root unknown	Relating to the saphenous vein in the thigh
vein	VANE		Latin *vein*	Blood vessel carrying blood toward the heart
venule	**VEN**-yule	S/ R/	Latin *small vein* -ule *small* ven- *vein*	Small vein leading from the capillary network

These also flow into the axillary vein.

As the axillary vein passes behind the clavicle, its name changes to the **subclavian vein.**

In the head and neck, the superficial veins outside the skull drain into the right and left **external jugular veins** *(Figure 8.21)*. From inside the cranial cavity, **venous sinuses** around the brain drain into the right and left **internal jugular veins.**

The external jugular veins empty into the subclavian veins. The internal jugular veins join with the subclavian veins on each side to form the **brachiocephalic veins.** The right and left brachiocephalic veins join together to form the **superior vena cava (SVC).** The SVC empties into the right atrium.

EXERCISES

*Build your knowledge of the elements and terms that make up the **language of the cardiovascular system**. All your answers can come from the above WAD. Fill in the blanks.*

1. The two suffixes in this WAD that both mean *small* are _____ and _____.

2. A small vein is a _____, and a small artery is an _____.

3. An axillary lymph node is located in the _____.

4. List two terms whose *different* suffixes both mean *pertaining to*.

   Terms are _____ and _____.

   Suffixes are _____ and _____.

5. The brachial pulse can be found in the _____.

6. List the four general terms in this WAD that are blood vessels: _____, _____,

   _____ and _____.

7. The jugular vein is in the _____ (location).

8. Recall your terms from Chapter 5—describe the location of the femur: _____

Keynote:

All blood vessel walls have three layers.

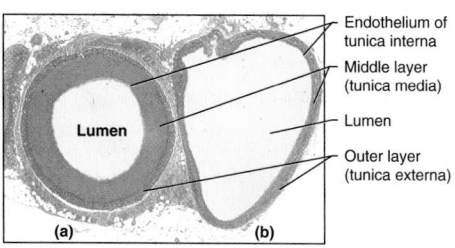

▲ FIGURE 8.22 Anatomy of an Artery and Vein. (*a*) Artery. (*b*) Vein.

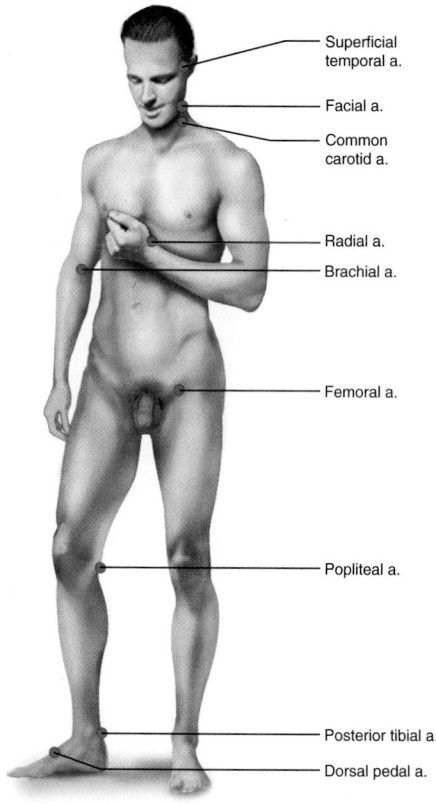

▲ FIGURE 8.23 Arterial Pulses.
(*a.* = artery)

Keynote

Vital signs (VS) measure temperature (T), pulse (P), respirations (R), and blood pressure (BP) to assess cardiorespiratory function.

Abbreviations	
BP	blood pressure
CVP	central venous pressure
VS	vital signs

Except for the capillaries and venules, all the blood vessel walls show a basic structure of three layers (*Figure 8.22*):

1. **Tunica intima (interna)**—the innermost layer of endothelial cells, with thin layers of fibrous and elastic connective tissue supporting them.

2. **Tunica media**—a middle layer of smooth muscle cells arranged circularly around the blood vessel. A membrane of elastic tissue separates the tunica media from the outer layer of the wall.

3. **Tunica adventitia (externa)**—an outer connective tissue layer of varying density and thickness.

The larger arteries near the heart, the aorta and its major branches, have to cope with large quantities of blood and fluctuating pressures between systole and diastole. Therefore, these arteries have a large number of elastic fibers and a relatively small number of muscle fibers.

The functions of the medium-size and smaller arteries are to regulate the blood supply to the different regions of the body and to ensure that the blood pressure in the arteries is at an appropriate level. The tunica media of these arteries contains 25 to 40 layers of smooth muscle to enable the muscles to contract (**vasoconstriction**) and to relax (**vasodilation**) to increase flow.

The function of the veins is to return the blood from the periphery to the heart in a low-pressure system. For example, by the time blood reaches the venules, its pressure has dropped from the 120 mm Hg of systole to around 15 mm Hg. By the time the blood is in the venae cavae, the **central venous pressure (CVP)** is down to around 4 to 5 mm Hg.

Veins have a much thinner tunica media than arteries, with few muscle cells and elastic fibers (*Figure 8.22*). They have a larger lumen and a thick tunica adventitia that merges with the connective tissue of surrounding structures. In the limbs, the veins are surrounded and massaged by muscles to squeeze the blood along the veins. One-way valves in the veins allow the blood to flow toward the heart but not away from the heart. They are shaped like and function like the semilunar valves of the heart.

Space Medicine

Normally, gravity helps the blood circulate in the lower limbs. When astronauts are weightless for long periods of time, blood pools in the central and upper areas of the body and there appears to be an excess blood volume. The kidney compensates by excreting more fluid, leading to a 10% to 20% decrease in blood volume and a low blood pressure. Astronauts compensate for this by wearing lower-body suction suits, which apply a vacuum force to draw blood into the lower limbs.

Arterial Pulses

The pulse is always part of a clinical examination because it can show heart rate, rhythm, and the state of the arterial wall by **palpation.** There are nine locations on each side of the body where large arteries are close to the surface and can be palpated (*Figure 8.23*).

The most easily accessible is the **radial artery** at the wrist, where the pulse is usually taken. The **brachial artery** at the elbow is used for taking blood pressure readings. All the pulse sites can be used as **pressure points** to temporarily reduce arterial bleeding in an emergency.

The two pulses that can be palpated in the feet are the **pedal** pulses, one in each foot.

Blood Pressure (BP)

Blood pressure is the force the blood exerts on arterial walls as it is pumped around the circulatory system by the left ventricle. The pressure is measured using a **sphygmomanometer** and a stethoscope.

WORD	PRONUNCIATION		ELEMENTS	DEFINITION
adventitia	ad-ven-**TISH**-ah		Latin *from outside*	Outer layer of connective tissue covering blood vessels or organs
intima	**IN**-tih-ma		Latin *inmost*	Inner layer of a structure, particularly a blood vessel
media	**ME**-dee-ah		Latin *middle*	Middle layer of a structure, particularly a blood vessel
palpate palpation (noun)	**PAL**-pate pal-**PAY**-shun	S/ R/	-ion *process* palpat- *touch, stroke*	To examine with the fingers and hands An examination with the fingers and hands
pedal	**PEED**-al	S/ R/	-al *pertaining to* ped- *foot*	Pertaining to the foot
radial	**RAY**-dee-al	S/ R/	-al *pertaining to* radi- *radius (forearm bone)*	Pertaining to the forearm
sphygmomanometer	**SFIG**-moh-mah-**NOM**-ih-ter	S/ R/CF R/CF	-meter *instrument to measure* sphygm/o- *pulse* -man/o- *pressure*	Instrument for measuring arterial blood pressure
tunica	**TYU**-nih-kah		Latin *coat*	A layer in the wall of a blood vessel or other tubular structure
vasoconstriction	**VAY**-soh-con-**STRIK**-shun	S/ R/CF R/	-ion *process* vas/o- *blood vessel* -constrict- *narrow*	Reduction in diameter of a blood vessel
vasodilation	**VAY**-soh-di-**LAY**-shun	S/ R/CF R/	-ion *process* vas/o- *blood vessel* -dilat- *open up*	Increase in diameter of a blood vessel
vital signs	**VI**-tal SIGNS		**vital** Latin *life* **signs** Latin *mark*	A procedure during a physical examination in which temperature (T), pulse (P), respirations (R), and blood pressure (BP) are measured to assess general health and cardiorespiratory function

EXERCISES

Match the definition in the left column with the correct medical term in the right column.

_____ 1. To examine by feeling with fingers and hands

_____ 2. Reduction in diameter of a blood vessel

_____ 3. Inner layer of a structure

_____ 4. Latin for *coat*

_____ 5. Outer tissue covering of an organ

_____ 6. Instrument to measure blood pressure

_____ 7. Pertaining to the foot

_____ 8. Increase in diameter of a blood vessel

_____ 9. Middle layer of a structure

_____ 10. Pertaining to the forearm

A. radial

B. vasodilation

C. adventitia

D. pedal

E. vasoconstriction

F. media

G. intima

H. sphygmomanometer

I. palpate

J. tunica

Mrs. Martha Jones, who had been referred to Dr. Bannerjee's cardiovascular clinic, has several circulatory problems related to her diabetes and obesity. She was diagnosed previously with hypertension, CAD, and diabetic retinopathy. She now has severe pain in her legs on walking.

Her ankle/brachial index (**ABI**), which measures the ratio of the blood pressure in her ankle to that in her arm, showed significant blockage of blood flow. Doppler studies confirmed this. This blockage produces the pain on walking (intermittent claudication). It is due to arteriosclerosis of the large arteries in her legs. Angiograms showed several atherosclerotic areas in her popliteal artery.

The ulcers on the edges of her big toes result from thickening of the walls of her capillaries and arterioles and the resulting poor circulation to her feet. Again, this is due to her diabetes.

In the venous system of her legs, the tender cordlike lesion is due to thrombophlebitis of a superficial vein in her left leg. Pain in the calf on flexion of the ankle (Homans sign) indicates that she may have a deep vein thrombosis (**DVT**). A venogram confirmed this diagnosis.

CIRCULATORY DISORDERS

Disorders of Veins

Thrombophlebitis is an inflammation of the lining of a vein (tunica intima), allowing clots (thrombi) to form.

Deep vein thrombosis (DVT) is thrombus formation in a deep vein, often due to reduced blood flow. Risk factors include immobility, surgery, prolonged travel, and contraception (estrogen). The increased pressure in the capillaries due to back-pressure from the blocked blood flow in the veins causes an increase in the flow of fluid from the capillaries to the interstitial spaces. The collection of fluid is called **edema.**

A major complication of thrombus formation is that a piece of the clot can break off and be carried in the bloodstream to lodge in a blood vessel in another organ and block blood flow. The piece that breaks off is called an **embolus.** It often lodges in the lungs, causing a pulmonary embolus *(see Chapter 9).*

Varicose veins are superficial veins that have lost their elasticity and appear swollen and tortuous *(Figure 8.24).* Their valves become incompetent, and blood flows backward and pools. Smaller, more superficial varicose veins are called **spider veins.** Varicose veins are associated with a family history, obesity, and prolonged standing. Treatments offered include laser technology and **sclerotherapy,** where solutions that scar **(sclerose)** the veins are injected into them. **Collateral** circulations develop to take the blood through alternative routes.

A **phlebotomist** is a technician who draws blood. The procedure is called **phlebotomy.**

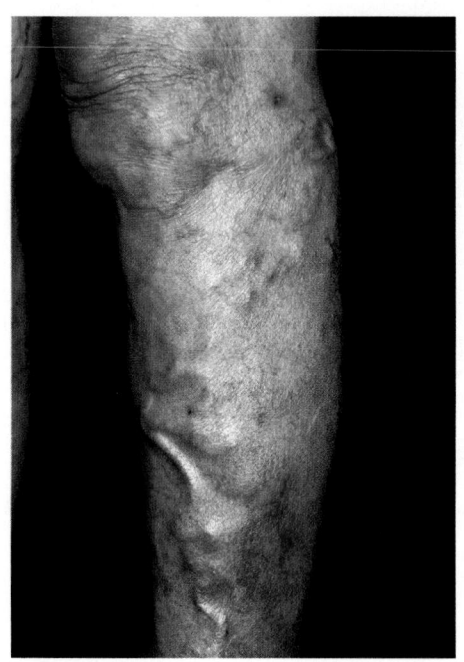

▲ **FIGURE 8.24** **Varicose Veins of Leg.**

Abbreviations

ABI	ankle/brachial index
DVT	deep vein thrombosis
PVD	peripheral vascular disease

Disorders of Arteries

An **aneurysm** is a localized dilation of an artery as a result of a localized weakness of the vessel wall. Common sites occur along the aorta, mostly the abdominal aorta. They can rupture, leading to severe bleeding and hypovolemic shock. Surgical repair consists of excision of the aneurysm and replacement with a synthetic graft.

Intracranial aneurysms, particularly at the base of the brain, are an important cause of bleeds into the cranial cavity *(see Chapter 10).*

Thromboangiitis obliterans (Buerger disease) is an inflammatory disease of the arteries with clot formation, usually in the legs. The occlusion of arteries and impaired circulation leads to intermittent claudication.

3. Which two heart chambers have a somewhat similar appearance?

    a. right and left ventricle

    b. right and left atrium

    c. left atrium and right ventricle

    d. right atrium and left ventricle

    e. right atrium and right ventricle

4. What is another spelling and pronunciation for *dilation?*

    a. dillation

    b. dilatation

    c. dillatation

    d. diletation

    e. dilletation

5. **Interstitial** means:

    a. space between the cells of a structure or organ

    b. cavity between the cells of a structure or organ

    c. fluid between the cells of a structure or organ

    d. membrane between the cells of a structure or organ

    e. wall between the cells of a structure or organ

D. **Build your knowledge of heart terms by working with the following word elements.** Fill in the table; then answer the questions in Exercise E on the next page.

Element	Type of Element (P, R, CF, S)	Meaning of Element
cardio		
ar		
logy		
gram		
logist		
vascul		
electro		
graph		
pulmon		

CARDIOVASCULAR SYSTEM

E. **Using elements in the chart in part D, form medical terms to fill in the blanks.**

1. A _____ is a specialist in the study of the heart.

2. In the abbreviation CPR, the "C" stands for _____.

3. The abbreviation ECG stands for _____.

4. The study of the heart is the specialty called _____.

5. The term that means *pertaining to the heart and blood vessels* is _____.

6. Instrument used for taking an ECG: _____

7. A specialist in the study of lung diseases: _____

F. **Label:** On the lines next to the statements below, write the medical term for the body part the statement refers to. Then write the medical term on the correct line in the illustration.

1. "Pacemaker of the heart": _____

2. Distribute electrical stimuli, which cause contraction of the ventricular myocardium: _____

3. Electrical gateway to the ventricles: _____

4. Supply both ventricles: _____

5. Superior and inferior venae cavae open into this atrium: _____

6. Electrical signals leaving the AV node reach the ventricles through this: _____

7. Blood from pulmonary veins flows into this atrium: _____

G. **Knowing your word elements will always help you to deconstruct a medical term.** Test your knowledge of word elements by defining the following medical terms.

Prefix: sub = _____

subclavian   _____

substernal   _____

sublingual   _____

subaortic   _____

Suffixes: Underline the suffix in each term; then write a brief definition of the term.

sonographer   _____

sonogram   _____

sonography   _____

sonograph   _____

H. **To better understand the peripheral circulations and their functions, complete the following mini-outline.**

The two major peripheral circulations are the:

1. _____

2. _____

Their functions are the same:

1. _____

2. _____

3. _____

4. _____

Study Hint
Use this outline for test review.

How are they different? Complete the table below to show in which circulation each event occurs.

Event	Pulmonary Circulation	Systemic Circulation
Oxygenated blood carried by		
Deoxygenated blood carried by		
Blood goes to all areas of the body		
Gas exchange occurs between lungs and blood		
Takes blood to left atrium		
Coronary circulation branches from here		
Removes carbon dioxide from blood		
Blood exits lung through these veins		
Ventricle pumps to aorta		

CARDIOVASCULAR SYSTEM

I. Build your knowledge of the heart's location and function by correctly answering the following questions.

1. Which of the following is *not* a function of the heart?

    a. pulmonary circulation

    b. maintain respiration

    c. systemic circulation

    d. regulate blood supply

    e. pump blood

2. The heart lies in the thoracic cavity between the lungs in an area called the:

    a. sternum

    b. mediastinum

    c. ventricle

    d. atrium

    e. vena cava

3. If the *base* of the heart is the upper end of the heart, what is the tip (or other end) of the heart called?

    a. tricuspid

    b. atrium

    c. aorta

    d. semilunar

    e. apex

4. The rate and force of heart contraction can be changed by:

    a. blood flow

    b. exercise

    c. body temperature

    d. all of the above

    e. none of the above

5. What is responsible for ensuring the one-way flow of blood in the heart?

    a. blood vessels

    b. pulmonary circulation

    c. coronary circulation

    d. valves

    e. blood pressure

J. Translate: Rewrite the sentences using medical terms instead of the abbreviations. Make sure you are communicating the same message either way. Check (✓) your spelling! Fill in the blanks.

1. The CVT started CPR after checking the patient's ECG. He paged the doctor STAT. Apparently, the patient had had an MI.

   _____

   _____

   _____

2. Because of the patient's PVD, the doctor ordered special stockings to prevent DVT.

   _____

   _____

   _____

3. ASD and VSD are holes in the walls of the chambers of the heart that allow blood to leak through.

   _____

   _____

   _____

4. Risk factors for CAD include hypertension, diabetes, obesity, and stress.

   _____

   _____

   _____

K. Challenge your knowledge of medical terminology and **provide the correct answers** to the following questions.

1. A *flat line* on an ECG is called _____.

2. *Death of tissue* is _____.

3. *Arrhythmia* is another term for _____.

4. An *abnormal sound* in the closure of a heart valve is a _____.

5. *Cardiomyopathy* can cause _____.

6. *Atherosclerotic plaques* are also called _____.

7. A *bypass* or diversion of fluid: _____

8. *Hollow tube* that allows passage of fluid into or out of a body cavity: _____

9. Agent that *increases* urine output: _____

10. *Main artery* of the neck: _____

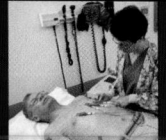

CHAPTER 8 REVIEW

CARDIOVASCULAR SYSTEM

L. Procedures: You have passed your certification examination and have been hired as the coder for the Cardiology Department in Fulwood Medical Center. You are coding the claims for the following tests performed in the department. How much do you know about cardiology testing? Match the letter to the numbered blank.

_____ 1. Thallium testing	A.	MRI
_____ 2. EKG, also known as	B.	through esophagus to record heart valves
_____ 3. Continuous ECG recorded on tape	C.	echocardiography
_____ 4. Cardiac stress testing	D.	detects patterns of pressure in the heart
_____ 5. TEE	E.	people unable to do physical exercise
_____ 6. Helps determine risk of CAD	F.	coronary angiogram
_____ 7. Event monitor	G.	exercise tolerance test
_____ 8. Sound waves study heart function	H.	sporadic symptoms
_____ 9. Electron beam CT	I.	lipid profile
_____ 10. Cardiac catheterization	J.	ECG
_____ 11. Radioactive substance injected	K.	Holter monitor
_____ 12. Can identify ischemic muscle	L.	identifies calcium in arteries
_____ 13. Dye injected to find heart blockage	M.	nuclear imaging

M. The diagnostic tests in part L may yield results that indicate a procedure should be performed. Match up the following cardiac procedures.

_____ 1. Catheter inflates and compresses plaque	A.	CABG
_____ 2. Converting an arrhythmia to normal rhythm	B.	rotational atherectomy
_____ 3. Prevents artery from closing up again	C.	CPR
_____ 4. Donor to recipient	D.	thrombolysis
_____ 5. Electrode used to destroy cells that produce arrhythmia	E.	PTCA
_____ 6. Sands away plaque	F.	cardioversion
_____ 7. Injection of clot-busting drugs	G.	heart transplant
_____ 8. Harvested healthy vessels replace blocked ones	H.	pacemaker implantation
_____ 9. Restores normal function to heart and lungs	I.	radiofrequency ablation
_____ 10. Artificial regulator of cardiac activity	J.	stent placement

N. **Recall and Review:** The following exercise on word elements contains some elements from this chapter and the previous chapter. Try to recall the previous elements without turning back in your book. Check the type of element; then write its meaning. Fill in the blanks.

Element	Prefix	Root/CF	Suffix	Meaning of Element
de	_____	_____	_____	_____
emia	_____	_____	_____	_____
erythro	_____	_____	_____	_____
hemato	_____	_____	_____	_____
inter	_____	_____	_____	_____
mal	_____	_____	_____	_____
scope	_____	_____	_____	_____
tri	_____	_____	_____	_____
um	_____	_____	_____	_____

O. **In Your Own Words:** Identify one procedure or type of service performed by the following occupations.

CVT: _____

phlebotomist: _____

cardiologist: _____

sonographer: _____

cardiovascular surgeon: _____

P. **Terminology Challenge:** Demonstrate your understanding of cardiac terminology by filling in the blanks.

1. What is the function of a *perfusionist?* _____

2. What is the difference between a *stent* and a *shunt?*

   stent: _____

   shunt: _____

3. A *dilated,* tortuous *vein* can also be called a _____.

4. What are the two terms for increase and decrease in the diameter of a blood vessel?

   Increase:_____ Decrease:_____

5. Name a function of a *sphygmomanometer* and a function of a *stethoscope*:

   Sphygmomanometer: _____

   Stethoscope: _____

CARDIOVASCULAR SYSTEM

Q. **The following procedures could all be performed by a cardiovascular surgeon.** First, slash the term into its elements. Use the suffix to help you analyze the meaning of the term. Write a brief description of the procedure on the line below. Fill in the blanks.

1. **ablation:** _____/ _____ / _____
   P   R/CF   S

   Description: _____

2. **angioplasty:** _____/ _____ / _____
   P   R/CF   S

   Description: _____

3. **endarterectomy:** _____/ _____ / _____
   P   R/CF   S

   Description: _____

4. **sclerotherapy:** _____/ _____ / _____
   P   R/CF   S

   Description: _____

5. **atherectomy:** _____/ _____ / _____
   P   R/CF   S

   Description: _____

R. **Test your knowledge of the heart by circling the correct answer.**

1. The long, flat bone forming the center of the anterior wall of the chest is the:

   a. mediastinum

   b. sternum

   c. myocardium

   d. apex

   e. pericardium

2. The area of cell death caused by the sudden blockage of a blood vessel is termed:

   a. fibrosis

   b. infarct

   c. coronary

   d. sinus

   e. visceral

3. The term **sinus rhythm** refers to:

   a. the AV node

   b. normal heartbeat

   c. dysrhythmias

   d. arrthythmias

   e. a pacemaker

4. Pathologic compression of the heart is known as:

   a. endocarditis

   b. prolapse

   c. tamponade

   d. regurgitation

   e. effusion

5. The abbreviations that represent cardiac diagnoses are:

   a. SOB and EKG

   b. MI and PAT

   c. CPR and CVT

   d. STAT and SA

   e. AED and ID

6. What is the purpose of the four valves in the heart?

   a. Blood flows in only one direction.

   b. Blood gets oxygenated.

   c. The heart muscle can rest between beats.

   d. They prevent infection.

   e. They are the gateway to the heart.

7. In the term **cardioversion,** the suffix *-ion* means:

   a. a structure

   b. a process

   c. to pour

   d. pertaining to

   e. small

CARDIOVASCULAR SYSTEM

S. Test your knowledge of the heart with the following questions.

1. Tissue heart valves can come from:

    a. pigs

    b. cows

    c. occasionally humans

    d. all of the above

    e. none of the above

2. Abnormality in valve closure produces:

    a. exudate

    b. infarct

    c. murmur

    d. necrosis

    e. fibrillation

3. The cordlike tendons that anchor the mitral and tricuspid heart valves to the floor of the ventricles are:

    a. semilunar

    b. intraventricular

    c. mesenteric

    d. chordae tendinae

    e. fibrotic

4. The pacemaker of heart rhythm is the:

    a. AV node

    b. bundle branch

    c. SA node

    d. coronary sinus

    e. PVC

5. **Marginal, interventricular,** and **circumflex** are all terms applied to heart:

    a. veins

    b. capillaries

    c. arteries

    d. tendons

    e. muscles

6. Components of a pacemaker:

   a. battery

   b. electronic circuits

   c. computer memory

   d. all of the above

   e. none of the above

7. The term **visceral** pertains to:

   a. an artery

   b. a vein

   c. a capillary

   d. the aorta

   e. an internal organ

8. Capillary exchange occurs by:

   a. infusion

   b. transfusion

   c. perfusion

   d. diffusion

   e. effusion

T. **Each of the following medical terms is defined—you need to fill in the missing element(s) to complete the word for the last column.** Fill in the chart.

Definition	Prefix	Root/CF	Suffix	Complete Medical Term
Increases urine production	di		ic	
Affects contractility of cardiac muscle			tropic	
Relating to autonomic nervous system		adren		
Ultrasound to record cardiac function		echo		
One who records sound waves		sono		
Agents that affect heart rate			tropic	
Surgical destruction of a tissue's function			ion	
Surgical intervention on a blood vessel		angio		

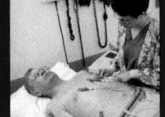

CHAPTER 8 REVIEW

CARDIOVASCULAR SYSTEM

U. **Knowledge of pharmacology is essential to be certain your patients are receiving the correct drugs for their conditions.** Listed below are six types of cardiac drugs in use. List the main function of each drug; then give an example of that type of drug.

Drug Type	Function of the Drug	Example
Vasodilators		
Inotropic drugs		
Anticoagulants		
Antiarrhythmic drugs		
Chronotropic drugs		
Diuretics		

V. Determine which type of drug listed in part U would be prescribed for the following conditions.

1. Patient has hypertension: _____

2. Patient suffers from atrial fibrillation: _____

3. Patient has excessive platelets: _____
    Critical thinking: Based on your knowledge of *Chapter 7*, what then is likely to form, and is that a problem?

    _____

    _____

4. Based on studies, patient has poor cardiac output: _____

5. Patient has tachycardia. This drug attempts to alter that rate: _____

6. Patient has CHF and needs a _____ to reduce fluid volume.

W. **Discussion Question: Regurgitation** means to *flow backward*. In this chapter, regurgitation through the heart valve is discussed. What previous chapter discusses regurgitation of another type? What body system is that present in? Describe that regurgitation as compared with cardiac regurgitation. How are they similar? How are they different? Write your notes below.

1. Previous chapter that discusses regurgitation: _____

2. Body system in question 1 above: _____

3. Describe the regurgitation in question 1, as opposed to cardiac regurgitation.

    Previous chapter regurgitation is _____

    _____.

    Cardiac regurgitation is _____

    _____.

4. How are they similar? _____

    _____

5. How are they different? _____

    _____

X. **The cardiac cycle can be heard through the stethoscope.** Apply the correct terms in the appropriate place to describe what happens in the chambers of the heart during the cardiac cycle. One term you will use twice. Three terms you will not use at all.

atrial diastole	**relax**	**heartbeat**	**atrial systole**	**ventricular systole**
atria	**ventricular diastole**	**contraction**	**contract**	**murmur**

1. When the atria _____, called _____ (atrial emptying), the ventricles _____, called _____ (or ventricular filling).

2. When the atria relax, called _____, the ventricles _____, called _____.

3. Then the atria and ventricles all relax briefly. This series of events is the complete cardiac cycle or _____.

Y. **The following elements are all roots or combining forms.** Write the meaning of the root/CF; then demonstrate its use with a medical term containing that element. Fill in the chart.

Root/Combining Form	Meaning of Root/CF	Medical Term Containing This Root/CF
coron		
cost		
diaphoret		
isch		
lun		
palpit		
resuscitat		
stetho		
tampon		
viscer		

Pick any two medical terms from the right column above, and create a sentence of patient documentation for each term.

Sentence 1:

_____

_____

_____

Sentence 2:

_____

_____

_____

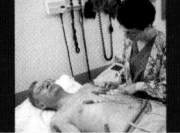

CARDIOVASCULAR SYSTEM

Z. **You are mentoring a new CVT who has just been hired in the Cardiology Department in Fulwood Medical Center.** Because you have been on the job for a while, you should be able to explain briefly the difference between:

1. *Heart valve stenosis* and *heart valve incompetency:*

_____

_____

_____

2. A *thrombus* and an *embolus:*

_____

_____

_____

3. *Essential hypertension, secondary hypertension,* and *malignant hypertension:*

_____

_____

_____

AA. **Translate from layman's language to medical terminology.** Provide a medical term for every underlined word or phrase. Fill in the blanks.

1. If any of the <u>heart</u> (_____) arteries become <u>blocked</u> (_____), the blood supply to a part of the <u>heart muscle</u> (_____) is cut off and the cells supplied by that artery are <u>dead</u> (_____) within minutes.

2. Aortic valve <u>narrowing</u> (_____) is common in the elderly when the valves become <u>hardened</u> (_____) due to <u>lipid deposits in the lining of an artery</u> (_____).

3. The <u>cause</u> (_____) of weakening of the heart muscle (_____) can be viral, unknown (_____), or alcoholic.

4. The other form of circulatory shock presents with <u>loss of blood volume</u> (_____), often from <u>excessive bleeding</u> (_____) or <u>water depletion</u> (_____).

5. <u>Inflammation of the lining of a vein</u> (_____) allows <u>clots</u> (_____) to form.

BB. **Cardiac terminology can be complex.** Test yourself on the following terms to demonstrate your understanding of the medical language. Use some answers more than once. This exercise will self-correct.

_____ 1. Fluid from tissue or capillary

_____ 2. Heart attack

_____ 3. Death of cells

_____ 4. Cut off blood supply

_____ 5. Blood goes from here to a capillary

_____ 6. Serous cells are here

_____ 7. Murmur signifies abnormal

_____ 8. Ischemia + necrosis =

_____ 9. Circumflex

_____ 10. Coronary

_____ 11. Attached inferiorly to diaphragm

_____ 12. Prevents backflow of blood

_____ 13. Opens into right atrium

R. artery

Y. exudate

C. valve

T. coronary sinus

E. parietal pericardium

U. necrosis

O. myocardial infarction

A. ischemia

CC. **Abbreviations are present throughout medical documentation, and you must be absolutely certain you are interpreting them correctly.** Fill in the correct abbreviation in the following patient documentation. All of the abbreviations contain some combination of the following letters. You will have to use some letters more than once.

A   C   D   F   H   I   M   P   S   V   O

1. Studies show that the patient has a hole in the interventricular septum, allowing blood to shunt from the higher-pressure left

   ventricle to the lower-pressure right ventricle. Abbreviation for the diagnosis: _____

2. The pediatric cardiologist was called to the Neonatal Unit because the baby's fetal blood vessel had not closed normally.

   He was diagnosed with _____.

3. The patient's arterial vessels have become dangerously narrowed due to his _____, and an angioplasty will be
   scheduled.

4. Due to her sedentary lifestyle, obesity, hypertension, and smoking history, the patient is at great risk for _____.

5. This patient's left ventricle is failing because it cannot pump out the blood it receives. He is going into _____.

6. Infant male was born with tetralogy of Fallot (_____). This is a form of _____.

7. This patient's ischemic attack resulted in occlusion of her coronary artery, and a (surgical procedure) _____
   followed.

CARDIOVASCULAR SYSTEM

CHAPTER SUMMARY EXERCISES

1. *Listen to the pronunciation of the medical terms as given by your instructor.*
2. *Circle the correct spelling of the medical term.*
3. *Match the correctly spelled terms to the brief descriptions below.*
4. *Write a sentence for each of the 10 terms that appear in this exercise.*

A. SPELLING COMPREHENSION: CIRCLE THE CORRECT SPELLING OF THE TERM.

1. ishemia	ishima	ischemia	iskemia	ischimia
2. dyuretic	diuretic	dyeretic	dieretic	diyuretic
3. regergitate	reguritate	regersitate	regurgitate	regugitate
4. resuscitation	resucitation	resusitation	risusitation	risusitation
5. thombolisis	thrombolysis	tombolisis	thrombylosis	tombolysis
6. dyastole	diastolye	dyastolie	diastole	diastolee
7. paretial	peretal	parietal	parital	partial
8. adventitia	advintitea	adventia	advinttia	adventetea
9. deaphoresis	diaphoresis	diaporesis	deaporesis	diaporisis
10. thrombopelpitis	thromblitis	thrombophlebitis	thrombuphelitis	thrombopelbitis

B. MATCH THE NUMBER OF THE CORRECT TERM IN PART A WITH THE BRIEF DESCRIPTION OF THE TERM BELOW.

_____ a. Revival from potential or apparent death

_____ b. Agent that increases urine output

_____ c. Relating to the wall of a cavity

_____ d. Deficiency of blood flow to an organ or tissue

_____ e. To flow backward

_____ f. Profuse sweating

_____ g. Inflammation of a vein with clot formation

_____ h. Destruction of a clot

_____ i. Outer connective tissue covering of a blood vessel or organ

_____ j. Relaxation of the heart chamber as it fills with blood

C. USING YOUR KNOWLEDGE OF TERMS 1–10 IN PART A AND THEIR CORRECT SPELLING, WRITE A BRIEF SENTENCE AS IT MIGHT APPEAR IN PATIENT DOCUMENTATION.

1. _____

2. _____

3. _____

4. _____

5. _____

6. _____

7. _____

8. _____

9. _____

10. _____

D. YOUR INSTRUCTOR WILL DIRECT YOU TO MCGRAW-HILL CONNECT. OPEN THE AUDIO GLOSSARY AND PRACTICE YOUR PRONUNCIATION OF THE TERMS IN PART A OF THIS EXERCISE.

E. AFTER READING CASE REPORT 8.2, ANSWER THE FOLLOWING QUESTIONS. BE PREPARED TO DISCUSS YOUR ANSWERS IN CLASS.

Case Report 8.2 (continued)

Mrs. Martha Jones, who had been referred to Dr. Bannerjee's cardiovascular clinic, has several circulatory problems related to her diabetes and obesity. She was diagnosed previously with hypertension, CAD, and diabetic retinopathy. She now has severe pain in her legs on walking.

Her ankle/brachial index (**ABI**), which measures the ratio of the blood pressure in her ankle to that in her arm, showed significant blockage of blood flow. Doppler studies confirmed this. This blockage produces the pain on walking (intermittent claudication). It is due to arteriosclerosis of the large arteries in her legs. Angiograms showed several atherosclerotic areas in her popliteal artery.

The ulcers on the edges of her big toes result from thickening of the walls of her capillaries and arterioles and the resulting poor circulation to her feet. Again, this is due to her diabetes.

In the venous system of her legs, the tender cordlike lesion is due to thrombophlebitis of a superficial vein in her left leg. Pain in the calf on flexion of the ankle (Homans sign) indicates that she may have a deep vein thrombosis (**DVT**). A venogram confirmed this diagnosis.

1. What weight problem is a complicating factor to Mrs. Jones's diabetes?

_____

2. What diagnoses are in Mrs. Jones's past medical history?

_____

3. What is the medical term for "severe pain in legs on walking"?

_____

4. What is an angiogram? _____

5. Explain in simple language what a DVT is. _____

_____

6. What diagnostic tests has Mrs. Jones had so far? _____

7. Where does retinopathy occur? _____

8. Name one circulatory problem Mrs. Jones has as a result of her diabetes.

_____

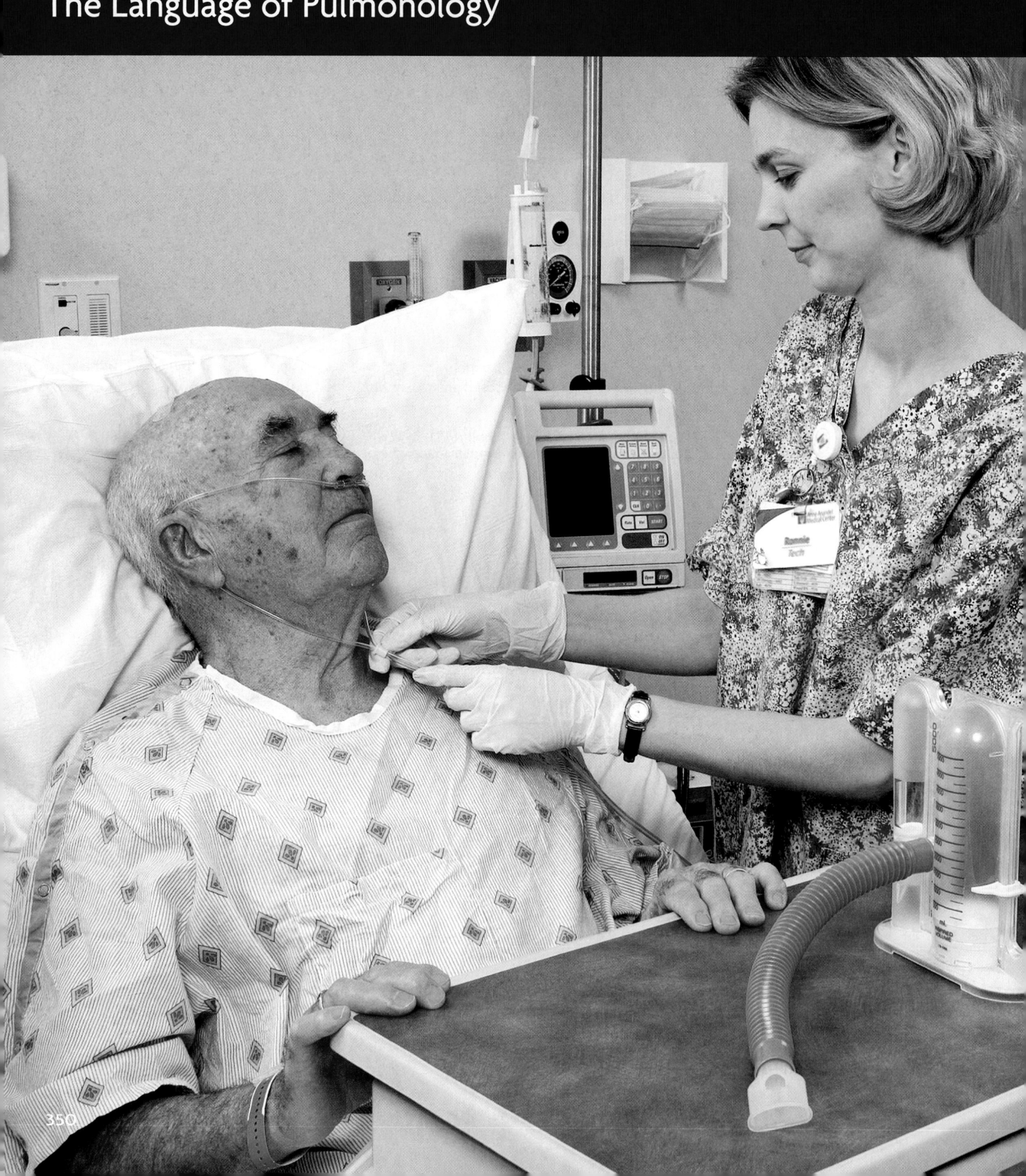

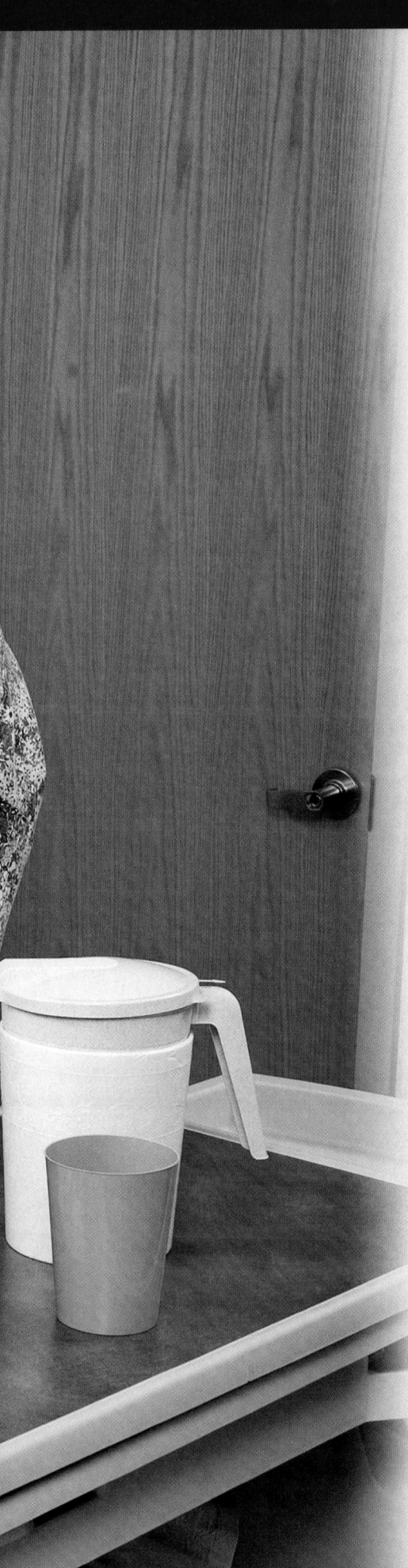

9

CASE REPORT 9.1

You are

. . . an advanced-level respiratory therapist (RT) working in the Acute Respiratory Care Unit of Fulwood Medical Center with **pulmonologist** Tavis Senko, MD.

Your patient is

. . . Mr. Jude Jacobs, a 68-year-old retired mail carrier, who is known to have chronic obstructive pulmonary disease (**COPD**) and is on continual oxygen by nasal prongs. He has smoked two packs per day for all his adult life.

Last night, he was unable to sleep because of increased shortness of breath and cough. His cough is productive of yellow **sputum.** He had to sit upright in bed to be able to breathe.

Vital signs are temperature (**T**) 101.6°F, pulse (**P**) 98, respirations (**R**) 36, blood pressure (**BP**) 150/90.

On examination, he is cyanotic and frightened and has nasal prongs. Air entry is diminished in both lungs, and there are **rales** (crackles) at both bases.

You have been ordered to draw blood for arterial blood gases (**ABGs**) and to measure the amount of air entering and leaving his lungs using **spirometry.**

Learning Outcomes

To provide optimal care to Mr. Jacobs, to determine what is causing his symptoms and signs, and to communicate with the other health professionals involved in his care, you need to be able to:

9.1 Apply the language of pulmonology to the anatomy and physiology of the respiratory system.

9.2 Comprehend, analyze, spell, and write the medical terms of pulmonology to communicate and document accurately and precisely in any health care setting.

9.3 Recognize and pronounce the medical terms of pulmonology so that you can communicate verbally with accuracy and precision in any health care setting.

9.4 Explain the effects of common respiratory disorders on health.

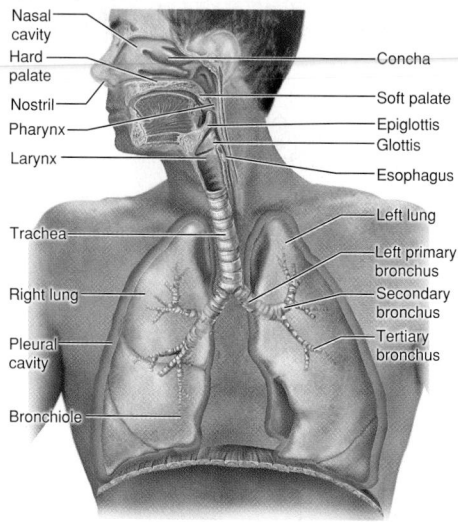

▲ FIGURE 9.1   The Respiratory System.

Labels (Figure 9.1):
Nasal cavity
Hard palate
Nostril
Pharynx
Larynx
Trachea
Right lung
Pleural cavity
Bronchiole
Concha
Soft palate
Epiglottis
Glottis
Esophagus
Left lung
Left primary bronchus
Secondary bronchus
Tertiary bronchus

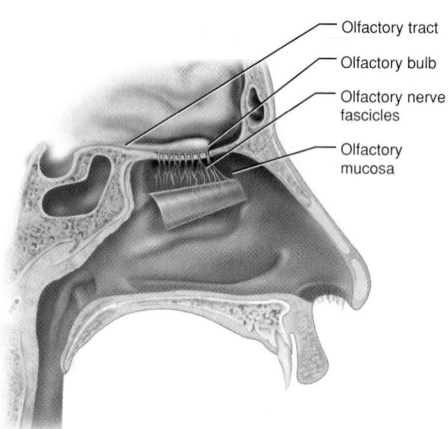

▲ FIGURE 9.2   Olfactory Region of Nose.

Labels (Figure 9.2):
Olfactory tract
Olfactory bulb
Olfactory nerve fascicles
Olfactory mucosa

Abbreviations

ABG	arterial blood gas
BP	blood pressure
COPD	chronic obstructive pulmonary disease
CO₂	carbon dioxide
O₂	oxygen
P	pulse
R	respiration
T	temperature

INTRODUCTION TO THE RESPIRATORY SYSTEM

It sounds like a good scheme. Humans and animals can breathe in oxygen (O_2) and breathe out carbon dioxide (CO_2); plants and trees can breathe in carbon dioxide and breathe out oxygen—and nature would stay in balance. Unfortunately, we humans have generated increasing amounts of carbon dioxide in the air by burning coal, oil, and natural gas and cutting down forests. We have disturbed the balance. In addition, we have created organic and inorganic chemicals and small particles of solid matter in the air that can damage the respiratory tract and be taken into our bodies to cause cancer, brain damage, and birth defects. These materials are called pollutants.

The **respiratory tract** *(Figure 9.1)* has six connected elements:

1. **Nose**
2. **Pharynx**
3. **Larynx**
4. **Trachea**
5. **Bronchi and bronchioles**
6. **Alveoli**

The term **respiration** has three meanings:

- **Ventilation,** which is the movement of air and its gases into and out of the lungs (inspiration and expiration).
- Exchange of gases between air and blood and between blood and interstitial fluids.
- Use of oxygen in cellular metabolism (internal respiration) *(see Chapter 2).*

The **functions** of the respiratory system are:

1. **Exchange of gases.** All the body cells need oxygen and produce carbon dioxide. The respiratory system allows oxygen from the air to enter the blood and carbon dioxide to leave the blood and enter the air.
2. **Regulation of blood pH.** This is accomplished by changing blood carbon dioxide levels *(see Chapter 2).*
3. **Protection.** The respiratory system protects against foreign bodies and against some microorganisms.
4. **Voice production.** Movement of air across the vocal cords makes speech and other sounds possible.
5. **Olfaction.** The 12 million receptor cells for smell are in a patch of epithelium the size of a quarter that is in the extreme superior region of the nasal cavity, the **olfactory region** *(Figure 9.2).* Each cell has 10 to 20 hairlike structures called **cilia** that project into the nasal cavity covered in a thin mucous film.

Because the **olfactory region** is right at the top of the nose, you often have to sniff the air right up there to stimulate the sense of smell. A dog has 4 billion receptor cells, which is why dogs can be trained to sniff for drugs, explosives, and dead bodies.

Many of your sensations of taste are influenced by your sense of smell. For example, without its aroma, coffee tastes only bitter. The same with peppermint. This is why, when you have a cold, much of your sense of taste is lost.

WORD	PRONUNCIATION		ELEMENTS	DEFINITION
alveolus alveoli (pl) alveolar (adj)	al-**VEE**-oh-lus al-**VEE**-oh-lee al-**VEE**-oh-lar		Latin *hollow sac*	Tiny air sac terminal element of the respiratory tract
bronchus bronchi (pl) bronchiole	**BRONG**-kuss **BRONG**-key **BRONG**-key-ole	S/ R/CF	Greek *windpipe* -ole *small* bronch/i- *bronchus*	One of two subdivisions of the trachea Increasingly smaller subdivisions of bronchi
cilium cilia (pl)	**SILL**-ee-um **SILL**-ee-ah		Latin *eyelash*	Hairlike motile projection from the surface of a cell
larynx laryngeal (adj)	**LAIR**-inks lah-**RIN**-jee-al		Greek *larynx*	Organ of voice production
olfaction olfactory (adj)	ol-**FAK**-shun ol-**FAK**-toh-ree		Latin *to smell*	Sense of smell Relating to the sense of smell
pharynx pharyngeal (adj)	**FAIR**-inks fair-**IN**-jee-al		Greek *throat*	Air tube from the back of the nose to the larynx
pulmonary	**PULL**-moh-**NAR**-ee	S/ R/	-ary *pertaining to* pulmon- *lung*	Pertaining to the lungs and their blood supply
pulmonology	**PULL**-moh-**NOL**-oh-jee	S/ R/CF	-logy *study of* pulmon/o- *lung*	Study of the lungs, or the medical specialty of disorders of the respiratory tract
pulmonologist	**PULL**-moh-**NOL**-oh-jist	S/	-logist *one who studies, specialist*	Medical specialist in pulmonary disorders
rale rales (pl)	RAHL RAHLS		French *rattle*	Crackle heard through a stethoscope when air bubbles through liquid in the lungs
respiration	**RES**-pih-**RAY**-shun	S/ P/ R/	-ation *process* re- *again* -spir- *to breathe*	Fundamental process of life used to exchange oxygen and carbon dioxide
respirator respiratory (adj)	**RES**-pir-**AY**-tor **RES**-pir-ah-**TOR**-ee	S/	-ator *person or thing that does something*	Another name for ventilator
spirometer	spy-**ROM**-eh-ter	S/ R/CF	-meter *measure* spir/o- *to breathe*	An instrument used to measure respiratory volumes
spirometry	spy-**ROM**-eh-tree	S/	-metry *process of measuring*	Use of a spirometer
sputum	**SPYU**-tum		Latin *to spit*	Matter coughed up and spat out by individuals with respiratory disorders
trachea	**TRAY**-kee-ah		Greek *windpipe*	Air tube from the larynx to the bronchi
ventilation	ven-tih-**LAY**-shun	S/ R/	-ation *process* ventil- *wind*	Movement of gases into and out of the lungs
ventilator	**VEN**-tih-**LAY**-tor	S/	-ator *person or thing that does something*	Device that breathes for the patient

EXERCISES

Latin/Greek/Other Terms: *Medical terms taken directly from Latin, Greek, or other languages do not deconstruct into prefix, root, or suffix elements the way other medical terms do. You simply have to know them for what they are. Match the medical term in the left column to the correct meaning in the right column. Fill in the blanks.*

_____ 1. rale

_____ 2. cilium

_____ 3. pharynx

_____ 4. sputum

_____ 5. olfaction

_____ 6. trachea

A. throat

B. spit

C. windpipe

D. eyelash

E. rattle

F. to smell

LESSON 9.1 Upper Respiratory Tract

OBJECTIVES

The **upper respiratory tract** consists of the nose, pharynx, and trachea. It is the first site that brings air and its pollutants inside your body. As health professionals, it's important that you understand the roles of the upper respiratory tract in trying to protect you, as well as enabling you to live by transporting oxygen into your body.

The information in this lesson will enable you to use correct medical terminology to:

9.1.1 Trace the flow of air from the nose through the pharynx and larynx.

9.1.2 Relate the function of any segment of the upper airway to its structure.

9.1.3 Define the protective mechanisms of the upper respiratory tract.

9.1.4 Describe how sound is produced.

9.1.5 Explain how smells are recognized.

9.1.6 Describe common disorders of the upper respiratory tract.

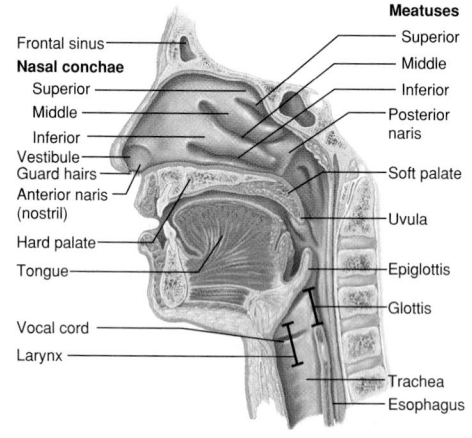

▲ **FIGURE 9.3** Upper Respiratory Tract.

Keynote

Your nose is the first line of defense against pollutants.

Abbreviation	
URI	upper respiratory infection

NOSE

When you breathe in air through your nose, the air goes through the nostrils (**nares**) into the **vestibule** of the **nasal cavity**. The nares are guarded by internal hairs to prevent the entry of large particles.

The nasal cavity is divided by the nasal **septum** into right and left compartments. On the lateral wall of each nasal cavity, three bony ridges called **conchae** (**turbinate bones**) stick out into each cavity. Beneath each **concha** is a passageway called a **meatus** *(Figure 9.3)*. The palate *(see Chapter 6)* forms the floor of the nose.

The nasal cavity is lined with a mucous membrane (mucosa) containing goblet cells that secrete mucus. Mucus forms a protective layer that can trap particles of dust and solid pollutants.

The **paranasal**, frontal, and maxillary **sinuses** open into the nose. Because they are hollow, the functions of these sinuses are to reduce the weight of the skull and to act as resonating chambers for the sounds of the voice. If your sinuses are congested, your voice loses its normal quality.

Functions of the Nose

- **Passageway for air.** The palate is the floor of the nasal cavity that separates it from the mouth and enables you to breathe even with food in your mouth.
- **Air cleanser.** The hairs in the vestibule trap some of the large particles in the air.
- **Air moisturizer.** Moisture from nasal mucus and from tears that drain into the cavity through the nasolacrimal duct *(see Chapter 4)* is added to the air.
- **Air warmer.** The blood flowing through the nasal cavity beneath the mucous membrane also warms the air. This prevents damage from the cold to the more fragile lower respiratory passages.
- **Sense of smell (olfaction).** The olfactory region recognizes some 4000 separate smells.

Disorders of the Nose

Common cold is a viral **upper respiratory infection (URI).** It is contagious, being transmitted from person to person in airborne droplets from coughing and sneezing. There is no proven effective treatment.

Rhinitis is an inflammation of the nasal mucosa, usually viral in origin. It is also called **coryza.**

Allergic rhinitis affects 15% to 20% of the population. There is swelling of the mucous membranes of the nose, pharynx, and sinuses, with a clear watery discharge.

Sinusitis is an infection of the paranasal sinuses, often following a cold. The infection can be bacterial, producing a **mucopurulent** discharge from the nose. Treatment with **antibiotics** and **decongestants** may be indicated.

WORD	PRONUNCIATION	ELEMENTS		DEFINITION
cautery	**KAW**-ter-ee		Greek *a branding iron*	Agent or device used to burn or scar a tissue
concha conchae (pl)	**KON**-kah **KON**-kee		Latin *shell*	Shell-shaped bone on the medial wall of the nasal cavity
coryza (also called rhinitis)	ko-**RYE**-zah		Greek *catarrh*	Viral inflammation of the mucous membrane of the nose
decongestant	dee-con-**JESS**-tant	S/ P/ R/	**-ant** *pertaining to* **de-** *take away* **-congest-** *accumulation of fluid*	Agent that reduces the swelling and fluid in the nose and sinuses
epistaxis	ep-ih-**STAK**-sis	S/ P/ R/	**-is** *condition* **epi-** *above, over* **-stax-** *fall in drops*	Nosebleed
meatus	me-**AY**-tus		Latin *a passage*	Passage or channel; also used to denote the external opening of a passage
mucopurulent	myu-koh-**PYUR**-you-lent	S/ R/CF R/	**-ent** *forming* **muc/o-** *mucus* **-purul-** *pus*	Mixture of pus and mucus
naris nares (pl) nasal	**NAH**-ris **NAH**-rez **NAY**-zal	 S/ R/	Latin *nostril* **-al** *pertaining to* **nas-** *nose*	Nostril Pertaining to the nose
paranasal	**PAR**-ah **NAY**-zal	P/	**para-** *adjacent to*	Adjacent to the nose
rhinitis (also called coryza) rhinoplasty	rye-**NI**-tis **RYE**-no-plas-tee	S/ R/CF S/	**-itis** *inflammation* **rhin/o-** *nose* **-plasty** *surgical repair*	Inflammation of the nasal mucosa Surgical procedure to change the size or shape of the nose
sinus sinusitis	**SIGH**-nus sigh-nyu-**SIGH**-tis	 S/ R/	Latin *cavity* **-itis** *inflammation* **sinus-** *sinus*	Cavity or hollow space in a bone or other tissue Inflammation of the lining of a sinus
turbinate	**TUR**-bin-ate		Latin *shaped like a top*	Another name for the nasal conchae on the lateral walls of the nasal cavity

Deviated nasal septum occurs when the partition between the two nostrils is pushed to one side, leading to a partially obstructed airway in one nostril.

Epistaxis is bleeding from the septum of the nose, usually from trauma. If pinching the nose or packing the nostril with gauze does not stop the bleeding, **cautery** (burning and scarring) with silver nitrate or electrical cautery is indicated.

Rhinoplasty is a surgical procedure to alter the size and/or shape of the nose.

EXERCISES

Elements: *Work with elements to build your knowledge of the* **language of pulmonology***. One element in each of the following medical terms is bold italic. Identify the type of element (P, R, CF, S) in the middle column; then write its meaning in the right column. Fill in the chart.*

Medical Term	Type of Element	Meaning of Element
epis*tax*is		
*rhin*itis		
muco*purul*ent		
*para*nasal		
*nas*al		

There are two elements in this list with the same meaning. What are they? _____ and _____

Both mean _____.

CASE REPORT 9.2

Mr. Gawlinski's wife states that he snores loudly and has 40 or 50 periods in the night when he stops breathing. The snoring is so loud that she cannot sleep even in the adjoining bedroom. Tye complains of being tired all day and not having the energy he needs for his job. The sleep study is being performed to confirm a diagnosis of obstructive sleep apnea.

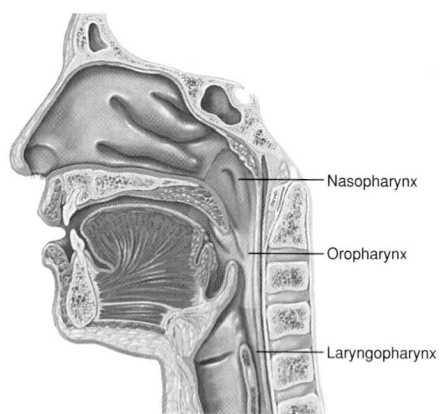

▲ **FIGURE 9.4   Regions of Pharynx.**

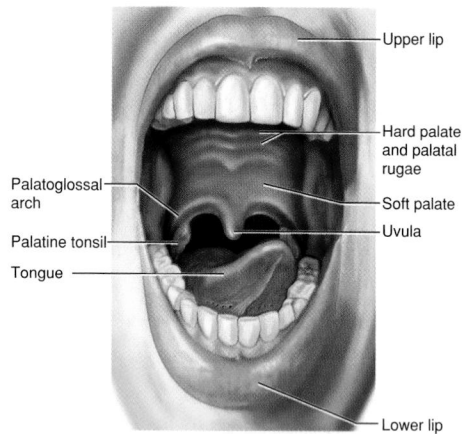

▲ **FIGURE 9.5   Soft Tissues at Back of Mouth.**

PHARYNX

The **pharynx** is a muscular funnel that receives air from the nasal cavity and food and drink from the oral cavity. It is divided into three regions *(Figure 9.4)*:

1. **Nasopharynx**—located at the back of the nose, above the soft palate and uvula. It is lined with a mucous membrane that includes goblet cells, which produce mucus. Mucus, including any trapped debris, is moved from the nasal cavity through the nasopharynx and swallowed. The posterior surface contains the **pharyngeal tonsil (adenoid).** Only air moves through this region.

2. **Oropharynx**—located below the soft palate and above the epiglottis. It contains two sets of tonsils called the palatine and lingual tonsils. Air, food, and drink all pass through this region.

3. **Laryngopharynx**—located below the tip of the epiglottis. This is the pathway to the esophagus. During swallowing, the epiglottis shuts off the trachea so that food cannot enter it. Only food and drink pass through the laryngopharynx.

Disorders of the Pharynx

Snoring   Twenty-five percent of normal adults are habitual snorers. The condition is most frequent in overweight males, and it becomes worse with age. The noises of **snoring** are made at the back of the mouth and nose where the tongue and upper pharynx meet the soft palate and uvula *(Figure 9.5)*. When there is obstruction to the free flow of air, these structures hit each other, and the vibration produces the sounds of snoring.

Obstructive Sleep Apnea   This is the condition Mr. Gawlinski has. He has bulky neck tissue from his football training regimen. Obstructive sleep apnea occurs when obstruction by the soft tissues at the back of the nose and mouth causes frequent episodes of gasping for breath followed by complete cessation of breathing **(apnea).** These episodes of stopped breathing can last for 10 to 30 seconds and occur many times every hour of sleep. The episodes reduce the level of oxygen in the blood **(hypoxia),** causing the heart to pump harder. After several years with this problem, hypertension and cardiac enlargement can occur.

Pharyngitis is an acute or chronic infection involving the pharynx, tonsils, and uvula. It is usually of viral origin in children.

Tonsillitis is an infection of the tonsils in the oropharynx by a virus or, in less than 20% of cases, a streptococcus.

Nasopharyngeal carcinoma is a rare form of cancer that occurs mostly in males between the ages of 50 and 60. Radiation and chemotherapy are used in treatment.

WORD ANALYSIS AND DEFINITION

S = Suffix   P = Prefix   R = Root   R/CF = Combining Form

WORD	PRONUNCIATION	ELEMENTS		DEFINITION
adenoid	**ADD**-eh-noyd	S/ R/	-oid *resembling* aden- *gland*	Single mass of lymphoid tissue in midline at the back of the throat
apnea	**AP**-nee-ah	P/ R/	a- *without* -pnea *breathe*	Absence of spontaneous respiration
hypoxia (**Note:** One of the two consecutive "o"s in the elements is deleted.)	high-**POCK**-see-ah	S/ P/ R/	-ia *condition* hypo- *below, deficient* -ox- *oxygen*	Below normal levels of oxygen in tissues, gases, or blood
laryngopharynx	lah-**RING**-oh-**FAIR**-inks	R/ R/CF	-pharynx *pharynx* laryng/o- *larynx*	Region of the pharynx below the epiglottis that includes the larynx
nasopharynx nasopharyngeal (adj)	**NAY**-zoh-**FAIR**-inks **NAY**-zoh-fair-**IN**-jee-al	R/ R/CF S/ R/	-pharynx *pharynx* nas/o- *nose* -eal *pertaining to* -pharyng- *pharynx*	Region of the pharynx at the back of the nose above the soft palate
oropharynx oropharyngeal (adj	**OR**-oh-fair-inks **OR**-oh-fair-**IN**-jee-al	R/ R/CF	-pharynx *pharynx* or/o- *mouth*	Region at the back of the mouth between the soft palate and the tip of the epiglottis
pharynx pharyngitis pharyngeal (adj)	**FAIR**-inks fair-in-**JI**-tis fah-**RIN**-jee-al	 S/ R/ S/	Greek *throat* -itis *inflammation* pharyng- *pharynx* -eal *pertaining to*	Air tube from the back of the nose to the larynx Inflammation of the pharynx
polysomnography	pol-ee-som-**NOG**-rah-fee	S/ P/ R/CF	-graphy *process of recording* poly- *many* -somn/o- *sleep*	Test to monitor brain waves, muscle tension, eye movement, and oxygen levels in the blood as the patient sleeps
snore	SNOR		Old English *snore*	Noise produced by vibrations in the structures of the nasopharynx
tonsil tonsillitis (note the double "ll") tonsillectomy	**TON**-sill ton-sih-**LIE**-tis ton-sih-**LEC**-toh-me	 S/ R/ S/	Latin *tonsil* -itis *inflammation* tonsill- *tonsil* -ectomy *surgical excision*	Mass of lymphoid tissue on either side of the throat at the back of the tongue Inflammation of the tonsils Surgical removal of the tonsils

EXERCISES

After reading Case Report 9.2 on the opposite page, answer the following questions. Be prepared to discuss your answers in class.

1. What are Mr. Gawlinski's symptoms? _____ .

2. Mr. Gawlinski underwent the diagnostic procedure of _____ .

3. If left untreated, his chronic obstructive sleep apnea could cause _____ .

4. Analyze the elements in *apnea,* and define it. _____

5. What causes Mr. Gawlinski's obstructive sleep apnea to occur?

_____

_____

6. The patient's sleep apnea can <u>reduce the level of oxygen in his blood</u>. What is the medical term for the underlined phrase? _____

7. In the term *electrodes,* the element *electro* refers to _____

8. Why is *polysomnography* done overnight?

_____

LARYNX

The flow of inhaled air moves on from the pharynx to the larynx, an enlargement of the airway located between the oropharynx and the trachea. The upper opening into it from the oropharynx is called the **glottis.**

The larynx has an outer casing of nine cartilages connected to each other by muscles and ligaments. The uppermost cartilage, the leaf-shaped **epiglottis,** guards the glottis. During the swallowing of food, the epiglottis is pushed down by the tongue to close the glottis and direct food into the esophagus that lies behind it *(Figure 9.6a).*

The **thyroid** cartilage, or "Adam's apple," is the largest cartilage and forms the anterior and lateral walls of the larynx. Below the thyroid cartilage the ring-shaped **cricoid** cartilage connects the larynx to the trachea *(Figure 9.6b).*

Inside the larynx, two pairs of horizontal ligaments stretch across the lateral walls. The superior pair are the **false vocal cords.** They play no role in sound production, but close the larynx during swallowing as reinforcement to the closing of the epiglottis. The inferior pair is the **true vocal cords** *(Figure 9.6b).* **Intrinsic** muscles control the cords.

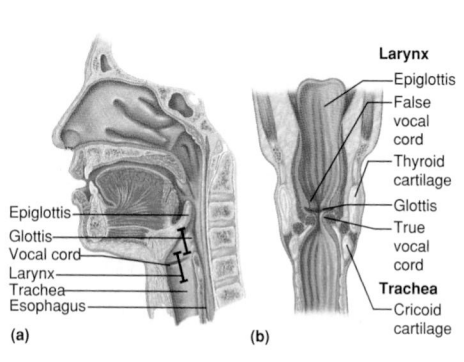

▲ **FIGURE 9.6 Larynx.** (*a*) Location. (*b*) Structure.

Functions of the Larynx

- The thyroid and cricoid cartilages maintain an open passage for the movement of air to and from the trachea.
- The epiglottis and vestibular folds prevent food and drink from entering the larynx *(Figure 9.7).*
- The vocal cords are the source of sound production.

Sound Production Air moving past the vocal cords makes them vibrate to produce sound. The force of the air moving past the vocal cords determines the loudness of the sound. The intrinsic muscles of the cords pull them closer together with varying degrees of tautness *(Figure 9.8).* A high-pitched sound is produced by taut cords and a lower pitch by more relaxed cords.

The male vocal cords are longer and thicker than the female, vibrate more slowly, and produce lower-pitched sounds.

The crude sounds produced by the larynx are transformed into words by the actions of the pharynx, tongue, teeth, and lips.

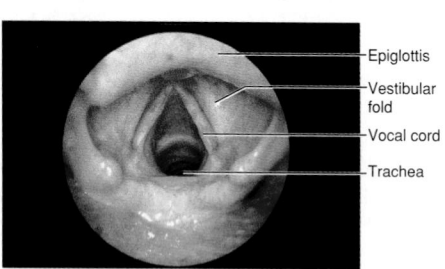

▲ **FIGURE 9.7 View of Larynx Using Laryngoscope.**

Disorders of the Larynx

Laryngitis is inflammation of the mucosal lining of the larynx, producing hoarseness and sometimes progressing to loss of voice **(aphonia).**

Epiglottitis is inflammation of the epiglottis. **Acute epiglottitis** is seen most commonly in children between ages 2 and 7 years and is caused by *Haemophilus influenzae type b* bacteria. Swelling in the epiglottis can cause acute airway obstruction and the need for **intubation.** It is preventable, using an available vaccine.

Croup (laryngotracheobronchitis) is a group of viral diseases in children age 3 months to 5 years. It causes inflammation and obstruction of the upper airway. It produces a characteristic cough that sounds like a seal barking. In severe cases, the child makes a high-pitched, squeaky inspiratory noise called **stridor.** Humidity is the initial treatment.

Papillomas or **polyps** are benign tumors of the larynx that result from overuse or irritation and are treated by surgical excision using a **laryngoscope.**

Carcinoma of the larynx produces a persistent hoarseness. Its incidence peaks in smokers in their fifties and sixties. Treatment can be radiation and/or chemotherapy.

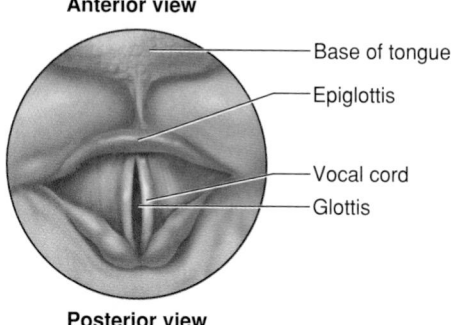

▲ **FIGURE 9.8 Vocal Cords Pulled Close and Taut.**

WORD	PRONUNCIATION		ELEMENTS	DEFINITION
aphonia	a-**FO**-nee-ah	S/ P/ R/	-ia *condition* a- *without* -phon- *voice*	Loss of voice
cricoid	**CRY**-koyd		Latin *a ring*	Ring-shaped cartilage in the larynx
croup (also called **laryn-gotracheobronchitis**)	KROOP		Old English *to cry out loud*	Infection of the upper airways in children; characterized by a barking cough
epiglottis epiglottitis glottis	ep-ih-**GLOT**-is ep-ih-**GLOT**-eye-tis **GLOT**-is	P/ R/ S/	epi- *above* -glott- *mouth of windpipe* -itis *inflammation* Greek *opening of larynx*	Leaf-shaped plate of cartilage that shuts off the larynx during swallowing Inflammation of the epiglottis The opening from the oropharynx into the larynx
intrinsic	in-**TRIN**-sik		Latin *on the inside*	Any muscle whose origin and insertion are entirely within the structure under consideration; for example, inside the vocal cords or the eye
intubation	**IN**-tyu-**BAY**-shun	S/ P/ R/CF	-tion *process* in- *in* -tub/a- *tube*	Insertion of a tube into the trachea
larynx laryngitis laryngoscope laryngotracheobronchi-tis (also called **croup**)	**LAIR**-inks lar-in-**JEYE**-tis lah-**RING**-oh-skope lah-**RING**-oh-**TRAY**-kee-oh-brong-**KI**-tis	S/ R/ S/ S/ R/CF R/CF R/	Greek *larynx* -itis *inflammation* laryng- *larynx* -scope *instrument for viewing* -itis *inflammation* laryng/o- *larynx* -trache/o- *trachea* -bronch- *bronchus*	Organ of voice production Inflammation of the larynx Hollow tube with a light and camera used to visualize or operate on the larynx Inflammation of the larynx, trachea, and bronchi
stridor	**STRY**-door		Latin *a harsh, creaking sound*	High-pitched noise made when there is respiratory obstruction in the larynx or trachea
thyroid	**THIGH**-royd		Greek *an oblong shield*	Gland in the neck, or a cartilage of the larynx
vocal	**VOH**-kal	S/ R/	-al *pertaining to* voc- *voice*	Pertaining to the voice

---

EXERCISES

Deconstruct: *For long or short medical terms, deconstruction into word elements is your key to solving the meaning of the term. Follow the directions, and fill in the blanks.*

1. laryngotracheobronchitis

Rewrite this term, and slash all its elements.

_____

2. Combine the meanings of the elements, and define the term.

Laryngotracheobronchitis means:

_____

_____

3. vocal

Slash this term into all its elements.

_____

4. Combine the meanings of the elements, and define the term.

Vocal means:

_____

> *Study Hint*
> Whether the term is 24 letters long or 5 letters long, the principle is the same. Know the meaning of the elements, and you will know the meaning of the term!

OBJECTIVES

Once the air you inhale has passed through the upper airway and many of the pollutants and impurities have been filtered out and swallowed into the digestive system, there still remain the major needs of getting oxygen into the blood and removing carbon dioxide from the blood. To do these, the inhaled air has to get down into the alveoli of the lungs, where these exchanges can occur.

In this lesson, you will learn to use correct medical terminology to:

9.2.1 **Trace the passage of air from the larynx into the alveoli and back.**

9.2.2 **Explain the exchange of oxygen from the air into the blood.**

9.2.3 **Explain the exchange of carbon dioxide from the blood into the air.**

9.2.4 **Describe the mechanics of ventilation.**

9.2.5 **Integrate the functions of the different elements of the lower airway with their structure.**

9.2.6 **Discuss the effects of common disorders of the lungs on overall health.**

TRACHEA

The flow of inhaled air now moves into the trachea (windpipe). This is a rigid tube that descends from the larynx to divide into the two main bronchi *(Figure 9.10a)*. The rigidity of the trachea is produced by 16 to 20 C-shaped rings of cartilage that form its anterior and lateral walls *(Figure 9.10b)*. The open part of the "C" faces posteriorly and is closed by the **trachealis** muscle.

LUNGS

The two lungs are the main organs of respiration and are located in the thoracic cavity. Each lung is a soft, spongy, conical organ with its base resting on the **diaphragm** and its apex above and behind the clavicle. Its outer, convex costal surface presses against the rib cage. Its inner, concave surface presses against the **mediastinum**.

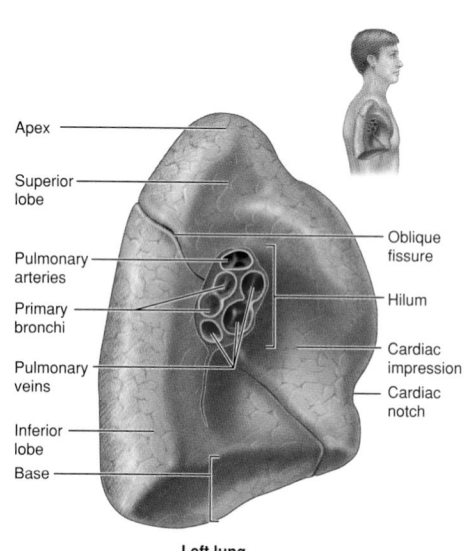

Apex
Superior lobe
Pulmonary arteries
Primary bronchi
Pulmonary veins
Inferior lobe
Base
Oblique fissure
Hilum
Cardiac impression
Cardiac notch

Left lung

▲ **FIGURE 9.9 Left Lung Hilum: Medial Surface.**

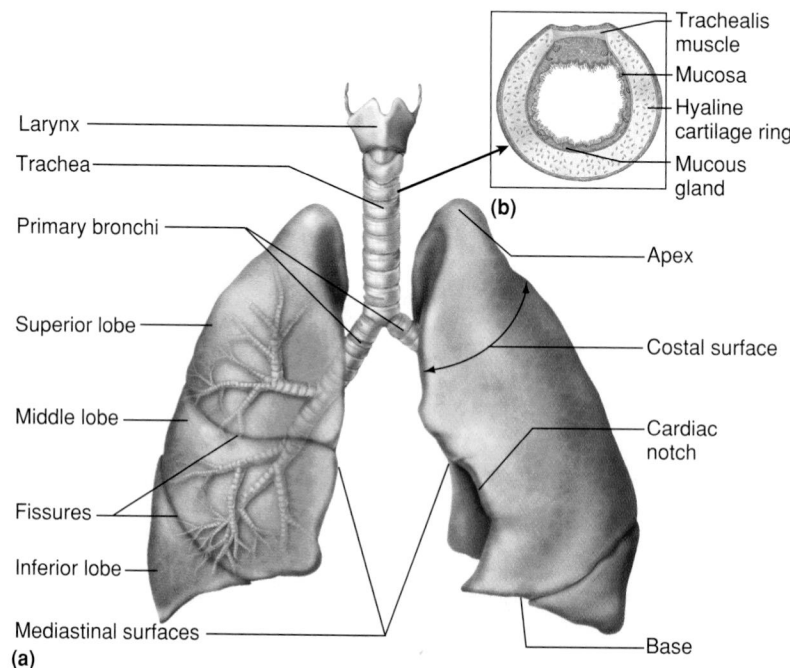

Trachealis muscle
Mucosa
Hyaline cartilage ring
Mucous gland
(b)

Larynx
Trachea
Primary bronchi
Superior lobe
Middle lobe
Fissures
Inferior lobe
Mediastinal surfaces
Apex
Costal surface
Cardiac notch
Base

▶ **FIGURE 9.10 Lower Respiratory Tract.**
(a) Gross anatomy. (b) C-shaped tracheal cartilage. **(a)**

WORD	PRONUNCIATION	ELEMENTS		DEFINITION
diaphragm diaphragmatic (adj)	**DIE**-ah-fram **DIE**-ah-frag-**MAT**-ic	S/ R/CF	Greek *diaphragm* -tic *pertaining to* diaphragm/a- *diaphragm*	Musculoligamentous partition separating the abdominal and thoracic cavities Pertaining to the diaphragm
fissure fissures (pl)	**FISH**-ur	S/ R/	-ure *result of* fiss- *split*	Deep furrow or cleft
hilum hila (pl)	**HIGH**-lum **HIGH**-lah		Latin *small area*	The site where the nerves and blood vessels enter and leave an organ
lobe lobar (adj)	LOBE **LOW**-bar	S/ R/	Greek *lobe* -ar *pertaining to* lob- *lobe*	Subdivision of an organ or other part
mediastinum mediastinal (adj)	**ME**-dee-ass-**TIE**-num **ME**-dee-ah-**STIE**-nal	S/ P/ R/	-um *tissue, structure* media- *middle* -stin- *partition*	Area between the lungs containing the heart, aorta, venae cavae, esophagus, and trachea
parenchyma	pah-**RENG**-kih-mah		Greek *to pour in beside*	Characteristic functional cells of a gland or organ that are supported by the connective tissue framework
stroma	**STROH**-mah		Greek *bed*	Connective tissue framework that supports the parenchyma of an organ or gland
trachealis	tray-kee-**AY**-lis	S/ R/CF	-alis *pertaining to* trach/e- *trachea*	Pertaining to the trachea

The right lung has three **lobes**—superior, middle and inferior. The left lung has two lobes, a superior and inferior *(Figure 9.10a)*. The lobes are separated from each other by **fissures**. The heart makes a concave impression in the left lung, known as the cardiac notch.

Each lung receives its bronchus, blood vessels, lymphatic vessels, and nerves through its **hilum** *(Figure 9.9)*. The lung's specific functional cells are called the lung **parenchyma** and are supported by a thin connective tissue framework called the **stroma**. This consists mostly of collagen and elastic fibers, and its elasticity is a factor in the lung's recoil after inhalation.

EXERCISES

Precision in communication means using the correct form of the medical term, as well as the correct spelling. Test your knowledge of plurals, adjectives, and spelling with this exercise. Circle the correct choice.

1. The area between the lungs containing the heart, aorta, venae cavae, esophagus, and trachea is the:

   mediastenum   medisternum   mediastinum   midiasternum

2. The patient was diagnosed with _____ pneumonia.

   lobe   lobular   lobar   lumbar

3. _____ is the term for the functional cells of an organ.

   perenchyma   parenchyma   perinchkima   perenkima

4. Since there is a hilum in each lung, collectively they are referred to as the:

   hilla   hila   hilia   hilea

5. The muscle separating the abdominal and thoracic cavities is the:

   diaphram   diaphragm   diahragm   diapragm

6. Removal of a lobe of a lung would be a:

   lobotomy   lobectomy   lobarectomy   lobarotomy

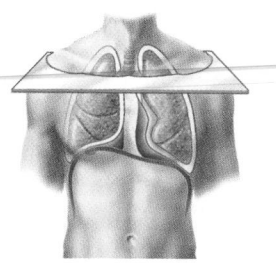

Pleurae

The surface of each lung is covered with a serous membrane called the **visceral pleura** *(Figure 9.11)*. At the hilum, the visceral pleura turns back on itself to form the **parietal pleura,** which lines the rib cage. The space between the visceral and parietal pleurae is called the **pleural cavity,** which contains a thin film of lubricant called the **pleural fluid.**

The functions of the **pleurae** and pleural fluid are to:

1. **Reduce friction.** The lubricant quality of the pleural fluid enables the lungs to expand (**inspiration**) and contract (**expiration**) with minimal friction.

2. **Assist in inspiration.** The pressure in the pleural cavity is lower than the pressure of the atmospheric air in the lungs. This assists the **inflation** of the lungs on inspiration.

3. **Separation.** The **pleurae, mediastinum,** and **pericardium** protect the organs inside them to prevent infections from spreading easily from one organ to another.

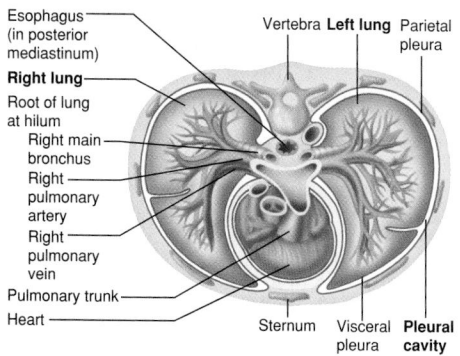

▲ **FIGURE 9.11   Pleural Cavity and Membranes: Superior View.**

TRACHEOBRONCHIAL TREE

As the inhaled air continues down the respiratory tract, the trachea divides and air flows into the right and left main (primary) bronchi, which enter each lung at the hilum. Like the trachea, the main bronchi are supported by C-shaped cartilages.

In turn, the main bronchi divide into a secondary (lobar) bronchus for each lobe. There are three secondary bronchi in the right lung and two in the left lung.

Each secondary bronchus divides into tertiary bronchi that supply segments of each lobe *(Figure 9.12)*.

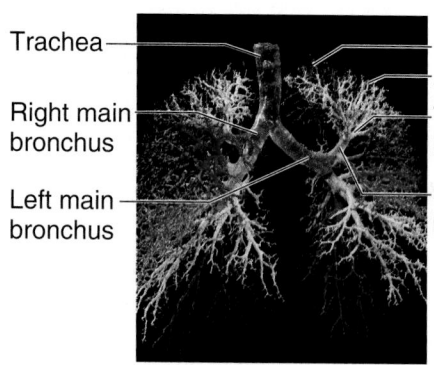

▲ **FIGURE 9.12   Latex Cast of Tracheobronchial Tree.**

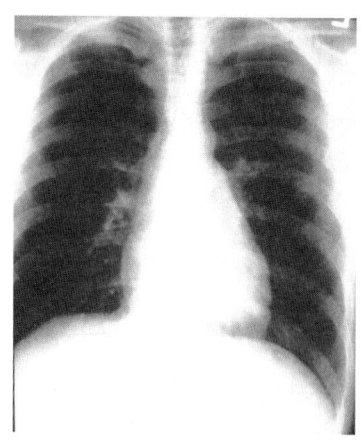

▲ **FIGURE 9.13   Normal Lungs with Air in Alveoli.**

WORD	PRONUNCIATION	ELEMENTS		DEFINITION
expiration (opposite of inspiration) (**Note:** The "s" is deleted from the root -spir- because the prefix ex- already has the "s" sound.)	**EKS**-pih-**RAY**-shun	S/ P/ R/	-ation *process* ex- *out* -spir- *to breathe*	Breathe out
inflate (verb) **inflation (noun)** (same as inspiration)	in-**FLAYT** in-**FLAY**-shun	S/ P/ R/	Latin *blow up* -ation *process* in- *into* -flate- *blow up*	Expand with air Process of expanding with air
inspiration (opposite of expiration)	in-spih-**RAY**-shun	S/ P/ R/	-ation *process* in- *into* -spir- *to breathe*	Breathe in
parietal	pah-**RYE**-eh-tal	S/ R/	-al *pertaining to* pariet- *wall*	Pertaining to the outer layer of the pericardium and other body cavities
pericardium	per-ih-**KAR**-dee-um	S/ P/ R/	-um *tissue, structure* peri- *around* -cardi- *heart*	The tissue covering the heart
pleura **pleurae (pl)** **pleural (adj)**	**PLUR**-ah **PLUR**-ee **PLUR**-al	S/ R/	Greek *rib, side* -al *pertaining to* pleur- *pleura*	Membrane covering the lungs and lining the ribs in the thoracic cavity Pertaining to the pleura
pleurisy **pleuritic (adj)**	**PLUR**-ih-see **PLUR**-it-ik	S/ S/	-isy *inflammation* -itic *pertaining to*	Inflammation of the pleura
surfactant	ser-**FAK**-tant	S/ R/ R/	-ant *pertaining to* surf- *surface* -act- *to do, perform*	A protein and fat compound that creates surface tension to hold lung alveolar walls apart

Bronchioles and Alveoli

The tertiary bronchi divide into **bronchioles,** which in turn divide into **terminal bronchioles** and then smaller respiratory bronchioles *(Figure 9.14)*. None of these bronchioles has cartilage in the walls, but smooth muscle enables them to dilate or constrict. These bronchioles in turn divide into thin-walled **alveoli.**

Each **alveolus** is a thin-walled sac supported by a thin **respiratory membrane** that allows the exchange of gases with the surrounding pulmonary capillary network *(Figure 9.14)*. About 5% of the **alveolar** cells secrete a detergent like substance called **surfactant** that keeps the alveolar sacs from collapsing *(Figure 9.13)*. There are approximately 300 million alveoli in the two lungs.

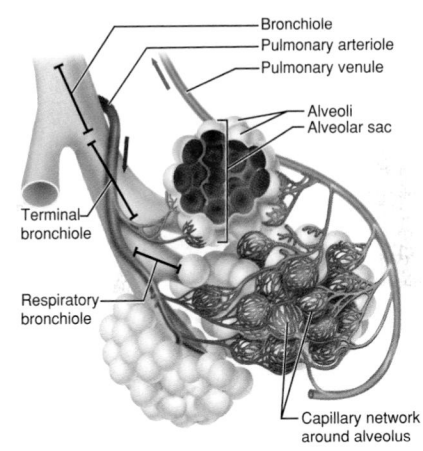

FIGURE 9.14 **Bronchioles and Alveoli.** ▶

EXERCISES

Make the WAD work for you. The following questions can all be answered with information you will find in this WAD. Insert the correct terms in the appropriate space.

1. A membrane covering the lung and lining the ribs is the _____. The plural of this term is _____.

   To describe the _____ membrane, you need the adjective form of this term.

2. The two opposite terms that relate to the breathing process are _____, which means _____,

   and _____, which means _____.

3. The root **spir** means to _____.

4. The purpose of **surfactant** is to _____

   _____.

5. **Parietal** pertains to the outer layer of the _____

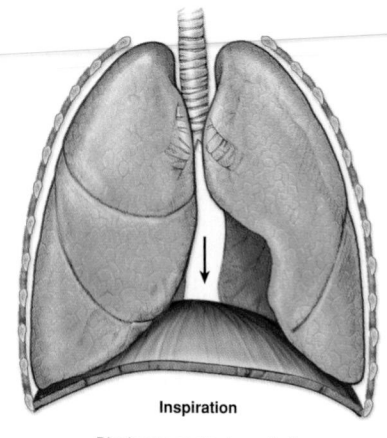

Inspiration

Diaphragm contracts; vertical
dimensions of thoracic cavity increase.

(a)

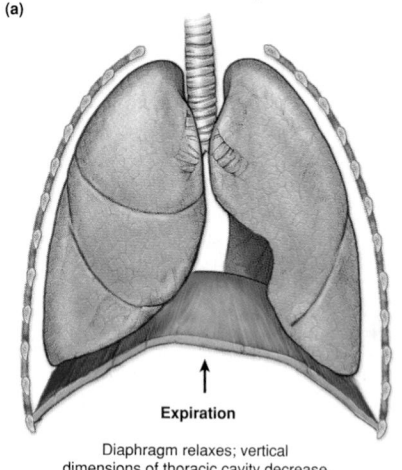

Expiration

Diaphragm relaxes; vertical
dimensions of thoracic cavity decrease.

(b)

▲ **FIGURE 9.15   Inspiration and Expiration.**

Abbreviation	
SOB	shortness of breath

RESPIRATION

Mechanics of Respiration

A resting adult breathes 10 to 15 times per minute, **inhales** about 500 mL of air during inspiration, and **exhales** it during expiration. The mission is to get air into and out of the alveoli so that oxygen can get into the blood and carbon dioxide can get out of the blood.

The diaphragm does most of the work. In inspiration it drops down and flattens to expand the thoracic cavity and reduce the pressure in the airways *(Figure 9.15a)*. In addition, the external intercostal muscles lift the chest wall up and out to further expand the thoracic cavity.

Expiration is a process of letting go. The diaphragm and the intercostal muscles relax, and the thoracic cavity springs back to its original size *(Figure 9.15b)*. If you want to blow out your birthday candles, you consciously contract your internal intercostal muscles and abdominal muscles to push the diaphragm up and expel the air rapidly.

Not all the inhaled air can get into the alveoli. The air that does not get into the alveoli and remains in the mouth, pharynx, trachea, and bronchi down to the respiratory bronchioles is said to be in the **anatomical dead space.**

Common Symptoms and Signs of Respiratory Disorders

1. **Coughing** is triggered by irritants in the respiratory tract. You close the glottis and contract the muscles of expiration to develop high pressure in the lower tract. Then you suddenly open the glottis to release an explosive blast of air.

   The irritants can be cigarette smoke (as with Mr. Jacobs) or infection or tumors (as in lung cancer). A productive cough produces sputum that can be swallowed or **expectorated.** Bloody sputum is called **hemoptysis.** Thick, yellow (purulent) sputum indicates infection. A nonproductive cough is dry and hacking.

   Abnormal amounts of mucus arising from the upper respiratory tract and expectorated are called **phlegm.**

2. **Dyspnea,** or **shortness of breath (SOB),** can be on exertion or, in severe disorders, at rest when all the respiratory muscles are used to exchange only a small volume of air.

   Dyspnea can result from airway obstruction. Wheezing associated with dyspnea is the sound of air being forced through constricted airways, as in asthma. Dyspnea can also be produced by fibrosis of lung tissues, when the lungs' **compliance** is reduced. Compliance is the ability of the lungs to expand on inspiration.

3. **Cyanosis** is seen when the blood has increased levels of **unoxygenated hemoglobin** and has a characteristic dark gray–blue color. It is best seen in the lips, whites of the eyes, mucous membranes, and nail beds where there is no skin pigmentation to mask it.
   - **Peripheral cyanosis** occurs when there is peripheral vasoconstriction. The reduced flow allows hemoglobin to yield more of its oxygen, leading to increased unoxygenated hemoglobin.
   - **Central cyanosis** occurs with inadequate blood oxygenation in the lungs as a result of impaired airflow or with impaired blood flow through the lungs.

4. **Changes in rate of breathing. Eupnea** is the normal, easy respiration—around 15 breaths per minute in a resting adult. Both **tachypnea** (rapid rate of breathing) and **hyperpnea** (breathing deeper and more rapidly than normal) are signs of respiratory difficulty, as is **bradypnea** (slow breathing).

5. **Sneezing** is caused by irritants in the nasal cavity. The glottis stays open while the soft palate and tongue block the flow of air from getting out. Then they suddenly release to let air burst out through the nose.

WORD ANALYSIS AND DEFINITION

WORD	PRONUNCIATION		ELEMENTS	DEFINITION
bradypnea (opposite of tachypnea)	brad-ip-**NEE**-ah	P/ R/	brady- *slow* -pnea *breathe*	Slow breathing
compliance	kom-**PLY**-ance	S/ R/	-ance *state of, condition* compli- *fulfill*	Measure of the capacity of a chamber or hollow viscus to expand; in this case, the lungs
cyanosis	sigh-ah-**NO**-sis	S/ R/	-osis *condition* cyan- *dark blue*	Blue discoloration of the skin, lips, and nail beds due to low levels of oxygen in the blood
cyanotic (adj)	sigh-ah-**NOT**-ik	S/ R/CF	-tic *pertaining to* cyan/o- *dark blue*	Marked by cyanosis
dyspnea	disp-**NEE**-ah	P/ R/	dys- *bad, difficult* -pnea *breathe*	Difficulty breathing
eupnea	yoop-**NEE**-ah	P/ R/	eu- *normal* -pnea *breathe*	Normal breathing
exhale	**EKS**-hail	P/ R/	ex- *out* -hale *breathe*	Breathe out
expectorate	ek-**SPEC**-toh-rate	S/ P/ R/	-ate *composed of* ex- *out* -pector- *chest*	Cough up and spit out mucus from the respiratory tract
hemoptysis	he-**MOP**-tih-sis	R/CF R/	hem/o- *blood* -ptysis *spit*	Bloody sputum
hyperpnea	high-perp-**NEE**-ah	P/ R/	hyper- *excessive* -pnea *breathe*	Deeper and more rapid breathing than normal
inhale	**IN**-hail	P/ R/	in- *in* -hale *breathe*	Breathe in
phlegm	FLEM		Greek *flame*	Abnormal amounts of mucus expectorated from the respiratory tract
tachypnea (opposite of bradypnea)	tak-ip-**NEE**-ah	P/ R/	tachy- *rapid* -pnea *breathe*	Rapid breathing

6. **Hiccups** are reflex spasms of the diaphragm, causing an involuntary inhalation followed by a sudden closure of the glottis that produces an audible sound—the "hic." The etiology is unknown, and there is no specific medical cure.

7. **Yawning** is a reflex that originates in the brainstem in response to hypoxia, boredom, or sleepiness. The exact mechanisms are not known.

EXERCISES

Build terms. *Knowing just one element will enable you to build more terms with the addition of other elements. Practice building your pulmonology terms with the following root and various prefixes. Fill in the blanks.*

1. The root *-pnea* means: _____ .

Add the following prefixes to the root -pnea to form new terms for questions 2 through 6.

tachy   brady   dys   eu   hyper

2. Difficult breathing   _____pnea

3. Deeper breathing than normal   _____pnea

4. Slow breathing   _____pnea

5. Normal breathing   _____pnea

6. Rapid breathing   _____pnea

> *Study Hint*
> Remember these prefixes—they can be applied to many other roots for new terms.

DISORDERS OF THE LOWER RESPIRATORY TRACT

Acute bronchitis can be viral or bacterial, leading to the production of excess mucus with some obstruction of airflow. A single episode resolves without significant residual damage to the airway.

Chronic bronchitis is the most common obstructive disease, due to cigarette smoking or repeated episodes of acute bronchitis. In addition to excess mucus production, cilia are destroyed. A pattern develops, involving chronic cough, dyspnea, and recurrent acute infections.

In advanced chronic bronchitis, hypoxia and **hypercapnia** (excess carbon dioxide) are produced, and heart failure follows.

Bronchiolitis, inflammation of the small airway bronchioles, occurs in the adult as the early and often unrecognized beginning of airway changes in cigarette smokers or those exposed to "secondhand smoke," inhaling the smoke produced by other peoples' cigarettes.

Bronchiolitis affects children under the age of 2 because their small airways become blocked very easily. The disease is viral and in severe cases can cause marked respiratory distress, with drawing in of the neck and intercostal spaces of the chest with each breath (known as **retractions**).

Pulmonary emphysema is a disease of the respiratory bronchioles and alveoli. These airways become enlarged, and the septa between the alveoli are destroyed, forming large sacs **(bullae)**. There is a loss of surface area for gas exchange. Because the septa contain elastic tissue that assists the lungs' recoil in exhalation, this becomes more difficult, and air is trapped in the bullae. This leads to **hyperinflation** of the lungs and the enlarged "barrel chest" shown by many patients with emphysema.

Chronic airway obstruction (CAO) is also called **chronic obstructive pulmonary disease (COPD).** This is a progressive disease, as Mr. Jacobs' history shows. It involves both chronic bronchitis and emphysema. A history of heavy cigarette smoking, with chronic cough and sputum production, is followed by exertional dyspnea. By the time his dyspnea was severe, irreversible lung damage *(Figure 9.16)* had led to emphysema, recurrent infections, and episodes of respiratory insufficiency. The insufficiency becomes permanent, and, as for Mr. Jacobs, oxygen is necessary round the clock. Right-sided heart failure **(cor pulmonale)** is the end-result of pulmonary hypertension and blood being backed up into the right ventricle *(see Chapter 8).*

Bronchiectasis is the abnormal dilatation of the small bronchioles due to repeated infections. The damaged, dilated bronchi are unable to clear secretions, so additional infections and more damage can occur.

Bronchial asthma is a disorder with recurrent acute episodes of bronchial obstruction as a result of constriction of bronchioles **(bronchoconstriction)**, **hypersecretion** of mucus, and inflammatory swelling of the bronchiolar lining. The airflow obstruction these produce is mainly during expiration, and the wheezing exhalation heard in asthma is the result of forcing air out of the lungs through constricted, swollen bronchioles *(Figure 9.17)*. Between attacks, breathing can be normal. The etiology of asthma is an allergic response to substances such as pollen, animal dander, or the feces of house dust mites.

Cystic fibrosis (CF) is caused by an increased viscosity of secretions from the pancreas, salivary glands, liver, intestine, and lungs. In the lungs, a particularly thick mucus obstructs the airways and causes repeated infections. Respiratory failure is the cause of death, often before the age of 30. The disorder is genetic *(see Chapter 21).*

Pulmonary edema is the collection of fluid in the lung tissues and alveoli. It is most frequently the result of left ventricular failure or mitral valve disease with **congestive heart failure (CHF).** Noncardiogenic pulmonary edema can result from sepsis, renal failure, disseminated intravascular coagulation *(see Chapter 7)*, and opiate or barbiturate poisoning *(see Chapter 10).*

During **auscultation** of the chest, the air bubbling through abnormal fluid in the alveoli and small bronchioles (as in pulmonary edema) produces a noise called rales. When the bronchi are partly obstructed and air is being forced past the obstruction, a high-pitched noise called a **rhonchus** is heard.

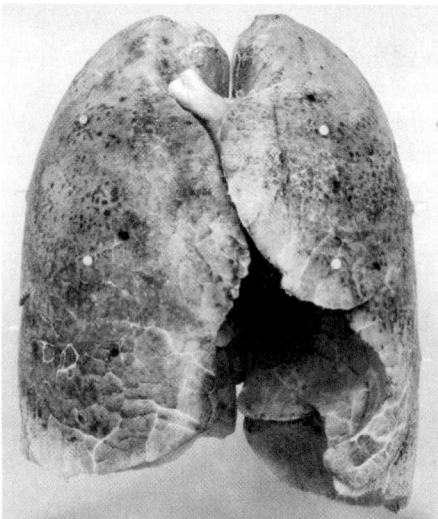

(a)

Heart

(b)

▲ **FIGURE 9.16 Whole Lungs.**
(a) Nonsmoker's lungs. (b) Smoker's lungs.

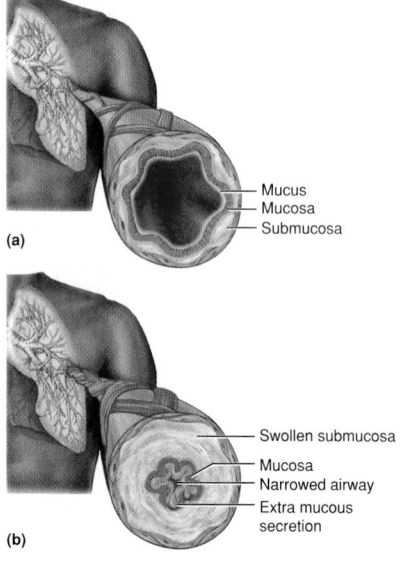

(a)

Mucus
Mucosa
Submucosa

(b)

Swollen submucosa
Mucosa
Narrowed airway
Extra mucous secretion

▲ **FIGURE 9.17   Bronchiole Diameter.**
(a) Normal airway. (b) Airway during an asthma attack.

WORD	PRONUNCIATION		ELEMENTS	DEFINITION
asthma asthmatic (adj)	**AZ**-mah az-**MAT**-ic		Greek *asthma*	Episodes of breathing difficulty due to narrowed or obstructed airways
auscultation	aws-kul-**TAY**-shun	S/ R/	-ation *process* auscult- *listen to*	Diagnostic method of listening to body sounds with a stethoscope
bronchiectasis	brong-kee-**ECK**-tah-sis	S/ R/CF	-ectasis *dilation* bronch/i- *bronchus*	Chronic dilation of the bronchi following inflammatory disease and obstruction
bronchiolitis (*Note:* This term has two suffixes—the "e" is dropped before the "i" in -itis.)	brong-kee-oh-**LYE**-tis	S/ S/ R/CF	-itis *inflammation* -ole *small* bronch/i- *bronchus*	Inflammation of the small bronchioles
bronchoconstriction	**BRONG**-koh-kon-**STRIK**-shun	S/ R/CF R/	-ion *process* bronch/o- *bronchus* -constrict- *to narrow*	Reduction in diameter of a bronchus
bulla bullae (pl)	**BULL**-ah **BULL**-ee		Latin *bubble*	Bubblelike dilated structure
cor pulmonale	KOR pul-moh-**NAH**-lee	R/ S/ R/	cor *heart* -ale *pertaining to* pulmon- *lung*	Right-sided heart failure arising from chronic lung disease
cystic fibrosis (CF)	**SIS**-tik fie-**BRO**-sis	S/ R/ S/ R/	-ic *pertaining to* cyst- *cyst* -osis *condition* fibr- *fiber*	Genetic disease in which excessive viscid mucus obstructs passages, including bronchi
emphysema	em-fih-**SEE**-mah	P/ R/	em- *in, into* -physema *blowing*	Dilation of respiratory bronchioles and alveoli
hypercapnia	**HIGH**-per-**KAP**-nee-ah	S/ P/ R/	-ia *condition* hyper- *excessive* -capn- *carbon dioxide*	Abnormal increase of carbon dioxide in the arterial bloodstream
hyperinflation	**HIGH**-per-in-**FLAY**-shun	S/ P/ P/ R/CF	-ion *process* hyper- *excessive* in- *in* -flat/e- *blow up*	Overdistension of pulmonary alveoli with air resulting from airway obstruction
hypersecretion	**HIGH**-per-seh-**KREE**-shun	S/ P/ R/	-ion *process* hyper- *excessive* -secret- *secrete*	Excessive secretion of mucus (or enzymes or waste products)
retraction	ree-**TRAK**-shun	S/ P/ R/	-ion *process* re- *back* -tract- *pull*	A pulling back, as a pulling back of the intercostal spaces and the neck above the clavicle
rhonchus rhonchi (pl)	**RONG**-kuss **RONG**-key		Greek *snoring*	Wheezing sound heard on auscultation of the lungs; made by air passing through a constricted lumen

Abbreviations

CAO chronic airway obstruction
CF cystic fibrosis
CHF congestive heart failure
COPD chronic obstructive pulmonary disease

EXERCISES

*These elements all appear in the **language of pulmonology**. Challenge your knowledge of these elements, and make the correct match. Fill in the blanks.*

_____ 1. re

_____ 2. auscult

_____ 3. capn

_____ 4. ole

_____ 5. osis

_____ 6. constrict

_____ 7. ion

_____ 8. tract

_____ 9. ectasis

_____ 10. bronchi

A. to narrow

B. process

C. pull

D. dilation

E. back

F. carbon dioxide

G. listen to

H. bronchus

I. small

J. condition

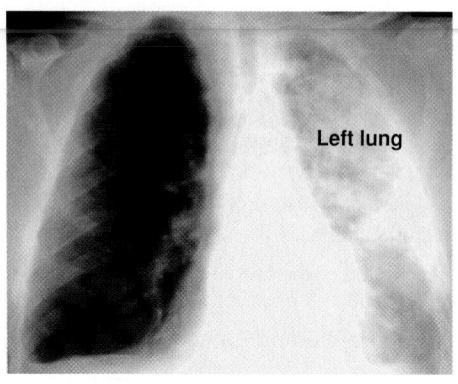

FIGURE 9.18 Chest X-Ray of Patient with Pneumonia in the Left Lung. A normal lung appears as a black space on an x-ray because its spongy structure is filled with air. In contrast, a pneumonic lung appears white or opaque on an x-ray as a result of accumulation of fluid and cells in the alveoli.

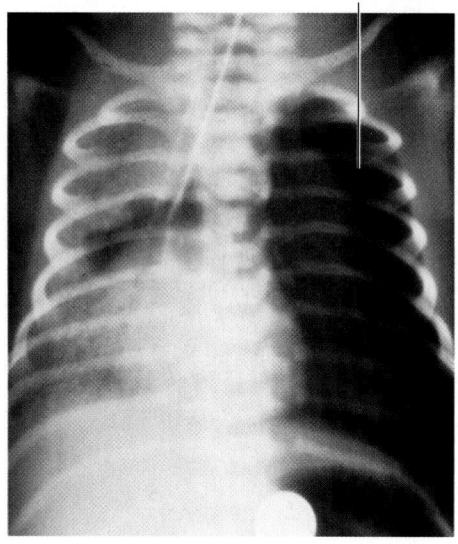

FIGURE 9.19 Left Pneumothorax. There are no lung markings seen in the area of the pneumothorax.

Abbreviations

ARDS acute respiratory distress syndrome
ARF acute respiratory failure
NRDS neonatal respiratory distress syndrome

DISORDERS OF THE LOWER RESPIRATORY TRACT (continued)

Pneumonia is an acute infection affecting the alveoli and lung parenchyma *(Figure 9.18)*. Bacterial infections focus on the alveoli, viral infections on the parenchyma. **Lobar pneumonia** is an infection limited to one lung lobe. **Bronchopneumonia** is used to describe an infection in the bronchioles that spreads to the alveoli.

When an area of the lung (**segment**) or a lobe becomes airless as a result of the infection, the lung is **consolidated.** When an area of the lung collapses as a result of bronchial obstruction, the condition is called **atelectasis.**

Pleurisy, an inflammation of the pleurae, can be a complication of pneumonia. This condition is very painful on breathing because the parietal pleura is very pain-sensitive. The inflammation often leads to an exudate accumulating in the pleural cavity. This is a **pleural effusion.** If the pleural effusion contains pus, it is called **empyema.** If it contains blood, it is called **hemothorax.** When pleural fluid is drawn off for therapeutic purposes or for laboratory analysis, the procedure is **aspiration** or **thoracentesis.**

Lung abscess can be a complication of bacterial pneumonia or cancer. Long-term antibiotics are used and surgical resection of the abscess may be required.

Pneumothorax is the entry of air into the pleural cavity *(Figure 9.19)*. The cause can be unknown (**spontaneous pneumothorax),** but it often results from trauma when a fractured rib, knife blade, or bullet lacerates the parietal pleura.

Thromboembolism is caused by an embolus, usually arising in the deep vein of the calf and lodging in a branch of the pulmonary artery. This cuts off the blood supply to an area of the lung. The symptoms are chest pain, dyspnea, tachypnea (increased respiratory rate), and a reduction in blood oxygen levels.

Acute respiratory distress syndrome (ARDS) is sudden life-threatening lung failure caused by a variety of underlying conditions, from major trauma to sepsis. The alveoli fill with fluid and collapse, and gas exchange is shut down. Hypoxia results. Mechanical ventilation has to be provided. The mortality is from 35% to 50%.

Neonatal respiratory distress syndrome (NRDS) is seen in premature babies whose lungs have not matured enough to produce surfactant. The alveoli collapse, and mechanical ventilation is needed to keep them open.

Chronic infections of the lung parenchyma are the result of prolonged exposure to infection or to occupational irritant dusts or droplets. These disorders are called **pneumoconioses.** Levels of dust inhalation overwhelm the airways' particle-clearing abilities; the dust particles accumulate in the alveoli and parenchyma, leading to fibrosis. **Asbestosis** from inhaling asbestos particles can lead to a cancer (**mesothelioma**) in the pleura. **Silicosis** from silica particles is called stone mason's disease. **Anthracosis** from coal dust particles is called coal miners' disease. **Sarcoidosis** is an idiopathic fibrotic disorder of the lung parenchyma.

Pulmonary tuberculosis is a chronic, infectious disease of the lungs *(see Chapter 20).*

Lung cancer, related to tobacco use, used to be a male disease, but now fatalities in women from lung cancer exceed those from breast cancer. Ninety percent of lung cancers arise in the mucous membranes of the larger bronchi and are called **bronchogenic carcinomas.** The tumor obstructs the bronchus, spreads into the surrounding lung tissues, and metastasizes to lymph nodes, liver, brain, and bone.

Flail chest occurs when a segment of the chest wall is separated from the rest of the thoracic cage. A free or separated segment occurs when there are two fractures in each of three adjoining ribs. This free segment flails and is unable to contribute to chest expansion. Flail chest is produced by blunt trauma, such as in a motor vehicle accident, and is associated with underlying damage to the lung.

Acute respiratory failure (ARF) is abnormal respiratory function resulting in inadequate tissue oxygenation or carbon dioxide elimination that is severe enough to impair vital organ functions. Causes of ARF include congestive heart failure (CHF); COPD; chest trauma with resultant flail chest; spinal cord injury; and neuromuscular disorders in which the muscles of respiration are weak or paralyzed. Endotracheal intubation and mechanical ventilation are used until the underlying cause is treated, if possible.

WORD	PRONUNCIATION	ELEMENTS		DEFINITION
anthracosis	an-thra-**KOH**-sis	S/ R/	-osis *condition* anthrac- *coal*	Lung disease caused by the inhalation of coal dust
asbestosis	as-bes-**TOE**-sis	S/ R/	-osis *condition* asbest- *asbestos*	Lung disease caused by the inhalation of asbestos particles
atelectasis	at-el-**ECK**-tah-sis	S/ R/	-ectasis *dilation* atel- *incomplete*	Collapse of part of a lung
bronchogenic	brong-koh-**JEN**-ik	S/ R/CF	-genic *creation* bronch/o- *bronchus*	Arising from a bronchus
bronchopneumonia	**BRONG**-koh-new-**MOH**-nee-ah	S/ R/ R/CF	-ia *condition* -pneumon- *air, lung* bronch/o- *bronchus*	Acute inflammation of the walls of smaller bronchioles with spread to lung parenchyma
empyema	**EM**-pie-**EE**-mah	S/ P/ R/	-ema *result* em- *in* -py- *pus*	Pus in a body cavity, particularly in the pleural cavity
hemothorax	he-moh-**THOR**-ax	R/CF R/	hem/o- *blood* -thorax *chest*	Blood in the pleural cavity
mesothelioma	**MEZ**-oh-thee-lee-**OH**-mah	S/ P/ R/CF	-oma *tumor, mass* meso- *middle* -thel/i- *lining*	Cancer arising from the cells lining the pleura or peritoneum
pneumonia	new-**MOH**-nee-ah	S/ R/	-ia *condition* -pneumon- *air, lung*	Inflammation of the lung parenchyma
pneumonitis (syn)	new-moh-**NI**-tis	S/	-itis *inflammation*	
pneumoconiosis	new-moh-koh-nee-**OH**-sis	S/ R/ R/CF	-osis *condition* -coni- *dust* pneum/o- *air, lung*	Fibrotic lung disease caused by the inhalation of different dusts
pneumothorax	new-moh-**THOR**-ax	R/CF R/	pneum/o- *air, lung* -thorax *chest*	Air in the pleural cavity
sarcoidosis (*Note:* Two suffixes.)	sar-koy-**DOH**-sis	S/ S/ R/	-osis *condition* -oid- *resembling* sarc- *sarcoma*	Granulomatous lesions of lungs and other organs; cause is unknown
silicosis	sil-ih-**KOH**-sis	S/ R/	-osis *condition* silic- *silicon*	Fibrotic lung disease from inhaling silica particles
thoracentesis (also called **pleural tap**)	**THOR**-ah-sen-**TEE**-sis	S/ R/	-centesis *to puncture* thora- *chest*	Insertion of a needle into the pleural cavity to withdraw fluid or air
thromboembolism	**THROM**-boh-**EM**-boh-lizm	S/ R/CF R/	-ism *condition* thromb/o- *blood clot* -embol- *plug*	A piece of detached blood clot (embolus) blocking a distant blood vessel
tuberculosis	too-**BER**-kyu-**LOW**-sis	S/ R/	-osis *condition* tubercul- *nodule, tuberculosis*	Infectious disease that can infect any organ or tissue

EXERCISES

Suffixes. *This WAD contains a lot of suffixes you will see again in later chapters for other medical terms. Confirm your knowledge of suffixes by filling in the chart with the correct meaning of the element.*

Suffix	Meaning of Suffix	Medical Term with This Suffix
-centesis		
-ectasis		
-ema		
-genic		
-ia		

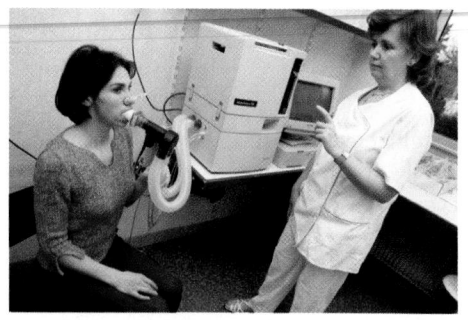

▲ FIGURE 9.20 Spirometer.

PULMONARY FUNCTION TESTS (PFTs)

A **spirometer** is a device used to measure the **volume** of air that moves in and out of the respiratory system *(Figure 9.20)*. You ask the patient to breathe in as deeply as possible and then breathe out as rapidly and completely as possible through the spirometer. The volume of air expired at the end of the test is the patient's **forced vital capacity (FVC).**

The spirometer also measures **flow rates.** The **forced expiratory volume in 1 second (FEV$_1$)** is the amount of air expired in the first second of the test.

In obstructive lung disorders such as asthma or COPD, the lumina of the airways are constricted and resistant to airflow. This will cause a reduction in the FEV$_1$.

In restrictive lung disorders in which the lung tissue is fibrotic or scarred and resists expansion, there will be a reduction in the FVC.

Keynote

Measure pulmonary function with spirometer, peak flow meter, and arterial blood gases.

Abbreviations

FEV$_1$	forced expiratory volume in 1 second
FVC	forced vital capacity
PEFR	peak expiratory flow rate
PFT	pulmonary function test

Case Report 9.1 (continued)

Mr. Jacobs' FEV$_1$ was only 40% of the predicted value for a man of his age, height, and weight. Mr. Jacobs' FVC was also reduced because of the fibrotic effects of repeated infections on his lung tissues reducing the volume in his airways. When he was off oxygen, Mr. Jacobs' oxygen levels were below 50% of normal. Even with nasal prongs and oxygen, his blood oxygen levels were only 75% of normal.

A **peak flow meter** records the greatest flow of air that can be sustained for 10 milliseconds on forced expiration, the **peak expiratory flow rate (PEFR).** It is of value in following the course of asthma and in postoperative care to monitor the return of lung function after anesthesia.

Arterial blood gases, the measurement of the levels of oxygen and carbon dioxide in the blood, are good indicators of respiratory function.

Pulmonary Pharmacology

- **Bronchodilators** relax the smooth muscles of the bronchioles. Examples are theophylline, beta$_2$-agonists (such as albuterol), and anticholinergics (such as ipratropium bromide).

- **Anti-inflammatory** drugs, such as corticosteroids, are best given by inhalation but can be used orally or intravenously in acute episodes of asthma or COPD.

- **Mucolytics** are agents that break up mucus to allow it to be cleared more effectively from the airways. Examples are guaifenesin (common in over-the-counter cough medications), potassium iodide, and *N*-acetylcysteine taken through a **nebulizer.**

- **Antibiotics** are used when a bacterial infection is present. Penicillin, erythromycin, cefotaxime, and flucloxacillin are frequently used.

- **Oxygen** is used in hypoxia and can be given by nasal **cannula** or by mask and intubation. Patients with severe, chronic COPD can be attached to a portable cylinder of oxygen.

WORD	PRONUNCIATION	ELEMENTS		DEFINITION
anti-inflammatory	**AN**-tee-in-**FLAM**-ah-tor-ee	S/ P/ R/	**-ory** *having the function of* **anti-** *against* **inflammat-** *set on fire*	Agent that reduces inflammation by acting on the body's response mechanisms without affecting the causative agent
bronchodilator	**BRONG**-koh-die-**LAY**-tor	S/ R/CF R/	**-or** *one who does* **bronch/o-** *bronchus* **-dilat-** *expand*	Agent that increases the diameter of a bronchus
cannula	**KAN**-you-lah		Latin *reed*	Tube inserted into a blood vessel or cavity as a channel for fluid
mucolytic	**MYU**-koh-**LIT**-ik	S/ R/CF R/	**-ic** *pertaining to* **muc/o-** *mucus* **-lyt-** *dissolve*	Agent capable of dissolving or liquefying mucus
nebulizer	**NEB**-you-liz-er	S/ R/	**-izer** *line of action* **nebul-** *cloud*	Device used to deliver liquid medicine in a fine mist
oxygen	**OCK**-see-jen	S/ R/	**-gen** *form, create* **oxy-** *oxygen*	The gas essential for life
spirometer	spy-**ROM**-eh-ter	S/ R/CF	**-meter** *measure* **spir/o-** *to breathe*	An instrument used to measure respiratory volumes

EXERCISES

Deconstruct each of these medical terms into basic elements. Define the elements; then use each in a sentence that is not a definition to demonstrate that you understand the term's meaning. Fill in the blanks.

Medical Term	Meaning of Prefix	Meaning of Root/CF	Meaning of Suffix
nebulizer			
spirometer			
mucolytic			
bronchodilator			

1. _____

2. _____

3. _____

4. _____

After reading Case Report 9.1 on the opposite page, answer the following questions. Be prepared to discuss your answers in class.

5. Substitute a medical term for the underlined word in the phrase "<u>repeated</u> (_____) infections."

6. Mr. Jacobs' oxygen levels (off oxygen) were below 50% of normal. What medical term would describe this condition?

_____

7. Mr. Jacobs' lung tissue is *fibrotic* because of repeated infections. What limits does fibrosis present to his lung function from now

on? _____

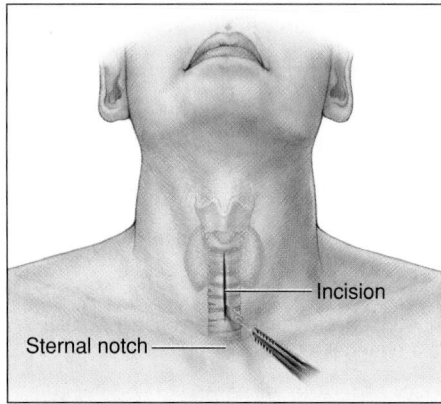

① Tracheotomy incision is made superior to sternal notch.

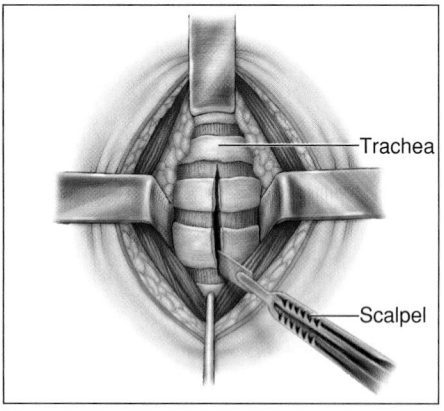

② Retractors separate the tissue, and an incision is made through the third and fourth tracheal rings.

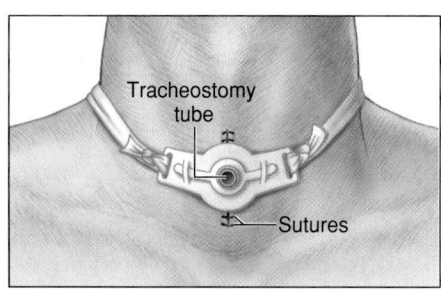

③ A tracheostomy tube is inserted, and the remaining incision is sutured closed.

▲ **FIGURE 9.21 Tracheostomy Procedure.**

Abbreviations

AP	anteroposterior
CPAP	continuous positive airway pressure
CT	computed tomography
CXR	chest x-ray
MRA	magnetic resonance angiography
PA	posteroanterior
PDT	postural drainage therapy
PEEP	positive end-expiratory pressure
PET	positron emission tomography

DIAGNOSTIC AND THERAPEUTIC PROCEDURES

Diagnostic Procedures

Chest x-ray (CXR) is a radiograph image of the chest taken in **anteroposterior (AP)**, **posteroanterior (PA)**, lateral, and sometimes oblique and lateral decubitus positions.

Computed tomography (CT), **angiography** of the pulmonary circulation using contrast materials, **magnetic resonance angiography (MRA)** to define emboli in the pulmonary arteries, and **ultrasonography** of the pleural space are chest imaging techniques in current use. **Positron emission tomography (PET)** can sometimes distinguish benign from malignant lesions.

Bronchoscopy is the insertion of a fiber-optic endoscope into the bronchial tree to visually examine it, take a tissue biopsy, or take a wash for secretions.

Mediastinoscopy is used to stage lung cancer and diagnose mediastinal masses. The mediastinoscope is inserted through an incision in the sternal notch.

Tracheal aspiration uses a soft catheter that allows brushings and washings to be performed to remove cells and secretions from the trachea and main bronchi. It can be passed through a tracheostomy or **endotracheal** tube or through the mouth or nose.

Thoracentesis is the insertion of a needle through an intercostal space to remove fluid from a pleural effusion for laboratory study or to relieve pressure. It is also called a **pleural tap.**

Thoracotomy is used to obtain an open biopsy of tissue from the lung, hilum, pleura, or mediastinum. It is performed through an intercostal incision under general anesthesia.

Therapeutic Procedures

Pulmonary rehabilitation includes education, breathing exercises and retraining, exercises for the upper and lower extremities, and psychosocial support.

Nutritional support is critical for patients who have difficulty breathing or who lose a lot of weight.

Immunizations are available against influenza and the pneumococcus bacterium, the most common cause of bacterial pneumonia.

Postural drainage therapy (PDT) uses gravity to promote drainage of secretions from lung segments by positioning and tilting the patient. Chest percussion (tapping) can help loosen, mobilize, and drain the retained secretions.

Continuous positive airway pressure (CPAP) is an attempt to keep the airway open by maintaining a positive pressure. A mask is fitted over the nose and mouth and attached to a ventilator. This can be used at night when sleeping or used in acute situations in COPD.

Positive end-expiratory pressure (PEEP) is a technique in ventilation to keep the alveoli from collapsing in conditions such as ARDS and NRDS.

Intubation uses an oropharyngeal airway in the unconscious patient during bag and mask ventilation to maintain an open airway. A tube is inserted to prevent the tongue from falling back to obstruct the airway and facilitates suctioning the airway. An **endotracheal intubation** involves the placement of a tube into the trachea. This allows patients to be placed on a ventilator and their breathing controlled.

Pulmonary resection is the surgical removal of lung tissue.

- **Wedge resection** is the removal of a small localized area of diseased lung.

- **Segmentectomy** is the removal of lung tissue attached to a bronchus.

- **Lobectomy** is the removal of a lobe.

- **Pneumonectomy** is the removal of an entire lung.

Tracheotomy is an incision made into the trachea (windpipe) so that a temporary or permanent opening into the windpipe, called a **tracheostomy,** is created (*Figure 9.21*). A tube is placed into the opening to provide an airway. A tracheostomy is used to maintain an airway when there is obstruction or paralysis in the respiratory structures above it.

Mechanical ventilation is a process by which gases are moved into and out of the lungs via a device that is set to meet the respiratory requirements of the patient. It requires that a tracheostomy or endotracheal tube be attached to the mechanical device (ventilator). It can augment or replace the patient's own ventilatory efforts.

WORD	PRONUNCIATION	ELEMENTS		DEFINITION
bronchoscope	**BRONG**-koh-skope	S/ R/CF	-scope *instrument for viewing* bronch/o- *bronchus*	Endoscope used for bronchoscopy
bronchoscopy	brong-**KOS**-koh-pee	S/	-scopy *to examine*	Examination of the interior of the tracheobronchial tree with an endoscope
endotracheal	en-doh-**TRAY**-kee-al	S/ P/ R/	-al *pertaining to* endo- *inside* -trache- *trachea*	Pertaining to being inside the trachea
lobectomy	low-**BECK**-toe-me	S/ R/	-ectomy *surgical excision* lob- *lobe*	Surgical removal of a lobe of the lungs
mediastinoscopy	**ME**-dee-ass-tih-**NOS**-koh-pee	S/ R/CF	-scopy *to examine* mediastin/o- *mediastinum*	Examination of the mediastinum using an endoscope
pneumonectomy	**NEW**-moh-**NEK**-toe-me	S/ R/	-ectomy *surgical excision* pneumon- *lung, air*	Surgical removal of a lung
resection resect (verb)	ree-**SEK**-shun ree-**SEKT**	S/ P/ R/	-ion *action* re- *back* -sect- *cut off*	Removal of a specific part of an organ or structure
segmentectomy	seg-men-**TEK**-toe-me	S/ R/	-ectomy *surgical excision* segment- *a section*	Surgical excision of a segment of a tissue or organ
thoracotomy	thor-ah-**KOT**-oh-me	S/ R/CF	-tomy *surgical incision* thorac/o- *chest*	Incision through the chest wall
tomography	toe-**MOG**-rah-fee	S/ R/CF	-graphy *process of recording* tom/o- *section*	Radiographic image of a selected slice or section of tissue
tracheostomy	tray-kee-**OST**-oh-me	S/ R/CF	-stomy *new opening* trache/o- *trachea*	Surgical opening into the windpipe, through which a tube can be inserted to assist breathing
tracheotomy	tray-kee-**OT**-oh-me	S/	-tomy *surgical incision*	Incision made into the trachea to create a tracheostomy
ultrasonography	**UL**-trah-soh-**NOG**-rah-fee	S/ P/ R/CF	-graphy *process of recording* ultra- *beyond* -son/o- *sound*	Delineation of deep structures using sound waves

EXERCISES

Put the following elements into the right combinations to form medical terms for the definitions provided. Some elements you will use more than once; some elements you will not use at all. Fill in the blanks.

endo-	-ectomy	trans-	bronch/o-	-trache/o-	mediastin/o-
lob-	-al	-ator	pharyng/e-	pneumon-	immuniz-
-ation	-son/o-	-tomy	-trache-	in-	-scopy
-sect-	tom/o-	re-	thorac/o-	-stomy	ventil-
-graphy	-ic	-stomy	hyper-	ultra-	-ion

1. Surgical removal of a lung _____

2. Examination of a bronchus _____

3. Radiographic image of a selected slice of tissue _____

4. Image of deep structures using sound waves _____

5. Pertaining to being inside the trachea _____

6. Removal of a specific part of an organ _____

7. Incision through the chest wall _____

8. New opening in the neck to the trachea _____

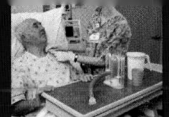

RESPIRATORY SYSTEM

CHALLENGE YOUR KNOWLEDGE

A. **Interpretation:** Use your knowledge of the **language of pulmonology** to understand the Case Report and answer the following questions. Fill in the blanks.

CASE REPORT

Mr. Jude Jacobs, a 68-year-old white retired mail carrier, is known to have COPD and is on continual oxygen by nasal prongs. He has smoked two packs a day for his adult life. Last night, he was unable to sleep because of increased shortness of breath and cough. His cough produced yellow sputum. He had to sit upright in bed to be able to breathe.

Vital signs are temperature (T) 101.6°F, pulse (P) 98, respirations (R) 36, blood pressue (BP) 150/90. On examination, he was cyanotic and frightened and had nasal prongs in his nose. Air entry is diminished in both lungs, and there are rales at both bases. You have been ordered to draw blood for arterial blood gases (ABGs) and to measure the amount of air entering and leaving his lungs using spirometry.

---

1. What disease appears in Mr. Jacobs' history?

   _____

2. Which particular symptom indicates Mr. Jacobs has an infection?

   _____

3. **Cyanotic** indicates an outward sign the physician can detect. What is it?

   _____

4. Rales heard through a stethoscope indicate the presence of what in the lungs?

   _____

5. What measure has been taken to restore the level of oxygen in Mr. Jacobs' blood?

   _____

6. What will be used to measure Mr. Jacobs' inspiration and expiration volumes?

   _____

7. Where in the Case Report can you substitute an abbreviation for a phrase?

   Abbreviation: _____ Means: _____

8. What are Mr. Jacobs' current symptoms and signs? _____

   _____

   _____

9. What is a lay term for *rales?* _____

10. What changes in his lifestyle does Mr. Jacobs do to help his breathing?

    _____

B. Deconstruct the following terms, and then answer the questions below.

Medical Term	Prefix	Root/CF	Suffix	Meaning of Term
empyema				
pneumoconiosis				
tachypnea				

Choose the correct preceding terms to complete the following sentences.

1. Rapid breathing is also called _____ .

2. Pleural effusion containing pus is also termed _____ .

3. Anthracosis is a form of _____ .

C. Terminology Challenge: Remembering terminology from a body system studied previously, explain the difference between the two terms below.

hemoptysis:

_____

hematemesis:

_____

What do both these terms have in common? _____

What two different body systems do they represent? _____ and _____

D. Pharmacology: For any body system, it is important to know the various types of medications and when they might be prescribed. Demonstrate your knowledge of pharmacology for the respiratory system by assigning the correct drug category in the right column to the statements in the left column. The first one is done for you.

__D__	1. Example: penicillin	A.	bronchodilators
_____	2. Relax smooth muscles of the bronchioles	B.	anti-inflammatories
_____	3. Corticosteroids	C.	mucolytics
_____	4. Example: potassium iodide	D.	antibiotics
_____	5. Used in hypoxia	E.	oxygen
_____	6. Used when a bacterial infection is present		
_____	7. Example: theophylline		
_____	8. Best given by inhalation		
_____	9. Administered by nasal cannula		
_____	10. Breaks up mucus		
_____	11. Can be administered using a nebulizer		

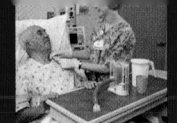

RESPIRATORY SYSTEM

E. **Roots:** Sometimes in medical terminology there can be two roots or combining forms with the same meaning. *Pneum/o-* and *pulmon/o-* are examples. These forms are not interchangeable—the medical term takes either one combining form or the other. Demonstrate your knowledge of the difference between the two elements by choosing the correct form for the terms listed below.

1. PFT is the abbreviation for what diagnostic test? _____

2. Acute infection affecting the alveoli and lung parenchyma: _____.

3. Presence of air in the pleural cavity is called _____.

4. A specialist in the study of the lung is called a _____.

5. Surgical removal of a lung: _____.

6. COPD is the abbreviation for what lung disease? _____

7. Sarcoidosis is a form of which disease? _____

8. Study of the lungs and lung diseases is _____.

F. **In Your Own Words:** Do you understand the following terms well enough to explain the difference to patients if they should ask?

What is the difference between:

1. inspiration:

   _____

   expiration:

   _____

   aspiration:

   _____

2. pneumothorax:

   _____

   hemothorax:

   _____

3. wedge resection:

   _____

   segmentectomy:

   _____

G. **Discussion Question:** Be prepared to discuss and define the **anatomical dead space.** Go online to see if you can find an illustration of this area to print out and use in your discussion. Describe the process of inspiration and how the lung inflates. Be prepared to name all the organs in the thoracic cavity. Outline your discussion below.

_____

_____

_____

_____

_____

_____

H. **Spelling:** The following terms come directly from Latin and Greek. A hint is given to you—choose the correct spelling. Circle the best answer.

1.	Reed	cannula	canula	canulla
2.	Passage	miatus	meatis	meatus
3.	Shell	conca	conka	concha
4.	Branding iron	cautiry	cautery	cautary
5.	Lack of breath	apenea	apnea	apnia
6.	Throat	pharynix	parynix	pharynx
7.	Ring	cricoid	crickoid	crecoid
8.	Creaking sound	strideor	stridore	stridor
9.	Oblong shield	thyrhoid	thiroyd	thyroid
10.	Nerves enter and leave this area	hylum	hilum	hylim

I. **Trace the Pathway:** The tracheobronchial tree begins with the trachea, which starts air on its pathway all the way down to the alveoli, where gas exchange can occur. Trace this path by sequentially lettering the following choices A through G. The first one is done for you.

1. Each secondary bronchus divides into tertiary bronchi.   _____

2. Terminal bronchioles divide into several alveoli.   _____

3. Bronchi enter the lung at the hilum.   _____

4. Bronchioles divide into terminal bronchioles.   _____

5. Main bronchi divide into a secondary bronchus for each lobe.   _____

6. Tertiary bronchi divide into bronchioles.   _____

7. At the carina, the trachea divides into right and left main bronchi.   _A_

RESPIRATORY SYSTEM

J. Interpretation: How well do you understand what the physician has written? Translate this physician's order into plain English without any abbreviations. Fill in the blanks.

This patient is to have AP and lateral CXRs, followed by a CT, MRI, and PET scan.

_____

_____

_____

K. Build Terms: The suffix *-itis* is one that you will meet over and over again in this book. Build the correct medical term to match its definition. Fill in the blanks.

1. inflammation of the bronchus   _____itis

2. inflammation of the organ of voice production   _____itis

3. inflammation of the tonsils   _____itis

4. inflammation of the throat   _____itis

5. inflammation of the nose   _____itis

6. inflammation of the epiglottis   _____itis

7. croup   _____itis

8. inflammation of the small bronchioles   _____itis

9. inflammation of the lung parenchyma   _____itis

L. Recall and Review: How well do you remember these word elements from the previous chapter? Try to answer without first looking back to check. Fill in the blanks.

Element	Type of Element (P, R, CF, S)	Meaning of Element
viscer		
inter		
um		
semi		
myo		

M. Language of Pulmonology: You are a new student in the Respiratory Therapy program. The following questions contain terminology you will use every day on the job. Answer the questions by circling the correct choice.

1. **Cyanosis** signals deficient oxygenation of blood and will turn nail beds:

   a. yellow

   b. red

   c. black

   d. white

   e. blue

2. The term **respiration** can mean:

   a. ventilation

   b. cellular metabolism

   c. exchange of gases

   d. a and c

   e. a, b, and c

3. Shell-shaped bone in the nose:

   a. meatus

   b. concha

   c. nares

   d. vestibule

   e. choana

4. Which medical term can be associated with mucopurulent discharge?

   a. pleurisy

   b. sinusitis

   c. epistaxis

   d. pneumonia

   e. nasal polyps

5. A segment of the chest wall separates from the rest of the thoracic cage in:

   a. pneumoconiosis

   b. epiglottitis

   c. flail chest

   d. thoracentesis

   e. ARF

6. **Cautery** can be performed electrically or chemically. What is its purpose?

   a. to burn a tissue

   b. to scar a tissue

   c. to stop bleeding

   d. all of the above

   e. none of the above

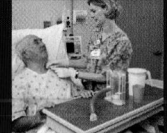
RESPIRATORY SYSTEM

N. Analyze: Knowledge of medical terms includes choosing the correct term for the meaning you want to convey either verbally or in documentation. Analyze the suffixes to help you choose the term. Use the following medical terms to fill in the statements, all relating to the bronchus.

bronchogenic	bronchi	bronchopneumonia	bronchioles	bronchiolitis
bronchus	bronchial asthma	bronchial	bronchitis	bronchiectasis

1. Greek word for *windpipe*: _____

2. Plural of the word in question 1: _____

3. Pertaining to the windpipe: _____

4. Tertiary bronchi divide into these: _____

5. Inflammation of the bronchus: _____

> **Study Hint**
> In the term **broncho-pneumonia**, the combining form is used, and it is one word. In the term **bronchial asthma,** the suffix *-al* makes it an adjective, and the two words are separated.

6. Abnormal dilation of bronchioles due to repeated infections: _____

7. Infection in the bronchioles that usually spreads to the alveoli: _____

8. Inflammation of the bronchioles: _____

9. Recurrent acute episodes of bronchial obstruction due to constriction: _____

10. Arising from a bronchus: _____

Now, using the word elements below, build new terms relating to the bronchus. Your root or combining form will still be bronch/o-.

malacia	stenosis	plasty
scope	pathy	pulmonary
staxis	scopy	dilator
dilation	gram	ostomy

1. An instrument used to see into the bronchus: _____

2. Drug meant to open bronchial passages: _____

3. A softening or deficiency in the wall of a bronchus: _____

4. Surgical procedure doing plastic repair on a bronchus: _____

5. Any disease of a bronchus: _____

6. Pertaining to the bronchus and the lung: _____

7. Widening the area of the bronchus: _____

8. Bleeding in the bronchus: _____

9. The procedure of viewing into the bronchus: _____

10. Constriction or narrowing of the bronchus: _____

11. The record obtained by bronchography: _____

12. Surgical creation of an opening into the bronchus: _____

O. **Objectives:** Meet lesson objectives by briefly explaining the following.

1. Relate the functions of the nose to its structure—in other words—why is the nose constructed the way it is to do the job it's supposed to do?

_____

_____

_____

_____

2. The lungs and the bloodstream work together to get oxygen into and carbon dioxide out of your body. Explain how this happens, using the terms *inspiration* and *expiration*.

_____

_____

_____

_____

3. Discuss the effects of common disorders of the lungs on overall health. Think of everyday life and how you would manage if your breathing was compromised.

_____

_____

_____

_____

4. In *Chapter 4* you read how sound is *heard* by the ear. Now describe how sound is *produced*. What organs are working to help you make sounds and form speech?

_____

_____

_____

_____

5. Explain how smells are recognized. What aids in their recognition? How does the brain get this information? Why are dogs so sensitive to smell and used to sniff out drugs, cadavers, and explosives?

_____

_____

_____

_____

6. Trace the flow of air from the nose to the alveoli. Be sure to include all the major respiratory organs the air travels through.

_____

_____

_____

_____

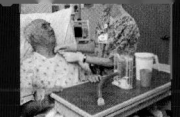
RESPIRATORY SYSTEM

P. Translate from medical language to layman's language. Take the following statement and translate it into layman's language. First, write a simple version of the medical terms in italics. Then reconstruct the sentence in language a nonmedical person could understand. Use your glossary or search online for any terms you can't recall. Fill in the blanks.

1. *Sarcoidosis* is an *idiopathic fibrotic* disorder of the lung *parenchyma*.

sarcoidosis _____

idiopathic _____

fibrotic _____

parenchyma _____

Sentence:

_____

_____

_____

Q. Abbreviations are meant to save time, but you must interpret them correctly. Write out the meaning for the abbreviations in the following sentences.

1. You have been ordered to draw blood for Mr. Jacobs' ABGs.

_____

2. Increased viscosity of secretions from the lungs leads to the conclusion that this patient has CF.

_____

3. PEEP is a technique in ventilation to keep the alveoli from collapsing.

_____

4. Patient suffers from dyspnea and is SOB.

_____

5. Mrs. White was prescribed medication for her URI.

_____

6. This patient has been on a ventilator for a week; provisional diagnosis is ARDS or ARF.

_____

7. PA view of the chest is all that is needed right now.

_____

8. Mrs. Black is experiencing CAO due to her COPD.

_____

R. **Test-Taking Skills:** Employ your test-taking skills when you answer multiple-choice questions. Start by immediately crossing off answers you know to be incorrect. With the choices you have left, one answer will clearly be the *best* choice. Circle the best choice.

1. The hairlike structures in the nasal cavity are called:

   a. polyps

   b. cilia

   c. adenoids

   d. bullae

   e. trachealis

2. What is the total number of lobes in *both* lungs?

   a. 4

   b. 5

   c. 6

   d. 2

   e. 3

3. What exactly is a lobe?

   a. an opening into an organ

   b. an exit from an organ

   c. a subdivision of an organ

   d. a blood reservoir in an organ

   e. a pathway through an organ

4. An instrument used to measure breathing volume is called:

   a. bronchoscope

   b. spirometer

   c. endoscope

   d. tenometer

   e. sphygmomanometer

5. What is a surfactant?

   a. creates surface tension

   b. a detergent like substance

   c. keeps alveolar sacs from collapsing

   d. all of the above

   e. none of the above

RESPIRATORY SYSTEM

S. **Test-Taking Skills:** Employ your test-taking skills when you answer multiple-choice questions. Start by immediately crossing off answers you know to be incorrect. With the choices you have left, one answer will clearly be the *best* choice. Circle the best choice.

1. The measure of the capacity of a chamber or hollow viscus to expand is called:

    a. expectorate

    b. idiopathic

    c. compliance

    d. postural drainage

    e. consolidation

2. What is another name for the nasal **conchae** on the lateral wall of each nasal cavity?

    a. meatus

    b. choana

    c. nares

    d. turbinates

    e. septum

3. A bubblelike structure is called a:

    a. bronchiole

    b. barbiturate

    c. bulla

    d. bronchus

    e. bradypnea

4. The sense of smell is:

    a. external respiration

    b. aspiration

    c. internal respiration

    d. exhalation

    e. olfaction

5. What is another term for heart failure?

    a. cyanosis

    b. conchae

    c. choana

    d. cor pulmonale

    e. chordae tendinae

6. Laryngeal polyps are:

   a. benign tumors of the larynx

   b. treated by excision

   c. papillomas

   d. all of the above

   e. none of the above

7. The medical term for the nostrils is:

   a. nares

   b. adenoids

   c. polyps

   d. tonsils

   e. papillomas

T. **Plurals:** Refresh your memory for the rules of plurals with this exercise. Check (✓) whether the given medical term is the singular or plural form. If it is singular, fill in the plural; if it is plural, fill in the singular form. Then write the meaning of the term. Fill in the chart.

Medical Term	Singular	Plural	Meaning of Medical Term
alveolus			
cilia			
rale			
conchae			
naris			

U. Translate the following sentence *from medical language* into language your patient can understand. Be sure to write out the abbreviations and use plain English for the other underlined terms.

   1. "Causes of ARF include CHF, COPD, chest trauma with resultant flail chest, spinal cord injury, and neuromuscular disorders in which the muscles of respiration are paralyzed."

   _____

   _____

   _____

   _____

   2. Translate the following sentence *from layman's language* into medical language for patient documentation. Be precise.

   "A piece of detached blood clot (_____) that blocks a distant blood vessel is caused by a clot (_____) usually arising in the deep vein of the calf and lodging in a branch of the lung (_____) artery."

   _____

   _____

   _____

   _____

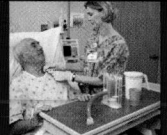
RESPIRATORY SYSTEM

CHAPTER SUMMARY EXERCISE

1. *Listen to the pronunciation of the medical terms as given by your instructor.*
2. *Circle the correct spelling of the medical term.*
3. *Match the correctly spelled terms to the brief descriptions below.*
4. *Write a sentence for each of the 10 terms that appear in this exercise.*

A. SPELLING COMPREHENSION: CIRCLE THE CORRECT SPELLING OF THE TERM.

1. oldfaction	olefaction	olfaction	olfarction	ofaction
2. hyperpipnea	hyperphnea	hypophnea	hyperpnea	hypopipnia
3. apnea	apenea	apnia	appnea	apneea
4. nubulizer	nebulizer	mebulizer	nebbulizer	nibulizer
5. mucuspurulent	mucousperulent	mucusprulent	mucopurulent	mucoperulent
6. barbiterate	barbiturate	berbiturate	barrbiturate	berbiturite
7. parencyma	parenchyma	parinchyma	parenckyma	peranchyma
8. expectorate	expicterate	expickerate	expextorate	expecturate
9. hyperoxia	hypoxia	hyperoxxia	hypoxxia	hypoxea
10. coriza	coryiza	corryiza	curiza	coryza

B. MATCH THE NUMBER OF THE CORRECT TERM IN PART A WITH THE BRIEF DESCRIPTION OF THE TERM BELOW.

a. Reduced oxygen in the blood _____

b. Cough up and spit out _____

c. Connective tissue framework in lungs _____

d. Delivers liquid medicine in a fine mist _____

e. Sense of smell _____

f. Deeper breathing than normal _____

g. Viral URI _____

h. CNS depressant _____

i. Cessation of breathing _____

j. Infected mucus coughed up _____

C. USING YOUR KNOWLEDGE OF TERMS 1–10 IN PART A AND THEIR CORRECT SPELLING, WRITE A BRIEF SENTENCE AS IT MIGHT APPEAR IN PATIENT DOCUMENTATION.

1. _____

2. _____

3. _____

4. _____

5. _____

6. _____

7. _____

8. _____

9. _____

10. _____

D. YOUR INSTRUCTOR WILL DIRECT YOU TO MCGRAW-HILL CONNECT. OPEN THE AUDIO GLOSSARY AND PRACTICE YOUR PRONUNCIATION OF THE TERMS IN PART A OF THIS EXERCISE.

E. MEET A LESSON OBJECTIVE BY DEFINING THE *PROTECTIVE MECHANISMS* OF THE UPPER RESPIRATORY TRACT. THINK ABOUT HOW THE BODY PROTECTS ITSELF. START BY LISTING THE ORGANS IN THE UPPER RESPIRATORY TRACT; THEN NAME A PROTECTIVE MECHANISM OF THAT ORGAN.

Organ   Protective Mechanism

1. _____   _____

2. _____   _____

3. _____   _____

4. _____   _____

5. _____   _____

6. _____   _____

Briefly discuss what happens if any one of the above mechanisms should fail.

7. If _____ fails, then _____

_____

_____

8. Would that failure then present a life-threatening emergency? _____

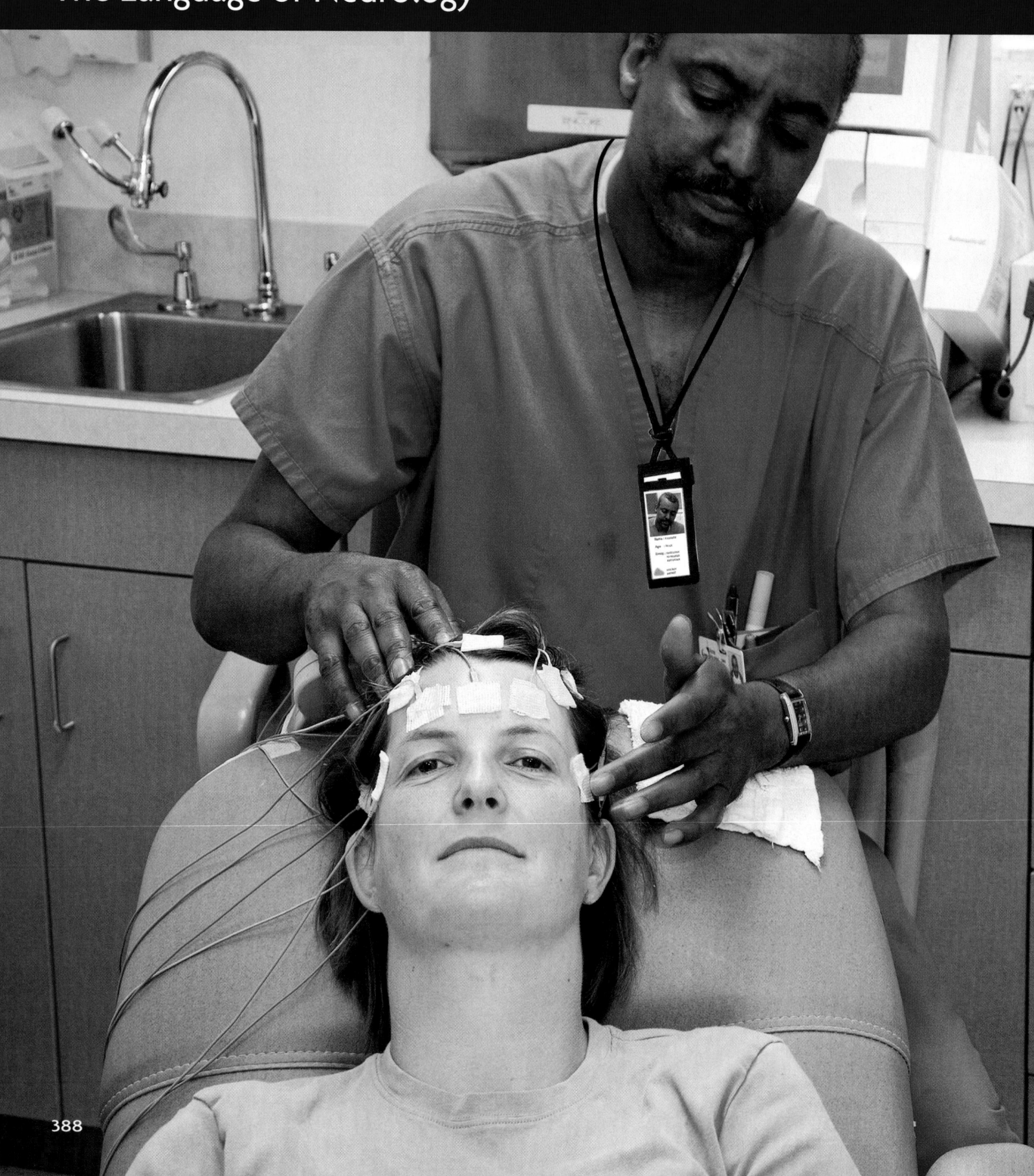

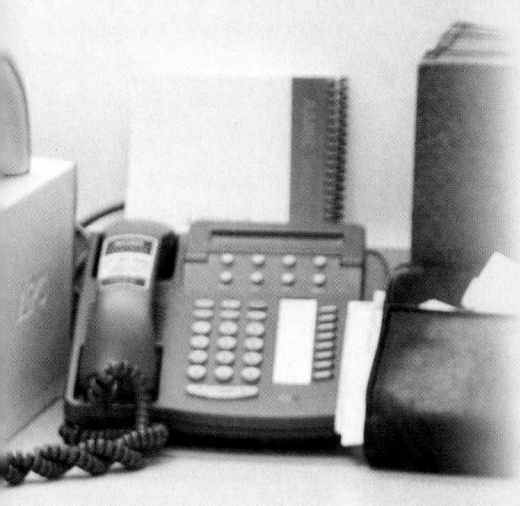

10

CASE REPORT 10.1

You are

...an **electroneurodiagnostic technologist** working with Gregory Solis, MD, a **neurosurgeon** at Fulwood Medical Center.

Your patient is

...Ms. Roberta Gaston, a 39-year-old woman, who has been referred by Raul Cardenas, MD, a **neurologist,** for evaluation for possible **neurosurgery.**

Ms. Gaston has had **epileptic seizures** since the age of 16. She has **generalized tonic-clonic seizures** occurring once a week. She also has daily minor spells when she stops interacting with her surroundings and blinks rhythmically for about 20 seconds, after which she returns to normal. Numerous **antiepileptic drugs,** including phenobarbital, valproic acid, and phenytoin, have been tried with no relief. She is not able to work and is cared for by her parents.

Her neurologic examination is normal. Her **EEG** (electroencephalogram) shows diffuse spike-and-wave discharges with a left-sided frontal predominance. Her **CT** (computed tomography) is normal. An **MRI** (magnetic resonance imaging) shows a 20-mm diameter mass adjacent to the anterior horn of her left **ventricle.** Continuous EEG/video monitoring showed **ictal** activity in the left frontal lobe.

Learning Outcomes

Your roles are to communicate with Ms. Gaston and her parents, communicate with other health professionals involved in her care, and maintain, review, and document her history. Also, you are to assist Dr. Solis with studies to identify the site and cause of her epilepsy and determine if surgery is needed.

To perform these roles you must be able to:

10.1 Apply the language of neurology to the anatomy and physiology of the nervous system.

10.2 Comprehend, analyze, spell, and write the medical terms of neurology so that you communicate and document accurately and precisely in any health care setting.

10.3 Recognize and pronounce the medical terms of neurology so that you communicate verbally with accuracy and precision in any health care setting.

10.4 Explain the effects of common disorders of the nervous system on health.

Functions and Structure of the Nervous System

Every time you stop to smell the roses, touch a petal, bend down, cut a stem, carry it indoors, place it in a vase, and admire its color, all of these sensations and actions are interpreted and controlled by your nervous system.

The trillions of cells in your body must communicate and work together for you to function effectively. This is done through your nervous system, and it is essential that you understand how this system operates. You can then understand how your body functions and maintains its homeostasis to respond to changes in your internal and external environments.

In this lesson, you will learn to use correct medical terminology to:

10.1.1 Describe the functions of the nervous system.

10.1.2 Relate the functions of the nervous system to the structures of its components.

10.1.3 List the subdivisions of the nervous system.

10.1.4 Define the basic cells of the nervous system.

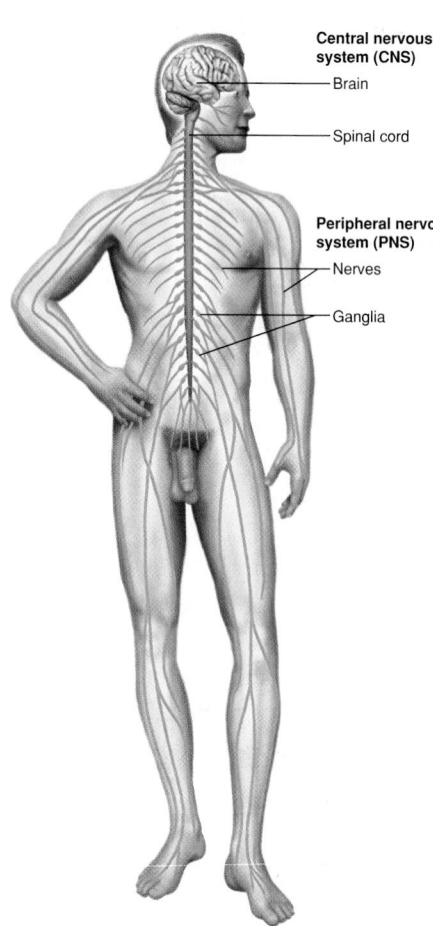

Central nervous
system (CNS)
— Brain
— Spinal cord

Peripheral nervous
system (PNS)
— Nerves
— Ganglia

▲ **FIGURE 10.1   The Nervous System.**

FUNCTIONS OF THE NERVOUS SYSTEM

1. **Sensory input** to the brain comes from receptors all over the body at both the conscious and subconscious levels *(Figure 10.1)*. Seeing the rose, touching it, smelling it, and noting your body position as you bend are external stimuli of which you are aware. Inside your body, internal stimuli about the amount of oxygen and carbon dioxide in your blood and other homeostatic variables are being continually processed at the subconscious level.

2. **Motor output** from the brain stimulates the skeletal muscles to contract and enables you to bend down, cut a stem, or move in any way. Smooth muscle in the walls of blood vessels contracts when stimulated by the nervous system. The production of sweat, saliva, and digestive enzymes is controlled by the nervous system.

3. **Evaluation and integration** occur in the brain and spinal cord to process the sensory input, initiate a motor response, and store the event in memory.

4. **Homeostasis** is maintained by the nervous system taking in internal sensory input and, for example, responding by stimulating the heart to deliver the correct volume of blood for oxygenation and removal of waste products.

5. **Mental activity** occurs in the brain so that you can think, feel, understand, respond, and remember.

   - The brain and spinal cord are called the **central nervous system (CNS)** *(Figure 10.1)*.
   - Nerves all over the body outside the CNS are called the **peripheral nervous system (PNS)** *(Figure 10.1)*.
   - The medical specialty of disorders of the nervous system is called **neurology.**
   - A specialist in neurology is called a **neurologist,** and a specialist who operates on the nervous system is a **neurosurgeon.**

Abbreviations	
EEG	electroencephalogram
CNS	central nervous system
CT	computed tomography
MRI	magnetic resonance imaging
PNS	peripheral nervous system

WORD	PRONUNCIATION	ELEMENTS		DEFINITION
afferent	**AF**-eh-rent		Latin *to bring to*	Conducting impulses inward *toward* the spinal cord or brain
autonomic	awe-toh-**NOM**-ik	S/ P/ R/	**-ic** *pertaining to* **auto-** *self* **-nom-** *law*	Not voluntary; pertaining to the self-governing visceral motor division of the peripheral nervous system
efferent	**EF**-eh-rent		Latin *to bring away from*	Conducting impulses outward *away from* the brain or spinal cord
ganglion ganglia (pl)	**GANG**-lee-on **GANG**-lee-ah		Greek *swelling*	Collection of nerve cell bodies outside the CNS
nerve nervous (adj)	NERV **NER**-vus		Latin *nerve*	A cord of fibers in connective tissue conduct impulses
neuron	**NYUR**-on		Greek *nerve*	Technical term for a nerve cell; consists of the cell body with its dendrites and axons
parasympathetic (*Note:* This term has two prefixes.)	par-ah-sim-pah-**THET**-ik	S/ P/ P/ R/	**-ic** *pertaining to* **para-** *beside* **-sym-** *together* **-pathet-** *suffering*	Pertaining to division of autonomic nervous system; has opposite effects of the sympathetic division
peripheral	peh-**RIF**-er-al	S/ R/	**-al** *pertaining to* **peripher-** *outer part*	Pertaining to the periphery or external boundary
plexus plexuses (pl)	**PLEK**-sus **PLEK**-sus-ez		Latin *braid*	A weblike network of joined nerves
somatic	soh-**MAT**-ik	S/ R/	**-ic** *pertaining to* **somat-** *body*	Pertaining to a division of peripheral nervous system serving the skeletal muscles
sympathetic	sim-pah-**THET**-ik	S/ P/ R/	**-ic** *pertaining to* **sym-** *together* **-pathet-** *suffering*	Pertaining to the part of the autonomic nervous system operating at the unconscious level
visceral	**VISS**-er-al	S/ R/	**-al** *pertaining to* **viscer-** *internal organs*	Pertaining to the internal organs

EXERCISES

*The nervous system has two major anatomical subdivisions, each with specialized functions. Keep in mind that there are systems and divisions of systems. Use the precise **language of neurology** to answer the following questions.*

1. This division carries signals to the skeletal muscles and is under voluntary control: _____

2. This system consists of the brain and spinal cord: _____

3. This division carries messages to the brain from the sensory organs: _____

4. The visceral motor division is also called the _____ system.

5. This division arouses the body for action: _____

6. This system consists of neurons, nerves, ganglia, and plexuses: _____

7. This division calms the body and slows the heartbeat: _____

8. Motor and sensory are further subdivisions of which system? _____

9. This division has efferent nerves to carry messages from the brain to muscles and organs: _____

10. Somatic nerves are in the _____ division of the _____ system.

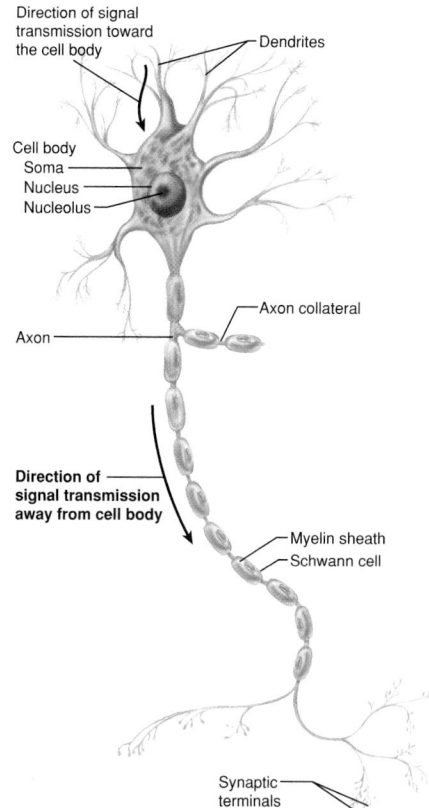

▲ FIGURE 10.4 Neuron.

Abbreviations	
C5	fifth cervical vertebra or nerve
T1	first thoracic vertebra or nerve

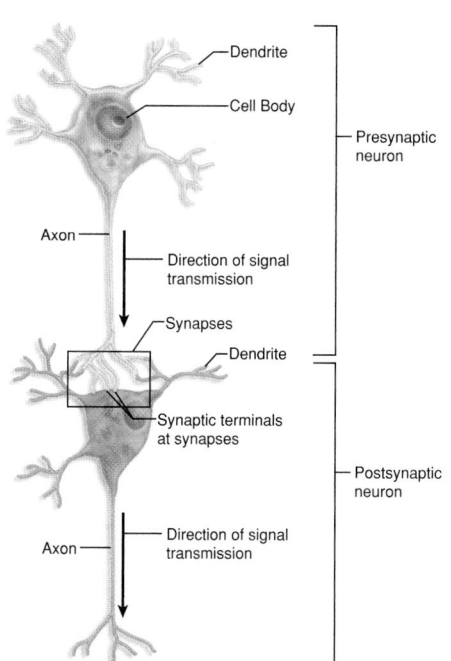

▲ FIGURE 10.5 Synapse.

CELLS OF THE NERVOUS SYSTEM

Neurons (nerve cells) receive stimuli and transmit impulses to other neurons or to receptors in other organs. Each neuron consists of a **cell body** and two types of processes or extensions, called **axons** and **dendrites** *(Figure 10.4)*.

Dendrites are short, highly branched extensions of the neuron's cell body. They conduct impulses toward the cell body. The more dendrites a neuron has, the more impulses it can receive from other neurons.

A single axon, or nerve fiber, arises from the cell body and carries impulses away from the cell body. Each axon has a constant diameter but can range in length from a few millimeters to a meter. The axon is covered in a fatty **myelin** sheath that is covered by a membrane called the **neurilemma.** The myelin sheath, like the plastic covering of electrical wire, enables the nerve impulse to travel faster.

The axon terminates in a network of small branches. Each branch ends in a **synaptic terminal** that forms a **synapse** (junction) with a dendrite from another neuron or with a receptor on a muscle cell or gland cell *(Figure 10.5)*. The synaptic knobs contain vesicles full of **neurotransmitters** that cross the synapse to stimulate or inhibit the receptor on a dendrite of another neuron or the cell of a muscle or gland. Examples of neurotransmitters are:

- **Acetylcholine**—stimulates muscle cells to contract.
- **Norepinephrine**—found in many areas of the brain and spinal cord; has a stimulatory effect that is increased by cocaine and amphetamines.
- **Serotonin**—found in many areas of the brain and spinal cord; involved with mood, anxiety, and sleep.
- **Dopamine**—confined to small areas of the brain; its absence is associated with **Parkinson disease.**
- **Endorphins**—found in areas around the brainstem; are the body's natural pain relievers.

Groups of cell bodies cluster together to form ganglia, and axons collect together to form nerves. Groups of nerves collect together to form a **plexus,** in which nerve fibers from different spinal nerves are sorted and recombined so that all the fibers (motor and sensory) going to a specific body part are located in a single nerve. The three plexuses are the **cervical plexus** to the neck, the **brachial plexus** to the arm, and the **lumbosacral plexus** to the pelvis and legs. *Figure 10.6* shows an example of a plexus, the brachial plexus, in which spinal nerves **C5** to **T1** unite to form three **roots** that go on to supply the motor and sensory functions of the arm. The labeling of nerves is addressed in a later lesson in this chapter.

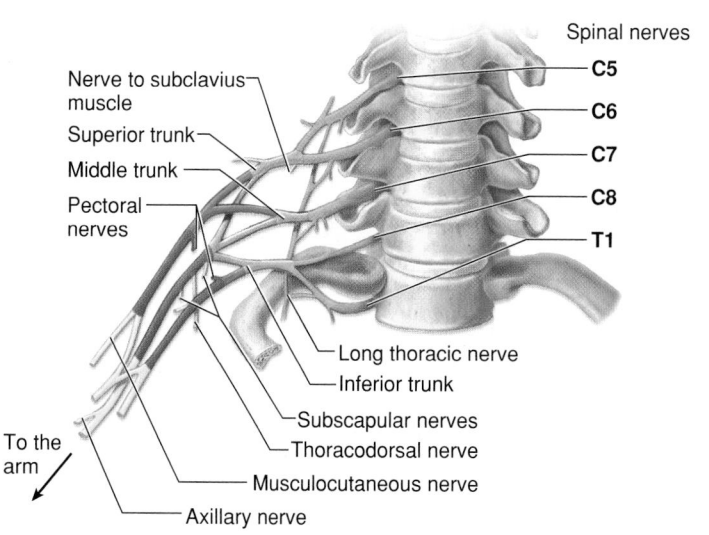

▲ FIGURE 10.6 Brachial Plexus.

WORD	PRONUNCIATION		ELEMENTS	DEFINITION
acetylcholine	**AS**-eh-til-**KOH**-leen	R/ R/	acetyl- *acetyl* -choline *choline*	Parasympathetic neurotransmitter
axon	**ACK**-son		Greek *axis*	Single process of a nerve cell carrying nervous impulses away from the cell body
dendrite	**DEN**-dright		Greek *looking like a tree*	Branched extension of the nerve cell body that receives nervous stimuli
dopamine	**DOH**-pah-meen		Precursor of norepinephrine	Neurotransmitter in some specific small areas of the brain
endorphin (***Note:*** The "m" of morphine is not used.)	en-**DOR**-fin	P/ R/	end- *within* -morphin *morphine*	Natural substance in the brain that has the same effect as opium
myelin	**MY**-eh-lin	S/ R/	-in *substance, chemical compound* myel- *spinal cord*	Material of the sheath around the axon of a nerve
neurilemma	nyu-ri-**LEM**-ah	S/ R/CF	-lemma *covering* neur/i- *nerve*	Covering of a nerve around the myelin sheath
neurotransmitter	**NYUR**-oh-trans-**MIT**-er	S/ R/CF P/ R/	-er *agent* neur/o- *nerve* -trans- *across* -mitt- *to send*	Chemical agent that relays messages from one nerve cell to the next
norepinephrine	**NOR**-ep-ih-**NEFF**-rin	P/ P/ R/ S/	nor- *normal* -epi- *upon, above* -nephr- *kidney* -ine *pertaining to*	Parasympathetic neurotransmitter
Parkinson disease	**PAR**-kin-son **DIZ**-eez		James Parkinson, British physician, 1755–1824	Disease of muscular rigidity, tremors, and a masklike facial expression
serotonin	ser-oh-**TOE**-nin	S/ R/CF R/	-in *chemical compound* ser/o- *serum, serous* -ton- *tension*	Neurotransmitter in the central and peripheral nervous systems
synapse synaptic (adj)	**SIN**-aps sih-**NAP**-tik	P/ R/	syn- *together* -apse *clasp*	Junction between two nerve cells, or a nerve fiber and its target cell; where electrical impulses are transmitted between the cells

EXERCISES   *Spelling is very important for every medical term. Choose the correct spelling in the **language of neurology**. Circle the best choice; then fill in the blanks.*

1. Junction between two nerve cells: synapses   sinapse   synapse

2. The material of the sheath around a nerve axon: myelin   mieline   myeline

3. Branched extension of the nerve cell body that receives an impulse: denderite   dendrite   dendryte

4. Chemical agent that relays messages: neutrontransmitter   neurontransmiter   neurotransmitter

5. Covering of a nerve around the sheath: neurilima   neurilemmia   neurilemma

Using the terms in the WAD, fill in the blanks in the following questions.

6. Which terms contain a prefix? _____

7. Which term contains a combining form and a suffix? _____

8. Which root means *the spinal cord*? _____

9. Which term contains two prefixes? _____

10. Name all the neurotransmitters in the WAD. _____

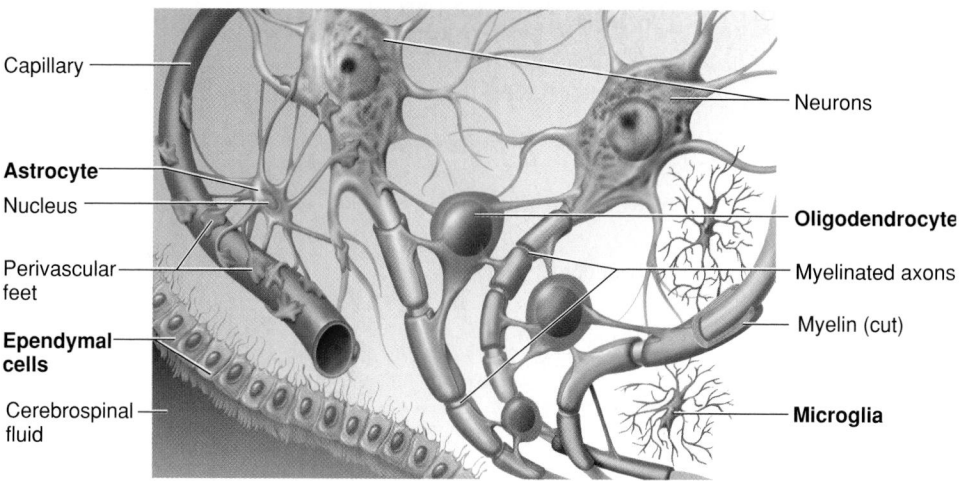

▲ FIGURE 10.7   Neuroglial Cells in the CNS.

NEUROGLIA

The trillion neurons in the nervous system are outnumbered 50 to 1 by the supportive **glial** cells (**neuroglia**). There are six types of neuroglia. Four are found in the CNS *(Figure 10.7)*:

1. **Astrocytes** are the most abundant glial cells. They are involved in the transportation of water and salts from capillaries to the neurons.
2. **Oligodendrocytes** form the myelin sheaths around axons in the brain and spinal cord. Axons that have myelin sheaths are called myelinated axons. Bundles of these axons appear white and create the **white matter** of the brain and spinal cord. Neuron cell bodies, dendrites, and synapses appear gray and create the **gray matter.**
3. **Microglia** phagocytize bacteria and cell debris.
4. **Ependymal cells** line the central canal of the spinal cord and the ventricles of the brain. They help regulate the composition of the **cerebrospinal fluid (CSF).**

Two types of neuroglial cells are found in the PNS:

1. **Schwann cells** form the myelin sheaths of the peripheral nerves that speed up signal conduction in the nerve fiber.
2. **Satellite cells** are found around the neuron cell bodies. Their function is unknown.

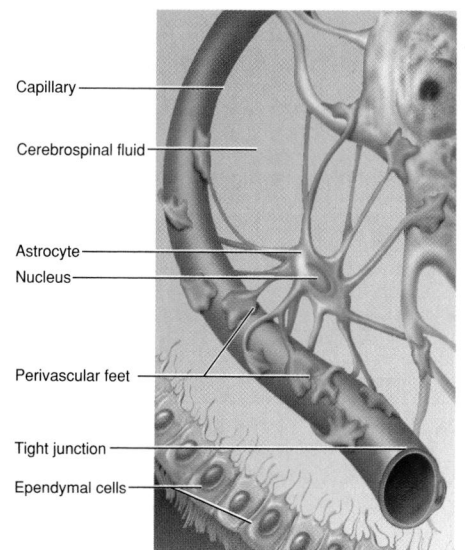

▲ FIGURE 10.8   Blood-Brain Barrier.

Abbreviations	
BBB	blood-brain barrier
CSF	cerebrospinal fluid

The **blood-brain barrier (BBB)** is a physical barrier between the capillaries that supply the CNS and most parts of the CNS. Astrocytes and the tight junctions between endothelial cells of the capillaries work together to prevent foreign substances, toxins, and infection from reaching the brain *(Figure 10.8).* Many medications are unable to pass this barrier, but alcohol gets through, producing its buzz and problems with coordination and **cognition.**

WORD	PRONUNCIATION	ELEMENTS		DEFINITION
astrocyte	**ASS**-troh-site	S/ R/CF	-cyte *cell* astr/o- *star*	Star-shaped connective tissue cell in the nervous system
blood-brain barrier (BBB)	BLUD BRAYN **BAIR**-ee-er			A selective mechanism that protects the brain from toxins and infections
cerebrospinal cerebrospinal fluid (CSF)	**SER**-eh-broh-**SPY**-nal	S/ R/CF R/	-al *pertaining to* cerebr/o- *brain* -spin- *spinal cord*	Pertaining to the brain and spinal cord Fluid formed in the ventricles of the brain; surrounds the brain and spinal cord
cognition cognitive (adj)	kog-**NIH**-shun **KOG**-nih-tiv		Latin *knowledge*	Process of acquiring knowledge through thinking, learning, and memory Pertaining to the mental activities of thinking and learninig
ependyma ependymal (adj)	ep-**EN**-dih-mah ep-**EN**-dih-mal		Greek *garment*	Membrane lining the central canal of the spinal cord and the ventricles of the brain
glia glial (adj) microglia	**GLEE**-ah **GLEE**-al my-**KROH**-glee-ah	 P/ R/	Greek *glue* micro- *small* -glia *glue, supportive tissue of the nervous system*	Connective tissue that holds a structure together Small nervous tissue cells that are phagocytes
neuroglia	nyu-roh-**GLEE**-ah	R/CF	neur/o- *nerve*	Connective tissue holding nervous tissue together
gray matter	GRAY **MATT**-er			Regions of the brain and spinal cord occupied by cell bodies and dendrites
oligodendrocyte	**OL**-ih-goh-**DEN**-droh-site	S/ P/ R/CF	-cyte *cell* oligo- *scanty* -dendr/o- *treelike*	Connective tissue cell of the central nervous system that forms a myelin sheath
Schwann cell	SHWANN SELL		Theodor Schwann, German anatomist, 1810–1882	Connective tissue cell of the peripheral nervous system that forms a myelin sheath
white matter	WITE **MATT**-er			Regions of the brain and spinal cord occupied by bundles of axons

EXERCISES

Identify the correct meaning for each element. Knowing the definitions of elements is your key to unlocking the meaning of medical terms. Match the element in the left column with its correct meaning in the right column.

_____ 1. oligo

_____ 2. glia

_____ 3. cerebro

_____ 4. astro

_____ 5. spin

_____ 6. cyte

_____ 7. dendro

_____ 8. al

_____ 9. neuro

_____ 10. micro

A. cell

B. nerve

C. small

D. spinal cord

E. treelike

F. scanty

G. brain

H. glue

I. star

J. pertaining to

LESSON 10.2 The Brain and Cranial Nerves

OBJECTIVES

Smelling the roses, seeing them, and touching them are recognized and interpreted in the brain, as are all sensations. The actions of bending down, cutting the rose stem, walking into the house, and placing it in a vase originate in the brain, as do all our voluntary actions. The integration of a sensory stimulus with a motor response occurs in the brain. The brain is the control center for many of the body's functions. The brain carries out the higher mental functions, such as reason, planning, forming ideas, and all aspects of memory.

The information in this lesson will enable you to:

10.2.1 Use correct medical terminology to describe the anatomy and physiology of the brain.
10.2.2 Identify the 12 pairs of cranial nerves and their functions.
10.2.3 Locate the major sensory and motor areas of the brain.
10.2.4 Describe how the brain is protected and supported.
10.2.5 Explain how common disorders of the brain and spinal cord affect health.

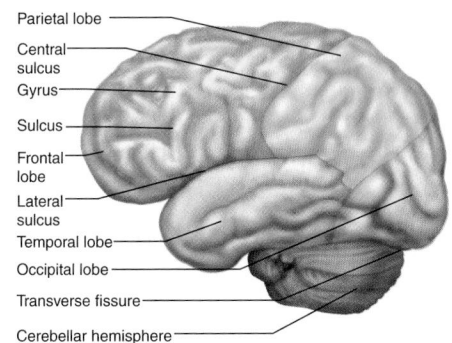

Parietal lobe
Central sulcus
Gyrus
Sulcus
Frontal lobe
Lateral sulcus
Temporal lobe
Occipital lobe
Transverse fissure
Cerebellar hemisphere

(a) Veiw from left side

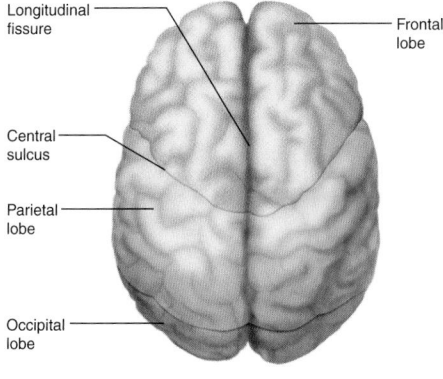

Longitudinal fissure
Frontal lobe
Central sulcus
Parietal lobe
Occipital lobe

(b) Veiw from above

▲ **FIGURE 10.9** Brain.

BRAIN

The adult brain weighs about 3 pounds. Its size and weight are proportional to body size, not intelligence.

The brain is divided into three major regions, the **cerebrum,** the **brainstem,** and the **cerebellum.**

The cerebrum is about 80% of the brain and consists of two **cerebral hemispheres** that are anatomically mirror images of each other *(Figure 10.9)*. They are separated by a deep longitudinal fissure, at the bottom of which they are connected by a bridge of nerve fibers called the **corpus callosum.**

On the surface of the cerebrum, numerous ridges **(gyri)** are separated by fissures called **sulci.**

Each cerebral hemisphere is divided into four lobes *(Figure 10.9a)*:

1. The **frontal lobe** is located behind the forehead. It forms the anterior part of the hemisphere. It is responsible for memory, intellect, concentration, problem solving, emotion, and the planning and execution of behavior, including voluntary motor control of muscles.

2. The **parietal lobe,** located above the ear, is posterior to the frontal lobe. The parietal lobe receives and interprets sensations of pain, pressure, touch, temperature, and body part awareness.

3. The **temporal lobe,** located behind the ear, is below the frontal and parietal lobes. The temporal lobe is involved in interpreting sensory experiences, sounds, and spoken words.

4. The **occipital lobe,** located at the back of the head, forms the posterior part of the hemisphere. The occipital lobe interprets visual images and the written word.

The cerebral hemispheres are covered by a thin layer of gray matter (unmyelinated nerve fibers) called the **cerebral cortex.** It is folded into the gyri, sulci, and fissures and contains 70% of all the neurons in the nervous system. Below the cerebral cortex is a mass of white matter, in which bundles of myelinated nerve fibers connect the neurons of the cortex to the rest of the nervous system.

WORD	PRONUNCIATION		ELEMENTS	DEFINITION
brainstem	BRAYN-STEM		Old English *brain* **stem** *support*	Region of the brain that includes the thalamus, pineal gland, pons, fourth ventricle, and medulla oblongata
cerebellum	ser-eh-**BELL**-um	S/ R/	-um *structure* cerebell- *little brain*	The most posterior area of the brain
cerebrum cerebral (adj)	**SER**-ee-brum **SER**-ee-bral		Latin *brain*	The major portion of the brain divided into two hemispheres (cerebral hemispheres) separated by a fissure
corpus callosum	**KOR**-pus kah-**LOW**-sum	R/ S/ R/	corpus *body* -um *structure* callos- *thickening*	Bridge of nerve fibers connecting the two cerebral hemispheres
cortex cortical (adj)	**KOR**-teks **KOR**-ti-kal		Latin *shell*	Gray covering of cerebral hemispheres
frontal lobe	**FRON**-tal LOBE	S/ R/	-al *pertaining to* front- *forehead* lobe Greek *lobe*	Area of brain behind the frontal bone
gyrus gyri (pl)	**JI**-rus **JI**-ree		Greek *circle*	Rounded elevation on the surface of the cerebral hemispheres
occipital lobe	ock-**SIP**-it-al LOBE	S/ R/	-al *pertaining to* occipit- *back of head*	Posterior area of cerebral hemispheres
parietal lobe	pah-**RYE**-eh-tal LOBE	S/ R/	-al *pertaining to* pariet- *wall*	Area of brain under the parietal bone
sulcus sulci (pl)	**SUL**-cuss **SUL**-sigh		Latin *furrow, ditch*	Groove on the surface of the cerebral hemispheres that separates gyri
temporal lobe	**TEM**-por-al LOBE	S/ R/	-al *pertaining to* tempor- *temple, side of head*	Posterior two-thirds of cerebral hemispheres

EXERCISES

Roots: *The lobes of the cerebral hemispheres share a common suffix* -al, *meaning* pertaining to. *It is the root that describe the exact location of the lobe in the cerebral hemispheres. Use your knowledge of roots to understand the anatomical location of the lobes. Fill in the blanks.*

1. _____ /al   Root means _____ .

   Lobe is located _____ .

   Lobe is responsible for _____ .

2. _____ /al   Root means _____ .

   Lobe is located _____ .

   Lobe is responsible for _____ .

3. _____ /al   Root means _____ .

   Lobe is located _____ .

   Lobe is responsible for _____ .

4. _____ /al   Root means _____ .

   Lobe is located _____ .

   Lobe is responsible for _____ .

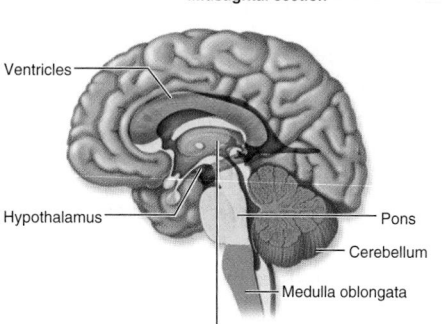

Midsagittal section

Ventricles

Hypothalamus

Pons

Cerebellum

Medulla oblongata

Thalamus

▲ **FIGURE 10.10 Lateral View of Functional Regions of Brain.**

FUNCTIONAL BRAIN REGIONS

Deep inside each cerebral hemisphere are spaces called **ventricles.** They contain the watery CSF, which circulates through the ventricles and around the brain and spinal cord. The CSF helps protect, cushion, and provide nutrition for the brain and spinal cord.

Underneath the cerebral hemispheres and the ventricles are important regions of the brain *(Figures 10.10 and 10.11):*

1. **Thalamus**—receives all sensory impulses and channels them to the appropriate region of the cortex for interpretation. As the sensory fibers carrying impulses pass through the thalamus, they **decussate** (cross over) so that the impulses from the left side of the body go to the right brain. Similarly, motor impulses coming from the right brain decussate and supply the left side of the body. In a stroke, if the lesion is in the right brain, the left side of the body will be affected, and vice versa.

2. **Hypothalamus**—regulates:
   a. Blood pressure
   b. Body temperature
   c. Water and electrolyte balance
   d. Hunger and body weight
   e. Sleep and wakefulness
   f. Movements and secretions of the digestive tract

3. **Basal nuclei**—are collections of gray matter lateral to the thalamus that aid in controlling the amplitude of our voluntary muscular movements and posture, as well as playing a part in emotion and cognition.

4. **Limbic system**—controls emotional experience, fear, anger, pleasure, and sadness. If your limbic system is destroyed, you go into a **comatose** state.

5. **Brainstem**—contains two major areas:
   a. The **pons,** which relays sensory impulses from peripheral nerves to higher brain centers.

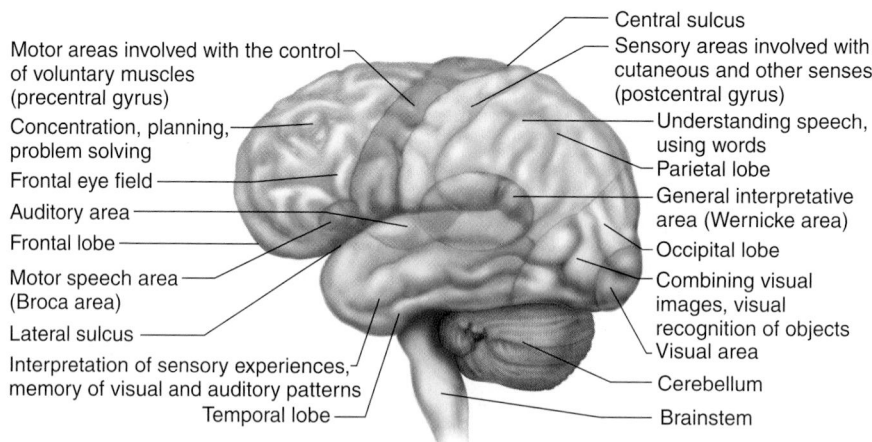

Motor areas involved with the control of voluntary muscles (precentral gyrus)

Concentration, planning, problem solving

Frontal eye field

Auditory area

Frontal lobe

Motor speech area (Broca area)

Lateral sulcus

Interpretation of sensory experiences, memory of visual and auditory patterns

Temporal lobe

Central sulcus

Sensory areas involved with cutaneous and other senses (postcentral gyrus)

Understanding speech, using words

Parietal lobe

General interpretative area (Wernicke area)

Occipital lobe

Combining visual images, visual recognition of objects

Visual area

Cerebellum

Brainstem

▲ **FIGURE 10.11 Cerebral Cortex, Functional Regions.**

WORD	PRONUNCIATION	ELEMENTS		DEFINITION
coma comatose	**KOH**-mah **KOH**-mah-toes		Greek *deep sleep, trance*	State of deep unconsciousness Being in a coma
decussate	**DEE**-kuss-ate		Latin *to make in the form of a cross*	Cross over like the arms of an "X"
hypothalamus	high-poh-**THAL**-ah-muss	S/ P/ R/	-us *pertaining to* hypo- *below* -thalam- *thalamus*	Area of gray matter forming part of the walls and floor of the third ventricle
hypothalamic	high-poh-tha-**LAM**-ik	S/	-ic *pertaining to*	Pertaining to the hypothalamus
limbic	**LIM**-bic		Latin *border*	Pertaining to the limbic system, an array of nerve fibers surrounding the thalamus
medulla oblongata	meh-**DULL**-ah ob-lon-**GAH**-tah	R/ S/ R/	medulla *middle* -ata *place* oblong- *elongated*	Most posterior subdivision of the brainstem, continuation of the spinal cord
pons	PONZ		Latin *bridge*	Part of the brainstem
reticulum reticular (adj)	reh-**TIK**-you-lum reh-**TIK**-you-lar	S/ R/ S/	-um *structure* reticul- *fine net* -ar *pertaining to*	Fine network of cells in the medulla oblongata
thalamus	**THAL**-ah-mus		Greek *inner room*	Mass of gray matter underneath the ventricle in each cerebral hemisphere
ventricle ventricular	**VEN**-trih-kel ven-**TRIK**-you-lar	S/ R/	-ar *pertaining to* ventricul- *ventricle*	A cavity of the heart or brain Pertaining to a ventricle
			Latin *belly*	

b. The **medulla oblongata,** within which nuclei of gray matter form centers to control vital visceral activities, such as:

  i. **Cardiac center**—regulates heart rate.

  ii. **Respiratory center**—regulates breathing.

  iii. **Vasomotor center**—regulates vasoconstriction and vasodilation of blood vessels.

  iv. **Reticular formation**—responds to sensory impulses by arousing the cerebral cortex into wakefulness.

The most posterior area of the brain, the cerebellum, coordinates skeletal muscle activity to maintain posture and balance.

Abbreviation

PET positron emission tomography

EXERCISES

Latin and Greek terms cannot be deconstructed into prefix, root, and suffix. You must know them for what they are. Test your knowledge of these terms with the following exercise. Match the terms in the left column to their correct meaning in the right column.

_____ 1. thalamus

_____ 2. decussate

_____ 3. limbic

_____ 4. coma

_____ 5. pons

A. deep sleep

B. bridge

C. inner room

D. border

E. cross over

TABLE 10.1 Mnemonic for the Cranial Nerves

Oh	(olfactory-I)
once	(optic-II)
one	(oculomotor-III)
takes	(trochlear-IV)
the	(trigeminal-V)
anatomy	(abducens-VI)
final	(facial-VII)
very	(vestibulocochlear-VIII)
good	(glossopharyngeal-IX)
vacations	(vagus-X)
are	(accessory-XI)
heavenly!	(hypoglossal-XII)

CRANIAL NERVES

To function, the brain must communicate with the rest of the body, and it does this through the spinal cord and the **cranial nerves.** Twelve pairs of cranial nerves arise from the base of the brain *(Figure 10.12)*. A mnemonic to assist memorizing their names is in Table 10.1.

The two pairs of nerves for smell and vision contain only sensory fibers. The other 10 pairs are mixed nerves containing sensory and motor and parasympathetic fibers. The cranial nerves have, from front to back, both names and numbers. The latter are always written in Roman numerals *(Table 10.2)*.

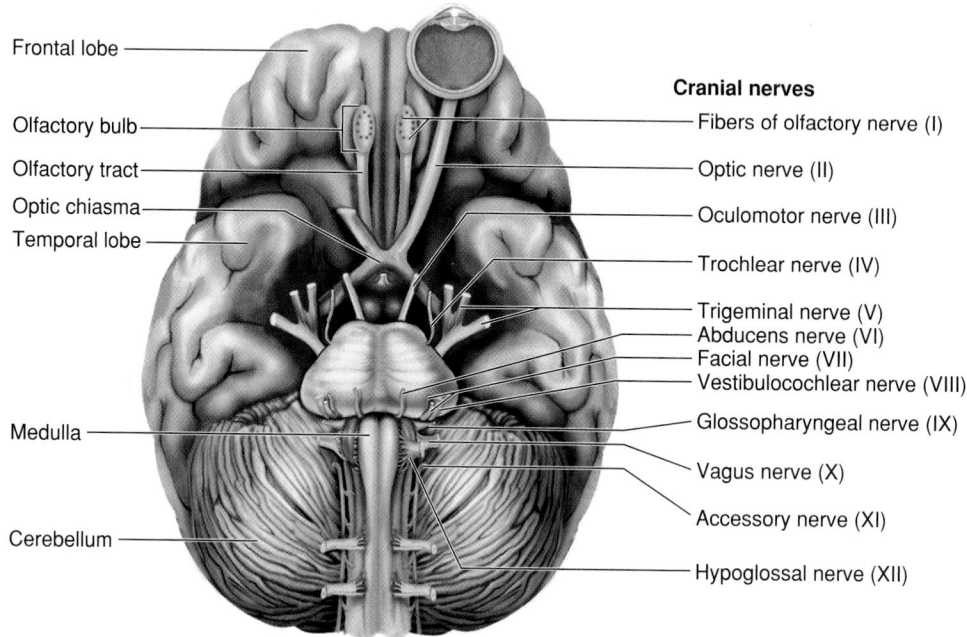

FIGURE 10.12 Cranial Nerves. ▶
Base of brain showing origins of the 12 cranial nerves.

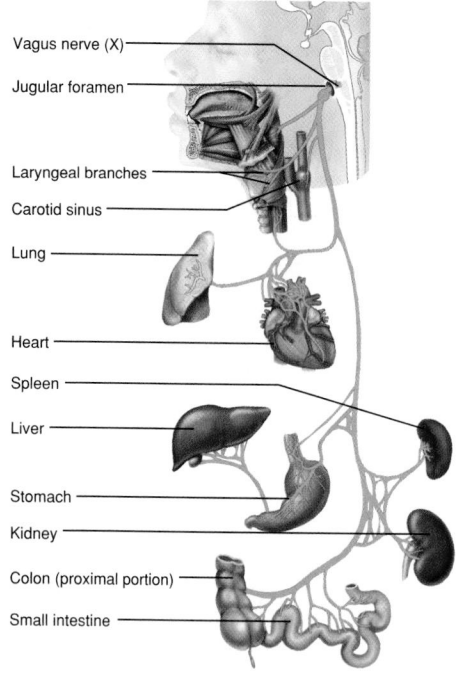

▲ **FIGURE 10.13 Left Vagus Nerve.**

TABLE 10.2 Cranial Nerves

Roman Numeral	Name	Description
I	**Olfactory** nerves	Sensory nerves for smell
II	**Optic** nerves	Sensory nerves for vision
III	**Oculomotor** nerves	Predominantly motor nerves for eye movement and pupil size
IV	**Trochlear** nerves	Predominantly motor nerves for eye movement
V	**Trigeminal** nerves	Sensory and motor nerves responsible for face, nose, and mouth sensations and for chewing
VI	**Abducens** nerves	Predominantly motor nerves responsible for eye movement
VII	**Facial** nerves	Mixed nerves associated with taste (sensory), facial expression (motor), and production of tears and saliva (parasympathetic fibers of motor nerves)
VIII	**Vestibulocochlear (auditory)** nerves	Predominantly sensory nerves associated with hearing and balance
IX	**Glossopharyngeal** nerves	Mixed nerves for sensation and swallowing in the pharynx
X	**Vagus** nerves	Mixed sensory and parasympathetic nerves supplying the pharynx, larynx (speech), and the viscera of the thorax and abdomen *(Figure 10.13)*
XI	**Accessory** nerves	Predominantly motor nerves supplying neck muscles, pharynx, and larynx
XII	**Hypoglossal** nerves	Predominantly motor nerves that move the tongue in speaking, chewing, and swallowing

WORD	PRONUNCIATION	ELEMENTS		DEFINITION
abducens	ab-**DYU**-senz		Latin *abduct, draw away from*	Sixth (VI) cranial nerve; responsible for eye movement
accessory	ack-**SESS**-oh-ree		Latin *move toward*	Eleventh (XI) cranial nerve; supplying neck muscles, pharynx, and larynx
auditory	**AW**-dih-tor-ee	S/ R/	-ory *having the function of* audit- *hearing*	Pertaining to the sense or the organs of hearing
cranial	**KRAY**-nee-al	S/ R/	-al *pertaining to* crani- *skull, cranium*	Pertaining to the skull
facial	**FAY**-shal		Latin *face*	Seventh (VII) cranial nerve; supplying the forehead, nose, eyes, mouth, and jaws
glossopharyngeal	**GLOSS**-oh-fah-**RIN**-jee-al	S/ R/CF R/	-eal *pertaining to* gloss/o- *tongue* -pharyng- *pharynx*	Ninth (IX) cranial nerve; supplying the tongue and pharynx
hypoglossal	high-poh-**GLOSS**-al	S/ P/ R/	-al *pertaining to* hypo- *below, under* -gloss- *tongue*	Twelfth (XII) cranial nerve; supplying muscles of the tongue
oculomotor	**OCK**-you-loh-**MOH**-tor	S/ R/CF R/	-or *doer* ocul/o- *eye* -mot- *move*	Third (III) cranial nerve; moves the eye
olfactory	ol-**FAK**-toh-ree	S/ R/	-ory *having the function of* olfact- *smell*	First (I) cranial nerve; carries information related to the sense of smell
optic	**OP**-tick		Greek *eye*	Second (II) cranial nerve; carries visual information
trigeminal	try-**GEM**-in-al	S/ P/ R/	-al *pertaining to* tri- *three* -gemin- *double, twin*	Fifth (V) cranial nerve, with its three different branches supplying the face
trochlear	**TROHK**-lee-are	S/ R/	-ar *pertaining to* trochle- *pulley*	Fourth (IV) cranial nerve; supplies one muscle of the eye
vagus	**VAY**-gus		Latin *to wander*	Tenth (X) cranial nerve; supplies many different organs throughout the body
vestibulocochlear (*Note:* This term starts with a combining form, not a prefix.)	ves-**TIB**-you-loh-**KOK**-lee-ar	S/ R/CF R/	-ar *pertaining to* vestibul/o- *vestibule of inner ear* -cochle- *cochlea*	Eighth (VIII) cranial nerve; carrying information for the senses of hearing and balance

EXERCISES

Elements: *Continue your work with elements to help build your knowledge of the **language of neurology**. One element in each of the following medical terms is set in bold. Identify the type of element (P, R, CF, S) in the middle column; then write the meaning of the element in the right column. Fill in the chart.*

> **Study Hint**
> Note that some terms can start with a root or combining form instead of a prefix.

Medical Term	Type of Element	Meaning of Element
glossopharyngeal		
hypoglossal		
trochlear		
oculomotor		
trigeminal		
auditory		
olfactory		
vestibulocochlear		

C1–C8	cervical spinal nerves
L1–L5	lumbar nerves
S1–S5	sacral nerves
T1–T12	thoracic spinal nerves

SPINAL CORD AND MENINGES

Spinal Cord

This part of the central nervous system consists of 31 segments, each of which gives rise to a pair of spinal nerves. These are the major link between the brain and the peripheral nervous system and are a pathway for sensory and motor impulses.

The spinal cord occupies the upper two-thirds of the vertebral canal, extending from the base of the skull to the first lumbar vertebra. From here, a group of nerve fibers continues down the vertebral canal and is called the **cauda equina.**

The spinal cord is divided into four regions *(Figure 10.14):*

1. The **cervical region** is continuous with the medulla oblongata. It contains the motor neurons that supply the neck, shoulders, and upper limbs through eight pairs of cervical spinal nerves (**C1–C8**).

2. The **thoracic region** contains the motor neurons that supply the thoracic cage, rib movement, vertebral column movement, and postural back muscles through 12 pairs of thoracic spinal nerves (**T1–T12**).

3. The **lumbar region** supplies the hips and front of the lower limbs through five pairs of lumbar nerves (**L1–L5**).

4. The **sacral region** supplies the buttocks, genitalia, and backs of the legs through five sacral nerves (**S1–S5**) and one coccygeal nerve.

A cross-section of the spinal cord *(Figure 10.15)* reveals that it has a core of gray matter shaped like a butterfly surrounded by white matter. In the center of the gray matter is the central canal that contains CSF. The gray matter contains the axons of sensory neurons bringing impulses into the cord and the neurons of motor nerves that send impulses out to skeletal muscles.

The white matter contains myelinated nerve fibers organized into **tracts** that conduct either sensory impulses up the cord to the brain or motor impulses down the cord from the brain.

All individual spinal nerves except C1 supply a specific segment of skin called a **dermatome.**

Meninges

The brain and spinal cord are protected by the cranium and the vertebrae, cushioned by the CSF, and covered by the **meninges** *(Figure 10.16).* The meninges have three layers:

1. **Dura mater**—the outermost layer, composed of tough connective tissue attached to the inner surface of the cranium but separated from the vertebral canal by the **epidural space,** into which **epidural injections** are introduced.

2. **Arachnoid mater**—a thin web over the brain and spinal cord. The CSF is contained in the subarachnoid space between the arachnoid and pia mater.

3. **Pia mater**—the innermost layer of the meninges, attached to the surface of the brain and spinal cord. It supplies nerves and blood vessels that nourish the outer cells of the brain and spinal cord.

To obtain a specimen of CSF, a **lumbar puncture (spinal tap)** is performed. A needle is inserted through the skin, back muscles, spinal ligaments of an **intervertebral space,** epidural space, dura mater, and arachnoid mater into the **subarachnoid space.** The CSF can then be aspirated *(Figure 10.17).*

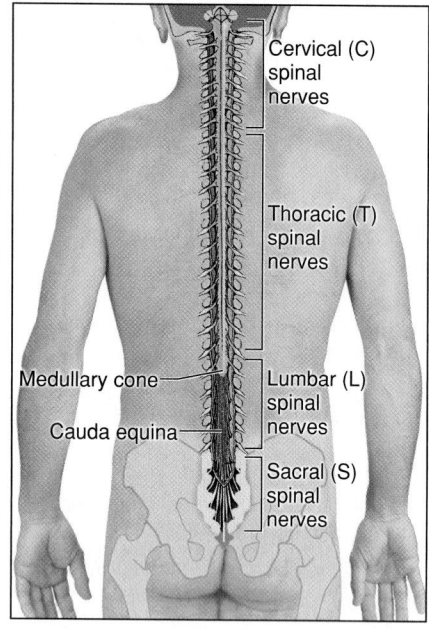

▲ **FIGURE 10.14   Spinal Cord Regions.**

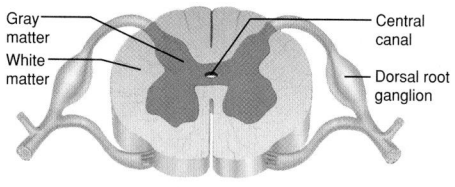

▲ **FIGURE 10.15   Cross-Section of Spinal Cord.**

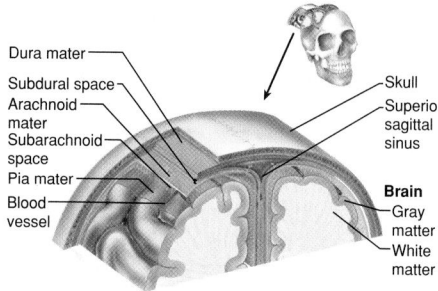

▲ **FIGURE 10.16   Meninges of Brain.**

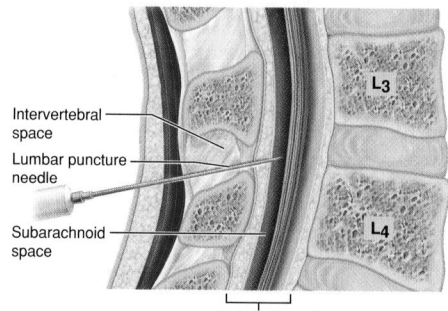

▲ **FIGURE 10.17   Lumbar Puncture (Spinal Tap).**

WORD ANALYSIS AND DEFINITION

S = Suffix   P = Prefix   R = Root   R/CF = Combining Form

WORD	PRONUNCIATION	ELEMENTS		DEFINITION
arachnoid mater	ah-**RACK**-noyd **MAY**-ter	S/ R/ R/	**-oid** *resembling* **arachn-** *cobweb, spider* **mater** *mother*	Weblike middle layer of the three meninges
cauda equina (***Note:*** Both these terms are stand-alone roots.)	**KAW**-dah eh-**KWY**-nah	R/CF R/CF	**caud/a** *tail* **equin/a** *horse*	Bundle of spinal nerves in the vertebral canal below the ending of the spinal cord
cervical (***Note:*** Cervical also is used to refer to a region of the uterus.)	**SER**-vih-kal	S/ R/	**-al** *pertaining to* **cervic-** *neck*	Pertaining to the neck region
dermatome	**DER**-mah-tome	S/ R/CF	**-tome** *instrument to cut* **derm/a-** *skin*	The area of skin supplied by a single spinal nerve; alternatively, an instrument used for cutting thin slices
dura mater (***Note:*** Both terms are stand-alone roots.)	**DYU**-rah **MAY**-ter	R/CF R/	**dur/a** *dura mater* **mater** *mother*	Hard, fibrous outer layer of the meninges
epidural **epidural space**	ep-ih-**DYU**-ral ep-ih-**DYU**-ral SPASE	S/ P/ R/	**-al** *pertaining to* **epi-** *above* **-dur-** *dura mater*	Above the dura Space between the dura mater and the wall of the vertebral canal or skull
intervertebral	in-ter-**VER**-teh-bral	S/ P/ R/	**-al** *pertaining to* **inter-** *between* **-vertebr-** *vertebra*	The space between two vertebrae
lumbar	**LUM**-bar		Latin *loin*	Pertaining to the region in the back and sides between the ribs and pelvis
meninges	meh-**NIN**-jeez		Greek *membrane*	Three-layered covering of the brain and spinal cord
pia mater (***Note:*** Both terms are stand-alone roots.)	**PEE**-ah **MAY**-ter	R/ R/	**pia** *delicate* **mater** *mother*	Delicate inner layer of the meninges
sacral	**SAY**-kral	S/ R/	**-al** *pertaining to* **sacr-** *sacrum*	In the neighborhood of the sacrum
spinal tap	**SPY**-nal TAP	S/ R/	**-al** *pertaining to* **spin-** *spine* **tap** Old English *to open*	Placement of a needle through an inter- tebral space into the subarachnoid space to withdraw CSF
subarachnoid space	sub-ah-**RACK**-noyd SPASE	S/ P/ R/	**-oid** *resembling* **sub-** *under* **-arachn-** *cobweb, spider*	Space between the pia mater and the arachnoid membrane
thoracic	**THOR**-ass-ik	S/ R/	**-ic** *pertaining to* **thorac-** *chest*	Pertaining to the chest (thorax)
tract	TRAKT		Latin *draw out*	Bundle of nerve fibers with common origin and destination

---

EXERCISES

Describe the location of these spinal nerves and what they affect in that body region. Do this in language your patient can understand.

1. Cervical: location _____   affect _____

2. Thoracic: location _____   affect _____

3. Lumbar: location _____   affect _____

4. Sacral: location _____   affect _____

LESSON 10.3 Disorders of the Nervous System

OBJECTIVES

When patients communicate with you as a health professional, they will often enhance your continual, ongoing learning by informing you of and reinforcing your knowledge about a specific disorder.

Information in this lesson will enable you to:

10.3.1 **Relate common disorders of the brain and cranial nerves to normal and abnormal anatomy and physiology.**

10.3.2 **Contrast the normal anatomy and physiology of the brain and cranial nerves with the abnormal anatomy and physiology that produce disorders.**

10.3.3 **Describe common disorders of the brain and cranial nerves.**

10.3.4 **Select the correct terminology to communicate about the brain and cranial nerves and their disorders with patients and other health professionals.**

You are

. . . a medical assistant working with Dr. Raoul Cardenas, a neurologist at Fulwood Medical Center.

Your patient is

. . . Mr. Lester Rood, a 75-year-old man who was diagnosed a year ago as having dementia.

CASE REPORT 10.2

Mr. Rood lives with his daughter, Judy, and she is with him today.

Patient Interview:

Mr. Lester Rood:

"How am I feeling? Scared stiff. Sometimes I don't know where I am. Most times I'm pretty sure I'm living with my daughter. I get so messed up. I can't cook anymore. I forget what I'm doing, can't get things straight. I find myself in the street and don't know how I got there. Judy has to help me shower and remind me to go to the bathroom. And it's only going to get worse. I don't want to be a burden. I used to have 100 people work for me. It's so frustrating, so frightening."

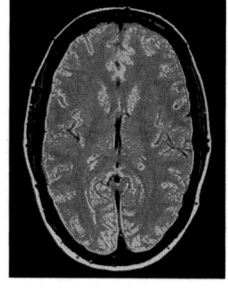
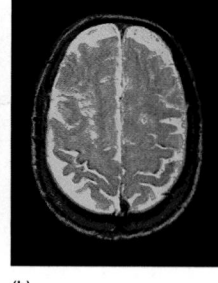

(a)   (b)

▲ **FIGURE 10.18** **Brain Sections.** *(a)* MRI scan of normal brain. *(b)* MRI scan of Alzheimer disease showing cerebral atrophy *(yellow).*

BRAIN

Dementia

Your **empathy** allowed Mr. Rood to talk without interruption. He reminded you that the symptoms of **dementia** include short-term memory loss, inability to solve problems, confusion, inappropriate behavior (such as wandering away), and impaired intellectual function that interferes with normal activities and relationships. In its early stages it is a very frightening and frustrating situation for the patient. It requires a lot of **sympathy** from family and caregivers.

Dementia is *not* a normal part of aging and is *not* a specific disease. It is a term used for a collection of symptoms that can be caused by a number of disorders affecting the brain.

Alzheimer disease is the most common form of dementia. It affects 10% of the population over 65 and 50% of the population over 85. Nerve cells in the areas of the brain associated with memory and cognition are replaced by abnormal clumps and tangles of a protein *(Figure 10.18).*

Vascular dementia is the second most common form of dementia. It can come on gradually when arteries supplying the brain become arteriosclerotic (narrowed or blocked), depriving the brain of oxygen, or can occur suddenly after a **stroke** *(see Chapter 7).*

Confusion is used to describe people who cannot process information normally. For example, they cannot answer questions appropriately, understand where they are, or remember important facts. Confusion is often part of dementia or delirium.

WORD	PRONUNCIATION	ELEMENTS		DEFINITION
Alzheimer disease	**AWLZ**-high-mer **DIZ**-eez		Alois Alzheimer, German neurologist, 1864–1915	Common form of dementia
confusion	kon-**FEW**-zhun	S/ R/	**-ion** *action, condition* **confus-** *bewildered*	Mental state in which environmental stimuli are not processed appropriately
conscious	**KON**-shus		Latin *to be aware*	Having present knowledge of oneself and one's surroundings
consciousness	**KON**-shus-ness	S/ R/	**-ness** *quality, state* **conscious-** *aware*	The state of being aware of and responsive to the environment
unconscious	un-**KON**-shus	P/	**un-** *not*	Not conscious, lacking awareness
delirium	de-**LIR**-ee-um	S/ R/	**-um** *structure* **deliri-** *confusion, disorientation*	Acute altered state of consciousness with agitation and disorientation; condition is reversible
dementia	dee-**MEN**-she-ah	S/ P/ R/	**-ia** *condition* **de-** *without* **-ment-** *mind*	Chronic, progressive, irreversible loss of the mind's cognitive and intellectual functions
empathy	**EM**-pah-thee	P/ R/	**em-** *into* **-pathy** *disease*	Ability to place yourself into the feelings, emotions, and reactions of another person
sympathy	**SIM**-pa-thee	P/	**sym-** *together*	Appreciation and concern for another person's mental and emotional state
stroke	STROHK		Old English *to strike*	Acute clinical event caused by an impaired cerebral circulation

Delirium is the sudden onset of disorientation, an inability to think clearly or pay attention. There is a change in the level of **consciousness**, varying from increased wakefulness to drowsiness. It is a mental state, not a disease. It can be part of dementia or a stroke.

Other conditions causing dementia are often treatable. They include:

- **Reactions to medications** (e.g., sedatives, antiarthritics).
- **Metabolic abnormalities** (e.g., hypoglycemia).
- **Nutritional deficiencies** (e.g., vitamins B_1 and B_6).
- **Emotional problems** (e.g., depression in the elderly).
- **Infections** (e.g., AIDS, encephalitis).

EXERCISES *Identify the elements in each medical term, and unlock the meaning of the word. Fill in the chart; then use one of the terms in a sentence of your choice that is not a definition.*

Medical Term	Meaning of Prefix	Meaning of Root/CF	Meaning of Suffix	Meaning of the Term
dementia				
sympathy				
unconscious				
delirium				
confusion				
empathy				

Sentence:

_____

_____

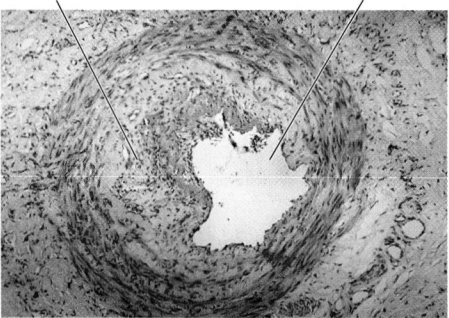

Atherosclerosis   Residual lumen of artery

(a)

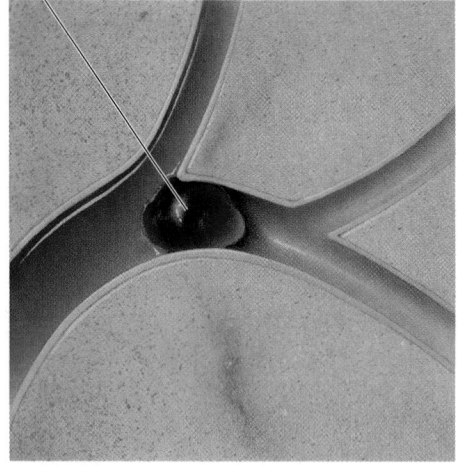

Embolus

(b)

▲ **FIGURE 10.19 Causes of Ischemic Strokes.** *(a)* Atherosclerosis in a cerebral artery leaving a small, residual lumen. *(b)* Embolus blocking an artery. Healthy tissue is on the left *(pink)*, blood-starved tissue is on the right *(blue)*.

Keynote

Risk factors for ischemic strokes are hypertension, diabetes mellitus, high cholesterol levels, cigarettes, and obesity.

Risk factors for hemorrhagic strokes are hypertension, cerebral **arteriovenous malformations,** and cerebral aneurysms.

One-third of people who have had a TIA will have more TIAs, and one-third will have a full-blown stroke later.

One in twenty people who suffer a TIA will have a stroke within 2 days.

Abbreviations	
AVM	arteriovenous malformation
CVA	cerebrovascular accident
TIA	transient ischemic attack
tPA	tissue plasminogen activator

CEREBROVASCULAR ACCIDENTS (CVAs) OR STROKES

A **stroke** (also known as a cerebrovascular accident, or **CVA**) occurs when the blood supply to a part of the brain is suddenly interrupted and thus brain cells are deprived of oxygen *(see Chapter 7)*. Some cells die; others are left badly damaged. With timely treatment, the damaged cells can be saved. There are two types of stroke:

1. Ischemic strokes account for 90% of all strokes and are caused by:

    a. **Atherosclerosis**—plaque in the wall of a cerebral artery *(Figure 10.19a)*.

    b. **Embolism**—blood clot in a cerebral artery originating from elsewhere in the body *(Figure 10.19b)*.

    c. **Microangiopathy**—occlusion of small cerebral arteries.

    Treatment of many acute ischemic strokes is by **thrombolysis** using clot busters such as **tissue plasminogen activator (tPA)** within 4½ hours of the stroke, with supportive measures followed by rehabilitation.

2. **Hemorrhagic strokes (intracranial hemorrhage)** occur when a blood vessel in the brain bursts or when a cerebral **aneurysm** or arteriovenous malformation (**AVM**) ruptures.

    Cerebral arteriography can determine the site of bleeding in hemorrhagic strokes, enabling surgery to be performed to stop the bleeding or to clip off the aneurysm or AVM.

Symptoms of Strokes

The symptoms of a stroke can include the sudden onset of numbness or weakness, especially on one side of the body; difficulty in walking, balance, or coordination; trouble speaking or understanding speech; trouble seeing in one or both eyes; dizziness; confusion; and severe headache.

Disability after Strokes

Although stroke is a disease of the brain, it can affect the whole body. A common residual disability is complete paralysis of one side of the body, called **hemiplegia.** If one side of the body is weak rather than paralyzed, the disability is called **hemiparesis.** Problems with forming and understanding speech and problems with awareness, attention, learning, judgment, and memory can remain after a stroke. Stroke patients may have difficulty controlling their emotions and may experience depression.

All of these disabilities require well-planned rehabilitation *(see Chapter 18)*.

Transient Ischemic Attack

Transient ischemic attacks (**TIAs**) are short-term, small strokes with symptoms lasting for less than 24 hours. If neurologic symptoms persist for more than 24 hours, then it is a full-blown stroke with brain cell damage and death.

The most frequent cause is a small **embolus** that occludes a small artery in the brain. Often, the embolus arises from a clot in the atrium in atrial fibrillation or from an atherosclerotic plaque in a carotid artery. If the impairment of blood supply lasts more than a few minutes, the affected nerve cells can die and cause permanent neurologic deficit.

Treatment is directed at the underlying cause. **Carotid endarterectomy** may be necessary if a carotid artery is significantly occluded with plaque.

WORD ANALYSIS AND DEFINITION

WORD	PRONUNCIATION		ELEMENTS	DEFINITION
aneurysm aneurysmal (adj)	**AN**-yur-izm an-yur-**RIZ**-mal		Greek *dilation*	Circumscribed dilation of an artery or cardiac chamber
arteriography	ar-teer-ee-**OG**-rah-fee	S/ R/CF	-graphy *process of recording* arteri/o- *artery*	X-ray visualization of an artery after injection of contrast material
arteriovenous malformation	ar-**TEER**-e-o-**VE**-nus mal-for-**MAY**-shun	S/ R/ S/ P/ R/	-ous *pertaining to* -ven- *vein* -ion *process* mal- *bad* -format- *to form*	An abnormal communication between an artery and a vein
carotid endarterectomy	kah-**ROT**-id **END**-ar-ter-**EK**-toe-me	R/ S/ P/ R/	carotid *large neck artery* -ectomy *surgical excision* end- *inside* -arter- *artery*	Surgical removal of diseased lining from the carotid artery to leave a smooth lining
hemiparesis	**HEM**-ee-pah-**REE**-sis	P/ R/	hemi- *half* -paresis- *weakness*	Weakness of one side of the body
hemiplegia	hem-ee-**PLEE**-jee-ah	S/ P/ R/	-ia *condition* hemi- *half* -pleg- *paralysis*	Paralysis of one side of the body
hemiplegic (adj)	hem-ee-**PLEE**-jik	S/	-ic *pertaining to*	Pertaining to or suffering from hemiplegia
microangiopathy	**MY**-kroh-an-jee-**OP**-ah-thee	S/ P/ R/CF	-pathy *disease* micro- *small* -angi/o- *blood vessel*	Disease of the very small blood vessels (capillaries)
thrombolysis thrombolytic (adj)	throm-**BOL**-ih-sis **THROM**-boh-**LIT**-ik	S/ R/CF	-lysis *dissolve* thromb/o- *clot*	Dissolving a thrombus (clot)

EXERCISES

Prefixes *are applicable to terms from various body systems and will appear repeatedly. Define the terms below; then define a term with the same prefix* **from a different body system or chapter.** *Fill in the blanks.*

1. **malformation** Prefix is _____ and means_____ .

   Definition of malformation: _____

   Term from a different body system/chapter with the same prefix: _____

   This term means _____ .

2. **endarterectomy** Prefix is _____ and means _____ .

   Definition of endarterectomy: _____

   Term from a different body system/chapter with the same prefix: _____

   This term means _____ .

3. **hemiparesis** Prefix is _____ and means _____ .

   Definition of hemiparesis:_____

   Term from a different body system/chapter with the same prefix: _____

   This term means _____ .

4. **microangiopathy** Prefix is _____ and means _____ .

   Definition of microangiopathy: _____

   Term from a different body system/chapter with the same prefix: _____

   This term means _____ .

CEREBRAL PALSY

Definition

Cerebral palsy (CP) is the term used to describe the motor **impairment** resulting from brain damage in an infant or young child, regardless of the cause or the effect on the child. It is not hereditary. In congenital CP, the cause is often unknown but can be brain malformations or maternal use of cocaine; CP developed at birth or in the neonatal period is usually related to an incident causing hypoxia of the brain.

Cerebral palsy causes delay in the development of normal milestones in infancy and childhood *(see Chapter 16)*.

The medical terminology of the classification and effects of CP is important, and it is used in many other conditions, including the after-effects of strokes. The technical terms that follow are labels used to describe the type and extent of a problem. They do not describe the individual.

Classification by Number of Limbs Impaired

- **Quadriplegia.** All four limbs are involved.
- **Diplegia.** All four limbs are involved, but the legs are affected more than the arms
- **Hemiplegia.** The arm and leg of one side of the body are affected.
- **Monoplegia.** Only one limb is affected, usually an arm.
- **Paraplegia.** Both lower extremities are involved.
- **Triplegia.** Three limbs are involved.

Classification by Movement Disorder

- **Spastic**—tight muscles that are resistant to being stretched. They can become overactive when used and produce clonic movements.
- **Athetoid**—difficulty in controlling and coordinating movements, leading to involuntary writhing movements in constant motion.
- **Ataxic**—a poor sense of balance and depth perception, leading to a staggering walk and unsteady hands.

Combined Classifications

- The classifications of movement disorder and number of limbs involved are combined; for example, **spastic diplegia.**

Treatment of Cerebral Palsy

A multidisciplinary team of health professionals is required to develop an individualized treatment plan and to involve the patients, families, teachers, and caregivers in decision making and planning.

Physical therapy is designed to prevent muscles from becoming weak or rigidly fixed with **contractures,** to improve motor development, and to facilitate independence. Speech therapy and psychotherapy complement physical therapy.

Muscle relaxants, such as diazepam, can reduce **spasticity** for short periods of time, and a variety of devices and mechanical aids ranging from muscle braces to motorized wheelchairs help overcome physical limitations.

Keynote

CP is caused by damage to the developing brain. Of all CP cases, 75% occur during pregnancy; 5%, during childbirth; and 15% during infancy up to age 3.

Spastic CP is the most common type, occurring in 70% to 80% of all cases.

Spastic CP can occur as spastic hemiplegia, spastic diplegia, and spastic quadriplegia.

Babies with very low birth weights are more likely to have CP.

WORD	PRONUNCIATION	ELEMENTS		DEFINITION
ataxia ataxic (adj)	a-**TAK**-see-ah a-**TAK**-sik	S/ P/ R/	**-ia** condition **a-** without **-tax-** coordination	Inability to coordinate muscle activity, leading to jerky movements
athetosis	ath-eh-**TOE**-sis	S/ R/	**-osis** condition **athet-** uncontrolled, without position	Slow, writhing involuntary movements
athetoid (adj)	**ATH**-eh-toyd	S/	**-oid** resembling	Resembling athetosis
contracture	kon-**TRAK**-chur	S/ R/	**-ure** result of, process **contract-** draw together	Muscle shortening due to spasm or fibrosis
diplegia diplegic (adj)	die-**PLEE**-jee-ah die-**PLEE**-jik	S/ P/ R/	**-ia** condition **di-** two **-pleg-** paralysis	Paralysis of all four limbs, with the two legs affected most severely
impairment	im-**PAIR**-ment	S/ R/	**-ment** action, state **impair-** worsen	Diminishing of normal function
monoplegia monoplegic (adj)	**MON**-oh-**PLEE**-jee-ah **MON**-oh-**PLEE**-jik	S/ P/ R/	**-ia** condition **mono-** one **-pleg-** paralysis	Paralysis of one limb
palsy	**PAWL**-zee		Latin *paralysis*	Paralysis or paresis from brain damage
paraplegia paraplegic (adj)	par-ah-**PLEE**-jee-ah par-ah-**PLEE**-jik	S/ P/ R/	**-ia** condition **para-** abnormal, beside **-pleg-** paralysis	Paralysis of both lower extremities
quadriplegia	kwad-rih-**PLEE**-jee-ah	S/ P/ R/	**-ia** condition **quadri-** four **-pleg-** paralysis	Paralysis of all four limbs
quadriplegic (adj)	kwad-rih-**PLEE**-jik	S/	**-ic** pertaining to	Pertaining to or suffering from quadriplegia
spasm	SPASM		Greek *spasm*	Sudden involuntary contraction of a muscle group
spastic (adj)	**SPAZ**-tik	S/ R/	**-ic** pertaining to **spast-** tight	Increased muscle tone on movement
triplegia triplegic (adj)	tri-**PLEE**-jee-ah tri-**PLEE**-jik	S/ P/ R/	**-ia** condition **tri-** three **-pleg-** paralysis	Paralysis of three limbs

EXERCISES

Prefixes: *Continue your work with prefixes of number. The following prefixes signify a number from one to four. List an English and a medical term that means that number. Try to think of terms from another chapter with that prefix. Fill in the blanks.*

1. monoplegia Prefix is_____ and means_____.

English word: _____

Medical term: _____

2. diplegic Prefix is _____ and means_____.

English word: _____

Medical term: _____

3. triplegia Prefix is _____ and means_____.

English word: _____

Medical term: _____

4. quadriplegia Prefix is _____ and means_____.

English word: _____

Medical term: _____

Case Report 10.1 (continued)

For Ms. Roberta Gaston, who was seen in Dr. Solis' neurosurgery clinic, the EEG did not localize an epileptic source. Therefore, deep brain electrodes were inserted into the region of the suspicious mass that showed on MRI. Seizures were recorded as arising in the mass itself. Dr. Solis performed a surgical resection of the mass, which was a **glioma.** Ms. Gaston has been seizure-free since the surgery a year ago.

EPILEPSY

Epilepsy is a chronic disorder in which clusters of neurons discharge their electrical signals in an abnormal rhythm. This disturbed electrical activity (a seizure) can cause strange sensations and behavior, convulsions, and loss of consciousness.

The causes of epilepsy are numerous, from abnormal brain development to brain damage.

An accepted classification of seizures is from the International League Against Epilepsy:

1. **Partial seizures** occur when the epileptic activity is in one area of the brain only. For example, the only symptom of an epileptic attack could be a series of involuntary jerking movements of a single limb.

2. **Generalized seizures:**
   a. **Absence seizures,** previously known as "**petit mal,**" begin between ages 5 and 10 years and may cease at puberty or continue through adult life. The child stares vacantly for a few seconds, apparently out of contact with surroundings. Recovery is quick. The child may be accused of daydreaming.
   b. **Tonic-clonic seizures,** previously called "**grand mal,**" are dramatic. The person experiences a **loss of consciousness (LOC),** breathing stops, the eyes roll upward, and the jaw is clenched. This "tonic" phase lasts for 30 to 60 seconds. It is followed by the "clonic" phase, in which the whole body shakes with a series of violent, rhythmic jerkings of the limbs. The seizures last for a couple of minutes, and consciousness returns.
   c. **Febrile seizures** are triggered by a fever in infants age 6 months to 5 years. Very few of these infants go on to develop epilepsy.

Status epilepticus occurs when the brain is in a state of persistent seizure. It is defined as one continuous seizure or recurrent seizures without regaining consciousness for 30 minutes or more. Many physicians believe that 5 minutes in this state is sufficient to damage neurons. Status epilepticus is a medical emergency and requires maintenance of the airway, breathing, and circulation and the intravenous administration of diazepam and anticonvulsant drugs.

Seizures may be followed by a period of diminished function in the area of brain surrounding the seizure focus. This transient neurologic deficit is called a **postictal state.**

Most epileptic disorders respond to **antiepileptic** medication, but occasionally brain surgery is required. The first-aid treatment during a seizure is to place the person in a reclining position on his or her side and to cushion the head. Do not try to keep the limbs from moving.

Tourette syndrome and other **tic disorders** are characterized by episodes of involuntary, rapid, repetitive, fixed movements of individual muscle groups. They occur with varying frequency and are associated with meaningless vocal sounds or meaningful words and phrases. The tics are probably genetic. There is no cure, but they can be treated pharmacologically with haloperidol or clonidine.

Narcolepsy is a chronic disorder caused by the brain's inability to regulate the sleep-wake cycle. Patients fall asleep during the day for a few seconds or up to an hour. It is associated with **cataplexy,** the sudden loss of voluntary muscle tone with brief episodes of total paralysis and vivid hallucinations. There is no cure, but it can be treated pharmacologically with stimulants.

Keynote

- Between 1% and 3% of the population will develop some form of epilepsy.
- Up to 50,000 Americans die each year from seizures and related causes, including drownings.

Abbreviation

LOC loss of consciousness

Keynote

Two-thirds of epileptic patients are manageable with medication and surgery; one-third are not.

- Status epilepticus is a medical emergency.
- First-aid treatment of a seizure is to place the person in a reclining position and cushion the head.

Keynote

The most common tic disorder is *transient tic disorder*, occurring in 10% of children during the early school years. It goes away within 1 year.

WORD	PRONUNCIATION	ELEMENTS		DEFINITION
antiepileptic	**AN**-tee-epih-**LEP**-tik	S/ P/ R/	**-tic** *pertaining to* **anti-** *against* **-epilep-** *seizure*	A pharmacologic agent capable of preventing or arresting epilepsy
cataplexy	**KAT**-ah-plek-see	P/ R/	**cata-** *down* **-plexy** *stroke*	Sudden loss of muscle tone with brief paralysis
glioma	gli-**OH**-mah	S/ R/	**-oma** *tumor, mass* **gli-** *glue*	Tumor arising in a glial cell
grand mal	**GRAHN MAL**	R/ R/	**grand** *big* **mal** *bad*	Old name for a generalized tonic-clonic seizure
narcolepsy	**NAR**-coh-lep-see	S/ R/CF	**-lepsy** *seizure* **narc/o-** *stupor*	Condition with frequent incidents of sudden, involuntary deep sleep
petit mal	peh-**TEE MAL**	R/ R/	**petit** *small* **mal** *bad*	Old name for an absence seizure
postictal	post-**IK**-tal	S/ P/ R/	**-al** *pertaining to* **post-** *after* **-ict-** *seizure*	Occurring after a seizure
status epilepticus	**STAT**-us ep-ih-**LEP**-tik-us	S/ R/ S/ R/	**-us** *pertaining to* **stat-** *standing still* **-ic** *pertaining to* **epilept-** *seizure*	A recurrent state of seizure activity lasting longer than a specific time frame (usually 30 minutes)
tic	TIK		French *tic*	Sudden, involuntary, repeated contraction of muscles
Tourette syndrome	tur-**ET SIN**-drome		Georges Gilles de la Tourette, French neurologist, 1857–1904	Disorder of multiple motor and vocal tics

After reading Case Report 10.1 on the opposite page, answer the following questions. Be prepared to discuss your answers in class.

1. Basically, what is a *seizure*? _____

_____

2. What do the electrodes measure? _____

3. Explain the phrase *"resection of the mass."* _____

_____

4. Define *glioma*. _____

5. These two terms have an element that means *electricity*: _____ and _____

6. What does the abbreviation MRI mean? _____

7. What is a *tic*? _____

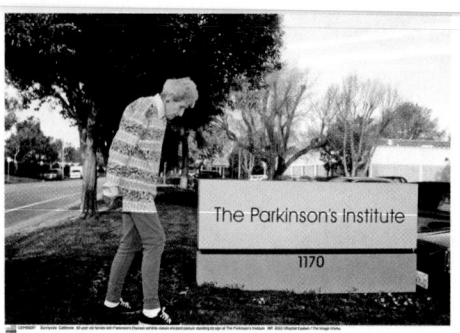

▲ **FIGURE 10.20 Stooped Posture of Parkinson Disease.**

Abbreviations

BSE	bovine spongiform encephalopathy
CJD	Creutzfeldt-Jakob disease
NMS	neurally mediated syncope
TB	tuberculosis

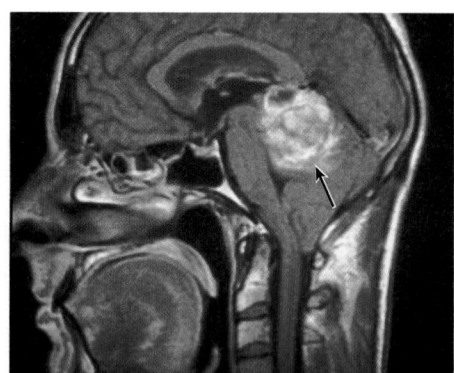

▲ **FIGURE 10.21 MRI Shows a Glioma** *(arrow).*

OTHER BRAIN DISORDERS

Parkinson disease is caused by the degeneration of neurons in the basic ganglia that produce a neurotransmitter called **dopamine.** Motor symptoms of abnormal movements, **tremor** of the hands, rigidity, a shuffling or **festinant** (hastening, falling-forward) gait, and weak voice appear *(Figure 10.20).* The symptoms gradually increase in severity. The cause is unknown, and there is no cure.

Huntington disease (also known as **Huntington chorea**) is a hereditary disorder starting with mild personality changes between the ages of 30 and 50. Involuntary, irregular, jerky **(choreic)** movements and muscle weakness follow, and dementia occurs in the later stages. A gene defect is on chromosome 4, but there is no known cure.

Creutzfeldt-Jakob disease (CJD) produces a rapid deterioration of mental function with difficulty in coordination of muscle movement. Some cases are linked to the consumption of beef from cattle with **mad cow disease (bovine spongiform encephalopathy, or BSE).** Damage to the brain is thought to be caused by an abnormal infectious protein called a **prion.**

Syncope (fainting or passing out) is a temporary loss of consciousness and posture. It is usually due to hypotension and the associated deficient oxygen supply (hypoxia) to the brain. This disorder is called **neurally mediated syncope (NMS).** In adults, it may be associated with cardiac arrhythmias and other diseases. The first-aid treatment is to place the person in a reclining position.

Migraine produces an intense throbbing, pulsating pain in one area of the head, often with nausea and vomiting. It can be preceded by an **aura,** visual disturbances such as flashing lights or temporary loss of vision. It occurs three times as often in women as men. There are multiple drugs used for prevention and treatment, with varying effectiveness. Stress management strategies *(see Chapter 24)* can also be of value.

Headache, in its chronic, recurrent form, is classified into three types:

1. **Vascular headaches,** of which migraine is the most common, are caused by blood vessels becoming dilated and distended, producing a throbbing type of pain. **Cluster headaches** with intense, episodic pain are associated with hypertension. Strokes can produce severe headache.

2. **Muscular,** in which there is tension of facial and neck muscles.

3. **Inflammatory,** associated with diseases of the meninges, sinuses, teeth, and ears.

Treatment is to eliminate the basic cause.

Cerebral edema is excess accumulation of water in the intra- or extracellular spaces of the brain. It is associated with trauma, tumors, inflammation, toxins (such as aspirin in **Reye syndrome;** *see Chapter 16*), ischemia, and malignant hypertension.

Encephalitis is inflammation of the parenchyma of the brain. It is usually caused by a virus such as human immunodeficiency virus (HIV), West Nile virus, herpes simplex, or the childhood diseases of measles, mumps, chickenpox, and rubella *(see Chapter 20).* It occurs most often in the elderly, those with compromised immune systems *(see Chapter 15),* and children.

Brain abscess is most often a direct spread of infection from sinusitis, otitis media, or mastoiditis *(see Chapter 4).* It can also be a result of bloodborne pathogens from lung or dental infections. Abscesses are also formed by exotic fungal or protozoan organisms in immunosuppressive diseases like AIDS (acquired immunodeficiency syndrome) and **tuberculosis (TB).** Protozoa are single-celled organisms that like to live in the damp. An example, *Trichomonas,* is sexually transmitted *(see Chapter 13).*

Brain tumors are most often secondary tumors that have metastasized from cancers in the lung, breast, skin, or kidney. **Primary brain tumors** arise from any of the glial cells and are called **gliomas** *(Figure 10.21).* The most malignant form of glioma is called **glioblastoma multiforme.**

Treatment is a combination of surgery, radiotherapy, and chemotherapy. The combination is necessary because even if you remove 99% of a tumor, there will be up to 1 billion cells remaining. A more recent therapy, **brachytherapy,** implants small radioactive pellets directly into the tumor. The radiation is released over time.

WORD ANALYSIS AND DEFINITION

WORD	PRONUNCIATION		ELEMENTS	DEFINITION
aura	AWE-rah		Greek *breath of air*	Sensory experience preceding an epileptic seizure or a migraine headache
bovine spongiform encephalopathy (also called **mad cow disease**)	**BO**-vine **SPON**-jee-form en-sef-ah-**LOP**-ah-thee	S/ R/ S/ R/CF S/ P/ R/	-ine *pertaining to* bov- *cattle* -form *appearance of* spong/i- *sponge* -pathy *disease* en- *in* -cephal/o- *head*	Disease of cattle (mad cow disease) that can be transmitted to humans, causing Creutzfeldt-Jakob disease
brachytherapy	bra-kee-**THAIR**-ah-pee	P/ R/CF	brachy- *short* -therapy *medical treatment*	Radiation therapy in which the source of irradiation is implanted in the tissue to be treated
chorea choreic (adj)	kor-**EE**-ah kor-**EE**-ik		Greek *dance*	Involuntary, irregular spasms of limb and facial muscles
Creutzfeldt-Jakob disease	**KROITS**-felt-**YAK**-op **DIZ**-eez		Hans Creutzfeldt (1885–1964) and Alfons Jakob (1884–1931), German neuropsychiatrists	Progressive incurable neurologic disease caused by infectious prions
festinant	**FES**-tih-nant		Latin *to hasten*	Shuffling, falling-forward gait
glioblastoma multiforme	**GLIE**-oh-blas-**TOE**-mah	S/ P/ R/ P/ R/CF	-oma *tumor* glio- *glue* -blast- *germ cell* multi- *many* -form/e *shape, appearance of*	A malignant form of brain cancer
Huntington disease (also called **Huntington chorea**)	**HUN**-ting-ton **DIZ**-eez kor-**EE**-ah		George Huntington, U.S. physician, 1851–1916	Progressive inherited, degenerative, incurable neurologic disease
migraine	**MY**-grain	P/ R/	mi- *derived from hemi; half* -graine *head pain*	Paroxysmal severe headache confined to one side of the head
prion	**PREE**-on		derived from *protein-infectious particle*	Small infectious protein particle
Reye syndrome	RAY **SIN**-drome		R. Douglas Reye, twentieth-century Australian pathologist	Encephalopathy and liver damage in children following an acute viral illness; linked to aspirin use
syncope	**SIN**-koh-peh		Greek *cutting short*	Temporary loss of consciousness and postural tone due to diminished cerebral blood flow
tremor	**TREM**-or		Latin *to shake*	Small, shaking, involuntary, repetitive movements of hands, extremities, neck, or jaw

EXERCISES

Apply the medical terminology you are learning in this chapter, and be prepared to discuss the following information about headaches.

1. What are the three types of headaches that reoccur in chronic form? _____, _____, and _____

2. What type of headache is associated with hypertension? _____

3. Muscular headaches result from tension in what part of the body? _____

4. What is the most common type of vascular headache? _____

5. Severe headache can be a symptom of impending _____.

TRAUMATIC BRAIN INJURY

Traumatic brain injury (TBI) causes damage to the brain. Over 1 million people are seen by medical doctors each year following a blow to the head. Of these, 50,000 to 100,000 will have prolonged problems affecting their work and their **activities of daily living (ADLs)**.

If you are driving your car at 50 miles per hour and are hit head-on, your brain goes from 50 miles per hour to zero instantly. Your soft brain tissue is propelled forward and squished against the front of your hard skull **(coup)**. Then the brain and the rest of your body rebound backward. The soft brain is then squished against the back of your rigid skull **(contrecoup)**. The squished front and back areas are at least bruised. This bruise is called a **contusion** (*Figure 10.22*).

If the process is more severe, blood vessels tear and blood flows into the brain. In addition, the brain itself can tear and cut brain connections and signals. In any injury, brain swelling can occur. Because the skull is hard and rigid, it cannot expand to cope with this extra volume. So the soft brain tissue is compressed, and some areas can stop working.

A mild head injury is called a **concussion.** You may feel dazed or have a period of confusion during which you do not recall the event that caused the concussion. In more severe cases, you may lose consciousness for a brief period of time and have no memory of the event. Repeated concussions have a cumulative effect, with loss of mental ability and/or traumatically induced Parkinson disease (as happened with professional boxer Muhammad Ali).

In more severe TBIs, the symptoms will depend on the area of the brain damaged. Some symptoms, such as difficulty with memory or concentration, irritability, aggression, **insomnia,** or depression, can be long-term. Traumatic brain injury has become a signature wound of the war in Iraq.

The residual effects of brain damage, whether due to trauma or stroke, have a terminology:

- **Impairment** is a deviation from normal function; for example, not being able to control an unwanted muscle movement.

- **Disability** is a restriction in the ability to perform a normal activity of daily living (ADL); for example, a 3-year-old who cannot walk independently.

- **Handicap** is defined as having a disability that prevents a child or adult from achieving a normal role in society commensurate with age and sociocultural setting; for example, a 16-year-old who cannot take care of personal toiletry and hygienic needs.

Shaken baby syndrome (SBS) is a type of TBI produced when a baby is violently shaken. The baby has weak neck muscles and a heavy head. Shaking makes the brain bounce back and forth in the skull, leading to severe brain damage. Other injuries include retinal hemorrhages, damage to the spinal cord, and fractures of the ribs and limb bones. This syndrome usually occurs in children younger than 2 years.

Abbreviations

ADLs	activities of daily living
PTSD	posttraumatic stress disorder
SBS	shaken baby syndrome
TBI	traumatic brain injury

▼ **FIGURE 10.22 Contusions Caused by Back-and-Forth Movement of Brain in Skull.**

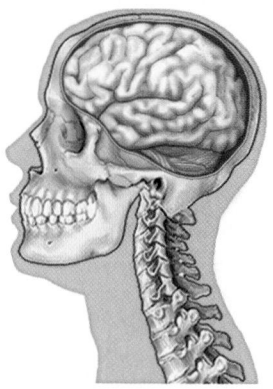

1. Position prior to impact.

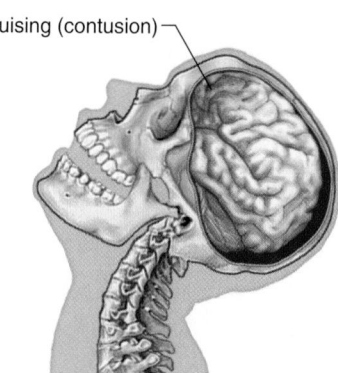

2. Impact from behind.

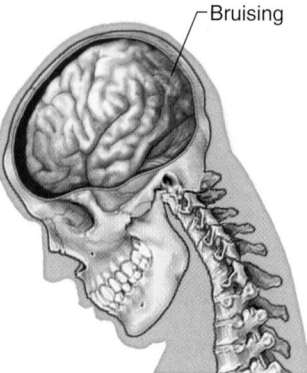

3. Contrecoup action.

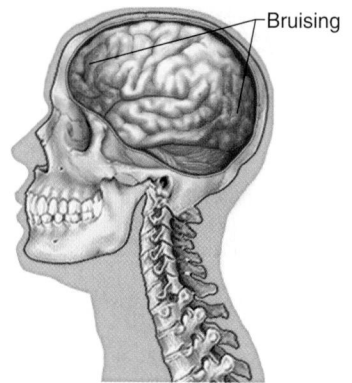

4. Subsequent coup-contrecoup injury.

WORD ANALYSIS AND DEFINITION

S = Suffix   P = Prefix   R = Root   R/CF = Combining Form

WORD	PRONUNCIATION	ELEMENTS		DEFINITION
activities of daily living (ADLs)	ak-**TIV**-ih-tees of **DAY**-lee **LIV**-ing	S/ R/ S/ R/ S/ R/	-ity *condition, state* activ- *movement* -ly *every* dai- *day* -ing *quality of* liv- *life*	Daily routines for mobility and personal care: bathing, dressing, eating, and moving
concussion	kon-**KUSH**-un	S/ R/	-ion *action, condition* concuss- *shake violently*	Mild head injury
contusion	kon-**TOO**-zhun	S/ R/	-ion *action, condition* contus- *bruise*	Bruising of a tissue, including the brain
coup	KOO		French *a blow*	Injury to the brain occurring directly under the skull at the point of impact
contrecoup	**KON**-treh-koo		French *counterblow*	Injury to the brain at a point directly opposite the point of original contact
disability	dis-ah-**BILL**-ih-tee	P/ R/	dis- *away from* -ability *competence*	Diminished capacity to perform certain activities or functions
handicap	**HAND**-ee-cap		French *assess before a race*	Condition that interferes with a person's ability to function normally
insomnia	in-**SOM**-nee-ah	S/ P/ R/	-ia *condition* in- *not* -somn- *sleep*	Inability to sleep

EXERCISES

Apply the correct medical language from this WAD to the sentences below. Remember to check your spelling when you are finished. Fill in the blanks.

1. A TBI can cause problems with the (abbreviation)_____ .

2. Rewrite sentence 1 without using the abbreviations. (Spell them out.)

   _____

   _____

3. Diminished capacity to perform certain activities or functions is a _____ .

4. A condition that interferes with a person's ability to function normally is a _____ .

5. A mild head injury can be termed a _____ .

6. Bruising of a tissue, including the brain, is a _____ .

7. List briefly some of the activities of daily living: _____

8. The two terms in this WAD that are diagnoses you might see on an Emergency Room record are _____ and

   _____ .

9. What is the difference between *insomnia* and *narcolepsy*? _____

   _____

10. What kind of brain injuries are likely to occur in a motor vehicle accident? _____

PAIN MANAGEMENT

Pain persisting longer than 3 months is said to be **chronic.** It can be caused by cancer, arthritis, fibromyalgia, low-back or neck problems, headache, or injuries that have not healed. Normal activities can be restricted or be impossible.

Among Americans, 6 million to 10 million are affected by fibromyalgia, 5 million are disabled by back problems, 8 million experience chronic neck and facial pain, and 40 million suffer from chronic recurrent headaches. In modern health care, chronic pain management has become essential and often uses a **multidisciplinary** approach. Pain management is now a board-certified subspecialty for **anesthesiologists.**

Medications are the cornerstone of pain management, and the following can be used based on the severity of the pain:

- Mild pain. **Analgesics,** such as acetaminophen, and **nonsteroidal anti-inflammatory drugs (NSAIDs),** such as ibuprofen, are used.

- Moderate pain. **Opiate** medications in combination with acetaminophen or NSAIDs are used. Some opiates used in combination medications are codeine, hydrocodone, and oxycodone. Examples are hydrocodone/acetaminophen (Vicodin), oxycodone/acetaminophen (Percocet), and oxycodone/aspirin (Percodan).

- Severe pain. Higher doses of opiates are used, often not as combination products. These include **morphine,** fentanyl, and oxy- and hydromorphone. The opiates can be taken orally, by patch, sublingually, by **intravenous (IV)** infusion, or by continuous delivery systems.

Central sensitization pain is a new concept describing how neurons in the spinal cord sending messages to the brain become excitable. They exaggerate the pain response in tissues they supply. The input can be somatic from skeletal muscles (as in fibromyalgia) or visceral (as in irritable bowel syndrome).

Interventional pain management, particularly for pain originating in the spine and spinal nerves, is being increasingly used. Examples are:

- **Epidural** or **facet nerve blocks.** Anesthetic or anti-inflammatory agents are injected into an area surrounding the pain-generating nerve.

- **Radiofrequency (RF) nerve ablation.** A probe heats the area around a pain-generating spinal nerve and temporarily deactivates it.

- **Spinal infusion pump.** Pain medications such as morphine are delivered through an indwelling catheter into the **intrathecal** CSF surrounding the spinal cord. A pump delivery device is inserted under the skin of the abdomen.

Phantom limb pain occurs following the **amputation** of a limb or part of a limb. Any stimulation of the remaining intact portion of the sensory pathway coming originally from the limb is interpreted by the brain as coming from the original limb. The pain can be severe and debilitating or just an insatiable urge to scratch an itch.

Referred pain occurs when pain in the viscera is felt in the skin or other superficial sites *(Figure 10.23)*. An example is the pain of a heart attack felt along the front of the left shoulder and down the underside of the left arm. This is because spinal cord segments **T1** to **T5** receive sensory input from the heart, as well as from the skin of the shoulder and arm. This input is transmitted to the brain. The brain cannot distinguish the true source of the pain. It assumes it is coming from the skin, which has more pain receptors than the heart and is injured more often.

Abbreviations	
IV	intravenous
NSAIDs	nonsteroidal anti-inflammatory drugs
RF	radiofrequency
T1	first thoracic vertebra or nerve
T5	fifth thoracic vertebra or nerve

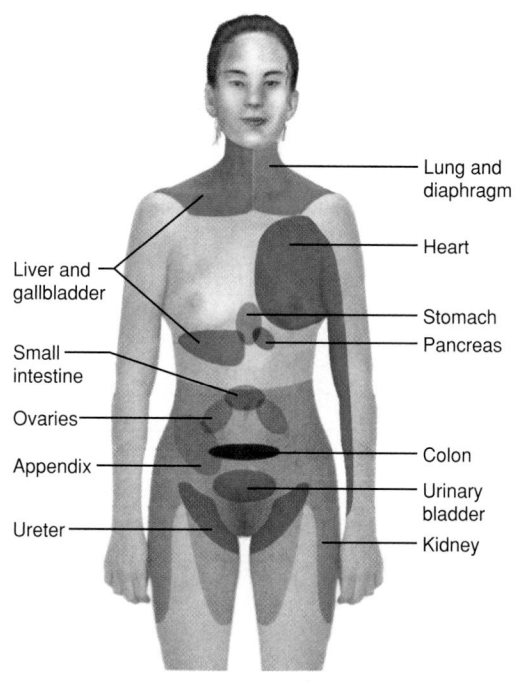

▲ FIGURE 10.23   Referred Pain.

WORD	PRONUNCIATION	ELEMENTS		DEFINITION
ablation	ab-**LAY**-shun	S/ P/ R/	-ion *action, condition* ab- *away from* -lat- *to take*	Removal of tissue to destroy its function
amputation	am-pyu-**TAY**-shun	S/ R/	-ation *process* amput- *to prune, lop off*	Process of removing a limb, part of a limb, a breast, or other projecting part
analgesia	an-al-**JEE**-ze-ah	S/ P/ R/	-ia *condition* an- *without* -alges- *sensation of pain*	State in which pain is reduced
analgesic	an-al-**JEE**-zic	S/	-ic *pertaining to*	Substance that produces analgesia
anesthesia	an-es-**THEE**-zee-ah	P/ R/CF	an- *without* -esthesi/a- *sensation, feeling*	Complete loss of sensation
anesthesiologist	**AN**-es-thee-zee-**OL**-oh-jist	S/	-logist *one who studies, specialist*	Medical specialist in anesthesia
anesthesiology	**AN**-es-thee-zee-**OL**-oh-jee	S/ P/ R/CF	-logy *study of* an- *without* -esthesi/o- *feeling, sensation*	Medical specialty related to anesthesia
anesthetic	an-es-**THET**-ic	S/ P/ R/	-ic *pertaining to* an- *without* -esthet- *sensation, perception*	An agent that causes absence of feeling or sensation
facet	**FAS**-et		French *little face*	Small area around a pain-producing nerve
intrathecal	**IN**-trah-**THEE**-kal	S/ P/ R/	-al *pertaining to* intra- *within* -thec- *sheath*	Within the subarachnoid or subdural space
intravenous	**IN**-trah-**VEE**-nuss	S/ P/ R/	-ous *pertaining to* intra- *within, inside* -ven- *vein*	Inside a vein
morphine	**MOR**-feen		Latin *god of dreams*	Derivative of opium used as an analgesic or sedative
multidisciplinary	mul-tee-**DIS**-ih-plin-**NAR**-ee	S/ P/ R/	-ary *pertaining to* multi- *many* -disciplin- *discipline, instruction*	Involving health care providers from more than one profession
opiate	**OH**-pee-ate		Latin *bringing sleep*	A drug derived from opium

EXERCISES

*Deconstruct the following **language of neurology**. Write the meaning of each element to see how it will aid you in understanding the meaning of the complete term. Fill in the chart.*

Medical Term	Meaning of Prefix	Meaning of Root/CF	Meaning of Suffix	Meaning of Term
intrathecal				
ablation				
analgesia				
anesthesia				
amputation				

Remember: Every term does not need a prefix!

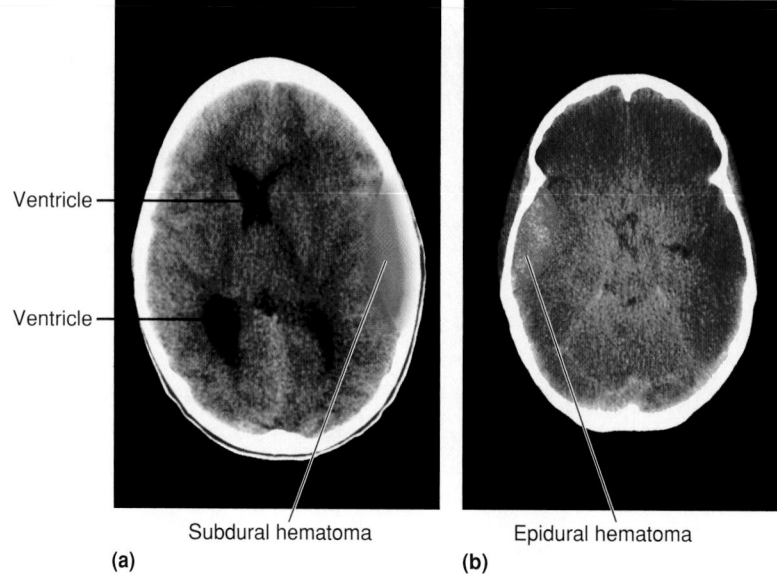

Ventricle

Ventricle

Subdural hematoma

Epidural hematoma

(a)

(b)

FIGURE 10.24 Hematomas. ▶
(a) CT scan with subdural hematoma compressing ventricles and pushing them laterally. (b) Epidural hematoma.

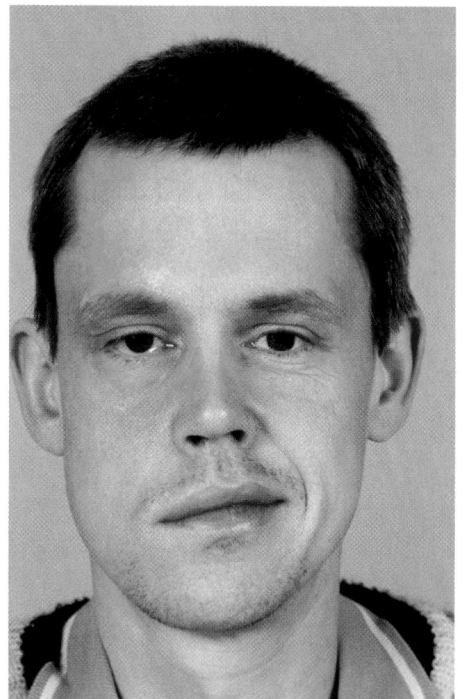

▲ **FIGURE 10.25 Bell Palsy of Left Side of Face.**

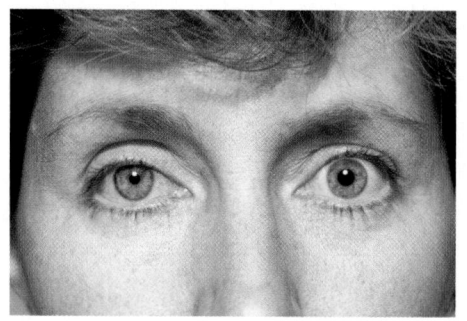

▲ **FIGURE 10.26 Horner Syndrome Showing Ptosis and Small Pupil of Right Eye.**

DISORDERS OF THE MENINGES

Subdural hematoma is bleeding into the subdural space outside the brain (*Figure 10.24a*). Most are associated with closed head injuries and bleeding from broken veins caused by violent rotational movement of the head. They have been seen following roller-coaster rides with high-speed turns that jerk and whip the head. Although the blood accumulation is slow, the bleeding must be stopped surgically.

Epidural hematoma is a pooling of blood in the epidural space outside the brain (*Figure 10.24b*). Most are associated with a fractured skull and bleeding from an artery that lies in the meninges. If the bleeding is not stopped surgically by **ligating** (tying off) the blood vessel, brain compression with severe neurologic injury or death can occur.

Meningitis is inflammation of the meninges covering the brain and spinal cord. Viral meningitis is the most common form and occurs at all ages. Bacterial meningitis is more common in the very young or very old. **Meningococcal meningitis** is contagious through droplet infection by coughing and sneezing (*see Chapter 20*) and through close living conditions, as in college dormitories. Vaccines are available to prevent most causes of meningitis (*see Chapter 20*).

Meningioma is a tumor originating in the arachnoid cells of the meninges, most commonly overlying the cerebral hemispheres. It is usually benign and produces a slow-growing, focal, spherical tumor. Symptoms can take years to develop. Surgical resection is usually curative.

DISORDERS OF THE CRANIAL NERVES

Bell palsy is a disorder of the seventh cranial nerve (facial nerve), causing a sudden onset of weakness or paralysis of facial muscles on one side of the face (*Figure 10.25*). Common symptoms are a **hemifacial** inability to smile, whistle, or grimace; drooping of the mouth with drooling of saliva; and inability to close the eye on the affected side. Early treatment with steroids and supportive measures is essential. The facial nerve can also be affected by trauma or tumors.

Trigeminal neuralgia (tic douloureux) is intermittent, shooting pain in the area of the face and head innervated by the fifth cranial nerve. The pain is abrupt (sudden), unilateral, often severe, and can affect any area of the face from the crown of the head to the jaw. Chewing or touching the affected area causes pain. Effective medications are carbamazepine and gabapentin.

Horner syndrome presents with a unilateral droopy eyelid (ptosis), small pupil, and decrease in perspiration on the face. It can occur in lung cancer and injuries to the head, neck, and cervical spinal cord (*Figure 10.26*).

WORD	PRONUNCIATION	ELEMENTS		DEFINITION
Bell palsy	BELL **PAWL**-ze		Charles Bell, 1774–1842, Scottish surgeon, anatomist, and physiologist	Paresis or paralysis of one side of face
hematoma	he-mah-**TOE**-mah	S/ R/	-oma *tumor, mass* hemat- *blood*	Collection of blood that has escaped from the blood vessels into tissue
hemifacial	hem-ee-**FAY**-shal	S/ P/ R/CF	-al *pertaining to* hemi- *half* -fac/i- *face*	Pertaining to one side of the face
Horner syndrome	**HOR**-ner **SIN**-drome		Johann Friedrich Horner 1831–1886, Swiss ophthalmologist	Disorder of the sympathetic nerves to the face and eye
ligate	**LIE**-gate		Latin *to tie, bind*	Tie off a structure, such as a bleeding blood vessel
meningioma	meh-**NIN**-jee-**OH**-mah	S/ R/CF	-oma *tumor, mass* mening/i- *meninges*	Tumor arising from the arachnoid layer of the meninges
meningococcal	meh-nin-goh-**KOK**-al	S/ R/CF R/	-al *pertaining to* mening/o- *meninges* -cocc- *spherical bacterium*	Pertaining to the *meningococcus* bacterium
meningitis	men-in-**JIE**-tis	S/	-itis *infection*	Acute infectious disease of children and young adults
neuralgia	nyu-**RAL**-jee-ah	S/ R/	-algia *pain* neur- *nerve*	Pain in the distribution of a nerve
subdural	sub-**DUR**-al	S/ P/ R/	-al *pertaining to* sub- *under* dur- *dura mater*	Located in the space between the dura mater and arachnoid membrane
tic douloureux (also called **trigeminal neuralgia**)	TIK duh-luh-**RUE**		douloureux French *painful tic*	Painful, sudden, spasmodic, involuntary contractions of the facial muscles supplied by the trigeminal nerve

EXERCISES

Suffixes can have more than one meaning, and only one of the meanings will apply to a particular term. In the following exercise, practice using the suffix -oma. Fill in the blanks; then fill in the chart.

1. The suffix -oma has two meanings: _____ and/or _____

2. In the term **hematoma**, the meaning of -oma is _____.

3. In the term **meningioma**, the meaning of -oma is _____.

4. Construct the term meaning *a nerve tumor.* _____

Now deconstruct the following medical terms into all their basic elements.

Medical Term	Prefix	Root/CF	Suffix
hematoma			
hemifacial			
meningioma			
neuralgia			

LESSON 10.4 Disorders of the Spinal Cord and Peripheral Nerves

OBJECTIVES

There are many disorders of the nervous system that affect the spinal cord and the peripheral nerves without affecting the brain. In this lesson, the information will enable you to:

10.4.1 **Discuss disorders of the spinal cord and peripheral nerves.**

10.4.2 **Distinguish between different diagnostic tests used for nervous system disorders.**

10.4.3 **Define methods by which nervous system medications influence disease processes.**

10.4.4 **Recognize common congenital disorders of the nervous system.**

10.4.5 **Select the correct terminology to communicate about the nervous system and its disorders with patients and other health professionals.**

You are

. . . Tanisha Colis, an electroneuro-diagnostic technologist working with Raul Cardenas, MD, a neurologist at Fulwood Medical Center.

Your patient is

. . . Mrs. Suzanne Kalish, a 42-year-old social worker employed by the medical center.

CASE REPORT 10.3

Mrs. Kalish has recently had an exacerbation of her symptoms due to multiple sclerosis **(MS)**. She is going to have a visual evoked potential **(VEP)** test, followed by an MRI of her brain and spinal cord.

Patient Interview:

Tanisha: "Good morning, Mrs. Kalish, I'm Tanisha Colis, the technologist who'll be performing your visual evoked potential test. How are you feeling?"

Mrs. Kalish: "I've been doing OK for the last 4 or 5 years. Then, a few weeks ago, I started dragging my right foot like a wounded witch. I've got to hang on to the walls to stay vertical. I'm tired out, can't come to work. It's a struggle to walk the few yards just to pick up the mail."

Tanisha: "The MRI you are going to have today will give us a lot of information about what's going on."

Mrs. Kalish: "My mind is going 'wheelchair, wheelchair, wheelchair.' Especially since in the last couple of days the vision in my right eye has got all blurred."

Tanisha: "That's the reason you are having the visual evoked potential test."

Mrs. Kalish: "I hate this disease. If I had cancer, I've got a chance. I'd fight it to the end, whatever that would be. Nobody's ever beat MS. You can only lose. It can be kind and leave you for a while, but it's never far away."

Tanisha: "Let me help you up, and we'll go get this test done."

Mrs. Kalish: "I can manage, thank you."

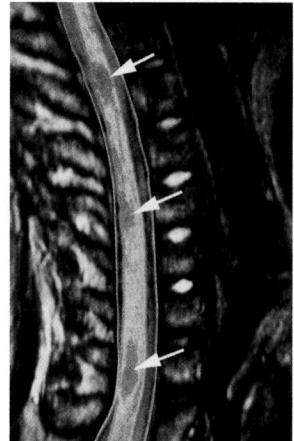

▲ **FIGURE 10.27 Multiple Sclerosis.**
Note areas of spinal cord where myelin sheath has been destroyed (arrows). Normal spinal cord is yellow.

DISORDERS OF THE MYELIN SHEATH OF NERVE FIBERS

When the myelin sheath surrounding nerve fibers is damaged, nerves do not conduct impulses normally. In newborns, many of their nerves have immature myelin sheaths, which is why some of their movements are jerky and uncoordinated.

Demyelination, the destruction of an area of the myelin sheath, can occur in the PNS caused by inflammation, vitamin B_{12} deficiency, poisons, and some medications.

Guillain-Barré syndrome is a disorder of the peripheral nerves in which the body makes antibodies against myelin, leading to loss of nerve conduction, muscle weakness, and **paresthesias** (changes in sensation). Treatment is with corticosteroids, and recovery of neurologic function is slow.

Demyelination of nerve fibers in the brain, spinal cord, and optic nerves can also occur. **Multiple sclerosis (MS)** is the most common of these demyelination disorders. As you can tell from Suzanne Kalish's story, MS is a chronic, progressive disorder. **Intermittent** myelin damage and scarring slows nerve impulses *(Figure 10.27)*. This leads to muscle weakness, pain, numbness, and vision loss. Because different nerve fibers are affected at different times, MS symptoms often worsen (**exacerbations**) or show partial or complete reduction (**remissions**). Mrs. Kalish is now in an exacerbation.

MS has an average age of onset between 18 and 35 years and is more common in women. Its cause is unknown, but it is thought to be an autoimmune disease.

WORD	PRONUNCIATION	ELEMENTS		DEFINITION
demyelination	dee-**MY**-eh-lin-**A**-shun	S/ P/ R/	-ation *process* de- *away from, without* -myelin- *myelin*	Process of losing the myelin sheath of a nerve fiber
encephalitis	en-**SEF**-ah-**LIE**-tis	S/ R/	-itis *inflammation* encephal- *brain*	Inflammation of brain cells and tissues
encephalomyelitis	en-**SEF**-ah-loh-**MY**-eh-lie-tis	R/CF R/	encephal/o- *brain* -myel- *spinal cord*	Inflammation of the brain and spinal cord
exacerbation (contrast remission)	ek-zas-er-**BAY**-shun	S/ R/	-ation *process* exacerbat- *increase, aggravate*	Period when there is an increase in the severity of a disease
Guillain-Barré syndrome	**GEE**-yan-bah-**RAY** **SIN**-drom		Georges Guillain (1876–1961) and Jean-Alexandre Barré (1880–1967), French neurologists	Disorder in which the body makes antibodies against myelin, disrupting nerve conduction
intermittent	**IN**-ter-**MIT**-ent	S/ P/ R/	-ent *end result* inter- *between* -mitt- *send*	Alternately ceasing and beginning again
modify	**MOD**-ih-fie		Latin *to limit*	Change the form or qualities of something
paresthesia paresthesias (pl)	par-es-**THEE**-ze-ah	S/ P/ R/	-ia *condition* par(a)- *abnormal* -esthes- *sensation, feeling*	Abnormal sensation; for example, tingling, burning, prickling
remission (contrast exacerbation)	ree-**MISH**-un	S/ P/ R/	-ion *action, condition* re- *back* -miss- *send*	Period when there is a lessening or absence of the symptoms of a disease

There is no known cure for MS, but recently developed **disease-modifying** drugs appear to have partial success in slowing down the accumulation of disabilities if started when the diagnosis is first made.

Other causes of demyelination in the CNS are injury, ischemia, toxic agents such as chemotherapy or radiotherapy, and congenital disorders such as **Tay Sachs disease** *(see Chapter 22).* After viral infections or vaccinations, **postinfectious encephalomyelitis** is a demyelination process, as is **HIV encephalitis,** which is seen in up to 30% of patients with AIDS.

Abbreviations

MS	multiple sclerosis
VEP	visual evoked potential

EXERCISES

Test yourself on the elements and terms in this WAD. Practice pronouncing the terms before you start the exercise. Circle the best answer.

1. **Guillain-Barré syndrome** disrupts:

   nerve conduction   blood flow   metabolism

2. In the term **paresthesia** the prefix means:

   between   abnormal   many

3. **Remission** is the opposite of:

   intermittent   exacerbation   demyelination

4. To **modify** something is to:

   dispose of it   change it   renew it

5. In the term **demyelination** the prefix means:

   away from   in front of   in between

6. Encephalomyelitis is inflammation of:

   brain   spinal cord   brain and spinal cord

Have you pronounced each word correctly? Did you listen to the audio glossary at McGraw-Hill Connect?

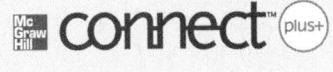

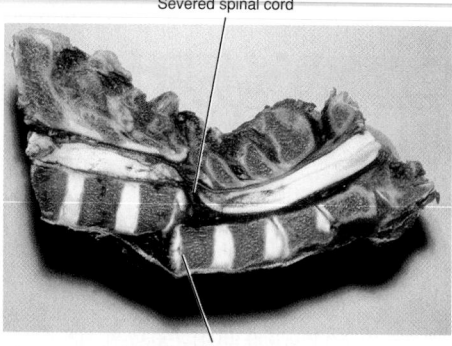

Severed spinal cord

(a) Fracture-dislocation of vertebra

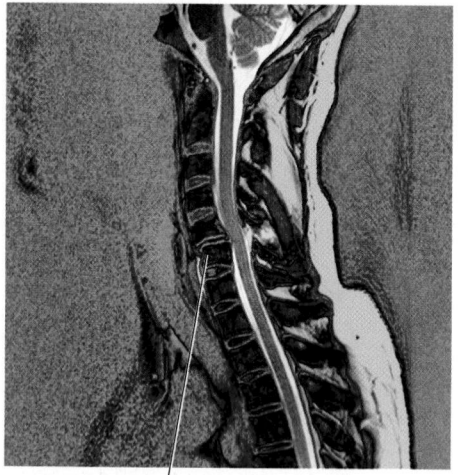

(b) Fractured vertebra

▲ **FIGURE 10.28 Spinal Cord Injuries.**
(a) Severed spinal cord from fracture-dislocation of vertebra. *(b)* Compressed spinal cord with vertebral fracture.

Keynote

PPS is rarely life-threatening, and the severity of residual weakness and disability relates to the severity of the original acute poliomyelitis.

Abbreviations

ALS	amyotrophic lateral sclerosis
polio	poliomyelitis
PPS	postpolio syndrome
SCI	spinal cord injury

DISORDERS OF THE SPINAL CORD

Trauma

The spinal cord is injured in three ways *(Figure 10.28):*

1. **Severed.**

2. **Contused.**

3. **Compressed,** by a broken or dislocated vertebra, bleeding, or swelling.

Because of its anatomy with nerve fibers and tracts going up and down, to and from the brain, injury to the spinal cord results in loss of function *below the injury.* For example, if the cord is injured in the thoracic region, the arms function normally, but the legs can be **paralyzed.** Both muscle control and sensation are lost.

If the spinal cord is severed, the loss is permanent. Contusions can cause temporary loss lasting days, weeks, or months. Compression injuries may require surgical intervention to relieve the pressure. Compression can also be due to a **herniated** disc.

The first goal of treatment is to prevent further damage, which is why you see football players being carried off the field strapped to a board and carefully padded to prevent even slight shifting of the spine.

Approximately half-a-million people in the United States have **spinal cord injuries (SCIs).** About 8000 new injuries occur each year; 82% involve males between the ages of 16 and 30. Quadriplegia is slightly more common than paraplegia.

Compression of the cord can also occur slowly from a tumor in the cord or spine. Cancer or osteoporosis can cause a vertebra to collapse and compress the cord.

- **Cervical spondylosis** is a disorder in which the discs and vertebrae in the neck degenerate, narrow the spinal canal, and compress the spinal cord and/or the spinal nerve roots.

- In **syringomyelia,** fluid-filled cavities grow in the spinal cord and compress nerves that detect pain and temperature. There is no specific cure.

Other Disorders

Acute transverse myelitis is a localized disorder of the spinal cord that blocks transmission of impulses up and down the spinal cord. People who have **Lyme disease, syphilis,** or **tuberculosis** *(see Chapter 20)* or those who inject heroin or amphetamines intravenously are at risk to develop this disorder. The disorder causes loss of sensation, muscle paralysis, and loss of bladder and bowel control. There is no specific treatment. Most people recover completely.

Subacute combined degeneration of the spinal cord is due to a deficiency of vitamin B_{12}. The sensory nerve fibers in the spinal cord degenerate, producing weakness, clumsiness, tingling, and loss of the position sense as to where limbs are. Treatment is injections of vitamin B_{12}.

Poliomyelitis (polio) is an acute infectious disease, occurring mostly in children, that is caused by the poliovirus. The virus can be asymptomatic in the nasopharynx and **gastrointestinal (GI)** tract. When it spreads to the nervous system, it replicates in the spinal cord and destroys motor neurons. Symptoms are progressive muscle **paralysis;** paralysis of the respiratory muscles can require mechanical ventilation using the **Drinker respirator** (iron lung). Poliomyelitis is preventable by vaccination and has almost been eradicated in the world.

Postpolio syndrome (PPS), in which people develop tired, painful, and weak muscles many years after recovery from polio, is classified as a motor neuron disorder.

Motor neuron disorders occur when motor nerves in the spinal cord and brain progressively deteriorate. This leads to muscle weakness that can progress to paralysis.

Amyotrophic lateral sclerosis (ALS, or Lou Gehrig disease) and its variants, **progressive muscular atrophy** and **primary lateral sclerosis,** are examples. There is no cure.

WORD	PRONUNCIATION	ELEMENTS		DEFINITION
amyotrophic	a-my-oh-**TROH**-fik	S/ P/ R/CF R/	-ic *pertaining to* a- *without* -my/o- *muscle* -troph- *nourishment,* *development*	Pertaining to muscular atrophy
atrophy	**AT**-roh-fee	P/ R/	a- *without* -trophy *development,* *nourishment*	Wasting or diminished volume of a tissue or organ
compression	kom-**PRESH**-un	S/ P/ R/	-ion *action, condition* com- *together* -press- *squeeze*	A squeezing together so as to increase density and/or decrease a dimension of a structure
herniation hernia (noun) herniate (verb)	**HER**-nee-ay-shun **HER**-nee-ah **HER**-nee-ate	S/ R/ S/	-ation *process* herni- *rupture* -ate *composed of*	Protrusion of an anatomical structure from its normal location
Lyme disease	LIME **DIZ**-eez		Named in 1977 after a group of children in Lyme, Connecticut	Disease transmitted by the bite of an infected deer tick
myelitis	**MY**-eh-**LIE**-tis	S/ R/	-itis *inflammation* myel- *spinal cord*	Inflammation of the spinal cord
paralyze	**PAR**-ah-lyze	P/ R/	para- *abnormal* -lyze *destroy*	To make incapable of movement
paralysis	pah-**RAL**-ih-sis	R/ R/	-lysis *destruction* -ly- *break down*	Loss of voluntary movement
paralytic (adj)	par-ah-**LYT**-ik	S/	-tic *pertaining to*	Pertaining to or suffering from paralysis
poliomyelitis polio (abbrev) postpolio syndrome (PPS)	**POE**-lee-oh-**MY**-eh-lie-tis post-**POE**-lee-oh **SIN**-drome	S/ R/ R/ P/ P/ R/	-itis *inflammation* polio- *gray matter* -myel- *spinal cord* post- *after* syn- *together* -drome *running*	Inflammation of the gray matter of the spinal cord, leading to paralysis of the limbs and muscles of respiration Progressive muscle weakness in a person previously affected by polio
spondylosis	spon-dih-**LOH**-sis	S/ R/	-osis *condition* spondyl- *vertebra*	Degenerative osteoarthritis of the spine
syringomyelia	sih-**RING**-oh-my-**EE**-lee-ah	S R R/CF	-ia *condition* myel- *spinal cord* syring/o- *tube, pipe*	Abnormal longitudinal cavities in the spinal cord that cause paresthesias and muscle weakness

EXERCISES

Meet a lesson objective by answering the following questions about the spinal cord. Fill in the blanks, and be prepared to discuss your answers in class.

1. What has happened to a *severed* spinal cord? _____

_____

2. If the spinal cord is *contused*, what does that mean? _____

_____

3. Briefly define a *compressed* spinal cord injury. _____

_____

4. Of the three injuries mentioned above, which one is permanent? _____

5. Where does loss of *function* occur in a spinal cord injury? _____

6. In the case of paralysis, what is lost? _____

DISORDERS OF THE PERIPHERAL NERVES

Neuropathy is used here as any disorder affecting one or more peripheral nerves.

Mononeuropathy is damage to a single peripheral nerve. Prolonged pressure on a nerve that runs close to the surface over a bony prominence is a common cause. Examples are:

- **Carpal tunnel syndrome.** The median nerve at the wrist is compressed between the wrist bones and a strong overlying ligament. Numbness, pain, and tingling of the thumb side of the hand are the symptoms. Incision of the ligament relieves the pressure.

- **Ulnar nerve palsy.** Nerve damage occurs as the ulnar nerve crosses close to the surface over the humerus at the back of the elbow. Pins-and-needles sensation and weakness in the hand result. Hitting the ulnar nerve is the cause of pain when you hit your "funny bone."

- **Peroneal nerve palsy.** Nerve damage occurs as the peroneal nerve passes close to the surface near the back of the knee. Compression of the nerve occurs in people who are bedridden or strapped in a wheelchair.

Polyneuropathy is damage to, and the simultaneous malfunction of, many peripheral nerves throughout the body.

Symptoms of acute polyneuropathy include muscle weakness and a pins-and-needles sensation or loss of sensation. The symptoms begin suddenly in the legs and work upward to the arms.

In diabetic chronic polyneuropathy, only sensation is affected, most commonly in the feet. Pins and needles, numbness, and a burning sensation are prominent.

When people with a neuropathy are unable to sense pain, they can injure a joint many times without feeling it. The joint malfunctions and can progress to being permanently destroyed. Joints involved in this **neuropathic joint disease** are called **Charcot joints.**

Herpes zoster (shingles) is an infection of peripheral nerves arising from a reactivation of the primary virus infection in childhood with **chickenpox (varicella).** During the primary infection of chickenpox, the virus gains entry into sensory dorsal root ganglia. Later in life, for unknown reasons, the virus produces the painful, unilateral dermatome rash of shingles *(Figure 10.29).*

Postherpetic neuralgia is acute dermatome pain persisting after the acute rash of shingles has subsided. It is debilitating and very difficult to treat *(see Chapter 3).*

Neuromuscular junction disorders occur where nerves connect with muscle fibers and interfere with the **neurotransmitter acetylcholine.** Examples are:

- In **myasthenia gravis** the immune system produces antibodies that attack the acetylcholine receptors on the muscle cells. The common symptoms are drooping eyelids; weak eye muscles, causing double vision; difficulty talking and swallowing; and muscle weakness in the limbs. Treatment is with a drug called **pyridostigmine,** which increases the amount of available acetylcholine.

- **Botulism** is a rare, life-threatening food poisoning caused by toxins from the bacterium *Clostridium botulinum.* These **neurotoxins** paralyze the muscles. In certain seasons, shellfish produce a similar neurotoxin.

- Certain **insecticides (organophosphates)** and nerve gases used in chemical warfare act on neuromuscular junctions.

- Nerve compression occurs when the space around a nerve is constricted. The pinched nerve becomes edematous and later fibrotic, and produces pain and paresthesias. Examples are sciatica when the sciatic nerve is compressed in the lower spine and carpal tunnel syndrome when the median nerve is compressed at the wrist.

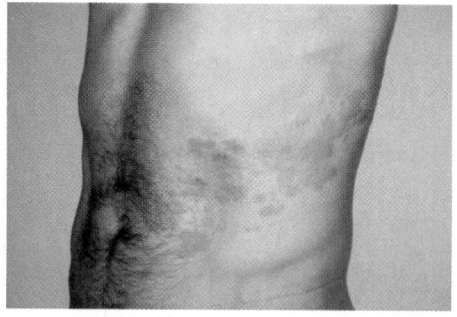

▲ **FIGURE 10.29** Herpes Zoster (Shingles).

Keynote

Herpes zoster occurs in people with depressed immune responses, HIV infection, or cancer and those on chemotherapy and/or radiation therapy, as well as for no apparent reason.

WORD	PRONUNCIATION	ELEMENTS		DEFINITION
botulism	**BOT**-you-lizm		Latin *sausage*	Food poisoning caused by the neurotoxin produced by *Clostridium botulinum*
Botox	**BO**-tox			Neurotoxin injected into muscles of the face to prevent the muscles from contracting and causing wrinkles
Charcot joint	**SHAR**-koh JOYNT		Jean-Martin Charcot, 1825–1893, French neurologist	Bone and joint destruction secondary to a neuropathy and loss of sensation
chickenpox (also called **varicella**)	**CHICK**-en-pocks		Disease originally considered a "chicken" (not dangerous) version of smallpox	Acute, contagious viral disease
Clostridium botulinum	klos-**TRID**-ee-um bot-you-**LIE**-num			Bacterium that causes food poisoning
insecticide	in-**SEK**-tih-side	S/ R/CF	-cide *kill* insect/i- *insect*	Agent that destroys insects
myasthenia gravis	my-as-**THEE**-nee-ah **GRA**-vis	S/ R/ P/ R/ R/	-ia *condition* my- *muscle* -a- *without* -sthen- *strength* gravis *serious*	Disorder of fluctuating muscle weakness
neuropathy neuropathic (adj) mononeuropathy polyneuropathy	nyu-**ROP**-ah-thee nyur-oh-**PATH**-ik **MON**-oh-nyu-**ROP**-ah-thee **POL**-ee-nyu-**ROP**-ah-thee	S/ R/CF P/ P/	-pathy *disease* neur/o- *nerve* mono- *one* poly- *many*	Any disease of the nervous system Disorder affecting a single nerve Disorder affecting many nerves
neurotoxin	**NYUR**-oh-tock-sin	R/ R/CF	-toxin *poison* neur/o- *nerve*	Agent that poisons the nervous system
organophosphate	**OR**-ga-no-**FOS**-fate	S/ R/CF R/	-ate *composed of* organ/o- *organic* -phosph- *phosphorus*	Organic phosphorus compound used as an insecticide
sciatica	sigh-**AT**-ih-kah		Greek *related to the hip joint*	Pain from compression of L5 or S1 nerve roots
sciatic (adj)	sigh-**AT**-ik			Pertaining to the sciatic nerve or sciatica

---

EXERCISES

Complete the definition with the correct medical language. Review this WAD for the elements you need to construct the term. Fill in the blanks.

> 💡 **Study Hint**
> Add the terms indicated by asterisks (*) to your list of prefixes designating numbers.

1. agent to destroy insects _____ /cide

2. Disorder affecting the nervous system   neuro/ _____

3. Disorder of fluctuating muscle weakness   my/a/sthen/ _____ _____

4. Agent that poisons the nervous system   _____ /toxin

5. Disorder affecting many nerves   _____ /neuro/ _____

6. What is another term for chickenpox?   _____

7. What is another term for botulism?   _____

8. Used as an insecticide   organo/phosph/ _____

9. Prefix meaning *affecting one** _____

10. Prefix meaning *affecting many** _____

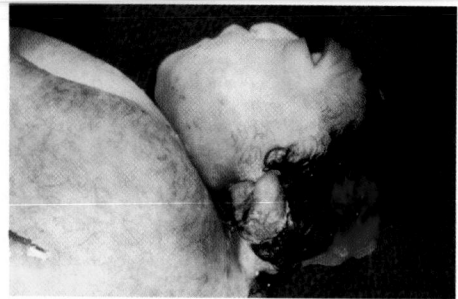

▲ FIGURE 10.30   Newborn with Anencephaly.

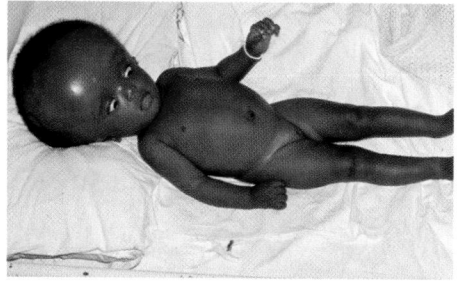

▲ FIGURE 10.31   Infant with Hydrocephalus.

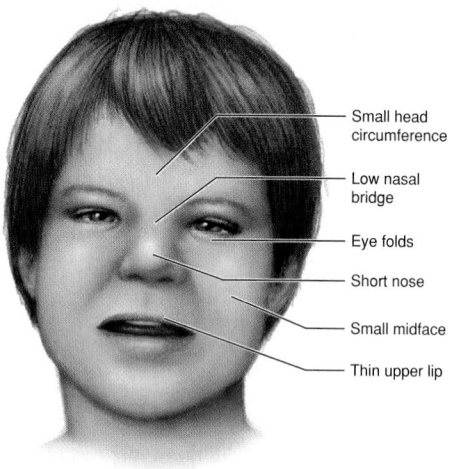

Small head circumference
Low nasal bridge
Eye folds
Short nose
Small midface
Thin upper lip

▲ FIGURE 10.32   Fetal Alcohol Syndrome.

Abbreviation	
FAS	fetal alcohol syndrome

CONGENITAL ANOMALIES OF THE NERVOUS SYSTEM

Some of the most devastating **congenital neurologic abnormalities** develop in the first 8 to 10 weeks of **gestation,** when the nervous system is in its early stages of formation. These malformations can be detected using **ultrasonography** and **amniocentesis** (*see Chapter 13*). Many can be prevented by the mother taking 4 mg/day of **folic acid** before conception and during early pregnancy.

A **teratogen** is an agent that can cause malformations of an embryo or fetus (*see Chapter 13*). It can be a chemical, virus, or radiation. Some teratogens are encountered in the workplace and include textile dyes, photographic chemicals, semiconductor materials, lead, mercury, and cadmium. One of the early uses of the drug thalidomide was to control morning sickness in pregnancy, but it caused severe limb and other deformities in the baby.

Anencephaly is absence of the cerebral hemispheres and is incompatible with life (*Figure 10.30*).

Microcephaly, decreased head size, is associated with small cerebral hemispheres and with moderate to severe motor and mental retardation.

Hydrocephalus, ventricular enlargement in the cerebral hemispheres with excessive CSF, is usually due to an obstruction that prevents the CSF from exiting the ventricles to circulate around the spinal cord (*Figure 10.31*). Treatment typically is to place a **shunt** to drain the CSF from the ventricles to either the peritoneal cavity or an atrium of the heart.

Fetal alcohol syndrome (FAS) can occur when a pregnant woman drinks alcohol. The child born with FAS has a small head, narrow eyes, and a flat face and nose (*Figure 10.32*). Intellect and growth are **impaired.** Fetal alcohol syndrome is the third most common cause of mental retardation in newborns.

Spina bifida occurs mostly in the lumbar and sacral regions (*Figure 10.33*). It is very variable in its presentation and symptoms. **Spina bifida occulta** has a small partial defect in the vertebral arch. The spinal cord or meninges does not protrude. Often the only sign is a tuft of hair on the skin overlying the defect.

In **spina bifida cystica,** no vertebral arch is formed. The spinal cord and meninges protrude through the opening and may or may not be covered with a thin layer of skin (*Figure 10.33a and b*). Protrusion of the meninges only is called a **meningocele;** protrusion of the meninges and spinal cord is called a **meningomyelocele.** Paralysis of the lower limbs may be present. The defect must be closed promptly to preserve spinal cord function and prevent infection. The cause of spina bifida is not known.

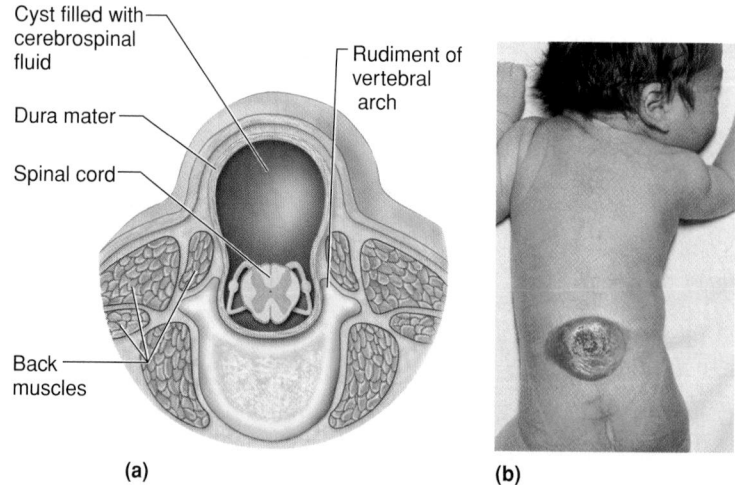

Cyst filled with cerebrospinal fluid
Dura mater
Spinal cord
Back muscles
Rudiment of vertebral arch

(a)   (b)

▲ FIGURE 10.33   **Spina Bifida Cystica.** (*a*) Cross-section of spinal cord. (*b*) Child with spina bifida cystica.

WORD	PRONUNCIATION		ELEMENTS	DEFINITION
anencephaly	AN-en-SEF-ah-lee	P/ R/	an- *without* -encephaly *condition of the brain*	Born without cerebral hemispheres
anomaly	ah-NOM-ah-lee		Greek *abnormality*	A structural abnormality
hydrocephalus	high-droh-SEF-ah-lus	S/ R/CF R/	-us *pertaining to* hydr/o- *water* -cephal- *head*	Enlarged head due to excess CSF in the cerebral ventricles
meningocele	meh-NING-oh-seal	S/ R/CF	-cele *hernia* mening/o- *meninges*	Protrusion of the meninges from the spinal cord or brain through a defect in the vertebral column or cranium
meningomyelocele	meh-NIN-goh-MY-el-oh-seal	S/ R/CF R/CF	-cele *hernia* -myel/o- *spinal cord* mening/o- *meninges*	Protrusion of the spinal cord and meninges through a defect in the vertebral arch of one or more vertebrae
microcephaly	MY-kroh-SEF-ah-lee	P/ R/	micro- *small* -cephaly *condition of the head*	An abnormally small head
spina bifida	SPY-nah BIH-fi-dah	R/CF P/ R/	spin/a *spine* bi- *two* -fida *split*	Failure of one or more vertebral arches to close during fetal development
spina bifida cystica	SIS-tik-ah	S/ R/	-ica *pertaining to* cyst- *cyst*	Meninges and spinal cord protruding through the absent vertebral arch and having the appearance of a cyst
spina bifida occulta	OH-kul-tah	R/	occulta *hidden*	The deformity of the vertebral arch is not apparent from the skin surface
teratogen	TER-ah-toe-jen	S/ R/CF	-gen *produce, create* terat/o- *monster, malformed fetus*	Agent that produces fetal deformities
teratogenic (adj) (*Note:* Has two suffixes.)	TER-ah-toe-jen-ik	S/	-ic *pertaining to*	Capable of producing fetal deformities

EXERCISES

Search and find the correct term for the element you are given. Circle the best answer.

1. Find the term with the prefix meaning *without:*

   hydrocephalus   anencephaly   impairment

2. Find the term with the root meaning *cyst:*

   meningocele   cystica   teratogen

3. Find the term with the root meaning *monster:*

   teratogen   spina   myelomeningocele

4. Find the term with the combining form meaning *water:*

   teratogenic   hydrocephalus   myelomeningocele

5. Find the term with the suffix meaning *hernia:*

   meningocele   hydrocephalus   anomaly

6. Find the term with the root meaning *split:*

   bifida   occulta   cystica

7. Find the term with the root meaning *head:*

   anomaly   hydrocephalus   meningocele

8. Find the term with the root meaning *hidden:*

   spina bifida   spina bifida cystica   spina bifida occulta

9. Find the term with the combining form meaning *spinal cord:*

   menigomyelocele   cystocele   meningocele

10. Find the term with the prefix meaning *small:*

   anencephaly   teratogenic   microcephaly

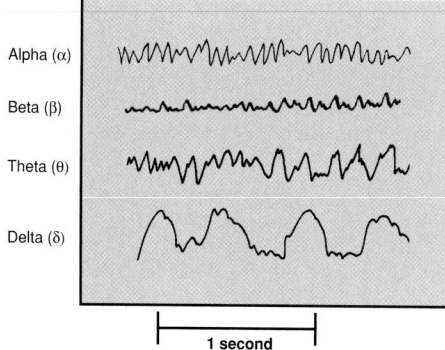

Alpha (α)

Beta (β)

Theta (θ)

Delta (δ)

1 second

▲ **FIGURE 10.34   Four Classes of Brain Waves on EEG.**

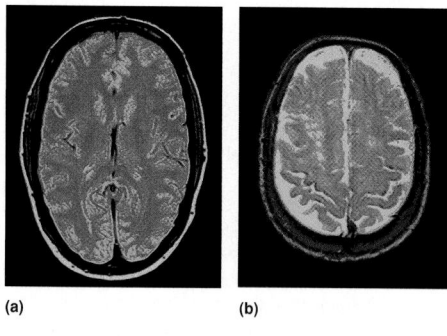

(a)   (b)

▲ **FIGURE 10.35   MRI Scans of Brain Sections.** *(a)* Scan of normal brain. *(b)* Scan of Alzheimer disease showing cerebral atrophy *(yellow).*

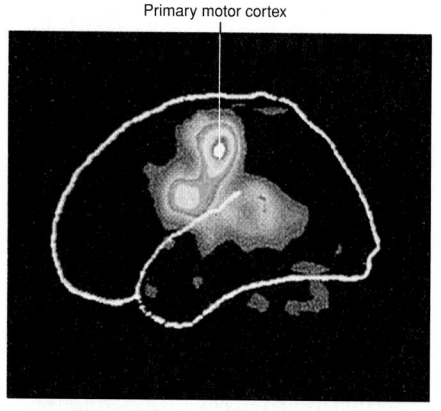

Primary motor cortex

▲ **FIGURE 10.36   PET Scan of the Brain Showing the Motor Cortex.**

DIAGNOSTIC PROCEDURES IN NEUROLOGY

Lumbar puncture (spinal tap) has been shown earlier. Laboratory examination of the CSF that shows white blood cells suggests meningitis. High protein levels indicate meningitis or damage to the brain or spinal cord. Blood suggests a brain hemorrhage or a traumatic tap.

Electroencephalography records the brain's electrical activity and helps identify seizure disorders, sleep disturbances, degenerative brain disorders, and brain damage *(Figure 10.34).*

Computed tomography (CT), a computer-enhanced x-ray technique, generates images of slices of the brain and can detect a wide range of brain and spinal cord disorders, including tumors, areas of dead brain tissue due to stroke, and birth defects.

Magnetic resonance imaging (MRI) produces highly detailed anatomical images of most neurologic disorders, including strokes, brain tumors, and myelin sheath damage *(Figure 10.35).*

Magnetic resonance angiography uses an injection of a radiopaque dye to produce images of blood vessels of the head and neck during MRI.

Cerebral angiography is an invasive procedure to inject a radiopaque dye into the blood vessels of the neck and brain. It can detect blood vessels that are partially or completely blocked, aneurysms, or arteriovenous malformations.

Color Doppler ultrasonography uses high-frequency sound (ultrasound) waves to show different rates of blood flow through the arteries of the neck or the base of the brain. This evaluates TIAs and the risk of a full-blown stroke.

Echoencephalography uses ultrasound waves to produce an image of the brain in children under the age of 2 because their skulls are thin enough for the waves to pass through them.

Positron emission tomography (PET) involves attaching radioactive molecules onto a substance necessary for brain function (for example, the sugar glucose). As the molecules circulate in the brain, the radioactive labels give off positively charged signals that can be recorded *(Figure 10.36).*

Myelography is the use of x-rays of the spinal cord that are taken after a radiopaque dye has been injected into the CSF by spinal tap. It has been replaced by MRI when that is available.

Evoked responses are a procedure in which stimuli for vision, sound, and touch are used to activate specific areas of the brain and their responses are measured with EEG or PET scans. This provides information about how that specific area of the brain is functioning in disorders such as MS.

Electromyography involves placing small needles into a muscle to record its electrical activity at rest and during contraction. It is used to provide information in disorders of muscles, peripheral nerves, and the **neuromuscular** junction.

Nerve conduction studies measure the speed at which motor or sensory nerves conduct impulses. The studies exclude disorders of the brain, spinal cord, and muscles and focus on the peripheral nerves.

WORD	PRONUNCIATION		ELEMENTS	DEFINITION
Doppler	DOP-ler		Johann Christian Doppler, 1803–1853, Austrian mathematician and physicist	Diagnostic instrument that sends an ultrasonic beam into the body
Doppler ultrasonography	DOP-ler UL-trah-soh-NOG-rah-fee	S/	-graphy *process of recording*	Imaging that detects direction, velocity, and turbulence of blood flow; used in workup of stroke patients
		P/	ultra- *beyond*	
color Doppler ultrasonography		R/CF	-son/o- *sound*	Computer-generated color image to show directions of blood flow
echoencephalography	EK-oh-en-sef-ah-LOG-rah-fee	S/	-graphy *process of recording*	Use of ultrasound in the diagnosis of intracranial lesions
		R/CF	ech/o- *sound wave*	
		P/	-en- *in*	
		R/CF	-cephal/o- *head*	
electroencephalogram (EEG)	ee-LEK-troh-en-SEF-ah-low-gram	S/	-gram *recording*	Record of the electrical activity of the brain
		R/CF	electr/o- *electricity*	
		R/CF	-encephal/o- *brain*	
electroencephalograph	ee-LEK-troh-en-SEF-ah-low-graf	S/	-graph *to write, record*	Device used to record the electrical activity of the brain
electroencephalography	ee-LEK-troh-en-SEF-ah-LOG-rah-fee	S/	-graphy *process of recording*	The process of recording the electrical activity of the brain
electromyography	ee-LEK-troh-my-OG-rah-fee	S/	-graphy *process of recording*	Recording of electrical activity in muscle
		R/CF	electr/o- *electricity*	
		R/CF	-my/o- *muscle*	
myelography	my-eh-LOG-rah-fee	S/	-graphy *process of recording*	Radiography of the spinal cord and nerve roots after injection of contrast medium into the subarachnoid space
		R/CF	myel/o- *spinal cord*	
nerve conduction study	NERV kon-DUK-shun STUD-ee	R/	nerve *nerve*	Procedure to measure the speed at which an electrical impulse travels along a nerve
		S/	-ion *action*	
		P/	con- *with, together*	
		R/	-duct- *lead*	
		R/	study *inquiry*	
neuromuscular	NYUR-oh-MUSS-kyu-lar	S/	-ar *pertaining to*	Pertaining to both nerves and muscles
		R/CF	neur/o- *nerve*	
		R/	-muscul- *muscle*	

EXERCISES

Meet a lesson objective by demonstrating your knowledge of diagnostic procedures in neurology. All the answers can be found on the opposite page. Fill in the blanks.

1. Which procedures can be considered *invasive* procedures? _____

_____

2. What makes a procedure *invasive?* _____

_____

3. Which procedures involve the use of injections of dye or radioactive molecules? _____

_____

4. Which procedures involve high-frequency sound waves? _____

_____

5. Which procedures measure electrical activity? _____

_____

You have now learned new terms related to diagnostic procedures in neurology!

Pharmacology of the Nervous System

The transmission of impulses from one neuron to another and from a neuron to a cell is achieved by **neurotransmitters at synaptic connections**. Drugs that affect the nervous system, called psychoactive drugs, target this synaptic mechanism.

Psychoactive drugs are able to change mood, behavior, cognition, and anxiety. They can be classified into several families:

1. Stimulants—**caffeine, nicotine, amphetamines**, and **cocaine**—enhance the stimulation provided by the **sympathetic nervous system**. They cause the level of **dopamine** to rise in the synapses, leading to the pleasurable effects associated with these drugs.

2. Sedatives—**ethanol** (beverage alcohol), **barbiturates**, and **meprobamate**—decrease the sensitivity of the postsynaptic neurons to quiet the nervous excitement. They also act on the sleep centers to induce sleep.

3. **Inhaled anesthetics** such as isoflurane act similarly to but are more powerfull than sedatives.

4. Opiates—**morphine, codeine, heroin, methadone**, and **oxycodone**—depress nerve transmission in the synapses of sensory pathways of the brain and spinal cord. They also inhibit centers in the brain controlling coughing, breathing, and intestinal motility. Codeine is used in cough medicines. Constipation is a side effect of all these drugs. Opiates are **addictive** because they produce **tolerance** and physical dependence.

5. **Opiate antagonists**, such as **naloxone** and **naltrexone**, prevent opiates from acting in the synapses. They can be used in drug overdose and to help recovering heroin addicts stay drug-free.

6. Tranquilizers, such as **chlorpromazine, haloperidol**, and the **benzodiazepines**, (Librium, Valium, Xanax), act like sedatives but without their sleep-inducing effect.

7. **Antidepressants** all increase the amount of **serotonin** at the synapses where it is a neurotransmitter. Zoloft and Prozac are examples.

8. **Antiepileptics** act in different ways on the synaptic junction to keep stimuli from passing across the synapse. Phenytoin and carbamazepine are examples.

9. **Psychedelics** distort sensory perceptions, particularly sight and sound. They can be natural plant products, such as mescaline, psilocybin, and dimethyltryptamine. They can be **synthetic**, such as **lysergic acid diethylamide (LSD)**, **methylenedioxymethamphetamine (MDMA** or "ecstasy"), and **phencyclidine (PCP** or "angel dust"). They increase the amount of serotonin in the synaptic junctions, and some have an additional amphetamine stimulation.

10. Marijuana has the active ingredient **tetrahydrocannabinol (THC)**. It produces the drowsiness of sedatives like alcohol, the dulling of pain like opiates, and, in high doses, the perception distortions of the psychedelics. Unlike the case with opiates or sedatives, tolerance does not occur.

Abbreviations

LSD   lysergic acid diethylamide
MDMA   methylenedioxymethamphetamine (ecstasy)
PCP   phencyclidine (angel dust)
THC   tetrahydrocannabinol (marijuana)

WORD	PRONUNCIATION	ELEMENTS		DEFINITION
addict	**AD**-ikt	P/ R/	**ad-** *to* **-dict** *consent, surrender*	Person with a psychologic or physical dependence on a substance or practice
addiction	ah-**DIK**-shun	S/	**-ion** *condition, action*	Habitual psychologic and physiologic dependence on a substance or practice
addictive	ah-**DIK**-tiv	S/	**-ive** *quality of, pertaining to*	Pertaining to or causing addiction
antagonist	an-**TAG**-oh-nist	S/ P/ R/	**-ist** *agent* **ant-** *against* **-agon-** *contest against*	An opposing structure, agent, disease, or process
antagonism	an-**TAG**-oh-nizm	S/	**-ism** *process, action*	Situation of opposing
marijuana	mar-ih-**HWAN**-ah		Mexican Spanish *María Juana*	Dried, flowering leaves of the plant *Cannabis sativa*
psychedelic	sigh-keh-**DEL**-ik	S/ R/CF R/	**-ic** *pertaining to* **psych/e-** *mind, soul* **-del-** *visible*	Agent that intensifies sensory perception
psychoactive	sigh-koh-**AK**-tiv	S/ R/CF R/	**-ive** *quality of, pertaining to* **psych/o-** *mind, soul* **-act-** *to do*	Able to alter mood, behavior, and/or cognition
sedative sedation	**SED**-ah-tiv seh-**DAY**-shun	S/ R/ S/	**-ive** *quality of, pertaining to* **sedat-** *to calm* **-ion** *condition, action*	Agent that calms nervous excitement State of being calmed
stimulant stimulate (verb) stimulation	**STIM**-you-lant **STIM**-you-late stim-you-**LAY**-shun	S/ R/	**-ant** *forming* **stimul-** *excite, strengthen*	Agent that excites or strengthens functional activity Arousal to increased functional activity
synthetic synthesis (noun)	sin-**THET**-ik **SIN**-the-sis	S/ P/ R/ S/	**-ic** *pertaining to* **syn-** *together* **-thet-** *place, arrange* **-esis** *abnormal condition*	Built up or put together from simpler compounds The process of building a compound from different elements
tolerance	**TOL**-er-ants	S/ R/	**-ance** *state of, condition* **toler-** *endure*	The capacity to become accustomed to a stimulus or drug
tranquilizer	**TRANG**-kwih-lie-zer	S/ R/	**-izer** *affects in a particular way* **tranquil-** *calm*	Agent that calms without sedating or depressing

EXERCISES

Deconstruct this language of neurology into its basic elements to help understand the meaning of the term. Write the elements between the slashes. The first one is done for you. Every term does not need every element, so you will have some blanks.

1. antagonist   _____*ant*_____ / _____*agon*_____ / _____*ist*_____

2. addict   _____ / _____ / _____

3. tranquilizer   _____ / _____ / _____

4. stimulant   _____ / _____ / _____

5. synthetic   _____ / _____ / _____

6. pyschedelic   _____ / _____ / _____

7. tolerance   _____ / _____ / _____

8. psychoactive   _____ / _____ / _____

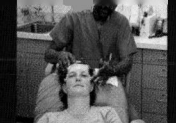

NERVOUS SYSTEM

CHALLENGE YOUR KNOWLEDGE

A. **Proofread your documentation.** The radiologist has just dictated the following report for a patient of the Fulwood Neurology Clinic. Before you print a final copy, always proofread the document for errors. Can you find the errors in the report? Circle the incorrect words in the report; then write the corrected words on the lines below, and include a brief definition for each correct word.

> ### CT SCAN OF THE HEAD
> CT of the head: CT of the head performed without IV contrast demonstrates mild dilutation of the venticular system. The sulcuses are also prominent. These findings are consistent with mild atrophie.
> No intracerbral hemorhage, subdaral, or epedural hemetoma is noted. No shift of the midline structures is noted.
> IMPRESSION: mild cerebral atrohy.

_____

_____

_____

_____

_____

_____

_____

_____

B. Analyze the following diagnostic procedures on the basis of their elements alone; then answer the questions. Fill in the blanks.

1. **echoencephalography**

   The combining form _____ tells me this is a diagnostic procedure on the _____.

2. **electromyography**

   The combining form _____ tells me this is a diagnostic procedure on the _____.

3. **myelography**

   The combining form _____ tells me this is a diagnostic procedure on the _____.

4. **electroencephalography**

   The combining form _____ tells me this is a diagnostic procedure on the _____.

5. Each of the four procedures listed above ends with the suffix _____, which means

   _____.

6. Change the suffix in each of these terms to *-gram*, which means the actual record produced by the diagnostic procedure. Write the new terms below._____

   _____

Use the terms in questions 1 to 6 to identify (define) the statements in questions 7 through 10. (*Hint:* In some cases you are asked for the *record,* and in some cases you are asked for the *recording.*) Be precise! Fill in the blanks.

7. Recording of electrical activity in muscle: _____

8. Use of ultrasound in the diagnosis of intracranial lesions: _____

9. Radiography of the spinal cord and nerve roots after injection of contrast medium into the subarachnoid space:

    _____

10. Record of the electrical activity of the brain: _____

Select any two of the diagnostic procedures in this exercise and describe their function or purpose.

11. Procedure: _____

     Purpose: _____

12. Procedure: _____

     Purpose: _____

C. **Roots and combining forms remain the core of a medical term.** Reinforce your knowledge of these elements with this exercise. Match the correct root or combining form in the left column to its meaning in the right column.

_____ 1. pathy

_____ 2. cephalo

_____ 3. algesia

_____ 4. syringo

_____ 5. audit

_____ 6. trophy

_____ 7. proto

_____ 8. pleg

_____ 9. somn

_____ 10. angio

A. hearing

B. first

C. sleep

D. blood vessel

E. tube, pipe

F. disease

G. development

H. head

I. sensation of pain

J. paralysis

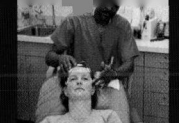

NERVOUS SYSTEM

D. Word Building Skills: Combine your knowledge of word elements and medical terminology construction, together with the power of your millions of brain cells, to answer the following questions.

1. In the term **neuralgia**, the suffix is _____, which means _____. If the element **ceph** means *head*, what does the term **cephalgia** mean? _____

   What does the term **arthralgia** mean? _____. If the element **caus** means *burning*, what is **causalgia**?

   _____

2. Exacerbation and remission are defined by their elements. Using their elements, explain the difference between these two processes.

   Exacerbation means _____ .

   Remission means _____ .

E. Similar but Different: The following medical terms contain a similar root, but the suffixes change the meaning of the terms. Use the correct form of these terms in the following sentences. Fill in the blanks.

neurosurgery   **neurologic**   **neurologist**   **neurosurgeon**   **neurology**

The _____ from the Fulwood _____ Department referred the patient to

a _____ for surgical consultation. The patient's _____ condition was deteriorating rapidly, and she would probably need _____ .

F. Plurals: Refresh your memory on the rules for plurals. Precision in communication depends on this. The singular form is given; circle the best answer for the plural form.

1. **ganglion:**   ganglius   ganglia   gangli

2. **plexus:**   plexuses   plexuia   plexui

3. **sulcus:**   sulces   sulci   sulcia

4. **gyrus:**   gyri   gryia   gryuses

G. Prefixes can be a very important part of medical terms. Challenge your knowledge of this chapter's prefixes by correctly filling in the following chart. You are given either the meaning or the prefix—complete the rest of the chart.

Prefix	Meaning of Prefix	Medical Term Containing This Prefix	Meaning of Medical Term
dis			
con			
	self		
re			
	together		
an			
de			

H. **Medical Language:** The nervous system is a complicated one and has a large range of vocabulary. Assess your knowledge of the nervous system by circling the correct answer in the questions below.

1. Abnormal movements marked by rapid contraction and relaxation of a muscle or muscle groups are called:

    a. compression

    b. clonic

    c. coma

    d. contusion

    e. concussion

2. Astrocytes, oligodendrocytes, microglia, ependymal, Schwann, and satellite are all terms relating to:

    a. capillaries

    b. tumors

    c. hematomas

    d. neuroglia

    e. ganglia

3. Body temperature is regulated by the:

    a. thalamus

    b. hypothalamus

    c. limbic system

    d. pons

    e. cerebellum

4. Centers that control vital visceral activities are located in the:

    a. pons

    b. corpus

    c. medulla oblongata

    d. hypothalamus

    e. CSF

NERVOUS SYSTEM

I. **Medical Language:** The nervous system is a complicated one and has a large range of vocabulary. Assess your knowledge of the nervous system by circling the correct answer in the questions below.

1. An agent capable of preventing or arresting epilepsy is called an:

   a. antidiuretic

   b. antibiotic

   c. antiepileptic

   d. antidepressant

   e. antibody

2. Administration of tPA is for:

   a. ALS

   b. thrombolysis

   c. seizures

   d. dementia

   e. meningitis

3. **Hypoglossal** refers to structures that can be found under the:

   a. diaphragm

   b. tongue

   c. jawbone

   d. bronchus

   e. alveoli

4. In simple terms, a **synapse** is a:

   a. malformation

   b. birth defect

   c. junction

   d. seizure

   e. vesicle

5. Implantation of radioactive pellets directly into a tumor is called:

   a. bradytherapy

   b. bradycardia

   c. brachytherapy

   d. brachial plexus

   e. none of the above

6. A state of deep unconsciousness is called:

   a. coma

   b. seizure

   c. sulcus

   d. dementia

   e. syncope

7. Groove that separates gyri:

   a. gyrus

   b. cortex

   c. fissure

   d. sulcus

   e. dermatome

8. The cerebral hemispheres are covered by a thin layer of gray matter called the:

   a. basal ganglia

   b. corpus callosum

   c. frontal lobe

   d. cerebral cortex

   e. cerebellum

9. The abbreviation for a short-term, small stroke is:

   a. EEG

   b. HACE

   c. TIA

   d. PET

   e. SBS

10. The medical term that means *pertaining to or caused by a seizure* is:

    a. clonic

    b. ictal

    c. tonic

    d. visceral

    e. synaptic

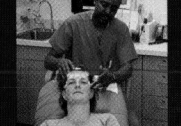

NERVOUS SYSTEM

J. **Terminology Challenge:** The difference in one or two letters makes for precision in medical language. *Brady-* and *brachy-* have two different meanings. Define them below, and give an example of their use in a term.

Brady- means _____. Example:_____

Brachy- means _____. Example:_____

K. **Recall and Review:** The following exercise on word elements contains some elements from this chapter and the previous chapter. Try to recall the previous elements without turning back in your book. Check the type of element; then write its meaning. Fill in the blanks.

Element	Prefix	Root/CF	Suffix	Meaning of Element
cyano	_____	_____	_____	_____
arachn	_____	_____	_____	_____
ar	_____	_____	_____	_____
pulmono	_____	_____	_____	_____
pleg	_____	_____	_____	_____
ectomy	_____	_____	_____	_____
purul	_____	_____	_____	_____
cervic	_____	_____	_____	_____
oro	_____	_____	_____	_____
plasty	_____	_____	_____	_____

L. **Abbreviations are helpful only if you know what they are meant to communicate.** Rewrite the following sentences without their abbreviations, but communicate the same message.

1. The patient's CVA has affected her PNS.

_____

_____

2. The BBB exists to protect brain tissue.

_____

_____

3. The patient's CSF will be tested today with a LP.

_____

_____

M. **In Your Own Words:** Translate into layman's terms these sentences directly from this chapter. How well do you understand what you read? Can you explain these sentences in nonmedical language? Rewrite each sentence in your own words.

1. Brain abscess is most often a direct spread of infection from sinusitis, otitis media, or mastoiditis.

   _____

   _____

   _____

2. Carotid endarterectomy may be necessary if a carotid artery is significantly occluded with plaque.

   _____

   _____

   _____

3. Risk factors for hemorrhagic strokes are hypertension, cerebral arteriovenous malformation, and cerebral aneurysms.

   _____

   _____

   _____

4. Cerebral angiography can detect blood vessels that are occluded, aneurysms, or arteriovenous malformations.

   _____

   _____

   _____

5. Anencephaly is absence of the cerebral hemispheres and is incompatible with life.

   _____

   _____

   _____

6. Some of the most devastating congenital neurologic anomalies develop in the first 8 to10 weeks of gestation.

   _____

   _____

   _____

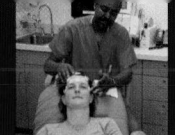

NERVOUS SYSTEM

N. Test-Taking Strategy Practice: Use your knowledge of medical terminology to insert the correct term in the appropriate statement. Not all answers will be used, and no answer will be used more than once.

hemiplegia	somatic	afferent
meningitis	meningioma	quadriplegia
festinant	comatose	visceral
neurotransmitters	dendrite	dementia

> *Study Hint*
> Start by answering the questions for which you are sure of the correct answer. Cross off the answer in the column after you insert it in the statement, and then answer the rest of the questions from the choices you have left. You will then be working with a smaller and smaller group of choices, which will make it easier to spot the correct answer.

1. _____ nerves carry signals from major organs such as the heart, lungs, stomach, and intestines.

2. State of deep unconsciousness: _____

3. A process or extension of a neuron is a(n) _____.

4. Shuffling gait: _____

5. Loss of the mind's cognitive functions: _____

6. Paralysis of all four limbs: _____

7. Chemicals that cross the synapse to another neuron are called _____.

8. _____ nerves carry signals from the skin, muscles, bones, and joints.

O. Precision of Medical Language: Medical language has many terms that look and sound similar. You must use the precise term in spoken and written medical communication and documentation. If a patient were to ask, you should be able to explain to him or her the difference between the pairs of words shown below. Write a short explanation for each.

1. *concussion* and *contusion:*

_____

_____

_____

2. *meningitis* and *meningioma:*

_____

_____

_____

3. *cerebellum* and *cerebrum:*

_____

_____

_____

P. **Construct the proper medical terms for the statements.** You have an assortment of prefixes, roots, combining forms, and suffixes with which to construct your terms. Fill in the blanks.

hydro	lepsy	
narco	lysis	esthesia
algia	occulta	a
neur/o	itis	para
an	trophy	post

1. Recurring episodes of falling asleep during the day: _____

2. Complete loss of sensation: _____

3. Pain in the distribution of a nerve: _____

4. Wasting away of tissue: _____

5. Derived from a word meaning *hidden:* _____

Brain Teaser: From previous chapters, what is the term for microscopic (hidden) blood in stool? _____

Q. **Diseases and Disorders:** The Fulwood Neurology Clinic treats patients with varied diseases and disorders of the nervous system. Are you familiar enough with their terminology and symptoms to match the correct disease or disorder with the appropriate statement for each patient? Circle the correct choice.

1. Patient has had a hemorrhagic stroke. Another name for this is:

   intercranial hemorrhage   intercerebral hemorrhage   intracranial hemorrhage

2. Patient bumped head on low doorway:

   concussion   seizure   convulsion

3. Patient has inflammation of the parenchyma of the brain:

   meningitis   encephalitis   vasculitis

4. Infection of the peripheral nerves arising from a reactivation of the chickenpox (varicella) virus:

   herpes simplex   shingles   post herpetic neuralgia

5. Infant has motor impairment resulting from brain damage at birth:

   Bell palsy   cerebral palsy   palsy

6. Patient had very bad dental infection that resulted in bloodborne pathogens lodging in her brain:

   brain tumor   brain abscess   brain hematoma

7. Patient complains of intermittent, shooting pain in the area of the face and head:

   trigeminal neuralgia   peripheral neuropathy   neuritis

NERVOUS SYSTEM

R. Latin and Greek terms do not deconstruct like some medical terms. Test your knowledge of these terms with this exercise. Match the terms in the left column to their correct meaning in the right column.

____1. epilepsy   A. stroke

____2. sulcus   B. braid

____3. efferent   C. swelling

____4. cerebrum   D. seizure

____5. ictal   E. brain

____6. plexus   F. ditch, furrow

____7. ganglion   G. away from

S. Pharmacology of Pain Management: Chronic pain management is a relatively new specialty of medicine. Medications are the cornerstone of this treatment. Demonstrate your knowledge of pain medications and their uses by filling in the chart. Place a checkmark (✓) in the correct column.

Medication	Mild Pain	Moderate Pain	Severe Pain
Percodan			
fentanyl			
Vicodin			
oxy- and hydromorphone			
continuous delivery system for drugs (pumps)			
hydrocodone			
acetaminophen			
oxycodone			
opiates combined with acetaminophen and NSAIDs			
NSAIDs			
morphine			

Prescribed For

Discussion questions:

1. Name a diagnosis for which pain medication would be prescribed. _____

   What type of medication might be prescribed? _____

2. Name three pain medications that are available OTC (over-the-counter; that is, available without a prescription) in any pharmacy.

   _____

   _____

T. **Diagnostic Testing:** You are responsible for scheduling diagnostic procedures for patients in the Neurology Clinic at Fulwood Medical Center. Practice your *language of neurology* by scheduling these patients appropriately, using the procedures listed below.

CT scan

myelography

evoked responses

electromyography

lumbar puncture or spinal tap

angiography

magnetic resonance imaging

nerve conduction studies

electroencephalogram

magnetic resonance angiography

Patient Needs/Symptoms:	Schedule Patient For:
Dr. Solis would like to measure the speed at which a patient's motor nerves conduct impulses.	
Doctor has ordered a recording of the electrical activity of the patient's brain.	
Dr. Solis suspects a tumor and needs to see a highly detailed anatomical image of the brain.	
Patient needs x-rays of the spinal cord taken after dye has been injected into it.	
Dr. Solis wants a sample of the patient's CSF.	
Patient has to schedule a study with contrast to image the cerebral blood vessels.	
Patient has a blocked carotid artery.	
Patient has possibly had a stroke; study will be looking for areas of dead brain tissue.	
Sensory stimuli will be used to activate specific areas of the brain and measure responses with EEG.	
Doctor wants to test and record the electrical activity of a patient's muscle at rest and during contractions	

U. **Precision in Documentation:** One of the five descriptions below is clearly the best choice for your answer—circle it, and explain why it is the best choice.

What type of tumors arise from glial cells?

tumors   primary tumors   secondary tumors   primary brain tumors   secondary brain tumors

The most precise description is _____ because _____

_____ .

NERVOUS SYSTEM

V. Label the following figure of the lateral aspect of the functional regions of the brain. On the blank lines, insert the correct number of the description of that area of the brain. Write the name of the area on the same line as the letter.

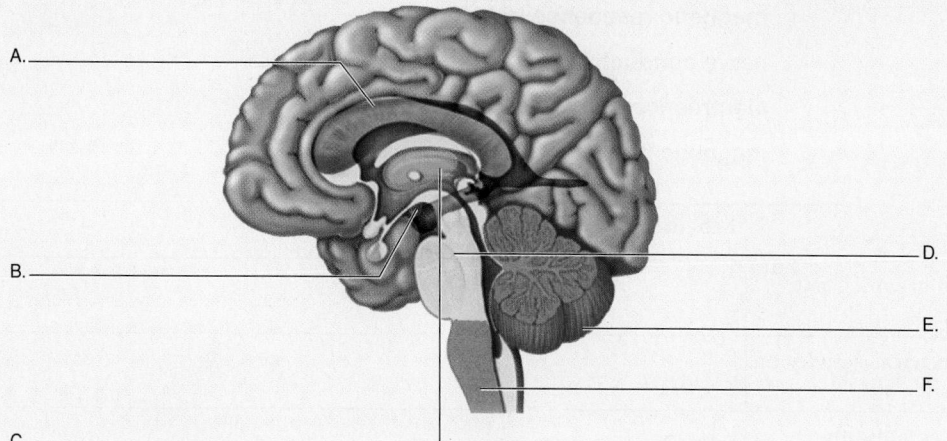

A._____

B._____

C._____

D._____

E._____

F._____

1. Regulates blood pressure and body temperature
2. Coordinates skeletal muscle activity to maintain posture and balance
3. Controls vital visceral activities
4. Spaces inside the cerebral hemisphere
5. Relays sensory impulses from peripheral nerves
6. Receives all sensory impulses and channels them to the cortex

CHAPTER SUMMARY EXERCISE

1. *Listen to the pronunciation of the medical terms as given by your instructor.*
2. *Circle the correct spelling of the medical term.*
3. *Match the correctly spelled terms to the brief descriptions below.*
4. *Write a sentence for each of the 10 terms that appear in this exercise.*

A. SPELLING COMPREHENSION: CIRCLE THE CORRECT SPELLING OF THE TERM.

1. synapse	sinapse	synipse	sinipse	synapsse
2. attetosis	athitoses	athitosis	athetosis	atetosis
3. Altheimer	Altzheimer	Alheimer	Alsheimer	Alzheimer
4. poleomielitis	polliomielitis	poliomyelitis	poliomielitis	poleomyelitis
5. serebelum	cerebellum	cerabelum	cerebelum	serabelum
6. perresthesia	paresthesia	peristhesia	parrestetia	peristesia
7. ketaplexy	cataprexie	ketaplexie	cataplexy	cateplexy
8. menninges	minengies	meninges	menningese	minenges
9. fantom	pantom	phantom	pantome	phantum
10. okcipital	ocipital	occipital	ocipitul	occipitule

B. MATCH THE NUMBER OF THE CORRECT TERM IN PART A WITH THE BRIEF DESCRIPTION OF THE TERM BELOW.

a. Posterior brain between midbrain and cerebral hemispheres _____

b. Three-layered covering of the brain and spinal cord_____

c. Inflammation of the gray matter of the spinal cord _____

d. Junction between two nerve cells _____

e. Abnormal sensation like tingling, burning _____

f. Slow, writing, involuntary movements _____

g. Sensation of a limb being present after amputation _____

h. Common form of dementia _____

i. Sudden loss of muscle tone with brief paralysis _____

j. Back of the head _____

C. USING YOUR KNOWLEDGE OF TERMS 1–10 IN PART A AND THEIR CORRECT SPELLING, WRITE A BRIEF SENTENCE AS IT MIGHT APPEAR IN PATIENT DOCUMENTATION.

1. _____

2. _____

3. _____

4. _____

5. _____

6. _____

7. _____

8. _____

9. _____

10. _____

D. YOUR INSTRUCTOR WILL DIRECT YOU TO MCGRAW-HILL CONNECT. OPEN THE AUDIO GLOSSARY AND PRACTICE YOUR PRONUNCIATION OF THE TERMS IN PART A OF THIS EXERCISE.

McGraw Hill **connect**™ (plus+)

E. SHOW YOUR COMPREHENSION OF THE LANGUAGE OF NEUROLOGY BY ANSWERING THE FOLLOWING QUESTIONS.

1. Interpret (rewrite) this physician's order without using the abbreviations: "Mr. Baker should be scheduled for an MRI and PET scan first thing in the AM." _____

_____

2. If a patient is suffering from PPS, what previous disease has he recovered from? _____

_____

3. What is a plexus? _____

_____

4. What is the logical term to complete this group: axon, dendrite, synapse _____

_____

5. Many medications are unable to pass the BBB, but one substance can get through. What is that substance? _____

6. Hypoglossal has the same meaning as _____ .

7. TIA and CVA are both abbreviations associated with _____ .

8. Quadriplegia, diplegia, hemiplegia, monoplegia, paraplegia, and triplegia *all* refer to _____ .

9. Translate into layman's language: "This transient neurologic deficit is called a postictal state." _____

_____

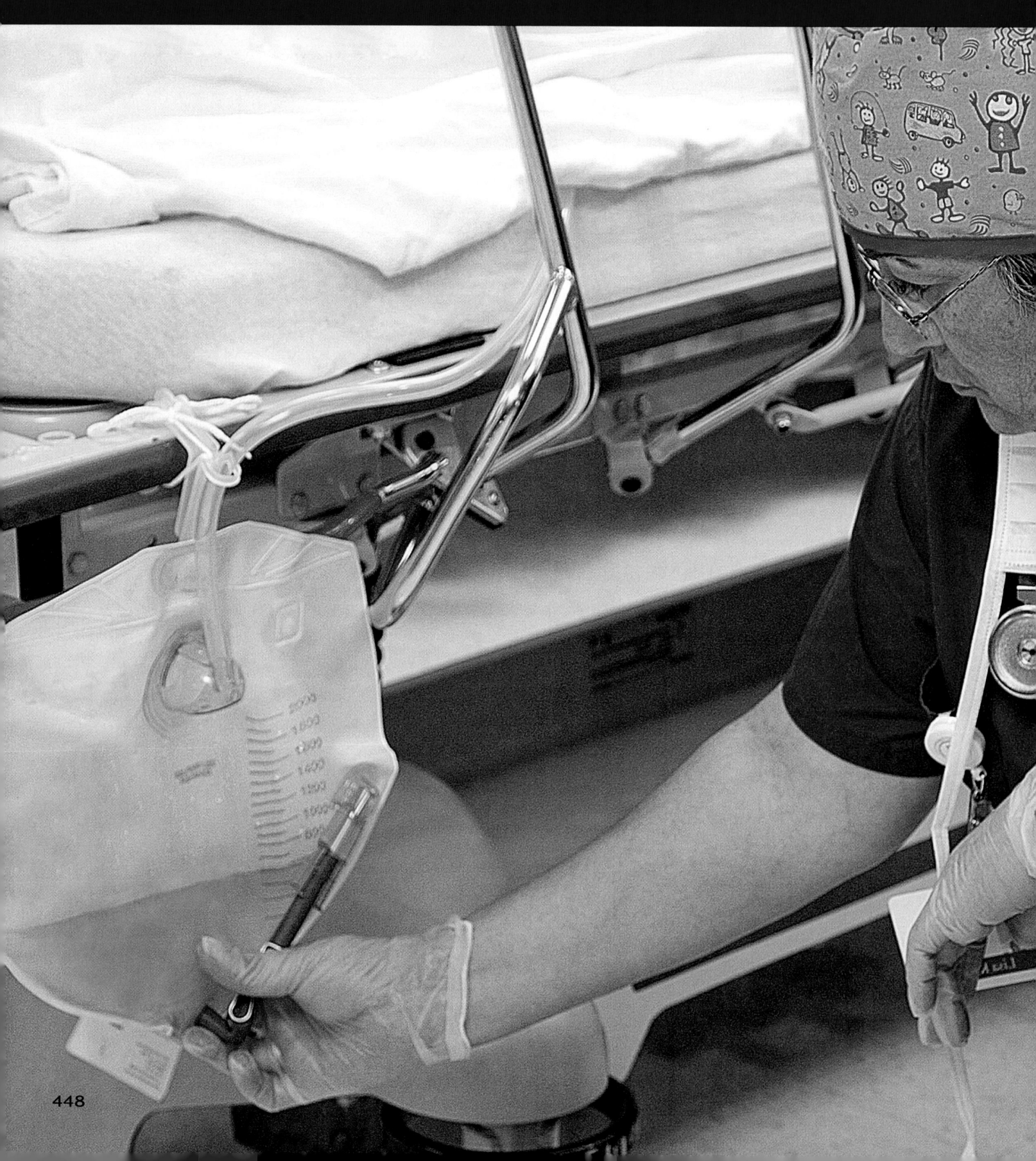

Urinary System
The Language of Urology

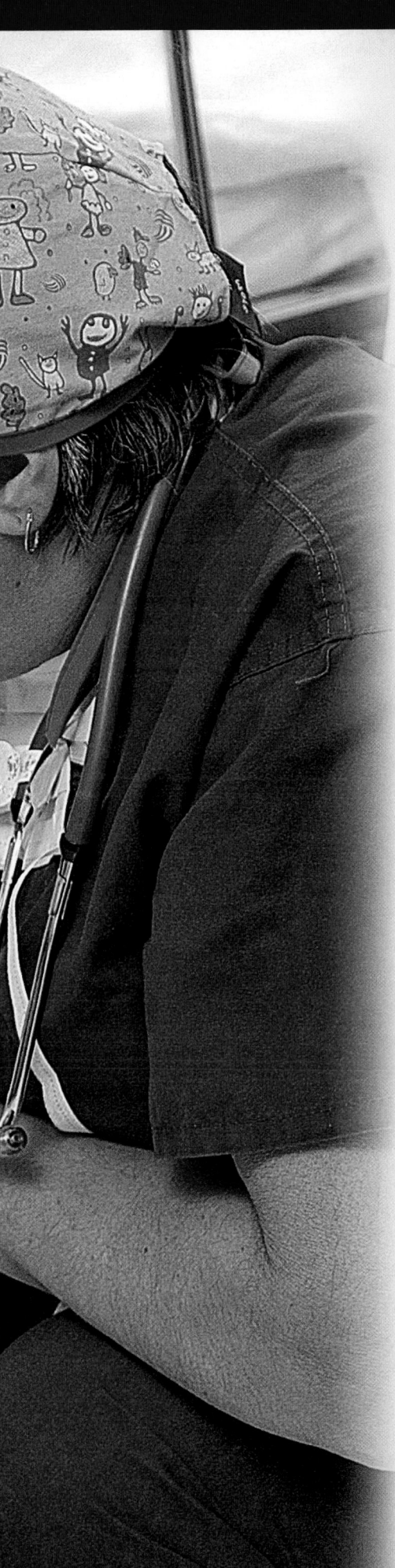

CASE REPORT 11.1

You are

. . . a surgical physician assistant working with **urologist** Phillip Johnson, MD, at Fulwood Medical Center.

Your patient is

. . . Mr. Nelson Hughes, a 58-year-old school principal. You are making your afternoon hospital visits to Dr. Johnson's patients. Earlier today you assisted at Mr. Hughes's surgery. A **laparoscopic radical nephrectomy** for a **TNM stage II renal** cell carcinoma (cancer) with no evidence of local invasion or lymph node involvement (metastasis) was performed.

Your job is to assess Mr. Hughes's postoperative state and determine whether postoperative complications exist.

Learning Outcomes

To define and understand these areas of concern, communicate with Dr. Johnson and the patient, and document Mr. Hughes's progress, you need to be able to:

11.1 Apply the language of **urology** to the anatomy and physiology of the urinary system.

11.2 Comprehend, analyze, spell, and write the medical terms of urology so that you communicate and document accurately and precisely in any health care setting.

11.3 Recognize and pronounce the medical terms of urology so that you communicate verbally with accuracy and precision in any health care setting.

11.4 Explain the effects of common urinary disorders on health.

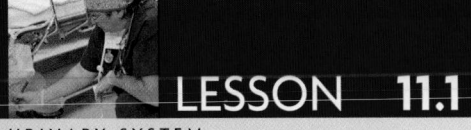
LESSON 11.1 Urinary System, Kidneys, and Ureters

OBJECTIVES

While the respiratory system *(see Chapter 9)* **excretes** carbon dioxide and water, the integumentary system *(see Chapter 3)* excretes water, inorganic salts, and lactic acid in sweat, and the digestive tract *(see Chapter 6)* excretes water, salts, lipids, bile pigments, and other wastes, the urinary system carries the major burden of excretion.

Within the urinary system, the kidneys are the agents that eliminate the waste products. If the kidneys fail to function, the other three systems of excretion are not able to replace them. Therefore, the kidney is a vital organ to be understood, and it brings with it a whole new set of terminology.

In this lesson, the information will enable you to:

11.1.1 **Identify the location and anatomical features of the kidney.**
11.1.2 **List the functions of the kidney.**
11.1.3 **Trace the flow of fluid through the renal filtration process.**
11.1.4 **Describe the functional anatomy of the ureters and urinary bladder.**
11.1.5 **Explain how common disorders of the kidneys and ureters affect health.**
11.1.6 **Apply correct medical terminology to the anatomy, physiology, and disorders of the kidneys, ureters, and urinary bladder.**

Keynote

The kidney is the major organ that eliminates the waste products of cellular metabolism.

Abbreviation

IVP	intravenous pyelogram
TNM	tumor-*node*-*metastasis* system of staging for cancer

Keynote

- **Urology** is the medical specialty of the diagnosis and treatment of diseases of the urinary system.
- A **urologist** is a medical specialist in the diagnosis and treatment of diseases of the urinary system.

URINARY SYSTEM

The urinary system *(Figure 11.1)* consists of six organs:

- Two **kidneys**
- A single **urinary bladder**
- Two **ureters**
- A single **urethra**

The process of removing metabolic waste is called **excretion**. It is an essential process in maintaining homeostasis *(see Chapter 2)*. The metabolic wastes include carbon dioxide from cellular respiration, excess water and electrolytes, **nitrogenous** compounds from the breakdown of proteins, and **urea**. If these wastes are not eliminated, they poison the whole body.

In the body's cells, protein is broken down *(see Chapter 2)* into amino acids. When an amino acid is broken down, **ammonia** is produced. Ammonia is extremely toxic to cells. The liver quickly converts it to the less toxic urea, which is excreted by the kidneys.

FIGURE 11.1 The Urinary System.
(*a*) Major organs. (*b*) Structures of the urinary system are visible in this colored IVP.

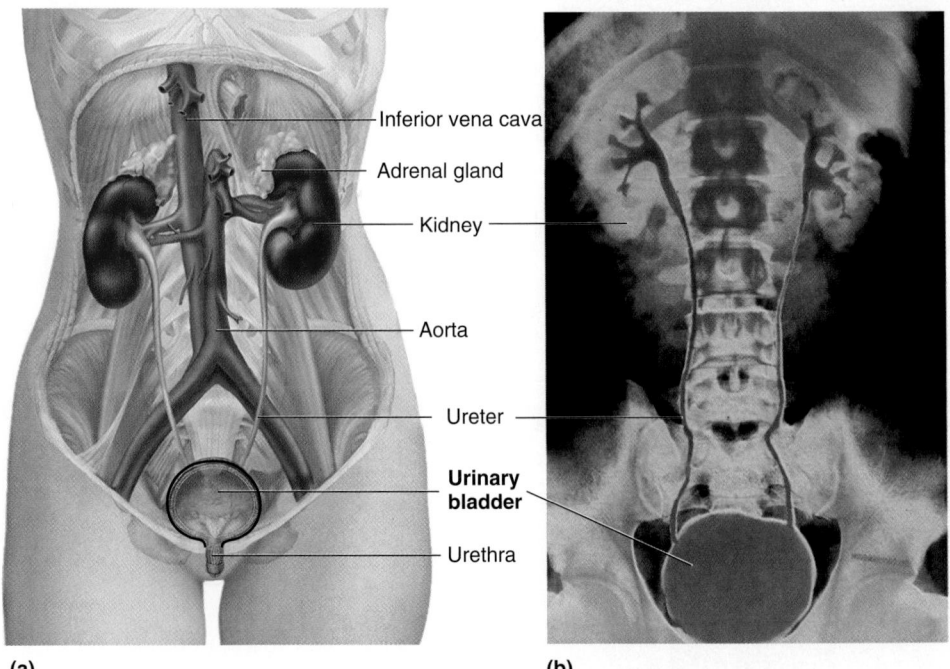

Inferior vena cava
Adrenal gland
Kidney
Aorta
Ureter
Urinary bladder
Urethra

(a) (b)

WORD	PRONUNCIATION	ELEMENTS		DEFINITION
ammonia	ah-**MOAN**-ih-ah	S/ R/	**-ia** *condition* **ammon-** *ammonia*	Toxic breakdown product of amino acids
bladder	**BLAD**-er		Old English *bladder*	Hollow sac that holds fluid; for example, urine or bile
excretion	eks-**KREE**-shun		Latin *remove*	Removal of waste products of metabolism out of the body
excrete (verb)	eks-**KREET**			To pass out of the body the waste products of metabolism
kidney	**KID**-nee		Greek *kidney*	Organ of excretion
nephrectomy	neh-**FREK**-toe-me	S/ R/CF	**-ectomy** *surgical excision* **nephr/o-** *kidney*	Surgical removal of a kidney
nephrology	neh-**FROL**-oh-jee	S/	**-logy** *study of*	Medical specialty of diseases of the kidney
nephrologist	neh-**FROL**-oh-jist	S/	**-logist** *one who studies, specialist*	Medical specialist in diseases of the kidney
nitrogenous	ni-**TROJ**-en-us	S/ R/CF R/	**-ous** *pertaining to* **nitr/o-** *nitrogen* **-gen-** *create*	Containing or generating nitrogen
radical	**RAD**-ih-cal		Latin *root*	Extensive, as in complete removal of a diseased part
renal	**REE**-nal	S/ R/	**-al** *pertaining to* **ren-** *kidney*	Pertaining to the kidney
urea	you-**REE**-ah		Greek *urine*	End product of nitrogen metabolism
urethra (**Note:** One "e" = one tube.)	you-**REE**-thra		Greek *urethra*	Canal leading from the bladder to outside (**Note:** The roots for **urethra** and **ureter** are different.)
urethral (adj)	you-**REE**-thral	S/ R/	**-al** *pertaining to* **urethr-** *urethra*	Pertaining to the urethra
urethritis	you-ree-**THRI**-tis	S/	**-itis** *inflammation*	Inflammation of the urethra
ureter (**Note:** Two "e's" = two tubes.)	you-**RET**-er		Greek *urinary canal*	Tube that connects the kidney to the urinary bladder (**Note:** The roots for **urethra** and **ureter** are different.)
ureteral (adj)	you-ree-**TER**-al	S/ R/	**-al** *pertaining to* **ureter-** *ureter*	Pertaining to the ureter
urine	**YUR**-in		Latin *urine*	Fluid and dissolved substances excreted by kidney
urinary (adj)	**YUR**-in-ary	S/ R/	**-ary** *pertaining to* **urin-** *urine*	Pertaining to urine
urinate (verb)	**YUR**-in-ate	S/	**-ate** *composed of, pertaining to*	To pass urine
urination	yur-ih-**NAY**-shun	S/	**-ation** *process*	The act of passing urine
urology	you-**ROL**-oh-jee	S/ R/CF	**-logy** *study of* **ur/o-** *urinary system*	Medical specialty of disorders of the urinary system
urologist	you-**ROL**-oh-jist	S/	**-logist** *one who studies*	Medical specialist in disorders of the urinary system
urological (adj)	yur-roh-**LOJ**-ik-al	S/	**-ical** *pertaining to*	Pertaining to urology

EXERCISES

The Same but Different: *More than one word element can have the same meaning. In this body system,* **nephr-** *and* **ren-** *both mean kidney. The elements are not interchangeable—one particular element will be used for a specific term. You need to know them individually. Fill in the blanks. Read carefully!*

1. Surgical removal of a kidney   _____/ _____ / _____

2. Medical specialist in kidney treatment   _____/ _____ / _____

3. Medical specialty in kidney diseases   _____/ _____ / _____

4. Pertaining to the kidney   _____/ _____ / _____

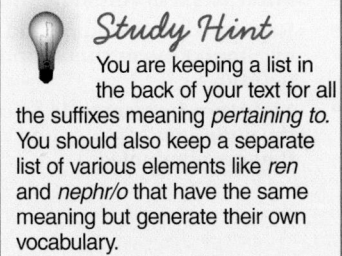

Study Hint

You are keeping a list in the back of your text for all the suffixes meaning *pertaining to*. You should also keep a separate list of various elements like *ren* and *nephr/o* that have the same meaning but generate their own vocabulary.

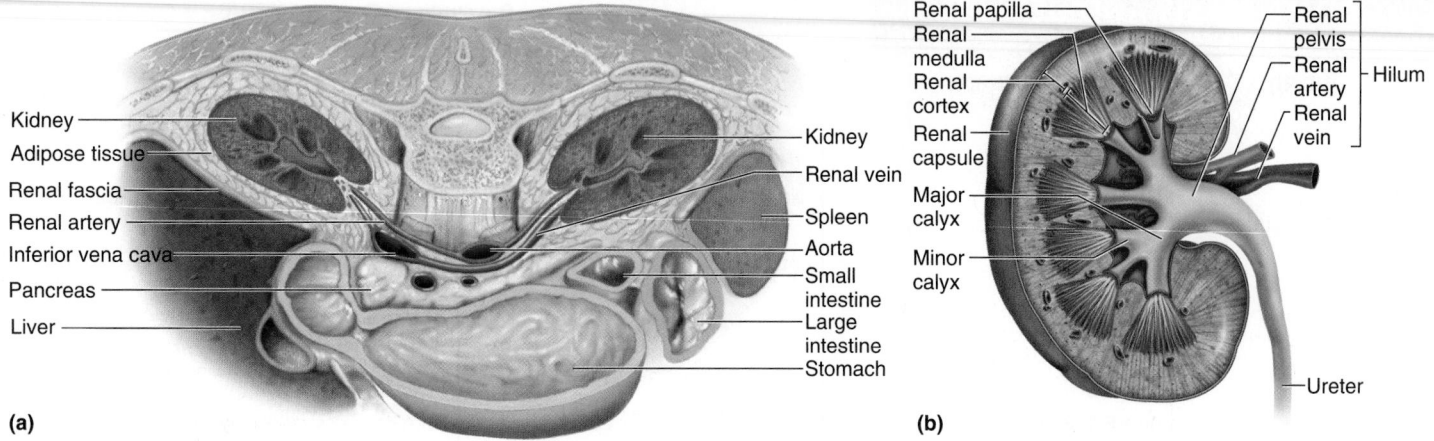

(a)

(b)

▲**FIGURE 11.2** **Kidney.** (*a*) Transverse section of abdomen showing position of kidneys. (*b*) Longitudinal section of a kidney.

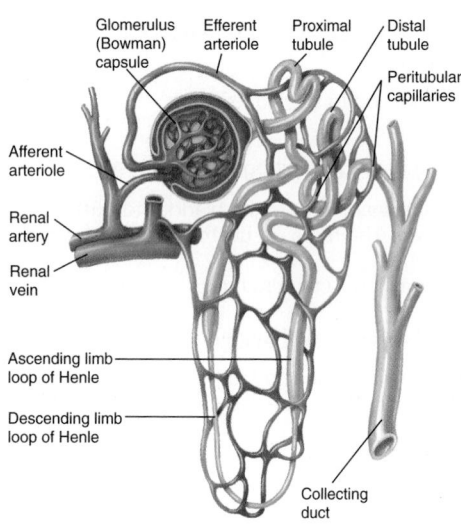

▲ **FIGURE 11.3** **Glomerulus and Renal Tubule.**

Keynote

Functions of the kidneys are to:

- **Filter** blood to eliminate wastes.
- **Regulate** blood volume and pressure by eliminating or conserving water as necessary.
- **Maintain homeostasis** by controlling the quantities of water and electrolytes that are eliminated.

ANATOMY AND PHYSIOLOGY OF THE KIDNEYS

Each kidney is a bean-shaped organ about the size of a clenched fist. It is located on either side of the vertebral column behind the peritoneum and lies against the deep muscles of the back. The left kidney is behind the spleen, and the right kidney behind and below the liver (*Figure 11.2a*).

Waste-laden blood enters the kidney at its **hilum** (*Figure 11.2b*) through the renal artery. Excess water, urea, and other waste products are **filtered** from the blood by the kidney, collected in the ureter, and carried off to the bladder. The filtered blood exits through the renal vein at the hilum.

Each kidney has three regions (*Figure 11.2b*):

- An outer renal **cortex**—contains the **nephrons,** the basic filtration unit.
- An inner renal **medulla**—contains the collecting ducts, which merge together to form about 30 papillary ducts, that enter into a **calyx.**
- A central renal **pelvis**—a funnel-shaped structure into which the calyces open that forms the ureter.

In the cortex, the renal artery divides into smaller and smaller arterioles, each of which enters a nephron and divides into a network of approximately 50 capillaries, known as a **glomerulus.** The glomerulus is encased in the **glomerular capsule (Bowman capsule).** Because the blood is under pressure and the capillaries and glomerular capsule are **permeable,** much of the fluid from the blood filters through the capillary wall and glomerular capsule into the renal tubule, which includes the **loop of Henle** (*Figure 11.3*).

This **filtrate** entering the renal tubule contains water, urea, glucose, electrolytes, amino acids, and vitamins. Red blood cells, platelets, and plasma proteins are too large to pass through the capillary membrane, and they remain in the blood.

Approximately 180 liters (45 gallons) of filtrate are formed each day. As the filtrate passes down the renal tubule, over 90% of the water is returned to the blood by **reabsorption.** Glucose and minerals are also returned to the blood. Some residual wastes in the blood are **secreted** from the blood into the tubule. These interchanges between the filtrate in the tubule and the blood are made possible by a mesh of capillaries that surrounds the renal tubule (*Figure 11.3*). The material that remains in the tubule is urine. It consists of excess water, electrolytes, and urea.

The renal tubules merge to form collecting ducts (*Figure 11.3*) that merge into the calyces and then form the **renal pelvis** and become the **ureter.**

Purified blood is returned from the **peritubular** mesh of capillaries to the circulatory system through the renal vein.

WORD	PRONUNCIATION		ELEMENTS	DEFINITION
calyx calyces (pl)	**KAY**-licks **KAY**-lih-sees		Greek *cup of a flower*	Funnel-shaped structure
cortex cortices (pl) cortical (adj)	**KOR**-teks **KOR**-tih-sees **KOR**-tih-kal	S/ R/	-ical *pertaining to* cort- *cortex*	Outer portion of an organ
filtrate	**FIL**-trate	S/ R/	-ate *composed of, pertaining to* filtr- *strain through*	That which has passed through a filter
filter	**FIL**-ter		Latin *to filter through felt*	A porous substance through which a liquid or gas is passed to separate out contained particles; or to use a filter
filtration	fil-**TRAY**-shun	S/	-ation *process*	Process of passing liquid through a filter
glomerulus glomeruli (pl) glomerular (adj)	glo-**MER**-you-lus glo-**MER**-you-lee glo-**MER**-you-lar		Latin *small ball of yarn*	Plexus of capillaries; part of a nephron
hilum hila (pl)	**HIGH**-lum **HIGH**-lah		Latin *small bit*	The part where the nerves and blood vessels enter and leave an organ
loop of Henle	LOOP of **HEN**-lee		Friedrich Henle, 1809–1885, German anatomist, pathologist, and histologist	Part of the renal tubule where reabsorption occurs
nephron	**NEF**-ron		Greek *kidney*	Filtration unit of the kidney; glomerulus + renal tubule
pelvis	**PEL**-vis		Latin *basin*	A cup-shaped cavity, as in the pelvis of the kidney
peritubular	**PER**-ih-too-**BYU**-lar	S/ P/ R/	-ar *pertaining to* peri- *around* -tubul- *small tube*	Surrounding the small renal tubules
permeable	**PER**-me-ah-bull	S/ R/CF	-able *capable of* perm/e- *pass through*	Allows passage of substances through a membrane
semipermeable impermeable	sem-ee-**PER**-me-ah-bull im-**PER**-me-ah-bull	P/ P/	semi- *half* im- *not, in*	Freely permeable to water but not to solutes Does not allow passage of anything
reabsorption (**Note:** This term has two prefixes.)	ree-ab-**SORP**-shun	S/ P/ P/ R/	-ion *process* re- *back* ab- *away from* -sorpt- *swallow*	The taking back into the blood of substances that had previously been filtered out from it
renin	**REE**-nin	S/ R/	-in *substance* ren- *kidney*	Enzyme secreted by the kidney that causes vasoconstriction

- **Secrete** the enzyme **renin.** If blood pressure falls in the kidney so that blood flow decreases, renin is produced and leads to widespread contraction of arterioles, which raises arterial pressure throughout the body.
- **Secrete** the hormone erythropoietin *(see page 273)*, which acts on the bone marrow to release red blood cells.
- **Synthesize vitamin D** to contribute to maintaining normal blood calcium levels.

Keynote

Kidneys remove waste products from the blood by a process of **filtration.**

The renal cortex contains about 1 million nephrons, the functional unit of the kidney.

A nephron is the combination of a glomerulus and the renal tubule.

EXERCISES   **Define and deconstruct** *the following medical terms into their basic elements. Write the name of the element on the line below the slash. Fill in the blanks.*

1. Passage of a substance through a membrane   _____ / _____ / _____

2. Enzyme that causes vasconstriction   _____ / _____ / _____

3. Surrounding the small renal tubules   _____ / _____ / _____

4. Blood reclaims previously filtered substances   _____ / _____ / _____

Abbreviations

EMT-P	emergency medical technician–paramedic
ESWL	extracorporeal shock wave lithotripsy
IV	intravenous
IVP	intravenous pyelogram
KUB	x-ray of abdomen to show **k**idneys, **u**reters, and **b**ladder
VS	vital signs

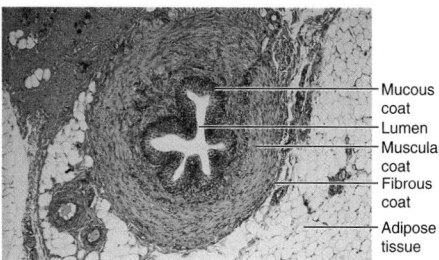

	Mucous coat
	Lumen
	Muscular coat
	Fibrous coat
	Adipose tissue

75×

▲ **FIGURE 11.4** **Cross-Section of a Ureter.**

Keynote

The muscle wall of the bladder acts as a sphincter around the ureters to prevent reflux of urine.

The presence of urine in the renal pelvis initiates peristalsis of the ureters.

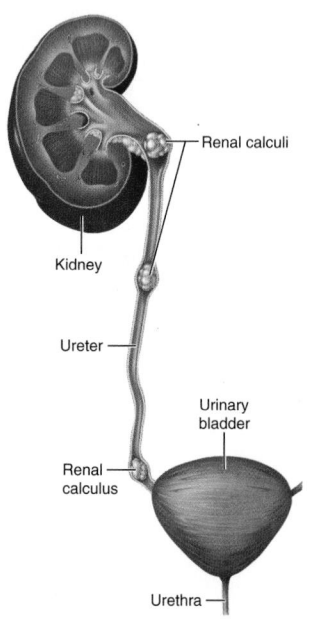

- Renal calculi
- Kidney
- Ureter
- Urinary bladder
- Renal calculus
- Urethra

▲ **FIGURE 11.5** **Renal Calculi.** Calculi can become lodged at different sites in the ureters.

CASE REPORT 11.2

Emergency Department, Fulwood Medical Center. 9/12/10

Justin Leandro, a 37-year-old construction worker, presented at 1520 hrs. He complained of a sudden onset of excruciating pain in his right abdomen and back an hour previously while at work. The pain is spasmodic and radiates down into his groin. He has vomited once and keeps having the urge to urinate but cannot. He has no previous medical history of significance.

Vital signs **(VS):** T 99.4°F, P 92, R 20, BP 130/86. Abdomen slightly distended, with tenderness in the right upper and lower quadrants and flank. A dipstick test showed blood in his urine.

Provisional diagnosis: stone in right ureter. An **IV** was started, 2 mg morphine sulfate given by IV push at 1540. He is going to x-ray stat for **KUB** and **IVP**.

Andrea Facundo, **EMT-P**. 1555 hrs.

URETERS

Each ureter *(Figure 11.4)* is a muscular tube, about 10 inches long (25.5 cm) and ¼ inch (0.6 cm) wide, that carries urine from the renal pelvis to the urinary bladder. It lies on the posterior abdominal wall, which is why Mr. Leandro had pain in his back. It passes behind the bladder and enters it on its posterior inferior surface, which is why the pain radiated into his groin.

Each ureter passes obliquely through the muscle wall of the bladder. As pressure builds in a filling bladder, the muscle wall compresses the ureter and prevents urine from being forced back up the ureter to the kidneys (**reflux**).

In addition to gravity, muscular peristaltic waves, originating in the renal pelvis, squeeze urine down the ureter and squirt it into the bladder. The peristaltic waves are intermittent, which is why Mr. Leandro's pain was **spasmodic**.

Case Report 11.2 (continued)

Mr. Leandro's KUB (x-ray of kidney, ureter, and bladder) showed a suspicious lesion halfway down his right ureter. An intravenous **pyelogram** (IVP) confirmed that this was a stone (renal calculus) blocking the ureter and showed the pelvis of the right kidney to be slightly dilated.

Mr. Leandro's stone was large enough to be lodged in the ureter, blocking the flow of urine and, because of the back flow pressure, leading to **hydronephrosis** of his kidney. Mr. Leandro was kept in the hospital overnight with IV pain medication but did not pass the stone. **ESWL** was successful in crumbling the stone. He urinated through a strainer so that the stone fragments could be recovered and chemically analyzed.

Kidney and Ureteral Stones (Nephrolithiasis)

Stones (**calculi**) begin in the pelvis of the kidney as a tiny grain of undissolved material, usually a mineral called calcium oxalate *(Figure 11.5)*. When the urine flows out of the kidney, the grain of material is left behind. Over time, more material is deposited and a stone is formed. The presence of stones is called **nephrolithiasis**.

Most stones enter the ureter while they are still small enough to pass down the ureter into the bladder and out of the body in urine. The passage of urine can be described as **urination, micturition,** or **voiding**.

Treatment options for renal calculi are:

- **Watchful waiting.** With pain medication to relieve symptoms, the hope is that the stone can be passed.

- **Extracorporeal shock wave lithotripsy (ESWL).** A machine called a **lithotripter** produces shock waves that crumble the stone into small pieces that can pass down the ureter.

WORD	PRONUNCIATION		ELEMENTS	DEFINITION
calculus calculi (pl)	**KAL**-kyu-lus **KAL**-kyu-lie		Latin *pebble*	Small stone
extracorporeal	**EKS**-trah-kor-**POH**-ree-al	S/ P/ R/CF	-al *pertaining to* **extra-** *outside, out of* **-corpor/e-** *body*	Outside the body
hydronephrosis	**HIGH**-droh-neh-**FRO**-sis	S/ P/ R/CF	-osis *condition* **hydro-** *water* **-nephr/o-** *kidney*	Dilation of pelvis and calyces of a kidney
hydronephrotic (adj)	**HIGH**-droh-neh-**FROT**-ik	S/	-tic *pertaining to*	Pertaining to or suffering from the dilation of the pelvis and calyces of the kidney
lithotripsy	**LITH**-oh-trip-see	S/ R/CF	-tripsy *to crush* **lith/o-** *stone*	Crushing stones by sound waves
lithotripter	**LITH**-oh-trip-ter	S/	-tripter *crusher*	Instrument that generates sound waves
nephrolithiasis	**NEF**-roe-lih-**THIGH**-ah-sis	S/ R/CF R/	-iasis *condition* **nephr/o-** *kidney* **-lith-** *stone*	Presence of a kidney stone
nephrolithotomy	**NEF**-roe-lih-**THOT**-oh-me	S/ R/CF R/CF	-tomy *surgical incision* **nephr/o-** *kidney* **-lith/o-** *stone*	Incision for removal of a renal stone
nephroscope	**NEF**-roe-skope	S/ R/CF	-scope *instrument for viewing* **nephr/o-** *kidney*	Endoscope to view the inside of the kidney
nephroscopy	neh-**FROS**-koh-pee	S/	-scopy *to view, examine*	Examination of the kidney
pyelogram	**PIE**-el-oh gram	S/ R/CF	-gram *a record, recording* **pyel/o-** *renal pelvis*	X-ray image of renal pelvis and ureters
reflux	**REE**-fluks	P/ R/	**re-** *back* **-flux** *flow*	Backward flow
spasmodic (**Note:** One "m" is taken out.)	spaz-**MOD**-ik	S/ R/ R/	-ic *pertaining to* **spasm-** *spasm* **-mod-** *nature, form*	Having intermittent spasms or contractions
ureteroscope	you-**REE**-ter-oh-scope	S/ R/CF	-scope *instrument for viewing* **ureter/o-** *ureter*	Endoscope to view the inside of the ureter
ureteroscopy	you-**REE**-ter-os-koh-pee	S/	-scopy *to view, examine*	Examination of the ureter

- **Ureteroscopy.** A small, flexible **ureteroscope** is passed through the urethra and bladder into the ureter. Devices can be passed through the endoscope to remove or fragment the stone.
- **Percutaneous nephrolithotomy.** A **nephroscope** is inserted through the skin and into the kidney to locate and remove the stone.
- **Open surgery.** A surgical incision is made to expose the ureter and remove the stone; this is rarely done.

EXERCISES

After reading both parts of Case Report 11.2 on the opposite page, answer the following questions. Be prepared to discuss your answers in class

Study Hint
Review the WAD again. Find the suffixes, _____ and _____, which both mean *pertaining to*. Add these to your list.

1. If Mr. Leandro's pain had a "sudden onset," is it acute or chronic? _____

2. What were Mr. Leandro's presenting symptoms?

    _____

    _____

3. What was the IV for? _____

4. What diagnostic tests did Mr. Leandro have? _____

5. What element in *hydronephrosis* indicates fluid is involved? _____

6. Is ESWL an invasive procedure? _____

Case Report 11.1 *(continued)*

Mr. Nelson Hughes had been well until a few months before his surgery when he noticed a vague, aching pain in his left loin. One week prior to surgery, he suddenly passed bright red urine. Urinalysis showed red blood cells (**hematuria**). Physical examination revealed an enlarged left kidney. Intravenous pyelogram (**IVP**) and other imaging tests showed a tumor 3 inches in diameter in the center of the left kidney. Bone scan was normal, indicating no metastases to bone.

Keynote

Of all renal cancers, 25% to 30% relate directly to smoking.

As little as 1 milliliter of blood will turn the urine red.

Keynote

Hematuria can be caused by a lesion anywhere in the urinary system.

Keynote

The acute form of glomerulonephritis has 100% recovery.

Acute interstitial nephritis causes 15% of cases of acute renal failure.

DISORDERS OF THE KIDNEYS

Renal cell carcinoma is the most common form of kidney cancer and occurs twice as often in men as in women. The cancer develops in the lining cells of the renal tubules, which is why Mr. Hughes had hematuria. Radical **nephrectomy** is the most common treatment for renal cell carcinoma.

Wilms tumor, or **nephroblastoma,** is a malignant kidney tumor of childhood, usually appearing between ages 3 and 8 years, that is treated effectively with a combination of surgery and chemotherapy.

Benign kidney tumors, such as **renal adenoma,** are usually asymptomatic, are discovered incidentally, and are not life-threatening.

Hematuria, blood in the urine, can be caused by lesions anywhere in the urinary system; this includes trauma (including long-distance running), infections, medications (such as quinine and phenytoin), and congenital diseases (such as sickle cell anemia). In **microscopic hematuria,** the urine is not red, and red blood cells can be seen only under a microscope or identified by a urine dipstick. Normal urine contains no blood. Excessive consumption of beets, rhubarb, and red food coloring can cause urine to be colored red. This is not hematuria. Also, in the collection of urine from a woman during menstruation, the urine can be contaminated with blood, giving the impression of hematuria.

Acute glomerulonephritis is an inflammation of the glomerulus. It damages the glomerular capillaries, allows protein and red blood cells to leak into the urine, and interferes with the clearance of waste products. In its acute form, it can develop rapidly after an episode of strep throat infection, most often in children. The *Streptococcus* bacteria do not invade the kidney but stimulate the immune system to overproduce antibodies that damage the glomeruli.

Chronic glomerulonephritis can occur with no history of kidney disease and present as kidney failure. It also occurs in **diabetic nephropathy** and can be associated with autoimmune diseases such as lupus erythematosus; HIV can cause glomerular disease even before developing into AIDS.

Nephrotic syndrome involves large amounts of protein leaking out into the urine, so the level of protein in the blood falls. In children it nearly always responds to treatment with steroids. The causes of nephrotic syndrome are described in *Table 11.1.* The most obvious symptom is fluid retention with edema of the ankles and legs. This is treated with **diuretics,** restriction of salt in the diet, and reduction of fluid intake.

Interstitial nephritis is an inflammation of the spaces between the renal tubules. Most often it is acute and temporary. It can be an allergic reaction to or a side effect of drugs such as penicillin or ampicillin, NSAIDs, and diuretics. Treatment is directed to the underlying disease. Temporary **dialysis** may be necessary.

Pyelonephritis is an infection of the renal pelvis. Most often it occurs as part of a total **urinary tract infection (UTI),** commencing in the urinary bladder. It has a high mortality rate in the elderly and in people with a compromised immune system *(see Chapter 15).* It requires aggressive antibiotic therapy.

WORD	PRONUNCIATION	ELEMENTS		DEFINITION
dialysis	die-**AL**-ih-sis	S/ P/	-lysis *to separate* dia- *complete*	An artificial method of filtration to remove excess waste materials and water from the body
diuretic (adj)	die-you-**RET**-ik	S/ P/ R/	-etic *pertaining to* di- *complete (from dia)* -ur- *urinary system*	Agent that increases urine output
diuresis (noun)	die-you-**REE**-sis	S/	-esis *abnormal condition*	Excretion of large volumes of urine
glomerulonephritis	glo-**MER**-you-low-nef-**RYE**-tis	S/ R/CF R/	-itis *inflammation* glomerul/o- *glomerulus* -nephr- *kidney*	Infection of the glomeruli of the kidney
hematuria	he-mah-**TYU**-ree-ah	S/ R/	-uria *urine* hemat- *blood*	Blood in the urine
interstitial	in-ter-**STISH**-al	S/ P/ R/	-ial *pertaining to* inter- *between* -stit- *space*	Pertaining to the spaces between cells in a tissue or organ
nephritis	neh-**FRY**-tis	S/ R/	-itis *inflammation* nephr- *kidney*	Inflammation of the kidney
nephropathy	neh-**FROP**-ah-thee	S/ R/CF	-pathy *disease* nephr/o- *kidney*	Any disease of the kidney
nephrotic syndrome	neh-**FROT**-ik **SIN**-drome	S/ R/CF	-tic *pertaining to* nephr/o- *kidney*	Glomerular disease with marked loss of protein
nephrosis (syn)	neh-**FRO**-sis	S/	-osis *condition*	
pyelonephritis	**PIE**-eh-loh-neh-**FRY**-tis	S/ R/CF R/	-itis *inflammation* pyel/o- *renal pelvis* -nephr- *kidney*	Inflammation of the kidney and renal pelvis
Wilms tumor	WILMZ **TOO**-mor		Max Wilms, 1867–1918, German surgeon	Cancerous kidney tumor of childhood
nephroblastoma (syn)	**NEF**-roh-blas-**TOE**-mah	S/ R/CF R/	-oma *tumor, mass* nephr/o- *kidney* -blast- *embryonic, immature cell*	

TABLE 11.1 Types of Nephrotic Syndrome

Disease (as Seen on Biopsy)	Description
Minimal change disease	Most common in children; responds to steroids
Focal segmental glomerulosclerosis (FSGS)	Cause unknown; little response to treatment
Membranous nephropathy	Cause unknown; may respond to immunosuppressive treatment
Diabetic	Occurs if blood sugar has been poorly controlled

EXERCISES

After reading Case Report 11.1 on the opposite page, answer the following questions. Be prepared to discuss your answers in class.

1. Define the term *loin*. Use a dictionary if you are not sure of the meaning.

_____

2. "Bright red urine" would indicate the presence of _____ in the urine.

3. What were Mr. Hughes' symptoms?

_____

4. What diagnostic tests has Mr. Hughes had so far?

_____

5. What is the good news for Mr. Hughes?

_____

Hypertension, with its high blood pressure, can damage the renal arterioles and glomeruli, causing them to thicken and narrow. This reduces their capability to remove wastes and excess water, which can cause the blood pressure to rise even more. If the cause of hypertension is not known, it is called **primary (or essential) hypertension** *(see Chapter 8).*

Polycystic kidney disease (PKD) is an inherited disease. Large, fluid-filled cysts grow within the kidneys and press against the kidney tissue. Finally, the kidneys cannot function effectively.

Acute renal failure (ARF) makes the kidneys suddenly stop filtering waste products from the blood. The signs and symptoms can include **oliguria** (reduction of urine output), **anuria** (cessation of urine output), confusion, seizures, coma.

The causes of acute renal failure include:

- **Severe burns, trauma,** or **complicated surgery**—with a drastic drop in blood pressure and the release of myoglobin from injured muscles *(see Chapter 5).* Myoglobin lodges in the renal tubules and blocks the flow of urine.

- **Drugs**—including pain medications such as aspirin and ibuprofen, antibiotics such as streptomycin and gentamicin, and contrast dyes used in angiography.

- **Toxins**—such as heavy metals (mercury is one) and excessive alcohol.

- **Systemic infections**—septicemia.

- **Blood disorders**—such as idiopathic thrombocytopenic purpura (ITP) or disseminated intravascular coagulation (DIC) *(see Chapter 7).*

In treatment of ARF, the goal is to treat the underlying disease. Dialysis may be necessary while the kidneys are healing.

Chronic renal failure (CRF), or **chronic kidney disease (CKD),** is a gradual loss of renal function. Symptoms and signs may not appear until kidney function is less than 25% of normal.

The causes of chronic renal failure include:

- **Diabetes**—type 1 and type 2 *(see Chapter 14)*—**hypertension, kidney diseases, lead poisoning.**

Azotemia is the buildup of nitrogenous waste products in the blood. **Uremia** is the complex of symptoms resulting from excess nitrogenous waste products in the blood, as seen in renal failure.

End-stage renal disease (ESRD) means the kidneys are functioning at less than 10% of their normal capacity. At this point, life cannot be sustained, and either dialysis or kidney **transplant** is needed.

Dialysis is an artificial method of removing waste materials and excess fluid from the blood. It is not a cure but can prolong life. There are several types of kidney dialysis:

- **Hemodialysis** *(Figure 11.6)* filters the blood through an artificial kidney machine (**dialyzer**). Most patients require 12 hours of hemodialysis a week, usually in three sessions.

- **Peritoneal dialysis** uses a dialysis solution that is infused into and drained out of your abdominal cavity through a small, flexible, **implanted** catheter. The dialysis solution extracts wastes and excess fluid from the network of capillaries in the peritoneal lining of the abdominal cavity.

- **Continuous ambulatory peritoneal dialysis (CAPD)** is performed by the patient at home through an implanted abdominal catheter *(Figure 11.7),* usually four times a day, 7 days a week.

- **Continuous cycling peritoneal dialysis** uses a machine to automatically infuse dialysis solution into and out of the abdominal cavity during sleep.

Keynote

Acute renal failure is usually reversible. Chronic renal failure has no cure.

Abbreviations

ARF   acute renal failure
CAPD continuous ambulatory peritoneal dialysis
CKD   chronic kidney disease; also known as chronic renal failure
CRF   chronic renal failure; also known as chronic kidney disease
ESRD end-stage renal disease
PKD   polycystic kidney disease

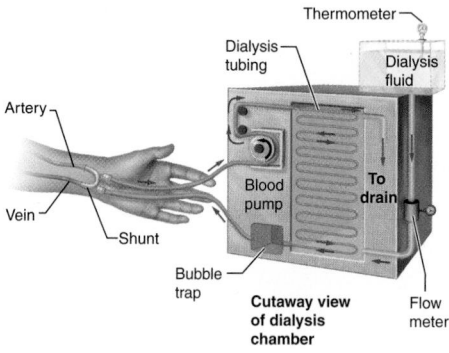

▲ **FIGURE 11.6   Hemodialysis.**

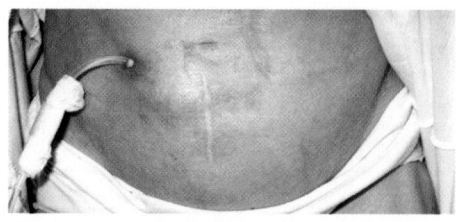

▲ **FIGURE 11.7   Continuous Ambulatory Peritoneal Dialysis.**

WORD	PRONUNCIATION	ELEMENTS		DEFINITION
anuria	an-**YOU**-ree-ah	P/ R/	**an-** *lack of, without* **-uria** *urine*	Absence of urine production
azotemia	azo-**TEE**-me-ah	S/ R/	**-emia** *blood condition* **azot-** *nitrogen*	Excess nitrogenous waste products in the blood
hemodialysis	**HE**-moh-die-**AL**-ih-sis	P/ R/CF R/	**-dia-** *complete* **hem/o-** *blood* **-lysis** *to separate*	An artificial method of filtration to remove excess waste materials and water directly from the blood
implant	im-**PLANT**	P/ R/	**im-** *in* **-plant** *insert or plant*	To insert material into tissues, or the material inserted into tissues
oliguria	ol-ih-**GYUR**-ee-ah	P/ R/	**olig-** *scanty* **-uria** *urine*	Scanty production of urine
polycystic	pol-ee-**SIS**-tik	S/ P/ R/	**-ic** *pertaining to* **poly-** *many* **-cyst-** *bladder, cyst*	Composed of many cysts
sibling	**SIB**-ling	S/ R/	**-ling** *small* **sib-** *relative*	Brother or sister
transplant	**TRANZ**-plant	P/ R/	**trans-** *across* **-plant** *insert, plant*	The act of transferring tissue from one person to another
uremia	you-**REE**-me-ah	S/ R/	**-emia** *blood condition* **ur-** *urinary system*	The complex of symptoms arising from renal failure

Kidney transplant provides a better quality of life than dialysis—if a suitable donor can be found. The donor has to match the recipient's blood type, cell surface proteins, and antibodies *(see Chapter 15)*. A **sibling** or a blood relative can often qualify as a donor. If not, tissue banks across the country can search for a kidney from an accident victim or a donor who has died.

EXERCISES

Build your knowledge of the elements contained in the **language of urology**. *Specific elements in each term are set in bold. Identify the type of element, and provide a meaning for the element. Fill in the blanks.*

Term	Type of Element (P, R, CF, S)	Meaning of Element	Meaning of Term
anuria	_____	_____	_____
hemodialysis	_____	_____	_____
azotemia	_____	_____	_____
transplant	_____	_____	_____
oliguria	_____	_____	_____
polycystic	_____	_____	_____
uremia	_____	_____	_____

Remember: Every element at the beginning of a medical term is not necessarily a prefix!

Give an example from this exercise: _____

LESSON 11.2 Urinary Bladder and Urethra

OBJECTIVES

The urinary bladder is a temporary storage place for urine before it is **voided** through the urethra. A moderately full bladder contains about 500 mL (1 pint). The maximum capacity of the bladder is around 750 to 800 mL (1.5 pints). **Urination,** emptying of the bladder, is also called **micturition.** While the urinary bladders in the male and female have the same structure and function, the male and female urethras have very different structures.

The information in this lesson will enable you to use correct medical terminology to:

11.2.1 Describe the structure and functions of the urinary bladder.

11.2.2 Contrast the differences in structure of the male and female urethras.

11.2.3 Explain the greater incidence of urinary tract infections in the female.

11.2.4 Discuss common disorders of the bladder and urethra.

You are

. . . a medical assistant working in the office of Dr. Susan Lee, a primary care physician at Fulwood Medical Center.

Your patient is

. . . Mrs. Caroline Dobson, a 32-year-old housewife. You have asked her to describe the reason for her visit to the office today.

CASE REPORT 11.3

Patient Interview:

Mrs. Dobson:

"Since yesterday afternoon I've had a lot of pain low down in my belly and in my lower back. I keep having to go to the bathroom every hour or so to pee. It's often difficult to start, and it burns as it comes out. I've had this problem twice before when I was pregnant with my two kids, so I've started drinking cranberry juice. I've been shivering since I woke up this morning, and the last urine I passed was pink. Was that due to the cranberry juice?"

At the end of this chapter you will be asked to document (using medical terminology) Mrs. Dobson's **history of her present illness (HPI)** and to detail any further questions you have for her.

Abbreviation

HPI history of present illness

URINARY BLADDER AND URETHRA

The **urinary bladder** is a hollow, muscular organ on the floor of the pelvic cavity, posterior to the pubic symphysis *(Figure 11.8)*. When the bladder is distended, it rises upward *(Figure 11.9)* and can be palpated above the symphysis pubis.

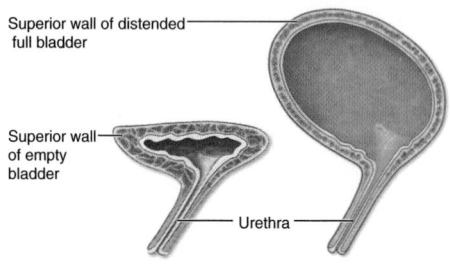

Superior wall of distended full bladder
Superior wall of empty bladder
Urethra

▲ **FIGURE 11.9** **Empty and Distended Bladder.**

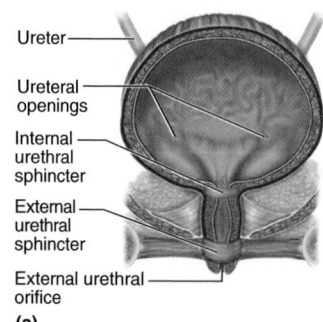

Ureter
Ureteral openings
Internal urethral sphincter
External urethral sphincter
External urethral orifice
(a)

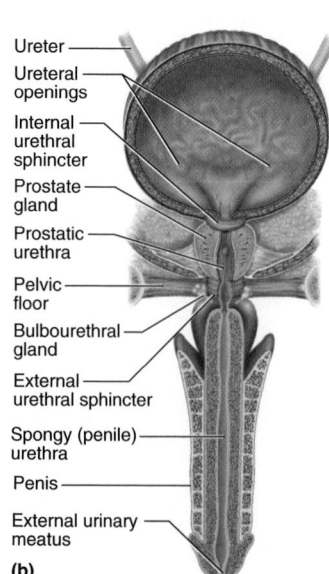

Ureter
Ureteral openings
Internal urethral sphincter
Prostate gland
Prostatic urethra
Pelvic floor
Bulbourethral gland
External urethral sphincter
Spongy (penile) urethra
Penis
External urinary meatus
(b)

▲ **FIGURE 11.8** **Urinary Bladder and Urethra.** (*a*) Female anatomy. (*b*) Male anatomy.

WORD	PRONUNCIATION	ELEMENTS		DEFINITION
enuresis	en-you-**REE**-sis	S/ R/	-esis *abnormal condition* enur- *urinate*	Bed-wetting; urinary incontinence
meatus	me-**AY**-tus		Latin *a passage*	The external opening of a passage
micturition	mik-choo-**RISH**-un	S/ R/	-ition *process* mictur- *pass urine*	Act of passing urine
micturate	**MIK**-choo-rate	S/	-ate *composed of, pertaining to*	Pass urine
reflex	**REE**-fleks		Latin *to bend back*	An involuntary response to a stimulus
sphincter	**SFINK**-ter		Greek *band*	Band of muscle that encircles an opening; when it contracts, the opening squeezes closed
urination	yur-ih-**NAY**-shun	S/ R/	-ation *process* urin- *urine*	The act of passing urine
void	VOYD		Latin *to empty*	To evacuate urine or feces

Urethra

The final passageway for the urine to escape to the outside is the urethra, a thin-walled tube that takes urine from the floor of the bladder to the outside. At the base of the bladder, the muscular wall is thickened to form the **internal urethral sphincter.** As the urethra passes through the skeletal muscles of the pelvic floor, the **external urethral sphincter** provides voluntary control of micturition.

In the female *(see Figure 11.8a)*, the urethra is only about 1.5 inches long, and it opens to the outside anterior to the vagina.

In the male *(Figure 11.8b)*, the urethra is 7 to 8 inches in length and passes through the penis.

In both the male and the female, the opening of the urethra to the outside is called the **external urinary meatus.**

Micturition

When the bladder contains about 200 mL of urine, stretch receptors in its wall trigger the **micturition reflex.** However, voluntary control of the external sphincter can keep that sphincter contracted and can hold urine in the bladder until you decide to urinate. Involuntary micturition during sleep in older children or adults is called **enuresis.**

EXERCISES

After reading Case Report 11.2 on the opposite page, answer the following questions. Be prepared to discuss your answers in class.

1. List all of Mrs. Dobson's "presenting" symptoms. (What symptoms does she have when she comes to the doctor?)

_____

_____

2. Has she ever had this condition before? If so, when? _____

3. Insert medical terms for the following phrases from the Case Report:

"in my **belly**"_____

"every hour or so to **pee**" _____

"I've been **shivering**" _____

4. If the last urine Mrs. Dobson passed was pink, what might be present in her urine now? _____

5. Right now, is this an acute or chronic condition for Mrs. Dobson?

_____

DISORDERS OF THE URINARY BLADDER AND URETHRA

Urinary Tract Infection

A **urinary tract infection (UTI)** occurs when bacteria invade and multiply in the urinary tract. The **portal** of entry for the bacteria is through the urethra. Because the female urethra is shorter than the male urethra and opens to the surface near the anus *(Figure 11.10)*, bacteria from the **gastrointestinal (GI)** tract, such as *Escherichia coli (E. coli)* can more easily invade the female urethra. This is why women are more prone than men to UTIs. Once UTIs have occurred, they often recur.

Infection of the urethra is called urethritis; infection of the urinary bladder is cystitis. If **cystitis** is untreated, infection can spread up the ureters to the renal pelvis, causing **pyelitis,** and carry on to reach the renal cortex and nephrons, causing **pyelonephritis.**

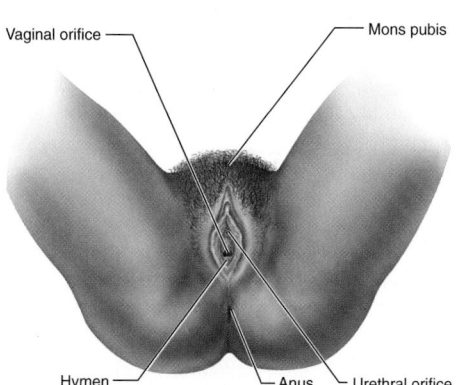

Vaginal orifice — Mons pubis

Hymen — Anus — Urethral orifice

▲ **FIGURE 11.10   Female External Genitalia.**

Case Report 11.3 (continued)

Mrs. Dobson described many of the symptoms of cystitis. She had **suprapubic** and low-back pain. She had increased **frequency** of micturition with **dysuria** and had difficulty in and burning on micturition. Her pink urine is probably hematuria.

The diagnosis can be made through urinalysis. Culture of the organism and testing of its sensitivity to different antibiotics enables appropriate antibiotic therapy to be prescribed. Cranberry juice makes the urine more acid.

Urinary Incontinence

Loss of control of your bladder is called **urinary incontinence.** The result is wet clothes. About 12 million adults in America have urinary incontinence. It is most common in women over the age of 50 years.

There are four types of urinary incontinence:

- **Stress incontinence.** Urine leaks because of sudden pressure on the lower stomach muscles when you cough, laugh, sneeze, lift something heavy, or exercise. It is most common in women, with previous pregnancy and childbirth being risk factors.

- **Urge incontinence.** The need to urinate comes on too fast for you to get to the toilet. It is often **idiopathic,** but can be associated with UTI, diabetes, stroke, Alzheimer and Parkinson disease, or bladder cancer.

- **Overflow incontinence.** Small amounts of urine leak from a bladder that is always full because you cannot empty it. This occurs when an enlarged prostate gland or tumor blocks the outflow of urine from the bladder and also occurs in spinal cord injuries and as a side effect of some medications.

- **Functional incontinence.** You have normal bladder control but cannot get to the toilet in time because of arthritis or any other disease that makes moving around difficult.

Treatment depends on the cause. If a medical or surgical problem is present, then the incontinence can go away when the problem is treated. **Bladder training** and **biofeedback** *(see Chapter 23)* lengthen the time between the urges to go to the toilet. **Kegel exercises** strengthen the muscles of the pelvic floor. Medications, for example, oxybutynin, are used for urge incontinence. Surgery can pull up the bladder and secure it if pelvic floor muscles are weak **(cystopexy).** Absorbent underclothing is available.

Urinary retention is the abnormal, involuntary holding of urine in the bladder. **Acute retention** can be caused by an obstruction in the urinary system; for example, an enlarged prostate in the male *(see Chapter 12)* or neurologic problems such as multiple sclerosis. It can be a side effect of anticholinergic drugs that include tricyclic antidepressants *(see Chapter 19).* **Chronic retention** can be caused by untreated obstructions in the urinary tract such as an enlarged prostate.

Keynote

Ten million doctor visits each year are for UTIs.

Aging itself is not a cause of urinary incontinence.

Incontinence is not a way of life. It can be helped.

Cigarette smoking contributes to more than 50% of bladder cancers.

Abbreviations

GI	gastrointestinal
E. coli	*Escherichia coli*
UTI	urinary tract infection

Keynote

Bladder cancer is more common in men than women. It is the fourth most common cancer in men and the eighth in women *(see Chapter 24).*

WORD	PRONUNCIATION	ELEMENTS		DEFINITION
cystitis	sis-**TIE**-tis	S/ R/	**-itis** *inflammation* **cyst-** *bladder*	Inflammation of the urinary bladder
cystopexy	**SIS**-toh-pek-see	S/ R/CF	**-pexy** *surgical fixation* **cyst/o-** *bladder*	Surgical procedure to support the urinary bladder
cystoscope	**SIS**-toh-skope	S/ R/CF	**-scope** *instrument for viewing* **cyst/o-** *bladder*	An endoscope inserted to view the inside of the bladder
cystoscopy	sis-**TOS**-koh-pee		**-scopy** *to examine*	The process of using a cystoscope
dysuria	dis-**YOU**-ree-ah	S/ P/ R/	**-ia** *condition* **dys-** *bad, difficult* **-ur-** *urinary system*	Difficulty or pain with urination
frequency	**FREE**-kwen-see	S/ R/	**-ency** *state of, quality of* **frequ-** *repeated, often*	The number of times something happens in a given time (e.g., passing urine)
idiopathic	**ID**-ih-oh-**PATH**-ik	S/ R/CF R/	**-ic** *pertaining to* **idi/o-** *personal, distinct* **-path-** *disease*	Pertaining to a disease of unknown etiology
incontinence	in-**KON**-tin-ence	S/ P/ R/	**-ence** *state of, quality of* **in-** *in* **-contin-** *hold together*	Inability to prevent discharge of urine or feces
incontinent	in-**KON**-tin-ent	S/	**-ent** *pertaining to, end result*	Denoting incontinence
Kegel exercises	**KEG**-al **EKS**-er-size-ez		Arnold Kegel, 1894–1981, American gynecologist	Contraction and relaxation of the pelvic floor muscles to improve urethral and rectal sphincter function
portal	**POR**-tal		Latin *gate*	The vein that brings blood from the intestines to the liver
pyelitis	pie-eh-**LYE**-tis	S/ R/	**-itis** *inflammation* **pyel-** *renal pelvis*	Inflammation of renal pelvis
retention	ree-**TEN**-shun		Latin *hold back*	A holding in of what should normally be discharged (e.g., urine)
suprapubic	**SOO**-prah-pyu-bik	S/ P/ R/	**-ic** *pertaining to* **supra-** *above* **-pub-** *pubis*	Above the symphysis pubis

Transitional cell carcinoma is the most common type of bladder cancer, arising in the transitional cells of the lining of the bladder. Its primary symptom is hematuria. It is diagnosed by:

- **Urinalysis** to detect microscopic hematuria.
- **NMP22®BladderChek®,** which detects elevated levels of a specific protein in the urine even in the early stages.
- **Imaging tests,** such as IVP, CT scan, MRI scan, and ultrasound.
- **Cystoscopy with biopsy,** which is the definitive test.

The cancer is **staged** using the **TNM system (tumor, node, metastasis)** *(see Chapter 22).*

EXERCISES   *After reading Case Report 11.3 on the opposite page, answer the following questions. Be prepared to discuss your answers in class.*

1. What organ in Mrs. Dobson's urinary system has become infected?

_____

2. What is the difference between a UTI and a URI?

UTI: _____   Body system: _____

URI: _____   Body system: _____

3. *Micturition* can also be termed _____ and _____.

4. Name two terms ending in *uria* that are Mrs. Dobson's symptoms.   _____/uria   and   _____/uria

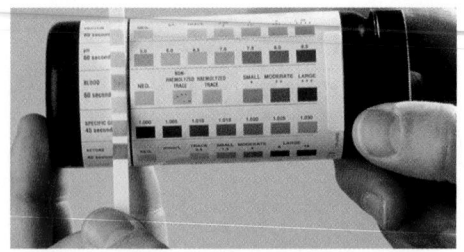

▲ **FIGURE 11.11 Urinalysis Dipstick Being Compared Against Color Chart on Container.**

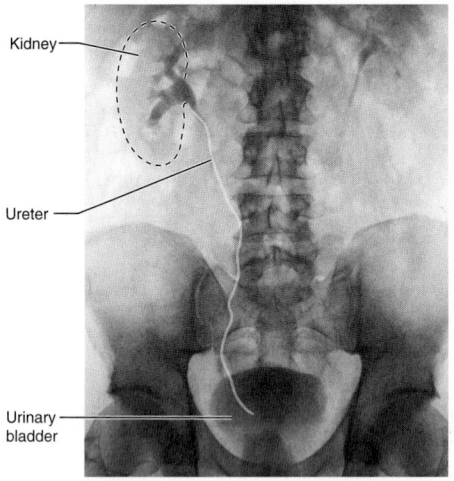

▲ **FIGURE 11.12 Intravenous Pyelogram (IVP).**

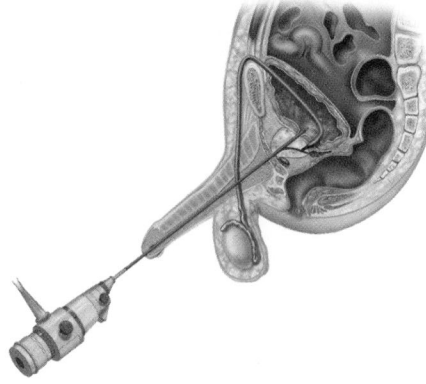

▲ **FIGURE 11.13 Cystoscopy.**

Abbreviations

RBC	red blood cell
SG	specific gravity
UA	urinalysis
VCUG	voiding cystourethrogram
WBC	white blood cell

DIAGNOSTIC PROCEDURES

Urinalysis

Dipstick (a plastic strip bearing paper squares of reagent) is the most cost-effective method of screening urine *(Figure 11.11).* After the stick is dipped in the urine specimen, the color change in each segment of the dipstick is compared to a color chart on the container. Dipsticks can screen for pH, specific gravity, protein, blood, glucose, ketones, bilirubin, **nitrite,** and leukocyte esterase (see below).

Routine urinalysis (UA) in the laboratory can include the following tests:

- **Visual observation** examines **color** and **clarity.** Normal urine is pale yellow or amber in color and clear. Cloudiness indicates excess cells or cellular material. Red and cloudy indicates red blood cells.
- **Odor** of normal urine has a slight "nutty" scent. Infected urine has a foul odor. **Ketosis** gives urine a fruity odor.
- **pH** measures how acidic or alkaline urine is *(see Chapter 2).*
- **Specific gravity (SG)** measures how dilute or concentrated the urine is.
- **Protein** is not detected normally in urine. Its presence **(proteinuria)** indicates infection or urinary tract disease.
- **Glucose** in the urine **(glycosuria)** is a spill over into the urine when the nephrons are damaged or diseased or blood sugar is high in uncontrolled diabetes.
- **Ketones** are present in the urine in **diabetic ketoacidosis** *(see Chapter 14)* or in starvation *(see Chapter 22).*
- **Leukocyte esterase** indicates the presence of white blood cells in the urine, which in turn can indicate a UTI.
- **Urine culture** from a clean-catch specimen *(see box)* is the definitive test for a UTI.

Microscopic urinalysis is performed on the solids deposited by centrifuging a specimen of urine. It can reveal:

- **Red blood cells (RBCs), white blood cells (WBCs),** and renal tubular epithelial cells stuck together to form **casts,** WBCs stuck together to form casts, and bacteria.

Other Diagnostic Procedures

- **KUB.** An x-ray of the abdomen shows the kidneys, ureters, and bladder.
- **Intravenous pyelogram (IVP).** A contrast material containing iodine is injected intravenously, and its progress through the urinary tract is then recorded on a series of rapid x-ray images *(Figure 11.12).*
- **Retrograde pyelogram.** Contrast material is injected through a urinary catheter into the ureters to locate stones and other obstructions.
- **Voiding cystourethrogram (VCUG).** Contrast material is inserted into the bladder through a catheter and x-rays are taken as the patient voids.
- **CT scan.** X-ray images show cross-sectional views of the kidneys and bladder.
- **MRI.** Magnetic fields are used to generate cross-sectional images of the urinary tract.
- **Ultrasound imaging.** High-frequency sound waves and a computer generate noninvasive images of kidneys.
- **Renal angiogram.** X-rays with contrast material are used to assess blood flow to the kidneys.
- **Cystoscopy.** A pencil-thin, flexible, tubelike optical instrument is inserted through the urethra into the bladder to examine directly the lining of the bladder and to take a biopsy if needed *(Figure 11.13).*

WORD	PRONUNCIATION	ELEMENTS		DEFINITION
cast	KAST		Latin *pure*	A cylindrical mold formed by materials in kidney tubules
cystourethrogram	sis-toh-you-**REETH**-roe-gram	S/ R/CF R/CF	**-gram** *a record* **cyst/o-** *bladder* **-urethr/o-** *urethra*	X-ray image during voiding to show structure and function of bladder and urethra
glycosuria (*Note:* The "s" is added to make the word flow.)	**GLYE**-koh-**SYU**-ree-ah	S/ R/CF R/	**-ia** *condition* **glyc/o-** *glucose* **-ur-** *urinary system*	Presence of glucose in urine
ketone	**KEY**-tone		Greek *acetone*	Chemical formed in uncontrolled diabetes or in starvation
ketosis	key-**TOE**-sis	S/ R/CF R/CF	**-sis** *condition* **ket/o-** *ketones* **-acid/o-** *acid, low pH*	Excess production of ketones
ketoacidosis	**KEY**-toe-as-ih-**DOE**-sis			Excessive production of ketones, making the blood acid
nitrite	**NI**-trite		Greek *niter, saltpeter*	Chemical formed in urine by *E. coli* and other microorganisms
proteinuria	pro-tee-**NYU**-ree-ah	R/ R/	**-uria** *urine* **protein-** *protein*	Presence of protein in urine
retrograde	**RET**-roh-grade	P/ R/	**retro-** *backward* **-grade** *going*	Reversal of a normal flow; for example, back from the bladder into the ureters
urinalysis	you-rih-**NAL**-ih-sis	S/ R/CF	**-lysis** *to separate* **urin/a-** *urine*	Examination of urine to separate it into its elements and define their kind and/or quantity

Methods of Urine Collection

- **Random collection** is taken with no precautions regarding contamination. It is often used for collecting samples for drug testing.

- **Early morning collection** is used to determine the ability of the kidneys to concentrate urine following overnight dehydration.

- **Clean-catch, midstream specimen** is collected after the external urethral meatus is cleaned. The first part of the urine is passed, and the sterile collecting vessel is introduced into the urinary stream to collect the last part.

- **Twenty-four-hour collection** is used to determine the amount of protein being excreted and to estimate the kidneys' filtration ability.

- **Suprapubic transabdominal needle aspiration** of the bladder is used in newborns and small infants to obtain a pure sample of urine.

- **Catheterization of the bladder** can be used as a last resort to obtain a urine specimen. A soft plastic or rubber tube (catheter) is inserted through the urethra into the bladder to drain and collect urine *(Figure 11.14)*.

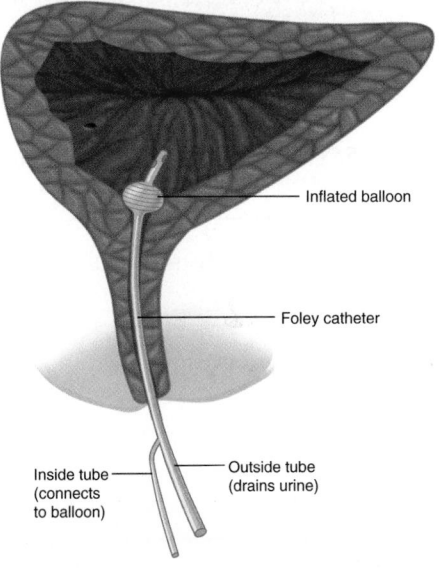

Inflated balloon

Foley catheter

Inside tube (connects to balloon)

Outside tube (drains urine)

▲ **FIGURE 11.14 Foley Catheter.**

EXERCISES

Apply your knowledge of medical language to this exercise. All the questions can be answered using terms from this spread. Circle the best answer.

1. An x-ray image taken during voiding:

    retrograde pyelogram   KUB   cystourethrogram

2. Presence of glucose in urine:

    hematuria   polyuria   glycosuria

3. Urine collection method to test for proteinuria:

    catheterization   24 hour   clean catch

4. Reversal of normal flow:

    reflex   retrograde   regenerate

5. Excessive ketones in the blood, making it acid:

    ketosis   ketoacidosis   ketone

6. Separate urine into its elements:

    urinalysis   cystourethrogram   retrograde pyelogram

URINARY SYSTEM
CHALLENGE YOUR KNOWLEDGE

A. Patient Documentation:

1. *Read the following case history aloud.*
2. *Go through the paragraph and underline all the medical terms.*
3. *Answer the questions.*

DOCUMENTATION

A 68-year-old female presents with hematuria, dysuria, and left-flank pain. I ordered a KUB and an IVP to ascertain the possibility or extent of obstruction. Test results indicate one large and several small calculi impacted in her left ureter just below the renal hilum. Patient would prefer ESWL, but surgical laparoscopy, I think, will offer better and quicker results to alleviate her pain. Patient will proceed with surgery tomorrow.

1. What are the patient's symptoms?

   _____

2. What diagnostic tests were performed?

   _____

3. What organs were checked in these tests?

   _____

4. What is the singular of calculi? _____

5. What does **impacted** mean?

   _____

6. What is obstructing the ureter?

   _____

7. Define ESWL.

   _____

8. What is a laparoscopy?

   _____

9. What type of doctor performs laparoscopy for renal calculi?

   _____

10. What is a preoperative diagnosis for this patient?

    _____

B. Brain Teaser: Taken directly from your text: "The peristaltic waves are intermittent, which is why Justin's pain was spasmodic."

1. Define **peristaltic.** _____

2. Which previous body system that you have already studied in this text also mentions peristalsis? _____

   Is it the same type of process?_____

C. **Elements:** Roots and combining forms may stay the same in similar terms, but you will notice that the suffix can change the entire meaning of the medical term. Insert the correct suffix on the line to provide the precise meaning. Pick the correct ending from among the following choices; you have more choices than you will need. Fill in the blanks.

-al	-iasis	-lysis	-scopy
-ectomy	-ion	-osis	-tomy
-emia	-logist	-pexy	-tripsy
-gen	-logy	-scope	-uria

1. Study of the kidney   nephro _____

2. Dilation of pelvis and calyces of a kidney   hydronephr _____ _

3. Instrument for viewing inside a kidney   nephro _____

4. Presence of a kidney stone   nephrolith _____

5. Process of eliminating waste products of metabolism   excret _____

6. Surgical removal of a kidney   nephr _____

7. Incision for removal of a kidney stone   nephrolitho _____

8. Separating urine for examination of elements   urina _____

9. Medical specialist in disorders of the urinary system   uro _____

10. Crushing a renal stone with sound waves   litho _____

11. Blood in the urine   hemat _____

12. Excess nitrogenous waste products in the blood   azot _____

D. **Seek and Find:** How many medical terms ending in *-itis* have you found in this chapter? List them here, and give a brief definition for each term. Fill in the blanks.

1. _____itis

    Definition: _____

2. _____itis

    Definition: _____

3. _____itis

    Definition: _____

4. _____itis

    Definition: _____

5. _____itis

    Definition: _____

6. _____itis

    Definition: _____

URINARY SYSTEM

E.   Documentation. Case Report 11.3 presents all the information you need to fill out the HPI (history of present illness) form for the patient's medical record. *You are translating the patient's own words into medical terminology.* First read the Case Report about Mrs. Dobson; then read the questions you need to answer. This will help you to fill in the blanks in the HPI form. The last part of the exercise involves asking Mrs. Dobson additional questions you think will provide helpful information for the doctor. Use the correct medical term whenever possible, and be prepared to define each term you use.

You are

. . . a medical assistant working in the office of Dr. Susan Lee, a primary care physician at Fulwood Medical Center.

Your patient is

. . . Mrs. Caroline Dobson, a 32-year-old housewife. You have asked her to describe the reason for her visit to the office today, 06/09/09.

CASE REPORT 11.3

Patient Interview:

Mrs. Dobson:

"Since yesterday afternoon I've had a lot of pain low down in my belly and in my lower back. I keep having to go to the bathroom every hour or so to pee. It's often difficult to start, and it burns as it comes out. I've had this problem twice before when I was pregnant with my two kids, so I've started drinking cranberry juice. I've been shivering since I woke up this morning, and the last urine I passed was pink. Was that due to the cranberry juice?"

Fulwood Medical Center
3333 Medical Parkway, Fulwood, MI 01234
555-247-6100

Medical record number: 123456_____   Date of visit: 06/09/09_____

Patient Name: _____   Patient age or DOB: _____

Physician: _____   Department: _____

History of Present Illness:

1. Onset (when did it begin?): _____

2. Location (where is the pain or problem?): _____

3. Duration (how long has patient had this pain?): _____

4. Severity (of pain—on a scale of 1 to 10, with 10 being the highest): _____

5. Timing (when does pain occur?): _____

6. Context (what can be associated with the pain/problem—standing, bending, fried

   foods?): _____

7. Modifying factors (does it get better or worse with anything the patient does?):

   _____

8. Is this a recurrent problem?_____

If so, when did it last occur?_____

What other additional questions could you ask Mrs. Dobson that would provide helpful information for Dr. Lee?

1.   _____

2.   _____

F. **Recall and Review:** One or more roots or combining forms can have the same meaning. Demonstrate that you can use these elements correctly. *Remember: They are not interchangeable.* One particular root or combining form goes with a specific suffix. Fill in the blanks.

1. Respiratory system: _____ and _____ both mean lung.

2. Urinary system: _____ and _____ both mean kidney.

Attach the following suffixes to the correct roots/combining forms for lung or kidney to form the exact medical terms. You will use some elements twice. Fill in the blanks.

-al	**-in**	**-ary**	**-logist**	**-ectomy**	**-itis**	**-otomy**	**-logy**

3. Pertaining to the lung _____

4. Removal of the lung _____

5. Inflammation of the lung _____

6. Study of the lung _____

7. Specialist in lung diseases _____

8. Incision into the kidney _____

9. Pertaining to the kidney _____

10. Removal of the kidney _____

11. Kidney enzyme that causes vasoconstriction _____

12. Inflammation of the kidney _____

13. Study of the kidney _____

14. Specialist in kidney diseases _____

G. **Short Answer:** You will often be called upon to express yourself in writing documentation. Practice writing clear, concise answers to the following questions. Always be sure to check your spelling!

1. Explain the body's process of reabsorption of water.

_____

_____

_____

_____

2. The kidneys secrete both an enzyme and a hormone. What are they called, and what are the functions of each?

Enzyme: _____

_____

_____

Hormone: _____

_____

_____

URINARY SYSTEM

H. **System Review:** Understanding the structure and function of the urinary system will give you a better grasp of the terminology. Circle the correct answers to the following questions.

1. Where does waste-laden blood enter the kidney?

   a. the fascia

   b. the glomerulus

   c. the hilum

   d. the renal vein

   e. the portal vein

2. The medical term to describe urine being forced back up the ureter to the kidneys is:

   a. reflux

   b. filtration

   c. excretion

   d. absorption

   e. micturition

3. What results if the kidney produces too much renin?

   a. hematuria

   b. oliguria

   c. primary hypertension

   d. anuria

   e. secondary hypertension

4. What is the end product of nitrogen metabolism?

   a. ammonia

   b. nitrogen

   c. urea

   d. nitrates

   e. renin

5. What do urethritis, cystitis, pyelitis, and pyelonephritis all have in common?

   a. infection

   b. inflammation

   c. the same suffix

   d. the same body system

   e. all of these

6. Each kidney is the size of a(n):

   a. orange

   b. golf ball

   c. clenched fist

   d. bean

   e. ping-pong ball

7. What protects the kidney?

   a. adipose tissue

   b. renal fascia

   c. renal capsule

   d. none of these

   e. all of these

8. The external opening of a passage is called:

   a. meatus

   b. urethra

   c. ureter

   d. bladder

   e. trigone

9. The glomerulus is encased in:

   a. a blood vessel

   b. a muscle

   c. renal fascia

   d. Bowman capsule

   e. urethra

10. Nephrotic syndrome leads to:

    a. acute renal failure

    b. primary hypertension

    c. secondary hypertension

    d. chronic renal failure

    e. oliguria

URINARY SYSTEM

I. **System Review:** Understanding the structure and function of the urinary system will give you a better grasp of the terminology. Circle the correct answers to the following questions.

1. *Muscular tube, about 10 inches long, that carries urine to bladder.* This describes:

   a. the ureter

   b. the urethra

   c. the portal vein

   d. the renal vein

   e. the aorta

2. Another name for a kidney stone:

   a. UTI

   b. calculus

   c. tumor

   d. hematuria

   e. lithotripsy

3. Water is returned to the blood by:

   a. excretion

   b. filtration

   c. resorption

   d. elimination

   e. reabsorption

4. What gets released from crushed muscles?

   a. myoglobin

   b. hemoglobin

   c. hematuria

   d. ammonia

   e. hormones

5. **Peritoneal** and **continuous cycling** are terms that apply to:

   a. incontinence

   b. azotemia

   c. dialysis

   d. nephrectomy

   e. transplants

J. **Terminology Challenge:** Medical terminology is full of words that sound and look similar but have very different meanings. Think about the following terms, and explain in plain language how they are different. **Notice** that these two terms differ by only one letter—this is where precision comes in! Fill in the blanks.

1. Reflex: _____

2. Reflux: _____

K. **Word elements remain your key for understanding a medical term.** Deconstruct the following medical terms into their basic elements; then write the meaning of the term. It will be visually helpful to you to put a slash (/) between each element in every term before you start. Fill in the chart.

Medical Term	Prefix	Root/CF	Suffix	Meaning of Term
hemodialysis				
hydronephrosis				
incontinence				
nephrectomy				
nephrolithiasis				
nephrolithotomy				
peritubular				
uremia				
nephropathy				
nephroblastoma				

L. **Plurals:** Precision in communication requires the correct use of the singular and/or plural form of the medical term. If the singular form is given in the left column, write in the plural form in the appropriate column, or vice versa. Be sure to define the term. Fill in the chart.

Medical Term	Singular	Plural	Meaning of Term
calculus			
calyces			
cortex			
glomeruli			
hila			

To finish this exercise, use any two terms from the chart in a sentence that is not a definition.

Sentence 1: _____

_____

Sentence 2: _____

_____

Precision in communication is the mark of a professional.

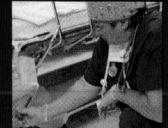
URINARY SYSTEM

M. **Common Denominator:** Each of the following groups of terms has something in common. Your knowledge of the terminology and functional anatomy of the urinary system will help you determine the common denominator for each group. Fill in the blanks.

1. filter, regulate, maintain, secrete, synthesize, detoxify

    All are _____ .

2. urination, micturition, voiding

    All are _____ .

3. sibling, blood relative, accident victim, cadaver

    All are _____ .

4. ESWL, ureteroscopy, percutaneous nephrolithotomy

    All are _____ .

5. stress, urge, overflow, functional

    All are _____ .

6. random, clean-catch, catheterization, early morning, 24-hour

    All are _____ .

N. **Matching:** Confirm that your knowledge of the **language of the urinary system** and its functions is accurate. Match the statements in the left column to the correct answers in the right column.

_____   1. Vessels and nerves enter and leave   **A.** uremia

_____   2. Outside the body   **B.** permeable

_____   3. Donor organ to recipient   **C.** azotemia

_____   4. Reversal of normal flow   **D.** flank

_____   5. Identified by dipstick   **E.** extracorporeal

_____   6. Loss of bladder control   **F.** dialyzer

_____   7. Disease state resulting from renal failure   **G.** radical

_____   8. Extensive removal of diseased part   **H.** incontinence

_____   9. Side of body between ribs and pelvis   **I.** hilum

_____   10. Artificial kidney machine   **J.** transplant

_____   11. Allows substance to pass through membrane   **K.** retrograde

_____   12. Excess waste products in blood   **L.** microscopic hematuria

O. **Differences:** Being able to explain how terms are different means you understand exactly what they mean. These terms all have the same suffix, but their other elements define them. Fill in the blanks.

1. A **nephroscopy** is _____ .

2. A **ureteroscopy** is _____ .

3. A **cystoscopy** is _____ .

4. The suffix in each term is _____ and means _____ .

P. Abbreviations are not helpful if you do not understand their meaning and cannot use them to communicate safely and effectively. The following abbreviations are from this chapter and earlier chapters. Demonstrate that you can put the appropriate abbreviation in the correct context. You will not use every abbreviation listed to fill in the blanks.

ARF	**ESWL**	**KUB**	**TNM**
BUN	**GRF**	**PKD**	**UA**
CRF	**IV**	**SG**	**UTI**
ESRD	**IVP**	**SPA**	**VCUG**

1. Dr. Lee ordered the _____ medication stat.

2. Patient informed me that there is a history of _____ in his family.

3. The patient with the kidney stone is scheduled for _____ early tomorrow morning.

4. Patient's renal carcinoma was staged using the _____ method.

5. Patient returns with her second _____ this month. Medication prescribed.

6. Dr. Johnson ordered the following radiologic diagnostic tests for the patient: _____, _____,

   and _____.

7. Patient's _____ progressed to _____,

   and _____ resulted.

Q. **Discussion Questions:** Discussions with patients require effort to get your thoughts organized about what you want to say. Prepare for these discussions by doing one of the following:

- Making a mini-outline of what you want to say.
- Making a list of keywords that will help your memory.
- Making a list of short notes to keep your thoughts on track—try to confine your list/outline to a large index card.

Use any of these methods to prepare a short discussion on one of the following topics:

1. The functions of the kidney: Pick any two functions of the kidney, and be prepared to explain what each function is, how important it is, what other systems may be involved with the function or impacted by it, what urinary structures are involved with the function, and so on. *Be sure that you can define/explain to your classmates any terms you use in your discussion.*

2. Trace the flow of fluid through the renal filtration process. This particular discussion may benefit from a simple illustration you might want to prepare. Research this on the Internet.

3. Explain the various methods of dialysis. Be prepared to explain which type of dialysis you would choose if you were in a condition where you needed it. Give reasons why this would be your choice rather than the other options. Search the Internet for illustrations of this type of dialysis. Perhaps you know someone who is on dialysis—interview the person.

Notes: _____

_____

_____

_____

_____

_____

_____

URINARY SYSTEM

R. **Roots and Combining Forms:** Form the foundation of a medical term. All these terms have the same suffix. Differentiate their meanings by analyzing the rest of the term. Every one of these terms could be a diagnosis for your next patient. Fill in the blanks.

Medical Term	Meaning of Prefix	Meaning of Root/CF	Meaning of Suffix
anuria			
dysuria			
glycosuria			
hematuria			
oliguria			
proteinuria			

Can you determine the meaning of these two terms after analyzing the rest of their elements?

1. If **py** means *pus*, then **pyuria** means_____ .

2. If **noct** means *night*, then **nocturia** means _____ .

S. **Tests and Procedures:** Patients with urinary problems will be sent for various renal function tests and diagnostic procedures that may result in a surgical procedure. Any of the following procedures might be ordered for your patient. Do you know their purpose? Be prepared to discuss which terms are tests and which are procedures.

_____ 1. Contrast material injected to locate stones

_____ 2. Used to collect bladder sample in newborns

_____ 3. Incision for removal of kidney stone

_____ 4. Crushing renal stone by sound waves

_____ 5. Assess blood flow to the kidneys

_____ 6. Tissue bank matches donor to recipient

_____ 7. Treatment for renal cell carcinoma

_____ 8. X-ray of the abdominal urinary organs

_____ 9. Viewing the bladder through a scope

_____ 10. Filters blood through an artificial kidney machine

A. dialysis

B. transplant

C. KUB

D. retrograde pyelogram

E. cystoscopy

F. nephrolithotomy

G. nephrectomy

H. needle aspiration

I. renal angiogram

J. lithotripsy

Study Hint

Create a study hint for yourself that will make it easy to remember exactly what an IVP is.

Write your hint here:

_____

_____

_____

_____

_____

T. **Labeling:** Demonstrate your knowledge of urinary anatomy and use of medical terminology by labeling the following diagram. The suffix in the term for each label tells you these diagnoses are all an *inflammation of* a particular part of the urinary system.

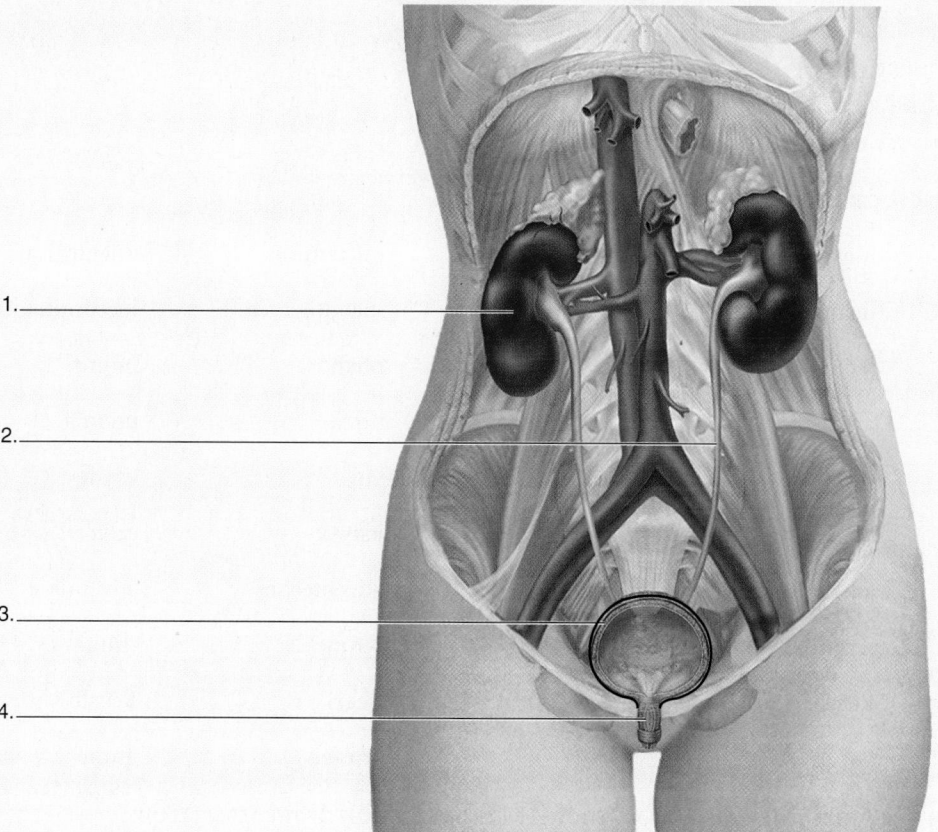

1._____

2._____

3._____

4._____

Diagnoses are lettered A through D in the table below.

1. Write the letter of the diagnosis and the term (from the left column below) on the line in the illustration that shows the part of the anatomy connected to that diagnosis.

2. In the left column of the table, write the layman's definition of the medical term.

Label these in the illustration:

Diagnosis	Layman's Terms
a. urethritis	
b. cystitis	
c. nephritis	
d. ureteritis	

Describe what part(s) of the urinary system are affected by:

1. glomerulonephritis: _____

2. pyelonephritis: _____

3. pyelitis: _____

URINARY SYSTEM

CHAPTER SUMMARY EXERCISE

1. *Listen to the pronunciation of the medical terms as given by your instructor.*
2. *Circle the correct spelling of the medical term.*
3. *Match the correctly spelled terms to the brief descriptions below.*
4. *Write a sentence for each of the 10 terms that appear in this exercise.*

A. SPELLING COMPREHENSION: CIRCLE THE CORRECT SPELLING OF THE TERM.

1. micktutrition	mictrition	mickterition	micterition	micturition
2. incontenince	incontenance	incontinence	incontinance	inccontinance
3. pilitis	pylitis	pyelitis	phylitis	pulitis
4. ureea	uria	urea	urrea	uremia
5. voyd	void	voyid	vuyde	voyde
6. kalyx	calyxx	calyx	kalyxx	calix
7. adventitia	adventishia	adventusa	adventechia	adventia
8. reninne	renine	renin	rynine	rinine
9. Kegelle	Kegele	Keggle	Kegel	Kegale
10. groin	groun	groan	grunne	grune

B. MATCH THE NUMBER OF THE CORRECT TERM IN PART A WITH THE BRIEF DESCRIPTION OF THE TERM BELOW.

a. Crease where thigh joins abdomen _____

b. Funnel-shaped structure _____

c. Causes vasoconstriction _____

d. End product of nitrogen metabolism _____

e. Inflammation of the renal pelvis _____

f. Act of passing urine _____

g. Outermost connective tissue layer of any structure _____

h. Exercises to strengthen muscles of pelvic floor _____

i. To evacuate urine or feces _____

j. Loss of control of the bladder _____

C. USING YOUR KNOWLEDGE OF TERMS 1–10 IN PART A AND THEIR CORRECT SPELLING, WRITE A BRIEF SENTENCE AS IT MIGHT APPEAR IN PATIENT DOCUMENTATION.

1. _____

2. _____

3. _____

4. _____

5. _____

6. _____

7. _____

8. _____

9. _____

10. _____

D. YOUR INSTRUCTOR WILL DIRECT YOU TO MCGRAW-HILL CONNECT. OPEN THE AUDIO GLOSSARY AND PRACTICE YOUR PRONUNCIATION OF THE TERMS IN PART A OF THIS EXERCISE.

E. AFTER READING CASE REPORT 11.1 BELOW, ANSWER THE FOLLOWING QUESTIONS. BE PREPARED TO DISCUSS YOUR ANSWERS IN CLASS.

You are

. . . a surgical physician assistant working with **urologist** Phillip Johnson, MD, at Fulwood Medical Center.

Your patient is

. . . Mr. Nelson Hughes, a 58-year-old school principal. You are making your afternoon hospital visits to Dr. Johnson's patients. Earlier today you assisted at Mr. Hughes's surgery. A **laparoscopic radical nephrectomy** for a **TNM stage II renal** cell carcinoma (cancer) with no evidence of local invasion or lymph node involvement (metastasis) was performed.

Your job is to assess Mr. Hughes's postoperative state and determine whether postoperative complications exist.

1. A *urologist* treats which organs in the urinary system?

   _____

2. Define:

   laparoscopic: _____

   radical: _____

   nephrectomy: _____

3. What does the abbreviation TNM stand for? _____

4. When does *postoperative* occur? _____

5. Why is "no evidence of metastasis" a good thing? _____

   _____

Note to student: A *urologist* can operate on any part of the urinary system. A *nephrologist* is not a surgeon, much like a *cardiologist* is not a surgeon. Both specialists <u>can diagnose the diseases but cannot provide surgical treatment</u> for them. The *nephrologist* will refer patients who need surgery to a *urologist* for the surgery, and a *cardiologist* will refer patients to a *cardiovascular* surgeon.

Male Reproductive System
The Language of Reproduction

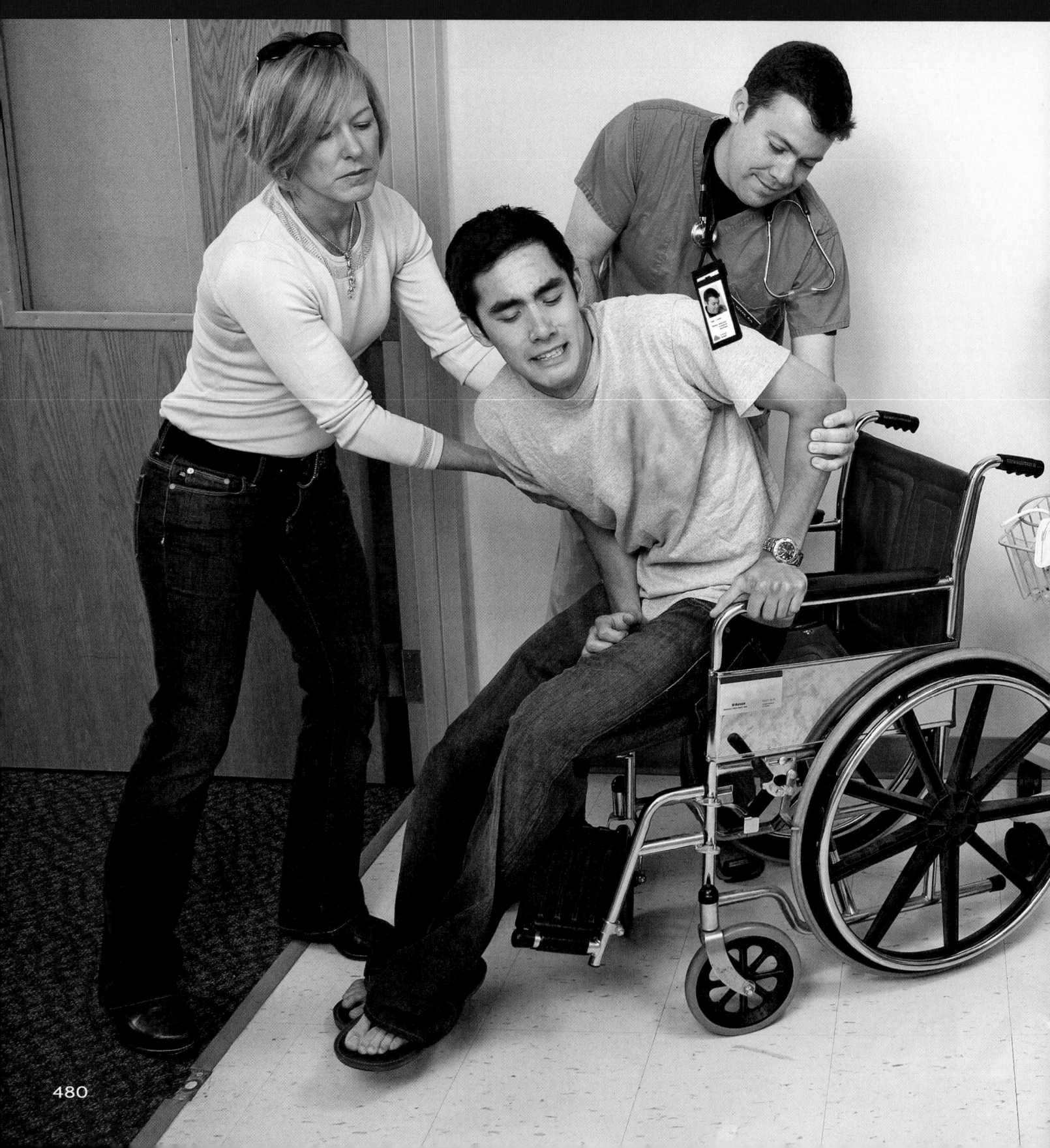

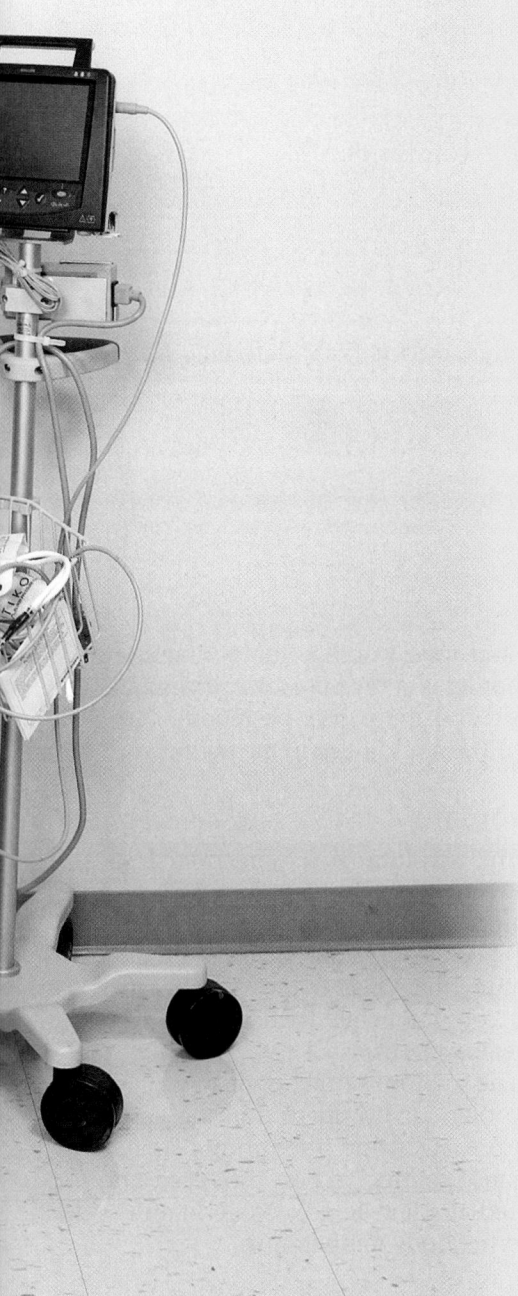

12

CASE REPORT 12.1

You are

...an EMT-P working in the Emergency Department at Fulwood Medical Center.

Your patient is

...Joseph Davis, a 17-year-old high school senior. He is brought in by his mother at 0400 hrs. He complains of **(c/o)** sudden onset of pain in his left **testicle** 3 hours earlier that woke him up. The pain is intense and has made him vomit. VS: T 99.2°F, P 88, R 15, BP 130/70. Examination reveals his left testicle to be enlarged, warm, and tender. His abdomen is normal to palpation.

At your request, Dr. Helinski, the emergency physician on duty, examines him immediately. He diagnoses a **torsion** of the patient's left testicle.

Learning Outcomes

As you set up the next stage of Joseph's treatment, there are immediate clinical decisions to be made. You will have to communicate clearly with Dr. Helinski and other health professionals and with Joseph and his mother. You must also document his care.

To participate effectively in all this, you must be able to:

12.1 Apply the language of urology to the anatomy and physiology of the male reproductive system.

12.2 Comprehend, analyze, spell, and write the medical terms of urology as they relate to the male reproductive system so that you communicate accurately and precisely in any health care setting.

12.3 Recognize and pronounce the medical terms of urology as they relate to the male reproductive system so that you communicate verbally with accuracy and precision in any health care setting.

12.4 Explain the effects of common disorders of the male reproductive system on health.

Male Reproductive System

OBJECTIVES

Unlike every other organ system, the reproductive system is not essential for an *individual human* to survive. However, without the reproductive system, the *human species* could not survive. The male reproductive system ensures the sexual **maturation** of each male, influences male behavior, and produces, maintains, and transports the male sex cells **(sperm cells)** to the female reproductive tract.

The information in this lesson will enable you to use correct medical terminology to:

12.1.1 Describe the anatomy and physiology of the male reproductive system.

12.1.2 Document the process of spermatogenesis.

12.1.3 List the functions of testosterone.

12.1.4 Explain the effects of common disorders of the testes on the health of the male.

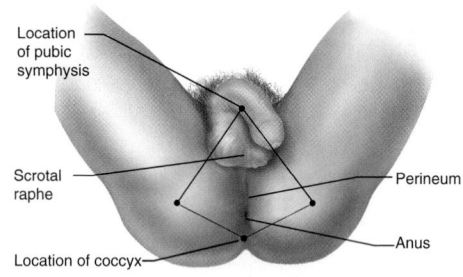

▲ **FIGURE 12.2   Male Perineum.**

Abbreviation	
c/o	complains of

MALE REPRODUCTIVE SYSTEM

The male reproductive organ system *(Figure 12.1)* consists of:

1. Primary sex organs or **gonads:** the **testes**

2. Secondary sex organs:

   a. **Penis**

   b. **Scrotum**

   c. System of ducts, including the **epididymis, ductus (vas) deferens,** and **urethra**

3. Accessory glands:

   a. **Prostate**

   b. **Seminal vesicles**

   c. **Bulbourethral (Cowper) glands**

Perineum

The **external genitalia** (the penis, scrotum, and testes) occupy the **perineum,** a diamond-shaped region between the thighs. Its border is at the pubic symphysis anteriorly and the coccyx posteriorly *(Figure 12.2)*. The anus is also in the perineum.

Scrotum

The **scrotum** is a skin-covered sac between the thighs. Its midline shows a distinct ridge called the **raphe.** It marks the position of the internal **median septum** that divides the scrotum into two compartments. Each compartment contains a testis.

The scrotum's function is to provide a cooler environment for the testes than that inside the body. This is because sperm are best produced and stored at a few degrees cooler than the internal body temperature.

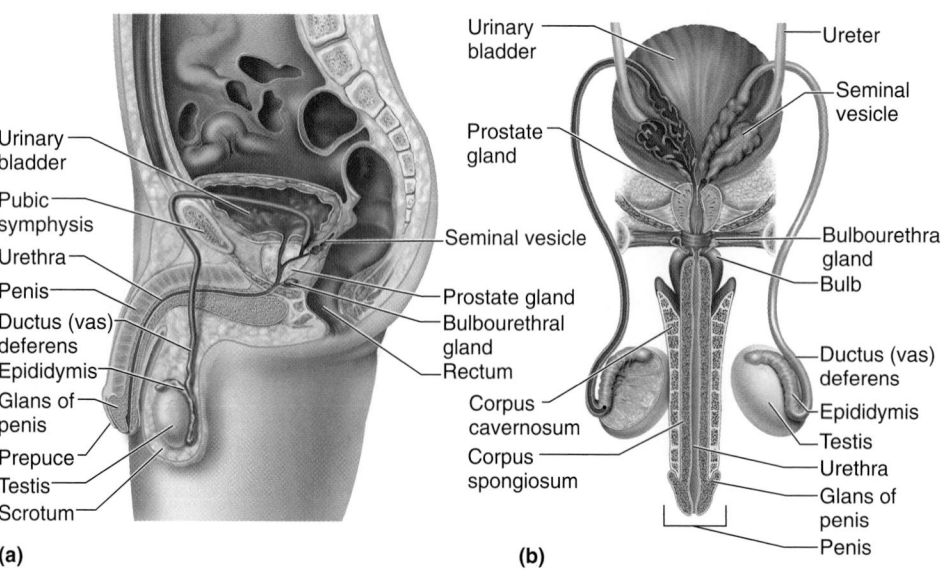

▲ **FIGURE 12.1   Male Reproductive System.** (*a*) Male pelvic cavity: midsagittal section. (*b*) Male reproductive organs.

WORD	PRONUNCIATION	ELEMENTS		DEFINITION
bulbourethral	**BUL**-boh-you-**REE**-thral	S/ R/CF R/	**-al** *pertaining to* **bulb/o-** *bulb* **-urethr-** *urethra*	Pertaining to the bulbous penis and urethra
ductus deferens vas deferens (syn)	**DUK**-tus **DEH**-fuh-renz VAS **DEH**-fuh-renz		**ductus** Latin *to lead* **deferens** Latin *carry away* **vas** Latin *blood vessel, duct*	Tube that receives sperm from the epididymis
epididymis	**EP**-ih-**DID**-ih-miss	P/ R/	**epi-** *above* **-didymis** *testis*	Coiled tube attached to the testis
genitalia	**JEN**-ih-**TAY**-lee-ah	S/ R/	**-ia** *condition* **genit-** *primary male or female sex organs*	External and internal organs of reproduction
genital	**JEN**-ih-tal	S/	**-al** *pertaining to*	Relating to reproduction or to the male or female sex organs
gonad gonads (pl)	**GO**-nad **GO**-nads		Greek *seed*	Testis or ovary
maturation	mat-you-**RAY**-shun	S/ R/	**-ation** *process* **matur-** *ripe, ready*	Process to achieve full development
penis penile	**PEE**-nis **PEE**-nile	S/ R/	Latin *tail* **-ile** *pertaining to* **pen-** *penis*	Conveys urine and semen to the outside Pertaining to the penis
perineum	**PER**-ih-**NEE**-um		Greek *perineum*	Area between thighs, extending from the coccyx to the pubis
perineal	**PER**-ih-**NEE**-al	S/ R/CF	**-al** *pertaining to* **perin/e-** *perineum*	Pertaining to the perineum
raphe	**RAY**-fee		Greek *seam*	Line separating two symmetrical structures
scrotum scrotal (adj)	**SKRO**-tum **SKRO**-tal	S/ R/	Latin *scrotum* **-al** *pertaining to* **scrot-** *scrotum*	Sac containing the testes Pertaining to the scrotum
semen	**SEE**-men		Latin *seed*	Penile ejaculate containing sperm and seminal fluid
seminal vesicle	**SEM**-in-al **VES**-ih-kull	S/ R/ S/ R/	**-al** *pertaining to* **semin-** *semen* **-le** *small* **vesic-** *sac containing fluid*	Sac of ductus deferens that produces seminal fluid
seminiferous	sem-ih-**NIF**-er-us	S/ R/CF R/	**-ous** *pertaining to* **semin/i-** *semen* **-fer-** *to bear*	Pertaining to carrying semen
testicle (also called **testis**) testicular	**TES**-tih-kul tes-**TICK**-you-lar	S/ R/	Latin *small testis* **-ar** *pertaining to* **testicul-** *testicle*	One of the male reproductive glands Pertaining to the testicle
testis testes (pl)	**TES**-tis **TES**-tez		Latin *testis*	A synonym for testicle
torsion	**TOR**-shun		Latin *to twist*	The act or result of twisting

EXERCISES

In Your Own Words: You could be working in the Emergency Department when this patient comes in. Using the information presented in Case Report 12.1, document the case in the patient's record. Use the following terms to fill in the blanks and answer the question.

testicular   **testes**   **testis**   **testicle**

This patient presented to the ED because of pain in his left _____. Both _____ were examined, but the left _____ was enlarged, warm, and tender. The emergency physician on duty diagnosed _____ torsion. Patient will be scheduled for surgery immediately.

1. Is a primary or secondary sex organ involved? _____

TESTES AND SPERMATIC CORD

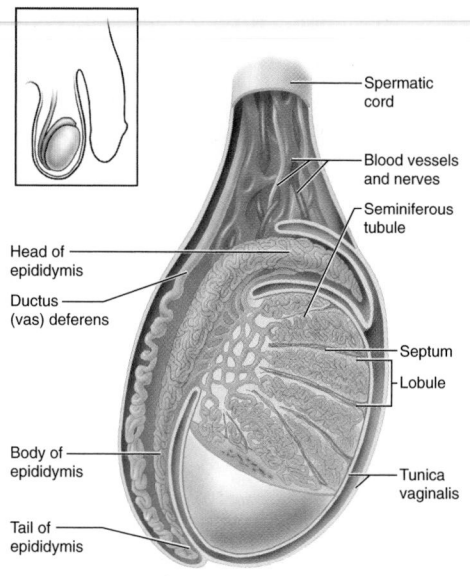

▲ **FIGURE 12.3** **The Testis and Associated Structures.**

Keynote

The male testes produce up to 100,000,000 sperm per day.

Abbreviation	
BMR	basal metabolic rate

In the adult male, each testis is a small, oval organ about 2 inches (5 cm) long and ¾ inch (2 cm) wide *(Figure 12.3)*. Each testis is covered by a serous membrane, the **tunica vaginalis,** which has an outer parietal layer and an inner visceral layer separated by serous fluid.

Inside the testis, thin septa subdivide the testis into some 250 lobules *(Figure 12.3)*. Each lobule contains three or four **seminiferous tubules** in which several layers of germ cells are in the process of becoming sperm.

Between the seminiferous tubules are the interstitial cells. They produce hormones called **androgens.**

Testosterone is the major androgen produced by the interstitial cells of the testes. It has the following effects:

- **Sustains** the male reproductive tract throughout adulthood.
- **Stimulates** spermatogenesis; testosterone levels peak at age 20, and then decline steadily to one-third of that level at age 65.
- **Inhibits** the secretion of female hormones.
- **Stimulates** the development of male secondary sex characteristics at puberty.
- **Enlarges** the spermatic ducts and accessory glands of the male reproductive system.
- **Stimulates** a burst of growth at puberty—including increased muscle mass, higher **basal metabolic rate (BMR),** and larger larynx (this effect deepens the voice).
- **Stimulates** erythropoiesis, giving men a higher red blood cell (RBC) count than women.
- **Stimulates** the brain to increase **libido** (sex drive) in the male.

Spermatic Cord

The blood vessels and nerves to the testis arise in the abdominal cavity. They pass through the inguinal canal, where they join with connective tissue to form a spermatic cord that suspends each testis in the scrotum *(see Figure 12.3)*. The left testis is suspended lower than the right. Within the cord are an artery, a plexus of veins, nerves, a thin muscle, and the ductus (vas) deferens (the passage into which sperm go when they leave the testis).

Spermatogenesis

Spermatogenesis is the process in which the germ cells of the seminiferous tubules mature and divide **(mitosis)** and then undergo two divisions called **meiosis.** The four daughter cells differentiate into **spermatids** and then **spermatozoa (sperm)** *(Figure 12.4)*. The germ cells have 23 pairs of chromosomes (a total of 46). Because of meiosis, each sperm has only 23 chromosomes that can combine at fertilization with the 23 chromosomes in a female **oocyte** (egg).

The mature sperm has a pear-shaped head and a long tail. The nucleus of the head contains 23 chromosomes.

The tail **(flagellum)** provides the movement as the sperm swims up the female reproductive tract.

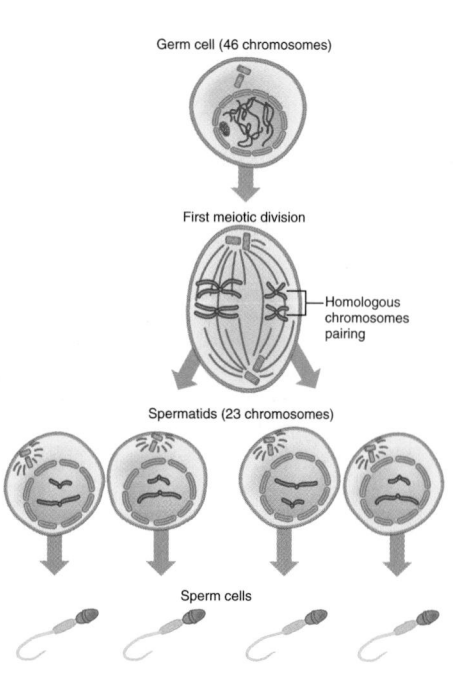

▲ **FIGURE 12.4** **Spermatogenesis.**

▲ **FIGURE 12.5** **Mature Sperm.**

WORD	PRONUNCIATION	ELEMENTS		DEFINITION
androgen	**AN**-droh-jen	S/ R/CF	**-gen** *form, create* **andr/o-** *masculine*	Hormone that promotes masculine characteristics
flagellum flagella (pl)	fla-**JELL**-um fla-**JELL**-ah		Latin *small whip*	Tail of a sperm
libido	li-**BEE**-doh		Latin *lust*	Sexual desire
meiosis	my-**OH**-sis	S/ R/	**-osis** *condition* **mei-** *lessening*	Two rapid cell divisions, resulting in half the number of chromosomes
mitosis	my-**TOE**-sis	S/ R/	**-osis** *condition* **mit-** *threadlike structure*	Cell division to create two identical cells, each with 46 chromosomes
oocyte	**OH**-oh-site	S/ R/CF	**-cyte** *cell* **o/o-** *egg*	Female egg cell
oogenesis	oh-oh-**JEN**-eh-sis	R/ S/	**-gen-** *origin, create* **-esis** *abnormal condition*	Development of female egg cell
puberty	**PYU**-ber-tee		Latin *grown up*	Process of maturing from child to young adult
seminiferous tubule	sem-ih-**NIF**-er-us **TU**-byul	S/ R/CF R/	**-ous** *pertaining to* **semin/i-** *semen* **-fer-** *to bear*	Coiled tubes in the testes that produce sperm
sperm (also called **spermatozoon**)	SPERM		Greek *seed*	Mature male sex cell
spermatozoa (pl)	**SPER**-mat-oh-**ZOH**-ah	S/ R/CF	**-zoa** *animals* **spermat/o-** *sperm*	Sperm (plural of spermatozoon)
spermatic (adj)	**SPER**-mat-ik	S/	**-ic** *pertaining to*	Pertaining to sperm.
spermatid	**SPER**-mah-tid	S/ R/	**-id** *having a particular quality* **spermat-** *sperm*	A cell late in the development process of sperm
spermatogenesis (**Note:** This term has no prefix or suffix.)	**SPER**-mat-oh-**JEN**-eh-sis	R/ R/CF	**-genesis** *origin, creation* **spermat/o-** *sperm*	The process by which male germ cells differentiate into sperm
testosterone	tes-**TOSS**-ter-own	S/ R/CF	**-sterone** *steroid* **test/o-** *testis*	Powerful androgen produced by the testes
tunica vaginalis	**TYU**-nih-kah vaj-ih-**NAHL**-iss	S/ R/	*tunica* Latin *coat* **-alis** *pertaining to* **vagin-** *sheath, vagina*	Covering, particularly of a tubular structure. The tunica vaginalis is the sheath of the testis and epididymis

EXERCISES

Deconstruction of medical terms is a tool for analyzing the meaning. In the following chart, you are given a medical term. Deconstruct the term into its root (or combining form) and suffix. Note that none of these terms have prefixes, and not all of the terms have a suffix. Write the element and its meaning in the appropriate column and the meaning of the term in the last column. The first one is done for you. Then answer the question at the end of the exercise.

Term	Root/CF	Suffix	Meaning of Element	Meaning of Term
vaginalis	*vagin*	*alis*	*sheath, pertaining to*	
testosterone				
androgen				
spermatid				
spermatogenesis				

In your opinion, which term is the most unusual in the above Word Analysis and Definition (WAD) box, and why? (**Hint:** Think of the elements.)

Keynote

The testis in testicular torsion will die in some 6 hours unless the blood supply is restored.

Case Report 12.1 (continued)

In the opening scenario to this chapter, Joseph Davis presented with typical symptoms and signs of testicular torsion. The affected testis rapidly became painful, tender, swollen, and inflamed. Emergency surgery was performed, and the testis and cord were manually untwisted through an incision in the scrotum. The testis was stitched to surrounding tissues to prevent a recurrence.

DISORDERS OF THE TESTES

Testicular torsion is the twisting of a testis on its spermatic cord. As the testis twists, the spermatic cord has to twist because it is fixed in the abdomen. The testicular artery in the twisted cord becomes blocked, and the blood supply to the testis is cut off. The condition occurs in men between puberty and age 25. In half the cases, it starts in bed at night.

Varicocele is a condition in which the veins in the spermatic cord become dilated and tortuous as varicose veins. If it is uncomfortable, it can be treated by surgically tying off the affected veins.

Hydrocele is a collection of excess fluid in the space between the visceral and parietal layers of the tunica vaginalis of the testis. It is most common after age 40. The diagnosis can be confirmed by transillumination, shining a bright light on the swelling to see the shape of the testis through the translucent excess fluid *(Figure 12.6)*. Surgical removal is performed for large hydroceles.

Spermatocele is a collection of sperm in a sac formed in the epididymis. It occurs in about 30% of men, is benign, and rarely causes symptoms. It does not require treatment unless it becomes bothersome.

Cryptorchism occurs when a testis fails to descend from the abdomen into the scrotum before the boy is 12 months old. In the **embryo,** the testes develop inside the abdomen at the level of the kidney. They must then migrate down the abdomen into the scrotum. As undescended testicles have a higher risk of infertility and cancer, **orchiopexy** is performed to bring the testis into the scrotum.

Epididymitis and **epididymoorchitis (orchitis)** are both inflammatory diseases. Epididymitis is inflammation of the epididymis; epididymoorchitis is inflammation of the epididymis and testis. Orchitis is usually a consequence of epididymitis. They are most commonly caused by a bacterial infection spreading from a urinary tract infection or infection of the prostate. They can also be caused by **sexually transmitted diseases (STDs),** such as gonorrhea or chlamydia *(see Chapter 20).*

A viral cause of orchitis is mumps. In males past puberty who develop mumps, 30% will develop orchitis, and 30% of those will develop resulting testicular atrophy. If the testicular infection is bilateral, **infertility** can result. Mumps is avoidable by immunization during childhood *(see Chapter 16).*

Testicular cancer usually develops in men younger than 40.

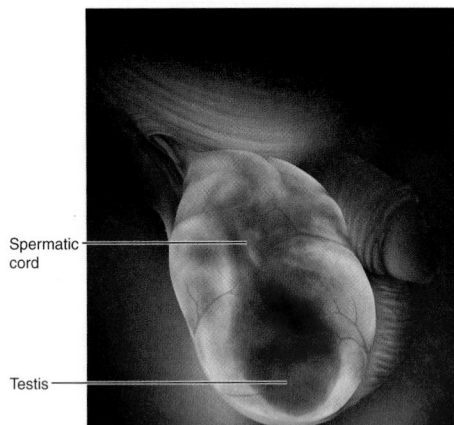

Spermatic cord

Testis

▲ **FIGURE 12.6   Transillumination of Hydrocele Showing Testis and Spermatic Cord.**

Case Report 12.2

Lance Armstrong, the world-renowned cyclist, presented with hemoptysis (coughing up blood). He had ignored a slight swelling of one testis, and the cancer in that testis had already metastasized to his lungs and brain. He required extensive chemotherapy, with brain surgery to remove several metastases.

Forty percent of testicular cancers are **seminomas,** made up of immature germ cells. Nonseminomas occur in different combinations of **choriocarcinoma, embryonal cell,** and **teratoma.** Lance Armstrong's cancer was 60% choriocarcinoma and 40% embryonal cell. The initial treatment for testicular cancer is surgical removal of the affected testis **(orchiectomy),** followed by chemotherapy and sometimes radiation therapy.

WORD	PRONUNCIATION	ELEMENTS		DEFINITION
choriocarcinoma	KOH-ree-oh-kar-sih-NOH-mah	S/ R/CF R/	-oma *tumor* chori/o- *membrane, chorion* -carcin- *cancer*	Highly malignant cancer in a testis or ovary
cryptorchism	krip-TOR-kizm	S/ P/ R/	-ism *condition* crypt- *hidden* -orch- *testicle*	Failure of one or both testes to descend into the scrotum
epididymis	ep-ih-DID-ih-mis	P/ R/	epi- *above* -didymis *testis*	Coiled tube attached to the testis
epididymitis	EP-ih-did-ih-MY-tis	S/	-itis *inflammation*	Inflammation of the epididymis
epididymoorchitis (syn: orchitis)	ep-ih-DID-ih-moh-or-KIE-tis	S/ P/ R/CF R/	-itis *inflammation* epi- *above* -didym/o- *testis* -orch- *testicle*	Inflammation of the epididymis and testicle
hydrocele	HIGH-droh-seal	S/ R/CF	-cele *cave, swelling* hydr/o- *water*	Collection of fluid in the space of the tunica vaginalis
infertility	in-fer-TIL-ih-tee	S/ P/ R/	-ity *condition* in- *not* -fertil- *able to conceive*	Failure to conceive
orchiectomy	or-key-ECK-toe-me	S/ R/CF	-ectomy *surgical excision* orch/i- *testicle*	Removal of one or both testes
orchitis (syn: epididymoorchitis) orchiopexy (*Note:* The letter "o" is added to make the word flow.)	or-KIE-tis OR-key-oh-PEK-see	S/ R/ S/ R/CF	-itis *inflammation* orch- *testicle* -pexy *surgical fixation* orch/i- *testicle*	Inflammation of the testis Surgical fixation of a testis in the scrotum
seminoma	sem-ih-NO-mah	S/ R/	-oma *tumor, mass* semin- *scatter seed*	Neoplasm of germ cells of a testis
spermatocele	SPER-mat-oh-seal	S/ R/CF	-cele *cave, swelling* spermat/o- *sperm*	Cyst of the epididymis that contains sperm
teratoma	ter-ah-TOE-mah	S/ R/	-oma *tumor, mass* terat- *monster, malformed fetus*	Neoplasm of a testis or ovary containing multiple tissues from other sites in the body
varicocele	VAIR-ih-koh-seal	S/ R/CF	-cele *cave, swelling* varic/o- *varicosity*	Varicose veins of the spermatic cord

EXERCISES   *After reading Case Report 12.2 on the opposite page, answer the following questions. Be prepared to discuss your answers in class.*

1. What element in *hemoptysis* confirms that the patient is coughing up blood?

_____

2. You learned in a previous chapter the medical term for *swelling*. Write it here:

_____

3. What does "already metastasized to his lungs and brain" mean for the patient?

_____

4. What is another medical term for *testis*? _____

5. What did the patient's follow-up treatment plan include? _____

_____

Spermatic Ducts and Accessory Glands

OBJECTIVES

The information provided in this lesson will enable you to:

12.2.1 **Trace the pathway taken by a sperm cell from a testis to its ejaculation.**

12.2.2 **Identify the structure and functions of the prostate and other male accessory glands.**

12.2.3 **Describe the origins, structure, and functions of semen.**

12.2.4 **Apply correct medical terminology to the anatomy and physiology of the spermatic ducts, the prostate, and other accessory glands.**

You are

. . . a surgical technologist **(LCC-ST)** working with **urologist** Phillip Johnson, MD, in the **Urology** Clinic at Fulwood Medical Center.

Your patient is

. . . Mr. Ronald Detrick, a 60-year-old man who has been referred to the Urology Clinic c/o having to get out of bed to urinate four or five times at night.

CASE REPORT 12.3

Mr. Detrick has difficulty starting urination, has a weak stream, and feels he is not emptying his bladder completely. His symptoms have been gradually worsening over the past year. He has lost interest in sex. His physical examination is unremarkable except that digital rectal examination **(DRE)** reveals a diffusely enlarged prostate with no nodules.

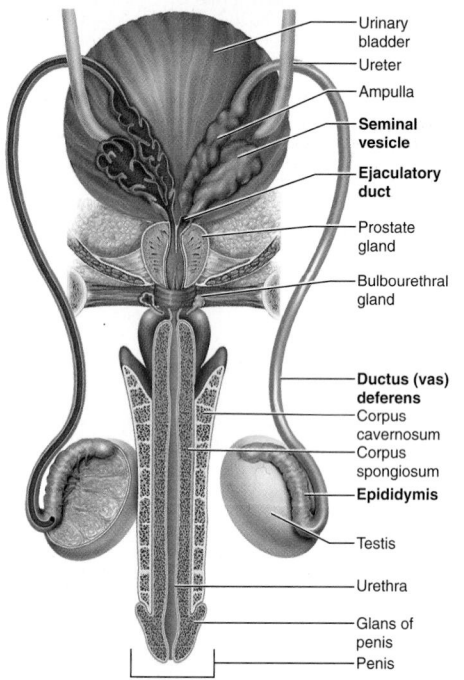

Urinary bladder
Ureter
Ampulla
Seminal vesicle
Ejaculatory duct
Prostate gland
Bulbourethral gland
Ductus (vas) deferens
Corpus cavernosum
Corpus spongiosum
Epididymis
Testis
Urethra
Glans of penis
Penis

▲ **FIGURE 12.7** **Components of Male Reproductive Ducts.**

Abbreviations

DRE	digital rectal examination
LCC-ST	Liaison Council on Certification for the Surgical Technologist

SPERMATIC DUCTS

The male prostate and urethra have both **urological** and **reproductive** functions, as the flow of urine and semen goes through both organs. Disorders of the prostate and urethra produce symptoms and signs that arise in both areas. This makes it essential to have knowledge of their anatomy, physiology, and terminology to be able to understand both functions.

Spermatic Ducts

As the sperm cells mature in the testes over a 60-day period, they move down the seminiferous tubules and pass into a network of tubules called the **rete testis.** From here, they move into the epididymis, into the ductus (vas) deferens, the ejaculatory duct, and finally the urethra to reach the outside of the body *(Figure 12.7)*.

The epididymis adheres to the posterior side of the testis. It is a single coiled duct in which the sperm are stored for 12 to 20 days until they mature and become **motile.** Stored sperm remain fertile for 40 to 60 days. If they become too old without being **ejaculated,** they disintegrate and are reabsorbed in the epididymis.

The ductus (vas) deferens is a muscular duct that travels up from the epididymis in the scrotum and through the inguinal canal *(see Chapter 5)* into the pelvic cavity *(Figure 12.7)*. Here the ductus turns medially and passes behind the urinary bladder and widens into a terminal **ampulla,** which joins with the duct of the seminal **vesicle.**

The **ejaculatory duct,** formed by the ductus deferens and seminal vesicle, is a short (¾-inch or 2-cm) duct that passes through the prostate gland and empties its contents of sperm and seminal fluid (semen) into the urethra.

WORD	PRONUNCIATION	ELEMENTS		DEFINITION
ampulla	am-**PULL**-ah		Latin *two-handled bottle*	Dilated portion of a canal or duct
ejaculate (*Note:* This term can be a verb or noun.)	ee-**JACK**-you-late	S/ R/	-ate *composed of, pertaining to* ejacul- *shoot out*	To expel suddenly, or the semen expelled in ejaculation
ejaculation	ee-**JACK**-you-**LAY**-shun	S/	-ation *process*	Process of expelling semen suddenly
motile	**MOH**-til	S/ R/	-ile *capable* mot- *to move*	Capable of spontaneous movement
motility (noun)	moh-**TILL**-ih-tee	S/	-ility *condition, state of*	The ability for spontaneous movement
reproductive	ree-pro-**DUC**-tiv	S/ P/	-ive *nature of, pertaining to* re- *again*	Relating to the process by which organisms produce offspring
reproduction (noun)	ree-pro-**DUC**-shun	R/ S/	-product- *lead forth* -ion *action, process*	
rete testis	**REE**-teh **TES**-tis		**rete** Latin *net* **testis** Latin *testis*	Network of tubules between the seminiferous tubules and the epididymis
urology	you-**ROL**-oh-jee	S/ R/CF	-logy *study of* ur/o- *urinary system*	Medical specialty of disorders of the urinary system
urologist	you-**ROL**-oh-jist	S/	-logist *one who studies, specialist*	Medical specialist in disorders of the urinary system
urological (adj)	yur-oh-**LOJ**-ih-kal	R/ S/	-log *study of* -ical *pertaining to*	Pertaining to urology
vesicle	**VES**-ih-kull		Latin *a blister*	Small sac containing liquid; for example, a blister or, in this case, semen

---

EXERCISES

Recall and Review: *Certain medical terms can appear in more than one body system. You need to know both applications of the same term. An example is given below as a series of questions that should help you learn to make various connections across the study material when you meet one of these terms.*

1. In this WAD, the Latin definition of **vesicle** is _____.

2. In what other *body system* would you see this term? _____

3. The specialist treating the body system in question 2 would be a _____ .

4. In what type of condition might a vesicle appear? _____

5. What is the role or function of a vesicle in this chapter's body system?

_____

_____

6. How are the uses of the term **vesicle** in these two body systems similar? Dissimilar?

_____

_____

_____

_____

Study Hint

"**SEVEN UP**" is used to remember the pathway of sperm.

S = seminiferous tubules
E = epididymis
V = vas deferens (now called ductus deferens)
E = ejaculatory duct
(N = nothing)
U = urethra
P = penis

ACCESSORY GLANDS

Seminal fluid contains components produced by all three accessory glands *(Figure 12.8)*. The functions of seminal fluid are to:

- **Provide nutrients** to the sperm as they are in the urethra and female reproductive tract.
- **Neutralize acid secretions** of the vagina (in which sperm cannot survive).
- **Provide hormones (prostaglandins)** that widen the opening of the cervix to enable sperm to enter more easily.
- **Provide the fluid vehicle** in which sperm can swim.

The two seminal vesicles are located on the posterior surface of the urinary bladder. The wall of each vesicle contains mucosal folds. They produce a viscous, yellowish, alkaline fluid that contains fructose and prostaglandins. Fructose is a sugar that provides energy for the sperm.

The single **prostate gland** is located immediately below the bladder and anterior to the rectum and surrounds the urethra and the **ejaculatory** duct. It is composed of 30 to 50 glands that open directly into the urethra. The glands secrete a slightly milky fluid that contains:

- **Citric acid,** a nutrient for sperm.
- **An antibiotic** that combats **urinary tract infections (UTIs)** in the male.
- **Clotting factors** that hold the sperm together in a sticky mass until **ejaculation.**
- **Prostate-specific antigen (PSA),** an enzyme that helps liquefy the sticky mass following ejaculation.

The two bulbourethral glands are located one on each side of the membranous urethra. Each gland has a short duct leading into the spongy (penile) urethra. The glands secrete a clear, slippery, alkaline mucus that protects the sperm as they pass through the urethra by neutralizing any residual acid urine. It also acts as a lubricant during sexual intercourse.

Semen is derived from the secretions of several glands:

- 5% comes from the testicles and epididymis.
- 50% to 80% comes from the seminal vesicles.
- 15% to 33% comes from the prostate gland.
- 2% to 5% comes from the bulbourethral glands.

Abbreviations

mL	milliliter
PSA	prostate-specific antigen
UTI	urinary tract infection

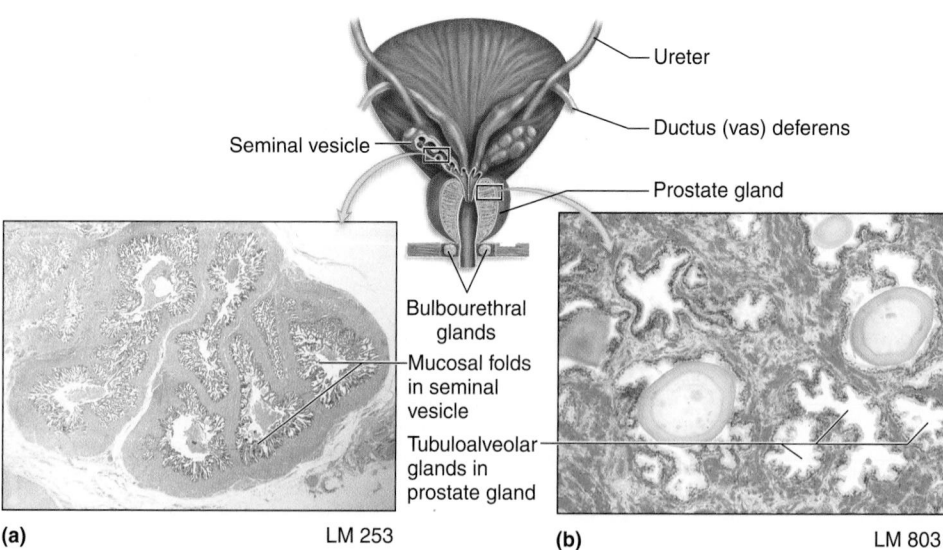

(a) LM 253   (b) LM 803

▲ **FIGURE 12.8   Accessory Glands of the Male Reproductive System.**
(a) Seminal vesicle. (b) Prostate gland.

WORD	PRONUNCIATION	ELEMENTS		DEFINITION
prostate	**PROS**-tate (***Note:*** *not* **PROS**-trate.)		Greek *one standing before*	Organ surrounding the beginning of the urethra
prostatic (adj)	pros-**TAT**-ik	S/ R/	-tic *pertaining to* prosta- *prostate*	Pertaining to the prostate
prostaglandin	**PROS**-tah-**GLAN**-din	S/ R/ R/	-in *chemical* prosta- *prostate* -gland- *gland*	Hormone present in many tissues, but first isolated from the prostate gland

EXERCISES

Elements: *Test your knowledge of the **language of reproduction**. Circle the best answer.*

1. PSA and prostaglandin:
   a. an enzyme and a hormone
   b. a hormone and an enzyme
   c. a hormone and an antibiotic
   d. a diagnostic test and an antibiotic
   e. none of the above

2. The two bulbourethral glands are located:
   a. near the ureters
   b. on each side of the membranous urethra
   c. behind the seminal vesicles
   d. on top of the prostate gland
   e. under the vas deferens

3. The suffix in the term **prostaglandin** tells you it is a:
   a. hormone
   b. enzyme
   c. protein
   d. chemical
   e. blood cell

4. The root for **prostatic** is:
   a. adeno-
   b. prosta-
   c. gland-
   d. ren-
   e. nephro-

5. Every term in this WAD is composed of:
   a. two roots
   b. a root and a combining form
   c. a root and a prefix
   d. at least one root and a suffix
   e. two prefixes and a root

6. In the abbreviation UTI, the "T" stands for:
   a. torsion
   b. testicle
   c. tract
   d. testosterone
   e. tunica

7. **Semen** is derived from the secretions of several glands:
   a. testicles, epididymis
   b. accessory glands
   c. thymus gland
   d. a, b, and c
   e. a and b only

8. The **prostate gland** is located:
   a. below the bladder and posterior to the rectum
   b. beside the bladder and anterior to the rectum
   c. below the bladder and anterior to the rectum
   d. beside the bladder and posterior to the rectum
   e. between the bladder and the kidney

9. What is a nutrient for sperm?
   a. alkaline mucus
   b. acid urine
   c. citric acid
   d. normal flora
   e. acid secretions of the vagina

10. In the abbreviation **PSA**, the "A" stands for:
    a. antidiuretic
    b. antibiotic
    c. antigen
    d. antibody
    e. allergen

11. What is the fluid vehicle for sperm?
    a. bloodstream
    b. lymph system
    c. plasma
    d. aqueous humor
    e. seminal fluid

12. What provides energy for sperm?
    a. citric acid
    b. prostaglandins
    c. fructose
    d. a and c
    e. none of these

DISORDERS OF THE PROSTATE GLAND

By the age of 20, the prostate weighs about 20 grams. It remains at that weight until age 45 to 50, when it begins to grow again. By age 80, some 90% of men have **benign prostatic hyperplasia (BPH)**. This is a noncancerous enlargement that compresses the prostatic urethra to produce symptoms of:

- Difficulty starting and stopping the urine stream.
- **Nocturia, polyuria,** and dysuria.

In some patients, surgical treatment by **transurethral resection of the prostate (TURP)** relieves the symptoms. An endoscope called a **resectoscope** is inserted into the urethra and used to remove the tissue surrounding and compressing the urethra.

Prostatic cancer affects more than 10% of men over the age of 50, and its incidence is increasing. It forms hard nodules in the periphery of the gland and is often asymptomatic in its early stages because it does not compress the urethra.

Screening for prostatic cancer is performed by:

- **Digital rectal exam.** The size and texture of the prostate is palpated by a finger inserted into the rectum.
- **Prostate-specific antigen (PSA)** levels in the blood. Even though cancer can be present when the level is zero, the benefit of the test is to see if levels rise rapidly over time.

Several treatment options involving radiotherapy are available *(see Chapter 24)*. Sometimes, a **radical prostatectomy,** with complete surgical removal of the prostate and surrounding tissues, is performed.

Prostatitis is inflammation of the prostate gland. It occurs in three main types:

Type I—an acute bacterial infection with fever, chills, frequency, dysuria, and hematuria.

Type 11—a chronic bacterial infection with less severe symptoms.

Type III—a chronic nonbacterial prostatitis in which the urinary symptoms are present but no bacteria can be detected. This is the most common type. Its etiology is unknown and treatment is difficult.

Male Infertility

Male infertility is the inability to conceive after at least 1 year of unprotected intercourse. The primary causes of infertility are:

1. Impaired sperm production:
   - **a.** Cryptorchism
   - **b. Anorchism** (absence of one or both testes)
   - **c.** Testicular trauma
   - **d.** Testicular cancer
   - **e.** Orchitis after puberty
2. Impaired sperm delivery:
   - **a.** Infections and blockage of spermatic ducts.
3. Testosterone deficiency **(hypogonadism):**
   - **a.** Medications to treat hypertension and/or high cholesterol.
   - **b.** Environmental endocrine disrupters that adversely affect the endocrine system; examples are phthalates in plastics and dioxins in paper production.

In the United States each year, 500,000 men choose to be made infertile **(sterile)** by having a **vasectomy.** Under local anesthesia, the ductus deferens is pulled through a small incision in the scrotum and cut in two places, a 1-centimeter segment is removed, and the ends are cauterized and tied. The site of the surgery makes the man infertile but still able to produce and ejaculate seminal fluid.

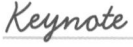
Keynote

Survival from prostate cancer is up to 80% if it is detected before it spreads outside the gland.

Abbreviations

BPH benign prostatic hyperplasia
TURP transurethral resection of the prostate
NIH National Institutes of Health

Keynote

Male infertility is involved in 40% of the 2.6 million infertile married couples in the United States (Data from the **National Institutes of Health [NIH]**).

Vasectomy is almost 100% successful in producing male sterility.

Keynote

Vasovasostomy is a microsurgical procedure to suture back together **(anastomosis)** the cut ends of the ductus deferens if requested following vasectomy.

WORD	PRONUNCIATION	ELEMENTS		DEFINITION
anastomosis anastomoses (pl)	ah-**NAS**-to-**MO**-sis	S/ R/	-osis *condition* anastom- *join together*	A surgically made union between two tubular structures
anorchism	an-**OR**-kizm	S/ P/ R/	-ism *condition* an- *without, lack of* -orch- *testicle*	Absence of testes
hyperplasia	high-per-**PLAY**-zee-ah	S/ P/ R/	-ia *condition* hyper- *excessive* -plas- *molding, formation*	Increase in the number of the cells in a tissue or organ
hypogonadism	**HIGH**-poh-**GOH**-nad-izm	S/ P/ R/	-ism *condition* hypo- *deficient* -gonad- *testes or ovaries*	Deficient gonad production of sperm or eggs or hormones
nocturia	nok-**TYU**-ree-ah	P/ R/	noct- *night* -uria *urine*	Excessive urination at night
polyuria	pol-ee-**YOU**-ree-ah	P/ R/	poly- *excessive* -uria *urine*	Excessive production of urine
prostatectomy	pross-tah-**TEK**-toe-me	S/ R/	-ectomy *surgical excision* prostat- *prostate*	Surgical removal of the prostate
prostatitis	pross-tah-**TIE**-tis	S/ R/	-itis *inflammation* prostat- *prostate*	Inflammation of the prostate
resectoscope	ree-**SEK**-toe-skope	S/ R/CF	-scope *instrument* resect/o- *cut off*	Endoscope for transurethral removal of lesions
sterile sterility	**STER**-isle steh-**RIL**-ih-tee	 S/ R/	Latin *barren* -ity *state, condition* steril- *barren*	Unable to fertilize or reproduce Inability to reproduce
vasectomy	vah-**SEK**-toe-me	S/ R/	-ectomy *surgical excision* vas- *duct*	Excision of a segment of the ductus deferens
vasovasostomy (also called **vasectomy reversal**)	**VAY**-soh-vay-**SOS**-toe-me	S/ R/CF	-stomy *new opening* vas/o- *duct*	Reanastomosis of the ductus deferens to restore the flow of sperm

EXERCISES

Recognition: *As you become more familiar with elements (especially suffixes), you will be able to recognize medical terms that are procedures and diagnoses. Practice with the terms in this WAD. Fill in the blanks.*

1. List all the terms in this WAD that could be a possible diagnosis for a patient.

_____

_____

2. List all the terms in this WAD that are a procedure.

_____

_____

_____

3. Which term in this WAD is an instrument?

_____

4. Which term or terms involve a surgical reconnection?

_____

LESSON 12.3 The Penis and Its Disorders

OBJECTIVES

The structure of the penis is specifically designed to meet its two main functions:

- **Deposit semen in the female vagina around the cervix.**
- **Enable urine to flow to the outside.**

It is essential that the anatomy, physiology, and terminology of the penis as related to performing these two functions be understood.

The information in this lesson will enable you to:

12.3.1 Apply correct medical terminology to the structure and functions of the penis.

12.3.2 Summarize the processes and functions of erection and ejaculation.

12.3.3 Describe common disorders of the penis and prepuce.

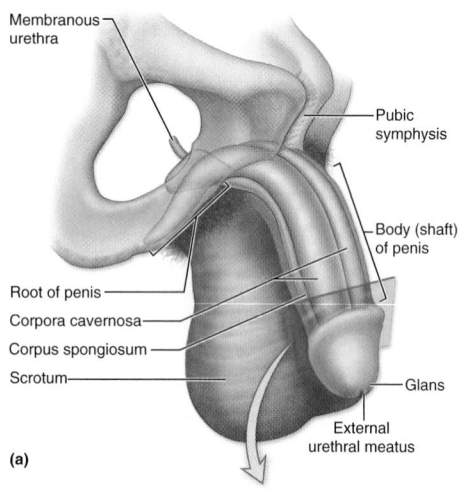

Membranous urethra
Pubic symphysis
Body (shaft) of penis
Root of penis
Corpora cavernosa
Corpus spongiosum
Scrotum
Glans
External urethral meatus
(a)

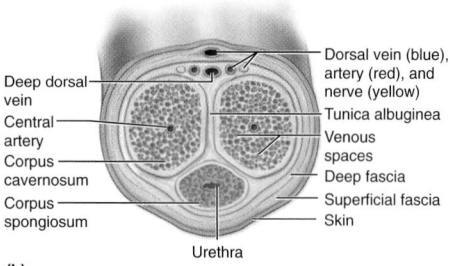

Deep dorsal vein
Central artery
Corpus cavernosum
Corpus spongiosum
Urethra
Dorsal vein (blue), artery (red), and nerve (yellow)
Tunica albuginea
Venous spaces
Deep fascia
Superficial fascia
Skin
(b)

▲ **FIGURE 12.9   Anatomy of Penis.**
(a) External anatomy. (b) Cross-sectional view.

Abbreviations

ED	erectile dysfunction
STD	sexually transmitted disease

Keynote

Erectile dysfunction occurs in some 20 million American men.

PENIS

The external, visible part of the penis comprises the **shaft** and the **glans,** at the tip of which the external urethral meatus is located. The skin of the penis is very loosely attached to the shaft to permit expansion during erection. The skin continues over the glans as the **prepuce** (foreskin). A ventral fold of tissue, the **frenulum,** attaches the skin to the glans. The glans and facing prepuce contain sebaceous glands that produce a waxy secretion called **smegma.**

The shaft of the penis contains three **erectile** vascular bodies *(Figure 12.9):*

- Paired **corpora cavernosa** are located dorsolaterally.
- A single **corpus spongiosum** is located inferiorly. It contains the urethra and goes on to form the glans.

The corpora cavernosa are composed of a network of venous sinuses surrounding a central artery. **Erection** occurs when the sinuses fill with blood, causing the erectile bodies to distend and become rigid. It is a parasympathetic nervous system response to stimulation.

Ejaculation occurs when the sympathetic nervous system stimulates the smooth muscle of the ductus deferens, ejaculatory ducts, and the prostate gland to contract. The seminal vesicles contract so that their fluids join to form semen. The internal urethral sphincter also contracts so that urine cannot enter the urethra and semen cannot enter the bladder.

Disorders of the Penis

Trauma to the penis can vary from being caught in a pants zipper to a fracture of an erect penis during vigorous sexual intercourse.

Peyronie disease is a marked curvature of the erect penis caused by fibrous tissue. Its etiology is unknown, and there is no successful treatment.

Priapism is a persistent, painful erection when blood cannot escape from the erectile tissue. It can be caused by drugs (such as epinephrine), blood clots, or spinal cord injury.

Cancer of the penis occurs most commonly on the glans and is rare in circumcised men. Circumcision also offers some protection against HIV infection.

Syphilis can cause flat pink or gray growths called **condylomata** or a sore called a **chancre.**

Other **STDs** can produce small, firm genital warts called **condylomata acuminata** or firm, dimpled growths called **molluscum contagiosum.** The STDs are discussed in detail in *Chapter 13.*

Erectile dysfunction (ED), or **impotence,** is the inability to have a satisfactory erection. **Premature ejaculation** occurs when a man ejaculates so quickly during intercourse that it causes embarrassment.

WORD	PRONUNCIATION		ELEMENTS	DEFINITION
balanitis	bal-ah-**NIE**-tis	S/ R/	-itis *inflammation* balan- *glans penis*	Inflammation of the glans and prepuce of the penis
circumcision	ser-kum-**SIZH**-un	S/ P/ R/	-ion *process, action* circum- *around* -cis- *to cut*	To remove part or all of the prepuce
contraception	kon-trah-**SEP**-shun	S/ P/ R/	-ion *process, action* contra- *against* -cept *to receive*	Prevention of conception
contraceptive	kon-trah-**SEP**-tiv	S/	-ive *quality of, nature of*	Agent that prevents conception
dorsum	**DOR**-sum		Latin *back*	Upper, posterior, or back surface
epispadias	ep-ih-**SPAY**-dee-as	S/ P/ R/	-ias *condition* epi- *above* -spad- *tear or cut*	Condition in which the urethral opening is on the dorsum of the penis
foreskin	**FOR**-skin	P/ R/	fore- *in front* -skin *skin*	Skin that covers the glans penis
hypospadias	high-poh-**SPAY**-dee-as	S/ P/ R/	-ias *condition* hypo- *below* -spad- *tear or cut*	Urethral opening more proximal than normal on the ventral surface of the penis
paraphimosis	**PAR**-ah-fi-**MOH**-sis	S/ P/ R/	-osis *condition* para- *abnormal* -phim- *muzzle*	Condition in which a retracted prepuce cannot be pulled forward to cover the glans
phimosis	fi-**MOH**-sis	S/ R/	-osis *condition* phim- *muzzle*	Condition in which the prepuce cannot be retracted
spermicide	**SPER**-mih-side	S/ R/CF	-cide *to kill* sperm/i- *sperm*	Agent that destroys sperm
spermicidal (adj)	**SPER**-mih-side-al	S/	-al *pertaining to*	Pertaining to the destruction of sperm
stricture	**STRICK**-shur		Latin *to draw tight*	Narrowing of a tube
urethrotomy	you-ree-**THROT**-oh-me	S/ R/CF	-tomy *surgical incision* urethr/o- *urethra*	Incision of a stricture of the urethra

EXERCISES   *Refine your knowledge of the **language of urology** by choosing the correct term to complete the statement. Circle the best choice. Be precise and watch the spelling!*

1. Inflammation of the glans and prepuce is:

   urethritis   cystitis   balanitis   hypospadias

2. Condition in which a retracted prepuce cannot be pulled forward to cover the glans:

   hypospadias   phimosis   spongiosum   paraphimosis

3. Incision of a stricture of the urethra:

   urethrectomy   urethroplasty   urethropexy   urethrotomy

4. To remove all or part of the prepuce:

   circumcision   circumscion   circummcision   circumsion

5. Skin that covers the glans penis:

   forskin   fourskin   forksin   foreskin

6. Narrowing of a tube:

   dilation   anastomosis   stricture   retraction

MALE REPRODUCTIVE SYSTEM

CHALLENGE YOUR KNOWLEDGE

A. Patient Documentation: Reread the Case Report from the beginning of this chapter

You are

. . . an EMT-P working in the Emergency Department at Fulwood Medical Center.

Your Patient Is

. . . Joseph Davis, a 17-year-old high school senior.

CASE REPORT 12.1

He is brought in by his mother at 0400 hrs. He complains of (c/o) sudden onset of pain in his left testicle 3 hours earlier that woke him up. The pain is intense and has made him vomit. VS: T 99.2°F, P 88, R 15, BP 130/70. Examination reveals his left testicle to be enlarged, warm, and tender. His abdomen is normal to palpation.

At your request, Dr. Helinski, the emergency physician on duty, examines him immediately. He diagnoses a torsion of the patient's left testicle.

Joseph Davis presented with typical symptoms and signs of testicular torsion. The affected testis rapidly became painful, tender, swollen, and inflamed. Emergency surgery was performed, and the testis and cord were manually untwisted through an incision in the scrotum. The testis was stitched to surrounding tissues to prevent a recurrence.

Dr. Helinski, the emergency physician on duty, has referred Joseph Davis to a surgeon for repair of his condition, and it is your duty to obtain from the patient's insurance company preapproval for the surgery. You must be prepared to furnish answers to the following questions the insurance company will ask. You make the telephone call to the 800 number listed on the patient's insurance card for preauthorization of hospitalization or surgery. You have answered all the usual insurance questions regarding the patient's subscriber ID number, group number, name of policyholder, and so on. The insurance company needs answers to the following clinical questions in order to preapprove the surgery. Fill in the blanks.

1. What is the patient's diagnosis? _____

2. With what symptoms did the patient present to the Emergency Department? _____

3. Is this condition the result of an accident? _____

4. What procedure is the surgeon going to perform? _____

5. Can you briefly describe this procedure?

   _____

6. Why is this procedure a surgical emergency?

   _____

On the basis of your answers, the insurance company representative has preapproved the surgery and one overnight stay in the hospital for the patient. Be sure to record the insurance company's preapproval reference number, the name of the person who gave it to you, and the date and time of your conversation.

B. "It's all Greek to me." Many urology terms are rooted in Latin or Greek. Fill in the chart with a check mark (✓) in the column for Latin or Greek origin; then give the meaning of the term.

Medical Term	Latin	Greek	Meaning
ampulla			
chancre			
deferens			
dorsum			
flagellum			

Medical Term	Latin	Greek	Meaning
libido			
prepuce			
septum			
torsion			
tunica			

C. **Short Answer:** To demonstrate that you really understand the processes and functions of components of the male urinary system, write a short answer that describes each of the following:

1. How a vasectomy renders a male sterile

_____

_____

_____

2. The primary causes of male infertility

_____

_____

_____

D. **Trace the pathway taken by a sperm cell from the testes to its ejaculation.** Number the following terms in the correct order. Fill in the blanks. *Remember your study hint!*

_____ a. epididymis

_____ b. urethra

_____ c. (nothing)

_____ d. seminiferous tubules

_____ e. ejaculatory duct

_____ f. ductus deferens

_____ g. penis

E. **Brain Teaser:** Taken directly from this chapter: "If it (a varicose vein in the spermatic cord) is uncomfortable, it can be treated by surgically tying off the affected veins." Rewrite this information in more precise medical language.

_____

_____

_____

_____

_____

MALE REPRODUCTIVE SYSTEM

F. Language of Urology: Every day on the job in the Urology Clinic you will be asked to apply the **language of urology** to the anatomy and physiology of the male reproductive system. Circle the correct choice.

1. The prostate, seminal vesicles, and bulbourethral glands are all:

   a. gonads

   b. primary sex organs

   c. accessory glands

   d. secondary sex organs

   e. none of the above

2. Surgical procedure that makes a male sterile:

   a. nephrectomy

   b. vasovasostomy

   c. orchiopexy

   d. vasectomy

   e. lithotripsy

3. Shining a bright light on a swelling to see the shape of the testes:

   a. maturation

   b. micturition

   c. vasoepididymostomy

   d. orchiopexy

   e. transillumination

4. Scarring that narrows the urethra is called:

   a. UTI

   b. urethral stricture

   c. ureteroscope

   d. urethrotomy

   e. urethropexy

5. The diamond-shaped region between the thighs is called:

   a. rete testis

   b. perineum

   c. median septum

   d. ductus deferens

   e. anal triangle

6. Androgens are:

   a. enzymes

   b. vitamins

   c. hormones

   d. special nerve cells

   e. flagellum

7. The penis, scrotum, and testes collectively are known as:

   a. primary sex organs

   b. accessory glands

   c. secondary sex organs

   d. external genitalia

   e. none of the above

8. Measured in a blood test to check for prostate cancer:

   a. BPH

   b. TURP

   c. BMR

   d. PSA

   e. ED

9. A female egg cell is called:

   a. flagellum

   b. spermatozoa

   c. spermatid

   d. oocyte

   e. varicocele

10. The distinct ridge in the scrotum is called the:

    a. dartos

    b. raphe

    c. hydrocele

    d. epididymis

    e. cavernosa

MALE REPRODUCTIVE SYSTEM

G. **Language of Urology:** Every day on the job in the Urology Clinic you will be asked to apply the **language of urology** to the anatomy and physiology of the male reproductive system. Circle the correct choice.

1. Transports the sperm away from the testes:

   a. spermatic cord

   b. autonomic nerves

   c. ductus deferens

   d. bulbourethral glands

   e. seminal vesicle

2. Suspends each testis in the scrotum:

   a. spermatic cord

   b. ductus deferens

   c. dartos muscle

   d. interstitial cells

   e. tunica

3. An endoscope that is inserted into the urethra to remove excess prostatic tissue is a:

   a. cystoscope

   b. ureteroscope

   c. resectoscope

   d. hysteroscope

   e. none of the above

4. The ductus deferens is also known as the:

   a. sustentacular cells

   b. seminiferous tubules

   c. tunica vaginalis

   d. tubuloalveolar glands

   e. vas deferens

5. **Hypogonadism** is a term meaning:

   a. undescended testis

   b. low sperm count

   c. testosterone deficiency

   d. male infertility

   e. premature ejaculation

H. Roots: The following medical terms all share the same root/combining form. Employ your knowledge of the other elements to determine the correct term for the sentence. First, slash (/) each term so that you can identify the elements. Then fill in the blanks.

| cryptorchism | orchitis | epididymoorchitis | orchiopexy | orchiectomy | anorchism |

1. Patient has inflammation of the epididymis and testicle on the right side. Diagnosis: _____

2. Patient was born without testes. Diagnosis: _____

3. Patient had one diseased testicle removed. Procedure: _____

4. Patient had testicular torsion repaired. Procedure: _____

5. Patient has inflammation of both testicles. Diagnosis: _____

6. Patient was born with an undescended right testicle. Diagnosis: _____

I. Study Review: Taking a test on any body system involves remembering a lot of information and terminology. Making short lists for yourself to study from is easier than trying to remember facts in paragraph context. There are three answers to each of the following questions. Fill in the blanks.

> *Study Hint*
> Use this exercise for a quick study review for a test.

1. Name the accessory glands.

   a. _____

   b. _____

   c. _____

2. Name three symptoms of BPH.

   a. _____

   b. _____

   c. _____

3. What are the three main types of prostatitis? (Specify acute or chronic.)

   a. _____

   b. _____

   c. _____

4. The shaft of the penis contains three erectile vascular bodies. Name them.

   a. _____

   b. _____

   c. _____

5. What are the three disorders that can affect the prepuce?

   a. _____

   b. _____

   c. _____

MALE REPRODUCTIVE SYSTEM

J. Terminology Challenge: Cryptorchism means *hidden* testicle because the testicle has failed to descend from the abdomen.

Find an element from a previous chapter that also means hidden.

1. The element _____ means _____.

2. Use this other element in a sentence.

_____

_____

_____

_____

K. Patient Education: Patients will always have questions that you must be able to answer professionally. How well could you explain to your patient the difference between:

1. The surgical procedures of *vasectomy* and *vasovasostomy*:

_____

_____

_____

2. A *radical prostatectomy* and a *TURP*:

_____

_____

_____

L. Recall and Review: How well do you remember these word elements from the previous chapter? Try to answer without first looking back to check. Fill in the blanks.

Element	Type of Element (P, R, CF, S)	Meaning of Element
ren	_____	_____
ex	_____	_____
peri	_____	_____
hydro	_____	_____
litho	_____	_____

M. Disorder or Disease: Complete the diagnosis documentation for the following patients. Fill in the blanks with the correct medical term for the disorder or disease mentioned in each statement.

1. Excess fluid has collected in the space between the visceral and parietal layers of the tunica vaginalis of the patient's right

   testis: hydro_____

2. Noncancerous enlargement compressing the prostatic urethra: benign _____ plasia

3. Marked curvature of the erect penis caused by fibrous tissue: _____ disease

4. Undescended testicles in a 10-month-old male: _____ism

5. Inability to have a satisfactory erection: _____ dys_____

6. Veins in the spermatic cord become tortuous and dilated: varico_____

7. Opening of the urethra is on the undersurface of the penis instead of at the head of the glans:

   hypo_____

8. Yeast infection of the glans and foreskin: _____itis

9. Foreskin is tight and cannot be retracted over the glans for cleaning: _____sis

10. Inflammation of the epididymis: _____itis

N. **Brain Teaser:** Why is a resectoscope also an endoscope?

_____

_____

O. **Abbreviations are another form of precise communication.** Demonstrate that you know the meanings of the abbreviations in this exercise. Circle the best answer.

1. Diagnosis for a type of prostate disease:

   a. BPH

   b. TURP

   c. PSA

2. Can produce condylomata acuminata:

   a. STD

   b. UTI

   c. ED

3. The abbreviation **BMR** relates to:

   a. metabolism

   b. bowel movement

   c. bulbourethral glands

4. **SET** refers to:

   a. a diagnostic test

   b. something you do yourself

   c. a surgical procedure

P. **Prefixes can be a critical clue to the meaning of a medical term.** Challenge your knowledge of prefixes with this exercise. Write the meaning of the prefix, a medical term containing that prefix, and the meaning of the medical term. Fill in the chart.

Prefix	Meaning of Prefix	Medical Term with Prefix	Meaning of Medical Term
an-			
circum-			
contra-			
crypt-			
epi-			
noct-			
para-			
poly-			

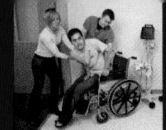

CHAPTER 12 REVIEW

MALE REPRODUCTIVE SYSTEM

CHAPTER SUMMARY EXERCISE

1. *Listen to the pronunciation of the medical terms as given by your instructor.*
2. *Circle the correct spelling of the medical term.*
3. *Match the correctly spelled terms to the brief descriptions below.*
4. *Write a sentence for each of the 10 terms that appear in this exercise.*

A. SPELLING COMPREHENSION: CIRCLE THE CORRECT SPELLING OF THE TERM.

1. gonad	gonnad	gonade	gunad	gunade
2. perikneal	perikneeal	perineal	perrineal	peraneal
3. coriocarcinoma	corriocarcinoma	choriacarcinoma	choriocarcinoma	corheacarcinoma
4. insemination	insemmination	insimination	insimmination	insimation
5. tortion	torsion	tortsion	tortcion	tostion
6. epidydimis	epidydimus	epididymis	epididymus	epodidymis
7. frinulum	frenullum	frenulum	frennulum	frenulumn
8. tistosterune	testosterine	testosterone	tistosterone	testosteron
9. priaprism	piaprism	priapism	prapism	piapresm
10. flagilla	flaggila	flagella	flaggela	flaggilla

B. MATCH THE NUMBER OF THE CORRECT TERM IN PART A WITH THE BRIEF DESCRIPTION OF THE TERM BELOW.

a. Androgen produced by testis _____

b. Highly malignant cancer in testis or ovary _____

c. Plural: tail of a sperm _____

d. The act or result of twisting _____

e. Deposition of semen in female reproductive tract _____

f. Pertaining to the area between the thighs _____

g. Testis or ovary _____

h. Structure on posterior surface of testis _____

i. Persistent, painful erection _____

j. Fold of mucous membrane _____

C. USING YOUR KNOWLEDGE OF TERMS 1–10 IN PART A AND THEIR CORRECT SPELLING, WRITE A BRIEF SENTENCE AS IT MIGHT APPEAR IN PATIENT DOCUMENTATION.

1. _____

2. _____

3. _____

4. _____

5. _____

6. _____

7. _____

8. _____

9. _____

10. _____

D. YOUR INSTRUCTOR WILL DIRECT YOU TO MCGRAW-HILL CONNECT. OPEN THE AUDIO GLOSSARY AND PRACTICE YOUR PRONUNCIATION OF THE TERMS IN PART A OF THIS EXERCISE.

Mc Graw Hill **connect**™ (plus+)

E. AFTER READING CASE REPORT 12.1, ANSWER THE FOLLOWING QUESTIONS. BE PREPARED TO DISCUSS YOUR ANSWERS IN CLASS.

CASE REPORT 12.1

You are

. . . an EMT-P working in the Emergency Department at Fulwood Medical Center.

Your patient is

. . . Joseph Davis, a 17-year-old high school senior. He is brought in by his mother at 0400 hrs. He complains of **(c/o)** sudden onset of pain in his left **testicle** 3 hours earlier that woke him up. The pain is intense and has made him vomit. VS: T 99.2°F, P 88, R 15, BP 130/70. Examination reveals his left testicle to be enlarged, warm, and tender. His abdomen is normal to palpation.

At your request, Dr. Helinski, the emergency physician on duty, examines him immediately. He diagnoses a **torsion** of the patient's left testicle.

Joseph Davis presented with typical symptoms and signs of testicular torsion. The affected testis rapidly became painful, tender, swollen, and inflamed. Emergency surgery was performed, and the testis and cord were manually untwisted through an incision in the scrotum. The testis was stitched to surrounding tissues to prevent a recurrence.

1. In nonmilitary time, when is 0400 hrs? _____

2. Joseph has "sudden onset of pain." Is that acute or chronic? _____

3. Interpret (spell out) each of the VS:

   T = _____

   P = _____

   R = _____

   BP = _____

4. What action is performed in *palpation?* _____

5. What is the difference between a *symptom* and a *sign?*

   Symptom: _____

   Sign: _____

6. In testicular tortion, what gets twisted? _____

7. What is the medical term for "stitched to surrounding tissues"? _____

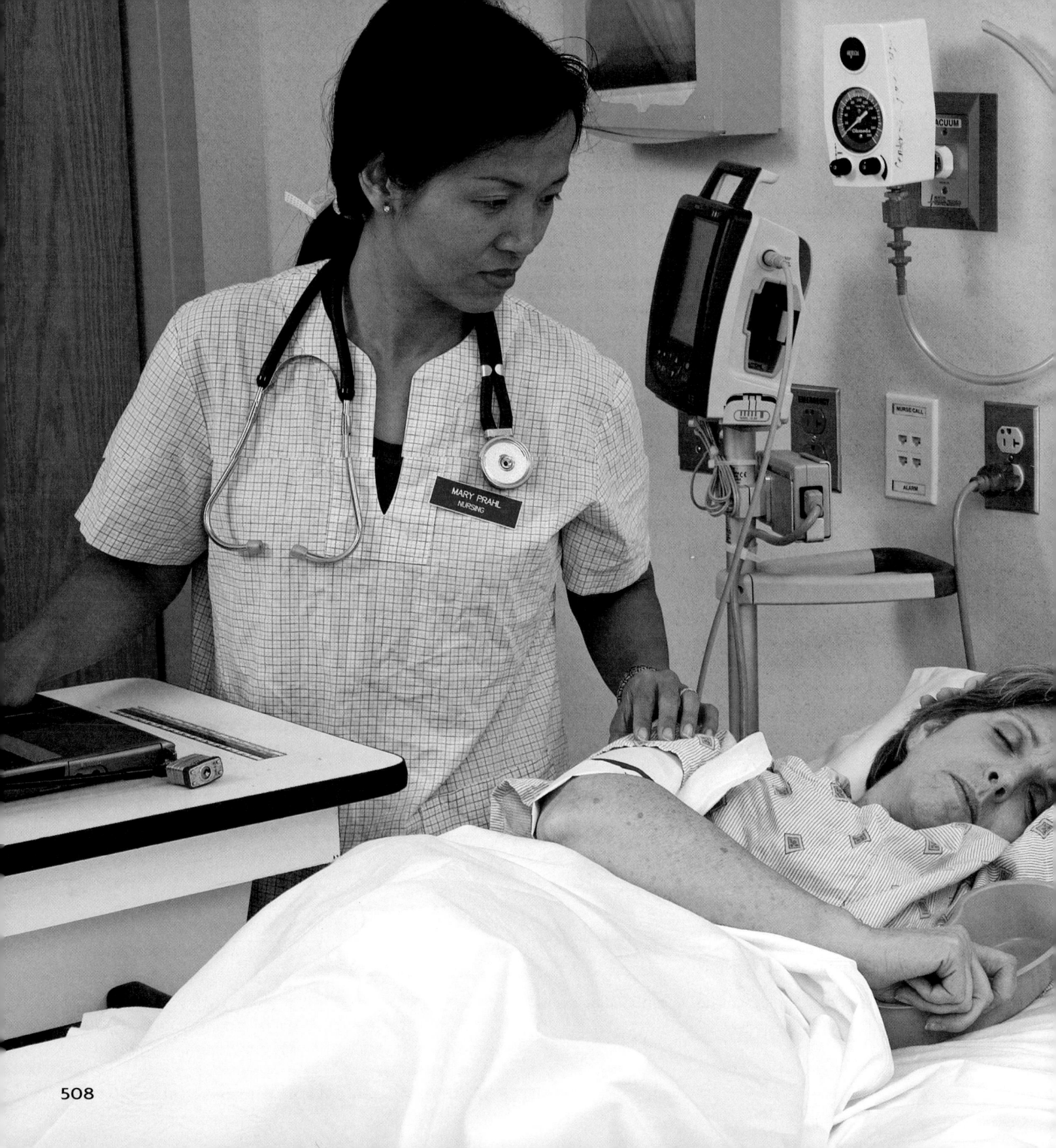

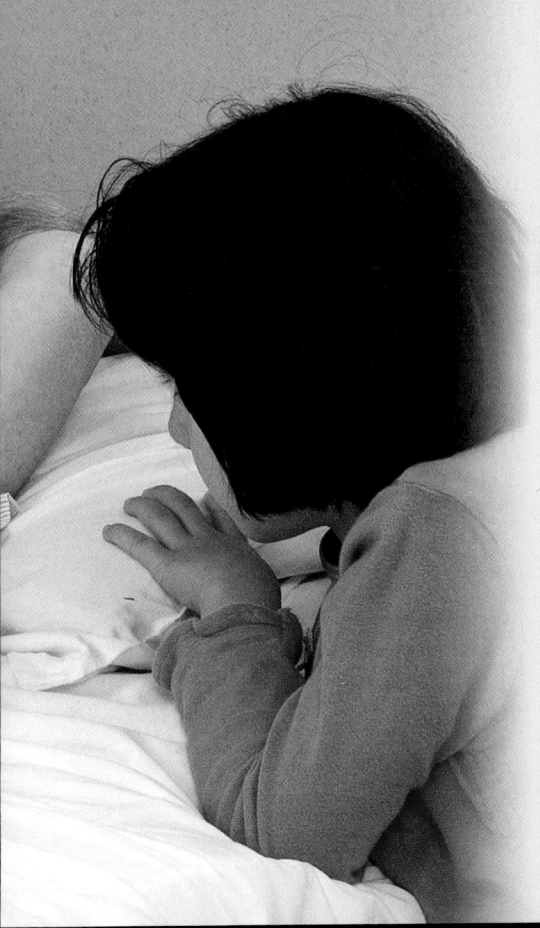

CASE REPORT 13.1

You are

. . . a **licensed practical nurse (LPN)** working in the Emergency Department at Fulwood Medical Center.

Your patient is

. . . Ms. Lara Baker, a 32-year-old single mother who works in the billing department of the medical center. You have been asked to take her vital signs. For the past couple of days she has had muscle aches and a feeling of general uneasiness that she had thought were due to her heavy menstrual period. In the past 3 hours, she has developed a severe headache with nausea and vomiting. A diffuse rash over her trunk that looks like sunburn is now spreading to her upper arms and thighs.

VS: T 104.2°F, P 120 and irregular, R 20, BP 86/50. As you took her VS, you noted that she did not seem to understand where she was. She was unable to pass a urine specimen.

For this patient, the treatment she receives in the next few minutes is vital for her survival. You have your supervising nurse and the emergency physician come to see her immediately. As you participate in this patient's care, clear communication among the team members is essential.

Learning Outcomes

The information in this chapter will enable you to:

13.1 Apply the language of **gynecology** to the anatomy and physiology of the female reproductive system.

13.2 Apply the language of **obstetrics** to the changes that occur in the female reproductive system during pregnancy and labor.

13.3 Recognize and pronounce the medical terms of gynecology and obstetrics as they relate to the female reproductive system so that you communicate verbally with accuracy and precision in any health care setting.

13.4 Comprehend, analyze, spell, and write the medical terms of gynecology and obstetrics as they relate to the female reproductive system in any health care setting.

13.5 Explain the effects of common **gynecologic** problems on health.

13.6 Understand the effects of common disorders of **pregnancy** on the mother and **fetus**.

13.7 Describe the structure and function of the female breast and the results of disorders of the breast.

LESSON 13.1 External Genitalia and Vagina

Both the female and male reproductive systems are dormant until **puberty,** when the gonads (**ovaries** in the female and **testes** in the male) begin to secrete significant quantities of sex hormones (**estrogen** and **progesterone** in the female, **androgens** in the male). In the female, the external **genitalia** become more prominent, pubic hair develops, the **vagina** becomes lubricated, and breast enlargement occurs. Understanding the anatomy and physiology of the mature external genitalia and vagina is an important introduction to the female **reproductive** system.

The information in this lesson will enable you to:

13.1.1 Identify the female external genitalia.

13.1.2 Describe the anatomy and physiology of the accessory glands.

13.1.3 Explain the structure and physiology of the erectile tissues.

13.1.4 Detail the anatomy and physiology of the vagina.

13.1.5 Apply correct medical terminology to the anatomy and physiology of the external genitalia and vagina.

13.1.6 Evaluate the effects of common disorders of the external genitalia and vagina on the health of the female.

EXTERNAL GENITALIA

The female external genitalia occupy most of the **perineum** and are collectively called the **vulva** *(Figure 13.1)*. The structures of the vulva include the:

- **Mons pubis**—a mound of skin and adipose tissue overlying the symphysis pubis. In **postpubescent** females it is covered with **pubic** hair.

- **Labia majora**—a pair of thick folds of skin, connective tissue, and adipose tissue. In postpubescent females, their outer surface is covered with coarse hair, and the inner surface has numerous sweat and sebaceous glands.

- **Labia minora**—a pair of thin folds of hairless skin immediately internal to the labia majora. Sebaceous glands are present on these folds, together with melanocytes *(see Chapter 3)* that give the folds a dark melanin pigmentation. Anteriorly, the labia minora join together to form the prepuce (hood) of the **clitoris.** Posteriorly they merge with the labia majora.

- **Clitoris**—a small erectile body capped with a glans. It has two corpora cavernosa surrounded by connective tissue. The clitoris contains many sensory nerve receptors.

Deep to the labia majora on either side of the vaginal orifice is an erectile body called the **vestibular bulb** *(Figure 13.1b)*. The two bulbs become congested with blood and more sensitive during sexual arousal. Posterior to the vestibular bulbs on each side of the vaginal orifice is a pea-size **Bartholin gland.** These glands secrete mucin, which lubricates the vagina. Secretion is increased during sexual arousal and intercourse.

Abbreviations

LPN	licensed practical nurse
GYN	gynecology
OB	obstetrics

Keynote

- **Obstetrics (OB)** is the medical specialty for the care of women during pregnancy and the **postpartum** period.

- Gynecology is the medical specialty for the care of the female reproductive system.

FIGURE 13.1   Female Perineum and Vulva. ▶
(*a*) Surface anatomy. (*b*) Subcutaneous structures.

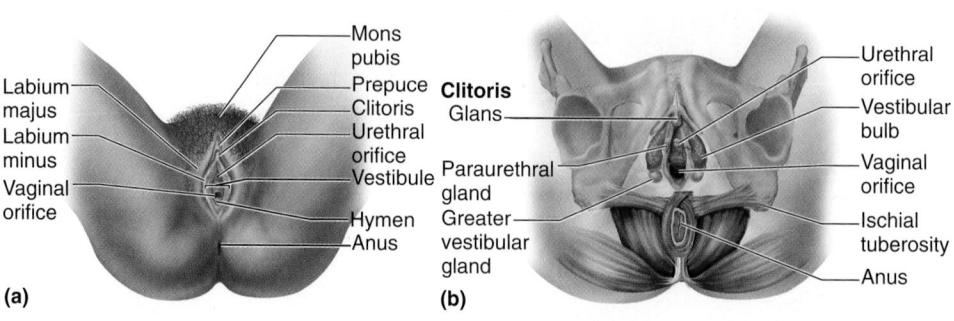

(a)   (b)

WORD ANALYSIS AND DEFINITION

WORD	PRONUNCIATION		ELEMENTS	DEFINITION
clitoris	**KLIT**-oh-ris		Greek *clitoris*	Erectile organ of the vulva
estrogen	**ES**-troh-jen	S/ R/CF	**-gen** *produce, create* **estr/o-** *woman*	Generic term for hormones that stimulate female secondary sex characteristics
gynecology	guy-nih-**KOL**-oh-jee	S/ R/CF	**-logy** *study of* **gynec/o-** *female*	Medical specialty for the care of the female reproductive system
gynecologist	guy-nih-**KOL**-oh-jist	S/	**-logist** *specialist*	Specialist in gynecology
labium labia (pl)	**LAY**-bee-um **LAY**-bee-ah		Greek *lip*	Fold of the vulva
majus majora (pl)	**MAY**-jus **MAY**-jora		Latin *greater*	Bigger or greater; for example, labia majora
minus minora (pl)	**MY**-nus **MY**-nora		Latin *smaller*	Smaller or lesser; for example, labia minora
mons pubis	MONZ **PYU**-bis		**mons** Latin *mountain* **pubis** Latin *pubic bone*	Fleshy pad with pubic hair, overlying the pubic bone
obstetrics (OB)	ob-**STET**-ricks		Latin *a midwife*	Medical specialty for the care of women during pregnancy and the postpartum period
obstetrician	ob-steh-**TRISH**-un	S/ R/	**-ician** *expert, specialist* **obstetr-** *midwifery*	Medical specialist in obstetrics
perineum perineal (adj)	**PER**-ih-**NEE**-um **PER**-ih-**NEE**-al		Latin *perineum*	Area between the thighs, extending from the coccyx to the pubis Pertaining to the perineum
postpartum	post-**PAR**-tum	P/ R/	**post-** *after* **-partum** *childbirth*	After childbirth
postpubescent	post-pyu-**BESS**-ent	S/ P/ R/	**-ent** *pertaining to, end result* **post-** *after* **-pubesc-** *to reach puberty*	After the period of puberty
progesterone (***Note:*** Two suffixes.)	pro-**JESS**-ter-own	S/ S/ P/ R/	**-one** *chemical substance, hormone* **-er-** *agent* **pro-** *before* **-gest-** *pregnancy*	Hormone that prepares uterus for pregnancy
puberty	**PYU**-ber-tee	S/ R/	**-ty** *quality, state* **puber-** *growing up*	Process of maturing from child to young adult capable of reproducing
pubis	**PYU**-bis		Latin *pubic bone*	Bony front arch of the pelvis of the hip; also called pubic bone
pubic (adj)	**PYU**-bik			Pertaining to the pubis
vulva vulvar (adj)	**VUL**-vah		Latin *a wrapper or covering*	Female external genitalia

EXERCISES

Latin and Greek terms cannot be further deconstructed into prefix, root, or suffix. You must know them for what they are. Match the meaning in the left column with the correct medical term in the right column.

_____ 1. A covering or wrapper

_____ 2. Pubic bone

_____ 3. Mountain

_____ 4. Lesser

_____ 5. Lip

_____ 6. Greater

A. labia

B. pubis

C. majora

D. vulva

E. minora

F. mons

VAGINA AND DISORDERS

The **vagina,** or birth canal, is a fibromuscular tube, 4 to 5 inches (10 to 13 cm) in length *(Figure 13.2).* It connects the vulva with the uterus. It has three main functions:

- Discharge of menstrual fluid
- Receipt of the penis and semen
- Birth of a baby

It is located between the rectum and the urethra. The urethra is embedded in its anterior wall. In the wall of the vagina around the urethra are several small **paraurethral (Skene) glands** that open into the urethra.

At its posterior end, the vagina extends beyond the cervix of the uterus to form blind spaces called the anterior and posterior **fornices.** The lower end of the vagina contains numerous transverse folds, or **rugae.** The rugae project into the vaginal orifice to form the **hymen,** which stretches across the orifice. The intact hymen contains one or two openings to allow the escape of menstrual fluid.

Bacterial vaginosis is the most common cause of vaginitis in women of childbearing age. Different types of invading bacteria outnumber the normal bacteria of the vagina. The main symptom is an abnormal vaginal discharge with a fishlike odor. Diagnosis is made by laboratory examination of a specimen taken by vaginal swab. Treatment is with antibiotics such as clindamycin or metronidazole.

Toxic shock syndrome is a life-threatening illness caused by toxins circulating in the bloodstream. Certain rare strains of bacteria produce these toxins. In the most common form of toxic shock syndrome, the bacteria are in the vagina of women, and their growth is encouraged by the presence of a superabsorbent **tampon** that is not changed frequently *(see Case Report 13.1).*

Vulvovaginal candidiasis is a common cause of genital itching or burning with a "cottage-cheese" **vaginal** discharge. It is caused by an overgrowth of the yeast fungus called *Candida* and can occur after taking antibiotics. Recent research has found that it is associated with vitamin D deficiency. Diagnosis is made by microscopic examination of a specimen taken by a vaginal swab. Treatment is with antifungal drugs that can be applied topically and used vaginally (miconazole or clotrimazole). If necessary, oral medications can be used (ketoconazole or fluconazole).

Allergic and irritative causes of **vulvovaginitis** can be found in vaginal hygiene products, spermicides, detergents, and synthetic underwear.

Vulvodynia is a chronic, lasting, severe pain around the vaginal orifice, which feels raw. Painful intercourse **(dyspareunia)** is common. The vulva may look normal or be slightly swollen. The etiology is unknown. Treatment varies from local anesthetics and creams to biofeedback therapy with exercises to the muscles of the pelvic floor. Surgical removal of the affected area **(vestibulectomy)** has been tried with variable results.

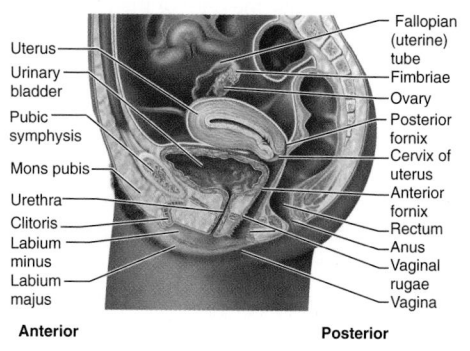

Uterus — Fallopian (uterine) tube — Fimbriae — Ovary — Posterior fornix — Cervix of uterus — Anterior fornix — Rectum — Anus — Vaginal rugae — Vagina

Urinary bladder — Pubic symphysis — Mons pubis — Urethra — Clitoris — Labium minus — Labium majus

Anterior · Posterior

▲ **FIGURE 13.2   Female Reproductive Organs.**

Keynote

Bacterial vaginosis is associated with increased risk of gonorrhea and HIV (human immunodeficiency virus) infection.

Seventy-five percent of adult women have at least one genital yeast infection in their lifetime.

Ten million office visits annually are for vulvodynia.

Keynote

Vaginal cancers are uncommon, comprising 1% to 2% of gynecologic malignancies. They can be effectively treated with surgery and radiation therapy.

Case Report 13.1 (continued)

In the opening Case Report to this chapter, Ms. Lara Baker presented to the Emergency Department with toxic shock syndrome. Because of her heavy period, she was using a superabsorbent tampon. She was admitted to intensive care. The **tampon** was removed and cultured, IV fluids and antibiotics were administered, and her kidney and liver functions were monitored. The causative organism was *Staphylococcus aureus.* She recovered well but had a second episode 6 months later.

WORD ANALYSIS AND DEFINITION

WORD	PRONUNCIATION		ELEMENTS	DEFINITION
Candida candidiasis (also called thrush)	KAN-did-ah kan-dih-DIE-ah-sis	S/ R/	Latin *dazzling white* -iasis *state of, condition* candid- *Candida, a yeast*	A yeastlike fungus Infection with the yeastlike fungus *Candida*
dyspareunia	dis-pah-RUE-nee-ah	S/ P/ R/	-ia *condition* dys- *painful* -pareun- *lying beside, sexual intercourse*	Pain during sexual intercourse
fornix fornices (pl)	FOR-niks FOR-nih-seez		Latin *arch, vault*	Arch-shaped, blind-ended part of the vagina behind and around the cervix
hymen	HIGH-men		Greek *membrane*	Thin membrane partly occluding the vaginal orifice
paraurethral	PAR-ah-you-REE-thral	S/ P/ R/	-al *pertaining to* para- *alongside* -urethr- *urethra*	Situated around the urethra
ruga rugae (pl)	ROO-ga ROO-jee		Latin *a wrinkle*	A fold, ridge, or crease
Skene glands (also called paraurethral glands)	SKEEN GLANZ		Alexander Skene, 1838–1900, New York gynecologist	Paraurethral glands in the anterior wall of the vagina
tampon	TAM-pon		French *plug*	Plug or pack in a cavity to absorb or stop bleeding
vagina	vah-JIE-nah		Latin *a sheath*	Female genital canal extending from the uterus to the vulva
vaginal (adj)	VAJ-in-al	S/ R/	-al *pertaining to* vagin- *vagina*	Pertaining to the vagina
vaginosis vaginitis	vah-jih-NOH-sis vah-jih-NIE-tis	S/ S/	-osis *condition* -itis *inflammation*	Any disease of the vagina Inflammation of the vagina
vestibulectomy	ves-tib-you-LEK-toe-me	S/ R/	-ectomy *surgical excision* vestibul- *entrance*	Surgical excision of the vulva
vulvodynia	vul-voh-DIN-ee-uh	S/ R/CF	-dynia *pain* vulv/o- *vulva*	Chronic vulvar pain
vulvovaginitis	VUL-voh-vaj-ih-NIE-tis	S/ R/CF R/	-itis *inflammation* vulv/o- *vulva* -vagin- *vagina*	Inflammation of the vagina and vulva
vulvovaginal (adj)	VUL-voh-VAJ-ih-nal	S/	-al *pertaining to*	Pertaining to the vulva and vagina

EXERCISES

After reading Case Report 13.1 on the opposite page, answer the following questions. Be prepared to discuss your answers in class.

1. What makes *toxic shock syndrome* life-threatening?

2. Is the causative agent for her condition a bacterium or a virus?

3. How do you know the correct answer in question 2 above?

4. Why does she require intensive care?

5. What was the patient's treatment plan?

Abbreviations

CDC	Centers for Disease Control and Prevention
PID	pelvic inflammatory disease
STD	sexually transmitted disease

SEXUALLY TRANSMITTED DISEASES

According to the **Centers for Disease Control and Prevention (CDC)**, 15 million cases of sexually transmitted diseases **(STDs)** are reported annually in the United States, with adolescents and young adults being at the greatest risk. Some of the common STDs are described below.

Chlamydia is known as the "silent" disease because up to 75% of infected women and men have no symptoms. When there are signs, a vaginal or penile discharge and irritation with dysuria are common. The diagnosis is made by laboratory testing of a **swab** from the cervix or male urethra. Highly accurate urine tests and DNA probes are now available.

Treatment is with oral antibiotics such as doxycycline, erythromycin, or azithromycin. Untreated, chlamydia can spread higher into the female reproductive tract and cause **pelvic inflammatory disease (PID).** It can be passed on to a newborn during childbirth, causing eye infections or pneumonia. It is a reason why antibiotic eyedrops are given to newborns.

Gonorrhea is spread by unprotected sex and can be passed on to a baby in childbirth, causing a serious eye infection. This is another reason why newborns are given eyedrops. Symptoms in both male and female adults may not be present. In the female, they can include a vaginal discharge, bleeding, and dysuria. Gonorrhea is also a cause of PID. Laboratory testing on a swab taken from the surface of the infected area can confirm the diagnosis; DNA probes are also available.

Gonorrhea can be treated with a single dose of an antibiotic such as cefixime; but its causative agent, *Neisseria gonorrhoeae*, is developing resistance to antibiotics.

Syphilis, caused by a **spirochete,** is transmitted sexually and can then spread through the bloodstream to every organ in the body. It is also transmitted among intravenous drug users who share needles. **Primary syphilis** begins 10 to 90 days after infection as an ulcer, a **chancre,** at the place of infection *(Figure 13.3)*. Four to ten weeks later, if the primary syphilis is not treated, **secondary syphilis** appears as a rash on the hands and soles of the feet, with swollen glands and muscle and joint pain. **Tertiary syphilis** can occur years after the primary infection and cause permanent damage to the brain with dementia. Because primary syphilis is curable with penicillin or other antibiotics, tertiary syphilis is rarely seen today. A pregnant woman with untreated syphilis can transmit the infection to her fetus before birth.

Chancroid is an ulcerative disease (not caused by a spirochete) and is without systemwide effects, unlike syphilis. It develops a chancre with swollen, tender lymph nodes in the groin. Antibiotics such as azithromycin and ceftriaxone are effective.

Trichomoniasis ("trich") is caused by the parasite *Trichomonas vaginalis.* Men can carry the infection in their urethra and almost never have symptoms. The vagina is the common site of infection in women. It can produce a frothy yellow-green discharge with irritation and itching of the vulva. Because it is a "ping-pong" infection that goes back and forth between partners, both individuals should be treated with metronidazole.

Molluscum contagiosum is caused by a virus that can be sexually transmitted; the resulting tumors are small, shiny bumps that have a milky-white fluid inside *(Figure 13.4)*. They can disappear and reappear anywhere on the body. Molluscum contagiosum is often seen in children and is not sexually transmitted in such cases. The lesions can be treated with podophyllin ointment, or liquid nitrogen and laser surgery can be used.

Keynote

Three million cases of chlamydia are recognized annually in the United States and could be prevented by using a **condom.**

Infection with gonorrhea can be prevented by using a **condom.**

Three million cases of trichomoniasis occur annually in the United States and could be prevented by using a **condom.**

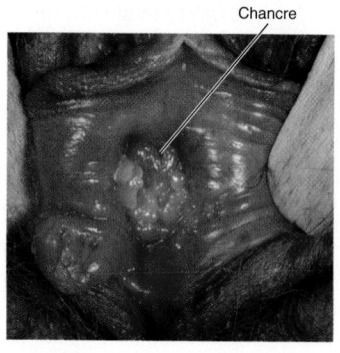

Chancre

▲ **FIGURE 13.3   Chancre of Primary Syphilis in Female.**

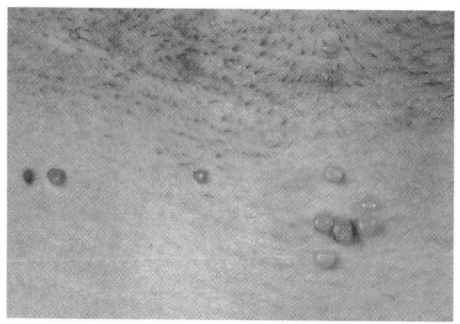

▲ **FIGURE 13.4   Molluscum Contagiosum.**

WORD	PRONUNCIATION		ELEMENTS	DEFINITION
chancre	**SHAN**-ker		Latin *cancer*	Primary lesion of syphilis
chancroid	**SHAN**-kroyd	S/ R	**-oid** *resembling* **chancr-** *chancre*	Infectious, painful, ulcerative STD not related to syphilis
chlamydia	klah-**MID**-ee-ah		Latin *cloak*	A species of bacteria causing a sexually transmitted disease
condom	**KON**-dom		Old English *sheath or cover*	A sheath or cover for the penis or vagina to prevent conception and infection
gonorrhea	gon-oh-**REE**-ah	S/ R/CF	**-rrhea** *flow or discharge* **gon/o-** *seed*	Specific contagious sexually transmitted infection
molluscum contagiosum (***Note:*** The "s" in contagiosum is added to make the word flow.)	moh-**LUS**-kum kon-**TAY**-jee-oh-sum	S/ R/ R/CF	**-um** *structure* **mollusc-** *soft* **contagi/o-** *transmissible by contact*	STD caused by a virus
spirochete	**SPY**-roh-keet	S/ R/CF	**-chete** *hair* **spir/o-** *spiral*	Spiral-shaped bacterium causing a sexually transmitted disease (syphilis)
swab	SWOB		Old English *to sweep*	Wad of cotton used to remove or apply something from/to a surface
syphilis	**SIF**-ih-lis		Possibly from Latin poem, "Syphilis Sive Morbus Gallicus," by Fracastorius Alteration	Sexually transmitted disease caused by a spirochete
Trichomonas trichomoniasis	trik-oh-**MOH**-nas **TRIK**-oh-moh-**NIE**-ah-sis	S/ R/CF R/	**-iasis** *condition* **trich/o-** *hair, flagellum* **-mon-** *single*	A parasite causing a sexually transmitted disease Infection with *Trichomonas vaginalis*

EXERCISES

Disease: *Test your knowledge of diseases. Anyone working in a gynecology clinic or internal medicine practice will have patients diagnosed with sexually transmitted diseases. Make the correct association between the name of the STD and its description by matching the statement in the left column with the medical term in the right column.*

_____   1. "Silent disease"

_____   2. Curable with penicillin

_____   3. Can be treated with single dose of antibiotic

_____   4. Chlamydia or gonorrhea can cause this

_____   5. Can cause dementia if untreated

_____   6. Appears as a rash with joint pain

_____   7. "Ping-pong" infection

_____   8. Ulcerative disease

A. secondary syphilis

B. trichomoniasis

C. chlamydia

D. primary syphilis

E. PID

F. tertiary syphilis

G. chancroid

H. gonorrhea

Note: These diseases can be particularly difficult to spell. Work with a fellow student. Ask your partner to spell these terms; then have your partner ask you to spell them. Master these terms now—they will surely be in a test question.

Spelling: _____

_____

_____

_____

_____

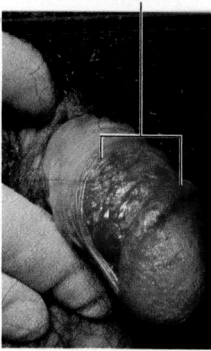

Vesicles

▲ **FIGURE 13.5   Genital Herpes Simplex in Male.**

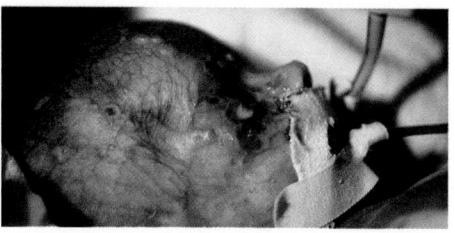

▲ **FIGURE 13.6   Premature Baby Born with Herpes Simplex Infection.**

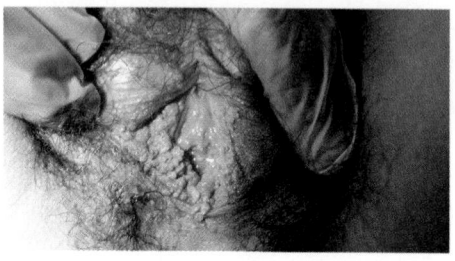

▲ **FIGURE 13.7   HPV in the Female Vulva.**

Abbreviations

AIDS   acquired immunodeficiency syndrome

C-section   cesarean section

ELISA enzyme-linked immunosorbent assay

HIV   human immunodeficiency virus

HPV   human papilloma virus

HSV   herpes simplex virus

Pap   Papanicolaou (Pap test, Pap smear)

SEXUALLY TRANSMITTED DISEASES (continued)

Genital herpes simplex is a disease caused by the virus **herpes simplex type 2 (HSV-2)** *(Figure 13.5)*. The sores are painful, and the disease can present with fever, joint pains, and enlarged, tender lymph nodes. The genital sores can recur throughout life. After the initial infection, the virus remains dormant in the dorsal root ganglia of nerves. Blisters around the mouth ("cold sores") are caused by a related virus, **herpes simplex type 1 (HSV-1).**

There is no cure for genital herpes. Three antiviral medications can provide clinical benefit by limiting the **replication** of the virus. These are acyclovir, valacyclovir, and famcyclovir. In people who have recurrent outbreaks, medication taken every day can reduce the recurrences by 70% to 80%.

Herpes of the newborn occurs when a pregnant woman with genital herpes sores delivers her baby vaginally and transmits the virus to the baby *(Figure 13.6)*. Because the baby's immune system is not well developed, the infection is destructive and can be fatal. If there is evidence of genital herpes lesions in the mother, the fetus should be delivered by **cesarean section (C-section).**

Human papilloma virus (HPV) causes genital warts in both men and women *(Figure 13.7)* and can also cause changes to the cells in the **cervix**. Some strains of the virus can increase a woman's risk for **cervical** cancer. More than 90% of abnormal **Pap** (papanicolaou) smears are caused by HPV infections. A vaccine is now available that can prevent lasting infections from the two human papilloma virus strains that cause 70% of cervical cancers and another two strains that cause 90% of genital warts. The vaccine will be offered to girls and women aged 9 to 26.

Medications such as podophyllin, trichloracetic acid, and Aldara cream can be applied to the warts, and cryotherapy or laser therapy can also be used. Because of the sites of the warts around the genitalia, condoms cannot provide complete protection.

Human immunodeficiency virus (HIV) is a virus that attacks the immune system and usually leads to **acquired immunodeficiency syndrome (AIDS).** Because HIV is carried in body fluids, it is transmitted during unprotected sex. Sharing needles can spread the virus. The virus can also pass from an infected pregnant woman to her unborn child, and she must take medications to protect the baby.

Symptoms often do not appear until years after the initial infection. The initial symptoms of HIV are similar to the flu. A person is diagnosed HIV-positive using a blood test that identifies antibodies to the virus **(ELISA)**, with a confirmatory Western blot *(see Chapter 20)*. The CDC considers an HIV-infected person with a CD4 count below 200 to have AIDS, whether the person is sick or well; CD4 cells, also known as helper T cells, play key roles in the body's defense mechanisms *(see Chapter 15)*.

There is no cure for HIV or AIDS, but combinations of anti-HIV medications are taken to stop the replication of the virus in the cells of the body and stop the progression of the disease *(see Chapter 20)*. Development of resistance to the drugs is a problem.

Human immunodeficiency virus damages the immune system, so infections will develop that the body would normally cope with easily. These are **opportunistic infections** and include herpes simplex, candidiasis, syphilis, and tuberculosis.

WORD ANALYSIS AND DEFINITION

WORD	PRONUNCIATION		ELEMENTS	DEFINITION
acquired immunodeficiency syndrome (AIDS)	ah-**KWIRED** **IM**-you-noh-de-**FISH**-en-see **SIN**-drome	S/ R/CF R/ P/ R/	**acquired** Latin *obtain* **-ency** *condition* **immun/o-** *immune response* **-defici-** *lacking, inadequate* **syn-** *together* **-drome** *running*	Infection with the HIV virus
cervix cervical (**Note:** This term also means *pertaining to the neck region.*)	**SER**-viks **SER**-vih-kal	S/ R/	Latin *neck* **-al** *pertaining to* **cervic-** *cervix*	Lower part of the uterus Pertaining to the cervix
cesarean section (also called **C-section**)	seh-**ZAH**-ree-an **SEK**-shun		Roman law under the Caesars required that pregnant women who died be cut open and the fetus extracted	Extraction of the fetus through an incision in the abdomen and uterine wall
herpes simplex virus (HSV)	**HER**-peez **SIM**-pleks **VIE**-rus		**herpes** Greek *spreading skin eruption*	Manifests with painful, watery blisters on the skin and mucous membranes
human immunodeficiency virus (HIV)	**HYU**-man **IM**-you-noh-dee-**FISH**-en-see **VIE**-rus	S/ R/CF R/ R/	**human** Latin *human being* **-ency** *condition* **immun/o-** *immune response* **-defici-** *lacking, inadequate* **virus** *poison*	Etiologic agent of acquired immunodeficiency syndrome (AIDS)
human papilloma virus (HPV)	**HYU**-man pap-ih-**LOW**-mah **VIE**-rus	S/ R/	**-oma** *tumor* **papill-** *pimple*	Causes warts on the skin and genitalia and can increase the risk for cervical cancer
opportunistic infection (**Note:** This term contains two suffixes.)	**OP**-or-tyu-**NIS**-tik in-**FEK**-shun	S/ S/ R/	**-ic** *pertaining to* **-ist-** *specialist in* **opportun-** *take advantage of*	An infection that causes disease when the immune system is compromised for other reasons
replication	rep-lih-**KAY**-shun	S/ R/	**-ation** *process* **replic-** *reply*	Reproduction to produce an exact copy

EXERCISES

Disease: Continue working with the medical terminology for sexually transmitted diseases. Make the correct association between the description of the disease in the left column and its medical term listed in the right column.

_____ 1. Causes cold sores around the mouth

_____ 2. Virus remains dormant

_____ 3. Virus attacks the immune system

_____ 4. No cure

_____ 5. Infections that would not normally develop

_____ 6. Not an inherited syndrome

_____ 7. Transmitted during vaginal delivery

_____ 8. Can be treated with laser or cryotherapy

A. herpes simplex type 2

B. AIDS

C. herpes of the newborn

D. HIV and AIDS

E. HPV

F. herpes simplex type 1

G. opportunistic

H. HIV

Abbreviations: *Take this opportunity to write out the meaning of any one of the abbreviations in this exercise.*

Ovaries, Fallopian (Uterine) Tubes, and Uterus

OBJECTIVES

The female gonads, the primary sex organs, are the ovaries. The female internal accessory organs include a pair of **fallopian (uterine) tubes**, a **uterus,** and a vagina. Women are born with all the eggs **(ova)** that they will release, but it is not until puberty that the eggs mature and start to leave the ovary. The ovarian hormones, estrogen and progesterone, are involved in **menstruation** and **pregnancy (PGY).** The pituitary gland at the base of the brain produces other hormones that control the functions of the ovaries, uterus, and breast *(see Chapter 14).*

These complex interactions are the core of the human reproductive system and an essential part of understanding the human body. The information in this lesson will enable you to:

13.2.1 **Describe the structure of an ovary.**

13.2.2 **Identify the major events of oogenesis.**

13.2.3 **List the functions of estrogen and progesterone.**

13.2.4 **Explain the control of the pituitary gland over the female reproductive system.**

13.2.5 **Detail the anatomy and physiology of the uterus and fallopian (uterine) tubes.**

13.2.6 **Apply correct medical terminology to the anatomy and physiology of the ovaries, fallopian (uterine) tubes, and uterus.**

13.2.7 **Evaluate the effects of common disorders of the ovaries, uterine tubes, and uterus on the health of the female.**

You are

. . . a certified health education specialist **(CHES)** employed by Fulwood Medical Center.

Your patient is

. . . Ms. Claire Marcos, a 21-year-old student referred to you by Anna Rusack, MD, a gynecologist.

CASE REPORT 13.2

Ms. Marcos has been diagnosed with **polycystic ovarian** syndrome, and your task is to develop a program of self-care as part of her overall plan of therapy.

From her medical record, you see that she presented with irregular, often missed menstrual periods since the beginning of puberty, persistent acne, patches of dark skin on the back of her neck and under her arms, loss of hair from the front of her scalp, and inability to control her weight. She is 5 feet 4 inches and weighs 150 pounds.

Her self-care program is to include exercise, diet, and regular use of birth control medication and metformin, both of which have been prescribed.

She has written out a list of questions that she hands to you. These include:

- Why are my periods so irregular?
- Why doesn't my acne respond to all the treatment I've had?
- Am I going bald?
- Will I be able to have children some day?
- Why am I taking birth control pills when I'm not sexually active?
- What are all these other health problems they say I'm at risk for?

At the end of this chapter you will be asked to answer these questions.

Abbreviations

CHES certified health education specialist
PGY pregnancy

WORD ANALYSIS AND DEFINITION

WORD	PRONUNCIATION		ELEMENTS	DEFINITION
fallopian tubes (also called **uterine tubes**)	fah-**LOW**-pee-an		Gabriello Fallopio, 1523–1562, Italian anatomist	Uterine tubes connected to the fundus of the uterus
menses	**MEN**-seez		Latin *month*	Monthly uterine bleeding
menstruation (syn of menses)	men-stru-**A**-shun	S/ R/CF	-ation *action* menstr/u- *menses*	
menstruate (verb)	**MEN**-stru-ate	S/	-ate *composed of, pertaining to*	The act of menstruation
menstrual (adj)	**MEN**-stru-al	S/	-al *pertaining to*	Pertaining to menstruation
ovary	**OH**-va-ree		Latin *egg*	One of the paired female egg-producing glands
ovaries (pl)	**OH**-vah-rees			
ovarian (adj)	oh-**VAIR**-ee-an	S/ R/	-an *pertaining to* ovari- *ovary*	Pertaining to the ovary
ovum (syn of **oocyte**)	**OH**-vum		Latin *egg*	Egg
ova (pl)	**OH**-va			
polycystic	pol-ee-**SIS**-tik	S/ P/ R/	-ic *pertaining to* poly- *many* -cyst- *cyst*	Composed of many cysts
pregnant	**PREG**-nant	S R/	-ant *forming, pertaining to* pregn- *with child, pregnant*	Having conceived
pregnancy	**PREG**-nan-see	S/	-ancy *state of*	State of being pregnant
gestation	jes-**TAY**-shun	S/ R/	-ion *condition, process* gestat- *gestation, pregnancy*	Period from conception to birth
uterus	**YOU**-ter-us		Latin *womb*	Organ in which an egg develops into a fetus
uterine (adj)	**YOU**-ter-ine			

EXERCISES

Elements: *Knowing the meaning of word elements is your best tool for building and analyzing medical terms. Choose from among the following word elements, and insert the correct element in the blank to complete the medical term. Then use any term from the WAD in a sentence of patient documentation.*

1. Pertaining to many cysts: _____cystic

   mono   poly   cyano   endo

2. Pertaining to the ovary: _____an

   gestat   ovari   menstru   pregn

3. This term is synonymous with *menstruation:* _____

   gynecology   gynecologic   menses   menstrual

4. Having conceived: _____ant

   pregn   gyneco   gestat   estra

5. From conception to birth: _____ion

   ovari   gestat   gyneco   menstru

6. Sentence: _____

   _____

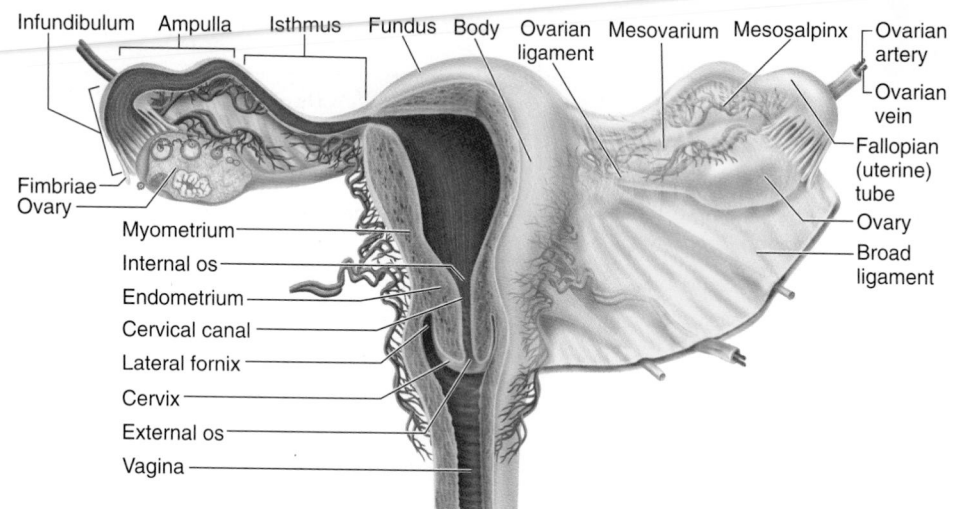

Infundibulum Ampulla Isthmus Fundus Body Ovarian ligament Mesovarium Mesosalpinx Ovarian artery

Fimbriae
Ovary

Myometrium
Internal os
Endometrium
Cervical canal
Lateral fornix
Cervix
External os
Vagina

Ovarian vein
Fallopian (uterine) tube
Ovary
Broad ligament

▲ **FIGURE 13.8** **Female Reproductive Tract.**

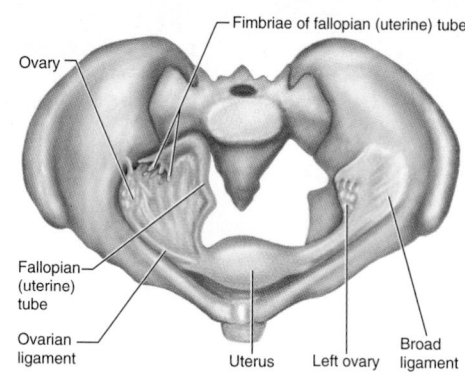

Ovary
Fimbriae of fallopian (uterine) tube
Fallopian (uterine) tube
Ovarian ligament
Uterus Left ovary Broad ligament

▲ **FIGURE 13.9** **Ovaries.** The ovaries are located on each side against the lateral walls of the pelvic cavity. The right fallopian (uterine) tube is retracted to reveal the ovarian ligament.

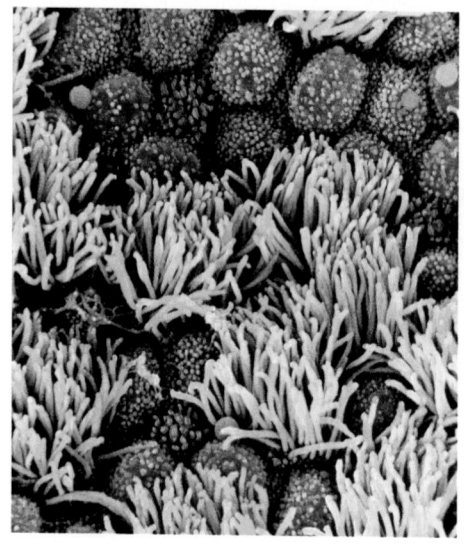

▲ **FIGURE 13.10** **Lining of Fallopian (Uterine) Tube.**

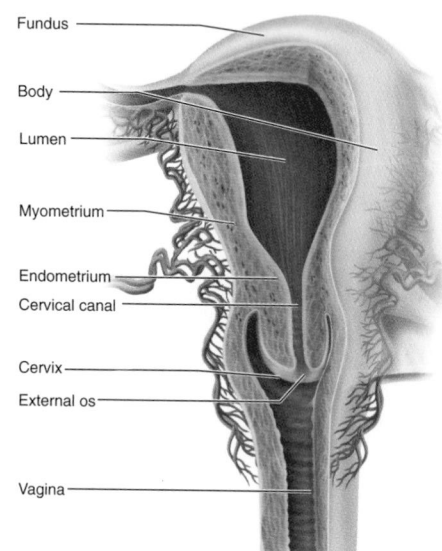

Fundus
Body
Lumen
Myometrium
Endometrium
Cervical canal
Cervix
External os
Vagina

▲ **FIGURE 13.11** **Uterus.**

ANATOMY OF THE FEMALE REPRODUCTIVE TRACT

Ovaries

Each ovary is an almond-shaped organ located in a shallow depression (ovarian fossa) in the lateral wall of the pelvic cavity *(Figure 13.8)*. The ovary is about 1 inch (2.5 cm) long and ½ inch (1.3 cm) in diameter. It is enclosed in a capsule called the tunica albuginea. Each ovary is held in place by ligaments that attach it to the pelvic wall and uterus *(Figure 13.9)*.

Fallopian (Uterine) Tubes

Each fallopian (uterine) tube is a canal about 4 inches (10 cm) long, extending from the uterus and opening to the abdominal cavity near the ovary. At the ovarian end, the outer one-third flares out into a funnel-shaped **infundibulum,** with finger-like folds called **fimbria.** At ovulation, the **fimbriae** enclose the ovary *(Figure 13.8)*.

The inner one-third approaching the uterus is called the **isthmus.** The tubes are supported by the broad ligament.

The wall of the tube has an inner layer of mucosal cells that secrete mucus. Some are ciliated *(Figure 13.10)*. The cilia beat toward the uterus and transport the egg down the uterine tube with peristaltic contractions, a journey that takes 3 or 4 days.

The ovaries and uterine tubes are called the **adnexa** of the uterus.

Uterus

The uterus *(Figure 13.11)* is a thick-walled, muscular organ in the pelvic cavity. It normally tilts forward **(anteverted)** over the urinary bladder. If it were to be tilted backward toward the rectum, its position would be **retroverted,** a condition found in 20% of women. Anatomically, it is divided into three regions:

- **Fundus**—the broad, curved upper region between the lateral attachments of the fallopian (uterine) tubes.
- **Body**—the midportion.
- **Cervix**—the cylindrical inferior portion that projects into the vagina.

The cavity of the uterus is triangular, with its upper two corners receiving the openings of the fallopian (uterine) tubes. Its lower end communicates with the vagina through the **cervical canal,** which has an **internal os** from the lumen and an **external os** into the vagina *(see Figure 13.11)*.

The cervical canal contains mucous glands; secretions of mucus help prevent the spread of infection from the vagina.

WORD	PRONUNCIATION		ELEMENTS	DEFINITION
adnexa (pl) adnexum (sing)	ad-**NEK**-sa ad-**NEK**-sum	S/ R/	Latin *connected parts* -um *mass* -adnex- *connected parts*	Parts accessory to an organ or structure
adnexal (adj)	ad-**NEK**-sal	S/	-al *pertaining to*	Pertaining to accessory structures; for example, structures alongside the uterus, fallopian tubes, and ovaries
anteverted	an-teh-**VERT**-ed	S/ P/ R/	-ed *pertaining to* ante- *before, forward* -vert *to turn*	Tilted forward
anteversion	an-teh-**VER**-shun	S/	-ion *condition, process*	Forward tilting of the uterus
endometrium	en-doh-**ME**-tree-um	S/ P/ R/CF	-um *tissue* endo- *within, inside* -metr/i- *uterus*	Inner lining of the uterus
endometrial (adj)	en-doh-**ME**-tree-al	S/	-al *pertaining to*	Pertaining to the inner lining of the uterus
fimbria fimbriae (pl)	**FIM**-bree-ah **FIM**-bree-ee		Latin *fringe*	A fringelike structure on the surface of a cell or a microorganism
fundus	**FUN**-dus		Latin *bottom*	Part farthest from the opening of a hollow organ
infundibulum infundibula (pl)	**IN**-fun-**DIB**-you-lum **IN**-fun-**DIB**-you-lah		Latin *funnel*	Funnel-shaped structure
isthmus	**IS**-mus		Greek *isthmus*	Part connecting two larger parts; in this case, the uterus to the uterine tube
myometrium	my-oh-**ME**-tree-um	S/ R/CF R/CF	-um *tissue* my/o- *muscle* -metr/i- *uterus*	Muscle wall of the uterus
os	OS		Latin *mouth*	Opening into a canal; for example, the cervix
perimetrium	per-ih-**ME**-tree-um	S/ P/ R/CF	-um *tissue* peri- *around* -metr/i- *uterus*	The covering of the uterus; part of the peritoneum
retroversion	reh-troh-**VER**-shun	S/ P/ R/	-ion *process, condition* retro- *backward* -vers- *turned*	The tipping backward of the uterus
retroverted	**REH**-troh-vert-ed	S/ R/	-ed *pertaining to* -vert *to turn*	Tilted backward

The wall of the uterus has three layers. From the outside, these are:

- The **perimetrium**—a continuation of the broad ligament.
- The **myometrium**—a thick layer of smooth muscle.
- The **endometrium**—the lining that sheds in menstruation.

The uterus is supported by the muscular floor of the pelvic outlet and by ligaments that extend to the pelvic wall from the uterus and cervix.

EXERCISES

*Demonstrate your understanding of the **language of gynecology** employed on this and the opposite page.*

1. Which two terms in the WAD are opposites, and what do they mean?

_____ means _____, and

_____ means _____ _____.

2. What is the "collective" (as a group) medical term for the ovaries and uterine tubes? _____

3. What is another name for the *uterine tube?* _____

4. Describe *peristaltic contractions.*

_____

5. Where else in the body does this action occur? _____

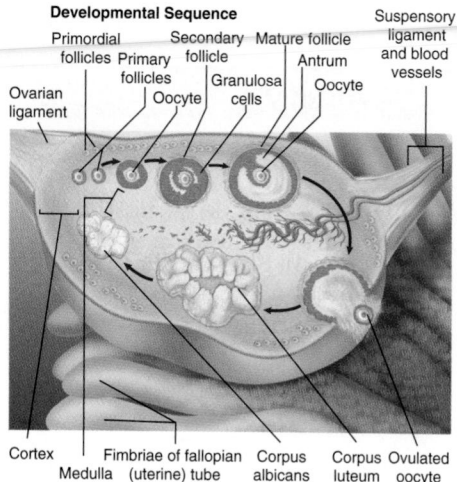

Developmental Sequence

Primordial follicles — Primary follicles — Secondary follicle — Mature follicle

Oocyte — Granulosa cells — Antrum — Oocyte

Ovarian ligament

Suspensory ligament and blood vessels

Cortex — Medulla — Fimbriae of fallopian (uterine) tube — Corpus albicans — Corpus luteum — Ovulated oocyte

▲ **FIGURE 13.12 Oogenesis.**
The development of the oocyte begins with the primordial follicles.

Keynote

Menarche cannot occur until a girl has reached at least 17% body fat.

High levels of estrogen and progesterone inhibit the secretion of GnRH. This is the basis for most forms of contraceptive medications.

Abbreviations

FSH	follicle-stimulating hormone
GnRH	gonadotropin-releasing hormone
LH	luteinizing hormone

OOGENESIS (EGG FORMATION)

During **prenatal** development, small groups of cells in the ovarian cortex form some 2 million **follicles.** These are a single large cell, the primary oocyte, surrounded by a layer of **follicular cells.** Many of these degenerate, a process called atresia.

At puberty, some 400,000 primary oocytes remain, each containing 23 pairs of chromosomes. They undergo meiosis to produce secondary oocytes, each containing 23 single chromosomes. As they mature, the follicular cells form a fluid-filled **primary follicle,** in which the egg is located *(Figure 13.12).* Surrounding the oocyte (egg) and lining the fluid-filled **antrum** of the follicle are **granulosa cells** that secrete estrogen.

At the beginning of the menstrual cycle, as many as 20 primary follicles can start the maturing process, but only one develops fully. The remainder degenerate. By the midpoint of the menstrual cycle, the mature follicle bulges out on the surface of the ovary and ruptures **(ovulation).** The oocyte and lining cells from the follicle can either be taken into the fallopian (uterine) tube or fall into the pelvic cavity and degenerate.

Ovarian Hormones

The ovaries of the sexually mature female secrete estrogens and progesterone.

Estrogens are produced in the ovarian follicles. Their sexual functions are to:

1. Convert girls into sexually mature women through **thelarche, pubarche,** and **menarche.**
2. Participate in the menstrual cycle *(see Figure 13.13).*
3. Participate in pregnancy when that occurs.

Progesterone is produced by the corpus luteum of the ovary and by the adrenal glands *(see Chapter 14).* Its sexual functions are to:

1. Prepare the lining of the uterus for implantation of the egg *(see Figure 13.13).*
2. Inhibit lactation during pregnancy.
3. Produce menstrual bleeding if pregnancy does not occur.

The synthesis and secretion of estrogen is stimulated by **follicle-stimulating hormone (FSH)** from the pituitary gland. FSH is controlled by the hypothalamic **gonadotropin-releasing hormone (GnRH).** Progesterone production is stimulated by **luteinizing hormone (LH)** from the pituitary gland, which is also stimulated by GnRH.

The ovaries also secrete small amounts of androgens, male hormones.

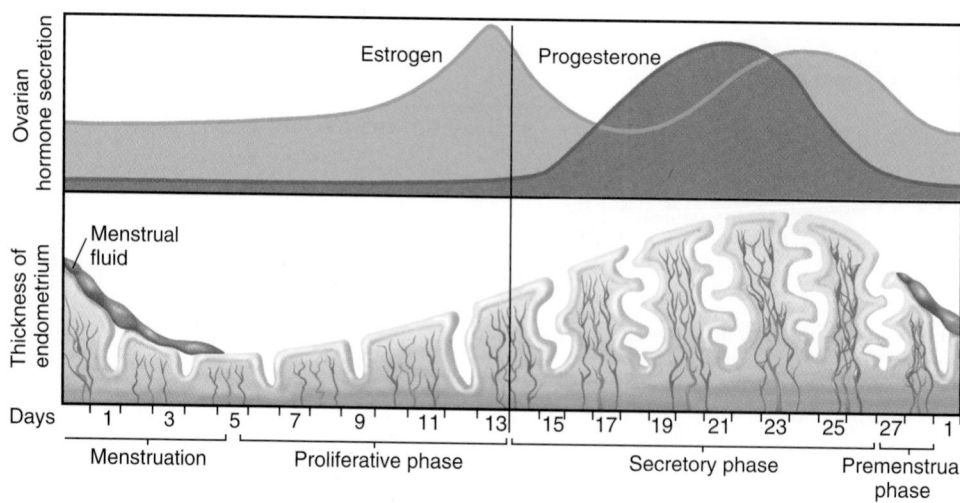

FIGURE 13.13 Menstrual Cycle. ▶

Ovarian hormone secretion — Estrogen — Progesterone

Thickness of endometrium — Menstrual fluid

Days 1 3 5 7 9 11 13 15 17 19 21 23 25 27 1

Menstruation — Proliferative phase — Secretory phase — Premenstrual phase

WORD	PRONUNCIATION		ELEMENTS	DEFINITION
antrum	**AN**-trum		Greek *cave*	A nearly closed cavity or chamber
follicle	**FOLL**-ih-kull		Latin *small sac*	Spherical mass of cells containing a cavity or a small cul-de-sac, such as a hair follicle
follicular (adj)	fo-**LIK**-you-lar	S/ R/	**-ar** *pertaining to* **follicul-** *follicle*	Pertaining to a follicle
gonadotropin	**GO**-nad-oh-**TROH**-pin	S/ R/CF	**-tropin** *nourishing* **gonad/o-** *gonad*	Hormone capable of promoting gonad function
granulosa cell	gran-you-**LOW**-sah SELL	S/ R/	**-osa** *like* **granul-** *small grain*	Cell lining the ovarian follicle
menarche	meh-**NAR**-key	S/ R/	**-arche** *beginning* **men-** *month, menses*	First menstrual period
ovulation	**OV**-you-**LAY**-shun	S/ R/	**-ation** *process* **ovul-** *egg*	Release of an oocyte from a follicle
ovulate (verb)	ov-you-**LATE**	S/	**-ate** *composed of, pertaining to*	To release an oocyte from a follicle
prenatal	pree-**NAY**-tal	S/ P/ R/	**-al** *pertaining to* **pre-** *before* **-nat-** *born*	Before birth
pubarche	pyu-**BAR**-key	S/ R/	**-arche** *beginning* **pub-** *pubis*	Development of pubic and axillary hair
thelarche	thee-**LAR**-key	S/ R/	**-arche** *beginning* **thel-** *breast, nipple*	Onset of breast development

EXERCISES

Deconstruct these medical terms into the meanings of their basic elements. This will help you learn the meaning of the term. Fill in the table, and answer the questions.

Medical Term	Meaning of Prefix	Meaning of Root/ CF	Meaning of Suffix	Meaning of Medical Term
pubarche				
follicular				
ovulation				
menarche				
prenatal				
thelarche				
granulosa				
gonadotropin				

Review the WAD before you fill in the blanks.

1. Find three terms in the WAD with the same suffix, and put these terms in the correct order of their occurrence:

   _____   _____   _____

2. Which term in this WAD is the name of a hormone? _____

3. The meaning of **prenatal** is _____ .

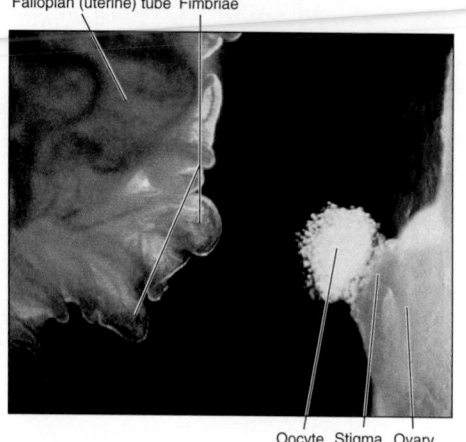

Fallopian (uterine) tube   Fimbriae

Oocyte   Stigma   Ovary

▲ **FIGURE 13.14   Ovulation.**

THE SEXUAL CYCLE

The sexual cycle averages 28 days in length. It begins with a 2-week follicular phase *(Figure 13.15)*. Menstruation occurs during the first 3 to 5 days.

After menstruation ends, the uterus starts to replace the endometrial tissue lost during menstruation. The developing ovarian follicles mature, and one of them ovulates around day 14 *(Figure 13.14)*. Around this time, the fimbriae of the uterine tube envelope and caress the ovary in time with the mother's heartbeat.

After ovulation, in the postovulatory phase, the endometrial lining continues to grow. The residual ovarian follicle becomes a **corpus luteum** containing **lutein** cells that are involved in progesterone production. Around day 24, the corpus luteum **involutes.** By day 26, it is an inactive scar called a **corpus albicans.** At this time, the arteries supplying the endometrium of the uterus contract. This leads to ischemia, tissue necrosis, and the start of menstruation.

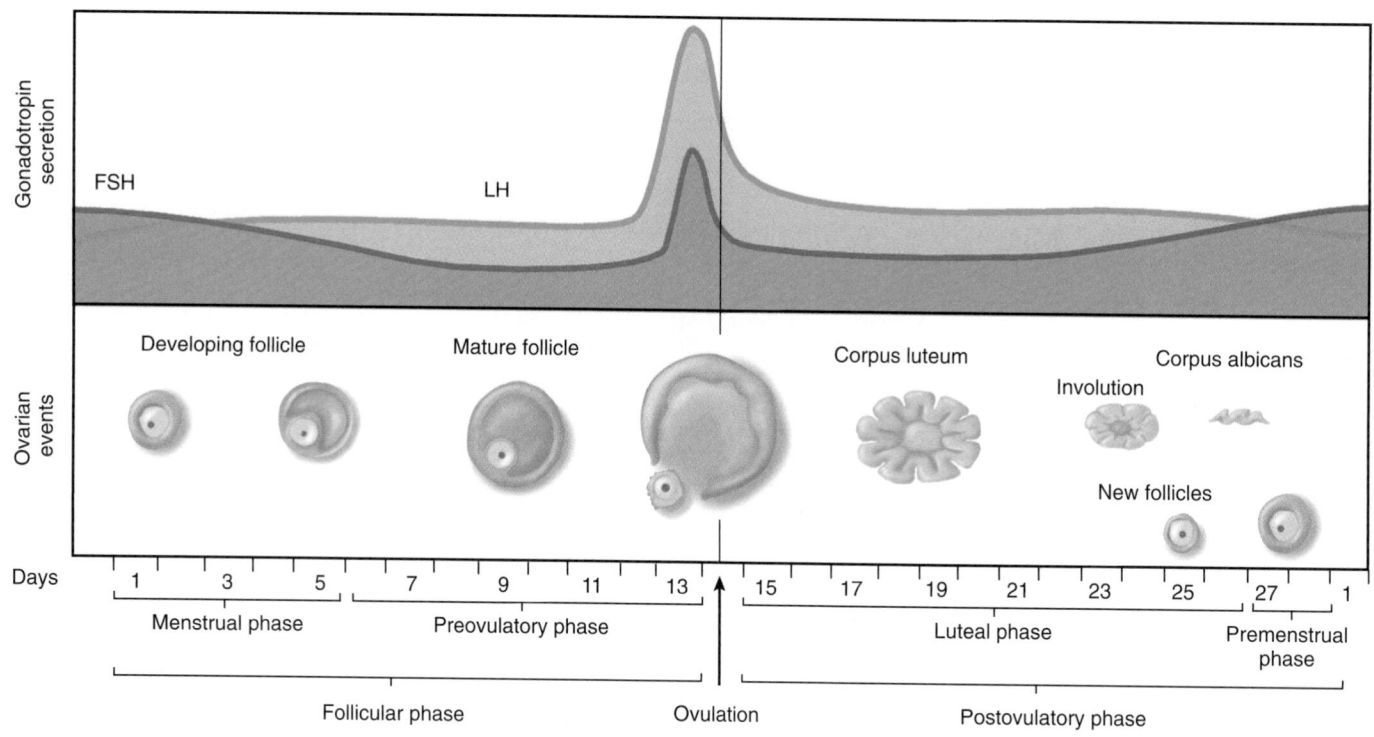

▲ **Figure 13.15   Ovarian Cycle.**

WORD	PRONUNCIATION	ELEMENTS		DEFINITION
corpus albicans corpus luteum	KOR-pus AL-bih-kanz KOR-pus LOO-teh-um		albicans Latin *white* luteum Latin *yellow*	An atrophied corpus luteum Yellow structure formed at the site of a ruptured ovarian follicle
involution involute (verb)	in-voh-LOO-shun	S/ P/ R/	-ion *process, condition* in- *in* -volut- *roll up, shrink*	A decrease in size or vigor
lutein	LOO-tee-in		Latin *saffron yellow*	Yellow pigment
luteal (adj)	LOO-tee-al	R/ S/	lute- *yellow* -al *pertaining to*	Pertaining to a corpus luteum

EXERCISES

*Employ the **language of gynecology** and your understanding of the female sexual cycle to match the phrases in the left column with the correct medical terminology in the right column.*

_____ 1. After menses ends, uterus replaces this

_____ 2. Formed where ovarian follicle ruptures

_____ 3. Envelope the ovary

_____ 4. Decreases in size

_____ 5. Averages 28 days in length

_____ 6. Inactive scar

_____ 7. Mature ovarian follicle does this

_____ 8. Cells involved in progesterone production

_____ 9. After ovulation

_____ 10. Menses occurs during first 3 to 5 days

A. sexual cycle

B. ovulates

C. lutein

D. corpus albicans

E. follicular phase

F. postovulatory phase

G. corpus luteum

H. endometrial tissue

I. involutes

J. fimbriae

A clear understanding of the medical terms used to explain the sexual cycle will help you answer the following questions:

11. Where is the *endometrial lining?* _____

12. What do *lutein cells* produce? _____

13. Is the answer in question 12 above a hormone or an enzyme? _____

14. When the corpus luteum *involutes*, what happens? _____

15. "When the arteries supplying the uterus contract, this leads to ischemia, tissue necrosis, and the start of menses." Explain this in layman's language to your patient.

_____

_____

Disorders of the Female Reproductive Tract

Use correct medical terminology to:

13.3.1 Describe disorders of the uterus, fallopian (uterine) tubes, and ovaries and their effects on a woman's health.

13.3.2 Discuss the etiologies of infertility and modern treatments for the condition.

13.3.3 Identify modern methods of contraception and their rates of success.

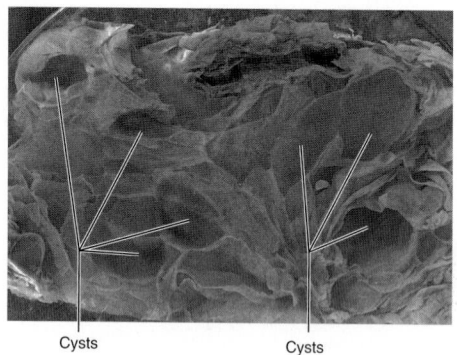

Cysts   Cysts

▲ **FIGURE 13.16** Polycystic Ovary.

Keynote

The peak incidence of ovarian cancer is in women in their fifties and sixties.

Abbreviations

NSAIDs	nonsteroidal anti-inflammatory drugs
PCOS	polycystic ovarian syndrome
PMS	premenstrual syndrome

Keynote

- More than 20,000 new cases of ovarian cancer are diagnosed in the United States each year.
- More than 15,000 deaths from ovarian cancer occur in the United States each year.
- Screening tests for ovarian cancer are in research trials.

Case Report 13.2 (continued)

When Ms. Claire Marcos first presented in the Gynecology Clinic, Dr. Rusack examined her abdomen and pelvis. Dr. Rusack was able to **palpate** both enlarged ovaries on vaginal examination. A vaginal ultrasound scan showed multiple small cysts in each ovary. Blood tests showed high levels of testosterone and luteinizing hormone. Dr. Rusack prescribed birth control pills because they contain estrogen and progesterone. These can correct the hormonal imbalance, regulate menses, and lower the level of testosterone to diminish acne and hair problems. Metformin was also prescribed.

DISORDERS OF THE OVARIES

Ovarian Cysts

An ovarian cyst is a fluid-filled sac in the ovary. Most cysts are normal and are called functional cysts. They follow ovulation and disappear within 3 months.

Polycystic ovarian syndrome (PCOS), in which multiple follicular cysts form in both ovaries *(Figure 13.16),* is the disorder diagnosed in Ms. Marcos. Because of the repeated cyst formation, no egg matures and is released, ovulation does not occur, and progesterone is not produced. Without progesterone, her menstrual cycle is irregular or absent.

The cysts produce androgens, which prevent ovulation and produce acne, the male-pattern hair loss from the front of the scalp, and weight gain. In addition, women with PCOS make too much insulin, which interferes with normal fat metabolism and prevents it being used for energy. This leads to difficulty in losing weight and causes patches of dark skin. Metformin, a medication that affects glucose and insulin metabolism, can help with the weight problems associated with PCOS.

Women with PCOS are also at increased risk for endometrial cancer, type 2 diabetes, high blood cholesterol, hypertension, and heart disease.

Ovarian cancer is the second most common gynecologic cancer after endometrial cancer, but it accounts for more deaths than any other gynecologic malignancy. Symptoms develop late and are usually vague. A mass in the abdomen may be detected during routine pelvic examination.

Treatment is to surgically remove the tumor and give chemotherapy. A majority of patients experience a recurrence. The 5-year survival rate is below 20%.

Primary amenorrhea occurs when a girl has not menstruated by age 16. This can occur with or without other signs of puberty. There are numerous possible causes: drastic weight loss from malnutrition, dieting, bulimia, or anorexia nervosa *(see Chapter 22),* extreme exercise, as in some young gymnasts, extreme obesity, chronic illness, congenital abnormalities of the uterus or vagina, and congenital hormonal disorders. Treatment is directed to the basic cause.

WORD	PRONUNCIATION	ELEMENTS		DEFINITION
amenorrhea	a-men-oh-**REE**-ah	S/ P/ R/CF	**-rrhea** *flow or discharge* **a-** *without* **-men/o-** *month, menses*	Absence or abnormal cessation of menstrual flow
dysmenorrhea	dis-men-oh-**REE**-ah	S/ P/ R/CF	**-rrhea** *flow or discharge* **dys-** *painful or difficult* **-men/o-** *month, menses*	Painful and difficult menstruation
menopause (***Note:*** This term has no suffix, only a combining form and a root.)	**MEN**-oh-paws	R/CF R/CF	**-paus/e** *cessation* **men/o-** *month, menses*	Permanent ending of menstrual periods
menopausal (adj)	**MEN**-oh-paws-al	S/	**-al** *pertaining to*	Pertaining to the menopause
palpate (verb) **palpation (noun)**	**PAL**-pate pal-**PAY**-shun	 S/ R/	Latin *to touch* **-ion** *process, action* **palpat-** *touch, stroke*	To examine with the fingers and hands Examination using the fingers and hands
premenstrual	pree-**MEN**-stru-al	S/ P/ R/	**-al** *pertaining to* **pre-** *before* **-menstru-** *menses*	Pertaining to the time immediately before the menses

Secondary amenorrhea occurs when a woman who has menstruated normally then misses three or more periods in a row and is not in her **menopause.** The causes include pregnancy (by far the most common cause); ovarian disorders such as PCOS; excessive weight loss; low body fat percentage; excessive exercise (e.g., in marathon runners); certain drugs, including antidepressants; and stress.

Primary dysmenorrhea, or **premenstrual syndrome (PMS),** refers to pain or discomfort associated with menstruation. The pain can begin 1 or 2 days before menses, peak on the first day of flow, and then slowly subside. The pain can be cramping or aching and be associated with headache, diarrhea or constipation, and urinary frequency. Treatment is with **nonsteroidal anti-inflammatory drugs (NSAIDs).** If these are ineffective, oral contraceptives are 80% to 90% effective.

Secondary dysmenorrhea is pain associated with disorders such as infection in the genital tract or endometriosis.

EXERCISES

Apply *your knowledge of the* **language of gynecology** *by choosing the correct answer to the following questions. Circle the best choice.*

1. The term **palpate** means to:

   excise   touch   incise

2. In the medical term **menopause,** the combining form means:

   menses   monthly   cycle

3. Gynecologic malignancy that accounts for the most deaths:

   cervical cancer   breast cancer   ovarian cancer

4. If this hormone is not present, the menstrual cycle is irregular or absent:

   estrogen   testosterone   lutein

5. Another medical term for PMS is:

   secondary amenorrhea   primary dysmenorrhea   secondary dysmenorrhea

6. In the medical term **dysmenorrhea,** *dys* means:

   dead   first   painful

7. What ceases after menopause?

   hemorrhaging   periods   egg production

8. In the medical term **amenorrhea,** the suffix means:

   monthly   blood   flow

9. Pick the term that contains a prefix, root, and suffix:

   menopause   palpate   amenorrhea

10. **Premenstrual** refers to something that happens:

   before menses   after menses   in the middle of menses

CASE REPORT 13.3 DOCUMENTATION

● **Fulwood Medical Center** ●
3333 Medical Parkway, Fulwood, MI 01234
555-247-6100

Progress Notes

Patient Name: CAROL Isbell Medical Record # 15826 Page # 1

Clinic: GYN Physician: DR. RUSACK

Date	**S** Subjective	**O** Objective	**A** Assess	**P** Plans

08/09/09 This 29-year-old patient c/o severe dysmenorrhea since the age of 15 and an inability to conceive after 2 yrs. of unprotected intercourse. Cramping pain in lower abdomen and low back begins a couple of days prior to her menses and continues for a couple of days after. OTC pain medications have no effect. Menstrual flow is always heavy; she uses tampons. Patient also c/o pelvic pain in the middle of her menstrual cycle and during intercourse.

Physical examination unremarkable, except for pelvic examination. Normal-sized anteverted uterus with several tender adnexal masses on each side.

Patient's ultrasound examinations showed enlarged, cystic ovaries, abnormal lesions attached to the fallopian tubes and deposits of abnormal tissue on the pelvic walls. A Pap smear is reported normal.

Laparoscopy is scheduled at 1100 hrs. on 08/12/09 to confirm a diagnosis of endometriosis and to remove abnormal tissue

Rusack

ORDER # **267116** ANDRUS CLINI-REC ® PRIMARY CARE CHARTING SYSTEM • © 1976 BIBBERO SYSTEMS, INC. • PETALUMA, CA
TO REORDER CALL TOLL FREE: (800) BIBBERO (800-242-9330) MFG IN U.S.A.

Endometriosis is said to affect 1 in 10 American women of childbearing age. The endometrium becomes implanted outside the uterus on the fallopian (uterine) tubes, the ovaries, and the pelvic peritoneum. The displaced endometrium continues to go through its monthly cycle. It thickens and bleeds; but because there is nowhere for the blood to go, it leads to cysts and scar tissue and produces pain. The etiology of endometriosis is unknown.

Salpingitis is an inflammation of the fallopian (uterine) tubes and is part of pelvic inflammatory disease (PID). A bacterial infection, often from an STD, spreads from the vagina through the cervix and uterus. Symptoms are lower abdominal pain, fever, and a vaginal discharge. Treatment is with appropriate antibiotics. If a pelvic abscess has developed, it may be necessary to remove the damaged tube (**salpingectomy**).

Keynote

Residual scarring of the fallopian tubes from salpingitis is a common cause of infertility.

WORD	PRONUNCIATION	ELEMENTS		DEFINITION
colpopexy	**KOL**-poh-peck-see	S/ R/CF	-pexy *surgical fixation* colp/o- *vagina*	Surgical fixation of the vagina
cystocele	**SIS**-toh-seal	S/ R/CF	-cele *swelling, hernia* cyst/o- *bladder*	Hernia of the bladder into the vagina
endometriosis	**EN**-doh-me-tree-**OH**-sis	S/ P/ R/CF	-osis *condition* endo- *within, inside* -metr/i- *uterus*	Endometrial tissue in the abdomen outside the uterus
hysterectomy	his-ter-**EK**-toe-me	S/ R/	-ectomy *surgical excision* hyster- *uterus*	Surgical removal of the uterus
pessary	**PES**-ah-ree		Greek *an oval stone*	Appliance inserted into the vagina to support the uterus
prolapse	pro-**LAPS**		Latin *a falling*	The falling or slipping of a body part from its normal position
rectocele	**REK**-toe-seal	S/ R/CF	-cele *swelling, hernia* rect/o- *rectum*	Hernia of the rectum into the vagina
salpingitis	sal-pin-**JIE**-tis	S/ R/	-itis *inflammation* salping- *fallopian tube*	Inflammation of the uterine tube
salpingectomy	sal-pin-**JECT**-oh-me	S/	-ectomy *surgical excision*	Surgical removal of fallopian tube(s)

Uterine Prolapse

The uterus is normally supported by the muscles, ligaments, and connective tissue of the pelvic floor. Difficult childbirth can weaken these tissues, so the uterus can descend into the vaginal canal. Aging, obesity, lack of exercise, chronic coughing, and chronic constipation are also thought to play a role in the development of the **prolapse** *(Figure 13.17)*.

Uterine prolapse can be accompanied by prolapse of the bladder and anterior vaginal wall, called a **cystocele**, or the rectum and posterior wall of the vagina, called a **rectocele**.

Treatment can be an individually fitted vaginal **pessary** inserted into the vagina to support the uterus. Surgical procedures such as **sacral colpopexy**, in which a mesh is inserted into the pelvic floor, or a **vaginal hysterectomy**, in which the uterus is removed through the vagina, achieve good results.

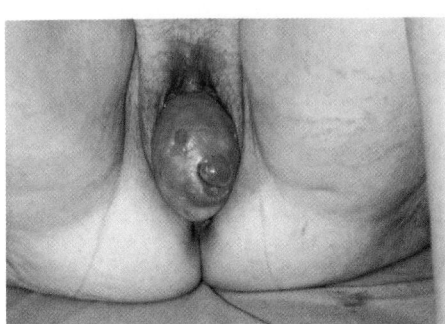

▲ **FIGURE 13.17   Prolapsed Uterus Protruding from the Vagina.**

EXERCISES

After reading the patient documentation on the opposite page, answer the following questions. Be prepared to discuss your answers in class.

1. What are the patient's chief complaints? _____

_____

2. What is a medical term for *inability to conceive?* _____

3. What are the two types of pain the patient complains about?

_____

4. Describe an *anteverted uterus.* _____

5. Where are the *adnexal masses?* _____

6. What is the medical term for this location? _____

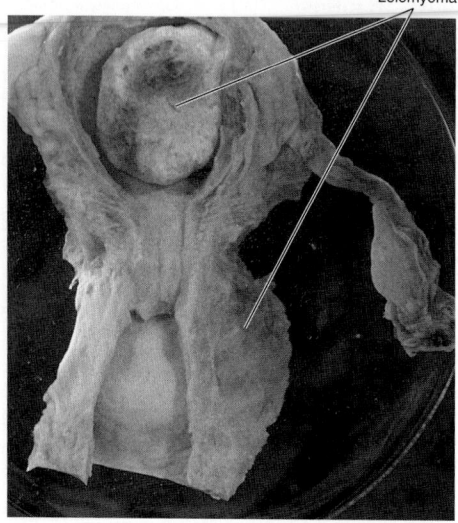

▲ FIGURE 13.18 Leiomyomas (Fibroids).
In this sectioned uterus a smaller rounded leiomyoma is present, causing a bulge in the uterine wall. The larger mass at the top is another leiomyoma projecting from the surface into the uterine cavity.

Abbreviations

D&C dilation and curettage
DUB dysfunctional uterine bleeding

Keynote

In postmenopausal women, the risk of heart disease becomes almost the same as it is in men.

Keynote

Menopause affects every woman differently: 50% never suffer any symptoms.

DISORDERS OF THE UTERUS AND FALLOPIAN TUBES (continued)

Uterine Fibroids

Fibroids are noncancerous growths of the uterus that appear during childbearing years. Three out of four women have them, but only one out of four women has symptoms from them.

The symptoms they can produce include:

- **Menorrhagia**—abnormally long, heavy menstrual bleeding.
- **Metrorrhagia**—irregular bleeding between menstrual periods.
- **Polymenorrhea**—too frequent periods (occur more often than every 21 days) and no ovulation in the cycle.
- Pelvic pressure and pain, low-back pain, urinary incontinence and frequency.

Uterine fibroids are also called **fibromyomas, leiomyomas,** or **myomas** *(Figure 13.18)*. They arise in the myometrium, producing a pale, firm, rubbery mass separate from the surrounding tissue. They vary in size from seedlings to large masses that distort the uterus. They can protrude into the uterine cavity, causing menorrhagia, or project outside the uterus and press on the bladder or rectum to produce symptoms.

Diagnostic studies include endometrial biopsy, transabdominal ultrasound, transvaginal ultrasound, hysterosonography, hysterosalpingography, hysteroscopy, computed tomography (CT), and magnetic resonance imaging (MRI).

Treatment options are numerous and include:

- **Expectant management** is watchful waiting.
- **Myomectomy** removes the fibroids surgically and leaves the uterus in place.
- **Hormone therapy** uses **GnRH agonists** to cause estrogen and progesterone levels to fall so that menstruation stops and fibroids shrink.
- **Hysterectomy** is major surgery and is considered by many gynecologists as a last resort.

Other Causes of Uterine Bleeding

Dysfunctional uterine bleeding (DUB) is a term applied when no cause can be found for a patient's menorrhagia. Treatment is with oral contraceptives. If that fails, **dilation and curettage (D&C)** may be effective. This procedure involves dilating the entrance to the uterus through the cervix so that a thin instrument can be inserted to scrape or suction away the lining of the uterus and take tissue samples. An alternative treatment is **endometrial ablation,** in which a heat-generating tool or a laser removes or destroys the lining of the uterus and prevents or reduces menstruation. Endometrial ablation and hysterectomy are used in women who have finished childbearing.

Endometrial polyps are benign extensions of the endometrium that can cause irregular and heavy bleeding. They can be removed by hysteroscopy or D&C.

Menopause

Menopause is diagnosed when a woman has not menstruated for a year and is not pregnant; she is in the "change of life." In this normal, natural, biological process of reproductive aging, levels of estrogen and progesterone start to decline around the age of 40. For most women, menstruation ceases between the ages of 45 and 55. Significant quantities of estrogen and progesterone are no longer secreted, so the endometrial lining of the uterus cannot grow and be shed as in a normal menstrual period.

Without estrogen and progesterone, the uterus, vagina, and breasts atrophy, and more bone is lost than is replaced. Blood vessels constrict and dilate in response to changing hormone levels and can cause hot flashes.

The risks, types, and benefits of hormone replacement therapy are an ongoing debate.

WORD	PRONUNCIATION	ELEMENTS		DEFINITION
ablation	ab-**LAY**-shun	S/ P/ R/	-ion *action, condition* ab- *away from* -lat- *to take*	Removal of tissue to destroy its function
agonist	**AG**-on-ist		Greek *contest*	Agent combines with receptors to initiate drug actions
curettage	kyu-reh-**TAHZH**	S/ R/	-age *related to* curett- *to cleanse*	Scraping of the interior of a cavity
dysfunctional	dis-**FUNK**-shun-al	S/ P/ R/	-al *pertaining to* dys- *painful, difficult* -function- *perform*	Having difficulty in performing
fibroid	**FIE**-broyd	S/ R/	-oid *resembling* fibr- *fiber*	Uterine tumor resembling fibrous tissue
fibromyoma	**FIE**-bro-my-**OH**-mah	S/ R/CF R/	-oma *tumor, mass* fibr/o- *fiber* -my- *muscle*	Benign neoplasm derived from smooth muscle containing fibrous tissue
leiomyoma (also called **fibroid**)	**LIE**-oh-my-**OH**-mah	S/ R/ R/CF	-oma *tumor, mass* -my- *muscle* lei/o- *smooth*	Benign neoplasm derived from smooth muscle
menorrhagia	men-oh-**RAY**-jee-ah	S/ R/CF	-rrhagia *excessive flow, discharge* men/o- *menses*	Excessive menstrual bleeding
metrorrhagia	**MEH**-troh-**RAY**-jee-ah	S/ R/CF	-rrhagia *excessive flow, discharge* metr/o- *uterus*	Irregular uterine bleeding between menses
myoma	my-**OH**-mah	S/ R/	-oma *tumor, mass* my- *muscle*	Benign tumor of muscle
myomectomy	my-oh-**MEK**-toe-me	S/ R/	-ectomy *surgical excision* -om- *tumor, body*	Surgical removal of a myoma (fibroid)
polymenorrhea	**POL**-ee-men-oh-**REE**-ah	S/ P/ R/CF	-rrhea *flow* poly- *many* men/o- *menses*	More than normal frequency of menses

EXERCISES

*Build the **language of gynecology** by completing the medical term with the correct element. Fill in the blanks.*

1. benign neoplasm derived from smooth muscle   leio/_____/_____

2. irregular bleeding between menses   metro/_____

3. removal of tissue to destroy its function   _____/_____/ion

4. uterine tumor resembling fibrous tissue   _____/oid

5. benign tumor of muscle   _____/oma

6. more than normal frequency of menses   _____/meno/_____

7. surgical removal of a fibroid   _____/ectomy

8. excessive menstrual bleeding   meno/_____

9. having difficulty in performing   _____/_____/al

10. scraping of the interior of a cavity   _____/age

*Note: Although the suffix **-oma** means tumor (or mass), it is not necessarily a malignancy. Fibromyomas, leiomyomas, and myomas are all benign neoplasms or tumors. This is an important distinction for coders especially to note.*

Abbreviations

LEEP	loop electrosurgical excision procedure
Pap	Papanicolaou (Pap test, Pap smear)

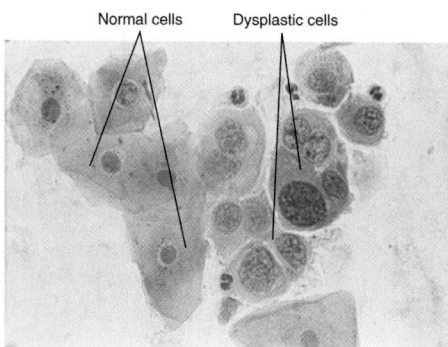

Normal cells   Dysplastic cells

LM 1603

▲ **FIGURE 13.19   Abnormal Pap Smear with Dysplastic Cells.**

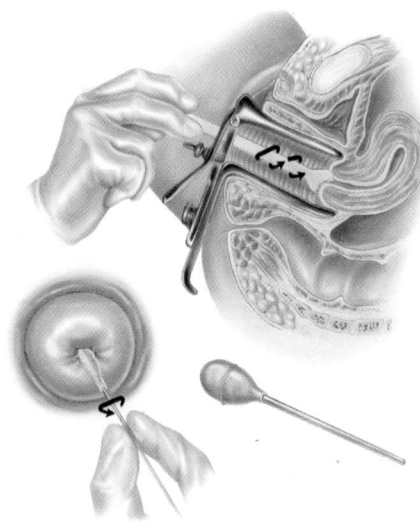

▲ **FIGURE 13.20   Pap Smear Being Performed.**

Endometrial Cancer

Endometrial cancer is the fourth most common cancer in women (after lung, breast, and colon cancer). Forty thousand new cases are diagnosed each year, mostly in women between ages 60 and 70. The most common symptom is vaginal bleeding after the menopause. It can also cause a vaginal discharge, pelvic pain, and dyspareunia. Higher levels than normal of estrogen are thought to be a risk factor for endometrial cancer.

Endometrial cancer is staged at the time of any surgical procedure into four groups, depending on its localization to the uterus or its spread outside. Surgery is the most common treatment. It can be a total hysterectomy, in which the uterus and cervix are removed, or a radical hysterectomy, in which the uterine tubes and ovaries are removed and a pelvic lymph node dissection is also done. If the cancer has spread to other parts of the body, progesterone therapy, radiation therapy, and chemotherapy are used.

Cervical Cancer

Cervical cancer is less common than endometrial cancer, but 50% of cases occur between ages 35 and 55. Some 10,000 new cases are diagnosed in the United States each year.

Early cervical cancer produces no symptoms or signs and may be found on routine Pap test (see below). In the precancerous stage, abnormal cells (**dysplasia**) are found only in the outer layer of the cervix.

Thirteen types of human papilloma virus (HPV) can convert these **dysplastic** cells to cancer cells (*Figure 13.19*). A vaccine has been developed that appears to make people immune to two of the most common types of HPV.

Treatment depends on the stage of the cancer. In preinvasive cancer, when it is only in the outer layer of the lining of the cervix, treatment can include:

- **Conization.** A cone-shaped piece of tissue from around the abnormality is removed with a scalpel.
- **Loop electrosurgical excision procedure (LEEP).** A wire loop carries an electrical current to slice off cells from the mouth of the cervix.
- **Laser surgery.** A laser beam is used to kill precancerous and cancerous cells.
- **Cryosurgery.** Freezing is used to kill the precancerous and cancerous cells.

In an invasive stage when cancer has invaded the cervix and beyond, treatment can include total or radical hysterectomy, chemotherapy, and radiation therapy.

Pap Test

In a Pap (Papanicolaou) test, the doctor brushes cells from the cervix (*Figure 13.20*). The cells are smeared onto a slide or rinsed into a special liquid and sent to the laboratory for examination. The test enables abnormal cells, precancerous or cancerous, to be detected. It is the most successful and accurate test for early detection of abnormalities and should be scheduled according to current guidelines:

- **Initial Pap test**—at age 21 or 3 years after starting sexual intercourse.
- **Age 21 to 65**—a regular Pap test every 3 years.
- **Age 65 to 70 onward**—if there have been no abnormal results, the test can be stopped.
- **Any abnormal result** at any age mandates working out the best schedule for follow-up testing with your doctor.

WORD	PRONUNCIATION	ELEMENTS		DEFINITION
conization	koh-nih-**ZAY**-shun	S/ R/	-ation *process* coniz- *cone*	Surgical excision of a cone-shaped piece of tissue
cryosurgery	cry-oh-**SUR**-jer-ee	S/ R/CF R/	-ery *process of* cry/o- *icy cold* -surg- *operate*	Use of liquid nitrogen or argon gas in surgery to freeze and kill abnormal tissue
dysplasia	dis-**PLAY**-zee-ah	S/ P/ R/	-ia *condition* dys- *painful, difficult* -plas- *molding*	Abnormal tissue formation
dysplastic (adj)	dis-**PLAS**-tic	S/	-tic *pertaining to*	Pertaining to abnormal tissue function
Pap test	PAP TEST		George Papanicolaou, 1883–1962, Greek-U.S. physician, anatomist, and cytologist	Examination of cells taken from the cervix

EXERCISES

Proofread the following sentences for errors in documentation. It may be an error of fact and/or spelling. Rewrite the correct form of the entire sentence on the lines below.

1. Cervixal cancer is more common than endometrial cancer.

_____

_____

2. The most common symptom of endometrial cancer is vaginal bleeding after mennopause.

_____

_____

3. Displasia is abnormal tissue formation.

_____

_____

4. Surgical excision of a wedge-shaped piece of tissue is colonization.

_____

_____

5. The Papanicolaou test should be examined by a citologist.

_____

_____

6. A total hysterectomy removes the uteris and the cervix.

_____

_____

Precision is everything!

FEMALE INFERTILITY

Approximately 20% of women now have their first child when they are aged 35 or older.

In 20% to 30% of female infertility problems, no identifiable cause is found.

Infertility is the inability to become pregnant after 1 year of unprotected intercourse. It affects 10% to 15% of all couples. The causes of infertility are due to:

- The female factor alone in 35%
- The male factor alone in 30%
- Male and female factors in 20%
- Unknown factors in 15%

In women, fertility begins to decrease as early as age 30, and pregnancy rates are very low after age 44.

Causes of Infertility

- **Infrequent ovulation** is responsible in 20% of female infertility problems; both ovulation and menses occur at intervals of longer than 1 month. Bulimia, anorexia nervosa, rapid weight loss, excessive exercise training, low body weight, obesity, and polycystic ovarian syndrome are among the causes.
- **Scarring of the fallopian (uterine) tubes** is responsible for 30% of female infertility problems. Scarring can result from previous surgery, previous tubal pregnancy, pelvic inflammatory disease, or endometriosis.
- **Structural abnormalities of the uterus** are responsible for 20% of female infertility problems. Fibroid tumors, uterine polyps, and scarring from infections, abortions, and miscarriages can all produce abnormalities of the uterus.

After a complete physical examination, including vagina and pelvic organs, other diagnostic tools include:

- **Hormone blood levels** of progesterone, estrogens, and FSH.
- **Hysterosalpingogram,** in which x-rays of the uterus and fallopian (uterine) tubes are taken after dye is injected into the uterus through a slender catheter.
- **Ultrasound** of the abdomen, which can show the shape and size of the uterus; and vaginal ultrasound, which can show the shape and size of the ovaries.
- **Hysteroscopy,** which can visualize the inside of the uterus and be used to take an endometrial biopsy and remove polyps or fibroids.
- **Laparoscopy,** which allows inspection of the outside of the uterus and ovaries and removal of any scar tissue blocking tubes.
- **Postcoital testing,** in which the cervix is examined soon after unprotected intercourse to see if sperm can travel through into the uterus.

Treatment is of any underlying cause arising from the results of the infertility evaluation. Infrequent ovulation can be treated with hormones to stimulate release of the egg. These include clomiphene citrate and injectable forms of FSH, LH, and GnRH.

Surgical procedures to initiate pregnancy include:

- **Intrauterine insemination.** Sperm are inserted directly into the uterus via a special catheter.
- **In vitro fertilization (IVF).** Eggs and sperm are combined in a laboratory dish, and two to four resulting embryos are placed inside the uterus. This can result in twins or triplets.

Keynote

The success rate for IVF is approximately 30% for each egg retrieval.

Abbreviation	
IVF	in vitro fertilization

WORD	PRONUNCIATION	ELEMENTS		DEFINITION
hysterosalpingogram	**HIS**-ter-oh-sal-**PING**-oh-gram	S/ R/CF R/CF	**-gram** *a record* **hyster/o-** *uterus* **-salping/o-** *fallopian tube*	Radiograph of uterus and uterine tubes after injection of contrast material
hysteroscopy	his-ter-**OS**-koh-pee	S/ R/CF	**-scopy** *view or examine* **hyster/o-** *uterus*	Visual inspection of the uterine cavity using an endoscope
infertility infertile (adj)	in-fer-**TIL**-ih-tee in-**FER**-tile	S/ P/ R/	**-ity** *condition* **in-** *not* **-fertil-** *able to conceive*	Inability to conceive over a long period of time
insemination inseminate (verb)	in-sem-ih-**NAY**-shun in-**SEM**-ih-nate	S/ P/ R/	**-ation** *process* **in-** *in* **-semin-** *scatter seed*	Introduction of semen into the vagina
intrauterine	**IN**-trah-**YOU**-ter-ine	S/ P/ R/	**-ine** *pertaining to* **intra-** *inside* **-uter-** *uterus*	Inside the uterine cavity
in vitro fertilization (IVF)	IN **VEE**-troh **FER**-til-eye-**ZAY**-shun	 S/ R/	**in vitro** *Latin in glass* **-ization** *process of creating* **fertil-** *able to conceive*	Process of combining sperm and egg in a laboratory dish and placing the resulting embryos inside the uterus
postcoital	post-**KOH**-ih-tal	S/ P/ R/	**-al** *pertaining to* **post-** *after* **-coit-** *sexual intercourse*	After sexual intercourse

EXERCISES

Build your knowledge of the meaning of elements. Write the correct element or term on the line to complete the term.

1. If it occurs after intercourse, it is _____coital.

   (pre   post)

2. Visual inspection of the uterine cavity using an endoscope is a _____scopy.

   (cysto   hystero)

3. Patient is unable to conceive and suffers from _____.

   (infertility   insemination)

4. Inside the uterine cavity is referred to as _____uterine.

   (intra   inter)

5. The process of combining sperm and egg in a laboratory dish is _____ fertilization.

   (intrauterine   in vitro)

6. Introduction of semen into the vagina is _____.

   (infertility   insemination)

7. A radiograph of the uterus and uterine tubes is a _____.

   (hysterogram   hysterosalpingogram)

8. Sperm can be _____ directly into the uterus via a catheter.

   (inseminated   insemination)

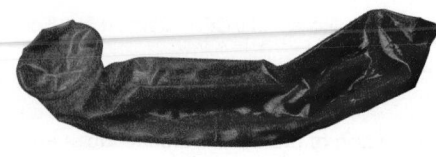

▲ **FIGURE 13.21   Female Condom.**

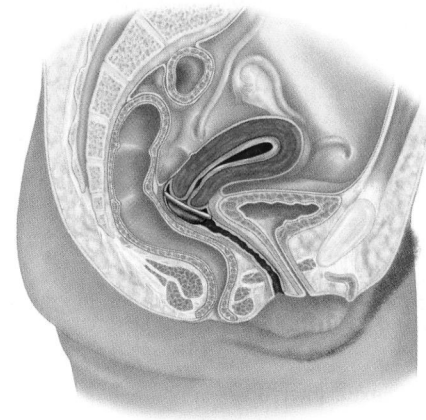

▲ **FIGURE 13.22   Diaphragm.**

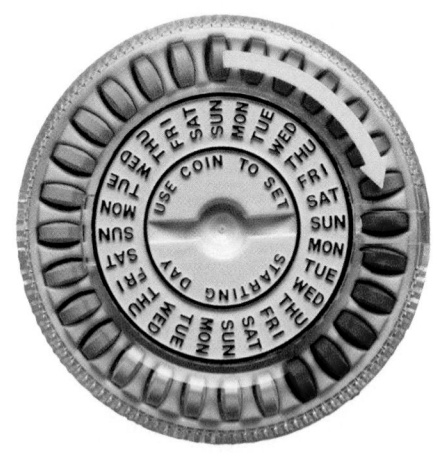

▲ **FIGURE 13.23   Oral Contraceptives.**

Keynote

Unprotected sex results in pregnancy 85% of the time.

Abbreviations	
IUD	intrauterine device
RU-486	mifepristone

CONTRACEPTION

Contraception is the prevention of pregnancy. Common methods of contraception include:

Behavioral Methods

- **Abstinence** is reliable if followed consistently.
- **Rhythm method** avoids intercourse near the time of expected ovulation, which is difficult to determine consistently. It has a 25% failure rate.
- **Coitus interruptus** involves the male withdrawing his penis before ejaculation. There is a 20% failure rate.

Barrier Methods

- **Male condom**—a sheath of latex or rubber rolled on over the erect penis.
- **Female condom**—a polyurethane sheath that fits into the vagina with a ring at one end to go over the cervix and a larger ring at the other end to go over the vulva *(Figure 13.21)*. Both male and female condoms help protect against STDs. They have a 5% to 10% failure rate.
- **Diaphragm** *(Figure 13.22)* **and cervical cap**—a latex or rubber dome inserted into the vagina and placed over the cervix. When used with a spermicide, they have a 5% to 10% failure rate for pregnancy.
- **Spermicidal foam and gel**—inserted into the vagina. Used on their own, they have a 25% failure rate.
- **Sponge**—a spermicidal-coated polyurethane barrier placed in the vagina to inhibit sperm. It has a 10% failure rate.

Intrauterine Devices

Intrauterine devices (IUDs) are T-shaped flexible plastic or copper devices inserted into the uterus and left in place for 1 to 4 years. Failure rate is less than 3%.

Hormonal Methods

- **Oral contraceptives** (birth control pills) utilize a mixture of estrogen and progesterone to prevent follicular development and ovulation *(Figure 13.23)*. They are taken orally and have a 5% failure rate, usually due to inconsistent pill taking.
- **Estrogen/progestin patches** deliver the hormones transdermally. Some are applied monthly, some weekly. Their failure rate is less than 1%.
- **Injected progestins,** such as Depo-Provera, are given by injection every 3 months. Their failure rate is less than 1%.
- **Implanted progestins,** such as Implanon, are contained in porous silicone tubes that are inserted under the skin and slowly release the progestin for up to 5 years. Their failure rate is less than 1%.
- **Morning-after pills,** such as Plan B, contain large doses of progestins to inhibit or delay ovulation. They are a backup when taken within 72 hours of unprotected intercourse. Their failure rate is around 10%.
- **Mifepristone (RU-486),** when taken with a prostaglandin, induces a miscarriage. It has an 8% failure rate.

Surgical Methods

- **Tubal ligation** ("getting your tubes tied") is performed with laparoscopy. Both fallopian (uterine) tubes are cut, a segment is removed, and the ends are tied off and cauterized shut. Failure rate is less than 1%. A **tubal anastomosis** is the procedure of rejoining the tubes if there is a subsequent change of mind.
- **Vasectomy** in the male is discussed in *Chapter 12.*

WORD	PRONUNCIATION	ELEMENTS		DEFINITION
anastomosis anastomoses (pl)	ah-**NAS**-to-**MO**-sis	S/ R/	-osis *condition* anastom- *join together*	A surgically made union between two tubular structures
coitus	**KOH**-it-us		Latin *come together*	Sexual intercourse
condom	**KON**-dom		Old English *sheath or cover*	A sheath or cover for the penis or vagina to prevent conception and infection
contraception	kon-trah-**SEP**-shun	S/ P/ R/	-ion *process* contra- *against* -cept- *receive*	Prevention of pregnancy
contraceptive	kon-trah-**SEP**-tiv	S/	-ive *quality of*	An agent that prevents conception
diaphragm (*Note:* Diaphragm also is the term for the muscle that separates the thoracic and abdominal cavities.)	**DIE**-ah-fram		Greek *partition or wall*	A ring and dome-shaped material inserted in the vagina to prevent pregnancy
ligature	**LIG**-ah-chur	S/	Latin *band, tie* -ion *process*	Thread or wire tied around a tubal structure to close it
ligation	lie-**GAY**-shun	R/	ligat- *tie up*	Use of a tie to close a tube
progestin	pro-**JESS**-tin	S/ P/ R/	-in *chemical compound* pro- *before* -gest- *produce, pregnancy*	A synthetic form of progesterone

EXERCISES

Review all the terms in this Word Analysis and Definition (WAD) box. With critical thinking, you will be able to answer the following questions using these terms. Fill in the blanks.

1. What is the Latin term for sexual intercourse? _____

2. If a patient has a tubal ligation and later changes her mind, what procedure is necessary to repair this? _____

   _____

   Briefly describe what this term means. _____

   _____

3. Write the two definitions of the word **diaphragm** and one sentence for each meaning.

   Definition 1: _____

   Sentence: _____

   _____

   Definition 2: _____

   Sentence: _____

   _____

4. A contraceptive works against something—what does it work against? _____

   _____

5. What is the medical term for a thread or wire that is used to close a tube? _____

LESSON 13.4 Obstetrics: Pregnancy and Childbirth

OBJECTIVES

The nuclei of the male and female cells unite; their chromosomes mingle. Fertilization **(conception)** is complete, and a **zygote** is formed. So begins the incredible, dramatic, and wondrous development of an embryo and a new human being. This process will be described in this lesson to enable you to:

13.4.1 **Specify the stages of embryonic development.**

13.4.2 **Describe the implantation of the embryo in the uterus.**

13.4.3 **List the functions of the placenta.**

13.4.4 **Identify the major events of fetal development.**

13.4.5 **Explain the process of childbirth.**

13.4.6 **Discuss some of the most common problems of fetal development and childbirth.**

13.4.7 **Recognize and use appropriately the medical terminology for embryonic and fetal development, pregnancy, and childbirth.**

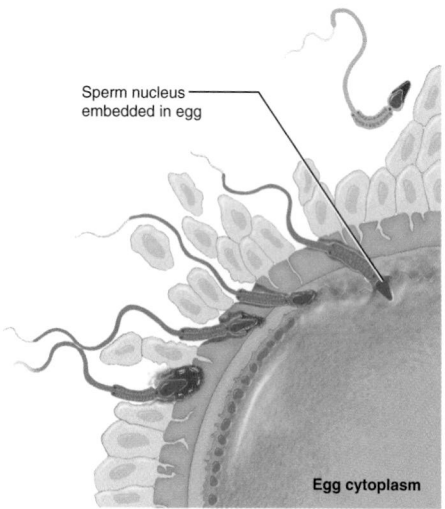

Sperm nucleus embedded in egg

Egg cytoplasm

▲ **FIGURE 13.24** **Fertilization.**

CONCEPTION

When released from the ovary, an egg takes 72 hours to reach the uterus, but it must be **fertilized** *(Figure 13.24)* within 12 to 24 hours to survive. Therefore, **fertilization** must take place in the distal third of the uterine tube.

Between 200 million and 600 million sperm are deposited in the vagina near the cervix. Many are destroyed by the acidity in the vagina or just drain out. Others fail to get through the cervical mucus. Approximately half the survivors will go up the wrong fallopian (uterine) tube. The journey through the uterus into the fallopian (uterine) tube takes about an hour. Some 2000 to 3000 sperm reach the egg. Several of these penetrate the outer layers of the egg and clear the path for the one sperm that will penetrate all the way into the egg cytoplasm to fertilize it *(Figure 13.24)*.

Implantation

While still in the uterine tube, the zygote divides, producing a ball of cells called a **morula** *(Figure 13.25)*. Within the morula, a fluid-filled cavity develops, and the morula becomes a **blastocyst**. A week after fertilization, the blastocyst enters the

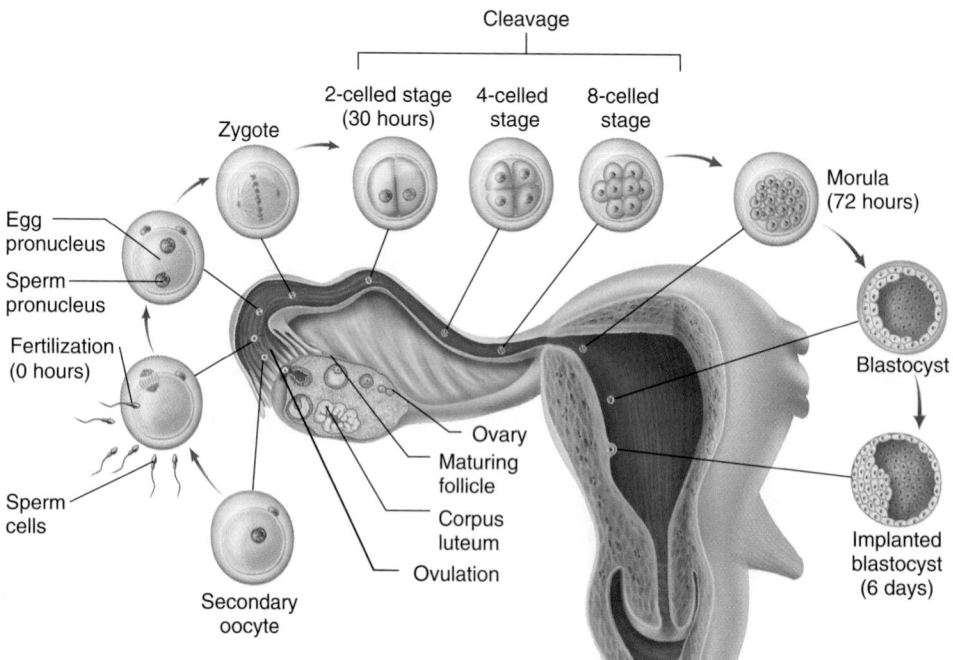

Cleavage

2-celled stage (30 hours)   4-celled stage   8-celled stage

Zygote

Egg pronucleus

Sperm pronucleus

Fertilization (0 hours)

Sperm cells

Secondary oocyte

Ovary

Maturing follicle

Corpus luteum

Ovulation

Morula (72 hours)

Blastocyst

Implanted blastocyst (6 days)

FIGURE 13.25 **Early Embryo Development.** ▶

WORD	PRONUNCIATION	ELEMENTS		DEFINITION
blastocyst	BLAS-toe-sist	S/ R/CF	-cyst *bladder* blast/o- *germ cell*	The developing embryo during the first 2 weeks
conception	kon-SEP-shun		Latin *something received*	Fertilization of the egg by sperm to form a zygote
dizygotic	die-zye-GOT-ik	S/ P/ R/	-ic *pertaining to* di- *two* -zygot- *yoked together*	Twins from two separate zygotes
fertilize	FER-til-ize		Latin *make fruitful*	To penetrate an oocyte with a sperm so as to impregnate
fertilization	FER-til-eye-ZAY-shun	S/ R/	-ation *process* fertiliz- *make fruitful*	Union of a male sperm and a female egg
implantation	im-plan-TAY-shun	S/ P/ R/	-ation *process* im- *in* -plant- *to plant*	Attachment of a fertilized egg to the endometrium
monozygotic	MON-oh-zye-GOT-ik	S/ P/ R/	-ic *pertaining to* mono- *one* -zygot- *yoked together*	Twins from a single zygote
morula	MOR-you-lah		Latin *mulberry*	Ball of cells formed from divisions of a zygote
placenta placental (adj)	plah-SEN-tah plah-SEN-tal		Latin *a cake*	Organ that allows metabolic interchange between the mother and fetus
zygote	ZYE-goat		Greek *joined together*	Cell resulting from the union of the sperm and egg

uterine cavity and burrows into the endometrium **(implantation).** A group of cells in the blastocyst, the inner cell mass, differentiate into the germ layers and form the embryo. Other cells from the blastocyst, together with endometrial cells, form the **placenta.**

Twins (and other multiple births) can be produced in two ways:

- **Dizygotic** twins are produced when two eggs are released by the ovary and fertilized by two separate sperm. They can be of different sexes and are only as genetically similar as other siblings would be.

- **Monozygotic** twins are produced when a single egg is fertilized and later two inner cell masses form within a single blastocyst, each producing an embryo. These twins share a single placenta, are genetically identical, are the same sex, and look alike.

EXERCISES

Meet a lesson objective by tracing the pathway of embryo implantation. You are given the terminology—put it in correct order of the implantation process.

placenta	morula	sperm	embryo
blastocyst	uterine tube	implantation	zygote
fertilization	egg	endometrium	

1. _____   7. _____

2. _____   8. _____

3. _____   9. _____

4. _____   10. _____

5. _____   11. _____

6. _____

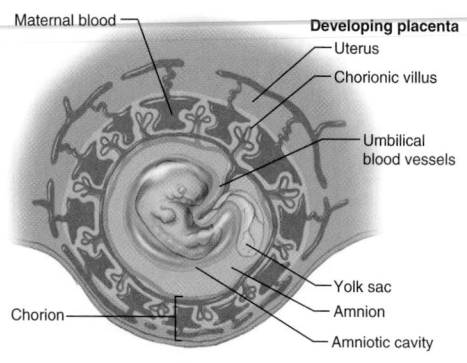

FIGURE 13.26 Embryo at 4.5 Weeks.

Maternal blood — **Developing placenta**
— Uterus
— Chorionic villus
— Umbilical blood vessels
Chorion —
— Yolk sac
— Amnion
— Amniotic cavity

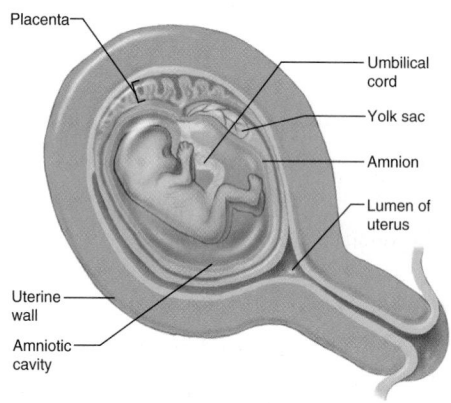

FIGURE 13.27 Embryo and Placenta at 13.5 Weeks.

Placenta —
— Umbilical cord
— Yolk sac
— Amnion
— Lumen of uterus
Uterine wall —
Amniotic cavity —

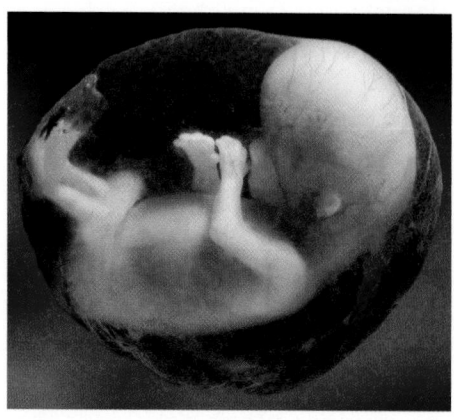

FIGURE 13.28 Developing Fetus at 20 Weeks.

EMBRYO AND FETUS

Embryo

From week 2 until week 8 is the **embryonic period,** in which most of the external structures and internal organs of the **embryo** are formed, together with the placenta, **umbilical** cord, **amnion, yolk sac,** and **chorion** *(Figure 13.26).* The **amnion** is a fluid-filled sac that protects the embryo. The yolk sac is a small sac arising from the ventral surface of the embryo. It contributes to the formation of the digestive tract and produces blood cells and future sex germ cells. The **chorion** forms the placenta by penetrating deeply into the endometrium. At the eighth week, all the organ systems are present; the embryo is just over 1 inch long and is now called a **fetus.**

The **placenta** is a disc of tissue that increases in size as pregnancy proceeds *(Figure 13.27).* The surface facing the fetus is smooth and gives rise to the **umbilical cord,** which contains two arteries and one vein. The surface attached to the uterine wall consists of treelike structures called **chorionic villi.** The cells of the villi keep the maternal and fetal circulations largely separate, but they are very thin and allow an exchange of gases, nutrients, and waste products to occur.

The functions of the placenta are to:

- **Transport nutrients** (such as glucose, amino acids, fatty acids, minerals) from mother to fetus.
- **Transport nitrogenous wastes** (such as ammonia, urea, creatinine) from fetus to mother, who can excrete them.
- **Transport oxygen** from mother to fetus and carbon dioxide from fetus to mother, who can excrete it.
- **Transport maternal antibodies** to the fetus.
- **Secrete hormones** (such as estrogen and progesterone) and allow maternal hormones to pass to the fetus.

Unfortunately, some undesirable items and many medications can also cross the placenta. These include the HIV and rubella viruses; the bacteria that cause syphilis; alcohol; nicotine and carbon monoxide from smoking; and drugs (for example, heroin and cocaine). All these have bad effects on the fetus.

Amniocentesis and **chorionic** villus sampling are performed to test for chromosomal abnormalities and genetic birth defects and are described in *Chapter 21.*

Fetus

The **fetal period** lasts from the eighth week until birth. At the eighth week, the heart is beating. By the twelfth week, the bones have begun to calcify, and the external genitalia can be differentiated as male or female. In the fourth month, downy hair called **lanugo** appears over the body. In the fifth month, skeletal muscles become active, and the baby's movements are felt between 16 and 22 weeks of gestation *(Figure 13.28).* A protective substance called **vernix caseosa** covers the skin. In the sixth and seventh months, weight gain is increased, and body fat is deposited.

At 38 weeks, the baby is at full term and ready for birth.

The length of pregnancy, the gestation, is often considered to be 40 weeks, which is the time from a woman's last menstrual period to birth. However, the woman does not become pregnant until she ovulates 2 weeks after her last period, so gestation is really 38 weeks. Gestation is also divided into **trimesters.** The first trimester is up to week 12, the second from week 13 to 24, and the third from week 25 to birth.

A pregnant woman is described as a **gravida.** A woman in her first pregnancy is a **primigravida.** A woman in her second pregnancy is a gravida 2. **Parity** relates to outcome of the pregnancy: Deliveries after the twentieth week are numbered successively as para 1, 2, 3, and so on. **Abortus** refers to losses of pregnancy before the twentieth week. The total of abortus and paras equals a woman's gravidity.

WORD ANALYSIS AND DEFINITION

WORD	PRONUNCIATION		ELEMENTS	DEFINITION
abortion	ah-**BOR**-shun	S/ R/	-ion *action, process* **abort-** *fail at onset*	Spontaneous or induced expulsion of an embryo or fetus from the uterus
abortus	ah-**BOR**-tus	S/	-us *pertaining to*	Product of abortion
amnion	**AM**-nee-on		Greek *membrane around fetus*	Membrane around the fetus that contains amniotic fluid
amniotic	am-nee-**OT**-ic	S/ R/CF	-tic *pertaining to* **amni/o-** *amnion*	Pertaining to the amnion
amniocentesis	**AM**-nee-oh-sen-tee-sis	S/	-centesis *puncture*	Removal of amniotic fluid for diagnostic purposes
chorion	**KOH**-ree-on		Greek *membrane*	The fetal membrane that forms the placenta
chorionic	koh-ree-**ON**-ick	S/ R/	-ic *pertaining to* **chorion-** *chorion*	Pertaining to the chorion
embryo	**EM**-bree-oh		Greek *a young one*	Developing organism from conception until the end of the second month
embryonic	em-bree-**ON**-ic	S/ R/CF	-nic *pertaining to* **embry/o-** *embryo*	Pertaining to the embryo
fetus	**FEE**-tus		Latin *offspring*	Human organism from the end of the eighth week after conception to birth
fetal	**FEE**-tal	S/ R/	-al *pertaining to* **fet-** *fetus*	Pertaining to the fetus
gravid	**GRAV**-id		Latin *pregnant*	Pregnant
gravida	**GRAV**-ih-dah		Latin *pregnant woman*	A pregnant woman
primigravida	pree-mih-**GRAV**-ih-dah	P/ R/	**primi-** *first* -gravida *pregnant woman*	First pregnancy
lanugo	la-**NYU**-go		Latin *wool*	Fine, soft hair on the fetal body
parity	**PAIR**-ih-tee		Latin *to bear*	Number of deliveries
para	**PAH**-rah		Latin *bring forth*	Abbreviation for number of deliveries
trimester	**TRY**-mes-ter		Latin *of 3 months' duration*	One-third of the length of a full-term pregnancy
umbilicus	um-**BIL**-ih-kus		Latin *navel*	Pit in the abdomen where the umbilical cord entered the fetus
umbilical	um-**BIL**-ih-kal	S/ R/	-al *pertaining to* **umbilic-** *umbilicus*	Pertaining to the umbilicus or the center of the abdomen
vernix caseosa	**VER**-nicks kay-see-**OH**-sah		**vernix** Latin *varnish* **caseosa** Latin *cheese*	Cheesy substance covering skin of the fetus
yolk sac	YOKE SACK		**yolk** Latin *yellow* **sac** Latin *pouch or bag*	Source of blood cells and future sex cells for the fetus

---

EXERCISES

Precision in documentation includes using the correct form (noun, verb, adjective) of the medical term. Practice precision in this written **language of obstetrics**. Fill in the blanks.

amniocentesis   amnion   amniotic

1. The _____ will be punctured in the procedure _____ in order to withdraw the

_____ fluid.

embryo   embryonic

2. The _____ stage of gestation means the _____ has formed in the first 8 weeks of human development.

umbilical   umbilicus

3. The medical term for navel is _____. The _____ cord enters the fetus in the abdomen.

Practice your precision in spelling, please!

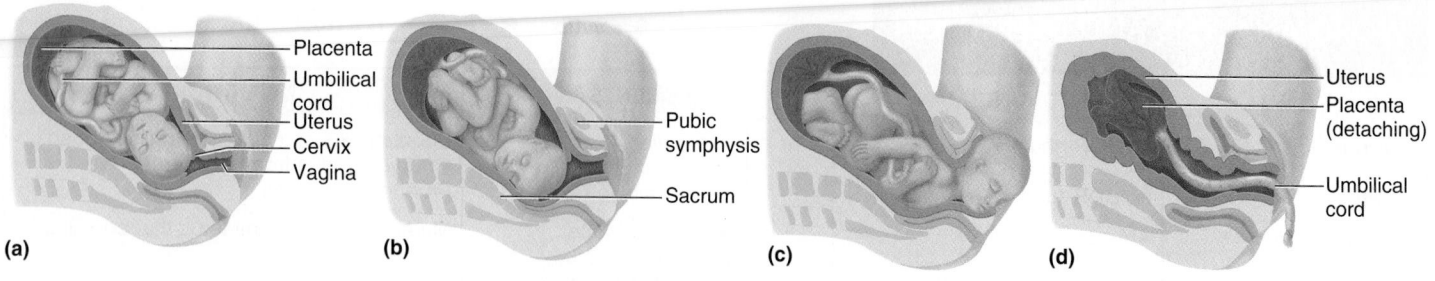

(a)   (b)   (c)   (d)

▲ **FIGURE 13.29   The Stages of Childbirth.** (*a*) First stage: Early dilation. (*b*) First stage: Late dilation. (*c*) Second stage: Expulsion of the fetus. (*d*) Third stage: Expulsion of the placenta.

PREGNANCY AND CHILDBIRTH

Hormones of Pregnancy

Human chorionic gonadotropin (HCG) is secreted by the blastocyst and the placenta. Its presence in the mother's blood and urine is the basis for laboratory and home pregnancy tests. It can be detected as early as 9 or 10 days after conception. Human chorionic gonadotropin stimulates the growth of the corpus luteum and its production of estrogen and progesterone.

Estrogen stimulates the mother's uterus to enlarge and her breasts to increase to twice their normal size. It makes the pelvic joints and ligaments more flexible so that the pelvic outlet widens for childbirth.

Progesterone is secreted by the corpus luteum and the placenta. It suppresses further ovulation, prevents menstruation, stimulates the proliferation of the endometrium to support the implantation, and inhibits contractions of the uterine muscle.

Follicle-stimulating hormone (FSH) and **luteinizing hormone (LH)** from the pituitary gland stimulate the maintenance of the corpus luteum and its estrogen and progesterone production.

Abbreviations

FSH	follicle-stimulating hormone
HCG	human chorionic gonadotropin
LH	luteinizing hormone

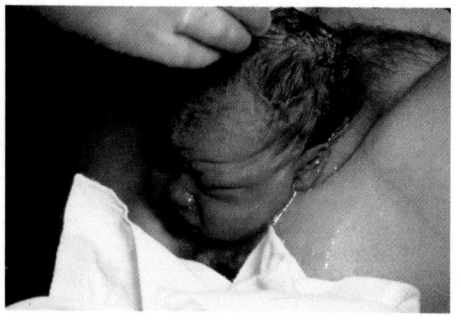

▲ **FIGURE 13.30   Delivery of Head.**

Childbirth

Labor contractions begin about 30 minutes apart. They have to be intermittent because each contraction shuts down the maternal blood supply to the placenta and therefore shuts down the blood supply to the fetus. Labor pains are due to ischemia of the myometrium.

Labor is divided into three stages, each of which is usually longer in a **primipara** (first-time birth) than in a **multipara** (two or more births).

First Stage—Dilation of the Cervix   This is the longest stage. It can be a few minutes in a multipara to more than 1 day in a primipara. **Dilation** is widening of the cervical canal to the same diameter as the baby's head *(Figure 13.29 a and b)*. At the same time the wall of the cervix becomes thinner, a process called **effacement.** During dilation, the fetal membranes rupture, and the "waters break" as amniotic fluid is released.

Second Stage—Expulsion of the Fetus   As the uterus continues to contract, additional pain is generated by the stretching of the cervix and vagina by the baby's head. When the head reaches the vaginal opening and stretches the vulva, the head is said to be **crowning** *(Figure 13.30)*. This process is sometimes helped by performing an **episiotomy,** making an incision in the perineum to prevent tearing.

After the baby is delivered, blood in the placental vein is drained into the baby, and the umbilical cord is clamped in two places and cut between the two clamps.

Third Stage—Expulsion of the Placenta   After the baby is delivered, the uterus continues to contract. It pushes the placenta off the uterine wall and expels it out of the vagina *(Figure 13.31)*.

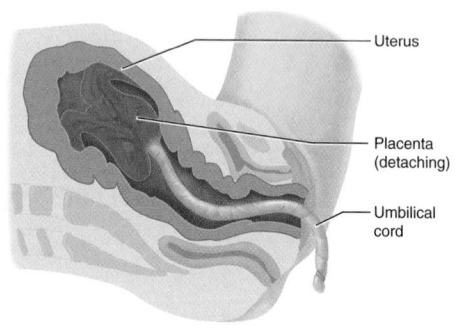

▲ **FIGURE 13.31   Placenta (Afterbirth) Detaching from Wall of Uterus.**

WORD	PRONUNCIATION		ELEMENTS	DEFINITION
autolysis	awe-**TOL**-ih-sis	P/ R/	**auto-** *self* **-lysis** *destruction*	Self-destruction of cells by enzymes within the cells
crowning	**KROWN**-ing	S/ R/	**-ing** *doing, quality of* **crown-** *crown*	During childbirth, when the maximum diameter of the baby's head comes through the vulvar ring
dilation	die-**LAY**-shun	S/ R/	**-ion** *process* **dilat-** *open out*	Stretching or enlarging of an opening
effacement	ee-**FACE**-ment	S/ R/	**-ment** *resulting state* **efface-** *wipe out*	Thinning of the cervix in relation to labor
episiotomy	eh-piz-ee-**OT**-oh-me	S/ R/CF	**-tomy** *surgical incision* **episi/o-** *vulva*	Surgical incision of the vulva
labor	**LAY**-bore		Latin *toil, suffering*	Process of expulsion of the fetus
lochia	**LOW**-kee-uh		Greek *relating to childbirth*	Vaginal discharge following childbirth
multipara	mul-**TIP**-ah-ruh	P/ R/	**multi-** *many* **-para** *to bring forth*	Woman who has given birth to two or more children
postpartum	post-**PAR**-tum	P/ R/	**post-** *after* **-partum** *childbirth*	After childbirth
primipara	pree-**MIP**-ah-ruh	P/ R/	**primi-** *first* **-para** *to bring forth*	Woman who has given birth for the first time
puerperium (***Note:*** This term is composed only of roots.)	pyu-er-**PEE**-ree-um	R/ R/	**puer-** *child* **-perium** *bringing forth*	Six-week period after birth in which the uterus involutes

Puerperium

The 6 weeks **postpartum** (after the birth) are called the **puerperium.** The uterus shrinks **(involution)** through self-digestion **(autolysis)** of uterine cells by their own lysosomal enzymes. This generates a vaginal discharge called **lochia** that lasts about 10 days.

EXERCISES *Several of these elements you have seen before, and you will certainly see them again in other terms. Learn it once, and recognize it all the time. Circle the best answer to the questions.*

1. The term that contains the prefix meaning *many* is:

   primipara   lochia   multipara

2. The term that contains the suffix meaning *incision* is:

   episiotomy   effacement   dilation

3. The term that contains the root meaning *to bring forth* is:

   primipara   involution   effacement

4. The term that contains the root meaning *child* is:

   lochia   multipara   puerperium

5. The term that contains the suffix meaning *process* is:

   effacement   episiotomy   involution

6. The term that contains the prefix meaning *first* is:

   multipara   puerperium   primipara

7. The term that contains the prefix meaning *self* is:

   multipara   autolysis   lochia

8. The term that contains the prefix meaning *after* is:

   primipara   postpartum   multipara

You are

. . . an obstetric assistant **(CNA)** working with Garry Joiner, MD, an obstetrician at Fulwood Medical Center.

Your patient is

. . . Mrs. Gloria Maggay, a 29-year-old housekeeper.

CASE REPORT 13.4

Mrs. Maggay's last menstrual period was 8 weeks ago, and she has a positive home pregnancy test. This is her first pregnancy. She has breast tenderness and mild nausea. For the past 2 days, she has had some cramping and right-sided, lower abdominal pain, and this morning she had vaginal spotting. Her VS are T 99°F, P 80, R 14, BP 130/70.

While you are waiting for Dr. Joiner to come and examine her, she complains of feeling faint and has a sharp, severe pain in her lower abdomen on the right side. Her pulse rate has increased to 92. You need to recognize what is happening.

Abbreviations	
CNA	certified nurse assistant
GDM	gestational diabetes mellitus
OR	operating room

Keynote

- Preeclampsia threatens the life of both mother and fetus.
- For the neonate, preeclampsia increases the risk of **perinatal mortality**.

DISORDERS OF PREGNANCY

Ectopic Pregnancy

If the fallopian (uterine) tube is obstructed, the fertilized egg will be prevented from moving into the uterus and will continue its development in the fallopian (uterine) tube. This is called an **ectopic pregnancy.** Tubal disorders that cause ectopic pregnancy include previous salpingitis, pelvic inflammatory disease, and endometriosis.

Case Report 13.4 (continued)

Mrs. Maggay's symptoms are those of an ectopic pregnancy. The sudden increase in the pain and the rise in pulse rate can indicate that the tube had ruptured and was hemorrhaging into the abdominal cavity. The gynecologist should see her immediately and, if necessary, take her to the **operating room (OR)** for laparoscopic surgery to stop the bleeding and evacuate the products of conception.

Preeclampsia and Eclampsia

Preeclampsia is a sudden, abnormal increase in blood pressure after the twentieth week of pregnancy, with proteinuria and edema.

Eclampsia is a life-threatening condition, characterized by the signs and symptoms of preeclampsia and with the addition of convulsions. Management involves immediate admission to the hospital with control of the mother's blood pressure. The baby is delivered as soon as the mother is stabilized, regardless of maturity.

Amniotic Fluid Abnormalities

Amniotic fluid abnormalities occur in the second trimester, when the fetus breathes in and swallows amniotic fluid. This promotes development of the gastrointestinal tract and lungs.

- **Oligohydramnios** is too little amniotic fluid. It is associated with an increase in the risk of birth defects and poor fetal growth. Its etiology is unknown.
- **Polyhydramnios** is too much amniotic fluid. It causes abdominal discomfort and breathing difficulties for the mother. It also is associated with **preterm delivery,** placental problems, and fetal growth.

Gestational Diabetes Mellitus

In some pregnant women, the amount of insulin they can produce decreases. This leads to **gestational diabetes mellitus (GDM)** and increased risk of preeclampsia. For the neonate, it increases the risk of **perinatal mortality.** Later in life, both mother and child are at increased risk for developing type 2 diabetes and obesity.

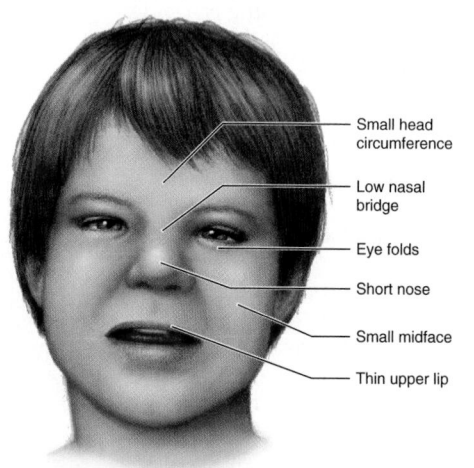

▲ **FIGURE 13.32   Fetal Alcohol Syndrome.**

Small head circumference
Low nasal bridge
Eye folds
Short nose
Small midface
Thin upper lip

WORD	PRONUNCIATION	ELEMENTS		DEFINITION
eclampsia	ek-**LAMP**-see-uh		Greek *a shining forth*	Convulsions in a patient with preeclampsia
ectopic	ek-**TOP**-ik	S/ R/	-ic *pertaining to* ectop- *on the outside, displaced*	Out of place, not in a normal position
hyperemesis	high-per-**EM**-ee-sis	P/ R/	hyper- *excessive* -emesis *vomiting*	Excessive vomiting
mortality	mor-**TAL**-ih-tee	S/ S/ R/	-al- *pertaining to* -ity *condition, state* mort- *death*	Fatal outcome or death rate
oligohydramnios	**OL**-ih-goh-high-**DRAM**-nee-os	P/ R/ R/	oligo- *too little, scanty* -hydr- *water* -amnios *amnion*	Too little amniotic fluid
polyhydramnios	**POL**-ee-high-**DRAM**-nee-os	P/	poly- *many*	Too much amniotic fluid
perinatal	per-ih-**NAY**-tal	S/ P/ R/	-al *pertaining to* peri- *around* -nat- *birth*	Around the time of birth
preeclampsia	pree-eh-**KLAMP**-see-uh	S/ P/ R/	-ia *condition* pre- *before* -eclamps- *shining forth*	Hypertension, edema, and proteinuria during pregnancy
preterm premature (syn)	**PREE**-term pree-mah-**TYUR**	P/ R/	pre- *before* -term *normal gestation*	Baby delivered before 37 weeks of gestation Occurring before the expected time; for example, an infant born before 37 weeks of gestation
teratogen	**TER**-ah-toe-jen	S/ R/CF R/	-gen *produce, create* terat/o- *monster, malformed fetus* -gen- *origin*	Agent that produces fetal deformities
teratogenesis teratogenic	**TER**-ah-toe-**JEN**-eh-sis **TER**-ah-toe-**JEN**-ik	S/ S/	-esis *condition* -ic *pertaining to*	Process involved in producing fetal deformities Capable of producing fetal deformities

Hyperemesis Gravidarum

Eighty percent of pregnant women experience some degree of "morning sickness." It is at its worst between 2 and 12 weeks and resolves in the second trimester. For a few women, nausea and vomiting persist. This is **hyperemesis gravidarum.** Severe cases may have to be admitted to the hospital for intravenous (IV) fluids.

Teratogenesis

Teratogenesis is the production of fetal abnormalities—**congenital malformations**—caused by a chemical agent taken by the mother early in pregnancy *(Figure 13.32)*. All medications readily cross the placenta. **Teratogens** include alcohol, isoretinoin (acne medication), valproic acid (anticonvulsant), and the rubella virus.

EXERCISES

After reading both parts of Case Report 13.4 on the opposite page, answer the following questions. Be prepared to discuss your answers in class.

1. What symptoms did Mrs. Maggay have when she came into the office?

_____

2. What symptoms did she develop while she was there?

_____

3. What does "the tube had ruptured" mean? _____

4. What is occurring if Mrs. Maggay is "hemorrhaging into the abdominal cavity"?

_____

5. What is the function of the laparoscope? _____

6. Why is this an emergency? _____

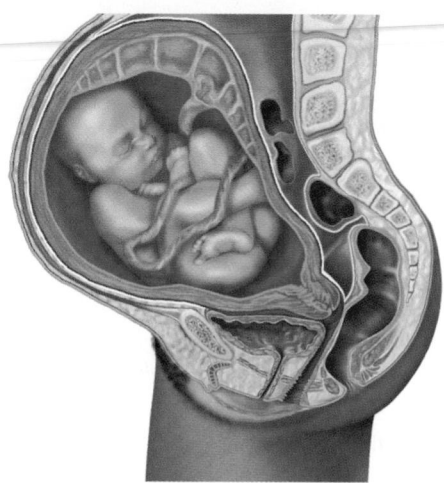

▲ FIGURE 13.33   Breech Presentation.

Abbreviations

PPH	postpartum hemorrhage
OB	obstetrics
RDS	respiratory distress syndrome

DISORDERS OF CHILDBIRTH

Fetal distress due to lack of oxygen is an uncommon complication of labor but is detrimental if not recognized. During labor, there is electronic fetal heart monitoring to determine whether the baby is in distress. Treatment is to give the mother oxygen or increase IV fluids. If distress persists, the baby is delivered as quickly as possible by **forceps extraction,** vacuum extractor, or cesarean section **(C-section).**

Abnormal position of fetus occurs when the baby at the beginning of labor is not in a head-first **(vertex)** presentation facing rearward. Abnormal positions include:

- **Breech.** The buttocks present *(Figure 13.33).*
- **Face.** The face instead of the top of the head presents.
- **Shoulder.** The shoulder and upper back are trying to exit the uterus first.

If the baby cannot be turned into a vertex presentation, a C-section is usually performed.

Prolapsed umbilical cord occurs when the cord precedes the baby down the birth canal. Pressure on the cord can cut off the baby's blood supply that is still being provided through the umbilical arteries.

Nuchal cord is the condition of having the cord wrapped around the baby's neck during delivery. This occurs in 20% of deliveries.

Premature rupture of the membranes occurs in 10% of normal pregnancies and increases the risk of infection of the uterus and fetus.

Gestational Classification

Every newborn **(neonate)** is either:

- **Premature**—less than 37 weeks gestation.
- **Full-term**—between 37 to 42 weeks gestation.
- **Postmature**—longer than 42 weeks gestation.

Prematurity occurs in about 8% of newborns. The earlier the baby is born, the more life-threatening problems occur.

Because their lungs are underdeveloped, premature babies can develop **respiratory distress syndrome (RDS),** also called **hyaline membrane disease.** The premature baby's lungs are not mature enough to produce **surfactant,** a mixture of lipids and proteins that keeps the alveoli from collapsing.

If their brain is underdeveloped, premature newborns can have inconsistent breathing with **apnea.** They are susceptible to bleeding into the brain. Their immune systems have low levels of antibodies to provide protection from infection.

An immature liver can impair the excretion of bilirubin *(see Chapter 6),* and premature babies become jaundiced. High levels of bilirubin can produce **kernicterus,** in which deposits of bilirubin in the brain cause brain damage.

Postmaturity is much less common than prematurity. Its etiology is unknown, but the placenta begins to shrink and is less able to supply sufficient nutrients to the baby. This leads to hypoglycemia; loss of subcutaneous fat; dry, peeling skin; and, if oxygen is lacking, fetal distress. The baby can pass stools **(meconium)** into the amniotic fluid. In its distress, the baby can take deep gasping breaths and inhale the meconium fluid. This leads to **meconium aspiration syndrome** and respiratory difficulty at birth.

Placental Disorders

Placenta abruptio is separation of the placenta from the uterine wall before delivery of the baby. The baby's oxygen supply is cut off, and fetal distress appears quickly. It is an obstetric (OB) emergency and usually a C-section is indicated.

Placenta previa is a low-lying placenta between the baby's head and the internal os of the cervix. It can cause severe bleeding during labor, and a C-section may be necessary.

Retained placenta means that all or part of the placenta and/or membranes remain behind in the uterus 30 minutes to an hour after the baby has been delivered. The expulsion of the placenta can happen naturally. The result of retained placenta is heavy uterine bleeding called **postpartum hemorrhage (PPH).** Manual removal of the retained product may be necessary under spinal, epidural, or general anesthesia *(Figure 13.34).*

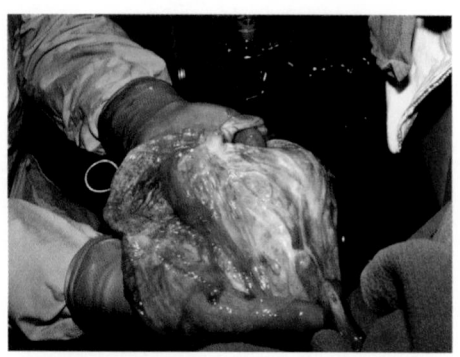

▲ FIGURE 13.34   Placenta (Afterbirth).

WORD	PRONUNCIATION		ELEMENTS	DEFINITION
abruptio	ab-**RUP**-she-oh		Latin *to break off*	Placenta abruptio is the premature detachment of the placenta
apnea	**AP**-nee-ah		Greek *lack of breath*	Absence of spontaneous respiration
breech	BREECH		Old English *trousers*	Buttocks-first presentation of fetus at delivery
forceps extraction	**FOR**-seps ek-**STRAK**-shun		Latin *a pair of tongs* Latin *to draw out*	Assisted delivery of the baby by an instrument that grasps the head of the baby
kernicterus	ker-**NICK**-ter-us	R/ R/	**kern-** *nucleus* **-icterus** *jaundice*	Bilirubin staining of basal nuclei of the brain
meconium	meh-**KOH**-nee-um		Greek *a little poppy*	The first bowel movement of the newborn
neonate	**NEE**-oh-nate	P/ R/CF	**neo-** *new* **-nat/e-** *born*	A newborn infant
neonatal (adj)	**NEE**-oh-**NAY**-tal	S/	**-al** *pertaining to*	Pertaining to the newborn infant or the newborn period
nuchal cord	**NYU**-kul KORD		**nuchal** French *the back (nape) of the neck*	Loop of umbilical cord around the fetal neck
postmature	post-mah-**TYUR**	P/ R/	**post-** *after* **-mature** *ripe, ready*	Infant born after 42 weeks of gestation
postmaturity	post-mah-**TYUR**-ih-tee	S/	**-ity** *condition*	Condition of being postmature
premature	pree-mah-**TYUR**	P/ R/	**pre-** *before, in front of* **-mature** *ripe*	Occurring before the expected time; for example, an infant born before 37 weeks of gestation
prematurity preemie (informal)	pree-mah-**TYUR**-ih-tee **PREE**-me	S/	**-ity** *condition, state*	Condition of being premature Premature baby
previa	**PREE**-vee-ah	P/ R/	**pre-** *before, in front of* **-via** *the way*	Anything blocking the fetus during its birth; for example, am abnormally situated placenta, *placenta previa*
surfactant	ser-**FAK**-tant		surface active agent	A protein and fat compound that creates surface tension to hold lung alveolar walls apart
vertex	**VER**-teks		Latin *whorl*	Topmost point of the vault of the skull

EXERCISES

Elements: *Real familiarity with obstetrical and reproductive terms means you can look at an element and identify it as either a prefix, root or combining form, or suffix. Identify each element by writing its type and meaning in the appropriate columns. The first one is done for you. Fill in the blanks.*

	Element	Type	Meaning
1.	post	*P*	*after*
2.	obstetr		
3.	kern		
4.	via		
5.	mature		
6.	pre		
7.	ician		
8.	icterus		
9.	ity		

OBJECTIVES

It is important to complete your understanding of reproduction by being able to use correct medical terminology to:

13.5.1 Describe the anatomy of the breast.

13.5.2 Differentiate the breast from the mammary gland.

13.5.3 Explain the physiology and mechanisms of lactation.

13.5.4 Discuss common disorders of the breast.

Keynote

There is no relationship between breast size and the ability to breastfeed.

Breastfeeding is not a reliable means of contraception. It has a failure rate of around 10%.

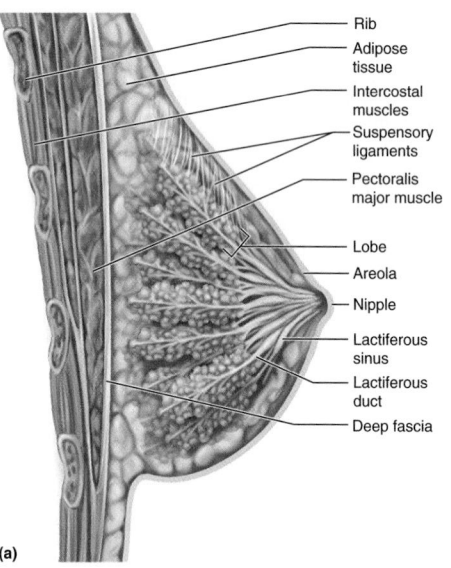

(a)

▲ **FIGURE 13.35   Anatomy of Lactating Breast.**

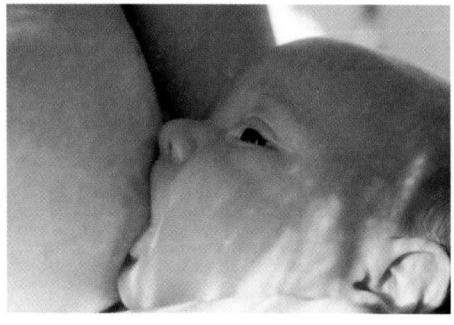

▲ **FIGURE 13.36   Breastfeeding.**

THE BREAST

Until the relatively recent introduction of bottles filled with liquid supplied by cows or soybeans, the milk produced by the female breast was essential for the survival of the human species. Nourishment of the infant remains the breast's major function, even though our culture has made the breast a visible, tangible, and beautiful symbol of femininity.

Anatomy of the Breast

The breasts of males and females are identical until puberty, when ovarian hormones stimulate the development of the breast in females. Adult males still have main milk ducts in their breasts.

Each adult female breast has a **body** located over the pectoralis major muscle and an **axillary tail** extending toward the armpit. The **nipple** projects from the breast and contains multiple openings of the main milk ducts. The reddish-brown **areola** surrounds the nipple. The small bumps on its surface are **areolar glands.** These are sebaceous glands, the secretions of which prevent chapping and cracking during breastfeeding.

Internally, the breasts are supported by **suspensory ligaments** that extend from the skin to the fascia overlying the pectoralis major muscle *(Figure 13.35)*.

The **nonlactating breast** consists mostly of adipose and connective tissues. It has a system of ducts that branch through the connective tissue and converge on the nipple.

Mammary Gland

When the **mammary gland** develops during pregnancy, it is divided into 15 to 20 lobes that contain the secretory **alveoli** that produce milk. Each lobe is drained by the main milk ducts, called **lactiferous ducts** *(see Figure 13.35)*. Immediately before opening onto the nipple, each lactiferous duct dilates to form a **lactiferous sinus** in which milk is stored before being released from the nipple.

Lactation

When the mammary gland develops during pregnancy, high estrogen levels cause the lactiferous ducts to grow and branch, and progesterone stimulates the budding of alveoli at the ends of the ducts. The alveoli are formed in grapelike clusters. The percentage of adipose and connective tissue diminishes.

In late pregnancy, the alveoli and ducts contain **colostrum.** This secretion contains more protein but less fat than human milk, but it also contains high levels of **immunoglobulins** *(see Chapter 15)* to give the newborn infant protection from infections. Colostrum is replaced by milk 2 or 3 days after the baby's birth, and this replacement is complete by day 5.

Milk production is mainly controlled by **prolactin,** a hormone from the pituitary gland. The other essential stimulus to milk production is the baby's sucking *(Figure 13.36)*, which stimulates prolactin production. In addition, the **sucking reflex** stimulates the pituitary gland to produce **oxytocin** *(see Chapter 15)*, which causes milk to be ejected from the alveoli into the duct system.

WORD	PRONUNCIATION		ELEMENTS	DEFINITION
apoptosis	AP-op-TOE-sis	R/ P/	-ptosis *drooping, falling* apo- *separation from, off*	Programmed normal cell death
areola areolar (adj)	ah-REE-oh-luh		Latin *small area*	Circular reddish area surrounding the nipple
colostrum	koh-LOSS-trum		Latin *foremilk*	The first breast secretion at the end of pregnancy
lactation	lak-TAY-shun	S/ R/CF	-ation *process* lact/i- *milk*	Production of milk
lactiferous lactate (verb)	lak-TIF-er-us	S/ R/	-ous *pertaining to* -fer- *to bear, carry*	Pertaining to or yielding milk
mammary	MAM-ah-ree	S/ R/	-ary *pertaining to* mamm- *breast*	Relating to the lactating breast
nipple	NIP-el		Old English *small nose*	Projection from the breast into which the lactiferous ducts open
oxytocin	OCK-see-toe-sin	S/ R/CF R/	-in *chemical compound* ox/y- *oxygen* -toc- *labor, birth*	Pituitary hormone that stimulates the uterus to contract
prolactin	pro-LAK-tin	S/ P/ R/	-in *chemical compound* pro- *before* -lact- *milk*	Pituitary hormone that stimulates production of milk

Milk production continues as long as the baby suckles at least twice daily, but in the United States only 20% of mothers are still breastfeeding at 6 months. The American Academy of Pediatrics recommends breastfeeding for 6 to 12 months.

After complete cessation of lactation, involution of the mammary gland occurs. The epithelial cells of the alveoli are lost through **apoptosis** (programmed cell death), the ducts shrink in size, and adipose and connective tissue return to being the major breast tissues.

EXERCISES

Spelling your documentation correctly is a mark of an educated professional. Read the following statements, and insert the correctly spelled term in the blanks.

1. (Prolectin/Prolactin) _____ is the pituitary hormone that stimulates production of milk.

2. The circular, reddish area surrounding the nipple is the (aireola/areola) _____.

3. After complete cessation of lactation, involution of the (mamery/mammary) _____ gland occurs.

4. (Oxitocin/Oxytocin) _____ is the pituitary hormone that stimulates the uterus to contract.

5. Programmed normal cell death is known as (apotosis/apoptosis) _____.

6. The first breast secretion at the end of pregnancy is known as (colestrium/colostrum) _____.

7. The projection from the breast into which the milk ducts open is the (nippel/nipple) _____.

8. (Laktiferous/Lactiferous) _____ means *pertaining to or yielding milk*.

9. The areolar glands are (cebaceous/sebaceous) _____ glands.

10. (Involation/Involution) _____ of the mammary glands occurs after breastfeeding stops.

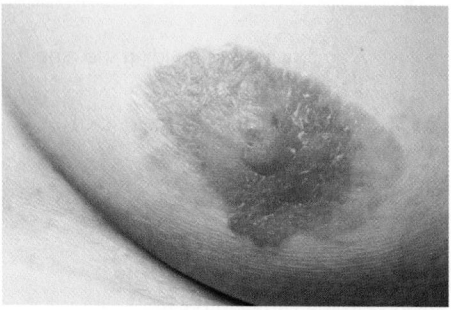

▲ **FIGURE 13.37 Paget Disease of the Nipple Is Associated with Breast Cancer.**

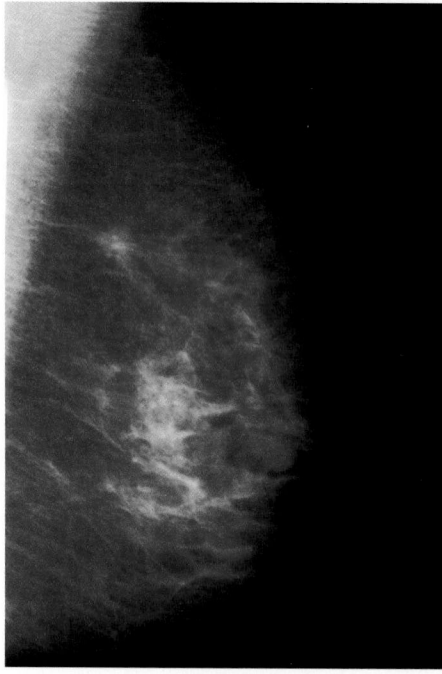

▲ **FIGURE 13.38 Fibrocystic Disease of the Breast.**

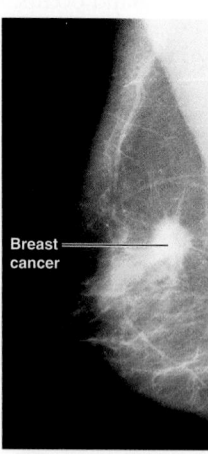

Breast cancer

▲ **FIGURE 13.39 Mammogram Showing Breast Cancer.**

DISORDERS OF THE BREAST

Mastitis, inflammation of the breast, can occur in association with breast-feeding if the nipple or areola is cracked or traumatized. It is usually segmental in one of the lobes of the breast and responds well to antibiotics. It is not an indication for stopping breastfeeding.

Mastalgia (breast pain) is the most common benign breast disorder. The pain can be associated with breast tenderness and be part of PMS. If the pain is not relieved by acetaminophen or NSAIDs, danazol or tamoxifen can be used for a short time.

Paget disease of the nipple presents as a scaling, crusting lesion of the nipple, sometimes with a discharge from the nipple *(Figure 13.37)*. It is indicative of an underlying cancer that has to be the focus of diagnosis and treatment.

Nipple discharge, particularly if it is from one breast and bloody, is an indication of an underlying disorder such as breast cancer and warrants investigation.

Fibroadenomas are circumscribed, small, benign tumors that can be either cystic or solid and can be multiple. They can be excised surgically.

Fibrocystic disease of the breast presents as a dense, irregular cobblestone consistency of the breast, often with intermittent breast discomfort *(Figure 13.38)*. It occurs in over 60% of all women and is considered by many doctors as a normal variant.

Breast cancer affects one in eight women in their lifetime. Risk factors include a family history, particularly if a woman carries either the **BRCA1** or **BRCA2** gene, the use of postmenopausal estrogen therapy, and an early menarche and late menopause.

Most breast cancers are discovered as a lump by the patient, which is why **monthly breast self-examinations (BSEs)** are so important. Another 40% are discovered on routine **mammogram** *(Figure 13.39)*. Routine **mammography** reduces breast cancer mortality by 25% to 30%.

Most breast cancers occur in the upper and outer quadrant of the breast. If cancer is suspected, biopsy should be planned. This is being performed more and more often as a **stereotactic biopsy,** a needle biopsy performed during mammography.

The surgical treatments for breast cancer include:

- **Excisional biopsy** to remove the breast tumor with a surrounding margin of normal breast tissue.

- **Lumpectomy** or **quadrantectomy,** which are breast-conserving surgeries.

- **Simple mastectomy** to remove the breast with skin and nipple *(Figure 13.40)*.

- **Modified radical mastectomy,** which is a simple mastectomy plus lymph node dissection.

- **Radical mastectomy,** with complete removal of breast tissue, pectoralis major muscle, and all associated lymph nodes.

Additional radiotherapy, combination chemotherapy, and Herceptin and Tamoxifen therapy are also used.

Procedures for postoperative breast reconstruction surgery *(Figure 13.41)* include submuscular silicone or saline implants and transfer of muscle from the latissimus dorsi *(see Chapter 5)*.

Breast cancer can metastasize to lymph nodes, lungs, liver, bone, brain, and skin.

Galactorrhea is the production of milk when a woman is not breastfeeding. Sometimes the cause cannot be found, but it can occur in association with hormone therapy, antidepressants, tumor of the pituitary gland *(see Chapter 14)*, and use of street drugs such as opiates and marijuana. In most cases, the milk production ceases with time.

Gynecomastia, enlargement of the breast, can be unilateral or bilateral and occur in both sexes. It is usually associated with either liver disease, marijuana, or drug therapy such as estrogens, calcium channel blockers, and antineoplastic drugs. It remits or disappears after the drug is withdrawn. Occasionally **suction lipectomy** and/or cosmetic surgery is needed.

WORD	PRONUNCIATION	ELEMENTS		DEFINITION
fibroadenoma	FIE-broh-ad-en-OH-mah	S/ R/ R/CF	-oma *tumor* -aden- *gland* fibr/o- *fiber*	Benign tumor containing much fibrous tissue
fibrocystic disease	fie-broh-SIS-tik DIZ-eez	S/ R/CF R/	-ic *pertaining to* fibr/o- *fiber* -cyst- *cyst*	Benign breast disease with multiple tiny lumps and cysts
galactorrhea	gah-LAK-toe-REE-ah	S/ R/CF	-rrhea *flow* galact/o- *milk*	Abnormal flow of milk from the breasts
gynecomastia	GUY-nih-koh-MAS-tee-ah	S/ R/CF R/	-ia *condition* gynec/o- *female* -mast- *breast*	Enlargement of the breast
lipectomy	lip-ECK-toe-me	S/ R/	-ectomy *surgical excision* lip- *fatty tissue*	Surgical removal of adipose tissue
lumpectomy	lump-ECK-toe-me	S/ R/CF	-ectomy *surgical excision* lump- *piece*	Removal of a lesion with preservation of surrounding tissue
mammogram	MAM-oh-gram	S/ R/CF	-gram *a record* mamm/o- *breast*	The record produced by x-ray imaging of the breast
mammography	mah-MOG-rah-fee	S/	-graphy *process of recording*	Process of x-ray examination of the breast
mastalgia	mass-TAL-jee-uh	S/ R/	-algia *pain* mast- *breast*	Pain in the breast
mastectomy	mass-TECK-toe-me	S/ R/	-ectomy *surgical excision* mast- *breast*	Surgical excision of the breast
mastitis	mass-TIE-tis	S/ R/	-itis *inflammation* mast- *breast*	Inflammation of the breast
quadrant quadrantectomy	KWAD-rant kwad-ran-TEK-toe-me	S/ R/	Latin *quarter* -ectomy *surgical excision* quadrant- *quarter*	One-quarter of a circle Surgical excision of a quadrant of the breast
stereotactic	STER-ee-oh-TAK-tic	S/ R/ R/CF	-ic *pertaining to* -tact- *orderly arrangement* stere/o- *three-dimensional*	Pertaining to a precise three-dimensional method to locate a lesion

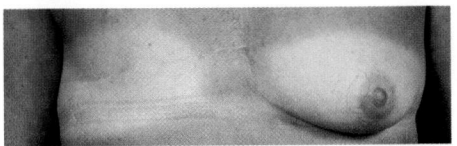

▲ **FIGURE 13.40   Same Patient as in *Figure 13.39* After Mastectomy.**

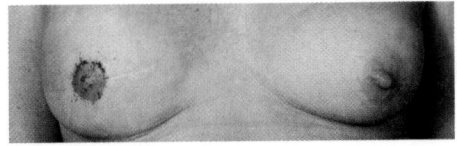

▲ **FIGURE 13.41   Same Patient as in *Figure 13.40* After Surgical Breast Reconstruction.**

EXERCISES

Build your knowledge of suffixes, which always provide a big clue to the meaning of a medical term. Review all the terms in this WAD; then answer the following questions. All of these questions can be answered by analyzing the elements in each term. Which of the terms in this WAD mean:

1. *surgical excision?* List them here. _____

2. *a glandular tumor?* _____

3. *condition of enlarged breasts?* _____

4. *precise, three-dimensional method to locate a lesion?* _____

5. *an inflammation of the breast?* _____

6. *breast pain?* _____

7. *an abnormal flow of milk?* _____

FEMALE REPRODUCTIVE SYSTEM

CHALLENGE YOUR KNOWLEDGE

A. **Patient Documentation:** The following mammogram report for a patient contains terminology you should understand after reading this chapter. Answer the questions about the report by filling in the blanks.

> **Exam:** Diagnostic bilateral mammogram
>
> **Reason for exam:** Discomfort in both breasts
>
> The glandular tissue is heterogeneously dense. There are scattered fibroglandular densities bilaterally. There is a benign-appearing curvilinear area of glandular tissue in the right lower inner breast. There are a few faint calcifications in the lower inner left breast and in the central left breast. Magnification views were performed of the left breast calcifications in two positions, and they have an appearance most consistent with benign process. There is no associated mass or distortion.
>
> **Impression:** Heterogeneously dense glandular tissue with focal glandular density in the medial aspect of the right breast and faint calcifications in the left breast. Probably benign.
>
> **Recommendation:** Comparison with prior films. If prior films are not available, recommend follow-up mammogram in 6 months. Findings were submitted to the patient in writing.

1. Define **bilateral**. _____

2. Deconstruct the term **fibroglandular** by putting slashes between each element.

   _____

3. Define **calcification**. Use a dictionary if needed.

   _____

4. Define **benign process**. Use a dictionary if needed.

   _____

5. Define **heterogeneously**. Use a dictionary if needed.

   _____

Discussion questions on this report and the breast:

6. Why does the radiologist recommend follow-up in 6 months if no previous films are available?

   _____

7. What is the difference between **mastitis** and **mastalgia**?

   _____

8. With what is **gynecomastia** usually associated?

   _____

9. Define **fibroadenoma**.

   _____

10. Does this patient's report show any malignancies? _____

B. Prefixes: The following medical terms all have the same prefix, but the rest of their elements make them entirely different terms. Analyze each medical term into its basic elements and meaning; then use the terms in sentences of your own making. Fill in the chart, and then write your sentences.

Medical Term	Prefix	Root/CF	Suffix	Meaning of Term
dysplasia				
dysmenorrhea				
dysplastic				
dysfunctional				
dyspareunia				

Sentences:

1. _____

2. _____

3. _____

4. _____

5. _____

C. Abbreviations: There are many abbreviations in this chapter, and they are of no use to you if you cannot interpret them correctly. Practice using abbreviations in this exercise. Everything in the sentence is spelled out—rewrite the sentence on the lines below, inserting abbreviations where appropriate.

1. Patient was advised to take naproxen sodium to relieve the symptoms of her premenstrual syndrome; she wishes to discontinue the birth control pills and try an intrauterine device for contraception instead.

   _____

   _____

2. The patient's untreated sexually transmitted disease, chlamydia, has progressed to pelvic inflammatory disease and needs immediate treatment.

   _____

   _____

3. Following a difficult labor and cesarean delivery, the patient suffered postpartum hemorrhage, and the infant is suffering from respiratory distress syndrome.

   _____

   _____

4. Patient has been referred to the Gynecology Clinic for a consultation regarding the need for a dilation and curettage.

   _____

   _____

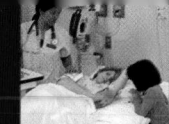
FEMALE REPRODUCTIVE SYSTEM

D. Terminology Challenge: Autolysis is a new term you learned in this chapter. It is composed of two elements you have encountered in previous chapters. Recall other terms you have already learned that have those elements.

Autolysis means _____ .

Other terms with the same elements and their meanings:

auto-: _____

-lysis: _____

E. Language of Gynecology: Demonstrate your knowledge of gynecologic terminology by answering the following multiple-choice questions. Circle the correct answer.

1. The mons pubis, labia majora and minora, and clitoris are collectively called the:

    a. prepuce

    b. hymen

    c. vulva

    d. vaginosis

    e. antrum

2. This procedure can be used to visualize the inside of the uterus, take a biopsy, and/or remove polyps or fibroids:

    a. cytoscopy

    b. hysteroscopy

    c. ureteroscopy

    d. bronchoscopy

    e. thoracoscopy

3. Painful intercourse:

    a. salpingitis

    b. dyspnea

    c. hyperemesis

    d. dyspareunia

    e. candidiasis

4. Thin membrane that partially occludes the vagina:

    a. fornix

    b. mons

    c. vestibule

    d. hymen

    e. clitoris

5. Irregular bleeding between menstrual periods is called:

   a. amenorrhea

   b. metrorrhagia

   c. polymenorrhea

   d. dysmenorrhea

   e. menorrhagia

6. The ovaries in the female and testes in the male can both be called:

   a. adnexa

   b. ova

   c. fornices

   d. rugae

   e. gonads

7. Which of the following is an STD?

   a. toxic shock syndrome

   b. vulvovaginal candidiasis

   c. dyspareunia

   d. all of these

   e. none of these

8. Human immunodeficiency virus damages the immune system, so infections will develop that the body would otherwise cope with easily. These infections are called:

   a. bacterial

   b. staph

   c. opportunistic

   d. strep

   e. viral

9. Chronic, lasting, severe pain around the vaginal orifice is a condition called:

   a. vulvitis

   b. vaginitis

   c. vulvodynia

   d. candidiasis

   e. endometriosis

FEMALE REPRODUCTIVE SYSTEM

F. **Language of Gynecology:** Demonstrate your knowledge of gynecologic terminology by answering the following multiple-choice questions. Circle the correct answer.

1. Inflammation of the fallopian (uterine) tubes is called:

    a. ureteritis

    b. uveitis

    c. hyperemesis

    d. endometriosis

    e. salpingitis

2. The process of egg formation is called:

    a. oophorectomy

    b. ova

    c. oogenesis

    d. oophocentesis

    e. ovulation

3. Estrogen, progesterone, and androgen are all:

    a. antigens

    b. enzymes

    c. hormones

    d. antibiotics

    e. vitamins

G. **The Same but Different:** More than one body part can be described using the same term, but the term may have obviously different meanings.

1. Find two different definitions for **cervix.**

    Definition: _____

    Definition: _____

    The term **cervix** can apply to these two different body systems:

    _____ and _____

2. The cervical canal **dilates** in labor. What else dilates in a different body system?

    _____

H. **Latin and Greek terms cannot be further deconstructed into prefix, root, combining form, or suffix.** You must know them for what they are. Test your knowledge of these terms with this exercise. Match the medical term in the left column with the correct meaning in the right column.

_____ 1. fornix   A. plug

_____ 2. menses   B. membrane

_____ 3. ruga   C. egg

_____ 4. ulcer   D. month

_____ 5. os   E. sheath

_____ 6. hymen   F. neck

_____ 7. ovary   G. arch, vault

_____ 8. vagina   H. mouth

_____ 9. cervix   I. ridge or crease

_____ 10. tampon   J. cancer

I. **Plurals of some medical terms can be difficult to convert from the singular because there are so many different rules for plurals.** Practice makes perfect in your ability to form the correct plural of the term. Fill in the plural column; then choose any one term, and write a sentence using that term.

Singular Term	Plural Term
cilium	
fimbria	
fornix	
infundibulum	
labium	
majus	
minus	
ovary	
ovum	
ruga	

Sentence: _____

_____

FEMALE REPRODUCTIVE SYSTEM

J. **Roots are the core foundation of every term.** Underline just the roots or combining forms in the following terms, and give their meanings.

1. amenorrhea _____

2. progesterone _____

3. leiomyoma _____

4. menstruation _____

5. antevert _____

6. endometrial _____

7. paraurethral _____

8. amniocentesis _____

9. perimetrium _____

10. hysterosalpingogram _____

K. **Dictionary: Tertiary** is a term used in connection with the disease syphilis. Using your dictionary or an online medical dictionary, look up its meaning.

tertiary: _____

Discuss: Prepare a brief discussion on the different stages of syphilis and its various signs, symptoms, and treatments. Write your discussion notes below.

_____

_____

_____

_____

L. **Recall and Review:** How well do you remember these word elements from the previous chapter? Try to answer without first looking back to check. Fill in the blanks.

Element	Type of Element (P, R, CF, S)	Meaning of Element
ous	_____	_____
hypo	_____	_____
orch	_____	_____
didymis	_____	_____
osis	_____	_____

M. **Language of Obstetrics:** Pregnancy has its own associated set of obstetric terms. Apply your knowledge of obstetric terms to answering the following questions. Circle the correct answer.

1. Where does fertilization actually take place?

   a. left ovary

   b. distal third of the fallopian (uterine) tube

   c. right ovary

   d. proximal third of the fallopian (uterine) tube

   e. uterus

2. During the first stage of labor, what is the process in which the wall of the cervix becomes thinner?

   a. crowning

   b. effacement

   c. delivery

   d. autolysis

   e. involution

3. A fertilized egg continues its development in the fallopian (uterine) tube instead of the uterus:

   a. preeclampsia

   b. postpartum

   c. eclampsia

   d. ectopic

   e. endometriosis

4. Protective covering for skin of fetus:

   a. estrogen

   b. lanugo

   c. vernix caseosa

   d. chorion

   e. morula

5. Woman who has given birth for the first time:

   a. multipara

   b. gravidarum

   c. primipara

   d. postpartum

   e. puerperium

FEMALE REPRODUCTIVE SYSTEM

N. **Language of Obstetrics:** Pregnancy has its own associated set of obstetric terms. Apply your knowledge of obstetric terms to answering the following questions. Circle the correct answer.

1. **Nuchal cord** is:

    a. only present in ectopic pregnancy

    b. wrapped around the baby's neck during delivery

    c. a congenital malformation

    d. only present in breech births

    e. present in 50% of births

2. What keeps the maternal and fetal blood circulations separated?

    a. umbilical cord

    b. amnion

    c. yolk sac

    d. cells of the villi

    e. placenta

3. Test for chromosomal abnormalities and genetic birth defects:

    a. teratogenesis

    b. hyperemesis

    c. dilation

    d. labor

    e. amniocentesis

4. When the head is just starting to push out of the vaginal opening, it is said to be:

    a. effacing

    b. crowning

    c. dilating

    d. ovulating

    e. none of these

5. Which undesirable item can cross the placenta into the fetus?

    a. rubella virus

    b. oxygen

    c. maternal antibodies

    d. glucose

    e. hormones

6. Pit in the abdomen where umbilical cord entered fetus:

    a. meatus

    b. navel

    c. yolk sac

    d. a and b

    e. none of these

7. Postpartum vaginal discharge is called:

    a. puerperium

    b. lochia

    c. polyhydramnios

    d. amniocentesis

    e. oligohydramnios

O. **Translation Please:** How well do you understand what you read? Use your knowledge of OB/GYN terminology to translate the following sentences taken directly from this chapter into layman's terms. Fill in the blanks.

1. "Gestation is divided into trimesters."

    _____

    _____

    _____

2. "Tubal ligation is performed with laparoscopy."

    _____

    _____

    _____

P. **Short Answer:** If you understand the terminology in these questions, you can explain it to someone else, as you will often have to do on the job. Fill in the blanks.

1. Explain how the difference of one word element changes the meanings of these words: conception   contraception

    _____

    _____

2. Explain what is meant by "an STD develops *resistance* to antibiotics."

    _____

    _____

3. A new patient's chart says she is "gravida 4, para 3." What does that mean?

    _____

    _____

    _____

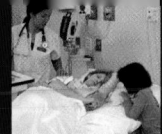

FEMALE REPRODUCTIVE SYSTEM

Q. **Patient Claire Marcos:** Go back and reread the scenario in Case Report 13.2. Now that you have completed this chapter, you should be able to answer her questions in language she will understand. Fill in the blanks.

1. Why are my periods so irregular?

   _____

   _____

2. Why doesn't my acne respond to all the treatment I've had?

   _____

   _____

3. Am I going bald?

   _____

   _____

4. Will I be able to have children some day?

   _____

   _____

5. Why am I taking birth control pills when I'm not sexually active?

   _____

   _____

6. What are all these other health problems they say I'm at risk for?

   _____

   _____

R. **Patient Education:** Breast cancer affects one in eight women in their lifetime. If a patient were to ask, could you give a brief description of each of the following surgical treatments for breast cancer?

1. excisional biopsy:

   _____

   _____

2. lumpectomy:

   _____

   _____

3. quadrantectomy:

   _____

   _____

4. simple mastectomy:

_____

_____

5. modified radical mastectomy:

_____

_____

6. radical mastectomy:

_____

_____

S. **Trace the Pathway of Conception.** The following phrases describe the process of fertilization. Number the items 1 to 8 to indicate the correct order of their occurrence.

_____ **a.** Nuclei of male and female cells unite.

_____ **b.** Morula becomes a blastocyst.

_____ **c.** Inner cell mass differentiates and forms embryo.

_____ **d.** Zygote produces morula.

_____ **e.** Ovary releases egg.

_____ **f.** All organ systems are present; embryo becomes fetus.

_____ **g.** Blastocyst implants in the endometrium.

_____ **h.** Zygote is formed.

Note: Notice how the various terms change, as what starts out as the "egg" progresses through different stages and terms to become the "fetus."

List those terms here: _____

_____

T. **Precision in Documentation:** The roots **recto-** and **retro-** can sound similar but have very different meanings. Demonstrate that you know the difference by using a term containing each element in sentences of your choice.

Sentence using a term containing **recto-**:

_____

_____

Sentence using a term containing **retro-**:

_____

_____

FEMALE REPRODUCTIVE SYSTEM

CHAPTER SUMMARY EXERCISE

1. *Listen to the pronunciation of the medical terms as given by your instructor.*
2. *Circle the correct spelling of the medical term.*
3. *Match the correctly spelled terms to the brief descriptions below.*
4. *Write a sentence for each of the 10 terms that appear in this exercise.*

A. SPELLING COMPREHENSION: CIRCLE THE CORRECT SPELLING OF THE TERM.

1. mensstuation	menstruation	menstuation	mensstruation	menstrruation
2. Falopian	fallopian	faloppian	fallopean	falopean
3. anteverted	antiverted	anteverrted	antiverrted	antevertted
4. postpubescent	postpubiscient	postpubescient	postpubisent	postpubessient
5. cotus	cottus	coitus	coituss	cutois
6. fimbeia	fimmbria	fembria	fimbrea	fembrea
7. dyspareeunia	dispareunia	dyspareunia	disspariunia	despariunia
8. liomioma	lyomyoma	leiomyoma	liomyoma	leomyoma
9. gonorhea	gonorrhea	gonnorhea	gonorhea	gonorheea
10. epesiotomy	episiotomy	eppesiotomy	epessiotomy	epeziotomy

B. MATCH THE NUMBER OF THE CORRECT TERM IN PART A WITH THE BRIEF DESCRIPTION OF THE TERM BELOW.

a. Pain during sexual intercourse _____

b. Synonym for menses _____

c. Uterine tubes _____

d. Fringelike structure _____

e. Contagious infection of genital mucosa _____

f. After the age of puberty _____

g. Tilted forward _____

h. Sexual intercourse _____

i. Benign neoplasm derived from smooth muscle _____

j. Surgical incision of the vulva _____

C. USING YOUR KNOWLEDGE OF TERMS 1–10 IN PART A AND THEIR CORRECT SPELLING, WRITE A BRIEF SENTENCE FOR EACH OF THE TERMS AS IT MIGHT APPEAR IN PATIENT DOCUMENTATION.

1. _____

2. _____

3. _____

4. _____

5. _____

6. _____

7. _____

8. _____

9. _____

10. _____

D. YOUR INSTRUCTOR WILL DIRECT YOU TO MCGRAW-HILL CONNECT. OPEN THE AUDIO GLOSSARY AND PRACTICE YOUR PRONUNCIATION OF THE TERMS IN PART A OF THIS EXERCISE.

McGraw Hill **connect**™ (plus+)

E. AFTER READING CASE REPORT 13.2, ANSWER THE FOLLOWING QUESTIONS. BE PREPARED TO DISCUSS YOUR ANSWERS IN CLASS.

You are

... a certified health education specialist **(CHES)** employed by Fulwood Medical Center.

Your patient is

... Ms. Claire Marcos, a 21-year-old student referred to you by Anna Rusack, MD, a gynecologist.

CASE REPORT 13.2

Ms. Marcos has been diagnosed with **polycystic ovarian** syndrome, and your task is to develop a program of self-care as part of her overall plan of therapy.

From her medical record, you see that she presented with irregular, often missed menstrual periods since the beginning of puberty, persistent acne, patches of dark skin on the back of her neck and under her arms, loss of hair from the front of her scalp, and inability to control her weight. She is 5 feet 4 inches and weighs 150 pounds.

Her self-care program is to include exercise, diet, and regular use of birth control medication and metformin, both of which have been prescribed.

She has written out a list of questions that she hands to you. These include:

- Why are my periods so irregular?
- Why doesn't my acne respond to all the treatment I've had?
- Am I going bald?
- Will I be able to have children some day?
- Why am I taking birth control pills when I'm not sexually active?
- What are all these other health problems they say I'm at risk for?

When Ms. Claire Marcos first presented in the Gynecology Clinic, Dr. Rusack examined her abdomen and pelvis. Dr. Rusack was able to **palpate** both enlarged ovaries on vaginal examination. A vaginal ultrasound scan showed multiple small cysts in each ovary. Blood tests showed high levels of testosterone and luteinizing hormone. Dr. Rusack prescribed birth control pills because they contain estrogen and progesterone. These can correct the hormonal imbalance, regulate menses, and lower the level of testosterone to diminish acne and hair problems. Metformin was also prescribed.

1. What diagnostic tests did Ms. Marcos have? _____

2. What is the medical term for *multiple small cysts?* _____

3. What was prescribed to restore Ms. Marcos' hormonal imbalance?

_____

4. What does a *gynecologist* specialize in?

_____

5. What did Dr. Rusack observe on *palpation?*

_____

6. Besides correcting the hormonal imbalance, what other conditions will Dr. Rusack's treatment plan address for the patient?

_____

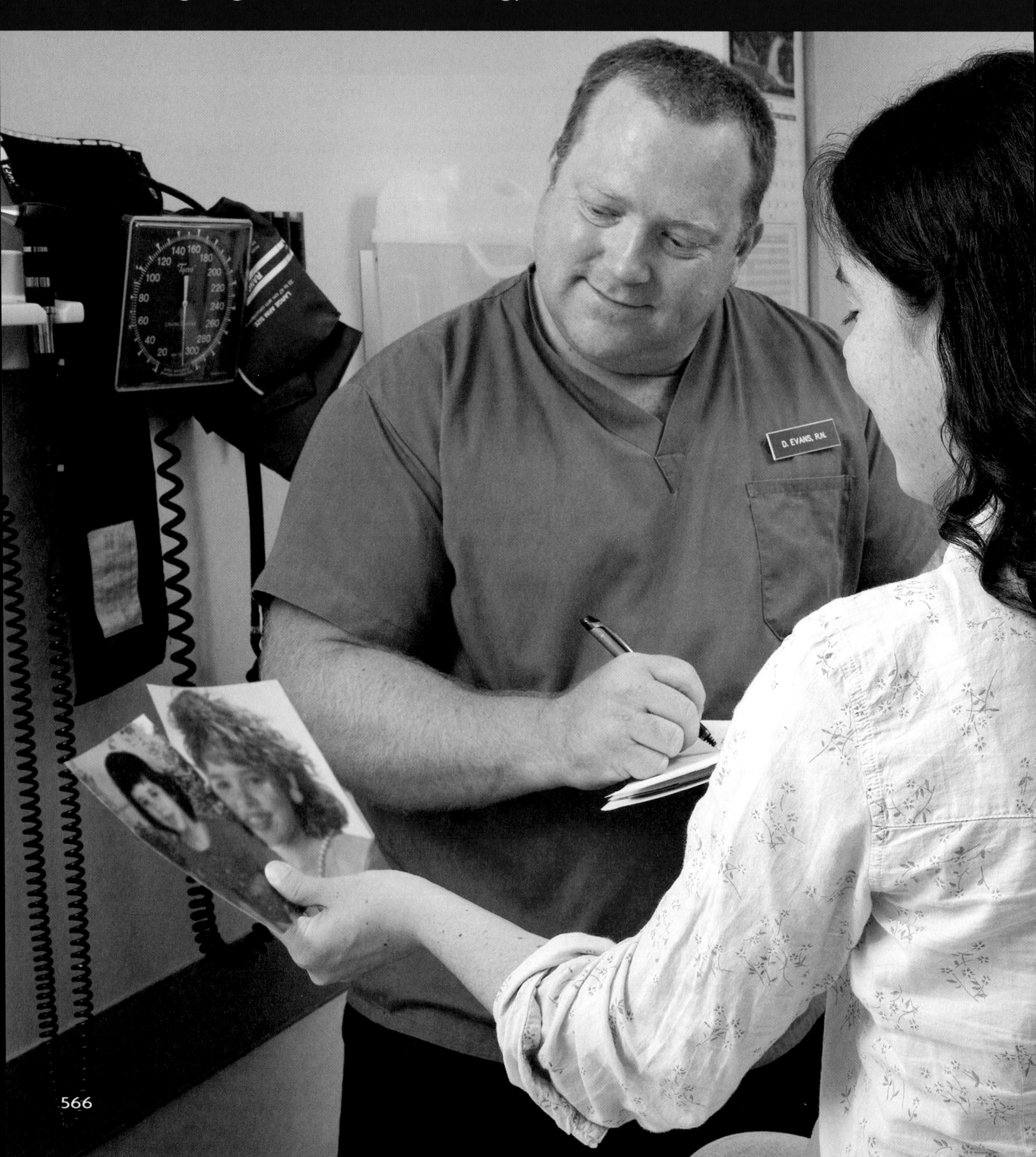

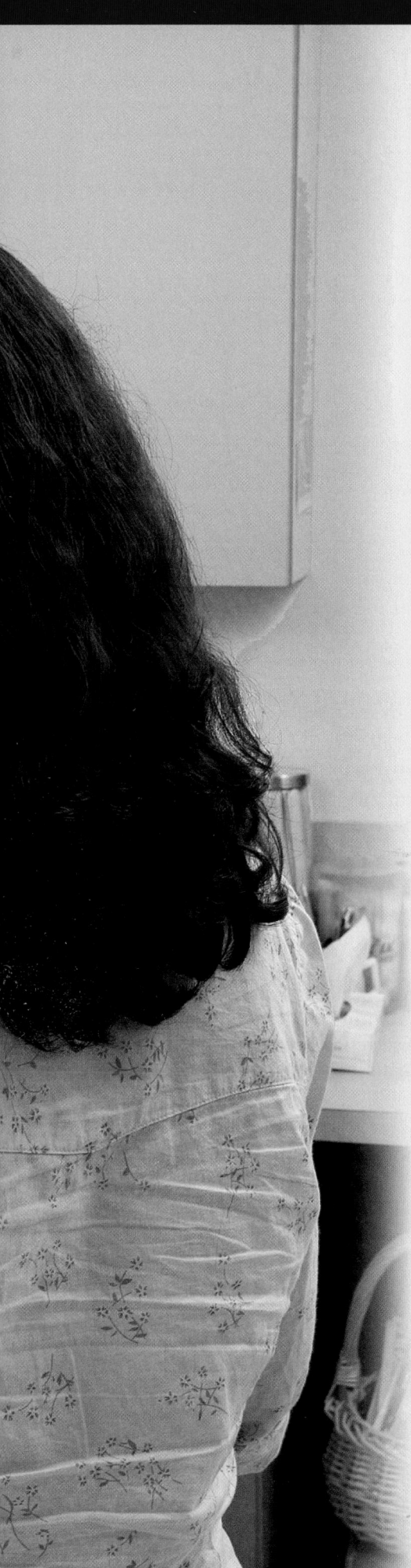

CASE REPORT 14.1

You are

. . . a registered nurse working with **endocrinologist** Sabina Khalid, MD, in the **Endocrinology** Clinic at Fulwood Medical Center.

Your patient is

. . . Mrs. Gina Tacher, a 33-year-old schoolteacher. She complains of coarsening of her facial features and enlargement of the bones of her hands. Over the past 10 years her nose and jaw have increased in size, and her voice has become husky. She has brought photos of herself at ages 9 and 16. She has no other health problems.

Keynote

A hormone is secreted by an organ and is carried by the bloodstream to act at distant target sites.

Learning Outcomes

The **endocrine system** is a communication system. The **hormones** it produces circulate in the bloodstream, giving them access to all other cells of the body. Hormones are blood-borne messengers secreted by endocrine glands. They are distributed anywhere that blood goes but affect only the target cells that have receptors for them; they alter the metabolism of these cells.

The information in this chapter enables you to:

14.1 Apply the language of endocrinology to the anatomy and physiology of the endocrine system.

14.2 Comprehend, analyze, spell, and write the medical terms of endocrinology so that you can communicate and document accurately and precisely in any health care setting.

14.3 Recognize and pronounce the medical terms of endocrinology so that you communicate verbally with accuracy and precision in any health care setting.

14.4 Explain the effects of common endocrine disorders on health.

Endocrine System Overview and Pituitary and Pineal Glands

OBJECTIVES

The information in this lesson will enable you to use correct medical terminology to:

14.1.1 **Name the glands that make up the endocrine system.**

14.1.2 **List the hormones produced by the hypothalamus and pituitary gland.**

14.1.3 **Explain the interactions between the hypothalamus and pituitary gland.**

14.1.4 **Identify the controls the hypothalamus and pituitary exert over other endocrine glands.**

14.1.5 **Specify the roles of the pineal gland.**

14.1.6 **Describe disorders of the hypothalamus, pituitary gland, and pineal gland.**

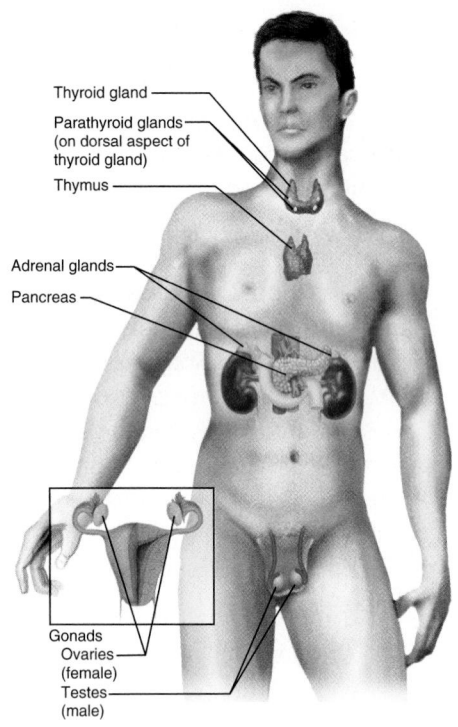

▲ **FIGURE 14.1 Major Endocrine Glands.**

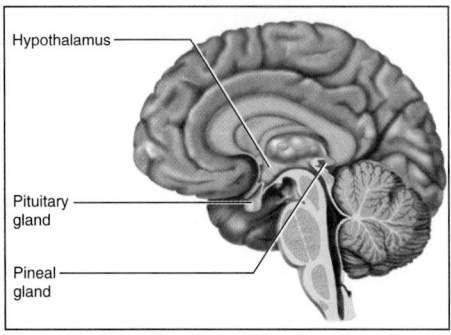

▲ **FIGURE 14.2 Hypothalamus, Pituitary Gland, and Pineal Gland.**

Abbreviations

ADH antidiuretic hormone
SAD seasonal affective disorder

ENDOCRINE SYSTEM

The endocrine system comprises several major organs *(Figure 14.1)*:

- Pituitary gland and the nearby hypothalamus
- Pineal gland
- Thyroid gland
- Parathyroid glands (4)
- Thymus gland
- Adrenal glands (2)
- Pancreas
- Gonads: testes (2) in the male; ovaries (2) in the female

In addition, endocrine cells found in tissues all over the body secrete hormones. Examples are:

- **Cells in the upper GI tract** secrete the hormone **gastrin,** which stimulates gastric secretions and the hormone **cholecystokinin,** which contracts the gallbladder *(see Chapter 6).*

- **Cells in the kidney** secrete **erythropoietin,** which stimulates erythrocyte production *(see Chapter 7).*

- **Fat cells** secrete **leptin,** which helps suppress appetite. Lack of it can lead to overeating and obesity *(see Chapter 17).*

- **Cells in tissues throughout the body** secrete **prostaglandins,** which act locally to dilate blood vessels, relax airways, stimulate uterine contractions in menstrual cramps or labor, and lower acid secretion in the stomach. When tissues are injured, prostaglandins promote an inflammatory response.

Hypothalamus

The hypothalamus *(Figure 14.2)* forms the floor and walls of the brain's third ventricle *(see page 400)* and produces eight hormones. Six of them are local hormones that regulate the production of hormones by the anterior pituitary gland *(see page 570)*. Two of them, oxytocin and **antidiuretic hormone (ADH),** are transported to the posterior pituitary, where they are stored until they are needed elsewhere in the body.

Pineal Gland

The pineal gland is located on the roof of the third ventricle of the brain, posterior to the hypothalamus *(Figure 14.2)*. It secretes **serotonin** by day and converts it to **melatonin** at night. The gland reaches its maximum size in childhood and may regulate the timing of puberty. It may also play a role in **seasonal affective disorder (SAD),** in which people are depressed in the dark days of winter.

WORD	PRONUNCIATION	ELEMENTS		DEFINITION
antidiuretic (*Note:* This term has two prefixes.)	**AN**-tih-die-you-**RET**-ik	S/ P/ P/ R/	**-ic** *pertaining to* **anti-** *against* **-di-** *complete* **-uret-** *urination*	An agent that decreases urine production
endocrine	**EN**-doh-krin	P/ R/CF	**endo-** *within* **-crin/e** *secrete*	Pertaining to a gland that produces an internal or hormonal secretion
endocrinology (*Note:* The "e" in -crine changes to "o" for easier pronunciation.)	**EN**-doh-krih-**NOL**-oh-jee	S/	**-logy** *study of*	Medical specialty concerned with the production and effects of hormones
endocrinologist	**EN**-doh-krih-**NOL**-oh-jist	S/	**-logist** *one who studies, specialist*	A medical specialist in endocrinology
hormone	**HOR**-mohn		Greek *to set in motion*	Chemical formed in one tissue or organ and carried by the blood to stimulate or inhibit a function of another tissue or organ
hormonal (adj)	hor-**MOHN**-al	S/ R/	**-al** *pertaining to* **hormon-** *chemical messenger*	Pertaining to a hormone(s) or the endocrine system
leptin	**LEP**-tin	S/ R/	**-in** *chemical compound* **lept-** *thin, small*	Hormone secreted by adipose tissue
melatonin	mel-ah-**TONE**-in	S/ R/ R/	**-in** *chemical compound* **mela-** *black* **-ton-** *tension, pressure*	Hormone formed by the pineal gland
oxytocin	**OCK**-see-toe-sin	S/ P/ R/	**-in** *chemical compound* **oxy-** *quick* **-toc-** *labor, birth*	Pituitary hormone that stimulates the uterus to contract
parathyroid	par-ah-**THIGH**-royd	S/ P/ R/	**-oid** *resemble* **para-** *beside* **-thyr-** *thyroid*	Endocrine glands embedded in the back of the thyroid gland
pineal	**PIN**-ee-al		Latin *like a pine cone*	Pertaining to the pineal gland
pituitary	pih-**TOO**-ih-tary	S/ R/	**-ary** *pertaining to* **pituit-** *pituitary*	Pertaining to the pituitary gland
prostaglandin	**PROS**-tah-**GLAN**-din	S/ R/CF R/	**-in** *chemical compound* **prost/a-** *prostate* **-gland-** *gland*	Hormone present in many tissues, but first isolated from prostate gland
seasonal affective disorder (*Note:* The abbreviation for this is SAD, which is how you feel with this disorder.)	see-**ZON**-al af-**FEK**-tiv dis-**OR**-der			Depression that occurs at the same time every year, often in winter
serotonin	ser-oh-**TOE**-nin	S/ R/CF R/	**-in** *substance* **ser/o-** *serum* **-ton-** *tension, pressure*	A neurotransmitter in the central and peripheral nervous systems

EXERCISES

Elements are listed in the left column. Place a check mark (✓) in the column identifying the type of element. Finish the exercise by writing the meaning of the element in the right column.

Element	Prefix	Root/CF	Suffix	Meaning of Element
di	_____	_____	_____	_____
anti	_____	_____	_____	_____
endo	_____	_____	_____	_____
mela	_____	_____	_____	_____
crine	_____	_____	_____	_____
oxy	_____	_____	_____	_____
toc	_____	_____	_____	_____
oid	_____	_____	_____	_____

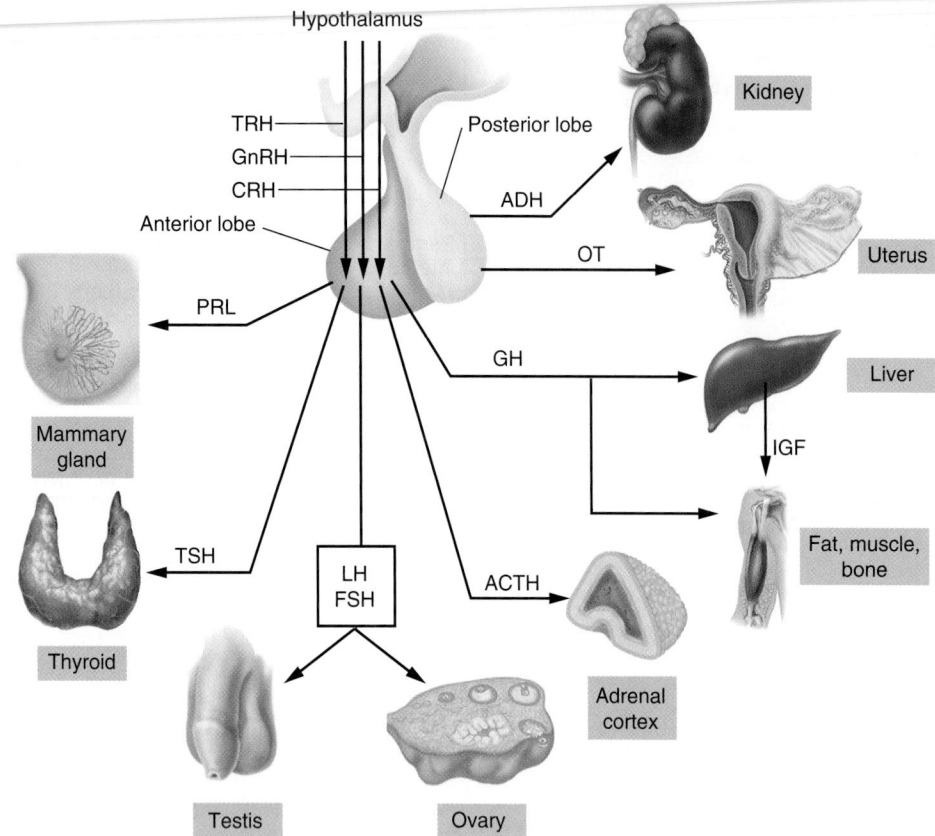

▲ FIGURE 14.3 Hormones of the Pituitary Gland and Their Target Organs.

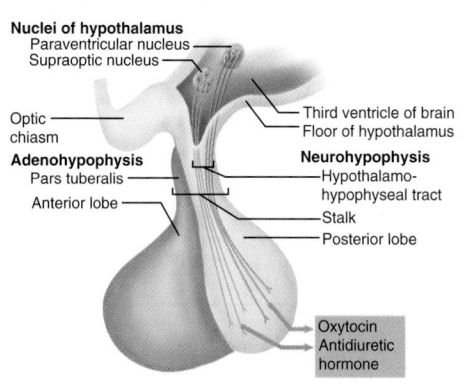

▲ FIGURE 14.4 Hormones of the Posterior Lobe of the Pituitary Gland.

Abbreviations	
ACTH	adrenocorticotropic hormone
ADH	antidiuretic hormone
FSH	follicle-stimulating hormone
GH	growth hormone
GnRH	gonadotropin-releasing hormone
LH	luteinizing hormone
OT	oxytocin
PRL	prolactin
TSH	thyroid-stimulating hormone

PITUITARY GLAND

While there is no single conductor of the endocrine orchestra in which each hormone plays its part in maintaining homeostasis, the pituitary gland and the hypothalamus work together and often influence the production of hormones in the other endocrine glands.

The pituitary gland **(hypophysis)** is suspended from the hypothalamus. The gland has two components:

1. A large anterior lobe called the **adenohypophysis.**
2. A smaller posterior lobe called the **neurohypophysis.**

Anterior lobe hormones are six in number *(Figure 14.3)*:

- **Follicle-stimulating hormone (FSH)** stimulates target cells in the ovaries to develop eggs and stimulates sperm production in the testes.
- **Luteinizing hormone (LH)** stimulates ovulation and the formation of a corpus luteum in the ovary *(see Chapter 13)* to secrete estrogen and progesterone. In the male, LH stimulates production of testosterone *(see Chapter 12).*

(FSH and LH are gonadotropins and are released under the control of GnRH of the hypothalamus *[see page 522]*.)

- **Thyroid-stimulating hormone (TSH),** or **thyrotropin,** stimulates the growth of the thyroid gland and the production of **thyroxine.**
- **Adrenocorticotropic hormone (ACTH),** or **corticotropin,** stimulates the adrenal glands to produce hormones called **corticosteroids.**
- **Prolactin (PRL)** stimulates the mammary glands after pregnancy to produce milk.
- **Growth hormone (GH),** or **somatotropin,** is produced in quantities at least a thousand times as great as any other pituitary hormone. It stimulates cells to enlarge and divide, particularly in childhood and adolescence.

Tropic hormones are hormones that stimulate other endocrine glands to produce their hormones. All of the anterior lobe hormones except PRL are tropic hormones.

Posterior lobe hormones are of two types. They are produced by nuclei in the hypothalamus and then stored in and released by the pituitary posterior lobe *(Figure 14.4)*:

- **Oxytocin (OT)** in childbirth stimulates uterine contractions and in lactation forces milk to flow down ducts to the nipple. In both sexes, its production increases during sexual intercourse to help give the feelings of satisfaction and emotional bonding.
- **Antidiuretic hormone (ADH)** reduces the volume of urine produced by the kidneys. It is also called **vasopressin.**

WORD	PRONUNCIATION	ELEMENTS		DEFINITION
adenohypophysis (*Note:* The prefix hypo- is part of **hypophysis,** which is a term in itself.)	**AD**-en-oh-hi-**POF**-ih-sis	R/ R/CF P/	**-physis** *growth* **aden/o-** *gland* **-hypo-** *below*	Anterior lobe of the pituitary gland
adrenal gland	ah-**DREE**-nal GLAND	S/ P/ R/	**-al** *pertaining to* **ad-** *near, toward* **-ren-** *kidney*	The suprarenal, or adrenal, gland on the upper pole of each kidney
adrenocorticotropic hormone	ah-**DREE**-noh-**KOR**-tih-koh-**TROH**-pik HOR-mohn	S/ R/CF R/CF	**-tropic** *stimulator* **adren/o-** *adrenal gland* **-cortic/o-** *cortisone, cortex*	Hormone of the anterior pituitary that stimulates the cortex of the adrenal gland to produce its own hormones
antidiuretic hormone (ADH) (also called **vasopressin**)	**AN**-tih-die-you-**RET**-ik **HOR**-mohn	S/ P/ P/ R/CF R/CF	**-tic** *pertaining to* **anti-** *against* **-di-** *complete* **-ur/e-** *urinary system* **hormon/e** *chemical messenger, hormone*	Posterior pituitary hormone that decreases urine output by acting on the kidney
corticosteroid	**KOR**-tih-koh-**STEHR**-oyd	S/ R/CF	**-steroid** *steroid* **cortic/o-** *cortisone, cortex*	A hormone produced by the adrenal cortex
corticotropin	**KOR**-tih-koh-**TROH**-pin	S/ R/CF	**-tropin** *stimulation* **cortic/o-** *cortisone, cortex*	Pituitary hormone that stimulates the cortex of the adrenal gland to secrete cortisone
hypophysis	high-**POF**-ih-sis	P/ R/	**hypo-** *below* **-physis** *growth*	Another name for the pituitary gland
neurohypophysis	**NYUR**-oh-high-**POF**-ih-sis	R/ R/CF P/	**-physis** *growth* **neur/o-** *nervous tissue* **-hypo-** *below*	Posterior lobe of the pituitary gland
prolactin	pro-**LAK**-tin	S/ P/ R/	**-in** *chemical compound* **pro-** *before* **-lact-** *milk*	Pituitary hormone that stimulates the production of milk
somatotropin (also called **growth hormone**)	**SO**-mah-toh-**TROH**-pin	S/ R/CF	**-tropin** *stimulation* **somat/o-** *the body*	Hormone of the anterior pituitary that stimulates growth of body tissues
thyroid	**THIGH**-royd		Greek *an oblong shield*	Endocrine gland in the neck, or a cartilage of the larynx
thyrotropin	thigh-roe-**TROH**-pin	S/ R/CF	**-tropin** *stimulation* **thyr/o-** *thyroid*	Hormone from the anterior pituitary gland that stimulates function of the thyroid gland
thyroxine	thigh-**ROCK**-sin	S/ R/ R/CF	**-ine** *pertaining to* **-ox-** *oxygen* **thyr/o-** *thyroid*	Thyroid hormone T$_4$, tetraiodothyronine
tropic (adj) **tropin** (noun)	**TROH**-pik **TROH**-pin		Greek *a turning*	Tropic hormones stimulate other endocrine glands to produce hormones
vasopressin (also called **antidiuretic hormone ADH**)	vay-soh-**PRESS**-in	S/ R/CF R/	**-in** *chemical compound* **vas/o-** *blood vessel* **-press-** *press, close*	Pituitary hormone that constricts blood vessels and decreases urine output

EXERCISES

Many hormones are known by their abbreviation. Match the description in the left column to the correct abbreviation in the right column.

_____ 1. Stimulates formation of corpus luteum   A. PRL

_____ 2. Stimulates production of corticosteroids   B. LH

_____ 3. Stimulates uterine contractions   C. GH

_____ 4. Stimulates ovaries to develop eggs   D. ACTH

_____ 5. Reduces volume of urine   E. TSH

_____ 6. Stimulates milk production   F. OT

_____ 7. Stimulates production of thyroxin   G. FSH

_____ 8. Stimulates cells to enlarge and divide   H. ADH

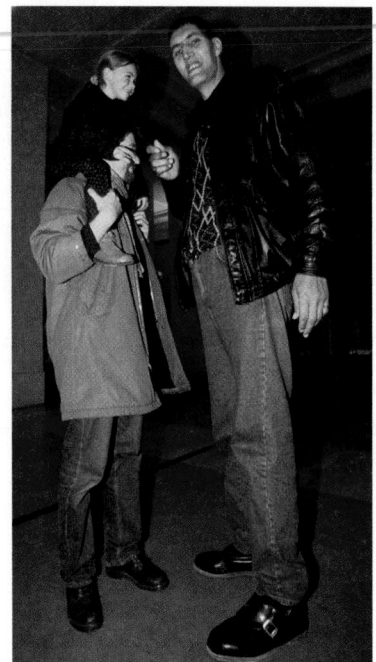

▲ FIGURE 14.5   Pituitary Gigantism.

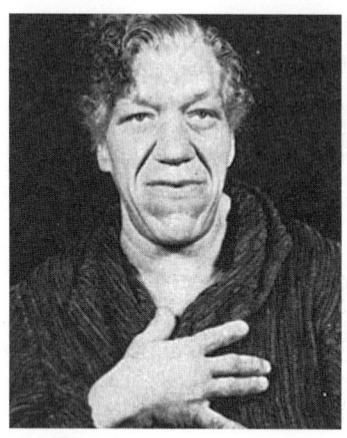

▲ FIGURE 14.6   Woman with Acromegaly, Age 52.

Case Report 14.1 (continued)

Dr. Khalid's examination of Mrs. Gina Tacher showed a protruding mandible **(prognathism)** and an enlarged, deeply grooved tongue. Her feet and hands are enlarged. She had noticed an increase in her shoe size and an inability to remove her wedding band. Her ribs are thickened, her heart is enlarged, and her BP is 140/90. Her body hair is dark and coarse, and she is sweating freely.

X-rays showed a thickened skull with enlarged nasal sinuses and thickened terminal phalanges of her hands. A diagnosis of **acromegaly** was made.

Computed tomography (CT) and magnetic resonance imaging (MRI) scans showed a tumor in the pituitary that occupies most of the sella turcica *(see Chapter 5)*.

Blood tests showed high levels of growth hormone and **insulin-like growth factor (IGF).**

DISORDERS OF PITUITARY HORMONES

Overproduction of Pituitary Hormones

Overproduction of growth hormone stimulates excessive growth of bones and muscles. It is almost always caused by a benign pituitary adenoma.

In children, the excessive production starts before the growth plates of the long bones have closed. The long bones grow enormously, producing **gigantism** *(Figure 14.5)*. Puberty can be delayed, genitalia may not develop fully, and diabetes can be a problem.

In adults, excessive growth hormone produces **acromegaly** *(Figure 14.6)*. This is the condition Mrs. Gina Tacher has.

Treatment of acromegaly is difficult. In Mrs. Tacher's case, surgery was able to remove much of the pituitary adenoma and was followed by radiation therapy.

A **prolactinoma** is a benign prolactin-secreting tumor of the pituitary gland in both men and women. It can lead to breast milk production in women who are not breast-feeding and produce scanty menstrual periods. In men it leads to breast milk production and impotence. The abnormal production of breast milk is called galactorrhea *(see Chapter 13)*.

Underproduction of Pituitary Hormones

Underproduction of growth hormone can be present at birth and leads to **pituitary dwarfism** *(Figure 14.7)*. The short stature becomes evident at around 1 year of age and is associated with episodes of hypoglycemia.

Hypopituitarism is uncommon. It can be caused by a pituitary tumor and cause a decline in the production of several hormones at the same time, a condition called **panhypopituitarism.**

Diabetes insipidus (DI) results from a decreased production of ADH, which helps regulate the amount of water in the body. (Diabetes mellitus is an entirely different disorder; *see Lesson 14.4.*) Antidiuretic hormone is produced in the hypothalamus and stored in the posterior pituitary lobe. Diabetes insipidus can result from insufficient production of ADH in the hypothalamus or failure of the pituitary gland to release it.

Symptoms begin with excessive urine production (polyuria) by day and by night. This leads to thirst and the need to drink up to 40 quarts of fluid per day.

In contrast to diabetes mellitus, urine in diabetes insipidus is dilute and does not contain sugar.

Treatment of diabetes insipidus is with vasopressin or desmopressin, synthetic modified forms of ADH. They are taken as a nasal spray several times daily, the dose being adjusted to maintain a normal urine output.

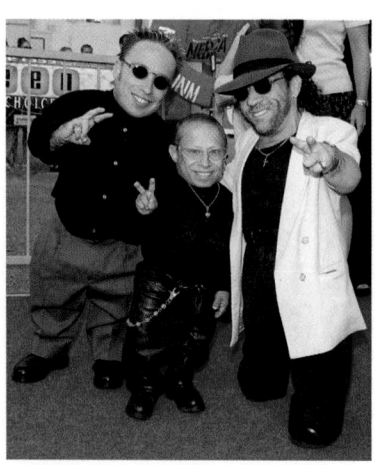

▲ FIGURE 14.7   Pituitary Dwarfism.

WORD	PRONUNCIATION	ELEMENTS		DEFINITION
acromegaly	ak-roe-**MEG**-ah-lee	P/ R/	**acro-** *highest point, extremity* **-megaly** *enlargement*	Enlargement of the head, face, hands, and feet due to excess growth hormone in an adult
diabetes insipidus	dye-ah-**BEE**-teez in-**SIP**-ih-dus	S/ P/ R/	**diabetes** Greek *siphon* **-us** *pertaining to* **in-** *not, without* **-sipid-** *flavor*	Excretion of large amounts of dilute urine as a result of inadequate ADH production
dwarfism	**DWORF**-izm	S/ R/	**-ism** *condition* **dwarf-** *miniature*	Short stature due to underproduction of growth hormone
gigantism	**JI**-gan-tizm	S/ R/	**-ism** *condition* **gigant-** *giant*	Abnormal height and size of entire body
hypopituitarism	**HIGH**-poh-pih-**TYU**-ih-tah-rizm	S/ P/ R/	**-ism** *condition* **hypo-** *deficient* **-pituitar-** *pituitary*	Condition of one or more deficient pituitary hormones
panhypopituitarism	pan-**HIGH**-poh-pih-**TYU**-ih-tah-rizm	S/ P/ P/ R/	**-ism** *condition* **-hypo-** *deficient* **pan-** *all* **-pituitar-** *pituitary*	Deficiency of all the pituitary hormones
prognathism	**PROG**-nah-thizm	S/ P/ R/	**-ism** *condition* **pro-** *before, in front* **-gnath-** *jaw*	Condition of a forward-projecting jaw
prolactinoma	pro-lak-tih-**NO**-muh	S/ P/ R/ S/	**-oma** *tumor* **pro-** *before, in front* **-lact-** *milk* **-in-** *chemical compound*	Prolactin-producing tumor

Abbreviations

DI	diabetes insipidus
IGF	insulinlike growth factor

EXERCISES

After reading Case Report 14.1 on the opposite page, answer the following questions. Be prepared to discuss your answers in class

1. Describe a *protruding mandible*. _____

2. What is the correct medical term for this condition? _____

3. What are the *signs* and *symptoms* Mrs. Tacher presented with?

   Signs (observable on the outside):

   _____

   Symptoms (felt by the patient on the inside):

   _____

4. Is her blood pressure elevated? _____

5. What diagnostic tests has Mrs. Tacher had? _____

6. In the diagnosis *acromegaly,* which element means *enlargement?* _____

7. What hormone does Mrs. Tacher have in excess? _____

8. Where are the *terminal phalanges?* _____

9. How has this condition affected her other body systems? (Be specific.) _____

Thyroid, Parathyroid, and Thymus Glands

OBJECTIVES

To understand what is happening in Case Report 14.2 and what treatment is being given, you will need to be able to use correct medical terminology to:

14.2.1 Describe the location and anatomy of the thyroid gland.
14.2.2 Explain how the three thyroid hormones are produced and secreted.
14.2.3 Specify the functions of the thyroid hormones.
14.2.4 Discuss common disorders of the thyroid gland.

In addition, information in this lesson will enable you to use correct medical terminology to:

14.2.5 Locate the positions of the parathyroid and thymus glands.
14.2.6 List the hormones produced by the parathyroid and thymus glands and state their functions.

You are

...an EMT working in the Emergency Room at Fulwood Medical Center at 0200 hours.

Your patient is

...Ms. Norma Leary, a 22-year-old college student living with her parents for the summer.

CASE REPORT 14.2

Ms. Leary is **emaciated,** extremely agitated, restless, and at times disoriented and confused. Her parents tell you that, in the past 3 or 4 days, she has been coughing and not feeling well. In the past 12 hours she has become feverish and been complaining of a left-sided chest pain. With questioning, the parents reveal that prior to this acute illness she had lost about 20 pounds in weight, although she was eating voraciously. Her VS are T 105.2°F, P 180 and irregular, R 24, BP 160/85.

You call for Dr. Hilinski STAT. On his initial examination, he believes that the patient is in **thyroid storm.** This is a medical emergency. There are no immediate laboratory tests that can confirm this diagnosis.

THYROID GLAND

The thyroid gland lies just beneath the skin of the neck and below the thyroid cartilage (Adam's apple). It is about 2 inches (5 cm) across and shaped like a bow tie. Two lobes extend up on either side of the trachea and are joined by an isthmus *(Figure 14.8)*.

The thyroid is a soft, very vascular organ composed mostly of small follicles lined with epithelial cells. These cells secrete the two thyroid hormones T_3 (**triiodothyronine**) and T_4 (**thyroxine**). The term **thyroid hormone** refers to T_3 and T_4 collectively.

Thyroid hormone acts in three interrelated ways:

- **Stimulates** almost every tissue in the body to produce proteins.
- **Increases** the amount of oxygen that cells use.
- **Controls** the speed at which the body's chemical functions proceed (metabolic rate).

The thyroid gland extracts **iodine** from the blood to produce T_3 and T_4. The hormones are produced in response to thyroid-stimulating hormone **(TSH)** from the anterior pituitary gland. The pituitary gland, in turn, increases or slows the release of TSH in response to the level of thyroid hormone in the blood.

The thyroid also produces the hormone **calcitonin** from the **C cells** found between the follicles. Calcitonin stimulates osteoblastic activity *(see Chapter 5)* to promote calcium deposition and bone formation. It is secreted in response to **hypercalcemia.**

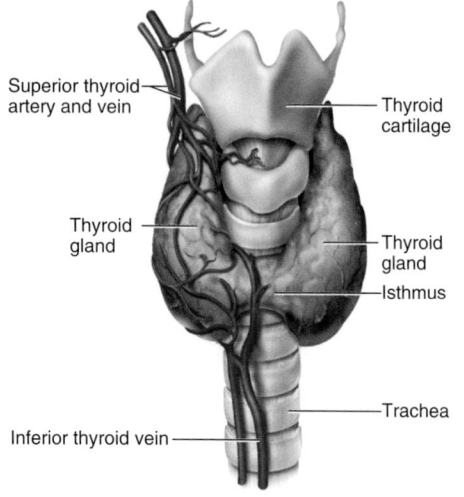

Superior thyroid artery and vein
Thyroid cartilage
Thyroid gland
Thyroid gland
Isthmus
Trachea
Inferior thyroid vein

▲ **FIGURE 14.8 Anatomy of the Thyroid Gland.**

Abbreviations

T₃	triiodothyronine
T₄	thyroxine (tetraiodothyronine)
TSH	thyroid-stimulating hormone

WORD ANALYSIS AND DEFINITION

WORD	PRONUNCIATION	ELEMENTS		DEFINITION
calcitonin	kal-sih-**TONE**-in	S/ R/CF R/	**-in** *chemical compound* **calc/i-** *calcium* **-ton-** *pressure, tension*	Thyroid hormone that moves calcium from blood to bones
emaciation emaciated (adv)	ee-may-see-**AY**-shun	S/ R/CF	**-ation** *process* **emac/i-** *make thin*	Abnormal thinness
hypercalcemia	**HIGH**-per-cal-**SEE**-me-ah	S/ P/ R/	**-emia** *condition of the blood* **hyper-** *above, excessive* **-calc-** *calcium*	Excessive level of calcium in the blood
iodine	**EYE**-oh-dine or **EYE**-oh-deen	S/ R/	**-ine** *pertaining to* **iod-** *violet, iodine*	Chemical element, the lack of which causes thyroid disease
thyroid storm	**THIGH**-royd STORM		**thyroid** *thyroid gland* **storm** *crisis*	Medical crisis and emergency due to excess thyroid hormones
thyroid hormone	**THIGH**-royd **HOR**-mohn		**thyroid** *thyroid gland* **hormone** *chemical messenger*	Collective term for the two thyroid hormones, T_3 and T_4
triiodothyronine	tri-**EYE**-oh-doh-**THY**-roh-neen	S/ P/ R/CF R/CF	**-ine** *pertaining to* **tri-** *three* **-iod/o-** *violet, iodine* **-thyr/o-** *thyroid gland*	Thyroid hormone T_3

EXERCISES

After reading Case Report 14.2 on the opposite page, answer the following questions. Be prepared to discuss your answers in class.

1. Describe someone who looks *emaciated*. _____

2. What *signs* are observable with this patient? _____

_____

3. What are Ms. Leary's *symptoms*? _____

_____

4. What additional symptoms developed in the last 24 hours before she came to the ER? _____

_____

5. What is unusual about her current weight? _____

_____

6. What is happening in Ms. Leary's body that makes it a *medical emergency*? _____

_____

7. Which other body systems are involved in her response in question 6 above? _____

_____

8. What does the abbreviation *STAT* mean? _____

_____

9. *Thyroid storm* is due to what?

_____

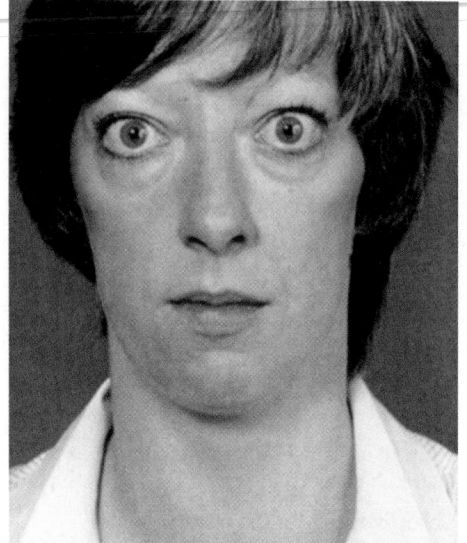

▲ **FIGURE 14.9 Hyperthyroidism May Cause the Eyes to Protrude (Exophthalmos).**

Case Report 14.2 (continued)

Thyroid storm is the condition Ms. Norma Leary presented with in the Emergency Department. It shows severely exaggerated effects of the thyroid hormones. This explains her hyperpyrexia, tachycardia, agitation, and delirium. The weight loss prior to her illness becoming acute was part of her undiagnosed Graves disease. Ms. Leary's immediate treatment included supplemental oxygen, intravenous (IV) fluids with dextrose solutions, ice packs and cooling blanket, propranolol, **antithyroid** medications, and oral iodine compounds.

DISORDERS OF THE THYROID GLAND

Hyperthyroidism (Thyrotoxicosis)

Whatever the cause of **hyperthyroidism,** the symptoms are those of increased body metabolism. These include tachycardia, hypertension, sweating, shakiness, anxiety, weight loss despite increased appetite, and diarrhea.

Graves disease is an autoimmune disorder *(see Chapter 15)* in which an antibody stimulates the thyroid to produce and secrete excessive quantities of thyroid hormones into the blood. It is associated with one or more symptoms of a **goiter** (enlarged thyroid gland), **exophthalmos,** and pretibial **myxedema.**

Exophthalmos, in which the eyes bulge outward *(Figure 14.9),* is caused by a substance that builds up behind the eyes. The same substance is occasionally deposited in the skin over the shins and called pretibial myxedema.

Thyroiditis is an inflammation of the thyroid gland. It presents in three forms:

- **Silent lymphocytic thyroiditis** is characterized by some thyroid enlargement and a **self-limiting** hyperthyroid phase of a few weeks, followed by recovery to the normal **euthyroid** state.
- **Subacute thyroiditis** has a history of an antecedent viral upper respiratory infection (URI) followed by signs of hyperthyroidism with a diffusely enlarged thyroid gland. It is self-limiting.
- **Hashimoto disease** is an autoimmune disease with lymphocytic infiltration of the gland. Hypothyroidism results, necessitating lifelong thyroid hormone replacement therapy.

Toxic thyroid adenoma is a nodule in the gland that produces thyroid hormones without stimulation by the pituitary's TSH. The nodule can be removed surgically.

Goiter *(Figure 14.10)* is an enlargement of the thyroid gland that, as it enlarges, can cause difficulty in swallowing and breathing. It can occur in any of the disorders listed above and also in pregnancy.

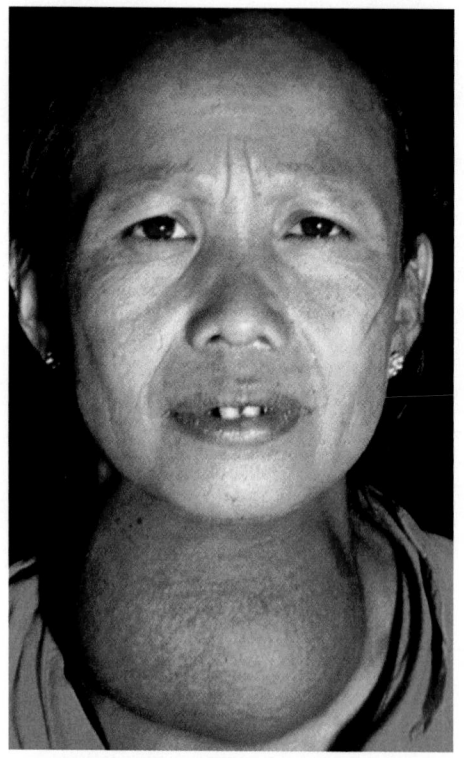

▲ **FIGURE 14.10 Woman with Goiter.**

WORD	PRONUNCIATION	ELEMENTS		DEFINITION
antithyroid	an-tee-**THIGH**-royd	P/ R/	**anti-** *against* **-thyroid** *thyroid*	A substance that inhibits production of thyroid hormones
euthyroid	you-**THIGH**-royd	P/ R/	**eu-** *good, normal* **-thyroid** *thyroid*	Normal thyroid function
exophthalmos	ek-sof-**THAL**-mos	P/ R/	**ex-** *out, out of* **-ophthalmos** *eye*	Protrusion of the eyeball
goiter	**GOY**-ter		Latin *throat*	Enlargement of the thyroid gland
Graves disease	GRAVZ **DIZ**-eez		Robert Graves, 1796–1853, Irish physician	Hyperthyroidism with toxic goiter
Hashimoto disease (also called **Hashimoto thyroiditis**)	hah-shee-**MOH**-toe diz-**EEZ**		Hakaru Hashimoto, 1881–1934, Japanese surgeon	Autoimmune disease of the thyroid gland
hyperthyroidism	high-per-**THIGH**-royd-ism	S/ P/ R/	**-ism** *condition, process* **hyper-** *excessive* **-thyroid-** *thyroid*	Excessive production of thyroid hormones
myxedema	miks-eh-**DEE**-muh	P/ R/	**myx-** *mucus* **-edema** *swelling*	Severe hypothyroidism
thyroidectomy	thigh-roy-**DEK**-toe-me	S/ R/	**-ectomy** *surgical excision* **thyroid-** *thyroid*	Surgical removal of the thyroid gland
thyroiditis	thigh-roy-**DIE**-tis	S/ R/	**-itis** *inflammation* **thyroid-** *thyroid*	Inflammation of the thyroid gland
thyrotoxicosis	**THIGH**-roe-toks-ee-**KOH**-sis	S/ R/CF R/CF	**-sis** *abnormal condition* **thyr/o-** *thyroid* **-toxic/o-** *poison*	Disorder produced by excessive thyroid hormone production

EXERCISES

Elements: *One word in each of the descriptions 1 through 7 is in bold. This is your clue to finding the correct medical term among the words below. Fill in the blanks.*

thyroiditis	euthyroid	antithyroid	exophthalmos	thyroidectomy	thyrotoxicosis	hyperthyroidism

1. **Excessive** production of thyroid hormones: _____

2. **Removal** of the thyroid gland: _____

3. **Inhibits** production of thyroid hormone: _____

4. Disorder produced by **excessive** thyroid hormone production: _____

5. **Normal** thyroid function: _____

6. **Inflammation** of the thyroid gland: _____

7. Protrusion of the **eye**ball: _____

After reading Case Report 14.2 on the opposite page, answer the following questions. Be prepared to discuss your answers in class.

8. Translate this sentence into layman's language:

   "This explains her hyperpyrexia, tachycardia, agitation and delirium."

   _____

   _____

   _____

9. What treatment was given to reduce the hyperpyrexia?

   _____

10. What is the *supplemental oxygen* helping?

    _____

DISORDERS OF THE THYROID GLAND (continued)

Hypothyroidism

Hypothyroidism results from an inadequate production of thyroid hormone, leading to a slowing of the body's metabolism. Primary hypothyroidism, in which no specific cause is found, affects 10% of older women. Severe hypothyroidism is called myxedema. In developing countries, a common cause is lack of iodine in the diet. In the United States, iodine is added to table salt to prevent hypothyroidism, and iodine is also found in dairy products and seafood.

Hypothyroidism causes the body to function slowly. Symptoms develop gradually. They include loss of hair; dry, scaly skin; puffy face and eyes; slow, hoarse speech; weight gain; constipation; and inability to tolerate cold *(Figure 14.11)*. If untreated, hypothyroidism can progress to coma, triggered by severe cold or other physical stresses.

Diagnosis of primary hypothyroidism is confirmed with a TSH blood level that is high. Treatment is to replace the thyroid hormone with synthetic T_4 (L-thyroxine), which is started in small doses.

Cretinism *(Figure 14.12)* is a congenital form of thyroid deficiency that severely retards mental and physical growth. If it is diagnosed and treated early with thyroid hormones, significant improvement can be achieved.

Thyroid cancer usually presents as a symptomless nodule in the thyroid gland.

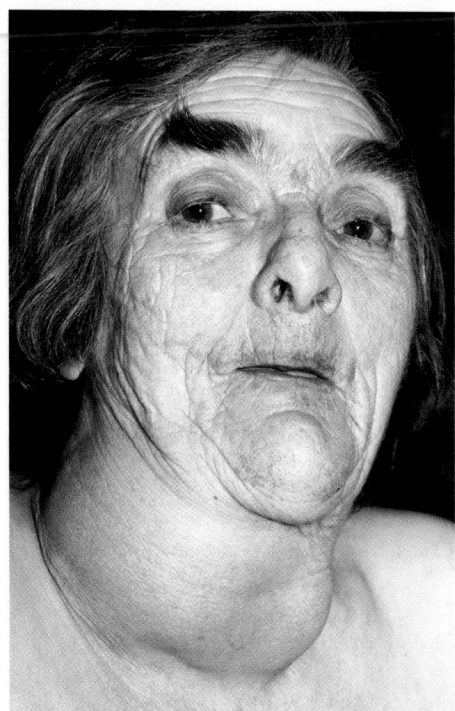

▲ **FIGURE 14.11 Elderly Woman with Hypothyroidism.**

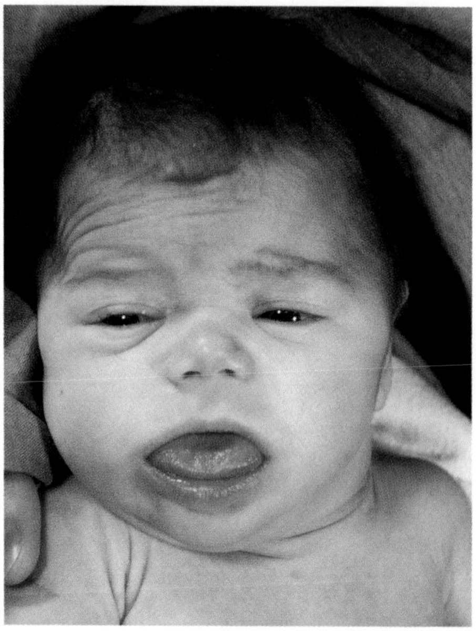

▲ **FIGURE 14.12 Infant with Cretinism.**

Thyroid Diagnostic Tests

TSH level in the blood: If the thyroid gland is overactive, the level of TSH is low.

Thyroid hormone levels in blood detail the activity of the gland: If the thyroid gland is overactive, thyroid hormones are generally high.

Antithyroid antibodies are associated with autoimmune inflammatory diseases of the thyroid.

Isotopic thyroid scans detail the nature of the thyroid enlargement and the function of the gland.

Serum calcitonin level is elevated in medullary carcinoma.

Fine needle aspiration biopsy distinguishes benign from malignant nodules.

Ultrasonography reveals the size of the gland and the presence of nodules.

Thyroid Pharmacology

Antithyroids prevent formation of thyroid hormones:

- Propylthiouracil inhibits the uptake of iodine and the conversion of T_4 to T_3.
- Methimazole inhibits the uptake of iodine.

Radioactive iodine taken orally reaches the thyroid through the bloodstream and destroys thyroid cells.

Thyroid replacements:

- L-thyroxine—this synthetic T_4 is a preferred replacement.
- Liothyronine sodium—this synthetic T_3 has a rapid turnover and has to be monitored frequently.

WORD	PRONUNCIATION		ELEMENTS	DEFINITION
cretin cretinism	**KREH**-tin **KREH**-tin-izm	S/ R/	French *cretin* -ism *condition, process* cretin- *cretin*	A person with severe congenital hypothyroidism Condition of severe congenital hypothyroidism
hypothyroidism	high-poh-**THIGH**-royd-ism	S/ P/ R/	-ism *condition, process* hypo- *deficient* -thyroid- *thyroid*	Deficient production of thyroid hormones
isotope isotopic (adj)	I-so-tope	P/ R/	iso- *equal* -tope *part*	Radioactive element used in diagnostic procedures
nodule	**NOD**-yule		Latin *small knot*	Small node or knotlike swelling
radioactive iodine	**RAY**-dee-oh-**AK**-tiv **EYE**-oh-dine	S/ R/CF R/	-ive *pertaining to* radi/o- *radiation* -act- *performance* iodine *nonmetallic element*	Any of the various tracers that emit alpha, beta, or gamma rays
ultrasonography	**UL**-trah-soh-**NOG**-rah-fee	S/ P/ R/CF	-graphy *recording* ultra- *beyond* -son/o- *sound*	Delineation of deep structures using sound waves

EXERCISES

*Certain kinds of tests are performed for the purpose of arriving at the correct diagnosis for treatment. Employ the **language of endocrinology** to fill in the blanks with the name of the test that is described.*

1. Associated with autoimmune inflammatory disease of the thyroid: _____

2. Blood test to measure activity of the thyroid gland: _____

3. Level becomes elevated in medullary carcinoma: _____

4. Levels in the blood are generally low if the thyroid gland is overactive: _____

5. Reveals the size of the gland and the presence of nodules: _____

6. Distinguishes benign from malignant nodules: _____

7. Detail the nature of the thyroid enlargement and the function of the gland: _____

Meet a lesson objective by correctly answering the following questions on a common disorder of the thyroid gland. Fill in the blanks.

8. What is the opposite of *hypothyroidism?* _____

9. What is the body's *metabolism?* _____

_____

10. Is *hypothyroidism* the result of an overactive or underactive thyroid gland? _____

_____

11. What confirms the diagnosis of *primary hypothyroidism?* _____

_____

12. What is the *congenital form of thyroid deficiency* that severely retards physical and mental growth? _____

_____

13. What is the *etiology of Hashimoto disease?* _____

_____

14. What is the medical term for *severe hypothyroidism?* _____

_____

OTHER ENDOCRINE GLANDS

Parathyroid Glands

The **parathyroid glands** are usually four in number and are partially embedded in the posterior surface of the thyroid gland *(Figure 14.13)*. They secrete **parathyroid hormone (PTH)** in response to hypocalcemia. Calcitonin and PTH are antagonistic: PTH stimulates osteoclasts to reabsorb bone and bring calcium back into the blood, while calcitonin takes calcium from the blood and stimulates osteoblasts to lay down bone *(see Chapter 5)*.

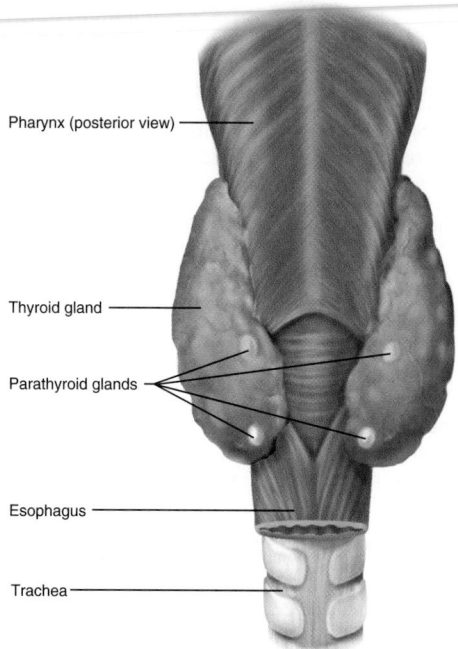

Pharynx (posterior view)

Thyroid gland

Parathyroid glands

Esophagus

Trachea

▲ **FIGURE 14.13 Site of Parathyroid Glands: Posterior View.**

Disorders of Parathyroid Glands

Hypoparathyroidism is a deficiency of PTH that lowers levels of blood calcium (hypocalcemia). Most symptoms are neuromuscular, ranging from tingling in the fingers to muscle cramps and the painful muscle spasms of **tetany** (*not* **tetanus**). A genetically engineered recombinant form of PTH is now available, but classic treatment for hypoparathyroidism still involves high-dose calcium and vitamin D supplements.

Hyperparathyroidism is an excess of PTH. It is seen more often than hypoparathyroidism and is usually caused by one of the four glands enlarging and secreting excess PTH in an unregulated manner. It leads to four major abnormalities:

1. Bones are depleted of calcium (osteopenia) and become brittle.
2. High blood calcium levels (hypercalcemia) lead to decreased bowel motility and constipation and to increased gastric acidity and heartburn.
3. Extra excretion of calcium in the urine leads to kidney stones (nephrolithiasis).
4. High blood calcium leads to mental symptoms such as depression and fatigue and can lead to coma.

Surgical removal of the enlarged gland is **curative.**

Abbreviation	
PTH	parathyroid hormone

Thymus Gland

The **thymus gland** is located in the mediastinum behind the sternum between the lungs and above the heart *(Figure 14.14)*. It is large in children and decreases in size until, in the elderly, it is mostly fibrous tissue. It secretes a group of hormones that stimulate the production of T lymphocytes *(see Chapter 15)*.

Disorders of Thymus Gland

DiGeorge syndrome is a genetic immunodeficiency disorder *(see Chapter 15)* in which the thymus is underdeveloped or absent at birth. Abnormalities of the thymus and parathyroid glands, heart, and facial structure are present, with few or no T lymphocytes. Transplantation of stem cells or thymus tissue can cure the immunodeficiency.

Thymomas, benign tumors, and **thymic carcinomas** are rare tumors that can be associated with myasthenia gravis *(see Chapter 10)* and other autoimmune syndromes, such as lupus erythematosus, and rheumatoid arthritis. Treatment is usually surgical removal of the tumor or the gland **(thymectomy),** followed by **adjuvant** radiotherapy.

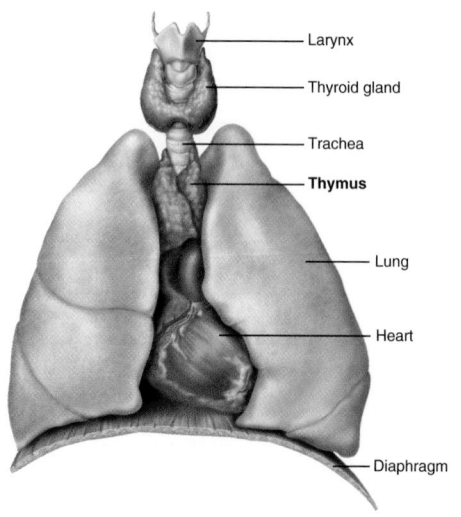

Larynx

Thyroid gland

Trachea

Thymus

Lung

Heart

Diaphragm

▲ **FIGURE 14.14 Position of Thymus Gland in Mediastinum.**

WORD	PRONUNCIATION	ELEMENTS		DEFINITION
adjuvant	**AD**-joo-vant	S/ R/	-ant *pertaining to* adjuv- *give help*	Additional treatment after a primary treatment has been used
antagonist (***Note:*** Two suffixes.)	an-**TAG**-oh-nist	S/ P/ R/	-ist *agent* ant- *against* -agon- *to fight*	An opposing structure, agent, disease, or process
antagonistic (adj)	an-**TAG**-oh-nist-ik	S/	-ic *pertaining to*	Having an opposite function
curative	**KYUR**-ah-tiv	S/ R/	-ive *quality of* curat- *to care for*	That which heals or cures
DiGeorge syndrome	dee-**JORJ SIN**-drome		Angelo M. DiGeorge, U.S. pediatrician, described syndrome in 1921	Congenital absence of the thymus gland
parathyroid	par-ah-**THIGH**-royd	S/ P/ R/	-oid *resembling* -para- *adjacent* -thyroid- *thyroid*	Endocrine glands embedded in the back of the thyroid gland
hyperparathyroidism	**HIGH**-per-para-**THIGH**-royd-ism	S/ P/	-ism *condition, process* hyper- *excessive*	Excessive levels of parathyroid hormone
hypoparathyroidism	**HIGH**-poh-para-**THIGH**-royd-ism	S/ P/ P/ R/	-ism *condition, process* hypo- *deficient* -para- *adjacent* -thyroid- *thyroid*	Deficient levels of parathyroid hormone
tetany tetanic (adj)	**TET**-ah-nee teh-**TAN**-ik		Greek *convulsive tension*	Severe muscle twitches, cramps, and spasms
thymectomy	thigh-**MEK**-toe-me	S/ R/	-ectomy *surgical excision* thym- *thymus gland*	Surgical removal of the thymus gland
thymoma	thigh-**MOH**-mah	S/ R/	-oma *tumor, mass* thym- *thymus gland*	Benign tumor of the thymus
thymus	**THIGH**-mus		Greek *sweetbread*	Endocrine gland located in the mediastinum

EXERCISES

*Meet a lesson objective by employing the **language of endocrinology** to answer the following questions.*

1. Locate the positions of the parathyroid and thymus glands.

   Parathyroid location: _____

   Thymus location: _____

2. List the hormone(s) produced by each gland, and state their function(s).

   Parathyroid gland:

   _____

   Function of the hormone(s) from the parathyroid gland:

   _____

   _____

   Thymus:

   _____

   Function of the hormone(s) from the *thymus:*

   _____

   _____

3. Translate the following sentence into language the patient can understand:

   "Hyperparathyroidism is an excess of PTH and can lead to osteopenia, hypercalcemia, and neophrolithiasis."

   _____

   _____

   _____

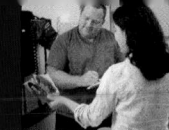

LESSON 14.3 Adrenal Glands and Hormones

OBJECTIVES

The information in this lesson will enable you to use correct medical terminology to:

14.3.1 **Locate the adrenal glands.**

14.3.2 **Differentiate between the adrenal cortex and medulla.**

14.3.3 **Identify the functions of the hormones produced by the cortex and medulla.**

14.3.4 **Detail how the body adapts to stress.**

14.3.5 **Explain common disorders of the adrenal glands.**

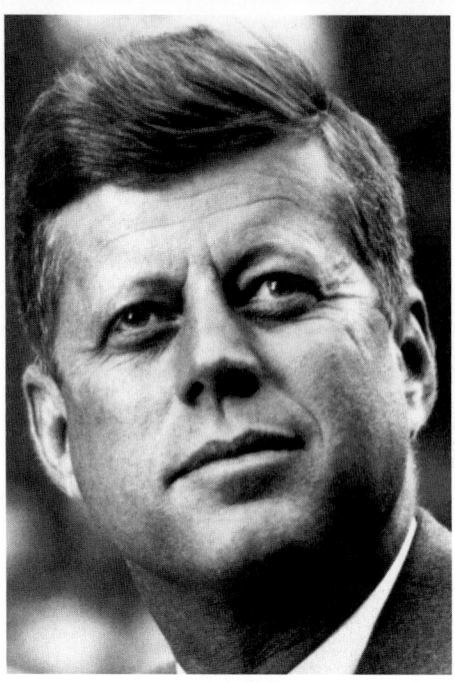

▲ **FIGURE 14.15** **John F. Kennedy.**

Abbreviation
DHEA dehydroepiandrosterone

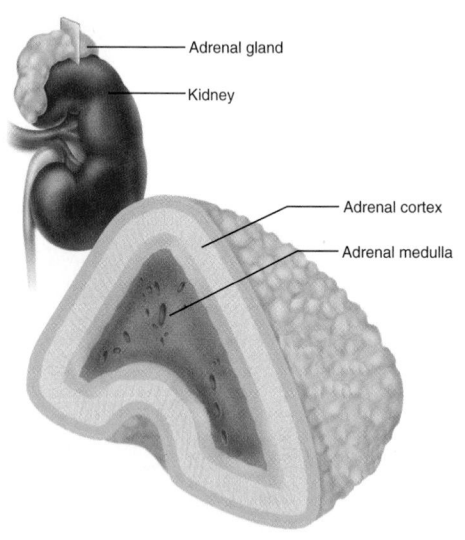

▲ **FIGURE 14.16** **Adrenal Gland.**

CASE REPORT 14.3

John Fitzgerald Kennedy (1917–1963) was elected president of the United States of America in 1960 at the age of 43, the youngest person elected to that office *(Figure 14.15)*. Since the age of 13, when he was diagnosed as having colitis, he had had health problems. At age 27, he had low-back pain necessitating lower-back surgery, and he was then diagnosed as having adrenal gland insufficiency **(Addison disease)** with osteoporosis of his lumbar spine. This required lower-back surgery on three more occasions. JFK received adrenal hormone replacement therapy for the rest of his life, together with pain medication for his low-back pain, until his assassination in Dallas, Texas, in 1963.

In medical retrospect, instead of colitis, he probably had celiac disease *(see Chapter 6)*, which has strong associations with Addison disease.

ADRENAL GLANDS

An **adrenal (suprarenal) gland** is anchored like a cap on the upper pole of each kidney *(Figure 14.16)*.

The outer layer of the gland, the **adrenal cortex,** synthesizes more than 25 steroid hormones known collectively as **adrenocortical hormones, corticosteroids,** or **corticoids.** There are three groups of corticosteroids:

1. Glucocorticoids—particularly **hydrocortisone (cortisol).** These hormones stimulate fat and protein catabolism and help regulate blood glucose levels, particularly as the body resists stress *(see next lesson)*. Hydrocortisone also has an anti-inflammatory effect and is used in ointments to relieve inflammation.

2. **Mineralocorticoids**—the principal one of which is called **aldosterone.** This hormone promotes sodium retention and potassium excretion by the kidneys.

3. **Sex steroids:**

    a. **Androgens**—principally **dehydroepiandrosterone (DHEA),** which is a weak androgen but is converted by other tissues into testosterone *(see Chapter 12)*.

    b. **Estrogens**—principally estradiol, which is produced in much smaller quantities than in the ovaries *(see Chapter 13)*.

The inner layer of the adrenal gland, the **adrenal medulla,** secretes hormones called **catecholamines,** principally **epinephrine (adrenaline)** and **norepinephrine.** These hormones prepare the body for physical activity. They raise blood pressure, increase circulation to muscles, increase pulmonary blood flow, and stimulate gluconeogenesis *(see Chapter 6)*.

WORD ANALYSIS AND DEFINITION

WORD	PRONUNCIATION	ELEMENTS		DEFINITION
Addison disease	**ADD**-ih-son **DIZ**-eez		Thomas Addison, 1793–1860, English physician	An autoimmune disease leading to decreased production of adrenocortical steroids
adrenal gland	ah-**DREE**-nal GLAND	S/ P/ R/	-al *pertaining to* ad- *to* -ren- *kidney*	The suprarenal, or adrenal, gland on the upper pole of each kidney
adrenaline (also called epinephrine)	ah-**DREN**-ah-lin	S/	-ine *pertaining to*	One of the catecholamines
adrenocortical	ah-dree-noh-**KOR**-tih-kal	S/ R/CF R/	-al *pertaining to* adren/o- *adrenal gland* -cortic- *cortex, cortisone*	Pertaining to the cortex of the adrenal gland
aldosterone	al-**DOS**-ter-own	S/ R/CF R/	-one *hormone* ald/o- *organic compound* -ster- *steroid*	Mineralocorticoid hormone of the adrenal cortex
catecholamine	kat-eh-**COAL**-ah-meen	S/ R/	-amine *nitrogen-containing* catechol- *benzene derivative*	Any major hormones in stress response; includes epinephrine and norepinephrine
corticoid (also called corticosteroid)	**KOR**-tih-koyd	S/ R/	-oid *resemble* cortic- *cortex, cortisone*	One of the steroid hormones produced by the adrenal cortex
cortisol (also called hydrocortisone)	**KOR**-tih-sol	S/ R/	-ol *chemical substance* cortis- *cortisone*	One of the glucocorticoids produced by the adrenal cortex; has anti-inflammatory effects
dehydroepian-drosterone (DHEA)	de-**HIGH**-droh-epee-an-**DROS**-ter-own	S/ P/ R/CF P/ R/ R/CF	-one *hormone* de- *without, change of* -hydr/o- *water* -epi- *above* -ster- *steroid* -andr/o- *male*	Precursor to testosterone; produced in the adrenal cortex
epinephrine (also called **adrenaline**)	ep-ih-**NEF**-rin	S/ P/ R/	-ine *pertaining to* epi- *above* -nephr- *kidney*	Main catecholamine produced by the adrenal medulla
glucocorticoid	glu-co-**KOR**-tih-koyd	S/ R/ R/CF	-oid *resemble* -cortic- *cortex, cortisone* gluc/o- *glucose*	Hormone of the adrenal cortex that helps regulate glucose metabolism
hydrocortisone (also called **cortisol**)	high-droh-**KOR**-tih-sohn	S/ R/CF R/	-one *hormone* hydr/o- *water* -cortis- *cortisone*	Potent glucocorticoid with anti-inflammatory properties
mineralocorticoid	**MIN**-er-al-oh-**KOR**-tih-koyd	S/ R/ R/CF	-oid *resemble* -cortic- *cortex, cortisone* mineral/o- *inorganic materials*	Hormone of the adrenal cortex that influences sodium and potassium metabolism
norepinephrine (also called **noradrenaline**)	**NOR**-ep-ih-**NEFF**-rin	S/ P/ P/ R/	-ine *pertaining to* nor- *normal* -epi- *above* -nephr- *kidney*	Parasympathetic neurotransmitter that is a catecholamine hormone of the adrenal gland

EXERCISES

Elements are the building blocks of medical terms. Match the elements in 1–10 to their correct meanings in A–J. Review the WAD before you begin the exercise.

____ 1. hydro

____ 2. adren/o

____ 3. oid

____ 4. epi

____ 5. ster

____ 6. andr/o

____ 7. gluc/o

____ 8. nor

____ 9. one

____ 10. nephr

A. normal

B. resemble

C. hormone

D. glucose

E. water

F. steroid

G. kidney

H. adrenal

I. above

J. male

DISORDERS OF ADRENAL GLANDS

Adrenal cortical hypofunction can be primary when the disorder is in the adrenal cortex (Addison disease) or secondary when there is a lack of ACTH from the pituitary gland.

Addison disease is caused mostly by idiopathic atrophy of the adrenal cortex. Production of the three groups of adrenocortical steroids is diminished or absent.

Decreased cortisol production leads to weakness, fatigue, diminished resistance to stress, increased susceptibility to infection, and weight loss.

Decreased aldosterone production leads to dehydration, decreased circulatory volume, hypotension, and circulatory collapse.

Replacement therapy in Addison disease is daily hydrocortisone **by mouth (PO)**. Additionally, fluorocortisone is given PO to replace aldosterone. **Intercurrent** infections require that the hydrocortisone dose be doubled. John F. Kennedy received replacement therapy from his late twenties until he died.

Acute adrenocortical insufficiency in patients with Addison disease is called an adrenal crisis. It can be precipitated by an infection or trauma and leads to peripheral vascular collapse and kidney failure. Treatment is with IV fluids and IV hydrocortisone.

Adrenal cortical hyperfunction is due to excessive production of the groups of the corticosteroids.

Hypersecretion of glucocorticoids produces **Cushing syndrome** (*Figure 14.17*). Clinical manifestations include "moon" **facies,** obesity of the trunk, muscle wasting and weakness, osteoporosis, kidney stones, and reduced resistance to infection. Most cases of Cushing syndrome are due to a pituitary tumor secreting too much ACTH, thereby causing the normal adrenal glands to produce too much cortisol. Other cases of Cushing syndrome are due to benign adenomas of the adrenal gland producing excess cortisol.

Pituitary tumors causing Cushing syndrome are removed surgically. Single, benign adrenal adenomas are removed by **laparoscopic adrenalectomy.**

Often, the symptoms of Cushing syndrome can be produced by therapeutic administration of excess cortisol medications (*Figure 14.18*).

Hypersecretion of aldosterone (aldosteronism, or **Conn syndrome)** leads to sodium retention and potassium loss with increased blood volume, hypertension, excessive thirst, and excessive urination. A benign adenoma **(aldosteronoma)** is the most common cause and can be removed by laparoscopic adrenalectomy.

Hypersecretion of androgens is called **adrenal virilism** or **adrenogenital syndrome.** In adult women, manifestations include **hirsutism,** baldness, acne, deepened voice, decreased breast size, and other signs of masculinization. If a tumor is found by CT or MRI scan, it can be removed surgically.

Pheochromocytoma is a tumor of the adrenal medulla that overproduces the catecholamines epinephrine and norepinephrine. It produces marked hypertension that is difficult to control, with severe headaches, tachycardia, palpitations, and feelings of impending death. Diagnosis is made by measuring the excess catecholamines in blood and 24-hour urine specimens. The tumor is located by standard CT or MRI scanning, or by performing a special scan using a labeled catecholamine analogue to highlight the tumor. It is removed by laparoscopic adrenalectomy.

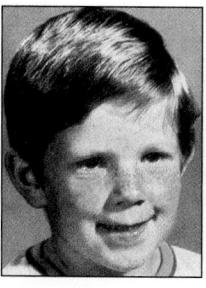
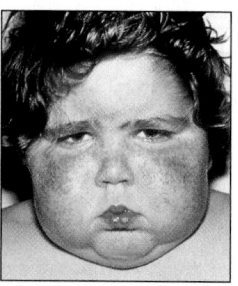

(a)   (b)

▲ **FIGURE 14.17 Cushing Syndrome.**
(*a*) Patient before onset of the syndrome.
(*b*) The same boy, only 4 months later, showing the "moon face" characteristic of Cushing syndrome.

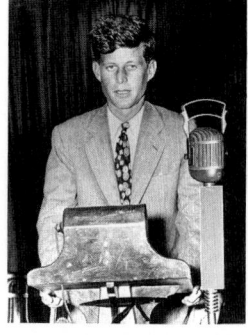
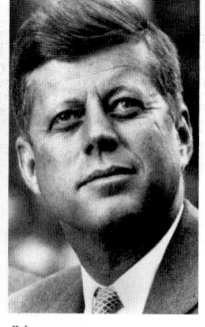

(a)   (b)

▲ **FIGURE 14.18 Treatment Effects of Excess Cortisol Medication May Mimic Symptoms of Cushing Syndrome.**

Keynote

Prolonged or repeated stress can cause physical illness.

Stress reduction techniques are an important part of modern life.

Stress

Is there an exam at the end of the week? Is the baby-sitter sick? You know what stress is and how it affects your physical and emotional well-being.

Your body reacts to stress in a consistent way called the stress response or general adaptation syndrome.

The initial response is an **alarm reaction** ("fight or flight") initiated by catecholamines that raise blood pressure and increase glucose production from stored

WORD	PRONUNCIATION		ELEMENTS	DEFINITION
adrenalectomy	ah-dree-nal-**ECK**-to-me	S/ S/ P/ R/	-al *pertaining to* -ectomy *surgical excision* ad- *to* -ren- *kidney*	Removal of part or all of an adrenal gland
adrenogenital syndrome	ah-**DREE**-no-**JEN**-it-al **SIN**-drome	S/ R/CF R/	-al *pertaining to* adren/o- *adrenal gland* -genit- *androgen*	Hypersecretion of androgens from the adrenal gland
aldosteronism (also called **Conn syndrome**)	al-**DOS**-ter-on-izm	S/ R/CF R/	-ism *condition, process* ald/o- *organic compound* -steron- *steroid*	Condition caused by excessive secretion of aldosterone
aldosteronoma	al-**DOS**-ter-on-oma	S/	-oma *tumor, mass*	Benign adenoma of the adrenal cortex
Conn syndrome (also called **aldosteronism**)	KON **SIN**-drom		Jerome W. Conn, 1907–1981, U.S. endocrinologist	Aldosteronism
Cushing syndrome	**KUSH**-ing **SIN**-drom		Harvey Cushing, 1869–1939, American neurosurgeon	Hypersecretion of cortisol (hydrocortisone) by the adrenal cortex
facies	**FASH**-eez		Latin *appearance*	Facial expression and features characteristic of a specific disease
hirsutism	**HER**-sue-tizm		Latin *shaggy*	Excessive body and facial hair
intercurrent	**IN**-ter-**KUR**-ent	S/ P/ R/	-ent *end result, pertaining to* inter- *among, between* -curr- *to run*	A disease attacking a person who already has another disease
pheochromocytoma	fee-oh-**KRO**-moh-sigh-**TOE**-muh	S/ P/ R/CF R/	-oma *tumor* pheo- *gray* -chrom/o- *color* -cyt- *cell*	Adenoma of the adrenal medulla secreting excessive catecholamines
virilism	**VIR**-ih-lizm	S/ R/	-ism *condition, process* viril- *masculine*	Development of masculine characteristics by a woman or girl

glycogen. This source of glucose is soon exhausted, and the feelings of anxiety, irritability, and insecurity are replaced by headache and back and neck pain due to the effects of the catecholamines on blood vessels and muscles.

If the stress is allowed to persist, the physical priority is to provide alternative fuels to provide energy. The adrenal gland increases its output of cortisol to stimulate glucose synthesis. Fatigue, indigestion, and diminished sex drive become dominant.

The third stage of a prolonged stress response is exhaustion when glycogen and fat stores have gone. The immune system cannot find the energy to continue functioning. This is when deep physical illness takes over. Body muscle wastes away, and heart and kidney failure or overwhelming infection are the end result.

EXERCISES

Language of Endocrinology: *The meaning of a word element never changes, regardless of the term that contains it. Demonstrate your knowledge of word elements by making the correct choice in the following multiple-choice questions.*

1. Based on its suffix, an **aldosteronoma** is a:
   a. condition
   b. facial hair
   c. tumor
   d. facial expression
   e. gland

2. In the term **pheochromocytoma**, the prefix is one of:
   a. size
   b. shape
   c. direction
   d. color
   e. gender

3. Circle the term with a root that means **masculine:**
   a. hirsutism
   b. aldosteronism
   c. facies
   d. virilism
   e. aldosteronoma

4. The suffix in this term means **surgical excision:**
   a. adrenalectomy
   b. virilism
   c. aldosteronoma
   d. facies
   e. pheochromocytoma

LESSON 14.4 Pancreas

OBJECTIVES

The information provided in this lesson will enable you to:

14.4.1 **Distinguish between the different cells of the pancreas and their secretions.**

14.4.2 **Identify the functions of the hormones produced by the pancreas.**

14.4.3 **Explain common disorders of the pancreatic hormones.**

You are

. . . a medical assistant working with Susan Lee, MD, in her primary care clinic at Fulwood Medical Center.

Your patient is

. . . Mrs. Martha Jones, who is here for her monthly checkup.

CASE REPORT 14.4

Mrs. Martha Jones is a 53-year-old type 2 diabetic on insulin, with diabetic retinopathy and diabetic neuropathy of her feet. Bariatric surgery has enabled her to reduce her weight from 275 to 156 pounds. The time is 0930 hrs.

She is complaining of having a cold and cough for the past few days. Now she is feeling drowsy and nauseous and has a dry mouth. As you talk with her, you notice that her speech is slurred. She cannot remember if she gave herself her morning insulin. Examination of her lungs reveals rales at her right base.

Her VS: T 97.8°F, P 120, R 20, BP 100/50. You perform her blood glucose measurement. The reading is 525 mg/dL (a recommended value 2 hours after breakfast is < 145 mg/dL).

At the end of this chapter you will be asked to document in SOAP format your encounter with her.

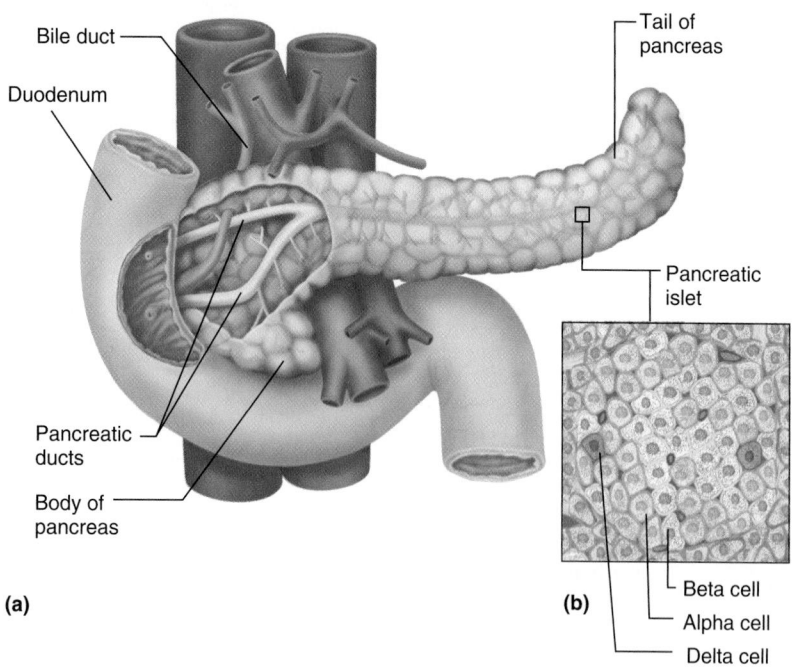

(a)

▲ **FIGURE 14.19** **Pancreas.** (*a*) General anatomy. (*b*) Alpha, beta, and delta cells.

Keynote

Glucagon is not the only hormone that raises blood glucose; epinephrine, cortisol, and growth hormone also have that effect. Insulin is the only hormone that lowers blood glucose.

PANCREAS

The location and structure of the pancreas are detailed in *Chapter 6.* Most of the pancreas is an exocrine gland that secretes digestive juices into the duodenum through a duct *(Figure 14.19).* Scattered throughout the pancreas are clusters of endocrine cells grouped around blood vessels. These clusters are called **pancreatic islets (islets of Langerhans).** Within the islets are three distinct cell types:

1. **Alpha cells**—secrete the hormone **glucagon** in response to a low blood glucose. Glucagon's actions are:

   a. In the liver, to stimulate **gluconeogenesis, glycogenolysis,** and the release of glucose into the bloodstream.

   b. In adipose tissue, to stimulate fat catabolism and the release of free fatty acids.

2. **Beta cells**—secrete **insulin** in response to a high blood glucose. Insulin has the opposite effects of glucagon:

   a. In muscle and fat cells, to encourage absorption of glucose and to store glycogen and fat.

   b. In the liver, to stimulate the conversion of glucose to glycogen and to inhibit the conversion of noncarbohydrates to glucose.

3. **Delta cells**—secrete **somatostatin,** which acts within the pancreas to inhibit the secretion of glucagon and insulin.

WORD ANALYSIS AND DEFINITION

WORD	PRONUNCIATION	ELEMENTS		DEFINITION
glucagon	GLU-kah-gon	S/ R/	-agon *contest* gluc- *glucose*	Pancreatic hormone that supports blood glucose levels
gluconeogenesis	GLU-ko-nee-oh-JEN-eh-sis	S/ P/ R/CF	-genesis *creation* -neo- *new* gluc/o- *glucose*	Formation of glucose from noncarbohydrate sources
glycogenolysis	GLYE-koh-jen-oh-LYE-sis	S/ R/CF R/CF	-lysis *break down* glyc/o- *glycogen* -gen/o- *to create*	Conversion of glycogen to glucose
insulin	IN-syu-lin	S/ R/	-in *chemical compound* insul- *island*	A hormone secreted by the islet cells of the pancreas
islets of Langerhans	EYE-lets of LAHNG-er-hahnz		Paul Langerhans, 1847–1888, German anatomist	Areas of pancreatic cells that produce insulin and glucagon
pancreas	PAN-kree-ass		Greek *sweetbread*	Lobulated gland, the head of which is tucked into the curve of the duodenum
pancreatic (adj)	pan-kree-AT-ik	S/ R/	ic *pertaining to* pancreat- *pancreas*	Pertaining to the pancreas
somatostatin	SO-mah-toe-STAT-in	S/ R/CF	-statin *inhibit* somat/o- *body*	Hormone that inhibits release of growth hormone and insulin

---

EXERCISES

After reading Case Report 14.4 on the opposite page, answer the following questions. Be prepared to discuss your answers in class.

1. What conditions appear in Mrs. Jones's past medical history?

_____

_____

2. What was the diagnosis that prompted Mrs. Jones to have *bariatric* surgery?

_____

3. What are the patient's chief complaints?

_____

_____

4. What *signs* are observable to the medical assistant and doctor?

_____

5. What are *rales?* _____

_____

   How are they detected? _____

_____

6. Where is the "right *base*" of the lung located?

_____

7. What can be said about Mrs. Jones's current blood glucose level?

_____

DISORDERS OF PANCREATIC HORMONES: DIABETES MELLITUS

Diabetes mellitus (DM) is a syndrome characterized by hyperglycemia resulting from an absolute or relative impairment of insulin secretion and/or insulin action. This leads to a disruption of carbohydrate, fat, and protein metabolism. It is the world's most prevalent metabolic disease and the leading cause of blindness, renal failure, and gangrene. There are four categories of diabetes mellitus:

1. **Type 1 diabetes,** also called **insulin-dependent diabetes mellitus (IDDM),** accounts for 10% to 15% of all cases of DM but is the predominant type of DM under the age of 30. When symptoms become apparent, 90% of the pancreatic insulin-producing cells have been destroyed by **autoantibodies.** The incidence of type 1 diabetes is increased in patients with Graves disease, Hashimoto disease, and Addison disease.

2. **Type 2 diabetes,** also called **non-insulin-dependent diabetes mellitus (NIDDM),** accounts for 85% to 90% of all cases of DM. Almost 7% of U.S. residents are diagnosed with type 2 diabetes. Not only is there some impairment of insulin response, but there is decreased insulin effectiveness in stimulating glucose uptake by tissues and in restraining hepatic glucose production. This is called **insulin resistance.** In addition to type 2 diabetes, insulin resistance leads to other common disorders such as obesity, hypertension, hyperlipidemia, and coronary artery disease. Type 2 diabetes can be secondary to Cushing syndrome, acromegaly, pheochromocytoma, and aldosteronism.

3. **Gestational diabetes** is seen in the latter half of 5% of pregnancies. While most cases of gestational diabetes resolve after the pregnancy, a woman who has this complication of pregnancy has a 30% chance of developing type 2 diabetes within 10 years.

4. **Mature-onset diabetes of youth (MODY)** is genetically inherited, occurs in thin individuals who are in their teens and twenties, and is comparable to type 2 diabetes in its severity.

Hypoglycemia is present when blood glucose is below 70 mg/dL. Hormonal defense mechanisms (glucagon and adrenaline) are activated as the blood glucose drops below 55mg/dL. Because brain metabolism depends primarily on glucose, the brain is the first organ affected by hypoglycemia. Impaired mental efficiency starts to be seen when the blood glucose falls below 65 mg/dL. It becomes very obvious (shakiness, anxiety, confusion, tremor) around 40 mg/dL, and below that figure seizures can occur. If the blood glucose falls below 10 mg/dL, the neurons become electrically silent, resulting in diabetic **coma.** Symptomatic hypoglycemia is sometimes called **insulin shock.**

Low blood glucose can be raised to normal in minutes by taking 3 to 4 ounces of orange, apple, or grape juice. Symptoms should begin to improve in 5 minutes, with full recovery in 10 to 15 minutes. In an emergency, if the patient is not able to take oral sugar, treatment is begun with a rapid IV **bolus** of 25 mL of 50% glucose solution, followed by an IV infusion of glucose.

WORD	PRONUNCIATION	ELEMENTS		DEFINITION
autoantibody	aw-toe-**AN**-tee-bod-ee	P/ P/ R/	auto- *self, same* -anti- *against* -body *body*	Antibody produced in response to an antigen from the host's own tissue
bolus	**BOH**-lus		Greek *a lump*	Single mass of a substance
coma	**KOH**-mah		Greek *deep sleep*	State of deep unconsciousness
diabetes mellitus	dye-ah-**BEE**-teez **MEL**-ih-tus		**diabetes** Greek *a siphon* **mellitus** Latin *sweetened with honey*	Metabolic syndrome caused by absolute or relative insulin deficiency and/or insulin ineffectiveness
diabetic (adj)	dye-ah-**BET**-ik	S/ R/	-ic *pertaining to* diabet- *diabetes*	Pertaining to or suffering from diabetes
hypoglycemia	**HIGH**-poh-glie-**SEE**-me-ah	S/ P/ R/	-emia *blood condition* hypo- *below, deficient* -glyc- *glucose*	Low level of glucose (sugar) in the blood
hypoglycemic (adj)	**HIGH**-poh-glie-**SEE**-mik	S/	-emic *in the blood*	Pertaining to or suffering from hypoglycemia

EXERCISES

Diabetes is the world's most prevalent metabolic disease. Many patients have diabetes as a concurrent condition with other health problems—which always makes it a consideration in treatment and prescribing medications. Test your knowledge of this disease by answering the following questions. Circle the correct choice.

1. Diabetes is the leading cause of:

   blindness   renal failure   gangrene   none of these   all of these

2. The first organ affected by hypoglycemia is the:

   kidney   heart   pancreas   brain   liver

3. The predominant type of DM in patients under the age of 30 is:

   type 1   type 2   non-insulin-dependent DM   gestational diabetes type 3

4. Impairment of insulin response and decreased insulin effectiveness are termed insulin:

   production   resistance   autoantibodies   control   conversion

5. Most cases of gestational diabetes resolve after:

   medication   treatment   testing   delivery   surgery

6. Symptomatic hypoglycemia is sometimes called:

   insulin resistance   coma   insulin shock   glucolysis   bolus

7. Type 1 diabetes is also known as:

   IDDM   NIDDM   hypoglycemia   hyperglycemia   coma

8. Insulin resistance can lead to:

   obesity   aldosteronoma   hirsutism   myxedema   virilism

9. Low blood glucose can be raised to normal with a:

   vitamin   hormone   enzyme   carbohydrate   electrolyte

10. What can raise blood glucose levels in type 2 diabetes?

   stress   dehydration   nausea   coughing   vomiting

Hyperglycemia causes damage to vascular endothelial cells at the microvascular and macrovascular levels.

Untreated hyperglycemia can progress to coma.

Diabetic ketoacidosis is a medical emergency.

DISORDERS OF PANCREATIC HORMONES: DIABETES MELLITUS (continued)

Hyperglycemia

The classic symptoms of hyperglycemia are *poly*uria (excessive urination), *poly*dipsia (excessive thirst), and *poly*phagia (excessive hunger), with unexplained weight loss.

Symptomatic hyperglycemia is how type 1 diabetes usually presents. Type 2 diabetes can be symptomatic or asymptomatic and is often found during a routine health examination.

Because of high glucose levels, hyperglycemia damages capillary endothelial cells in the retina, renal glomerulus, and neurons and Schwann cells in peripheral nerves. Of all diabetics, 85% develop some degree of diabetic retinopathy, while 30% develop diabetic nephropathy, which can progress to end-stage renal disease *(see Chapter 11)*. Diabetic neuropathy causes sensory defects with numbness, tingling, and **paresthesias** in the stocking-glove distribution.

In larger blood vessels, the hyperglycemia contributes to endothelial cell lining damage and atherosclerosis. Coronary artery disease and peripheral vascular disease with claudication *(see Chapter 8)* are complications. Hyperglycemia is the most common cause of foot ulcers and then gangrene of the lower extremity, sometimes necessitating amputation. The risk of infection is increased by the cellular hyperglycemia and the circulatory deficits.

The complications of hyperglycemia can be kept at bay by strict control of blood glucose levels.

Diabetic ketoacidosis (DKA) is a state of marked hyperglycemia with dehydration, **metabolic acidosis,** and **ketone formation.** It is seen mostly in type 1 diabetes and is usually the result of a lapse in insulin treatment, acute infection, or trauma that renders the usual insulin treatment inadequate.

It presents with polyuria, vomiting, and lethargy and can progress to coma. **Acetone** (a ketone) can be smelled on the breath. Diabetic ketoacidosis is a medical emergency and requires rapid fluid volume expansion, correction of the hyperglycemia, prevention of hypokalemia, and treatment of any infection. There is a 2% to 5% mortality from circulatory collapse.

Diabetic coma, a severe medical emergency, has three causes, which have been described above:

- **Diabetic ketoacidosis.**

- **Hyperglycemia** with dehydration, but not the ketosis and acidosis of DKA. This condition is called **hyperosmolar coma.** This is the condition that Mrs. Jones presented with. She was on the edge of going into a coma.

- **Hypoglycemic coma.**

  A blood glucose test will differentiate hypoglycemia from the other two causes.

Case Report 14.4 (continued)

Mrs. Martha Jones is in the early stages of a hyperglycemic nonketotic (hyperosmolar) coma, probably initiated by a right lower lobe pneumonia. A urine specimen was obtained. Dr. Lee was notified. Blood was taken for a full chemistry panel, and arterial blood gases were drawn. An IV infusion bolus of 550 mL of isotonic sodium chloride was given, followed by 1.5 liters of isotonic **saline** over the next 2 hours. Mrs. Jones was given 10 units of regular insulin IV and admitted to the hospital.

WORD	PRONUNCIATION		ELEMENTS	DEFINITION
acetone	**ASS**-eh-tone		Latin *vinegar*	Ketone that is found in blood, urine, and breath when diabetes mellitus is out of control
hyperglycemia	**HIGH**-per-gly-**SEE**-me-ah	S/ P/ R/	-emia *blood condition* hyper- *above* -glyc- *glucose*	High level of glucose (sugar) in blood
hyperglycemic (adj)	**HIGH**-per-gly-**SEE**-mik	S/	-emic *in the blood*	Pertaining to high blood sugar
hyperosmolar	**HIGH**-per-os-**MOH**-lar	S/ P/ R/	-ar *pertaining to* hyper- *above* -osmol- *concentration*	Marked hyperglycemia without ketoacidosis
ketoacidosis	**KEY**-toe-ass-ih-**DOE**-sis	S/ R/ R/CF	-osis *condition* -acid- *acid* ket/o- *ketone*	Excessive production of ketones, making the blood acid
ketone	**KEY**-tone		Greek *acetone*	Chemical formed in uncontrolled diabetes or in starvation
ketosis (**Note:** With the "o" in ket/o- preceding the "o" in -osis, one "o" drops out for simpler pronunciation.)	key-**TOE**-sis	S/ R/	-osis *condition* ket/- *ketone*	Excessive production of ketones
metabolic acidosis	met-ah-**BOL**-ik ass-ih-**DOE**-sis	S/ R/ S/ R/	-ic *pertaining to* metabol- *change* -osis *condition* acid- *acid*	Decreased pH in blood and body tissues as a result of an upset in metabolism
paresthesia paresthesias (pl)	par-es-**THEE**-ze-ah par-es-**THEE**-ze-as	S/ P/ R/	-ia *condition* par- *abnormal* -esthes- *sensation*	An abnormal sensation; for example, tingling, burning, pricking
polydipsia	pol-ee-**DIP**-see-ah	S/ P/ R/	-ia *condition* poly- *many, much* -dips- *thirst*	Excessive thirst
polyphagia	pol-ee-**FAY**-jee-ah	S/ P/ R/	-ia *condition* poly- *many, much* -phag- *to eat*	Excessive eating
polyuria	pol-ee-**YOU**-ree-ah	S/ P/ R/	-ia *condition* poly- *many, much* -ur- *urinary system*	Excessive production of urine
saline	**SAY**-leen		Latin *salt*	Salt solution, usually sodium chloride

EXERCISES

After reading Case Report 14.4 on the opposite page, answer the following questions. Be prepared to discuss your answers in class.

1. *Hyperglycemic* means that the level of _____ is too high in the patient's blood.

2. *Hyperosmolar coma* is the same thing as _____ .

3. What are the three classic symptoms of *diabetes mellitus,* and what do they describe?

   a._____ is _____ .

   b._____ is _____ .

   c._____ is _____ .

4. What diagnostic tests were performed on Mrs. Jones? _____

5. What is a *coma?* _____

6. What does *ketoacidosis* signify? _____

   _____

7. What was the treatment plan for this patient?

   _____

   _____

Abbreviations

BUN	blood urea nitrogen
ECG	electrocardiogram
Hb A1c	glycosylated hemoglobin (hemoglobin A one-C)
NPH	neutral protamine Hagedorn insulin
OGTT	oral glucose tolerance test
U	unit

Criteria for the Diagnosis of Diabetes Mellitus

The accepted **criteria** for the diagnosis of DM include either a fasting (8 hours) plasma glucose of 126 mg/dL or greater or symptoms (polyuria, polydipsia, polyphagia, unexplained weight loss) and a random plasma glucose of 200 mg/dL or higher.

An **oral glucose tolerance test (OGTT)** is used occasionally in diagnosing type 2 diabetes.

Treatment of Diabetes Mellitus

The basic principle of diabetes treatment is to avoid hyperglycemia and hypoglycemia. The following are the areas of treatment:

- **Diet and exercise.** To achieve weight reduction of 2 pounds per week in overweight type 2 patients is essential. For insulin-treated diabetics, detailed diet management restricts variations in timing, size, and content of meals.

- **Patient education.** Patients are taught to understand the disease process, to recognize the indications for seeking immediate medical care, and to follow a regimen of foot care.

- **Plasma glucose monitoring.** This is an essential skill that all diabetics must learn. Patients on insulin must learn to adjust their insulin doses. Home glucose analyzers use a drop of blood obtained by a spring-powered lancet from the fingertip or forearm. The frequency of testing is varied individually. Insulin-treated patients should test their plasma glucose before meals, 2 hours after meals, and at bedtime.

- **Routine physician visits.** The patient is assessed for symptoms or signs of complications. Skin condition, pulses, and sensation in feet are tested. Urine is tested for **microalbuminuria** using **immunoassays**. This detects smaller increases in urinary albumin than does conventional urine testing.

- **Periodic laboratory evaluation.** This includes **blood urea nitrogen (BUN)** and serum creatinine (kidney function), lipid profile, **electrocardiogram (ECG)**, and an annual complete ophthalmologic evaluation.

Glycosylated hemoglobin (Hb A1c) is used to monitor plasma glucose control during the preceding 1 to 3 months. It is formed at rates that increase with plasma glucose levels. Normal Hb A1c is less than 6%. In poor control, the value is 9% to 12%. It is also part of a periodic laboratory evaluation.

Fructosamine is formed by glucose combining with plasma protein and reflects plasma glucose control over the preceding 1 to 3 weeks. A standard reference range for this test is not available.

Insulin preparations routinely contain 100 U/mL **(U-100 insulin)**. The insulin is injected subcutaneously using disposable syringes that hold 0.5 mL. In addition, already prepared mixtures of intermediate and regular insulins in different ratios are available. An **insulin pen** is an injection device that holds several days' dosage.

Continuous subcutaneous insulin infusion is given by a battery-powered, programmable pump that provides continuous insulin through a small needle in the abdominal wall.

Pharmacology: Classes of Insulin

Insulin Type	Onset of Action*	Peak of Action*	Duration of Action*	Examples
Rapid acting	15 min	30–60 min	3–5 hr	Humalog, NovoLog
Regular acting	30–60 min	100–120 min	5–8 hr	Humulin R, Novolin R
Intermediate acting (NPH)	1–3 hr	7–8 hr	18–24 hr	Humulin N, Novolin N
Long acting	4–8 hr	minimal peak effects	16–24 hr	Lantus, Levemir

*min = minutes; hr = hours.

WORD	PRONUNCIATION	ELEMENTS		DEFINITION
criterion criteria (pl)	kri-**TEER**-ee-on kri-**TEER**-ee-ah		Greek *a standard*	Standard or rule for judging
fructosamine	**FRUK**-toe-sah-meen	S/ R/	-amine *nitrogen-containing* fructos- *fruit sugar*	Organic compound with fructose as its base
glycosylated hemoglobin (Hb A1c)	**GLYE**-koh-sih-lay-ted **HE**-moh-**GLOW**-bin	R/CF S/	glyc/o- *glucose* -sylated *linked*	Hemoglobin A fraction linked to glucose; used as index of glucose control
immunoassay	**IM**-you-noh-**ASS**-ay	R/ R/CF	-assay *evaluate* immun/o- *immune* *response*	Biochemical test to measure the amount of a substance in a liquid using the reaction of an antibody to its antigen
microalbuminuria	**MY**-kroh-al-byu-min-**YOU**-ree-ah	S/ P/ R/ R/	-ia *condition* micro- *small* -albumin- *albumin* -ur- *urinary system*	Presence of very small quantities of albumin in urine that cannot be detected by conventional urine testing
synergist synergistic (adj)	**SIN**-er-jist	S/ P/ R/	-ist *specialist* syn- *together* -erg- *work*	Agent or process that aids the action of another

Oral Diabetic Pharmacology

Oral antidiabetic drugs are used for type 2 but not type 1 diabetes. These drugs include:

- **Metformin** acts by decreasing hepatic glucose production. It also promotes weight loss and decreases lipid levels. It is **synergistic** in combination with sulfonylureas.

- **Sulfonylureas** act by stimulating the beta cells to secrete insulin.

- **Thiazolidinediones,** such as pioglitazone, improve insulin sensitivity in skeletal muscle and suppress hepatic glucose production. They are used in type 2 DM patients to help insulin work more effectively.

EXERCISES

Medications: *Diabetics will deal with medications for the rest of their lives. Match the statement to the correct drug by placing a check mark (✓) in the column with the appropriate drug name. Then fill in the blanks below.*

Statement	Metformin	Sulfonylureas	Thiazolidinediones
Act by stimulating the beta cells to secrete insulin			
Improves insulin sensitivity in skeletal muscle			
Suppresses hepatic glucose production			
Can be used in combination with other drugs			
Promotes weight loss			
Allows insulin to work more effectively in type 2 DM patients			
Decreases lipid levels			
Pioglitazone is an example			

1. Oral antidiabetic drugs are used for type _____ diabetes but not type _____ .

2. Name the four major types of insulin preparations:

   a. _____   c. _____

   b. _____   d. _____

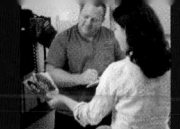
ENDOCRINE SYSTEM

CHALLENGE YOUR KNOWLEDGE

A. **Written Communication:** Reread the Case Report on Dr. Lee's patient, Martha Jones. *As you read the report for the second time, try highlighting the important terminology you will use to write your SOAP note.*

CASE REPORT 14.4

Your patient is

. . . Mrs. Martha Jones, who is here for her monthly checkup. She is a 53-year-old type 2 diabetic on insulin, with diabetic retinopathy and diabetic neuropathy of her feet. Bariatric surgery has enabled her to reduce her weight from 275 to 156 pounds. The time is 0930 hrs.

She is complaining of having a cold and cough for the past few days. Now she is feeling drowsy and nauseous and has a dry mouth. As you talk with her, you notice that her speech is slurred. She cannot remember if she gave herself her morning insulin. Examination of her lungs reveals rales at her right base.

Her VS: T 97.8°F, P 120, R 20, BP 100/50. You perform her blood glucose measurement. The reading is 525 mg/dL (a recommended value 2 hours after breakfast is < 145 mg/dL).

Mrs. Martha Jones is in the early stages of a hyperglycemic, nonketotic coma, probably initiated by a right lower lobe pneumonia. A urine specimen was obtained. Dr. Lee was notified. Blood was taken for a full chemistry panel, and arterial blood gases were drawn. An IV infusion bolus of 550 mL of isotonic sodium chloride was given, followed by 1.5 liters of isotonic saline over the next 2 hours. She was given 10 units of regular insulin IV and was admitted to the hospital.

During your career, any documentation you write will be read by other health care personnel. This is an official document for the patient's chart and must be professional-looking—writing must be legible and neat, and all spelling must be correct.

This part of the exercise is for organizing your thoughts about what to write on the actual documentation. To obtain the form to use after you have completed this exercise, go to CONNECT and print out a blank SOAP form. Transfer your notes from this exercise to the official form, and hand it in to your instructor. Organize your notes in the following manner:

S (subjective)   What are the patient's chief complaint and symptoms at this visit (from the patient's own words)?

_____

_____

_____

_____

O (*objective*)   What can be observed or measured by examination of the patient?

_____

_____

_____

_____

A (*assessment*)   What measures (tests, etc.) were taken to determine the cause of this patient's problem? What is the possible or tentative diagnosis?

_____

_____

_____

_____

P (*plan*)   What is being done for this patient now to alleviate her complaint?

_____

_____

_____

_____

B. **Prefixes:** Practice the prefixes contained in endocrine terminology. Write the meaning of each of the prefixes listed below; then give an example of a medical term that begins with that prefix. Finally, pick any three terms, and use each in a sentence of patient documentation.

Prefixes	Meaning of Prefix	Medical Term Using This Prefix
ad-		
anti-		
endo-		
eu-		
ex-		
in-		
iso-		
pan-		
par-		
para-		
pheo-		
pro-		

1. _____

_____

2. _____

_____

3. _____

_____

ENDOCRINE SYSTEM

C. **Diseases and Disorders:** Identify the diseases and disorders of the endocrine system as described in the following statements. Special attention to the prefixes will aid you in matching your correct choice.

_____ 1. Autoimmune disease with lymphocytic infiltration manifesting with hypothyroidism   A. Graves disease

_____ 2. Congenital form of thyroid deficiency   B. thyroid cancer

_____ 3. Excess of PTH   C. hypoparathyroidism

_____ 4. Severe hypothyroidism   D. thyroiditis

_____ 5. Presents as symptomless thyroid nodule   E. Hashimoto disease

_____ 6. Inflammation of the thyroid gland   F. goiter

_____ 7. Hyperthyroidism associated with a goiter   G. exophthalmos

_____ 8. Deficiency of PTH   H. hyperparathyroidism

_____ 9. Enlargement of the thyroid gland   I. myxedema

_____ 10. Eyes bulging outward   J. cretinism

D. **Terminology Construction:** Construct the **language of endocrinology**. Build the term for the definition provided. Fill in the blanks.

1. Hormone formed by the pineal gland   _____ / _____ / _____

2. Protrusion of the eyeball   _____ / _____ / _____

3. Hormone produced by the adrenal cortex   _____ / _____ / _____

4. Deficiency of all the pituitary hormones   _____ / _____ / _____

5. Another name for the pituitary gland   _____ / _____ / _____

6. Stimulates the uterus to contract   _____ / _____ / _____

7. Removal of part or all of the adrenal gland   _____ / _____ / _____

8. Prolactin-producing tumor   _____ / _____ / _____

9. Waxy, nonpitting edema of skin   _____ / _____ / _____

10. Excessive growth hormone produces enlarged hands and feet   _____ / _____ / _____

E. **Translation:** Rewrite the following sentence—without any abbreviations—into language a patient can understand. Review any terms you need to before you start writing.

"ADH, also called vasopressin, causes vasoconstriction in small arterioles, usually insufficient to cause hypertension."

_____

_____

_____

_____

F. **Recall and Review:** How well do you remember these word elements from the previous chapter? Try to answer without first looking back to check. Fill in the blanks.

Element	Type of Element (P, R, CF, S)	Meaning of Element
estr/o	_____	_____
poly	_____	_____
vert	_____	_____
ovari	_____	_____
pro	_____	_____

G. **Language of Endocrinology:** Knowing the endocrine system will aid you in understanding the overall body process of *homeostasis.* Apply the ***language of endocrinology*** to the following questions about the anatomy and physiology of the endocrine system; circle the correct answer.

1. Which of the following is not a part of the endocrine system?

   a. pancreas

   b. pituitary

   c. pineal

   d. parathyroid

   e. palatine

2. The abnormal production of breast milk is called:

   a. dysmenorrhea

   b. polydipsia

   c. galactorrhea

   d. dysphagia

   e. menorrhagia

3. The speed at which the body's chemical functions proceed is called:

   a. cardiac rate

   b. vasoconstriction

   c. metabolic rate

   d. blood pressure

   e. homeostasis

4. The only hormone that lowers blood glucose is:

   a. glucagon

   b. cortisol

   c. aldosterone

   d. corticosterone

   e. insulin

ENDOCRINE SYSTEM

H. Language of Endocrinology: Apply the *language of endocrinology* to the following questions about the anatomy and physiology of the endocrine system; circle the correct answer.

1. A congenital form of thyroid deficiency that severely retards mental and physical growth is:

   a. goiter

   b. thyroid adenoma

   c. cretinism

   d. pretibial myxedema

   e. hyperthyroidism

2. **Tetany** is:

   a. lockjaw

   b. painful muscle spasm

   c. protrusion of the eyeball

   d. enlargement of the thyroid gland

   e. excessive production of thyroid hormones

3. A condition produced by a pituitary tumor that causes a decline in the production of several hormones at the same time is called:

   a. hypopituitarism

   b. hyperpituitarism

   c. panhypopituitarism

   d. prolactinoma

   e. diabetes mellitus

4. Another name for **epinephrine** is:

   a. corticosteroid

   b. corticosterone

   c. adrenalin

   d. hydrocortisone

   e. cortisol

5. The pineal gland secretes **serotonin** by day and converts it to _____ at night.

   a. melatonin

   b. a vasodilator

   c. vasopressin

   d. prolactin

   e. an enzyme

6. This term can be used to describe the location of the adrenal gland:

   a. infrarenal

   b. interrenal

   c. intrarenal

   d. hyporenal

   e. suprarenal

7. In the term **paresthesia,** the root means:

   a. obese

   b. sensation

   c. movement

   d. abnormally thin

   e. body

8. **Hypophysis** is the term for the:

   a. pituitary gland

   b. thyroid gland

   c. pineal gland

   d. parathyroid gland

   e. thymus gland

9. Condition of a forward-projecting jaw is called:

   a. hypercalcemia

   b. goiter

   c. exophthalmos

   d. prognathism

   e. myxedema

10. A fine needle aspiration biopsy would be done to:

   a. measure size of nodule

   b. determine place of nodule

   c. count numbers of nodules

   d. reduce size of nodule

   e. determine possible pathology of nodule

ENDOCRINE SYSTEM

I. **Hormones:** Hormones are bloodborne messengers secreted by endocrine glands. Each has a specific function, as stated below. Correctly use the following terms or abbreviations to fill in the blanks.

ACTH	**FSH**	**somatotropin**	**PRL**	**tropic**
insulin	glucocorticoid	melatonin	**LH**	thyrotropin

1. Hormone that stimulates the growth of the thyroid gland: _____

2. Hormones that stimulate other endocrine glands to produce hormones: _____

3. Hormone that stimulates ovulation and testosterone production: _____

4. Hormone of the adrenal cortex that helps regulate glucose metabolism: _____

5. Hormone that stimulates cells to enlarge and divide: _____

6. Hormone produced by the islet cells of the pancreas: _____

7. Hormone of the anterior pituitary that stimulates cortex of adrenal gland to produce its own hormones: _____

8. Hormone that stimulates target cells in the ovaries and testes: _____

9. Hormone formed by pineal gland: _____

10. Hormone that stimulates the mammary glands after pregnancy to produce milk: _____

J. **Latin and Greek Terms:** Latin and Greek terms cannot be further deconstructed into prefix, root, or suffix. You must know them for what they are. Test your knowledge of these terms with the following exercise. Match the meaning in the left column with the correct medical term in the right column. Use any one medical term (A–J) in a sentence of patient documentation.

_____	1.	Oblong shield	A.	tetany
_____	2.	Island	B.	coma
_____	3.	Deep sleep	C.	tropic
_____	4.	Stimulation, change	D.	thyroid
_____	5.	Insulin deficiency	E.	insulin
_____	6.	A lump	F.	facies
_____	7.	Convulsive tension	G.	hirsutism
_____	8.	Appearance	H.	bolus
_____	9.	Shaggy or hairy	I.	hormone
_____	10.	To set in motion	J.	diabetes

Sentence:

_____

_____

_____

K. Terminology Challenge: An element may have more than one meaning. For example, **hypo-** can mean either *below* (location) or *deficient* (less in quantity or number). The following five terms all start with **hypo-**. Write the meaning of each term, and check mark (✓) whether the prefix in this case means *below* or *deficient*. Fill in the chart.

Medical Term	Prefix Means *below*	Prefix Means *deficient*	Meaning of Term
hypoglycemia			
hypothyroidism			
hypothalamus			
hypopituitarism			
hypophysis			

L. Plurals: Enhance your command of plurals in medical terminology by completing this exercise. Circle the best choice for the correct form of the plural in the sentence.

1. Patient complains of multiple (paresthesiae/paresthesias) on her left side.

2. There are several (criterion/criteria) by which to judge this patient's recovery.

3. (Catecholamines/Catecholamina) are major elements in stress response.

4. Insulin sensitivity in skeletal muscle is improved by (thiazolidinediones/thiazolidinedionia).

M. Deconstruction: Deconstruct these medical terms into the meanings of their basic elements. Demonstrate that you understand the meanings by using one term in a sentence of patient documentation. Fill in the chart.

Medical Term	Meaning of Prefix	Meaning of Root(s)/CF	Meaning of Suffix	Meaning of Medical Term
polyuria				
parathyroid				
vasopressin				
panhypopituitarism				
prognathism				
polydipsia				
euthyroid				
autoantibody				
hypoglycemia				
polyphagia				
endocrinology				
paresthesia				

Sentence:

_____

_____

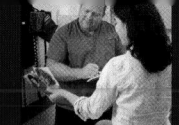

ENDOCRINE SYSTEM

N. Discussion: Team up with another student to do some research on *plasma glucose monitoring*. Prepare a brief presentation for the class.

1. Discuss how this monitoring is done and why it is so important for diabetics to do this regularly.

2. Look on the Internet for pictures of equipment used for this purpose.

3. Discuss what can happen to diabetic individuals who do not keep careful track of their glucose levels.

4. Mention how this monitoring will affect their daily lives and medication.

Your instructor may ask you to hand this in as an assignment instead of a presentation.

O. Diagnostic Tests: Diagnostic tests are performed specifically to test for certain thyroid problems. Circle the best choice for the designated test.

1. Reveals the size of the gland and presence of nodules:

   MRI   CT   ultrasound

2. Blood test for detailed activity of the gland:

   TSH level   ADH level   OGTT level

3. Details nature of enlargement and function of the gland:

   isotopic thyroid scan   x-ray   MRI

4. Distinguishes benign from malignant lesions:

   fine needle aspiration biopsy   ADH level in blood   ultrasound

P. Elements: Use your knowledge of word elements to answer the following questions about hormones in other body systems. Fill in the blanks.

1. Based on its root, the hormone gastrin would have a connection with which body organ? _____

2. Based on its root, the hormone cholecystokinin has an effect on which body organ? _____

3. Both of the above organs are part of which body system that you have already studied? _____

4. Based on its root, the hormone erythropoietin stimulates production of _____. This hormone is

   secreted by the (organ) _____, which is part of the _____ system.

Continue working with elements as clues in the following terms. From among this bank of terms, choose the correct terms to fit the descriptions. Some blanks may need more than one term, and there are extra terms you will not use. Fill in the blanks.

acromegaly	iodine	microalbuminuria	serotonin	hypoglycemia
thyroidectomy	prolactinoma	galactorrhea	adrenalectomy	antidiuretic
prolactin	panhypopituitarism	melatonin	gigantism	pheochromocytoma

5. Term(s) connected to urine:

   _____

6. Blood condition:

   _____

7. Procedure(s):

   _____

8. Term(s) connected to milk:

9. Excessive growth:

_____

10. Term(s) that contain a color:

_____

Q. **Abbreviations:** This exercise contains all the letters you need to form the correct abbreviations for the terms described. Fill in the blanks.

   A   D   G   H   I   K   M   N   O   P   S   T

1. Stored in the posterior pituitary: _____

2. Type 2 diabetes: _____

3. Thyrotropin: _____

4. Somatotropin: _____

5. Secreted in response to hypocalcemia: _____

6. Type 1 diabetes: _____

7. Winter depression: _____

8. Marked hyperglycemia with dehydration: _____

9. Used occasionally to diagnose type 2 diabetes: _____

10. Disorder caused by insulin deficiency: _____

R. **Brain Teaser:** The alarm reaction ("fight or flight") triggers other body systems to kick into action along with the endocrine response. Based on the chapters you have already read, what other systems come into action, and how do they perform? Write your thoughts on the lines below.

_____

_____

_____

S. **Precision in Communication:** Because of errors in communication, these patients were sent to the wrong specialists! Find the errors and correct the sentences.

Underline the incorrect medical terminology in the following sentences.

1. Because of this patient's *neuropathy*, I am referring him to a kidney specialist.

   This sentence should have read:

   Because of _____

   _____ .

2. Because of this patient's *diabetic retinopathy*, I am referring her to an orthopedist.

   This sentence should have read:

   Because of _____

   _____ .

You are ultimately responsible for everything you communicate regarding patient care!

ENDOCRINE SYSTEM

CHAPTER SUMMARY EXERCISE

1. *Listen to the pronunciation of the medical terms as given by your instructor.*
2. *Circle the correct spelling of the medical term.*
3. *Match the correctly spelled terms to the brief descriptions below.*
4. *Write a sentence for each of the 10 terms that appear in this exercise.*

A. SPELLING COMPREHENSION: CIRCLE THE CORRECT SPELLING OF THE TERM.

1. hypophysis	hypopersis	hypopisis	hypophsis	hypophses
2. hersutism	hirsutism	herrsutism	hirssutism	hirsutesm
3. emaciated	emmaciated	imaciated	immaciated	emacciated
4. prolacktinomma	prolactinoma	prolictinoma	proliktinoma	prolacktinnoma
5. gooter	gutter	goiter	goiiter	guiter
6. isotope	issotope	eisotope	eissotope	isutope
7. thyroidtoxicosis	thyrotoxicosis	thyroidtoxicossis	thyrodtoxicosis	throidtoxicosis
8. myxxedema	mixxedema	mexidema	myxedema	mixedema
9. uthyroid	euthyroid	euuthroid	uthroid	utthryoid
10. insepidus	insippidus	inseppidus	insipidus	insipides

B. MATCH THE NUMBER OF THE CORRECT TERM IN PART A WITH THE BRIEF DESCRIPTION OF THE TERM BELOW.

a. Normal thyroid function _____

b. Excessive body and facial hair _____

c. Enlargement of thyroid gland _____

d. Another term for pituitary gland _____

e. Radioactive element used in diagnostic procedures _____

f. Nonpitting edema _____

g. Can appear in both men and women _____

h. Abnormally thin _____

i. Results from decreased production of ADH _____

j. Disorder produced by excessive thyroid
   hormone production _____

C. USING YOUR KNOWLEDGE OF TERMS 1–10 IN PART A AND THEIR CORRECT SPELLING, WRITE A BRIEF SENTENCE FOR EACH OF THE TERMS AS IT MIGHT APPEAR IN PATIENT DOCUMENTATION.

1. _____

2. _____

3. _____

4. _____

5. _____

6. _____

7. _____

8. _____

9. _____

10. _____

D. YOUR INSTRUCTOR WILL DIRECT YOU TO MCGRAW-HILL CONNECT. OPEN THE AUDIO GLOSSARY AND PRACTICE YOUR PRONUNCIATION OF THE TERMS IN PART A OF THIS EXERCISE.

McGraw Hill **connect**™ plus+

E. AFTER READING CASE REPORT 14.3, ANSWER THE FOLLOWING QUESTIONS. BE PREPARED TO DISCUSS YOUR ANSWERS IN CLASS.

CASE REPORT 14.3

John Fitzgerald Kennedy (1917–1963) was elected president of the United States of America in 1960 at the age of 43, the youngest person elected to that office *(Figure 14.15)*. Since the age of 13, when he was diagnosed as having colitis, he had had health problems. At age 27, he had low-back pain necessitating lower-back surgery, and he was then diagnosed as having adrenal gland insufficiency **(Addison disease)** with osteoporosis of his lumbar spine. This required lower-back surgery on three more occasions. JFK received adrenal hormone replacement therapy for the rest of his life, together with pain medication for his low-back pain, until his assassination in Dallas, Texas, in 1963.

In medical retrospect, instead of colitis, he probably had celiac disease *(see Chapter 6)*, which has strong associations with Addison disease.

1. Define *colitis*. _____

2. What is another term for *adrenal gland insufficiency?* _____

3. The disease in question 2 above falls under which generalized group of diseases?

_____

4. Where are the adrenal glands located?

_____

5. What is *osteoporosis?*

_____

6. Describe the location of the *lumbar spine.* _____

_____

7. What was JFK's treatment plan? _____

_____

8. What diagnosis most likely was the correct one, and what body system does it represent?

Diagnosis: _____

Body system: _____

Lymphatic and Immune Systems
The Language of Immunology

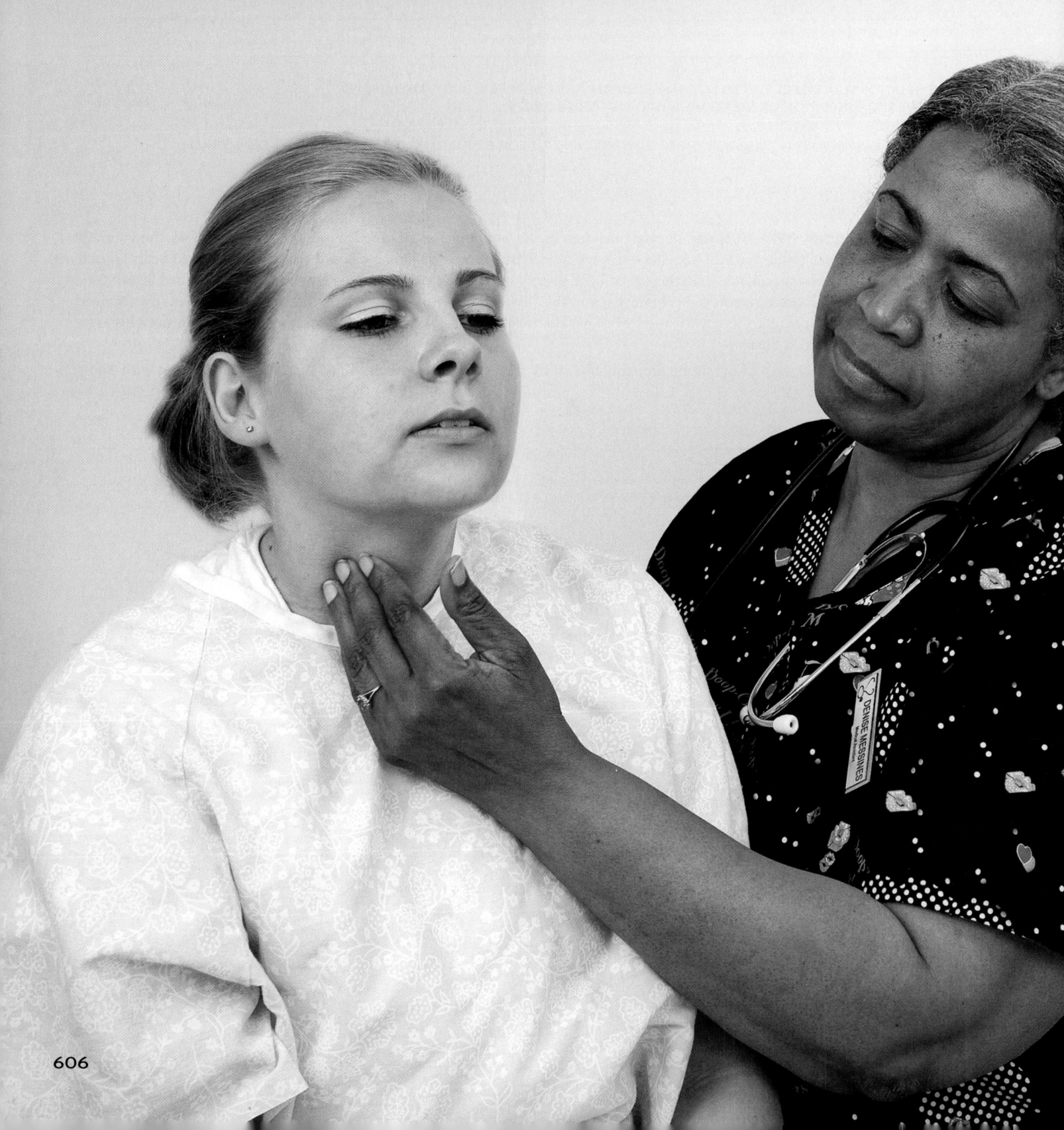

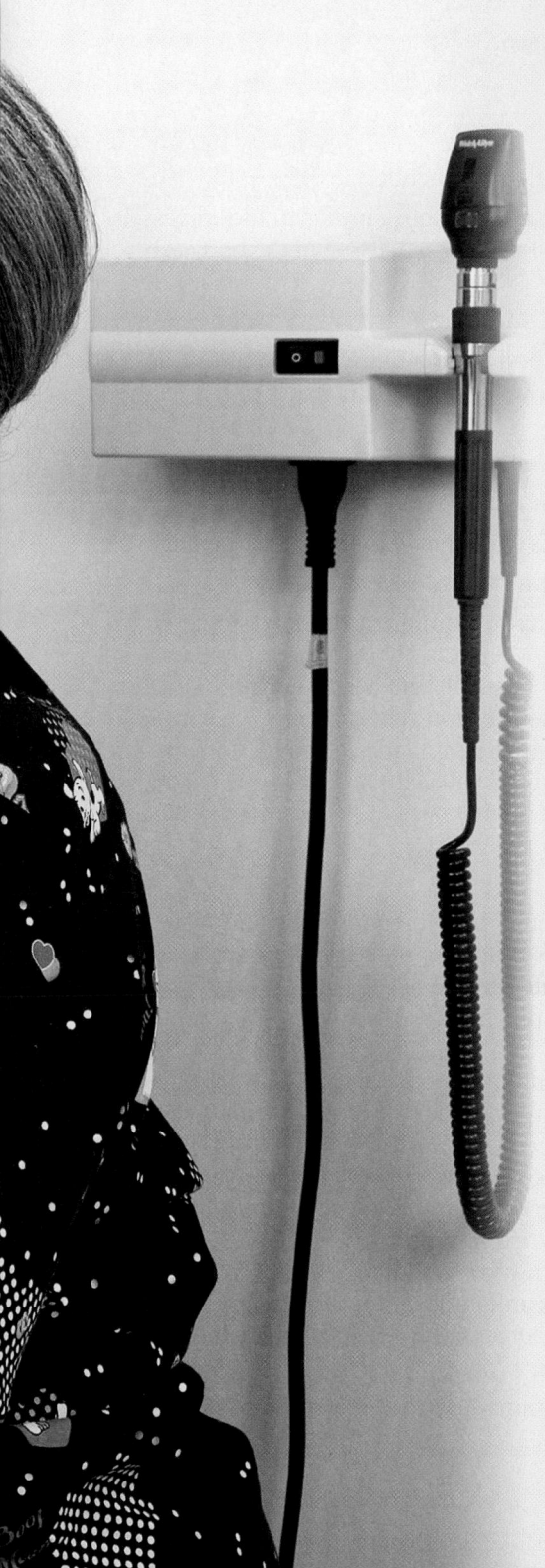

CASE REPORT 15.1

You are

. . . a medical assistant working with Susan Lee, MD, in her primary care clinic.

Your patient is

. . . Ms. Anna Clemons, a 20-year-old waitress, who is a new patient. She has noticed a lump in her right neck. On questioning, you elicit that she has lost about 8 pounds in weight in the past couple of months, has felt tired, and has had some night sweats.

Her vital signs are normal. There are two firm, enlarged lymph nodes in her right neck. Physical examination is otherwise unremarkable.

The body has three lines of defense mechanisms against foreign organisms **(pathogens)**, cells **(cancer)**, and molecules **(pollutants** and **allergens):**

    1. Physical mechanisms—the skin and mucous membranes, chemicals in perspiration, saliva and tears, hairs in the nostrils, cilia and mucus to protect the lungs.

    2. Cellular mechanisms—based on defensive cells (lymphocytes) that directly attack suspicious cells such as cancer cells, transplanted tissue cells, or cells infected with viruses or parasites.

    3. Humoral defense mechanisms—based on **antibodies** that are found in body fluids and bind to bacteria, toxins, and extracellular viruses, tagging them for destruction.

Learning Outcomes

The physical mechanisms of defense are discussed in the individual body system chapters. The lymphatic and immune systems form the core of this chapter, in which the material is designed to enable you to:

15.1 Apply the language of immunology to the anatomy and physiology of the lymphatic and immune systems.

15.2 Comprehend, analyze, spell, and write the medical terms of immunology so that you communicate and document accurately and precisely in any health care setting.

15.3 Recognize and pronounce the medical terms of immunology so that you can communicate verbally with accuracy and precision in any health care setting.

15.4 Explain the effects of common lymphatic and immune system disorders on health.

OBJECTIVES

As part of your defense mechanisms, the lymphatic system and its fluid provide surveillance and protection against foreign materials.

In this lesson the information provided will enable you to use correct medical terminology to:

15.1.1 Describe the anatomy and flow of the lymphatic system.

15.1.2 List the functions of the lymphatic system.

15.1.3 Identify the major cells of the lymphatic system and their functions.

15.1.4 Detail the anatomy and functions of the lymph nodes, tonsils, thymus gland, and spleen.

15.1.5 Explain the effects of common disorders of the lymphatic system on health.

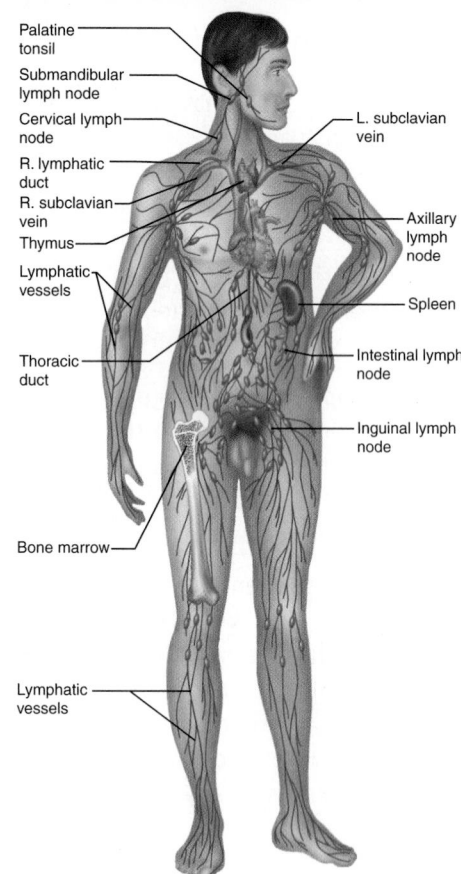

▲ **FIGURE 15.1 The Lymphatic System.**
(R. = right; L. = left)

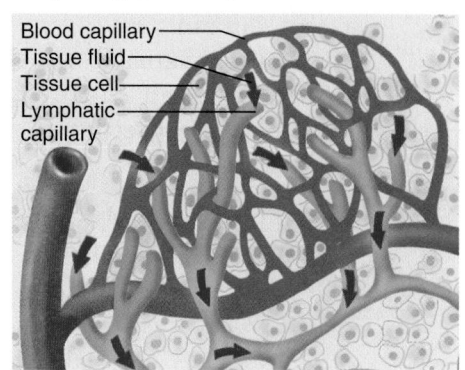

▲ **FIGURE 15.2 Lymphatic Flow.**

LYMPHATIC SYSTEM

The lymphatic system *(Figure 15.1)* has three components:

1. A network of thin **lymphatic capillaries and vessels,** similar to blood vessels, that penetrates into the interstitial spaces of nearly every tissue in the body except cartilage, bone, red bone marrow, and the CNS.

2. A group of tissues and organs that produce **immune cells.**

3. **Lymph,** a clear colorless fluid similar to blood plasma but whose composition varies from place to place in the body. It flows through the network of lymphatic capillaries and vessels.

The lymphatic system has three functions:

1. **Absorb** excess interstitial fluid and return it to the bloodstream.

2. **Remove** foreign chemicals, cells, and debris from the tissues.

3. **Absorb** dietary lipids from the small intestine *(see Chapter 6).*

The lymphatic network begins with **lymphatic capillaries** that are closed-ended tubes nestled among blood capillary networks *(Figure 15.2).* The lymphatic capillaries are designed to let interstitial fluid enter, and the interstitial fluid becomes lymph. In addition, bacteria, viruses, cellular debris, and traveling cancer cells can enter the lymphatic capillaries with the interstitial fluid. The lymphatic capillaries converge to form the larger lymphatic collecting vessels. These resemble small veins and have one-way valves in their lumen. They travel alongside veins and arteries.

Lymph Nodes

At irregular intervals, the collecting vessels enter into the part of the lymphatic network called **lymph nodes.** There are hundreds of lymph nodes stationed all over the body *(Figure 15.1).* They are especially concentrated in the neck, axilla, and groin. Their functions are to filter impurities from the lymph and alert the immune system to the presence of pathogens.

The lymph moves slowly through the node *(Figure 15.3),* which filters the lymph and removes any foreign matter. On its journey back to the bloodstream, lymph passes through several nodes *(Figure 15.1)* and becomes cleansed of most foreign matter. Macrophages in the lymph nodes ingest and break down the foreign matter and display fragments of it to **T cells** *(see page 610).* This alerts the immune system to the presence of an invader. Lymph leaves the nodes again when it enters into the efferent collecting vessels. All these lymph vessels move lymph toward the thoracic cavity.

Collecting vessels merge into **lymphatic trunks** that drain lymph from a major body region. In turn, these lymphatic trunks merge into two large **lymphatic ducts:**

1. The **right lymphatic duct** receives lymph from the right arm, right side of the thorax, and right side of the head and drains into the **right subclavian vein** *(Figure 15.1).*

WORD	PRONUNCIATION	ELEMENTS		DEFINITION
allergen (*Note:* The duplicate letter "g" is deleted to better form the word.)	**AL**-er-jen	S/ R/ R/	**-gen** *to produce* **all-** *different, strange* **-erg-** *work*	Substance producing a hypersensitivity (allergic) reaction
antibody **antibodies** (pl)	**AN**-tih-body **AN**-tih-bod-ees	P/ R/	**anti-** *against* **-body** *substance, body*	Protein produced in response to an antigen
immune **immunity**	im-**YUNE** im-**YUNE**-nih-tee	S/ R/	Latin *protected from* **-ity** *condition* **immun-** *immune response*	Protected from an infectious disease State of being protected
immunology	im-you-**NOL**-oh-jee	S/ R/CF	**-logy** *study of* **immun/o-** *immune response*	The science and practice of immunity and allergy
immunologist	im-you-**NOL**-oh-jist	S/	**-logist** *one who studies, specialist*	Medical specialist in immunology
immunize	**IM**-you-nize	S/ R/	**-ize** *affect in a specific way* **immun-** *immune response*	Make resistant to an infectious disease
immunization	im-you-nih-**ZAY**-shun	S/	**-ization** *process of affecting in a specific way*	Administration of an agent to provide immunity
immunoglobulin	**IM**-you-noh-**GLOB**-you-lin	R/CF R/ S/	**immun/o-** *immune response* **-globul-** *protein* **-in** *chemical compound*	Specific protein evoked by an antigen. All antibodies are immunoglobulins
lymph	LIMF		Latin *clear spring water*	A clear fluid collected from tissues and transported by lymph vessels to the venous circulation
lymphatic	lim-**FAT**-ik	S/ R/	**-atic** *pertaining to* **lymph-** *lymph*	Pertaining to lymph or the lymphatic system
node	NOHD		Latin *a knot*	A circumscribed mass of tissue
pathogen	**PATH**-oh-jen	S/ R/CF	**-gen** *to produce* **path/o-** *disease*	A disease-causing microorganism
pollutant	poh-**LOO**-tant	S/ R/	**-ant** *pertaining to* **pollut-** *unclean*	Substance that makes an environment unclean or impure

2. The **thoracic duct** on the left, the largest lymphatic vessel, receives lymph from both sides of the body below the diaphragm and from the left arm, left side of the head, and left thorax. It begins in the abdomen at the level of the second lumbar vertebra (L2) and passes up through the diaphragm and mediastinum to empty into the **left subclavian vein** (*see Figure 15.1*).

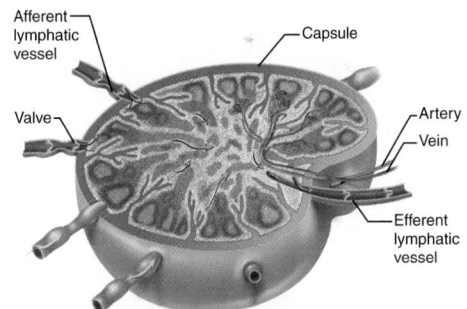

▲ **FIGURE 15.3** **Lymph Node.**

EXERCISES

Precision in usage is important if you want to communicate correct information. These seven terms all contain a common root/combining form. Insert the correct term in each sentence.

immune   **immunity**   **immunization**   **immunology**

immunologist   **immunoglobulin**

1. One who specializes in _____ (the study of the science of immunity and allergy) is termed

    an _____ (type of specialist).

2. An _____ is a class of protein that functions as an antibody.

3. The _____ system is a group of specialized cells in different parts of the body that recognize foreign substances and neutralize them.

4. A prior _____ (vaccination) obtained before she went overseas boosted her _____ (status of being immune) to the disease.

LYMPHATIC TISSUES AND CELLS

Abbreviations	
CD	cluster of differentiation
Ig	immunoglobulin

Many organs have a sprinkling of lymphocytes in their connective tissues and mucous membranes, particularly in passages that open to the exterior—the respiratory, digestive, urinary, and reproductive tracts—where invaders have access to the body.

In some organs, lymphocytes and other cells form dense clusters called **lymphatic follicles.** These are constant features in lymph nodes, the tonsils, and the ileum.

Lymphatic Tissues

Lymphatic tissues are composed of a variety of cells that include:

1. **T lymphocytes (T cells).** The "T" stands for *thymus,* where they mature. T lymphocytes make up 75% to 85% of body lymphocytes. There are several types of T cells:

   a. **Cytotoxic or "killer" T cells** destroy target cells. Their cell membrane holds a **coreceptor** that can recognize a specific antigen. Coreceptors are named with the letters "CD" **(cluster of differentiation)** followed by a number, for these cells, CD8.

   b. **Helper T cells** contain the CD4 coreceptor and are called CD4 cells. They begin the defensive response against a specific antigen.

   c. **Memory T cells** arise from cytotoxic T lymphocytes that have previously destroyed a foreign cell. If they encounter the same antigen, they can now quickly kill it without initiation by a helper T cell.

   d. **Suppressor T cells** suppress activation of the immune system. Failure of these cells to function properly may result in autoimmune diseases.

2. **B lymphocytes (B cells).** These cells mature in the bone marrow. B lymphocytes make up 15% to 25% of lymphocytes. They are activated by helper T cells, respond to a specific antigen, and cause the production of antibodies called **immunoglobulins (Ig).** The mature B cells are called **plasma cells** and secrete large quantities of antibodies that immobilize, neutralize, and prepare the specific antigen for destruction.

3. **Null cells.** These are large granular lymphocytes that are natural killer cells but lack the specific surface markers of the T and B lymphocytes

4. **Macrophages.** These cells develop from monocytes that have migrated from blood. They ingest and destroy tissue debris, bacteria, and other foreign matter **(phagocytosis).**

LYMPHATIC ORGANS

Spleen

The **spleen,** a highly vascular and spongy organ, is the largest lymphatic organ. It is located in the left upper quadrant of the abdomen below the diaphragm and lateral to the kidney *(Figure 15.4).*

The spleen contains two basic types of tissue:

1. **White pulp**—a part of the immune system that produces T cells, B cells, and macrophages. The blood passing through the spleen is monitored for antigens. Antibodies are produced, and the foreign matter is removed.

2. **Red pulp**—acts as a reservoir for erythrocytes, platelets, and macrophages that remove old and defective erythrocytes.

Thus, the functions of the spleen are to:

- **Phagocytize bacteria** and other foreign materials.
- **Initiate an immune response** when antigens are found in the blood.
- **Phagocytize old, defective erythrocytes** and platelets (hemolysis).
- **Serve as a reservoir** for erythrocytes and platelets.

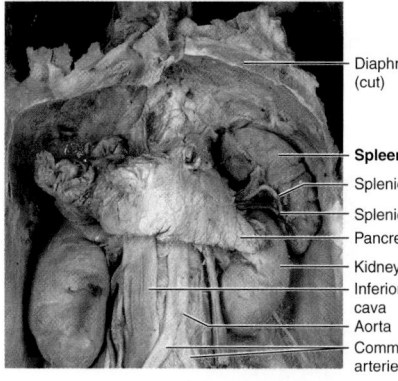

Diaphragm (cut)

Spleen
Splenic artery
Splenic vein
Pancreas
Kidney
Inferior vena cava
Aorta
Common iliac arteries

▲ **FIGURE 15.4   Position of Spleen.**

WORD	PRONUNCIATION	ELEMENTS		DEFINITION
adenoid	**ADD**-eh-noyd	S/ R/	-oid *resemble* aden- *gland*	Single mass of lymphoid tissue in the midline at the back of the throat
coreceptor	koh-ree-**SEP**-tor	S/ P/ R/	-or *a doer* co- *with, together* -recept- *receive*	Cell surface protein to enhance the sensitivity of an antigen receptor
follicle	**FOLL**-ih-kull		Latin *a small sac*	Spherical mass of cells containing a cavity or a small cul-de-sac, such as a hair follicle
macrophage	**MAK**-roh-fayj	P/ R/CF	macro- *large* -phag/e *to eat*	Large white blood cell that removes bacteria, foreign particles, and dead cells
null cells	NULL SELLS		**null** Latin *none*	Lymphocytes with no surface markers, unlike T cells or B cells
phagocyte	**FAG**-oh-site	S/ R/CF	-cyte *cell* phag/o- *to eat*	Blood cell that ingests and destroys foreign particles and cells
phagocytize (verb) phagocytosis phagocytic (adj)	**FAG**-oh-site-ize **FAG**-oh-sigh-**TOE**-sis fag-oh-**SIT**-ik	S/ S/ S/	-ize *action* -osis *condition* -ic *pertaining to*	Ingest foreign particles and cells Process of ingestion and destruction Pertaining to phagocytes or phagocytosis
plasma cell	**PLAZ**-mah SELL		**plasma** Greek *something formed*	Cell derived from B lymphocytes and active in formation of antibodies
spleen	SPLEEN		Greek *spleen*	Vascular, lymphatic organ in the left upper quadrant of the abdomen
splenectomy splenomegaly (**Note:** The "ee" in **spleen** becomes "e" for easier pronunciation.)	sple-**NECK**-toe-me sple-noh-**MEG**-ah-lee	S/ R/CF S/	-ectomy *surgical excision* splen/o- *spleen* -megaly *enlargement*	Surgical removal of the spleen Enlarged spleen
tonsil tonsillectomy tonsillitis	**TON**-sill ton-sih-**LEC**-toh-me ton-sih-**LIE**-tis	S/ R/ S/	Latin *tonsil* -ectomy *surgical excision* tonsill- *tonsil* -itis *inflammation*	Mass of lymphoid tissue on either side of the throat at the back of the tongue Surgical removal of the tonsils Inflammation of the tonsils

Tonsils

The **tonsils** *(see Chapter 9)* are two masses of lymphatic tissue located at the entrance to the oropharynx, where they entrap inhaled and ingested pathogens. **Adenoids** are similar tissue on the posterior wall of the nasopharynx *(see Chapter 9)*. The tonsils and adenoids form lymphocytes and antibodies, trap bacteria and viruses, and drain them into the tonsillar lymph nodes for elimination. They can become infected themselves.

Thymus Gland

The thymus gland has both endocrine *(see Chapter 14)* and lymphatic functions. T cells develop and mature in it and are released into the bloodstream. The thymus is largest in infancy and childhood and reaches its maximum size at puberty. It then regresses and is eventually replaced by fibrous and adipose tissue *(Figure 15.5)*.

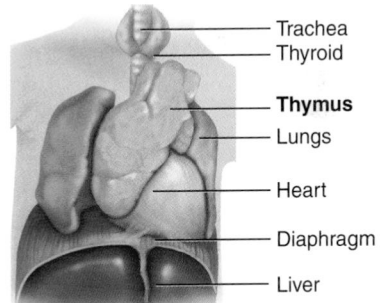

▲ **FIGURE 15.5   Large Thymus in an Infant.**

EXERCISES

Elements. Knowledge of elements is your best key to understanding medical terminology. Reinforce that knowledge with this exercise. Circle the best choice.

1. In the term **adenoid,** one element means:

   tissue   organ   gland

2. The prefix in **macrophage** identifies:

   color   location   size

3. The suffix in **phagocyte** means:

   cyst   cell   mass

4. The prefix *co-* means:

   next to   with   under

5. The root *-phage* means:

   flow   eat   produce

6. This suffix means *enlargement*:

   oid   megaly   ectomy

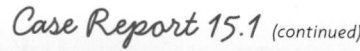

Case Report 15.1 (continued)

Ms. Clemons has cancerous nodes in her neck. They were not caused by metastatic cancer but by a cancer of the lymph nodes called Hodgkin lymphoma (below).

DISORDERS OF THE LYMPHATIC SYSTEM

Physicians routinely palpate accessible lymph nodes in the neck (**cervical nodes**), axilla (**axillary nodes**), and groin (**inguinal nodes**) for enlargement and tenderness. Their presence indicates disease in the tissues drained by the lymph nodes. Cancerous lymph nodes are enlarged, firm, and usually painless.

Infections in the lymph nodes cause them to be swollen and tender to the touch, a condition called **lymphadenitis.** All lymph node enlargements are collectively called **lymphadenopathy.** When lymph nodes are removed, it is called **lymphadenectomy.**

Lymphoma is a malignant neoplasm of the lymphatic organs, usually the lymph nodes. The disorder usually presents as an enlarged, nontender lymph node, often in the neck or axilla.

Lymphomas are grouped into two categories:

1. **Hodgkin lymphoma**—characterized by the presence of abnormal, cancerous B cells called **Reed-Sternberg cells.** These are large cells with two nuclei resembling the eyes of an owl *(Figure 15.6)*. The cancer spreads in an orderly manner to adjoining lymph nodes. This enables the disease to be staged, depending on how far it has spread. Diagnostic procedures include biopsy of an enlarged node to look for Reed-Sternberg cells, x-rays, computed tomography (CT) and magnetic resonance imaging (MRI) scans, **lymphangiogram,** and bone marrow biopsy. Treatment options include radiation, chemotherapy, and an autologous bone marrow transplant.

2. **Non-Hodgkin lymphomas**—occur much more frequently than Hodgkin lymphoma. They include some 30 different disease entities in 10 different subtypes. Treatment depends on the rate of growth of the disease and varies from careful observation through chemotherapy and radiation to bone marrow transplantation.

Tonsillitis, inflammation of the tonsils and adenoids, occurs mostly in the first years of life. The infection can be viral or bacterial (usually streptococcal). It produces enlarged, tender lymph nodes under the jaw. A rapid strep test can determine if *Streptococcus* is the cause, in which case a full course of antibiotics is indicated. The infection can be recurrent, and tonsillectomy is sometimes performed.

Splenomegaly, an enlarged spleen, is not a disease in itself but the result of an underlying disorder. However, when the spleen enlarges, it traps and removes an excessive number of blood cells and platelets (**hypersplenism**) and reduces the number of blood cells and platelets in the bloodstream.

The potential causes of splenomegaly are numerous and include infections such as infectious mononucleosis; lymphomas; anemias such as sickle cell anemia; and storage diseases such as Gaucher disease.

Diagnosis and treatment focus on the underlying cause. Occasionally splenectomy is necessary.

Ruptured spleen is a common complication from car accidents or other trauma when the abdomen and rib cage are damaged. Intra-abdominal bleeding from the ruptured spleen can be extensive, with a dramatic fall in blood pressure, and is a surgical emergency requiring splenectomy.

After splenectomy, patients are very susceptible to infection, but function very well without the organ.

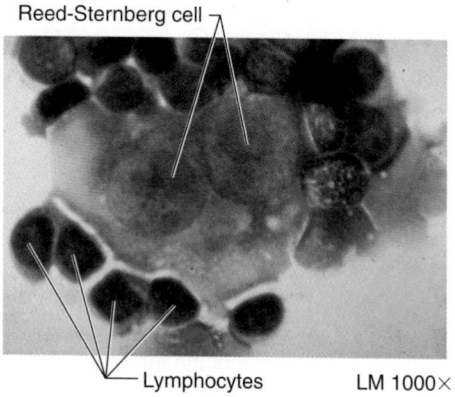

Reed-Sternberg cell

Lymphocytes   LM 1000×

▲ **FIGURE 15.6   Reed-Sternberg Cell.**

WORD	PRONUNCIATION	ELEMENTS		DEFINITION
Hodgkin lymphoma	**HOJ**-kin lim-**FO**-muh		Thomas Hodgkin, 1798–1866, British physician	Disease marked by chronic enlargement of lymph nodes spreading to other nodes in an orderly way
hypersplenism (Note the one "e.")	high-per-**SPLEN**-izm	S/ P/ R/	**-ism** *condition, process* **hyper-** *excessive* **-splen-** *spleen*	Condition in which the spleen removes blood components at an excessive rate
inguinal	**IN**-gwin-al	S/ R/	**-al** *pertaining to* **inguin-** *groin*	Pertaining to the groin
lymphadenectomy	lim-**FAD**-eh-**NECK**-toe-me	S/ R/	**-ectomy** *surgical excision* **lymphaden-** *lymph node*	Surgical excision of a lymph node
lymphadenitis **lymphadenopathy**	lim-**FAD**-eh-neye-tis lim-**FAD**-eh-**NOP**-ah-thee	S/ S/ R/CF	**-itis** *inflammation* **-pathy** *disease* **lymphaden/o** *lymph node*	Inflammation of a lymph node Any disease process affecting a lymph node
lymphangiogram	lim-**FAN**-jee-oh-gram	S/ R/CF	**-gram** *recording* **lymphangi/o-** *lymphatic vessels*	Radiographic images of lymph vessels and nodes following injection of contrast material
lymphedema	**LIMF**-e-dee-mah	R/ R/	**lymph-** *lymph* **-edema** *edema*	Tissue swelling due to lymphatic obstruction
lymphoma	lim-**FO**-muh	S/ R/	**-oma** *tumor* **lymph-** *lymph*	Any neoplasm of lymphatic tissue

Lymphedema is localized, nonpitting fluid retention caused by a compromised lymphatic system, often after surgery or radiation therapy. It can also be primary, where the cause is unknown.

EXERCISES

Language of Immunology: *Work with these six terms from the* **language of immunology.** *Their roots/combining forms are similar, and their suffixes help define them. First deconstruct each of the terms in the table. Then use those terms to answer the following questions.*

Medical Term	Meaning of Prefix	Meaning of Root/ CF	Meaning of Suffix	Meaning of Medical Term
lymphoma				
lymphadenectomy				
lymphadenopathy				
lymphangiogram				
lymphedema				
lymphadenitis				

Using the terms from this table, answer the following questions.

1. List the terms that can be billed as a diagnosis: _____

2. Write the term that is a *surgical* procedure: _____

3. Write the term that is a *radiological* procedure: _____

4. List the terms that concern lymph nodes: _____

5. Find the term that concerns lymphatic vessels. (**Hint:** Check the elements.) _____

OBJECTIVES

The study of the immune system is called **immunology.** The medical specialist involved in the study and research of the immune system and in treating disorders of the immune system is called an **immunologist.** The information in this lesson will enable you to use correct medical terminology to:

15.2.1 **Define the immune system and its specificity.**

15.2.2 **Contrast cellular and humoral immunity.**

15.2.3 **Describe the life histories of B cells and T cells.**

15.2.4 **Explain the structure and actions of antibodies.**

15.2.5 **Discuss some common disorders of the immune system, including HIV and AIDS.**

You are

. . . a laboratory technician working the night shift at Fulwood Medical Center.

Your patient is

. . . Mr. Michael Cowan, a 40-year-old homeless man and drug addict, who has presented to the Emergency Department with a high fever for which no cause is obvious on clinical examination.

CASE REPORT 15.2

You are called to the Emergency Room to take blood from Mr. Cowan. You have inserted the needle into an antecubital vein, and he starts jerking his arm around and trying to get off the gurney. In the struggle, the needle comes out of the vein and pricks your hand through your glove.

As you immediately *flush* and *clean* the wound, *report* the incident, seek *immediate medical attention*, and go through your *initial medical evaluation*, it is essential that you have knowledge about your immune system and its response to the potential infection. Then you can make *informed decisions* about your treatment and future employment.

You will be asked to fill out your incident report at the end of this chapter.

THE IMMUNE SYSTEM

The immune system is a group of specialized cells in different parts of the body that recognize foreign substances and neutralize them. It is the third line of defense listed at the beginning of this chapter. When the immune system is functioning correctly, it protects the body against bacteria, viruses, cancer cells, and foreign substances. When the immune system is weak, it allows pathogens (including the viruses that cause common colds and "flu") and cancer cells to successfully invade the body.

Three characteristics distinguish immunity from the first two lines of defense:

1. **Specificity.** The immune response is directed against a particular pathogen. Immunity to one pathogen does not confer immunity to others. Specificity has one disadvantage. If a virus or a bacterium changes a component of its genetic code, it will lead to a change in the structure and/or physiology of the microorganism, which then is no longer recognized by the immune system. This **mutation** occurs, for example, with bacteria in response to antibiotics and in HIV's response to anti-HIV drugs (development of **resistance**).

2. **Memory.** When exposure to the same identical pathogen occurs again, the immune system recognizes the pathogen and has its responses ready to act quickly.

3. **Discrimination.** The immune system learns to recognize agents **(antigens)** that represent **"self"** and agents that are **"nonself"** (foreign). Most of this recognition is developed prior to birth. A variety of disorders occur when this discrimination breaks down. They are known as **autoimmune** disorders.

Keynote

The immune system is not an organ system but a group of specialized cells.

Receptors on the surface of T cells and B cells recognize specific nonself antigens.

WORD	PRONUNCIATION	ELEMENTS		DEFINITION
antigen	**AN**-tee-gen	P/ R/	**anti-** *against* **-gen** *produce, create*	Substance capable of triggering an immune response
autoimmune	aw-toe-im-**YUNE**	P/ R/	**auto-** *self, same* **-immune** *immune response*	Immune reaction directed against a person's own tissue
discrimination	**DIS**-krim-ih-**NAY**-shun	S/ P/ R/	**-ation** *process* **dis-** *away from, apart* **-crimin-** *distinguish*	Ability to distinguish between different things
hapten	**HAP**-ten		Greek *to fasten or bind*	Small molecule that has to bind to a larger molecule to form an antigen
mutation	myu-**TAY**-shun		Latin *to change*	Change in the chemistry of a gene
resistance	ree-**ZIS**-tants	S/ R/	**-ance** *state of, condition* **resist-** *to withstand*	Ability of an organism to withstand the effects of an antagonistic agent
resistant	ree-**ZIS**-tant	S/	**-ant** *pertaining to*	Able to resist
specific	speh-**SIF**-ik	S/ R/	**-ic** *pertaining to* **specif-** *species*	Relating to a particular entity
specificity	spes-ih-**FIS**-ih-tee	S/	**-ity** *condition, state*	State of having a fixed relation to a particular entity

An **antigen** is any molecule that triggers an immune response. Some antigens are free molecules, such as toxins. Others are components of a cell membrane or a bacterial cell wall. Most antigens are large, complex molecules with a unique structure. It is this uniqueness that enables your body to distinguish its own (self) molecules from foreign (nonself) molecules.

Some small foreign molecules, called **haptens,** are too small to generate their own antigenic response; they attach themselves to host molecules, forming large, unique complexes that the body recognizes as foreign.

Keynote

Haptens are found in cosmetics, detergents, dust particles, industrial chemicals, poison ivy, and animal dander.

EXERCISES

Build your knowledge of elements and their meaning by matching the element in the left column with the definition in the right column. One answer will be used twice.

_____ 1. crimin

_____ 2. ity

_____ 3. specif

_____ 4. ant

_____ 5. dis

_____ 6. ation

_____ 7. ic

_____ 8. ance

A. species

B. away from

C. distinguish

D. process

E. pertaining to

F. condition, state

G. state of

After reading Case Report 15.2 on the opposite page, answer the following questions. Be prepared to discuss your answers in class.

9. Where is the location of the *antecubital vein?* _____

10. What is the immediate danger after the needle has pricked you through your glove? _____

11. How do you "flush" a wound? _____

12. Why must this incident be reported? _____

IMMUNITY

Immunity is classified biologically into two types, though both mechanisms often respond to the same antigen:

1. **Cellular (cell-mediated) immunity** is a direct form of defense based on the actions of lymphocytes to attack foreign and diseased cells and destroy them. The many different types of T cells, B cells, and macrophages described in the previous lesson of this chapter are involved in this style of attack.

2. **Humoral (antibody-mediated) immunity** is an indirect form of attack that employs antibodies produced by plasma cells, which have been developed from B cells. The antibodies bind to an antigen and thus tag them for destruction.

These antibodies are called **immunoglobulins (Igs)**, defensive gamma globulins in the blood plasma and body secretions. There are five classes of antibodies:

- **IgG** makes up about 80% of the antibodies. It is found in plasma and tissue fluids. It crosses the placenta to give the fetus some immunity.

- **IgA** makes up about 13% of the antibodies. It is found in exocrine secretions such as breast milk, tears, saliva, nasal secretions, intestinal juices, bile, and urine.

- **IgM** makes up about 6% of antibodies. It develops in response to antigens in food or bacteria.

- **IgD** is found on the surface of B cells and acts as a receptor for antigens.

- **IgE** is found in exocrine secretions along with IgA, and also in the serum.

Once released by plasma cells, the antibodies function in several ways to make antigens harmless, including:

- **Neutralization.** An antibody binds to the antigen and masks it.

- **Agglutination.** An antibody binds to two or more bacteria to prevent them from spreading through the tissues.

- **Precipitation.** Antibodies create an antigen-antibody complex that is too heavy to stay in solution. The complex precipitates (drops out of solution) and can be ingested and destroyed by phagocytes.

- **Complement fixation.** The complement system is a group of 20 or more proteins continually present in blood plasma; IgG and IgM bind to foreign cells, initiating the **binding of complement** to the cell and leading to its destruction. Complement fixation is the major defense mechanism against bacteria and mismatched blood cells.

Based on the production or acquisition of antibodies, four classes of immunity can be described:

1. **Natural active immunity**—the production of your own antibodies as a result of normal maturation, pregnancy, or an infection.

2. **Artificial active immunity**—the production of your own antibodies as a result of **vaccination** or **immunization**. A vaccine consists of either killed or **attenuated** (weakened) pathogens (antigens).

3. **Natural passive immunity**—a temporary immunity that results from acquiring antibodies from another individual. This occurs for the fetus through the placenta (IgG) or for the infant through breast milk (IgA).

4. **Artificial passive immunity**—a temporary immunity that results from the injection of an **immune serum** from another individual or an animal. Immune serum is used to treat snakebite, tetanus, and rabies.

Keynote

The immune system is thought to be able to produce some 2 million different antibodies.

Antibodies do not actively destroy an antigen. They render it harmless and mark it for destruction by phagocytes.

Abbreviations

IgA	immunoglobulin A
IgD	immunoglobulin D
IgE	immunoglobulin E
IgG	immunoglobulin G
IgM	immunoglobulin M

Keynote

Antibodies can be produced naturally in response to an antigen or artificially in response to immunizations and vaccines.

S = Suffix   P = Prefix   R = Root   R/CF = Combining Form

WORD	PRONUNCIATION	ELEMENTS		DEFINITION
agglutination	ah-glue-tih-**NAY**-shun	S/ R/	-ation *process* **agglutin-** *sticking together, clumping*	Process by which cells or other particles adhere to each other to form clumps
agglutinate (verb)	ah-**GLUE**-tin-ate	S/	-ate *composed of, pertaining to*	Stick together to form clumps
attenuate	ah-**TEN**-you-ate	S/	-ate *composed of, pertaining to*	Weaken the ability of an organism to produce disease
attenuated (adj)	ah-**TEN**-you-a-ted	R/ S/	**attenu-** *to weaken* -ated *process*	Weakened
complement	**KOM**-pleh-ment		Latin *that which completes*	Group of proteins in serum that finish off the work of antibodies to destroy bacteria and other cells
humoral immunity	**HYU**-mor-al im-**YOU**-nih-tee	S/ R/ S/ R/	-al *pertaining to* **humor-** *fluid* -ity *condition* **immun-** *immune response*	Defense mechanism arising from antibodies in the blood
immune serum (also called **antiserum**)	im-**YUNE SEER**-um		**immune** Latin *protected from* **serum** Latin *whey*	Serum taken from another human or animal that has antibodies to a disease
vaccine vaccinate (verb)	**VAK**-seen **VAK**-sin-ate	S/	Latin *relating to a cow* -ate *composed of, pertaining to*	Preparation to generate active immunity To administer a vaccine
vaccination	vak-sih-**NAY**-shun	R/ S/	**vaccin-** *giving a vaccine* -ation *process*	Administration of a vaccine

EXERCISES

*Organize the important information about immunity. The **language of immunology** will help you understand the questions and provide the answers. Refer to this exercise for test review. Fill in the blanks.*

1. Name the two types of immunity, and explain how they function.

   a. _____

   b. _____

2. Which of the types of immunity in question 1 is a direct defense, and which is an indirect form of attack?

   Direct: _____

   Indirect: _____

3. What type of cells produce antibodies? _____

4. Are antibodies produced in direct or indirect defense? _____

5. What is the correct term for these particular antibodies? _____

6. What are the main functions of antibodies?

   a. _____

   b. _____

   c. _____

   d. _____

7. In a previous chapter the process of *agglutination* was described in relation to different cells. Define that process, and compare it to this process of agglutination. (**Hint:** What is it that is clumping together?) _____

_____

DISORDERS OF THE IMMUNE SYSTEM

Hypersensitivity is an excessive immune response to an antigen that would normally be tolerated. Hypersensitivity includes:

- **Allergies,** reactions to environmental antigens such as pollens, molds, and dusts; to foods such as peanuts, shellfish, and eggs; to plants like poison ivy; and to drugs such as penicillin; as well as asthmatic reactions to inhaled antigens (see below).
- Abnormal reactions to your *own* tissues (autoimmune disorders).
- Reactions to tissues **transplanted** from *another* person (**alloimmune disorders).**

In most allergic (hypersensitivity) reactions, allergens (antigens) bind to IgE on the membranes of basophils and mast cells *(see Chapter 7)* and, within seconds of exposure, stimulate the cells to produce **histamine.** This triggers vasodilation, increased capillary permeability, and smooth muscle spasms. The symptoms produced by these changes include edema, mucus hypersecretion and congestion, watery eyes, hives **(urticaria),** and sometimes cramps, diarrhea, and vomiting.

Anaphylaxis is an acute, immediate, and severe allergic reaction. It can be relieved by antihistamines.

Anaphylactic shock is more severe and is characterized by dyspnea due to bronchiole constriction, circulatory shock, and sometimes death. It is a life-threatening medical emergency and requires immediate epinephrine and circulatory support.

Asthma is triggered by allergens (as listed above) and by air pollutants, drugs, and emotions. These all stimulate plasma cells to secrete IgE, which binds to cells in the respiratory mucosa and releases a mixture of histamine and interleukins. Within minutes, the bronchioles constrict spasmodically (bronchospasm), leading to the wheezing and coughing of asthma.

Autoimmune disorders are an overvigorous response of the immune system in which the immune system fails to distinguish self-antigens from foreign antigens. These self-antigens produce autoantibodies that attack the body's own tissues. This type of response occurs, for example, in lupus erythematosus, type 1 diabetes, multiple sclerosis, rheumatoid arthritis, and psoriasis.

Immunodeficiency disorders are a deficient response of the immune system in which it fails to respond vigorously enough. They are in three categories:

1. **Congenital** (inborn)—caused by a genetic abnormality that is often sex-linked *(see Chapter 21),* with boys affected more often than girls. An example from among the 20 or more congenital immunodeficiency diseases is **inherited combined immunodeficiency disease,** in which there is an absence of both T cells and B cells. Affected children are very susceptible to opportunistic infections and must live in protective sterile enclosures *(Figure 15.7).*
2. **Immunosuppression**—is a common side effect of corticosteroids in treatment to prevent transplant rejection and in chemotherapy treatment for cancer. These drugs reduce the numbers of all lymphocytes, making it possible for opportunistic infections to invade the body.
3. **Acquired immunodeficiency**—results from diseases such as **acquired immunodeficiency syndrome (AIDS)** that involve a severely depressed immune system from infection with the **human immunodeficiency virus (HIV).**

Immunology of Transplantation

The success of any organ transplantation is based on control of the recipient's immune system to prevent rejection of the **allograft,** tissue from another individual of the same species.

Transplant immunity is designed to cause rejection, and both cellular and humoral defense mechanisms are involved. To try to prevent this, recipient and donor must match at both the HLA and ABO *(see Chapter 7)* types. A combination of immunosuppressive drugs is used to control graft rejection, but the drugs have adverse side effects on the recipient. One combination is corticosteroids with cyclosporine or FK506. Other drugs are in clinical trials.

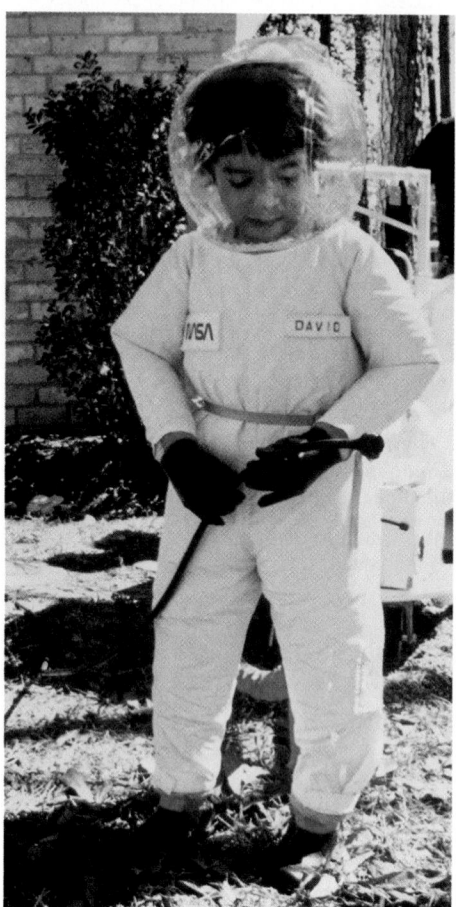

▲ **FIGURE 15.7   Boy with Combined Immunodeficiency Disease in Protective Sterile Enclosure.**

Abbreviations

AIDS	acquired immunodeficiency syndrome
CMV	cytomegalovirus
HIV	human immunodeficiency virus

Keynote

Because of the use of immunosuppressive drugs, 75% of all solid-organ transplants will be newly affected with cytomegalovirus (CMV) following organ transplantation.

WORD ANALYSIS AND DEFINITION

WORD	PRONUNCIATION		ELEMENTS	DEFINITION
allogen	**AL**-oh-jen	S/	-gen *producing*	Antigen from someone else in the same species
allogenic (adj)	al-oh-**JEN**-ik	P/	allo- *strange, different*	
allograft	**AL**-oh-graft	S/	-graft *tissue for transplant*	Skin graft from another person or cadaver
alloimmune	**AL**-oh-im-**YUNE**	P/	allo- *strange, different*	Reaction directed against foreign tissue
		R/	-immune *immune response*	
anaphylaxis	**AN**-ah-fih-**LAK**-sis	P/	ana- *away from*	Immediate severe allergic response
		R/	-phylaxis *protection*	
anaphylactic (adj)	**AN**-ah-fih-**LAK**-tik	S/	-tic *pertaining to*	Pertaining to anaphylaxis
		R/	-phylac- *protect*	
histamine	**HISS**-tah-mean	R/	hist- *derived from histidine*	Compound liberated in tissues as a result of injury or an allergic response
		R/CF	–amin/e *nitrogen compound*	
antihistamine	an-tee-**HISS**-tah-mean	P/	anti- *against*	Drug used to treat allergic symptoms because of its action antagonistic to histamine
hypersensitivity	**HIGH**-per-sen-sih-**TIV**-ih-tee	S/	-ity *condition*	Exaggerated abnormal reaction to an allergen
		P/	hyper- *excessive*	
		R/	-sensitiv- *feeling*	
immunodeficiency	**IM**-you-noh-dee-**FISH**-en-see	S/	-ency *quality*	Failure of the immune system
		R/CF	immun/o- *immune response*	
		R/	-defici- *failure*	
immunosuppression	**IM**-you-noh-suh-**PRESH**-un	S/	-ion *process*	Suppression of the immune response by an outside agent, such as a drug
		R/CF	immun/o- *immune response*	
		R/	-suppress- *pressed under*	
transplant	**TRANZ**-plant	P/	trans- *across*	The tissue or organ used, or the act of transferring tissue from one person to another
		R/	-plant *plant*	
transplantation	**TRANZ**-plan-**TAY**-shun	S/	-ation *process, action*	The moving of tissue or an organ from one person or place to another
urticaria	ur-tee-**KARE**-ee-ah		Latin *nettle*	Rash of itchy wheals (hives)

EXERCISES

Build more medical vocabulary for immunology. Complete the construction of the medical term by using the following elements to fill in the blanks.

hyper	defici	phylaxis	auto	suppress	graft
ion	anti	sensitiv	trans	allo	gen

1. Exaggerated, abnormal reaction to an antigen _____/_____/ity

2. Immune reaction directed against self _____/immuno

3. Immediate, severe, allergic response ana/_____

4. Skin from another person or cadaver allo/_____

5. Failure of the immune system immuno/_____/ency

6. Transferring tissue or organ from one person to another _____/plant

7. Antigen from someone else in the same species allo/_____

8. Reaction against foreign tissue _____/immune

9. Drug used to treat allergic symptoms _____/histamine

10. Suppression of the immune response *caused by an outside agent* immuno/_____/_____

You are

... a medical assistant working with Henry Vandenberg, MD, in the AIDS Clinic at Fulwood Medical Center.

Your patient is

... Mr. Eugene Holman, a 40-year-old male who is known to be **HIV-positive (HIV+)** and has been receiving treatment with efavirenz, zidovudine, and lamivudine.

CASE REPORT 15.3

However, in the past couple of months, he has not been taking his medication regularly. In the previous week, he has noticed a progressive shortness of breath and a nonproductive cough. VS are T 102°, P 120, R 32, BP 110/60. He is anxious and dyspneic but not cyanotic. His breath sounds are clear, with no rales or rhonchi heard. You have called Dr. Vandenberg to see him.

Mr. Holman's chest x-ray showed bilateral, diffuse, fluffy infiltrates spreading out from the hila. Bronchial **lavage** with laboratory examination showed *Pneumocystis jiroveci*. His CD4 count was 140. Mr. Holman had developed an opportunistic infection, which is now thought to be a fungus.

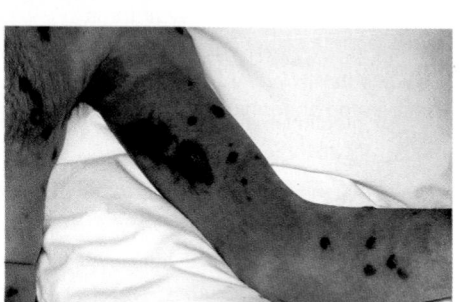

▲ **FIGURE 15.8 Lesions of Kaposi Sarcoma.**

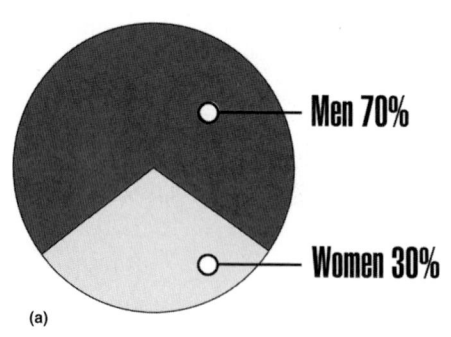

— **Men 70%**

— **Women 30%**

(a)

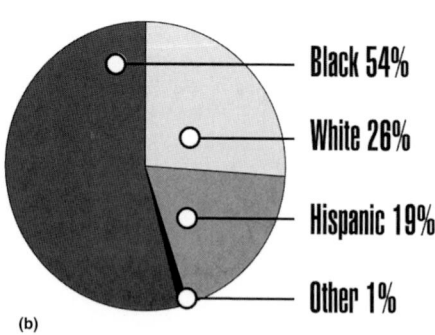

— **Black 54%**

— **White 26%**

— **Hispanic 19%**

— **Other 1%**

(b)

▲ **FIGURE 15.9 New HIV Infections Each Year in the United States.**
(a) By gender. (b) By race.

HIV AND AIDS

Human immunodeficiency **virus** is one of a group of viruses known as **retroviruses.** Like other viruses, it can replicate only inside a living host cell *(see Chapter 20)*; HIV invades helper T (CD4) cells and cells in the upper respiratory tract and CNS. Inside the cell, the virus generates new DNA and can stay **dormant** in the cell for months or years. When it is activated, the new viruses emerge from the dying host cell and attack more CD4 cells. This dormant phase (**incubation**) can range from a few months to 12 years.

The CD4 cells are the central coordinators for the immune response. As the virus destroys more and more cells, the CD4 count falls, and antibodies cannot be produced. Symptoms appear, including chills, fever, night sweats, fatigue, weight loss, and lymphadenitis.

When CD4 cells are very low, **opportunistic infections** by bacteria, viruses, and fungi can occur. These infections include toxoplasmosis, pneumocystis, tuberculosis, herpes simplex, cytomegalovirus, and candidiasis. If HIV invades the brain, it causes dementia. Cancers can also invade, and a form of malignancy called **Kaposi sarcoma** *(Figure 15.8)* is often seen in association with AIDS.

Human immunodeficiency virus is found in blood, semen, vaginal secretions, saliva, tears, and breast milk of infected mothers.

The most common means of transmission of HIV are:

- **Sexual intercourse** (vaginal, oral, anal).
- **Sharing needles** for drug use.
- **Contaminated blood products.** (All donated blood is now tested for HIV.)
- **Transplacental** (from an infected mother to her fetus).

The virus survives poorly outside the human body. It is destroyed by laundering, dishwashing, chlorination, disinfectants, alcohol, and germicidal skin cleansers.

About 1% of HIV's genes mutate every year. This makes the development of natural immunity and the production of a vaccine difficult, so new infections continue to occur *(Figure 15.9)*.

HIV Testing

HIV antibody blood test takes between 3 weeks and 3 months after infection to become positive.

CD4-cell count. The normal CD4 count is from 600 to 1200 cells/μL of blood; AIDS patients have counts below 200/μL. Below this figure, opportunistic infections occur, as they did with Mr. Holman.

Viral load count measures the quantity of HIV in the blood. If there are 50 to 200 copies of the virus present, the test will be reported as "undetectable." A 5000 count is very low. The count can rise to several hundred thousand.

There are more than 20 approved anti-HIV (antiretroviral) drugs available and many more in research and development.

WORD ANALYSIS AND DEFINITION

S = Suffix   P = Prefix   R = Root   R/CF = Combining Form

WORD	PRONUNCIATION	ELEMENTS		DEFINITION
dormant	DOR-mant	S/ R/	-ant *forming* dorm- *sleep*	Inactive
incubation	in-kyu-BAY-shun	S/ R/	-ation *process* incub- *sit on, hatch*	Process to develop an infection
Kaposi sarcoma	ka-POH-see sar-KOH-mah		Moritz Kaposi, 1837–1902, Hungarian dermatologist	A malignancy often seen in AIDS patients
lavage	lah-VAHZH		Latin *to wash*	Washing out of a hollow cavity, tube, or organ
opportunistic	OP-or-tyu-NIS-tik	S/ S/ R/	-ic *pertaining to* -ist- *agent* opportun- *take advantage of*	An organism or a disease in a host with lowered resistance
retrovirus	REH-troh-vie-rus	P/ R/	retro- *backward* -virus *poison*	Virus that replicates in a host cell by converting its RNA core into DNA
virus viral (adj)	VIE-rus VIE-ral	 S/ R/	Latin *poison* -al *pertaining to* vir- *virus*	Group of infectious agents that require living cells for growth and reproduction

EXERCISES

After reading Case Report 15.3 on the opposite page, answer the following questions. Be prepared to discuss your answers in class.

1. Explain this sentence to Mr. Holman: "Mr. Holman's CXR showed bilateral, diffuse, fluffy infiltrates spreading out from the hila."

   "Mr. Holman, your _____

   _____."

2. What was the purpose of the *bronchial lavage?* _____

   _____

3. What was found on laboratory examination of the *bronchial washings?* _____

   _____

4. What type of *opportunistic infection* do the doctors think Mr. Holman has? _____

5. The diagnosis of *Pneumocystis jiroveci* places this infection in Mr. Holman's (specific organ) _____ .

6. Which vital sign could indicate that Mr. Holman has an infection going on in his system? _____

7. What does an *opportunistic infection* take advantage of? _____

8. What is the underlying cause of this infection occurrence? _____

A. **Incident Report:** Use the appropriate information from this report to fill in the blanks in the incident report below. You are granted creative license (use your imagination) to fill in the rest of the report in your own words.

Your patient is

. . . Mr. Michael Cowan, a 40-year-old homeless man and drug addict, who has presented to the Emergency Department with a high fever for which no cause is obvious on clinical examination.

You are called to the Emergency Room to take blood from Mr. Cowan. You have inserted the needle into an antecubital vein, and he starts jerking his arm around and trying to get off the gurney. In the struggle, the needle comes out of the vein and pricks your hand through your glove.

(As you immediately *flush and clean* the wound, *report the incident,* seek immediate *medical attention,* and go through your *initial medical evaluation,* it is essential that you have knowledge about your immune system and its response to the potential infection. Then you can make *informed decisions* about your treatment and future employment.)

Fulwood Medical Center
3333 Medical Parkway, Fulwood, MI 01234
555-247-6100

Department of Employee Health: Incident Report

Staff member's name: *Jane/John Doe* _____ Department: _____

Date of occurrence: _____ Date Report filed: _____

Location of incident: _____

Describe the incident in your own words: _____

_____

_____

_____

What is the specific nature of the injury? _____

Was any immediate action taken in the department at the time of the incident?

Yes_____ No_____

If "yes," please describe what action was taken: _____

_____

_____

_____

Were you engaged in patient care at the time of the incident? Yes_____ No_____

If so, give name of patient: _____

Were gloves worn by the employee? Yes_____ No_____

Was the glove penetrated? Yes_____ No_____

Were there any witnesses to the incident? Yes_____ No_____

If yes, please provide their names and departments:

_____

_____

Did you seek immediate medical attention? Yes_____ No_____

If so, where? _____

Name of physician who treated you: _____

Was this incident reported to your immediate supervisor? Yes_____ No_____

Date reported to supervisor: _____

Name of supervisor: _____

Signature of employee: _____ Date: _____

Received by Employee Health Department:

Signature _____ Date _____

B. **Correct spelling of medical terms is *always important*.** Listed below are two examples of medical terms for which the variation is not always spelled the same as the original term. Fill in the blanks with the correctly spelled medical terms.

Example 1:

Lymphatic organ in LUQ of abdomen   _____

Excision/removal of this organ   _____

Enlargement of this organ due to an underlying disorder   _____

Excessive number of RBCs and platelets in this organ   _____

What is the difference you notice in the spelling of these four terms?

_____

_____

Example 2:

Lymphoid tissue on either side of the throat   _____

Inflammation of this tissue   _____

Removal of this tissue   _____

What is the difference you notice in the spelling of these three terms?

_____

_____

C. **Immune System:** Build your knowledge of the immune system and its components by correctly matching the definition in the left column with the medical term in the right column. Fill in the blanks.

_____   1. Molecule that triggers an immune response   A. mutation

_____   2. Major defense mechanism against bacteria   B. agglutination

_____   3. Preparation for active development of antibodies C. hapten

_____   4. Weakened ability to produce disease   D. hypersensitivity

_____   5. Change in the chemistry of a gene   E. immunoglobulins

_____   6. Often appears after surgery or radiation therapy F. antigen

_____   7. Excessive immune response to an antigen   G. lymphedema

_____   8. Small molecule has to bind to a larger molecule   H. attenuate

_____   9. Cells clumping together   I. vaccine

_____ 10. Antibodies produced by humoral immunity   J. complement fixation

LYMPHATIC AND IMMUNE SYSTEMS

D. Terminology Challenge: In a previous chapter, you used the term **prophylaxis.** Define the difference between **prophylaxis** and **anaphylaxis,** which you have learned in this chapter. Then use each term in a sentence of your choice.

prophylaxis

Definition: _____

_____

_____

Sentence: _____

_____

_____

anaphylaxis

Definition: _____

_____

_____

Sentence: _____

_____

_____

E. Elements: With the exception of Greek and Latin terms that do not deconstruct, most medical terms from any body system can typically be reduced into their basic elements for analysis. Deconstruct the following medical terms into their basic elements to analyze the meanings for the *language of immunology.* The first one is done for you. Fill in the table. When you have finished filling in the table, use any two terms in a sentence of your choice.

Medical Term	Prefix	Root/CF	Suffix	Meaning of Elements
coreceptor	*co*	*recept*	*or*	*with, receive, a doer (someone/something that does)*
phagocytosis				
dormant				
hypersplenism				
tonsillitis				
anaphylaxis				
retrovirus				

Define any two terms based on their elements:

1. _____ –

_____

2. _____

_____

F. **Dictionary/Glossary Exercise:** Look up the word **reservoir**. Define it, and then give a brief explanation as to how the spleen functions as a reservoir.

Definition of **reservoir:** _____ –

Spleen as a reservoir:

_____

_____

G. **Analyze:** Medical language has many terms that appear similar but have unique meanings all their own. If you can analyze similar terms, you will understand the difference and be able to explain it to your patient. Fill in the blanks.

1. **alloimmune**

Prefix: _____   Means: _____

Root: _____   Means: _____

autoimmune

Prefix: _____   Means: _____

Root: _____   Means: _____

Explain to your patient the difference between *alloimmune* and *autoimmune*.

_____

_____

2. **immunodeficiency**

Root: _____   Means: _____

CF: _____   Means: _____

Suffix: _____   Means: _____

immunosuppression

Root: _____   Means: _____

CF: _____   Means: _____

Suffix: _____   Means: _____

Explain to your patient the difference between *immunodeficiency* and *immunosuppresion*.

_____

_____

H. Discussion: You may choose from either topic for your discussion/presentation.

1. There are four classes of immunity described in this chapter: natural active, artificial active, natural passive, and artificial passive. Pick any two of these classes, and compare and contrast them. How do you acquire these immunities? Give examples. Prepare a 5-minute class presentation on your topic. *You should be able to define any medical terms you use in your presentation.* Hand in your notes and outline of your presentation to the instructor.

2. Your body has three lines of defense mechanisms against foreign organisms that may harm you. Answer these questions: Which types of organisms seek to harm you, and what are the three lines of defense your body puts up? Give examples of each type of defense mechanism, and explain how they act against foreign organisms. Prepare a 5-minute class presentation on your topic. *You should be able to define any medical terms you use in your presentation.* Hand in your notes and outline of your presentation to the instructor.

I. Language of Immunology: Challenge your knowledge of the immune system and employ the *language of immunology* to answer the following questions. Circle the correct choice.

1. Choose the correct pair of spellings:

   a. tonsel   tonselectomy

   b. tonsil   tonsillectomy

   c. tonssil   tonsilectomy

   d. tonsill   tonsilectomy

   e. tonnsil   tonsillectomy

2. This triggers vasodilation in an allergic response:

   a. interferon

   b. complement fixation

   c. histamine

   d. hormones

   e. antihistamine

3. The largest lymphatic vessel is the:

   a. thoracic duct

   b. lymph node

   c. spleen

   d. lymphatic duct

   e. aorta

4. Kaposi sarcoma is a form of:

   a. lymphadenitis

   b. malignancy

   c. lymphadenopathy

   d. lung cancer

   e. lymphoma

5. Ingestion and destruction of tissue debris and bacteria is called:

    a. lymphadenitis

    b. phagocytosis

    c. lymphadenopathy

    d. agglutination

    e. osmosis

6. Life-threatening medical emergency that cannot be relieved by antihistamines:

    a. asthma

    b. anaphylaxis

    c. Kaposi sarcoma

    d. anaphylactic shock

    e. urticaria

7. An allergic reaction is one of:

    a. hypoglycemia

    b. hypersensitivity

    c. hypotension

    d. hyperglycemia

    e. hypertension

8. White pulp and red pulp can be found in the:

    a. lymph nodes

    b. spleen

    c. lymph vessels

    d. none of these

    e. all of these

9. *Elevated body temperature* is another name for:

    a. pathogen

    b. pyrexia

    c. precipitation

    d. protease

    e. phagocytosis

LYMPHATIC AND IMMUNE SYSTEMS

J. Language of Immunology: Challenge your knowledge of the immune system and employ the *language of immunology* to answer the following questions. Circle the correct choice.

1. Which disease is likely to cause enlarged lymph nodes under the jaw?

    a. tonsillitis

    b. lymphoma

    c. hypersplenism

    d. asthma

    e. urticaria

2. Abnormal, cancerous B cells are known as:

    a. macrophages

    b. osteoblasts

    c. Reed-Sternberg cells

    d. killer cells

    e. phagocytes

3. Lymph nodes accessible for palpation are in the:

    a. neck

    b. axilla

    c. groin

    d. all of these

    e. only a and c

4. Lymphatic capillaries and vessels do not penetrate:

    a. the liver

    b. the CNS

    c. the thoracic duct

    d. the left subclavian vein

    e. the tonsils

5. Immunosuppressive drugs are given after:

    a. organ transplant

    b. anaphylactic shock

    c. retrovirus

    d. opportunistic infection

    e. viral load count

6. Serum used to treat a snakebite is an example of:

    a. natural active immunity

    b. artificial active immunity

    c. natural passive immunity

    d. artificial passive immunity

    e. none of the above

K. **Recall and Review:** How well do you remember these word elements from the previous chapter? Try to answer without first looking back to check. Fill in the blanks.

Element	Type of Element (P, R, CF, S)	Meaning of Element
melan	_____	_____
ren	_____	_____
vas/o	_____	_____
megaly	_____	_____
pro	_____	_____

L. **Prefixes:** All of the following terms are lacking their prefix. After you have entered the prefix *on* the line, write the meaning of the prefix *under* the line. Fill in the blanks.

    1. Reaction directed against foreign tissue   _____/immune

    2. Substance produced in response to an antigen   _____/body

    3. Surface protein that enhances sensitivity of antigen receptor   _____/recept/or

    4. Spleen removes blood components at an excessive rate   _____splen/ism

    5. Virus that converts its RNA core to DNA in a host cell   _____/virus

M. **Translation:** First, use your knowledge of medical terminology to understand the statement. Then organize your thoughts and formulate your answer in layman's terms that a patient could understand. Write an explanation of each sentence on the lines below.

    1. Pyrexia is a defense mechanism because it inhibits reproduction of bacteria and viruses and accelerates tissue repair.

         _____

         _____

    2. Intra-abdominal hemorrhage from the ruptured spleen can be extensive, with dramatic hypotension, and is a surgical emergency requiring splenectomy.

         _____

         _____

LYMPHATIC AND IMMUNE SYSTEMS

N. Suffixes: Use your knowledge of word elements from this and previous chapters. Take a basic root/combining form, add a variety of suffixes, and change the meaning different ways to form six new terms. Fill in the chart, and then fill in the blanks.

Root/CF	Suffix	Meaning of Term
lymphaden		Neoplasm of lymphatic tissue
lymphaden		Inflammation of a lymph node
lympho		Small white blood cell with large nucleus
lymphaden		Removal of a lymph node
lymph		Pertaining to lymph
lymphadeno		Any disease process affecting a lymph node

1. Which of the above terms would be found in a surgeon's dictation? _____

2. Which of the above terms would a pathologist use? _____

3. Which term would an oncologist use in dictation? _____

4. Which of the above terms is a diagnosis? (There is more than one term.) _____

_____

O. Patient Documentation: Apply your knowledge of medical language to the following Case Report about Mr. Holman.

- Read the complete report.

Your patient is

... Mr. Eugene Holman, a 40-year-old male who is known to be HIV-positive and has been receiving treatment with efavirenz, zidovudine, and lamivudine. However, in the past couple of months, he has not been taking his medication regularly. In the previous week, he has noticed a progressive shortness of breath and a nonproductive cough. VS are T 102°F, P 120, R 32, BP 110/60. He is anxious and dyspneic but not cyanotic. His breath sounds are clear, with no rales or rhonchi heard. You have called Dr. Vandenberg to see him.

Mr. Holman's chest x-ray showed bilateral, diffuse, fluffy infiltrates spreading out from the hila. Bronchial lavage with laboratory examination showed *Pneumocystis jirovec*. His CD4 count was 140. Mr. Holman had developed an opportunistic infection, which is now thought to be a fungus.

- Read it a second time, underlining the medical terminology that will help you answer the questions.

1. What is the meaning of the abbreviation HIV? _____

_____

2. For what reason might Mr. Holman not be taking his medication? _____

_____

3. What symptoms did Mr. Holman note in the previous week? _____

_____

4. How could the physician tell the patient was not cyanotic? _____

_____

5. What does **dyspneic** mean? _____

_____

6. If a cough is *nonproductive,* what does that mean? _____

_____

7. Describe rales: _____

_____

8. Describe rhonchi: _____

_____

9. How does the physician assess for rales and rhonchi? _____

_____

10. Mr. Holman's infiltrate was bilateral—what does that mean? _____

_____

11. What procedure did Mr. Holman undergo? _____

_____

12. Why does this patient have an opportunistic infection? _____

_____

13. There are two other abbreviations that could have been inserted in this Case Report but were not. Rewrite the sentences that could contain additional abbreviations. _____

_____

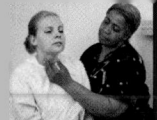

LYMPHATIC AND IMMUNE SYSTEMS

P. **Immunology Terminology:** Increase your knowledge of the *language of immunology.* The element's meaning is given to you in the left column. List the element and identify the type of element in the appropriate columns. In the right column, give an example of a medical term containing the element. Complete the exercise by defining any five terms you have written in the right column.

Meaning of Element	Element	Type of Element (P, R, CF, S)	Medical Term Containing This Element
strange, other			
tissue			
across			
backward			
sleep			
fluid			
against			
large			
with			
condition			
disease			
lymphatic vessels			

1. _____ Definition: _____

2. _____ Definition: _____

3. _____ Definition: _____

4. _____ Definition: _____

5. _____ Definition: _____

Q. Patient Education: Explain to your patients, in words they can understand, the difference among:

edema: _____

_____

_____

peripheral edema: _____

_____

_____

pitting edema: _____

_____

_____

lymphedema: _____

_____

_____

R. Latin and Greek elements cannot be further deconstructed into prefix, root, or suffix. You must know them for what they are. Test your knowledge of these elements with this exercise. Match the meaning in the left column with the correct medical term in the right column.

_____ 1. Protected from   A. medial

_____ 2. That which completes   B. hapten

_____ 3. None   C. lymph

_____ 4. To fasten or bind   D. lavage

_____ 5. Divide in the middle   E. mutate

_____ 6. A knot   F. complement

_____ 7. To change   G. edema

_____ 8. To wash   H. immune

_____ 9. Swelling   I. null

_____ 10. Clear fluid   J. node

Complete the exercise by using any three medical terms (answers A–J) in sentences of patient documentation.

1. _____

_____

2. _____

_____

3. _____

_____

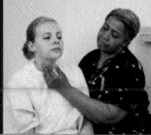

CHAPTER 15 REVIEW

LYMPHATIC AND IMMUNE SYSTEMS

CHAPTER SUMMARY EXERCISE

1. *Listen to the pronunciation of the medical terms as given by your instructor.*
2. *Circle the correct spelling of the medical term.*
3. *Match the correctly spelled terms to the brief descriptions below.*
4. *Write a sentence for each of the 10 terms that appear in this exercise.*

A. SPELLING COMPREHENSION: CIRCLE THE CORRECT SPELLING OF THE TERM.

1. pagocyossis	phaggocytosis	pagocytosis	phagocytosis	phagocytossis
2. pirexia	pyrexxia	pyirexia	phirexia	pyrexia
3. attenuated	atenuated	atinuated	attinuated	ateenuated
4. addenoid	adinoid	adenoid	adennoid	adinoyd
5. lypedema	lymphedema	lynphedema	lympedema	lyfedemia
6. imunization	immunisation	imunnization	immunization	imunisation
7. anapylaxis	annaphylasix	anaphylaxis	anaphylasis	anaphylasix
8. vacination	vacation	vacinnation	vaccination	vackination
9. imunoglobulin	immunogobulin	imunogobulin	immunoglobulin	imunnogobulin
10. interstitial	intersisteal	insterstial	interstissial	interstittial

B. MATCH THE NUMBER OF THE CORRECT TERM IN PART A WITH THE BRIEF DESCRIPTION OF THE TERM BELOW.

a. Act of administering a vaccine _____

b. Tissue swelling due to lymphatic obstruction _____

c. Obtaining immunity by administration of a killed agent _____

d. Fever _____

e. Fluid that surrounds cells _____

f. To ingest foreign bacteria _____

g. Lymphatic tissue in the nasopharynx _____

h. Weakens ability of organism to produce disease _____

i. Immediate, severe allergic response _____

j. Protein of an antibody _____

C. USING YOUR KNOWLEDGE OF TERMS 1–10 IN PART A AND THEIR CORRECT SPELLING, WRITE A BRIEF SENTENCE AS IT MIGHT APPEAR IN PATIENT DOCUMENTATION.

1. _____

2. _____

3. _____

4. _____

5. _____

6. _____

7. _____

8. _____

9. _____

10. _____

D. YOUR INSTRUCTOR WILL DIRECT YOU TO MCGRAW-HILL CONNECT. OPEN THE AUDIO GLOSSARY AND PRACTICE YOUR PRONUNCIATION OF THE TERMS IN PART A OF THIS EXERCISE.

E. AFTER READING CASE REPORT 15.1, ANSWER THE FOLLOWING QUESTIONS. BE PREPARED TO DISCUSS YOUR ANSWERS IN CLASS.

CASE REPORT 15.1

You are

. . . a medical assistant working with Susan Lee, MD, in her primary care clinic.

Your patient is

. . . Ms. Anna Clemons, a 20-year-old waitress, who is a new patient. She has noticed a lump in her right neck. On questioning, you elicit that she has lost about 8 pounds in weight in the past couple of months, has felt tired, and has had some night sweats. Her vital signs are normal. There are two firm, enlarged lymph nodes in her right neck. Physical examination is otherwise unremarkable.

Ms. Clemons has cancerous nodes in her neck. They were not caused by metastatic cancer but by a cancer of the lymph nodes called Hodgkin lymphoma.

1. What outward sign does the patient have? _____

2. What is the patient's chief complaint? _____

_____

3. Did the patient present with a temperature? _____

4. What is the medical term for *enlarged lymph nodes?* _____

5. What findings were present on physical examination? _____

6. The cancerous nodes were not caused by *metastatic cancer*. What does this mean? _____

_____

7. What are some of the diagnostic tests used to confirm this disease? _____

_____

8. What is the surgical procedure to remove malignant lymph nodes? _____

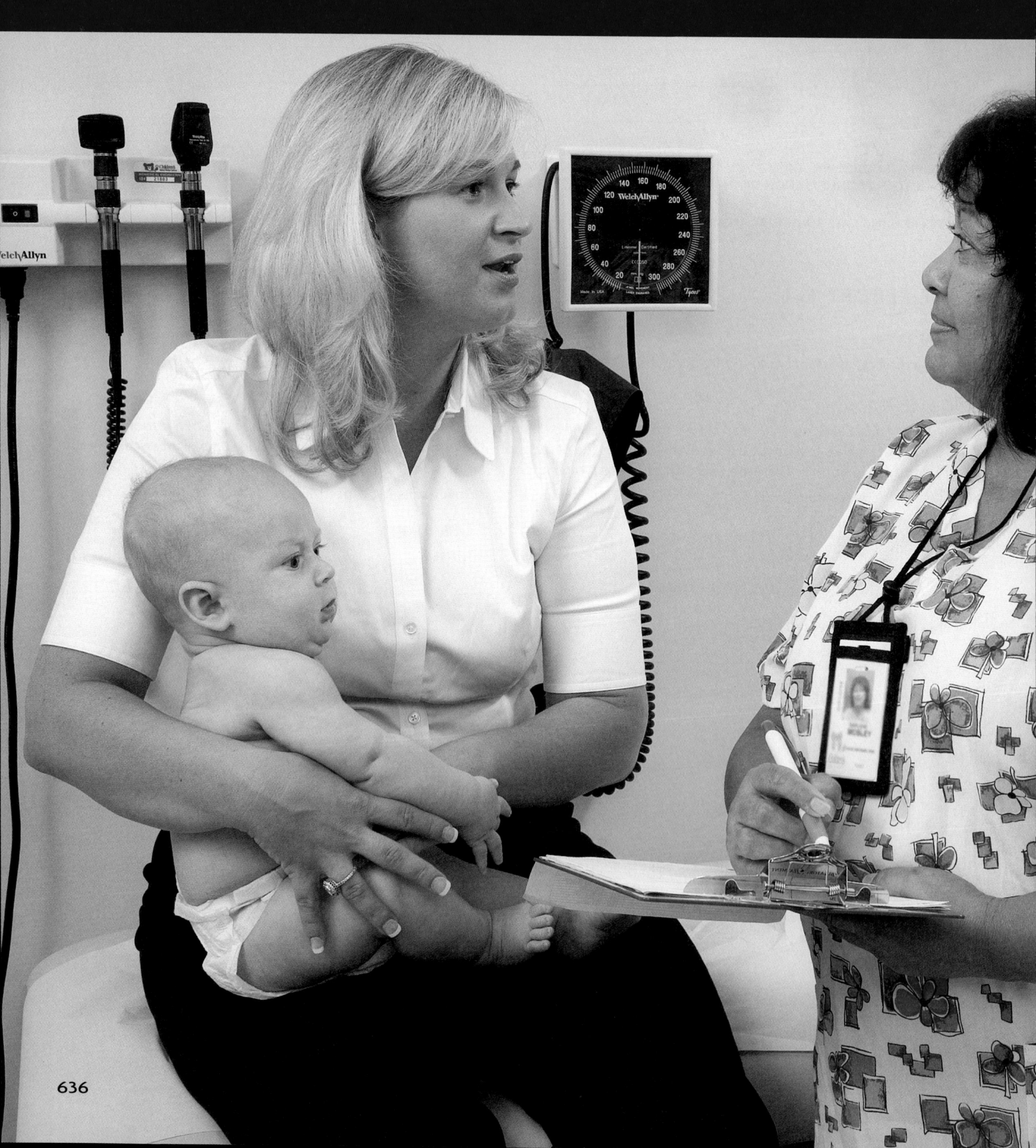

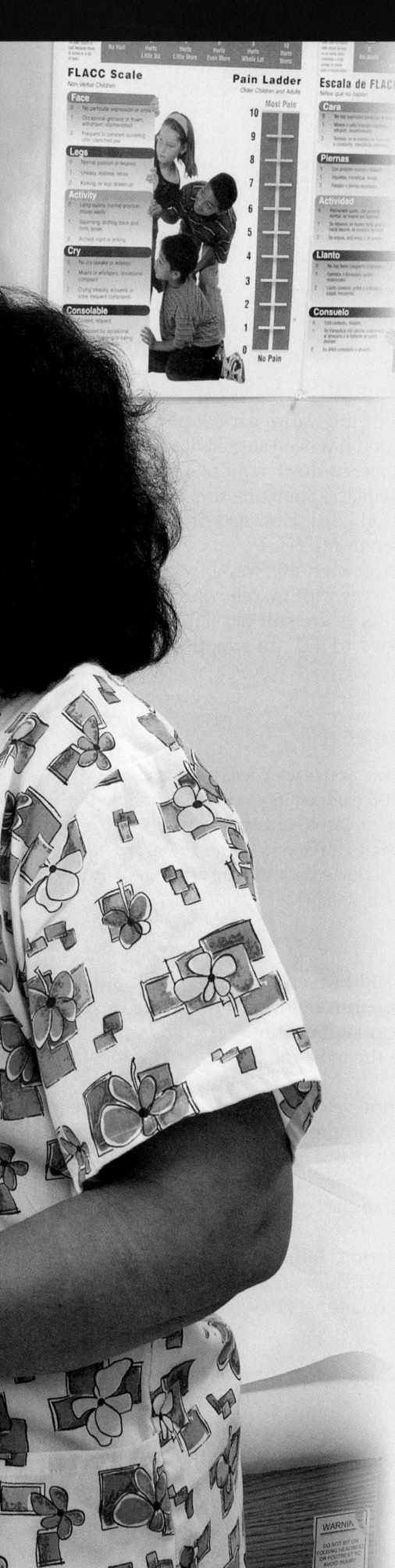

CASE REPORT 16.1

You are

. . . a pediatric medical assistant working with Sandra Mendes, MD, a **pediatrician** at Fulwood Medical Center. You are working in her well-baby clinic.

Your patients are

. . . 8-week-old Carol Hotteling and her mother, Mrs. Anna Hotteling, a 35-year-old executive in a book publishing company. Mrs. Hotteling's first baby was born normally at term and weighed 7 pounds 2 ounces. She had normal Apgar scores. Carol had persistent jaundice when seen at 2 weeks of age. She is being breastfed. Using holidays and sick leave, her mother has managed to obtain 3 months' leave of absence from work.

You ask Mrs. Hotteling if she has any concerns.

Learning Outcomes

To understand the growth and development of children, adults, and the elderly and communicate about this with your employer, other health professionals, and patients, you need to be able to:

16.1 Apply the languages of **pediatrics** and **gerontology** to the anatomy, physiology, and psychology of human growth and development.

16.2 Comprehend, analyze, spell, and write the medical terms of pediatrics and gerontology so that you communicate and document accurately and precisely in any health care setting.

16.3 Recognize and pronounce the medical terms of pediatrics and gerontology so that you communicate verbally with accuracy and precision in any health care setting.

16.4 Explain the effects of disorders in growth and development on health.

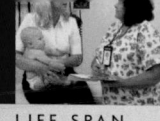

LESSON 16.1 Neonatal Period

OBJECTIVES

To be able to understand where **neonates** are in their development and to talk to mothers and other health professionals about this, you need to be able to use correct medical terminology as you:

16.1.1 **Describe the anatomical and physiological adaptations that occur at birth.**

16.1.2 **Discuss the normal neonatal development of anatomical, physiological, and psychological functions.**

16.1.3 **Explain congenital anomalies that interfere with normal anatomical and physiological development.**

16.1.4 **Recognize common causes of disorders in growth and development in the neonatal period.**

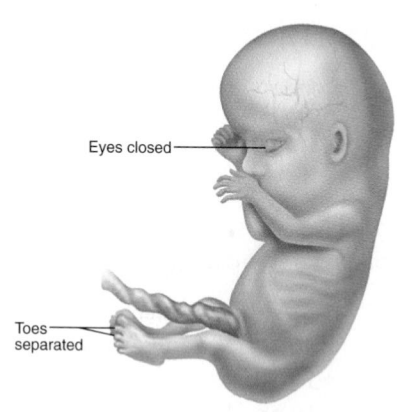

Eyes closed

Toes separated

▲ **FIGURE 16.1 Fetus at 8 Weeks (56 Days).**

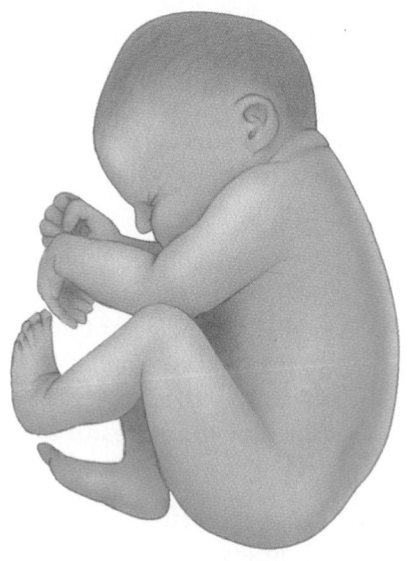

▲ **FIGURE 16.2 Full-Term Infant (38 Weeks).**

Abbreviation

SIDS sudden infant death syndrome

NEONATAL ADAPTATIONS

"It's incredibly disturbing to be pushed out of the warm, dark, liquid environment in which I've lived for 9 months. All my food has been supplied, and I've had nobody else to interact with. Suddenly, I'm squeezed down a narrow passage that hurts my head, out into a brightly lit, dry, noisy place. Someone says 'breathe' and cuts off my source of nourishment, my **umbilical cord.** How *do* I breathe? Where *do* I find the right food? What's going to happen to me next?"

"I'm not even fully developed. I've got to change the way blood circulates through me so that I can get this stuff called oxygen to my cells on my own. My liver and kidneys aren't fully functional, my bones are still developing, and my nervous system isn't mature. What am I expected to *do?* Am I supposed to know **innately** what it's all about?"

Case Report 16.1 (continued)

Mrs. Anna Hotteling, the mother, has several areas of concern. A friend's baby recently died of **SIDS (sudden infant death syndrome).** How can she prevent this for her child? Carol wants to feed every 2 to 3 hours day and night, and she (Anna) is exhausted. How long will this go on, and for how long should she continue breastfeeding? Mrs. Hotteling also wants to know what her baby can see and how she should communicate with her.

Fetal life is a preparation for birth. At the end of the first 8 weeks of fetal life, all the organ systems are in place *(Figure 16.1)*. From then until birth, the organs grow and acquire the functional capabilities to support life outside the mother. Sometimes a part of this process will fail, and the fetus can have a developmental abnormality.

At birth, normal organ development is not yet complete, but the neonate suddenly has to **adapt** to a totally different environment *(Figure 16.2)*. Each of the organ systems has to adapt to the new environment and then go on to complete its development during childhood. This developmental process is why children are not just "little adults," and why there is a specialty of **pediatrics** practiced by **pediatricians.**

The first 4 weeks after birth, the **neonatal period,** is the time for the most rapid adaptations of the organ systems. In this lesson, you will review normal adaptations in the neonatal period and see what effects failure of development and failure of adaptation can have on the neonate.

WORD ANALYSIS AND DEFINITION

WORD	PRONUNCIATION	ELEMENTS		DEFINITION
adaptation adapt (verb)	ad-ap-**TAY**-shun ad-**APT**	S/ R/	-ation *process* adapt- *to adjust*	Change in function or structure of an organ to meet new conditions
congenital	kon-**JEN**-ih-tal	S/ P/ R/	-al *pertaining to* con- *with, together* -genit- *birth*	Present at birth, either inherited or due to an event during gestation up to the moment of birth
geriatrics (**Note:** This term consists only of two roots.)	jer-ee-**AT**-riks	R/ R/	-iatrics *healing, field of medicine* ger- *old age*	Medical specialty that deals with the problems of old age
gerontology	jer-on-**TOL**-oh-jee	S/ R/CF	-logy *study of* geront/o- *old age*	Study of the process and problems of aging
gerontologist	jer-on-**TOL**-oh-jist	S/	-logist *one who studies, specialist*	Medical specialist in gerontology
innate innately (adj)	ih-**NATE**	P/ R/CF	in- *in* -nat/e *birth, born*	Present at birth; arising from the intellect
neonate	**NEE**-oh-nate	P/ R/CF	neo- *new* -nat/e *birth, born*	A newborn infant
neonatal (adj)	**NEE**-oh-**NAY**-tal	S/	-al *pertaining to*	Pertaining to the newborn infant or the newborn period
pediatrics	pee-dee-**AT**-riks	S/ R/ R/	-ics *knowledge* -iatr- *medical treatment* ped- *child*	Medical specialty of treating children during development from birth through adolescence
pediatrician	**PEE**-dee-ah-**TRISH**-an	S/	-ician *expert, specialist*	Medical specialist in pediatrics
umbilicus	um-**BIL**-ih kus		Latin *navel*	Pit in the abdomen where the umbilical cord entered the fetus
umbilical	um-**BIL**-ih-kal	S/ R/	-al *pertaining to* umbilic- *umbilicus, navel*	Pertaining to the umbilicus or the center of the abdomen

EXERCISES

Spelling: *Test your ability to recognize and correctly spell the following medical terms, which come from the **languages of pediatrics and gerontology**. The correct term is given to you in a word scramble in the left column—unscramble the term, and write it on the blank. A brief definition is given in the middle column to help you determine the correct term you need. Remember: The answer is not acceptable unless it is spelled correctly!*

1. otsoitlngrgeo   Medical specialist who treats aged population   _____

2. onteane   Newborn infant   _____

3. olgninaetc   Born with   _____

4. eirciatpdain   Medical specialist in treating children   _____

5. datintaapo   Change in organ function to meet new conditions   _____

6. itnaen   Present at birth   _____

7. iumlbcsui   Site where umbilical cord enters fetus   _____

8. ontgyrogleo   Study of the aging process   _____

9. dpata   To meet new conditions   _____

Employ the ***languages of pediatrics and gerontology*** in communication. Choose any two of the above terms and write a brief sentence for each term that is *not a definition.*

10. _____

11. _____

NEONATAL ADAPTATIONS (continued)

Immediately after birth, the neonate is evaluated for her **Apgar score** at 1 minute and 5 minutes of life. The Apgar score gives health care providers an immediate assessment of the baby's condition at birth. The five parameters of *Activity*, *Pulse*, *Grimace*, *Appearance*, and *Respiration* are scored on a three-point scale: 0 (poor), 1, or 2 (normal). Total scores obtainable are between 0 and 10 *(Table 16.1)*. A score of 7 or above is normal. Below 7, the baby needs special immediate care, including oxygen and further airway **suctioning**.

The Apgar score does not predict long-term health, intellectual status, or outcome.

Cardiovascular System Adaptations

The **cardiovascular system (CVS)** changes from being dependent on the **placenta** and **umbilical cord** to provide oxygen and nutrients and to remove carbon dioxide and fetal wastes to being independent. The fetal heart pumps blood to the placenta through two umbilical arteries. Blood flows back to the fetus by a single umbilical vein. At birth, the two major divisions, the pulmonary and systemic circuits, become separate and operational.

Congenital cardiovascular defects or **malformations** are present in about 1% of births. Before birth an open vessel **(ductus arteriosus)** connects the aorta and pulmonary artery. Normally this closes within a few hours of birth. When it doesn't close, a **patent ductus arteriosus (PDA)** allows blood that should flow through the aorta to nourish the body to return to the lungs *(see Chapter 8)*. Children with a PDA may grow slowly, tire easily, and catch pneumonia. A small patent ductus can close spontaneously. Medication with indomethacin can constrict the muscle in the wall. A plug can be inserted in the lumen of the PDA by using a **transcatheter**. The ductus can be closed by surgically tying it.

Septal defects occur when the baby is born with an opening in the septum (wall) that separates the right and left sides of the heart ("hole in the heart"). An opening between the two upper chambers is called an **atrial septal defect (ASD)**. An opening between the two lower chambers is called a **ventricular septal defect (VSD)** *(see Chapter 8)*. Small defects often close spontaneously during the first year of life. If not, the defects can be closed by open-heart surgery.

Cyanotic heart defects occur when insufficient blood is being pumped to the lungs, so the blood being pumped to the body contains less oxygen than the tissues need. Neonates with this defect are called "blue babies" because of their cyanotic blue skin *(Figure 16.3)*. An example is the **tetralogy of Fallot (TOF)**, in which four heart defects all shunt blood away from the lungs. Children with TOF do not grow normally, are dyspneic, and require open-heart surgery to correct the defects.

Abbreviations

ASD	atrial septal defect
CVS	cardiovascular system
PDA	patent ductus arteriosus
TOF	tetralogy of Fallot
VSD	ventricular septal defect

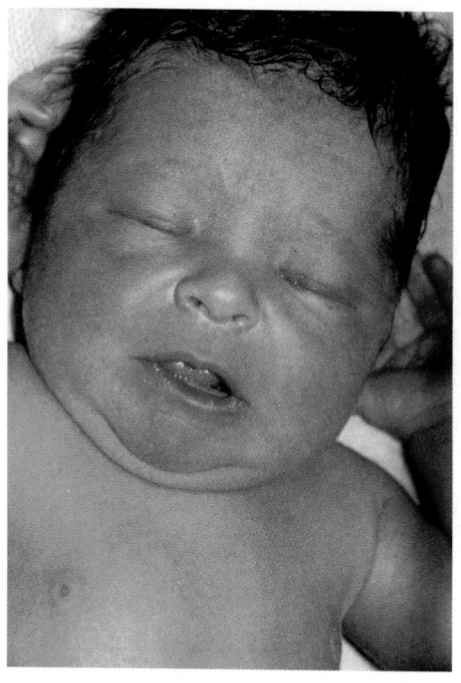

▲ **FIGURE 16.3 Cyanotic ("Blue") Baby.**

TABLE 16.1 Apgar Scoring

Apgar Sign		0	1	2
A	**Activity (muscle tone)**	Limp, no movement	Limbs flexed, little movement	Active spontaneous movement
P	**Pulse**	No pulse	Below 100 beats per minute	Above 100 beats per minute
G	**Grimace (responsiveness)**	No response to airway suction	Grimace only to airway suction	Pulls away from airway suction
A	**Appearance (skin color)**	Blue-gray all over	Pink, except hands and feet are bluish	Pink all over
R	**Respiration**	No breathing	Weak cry, gasping	Strong cry, normal breathing effort and rate

WORD	PRONUNCIATION	ELEMENTS		DEFINITION
Apgar score	**AP**-gar SKOR		Virginia Apgar, 1909–1974, U.S. anesthesiologist	Evaluation of newborn status
cyanosis	sigh-ah-**NO**-sis	S/ R/	-osis *condition* cyan- *dark blue*	Blue discoloration of the skin, lips, and nail beds due to low levels of oxygen in the blood
cyanotic (adj)	sigh-ah-**NOT**-ik	S/ R/CF	-tic *pertaining to* cyan/o- *dark blue*	Marked by cyanosis
defect defective (adj)	**DEE**-fect dee-**FEK**-tiv		Latin *to lack or fail*	An absence, malformation, or imperfection Imperfect
ductus arteriosus	**DUK**-tus ar-**TEER**-ih-**OH**-sus		Latin *duct that connects two arteries*	Fetal vessel that connects the descending aorta with the left pulmonary artery
Fallot	fah-**LOW**		Étienne-Louis A. Fallot, 1850–1911, French physician	First described this tetralogy of congenital heart defects
malformation	**MAL**-for-**MAY**-shun	S/ P/ R/	-ion *condition* mal- *bad* -format- *to form*	Failure of proper or normal development
patent	**PAY**-tent		Latin *lie open*	Open
placenta	plah-**SEN**-tah		Latin *a cake*	Organ that allows metabolic interchange between the mother and fetus
suction suctioning	**SUK**-shun		Latin *sucking*	Use of a catheter to clear the upper airway or other tubes
tetralogy	teh-**TRAL**-oh-jee	S/ P/	-logy *study of* tetra- *four*	A set of four congenital heart defects
transcatheter	trans-**KATH**-eh-ter	S/ P/ R/	-er *agent* trans- *across* -cathet- *catheter*	Catheter with a self-expanding mushroom device that is placed and left inside the PDA

EXERCISES

Patient Documentation: *Incorporate your knowledge of abbreviations from this lesson into the following patient documentation. Fill in the blanks, using the following choices. Use each answer only once.*

ASD	TOF	VSD	PDA

1. Diagnostic testing confirms _____, which is an opening between the two lower chambers of the infant's heart. Patient will be scheduled for open-heart surgery early next week.

2. Admitting diagnosis: "blue baby," cyanotic heart defect. _____

3. The septal defect in this infant has been confirmed as being between the two upper heart chambers. _____

4. Child has a history of failure to thrive and tires easily. Possible diagnosis is _____. I am referring him to a pediatric cardiologist.

*Use your knowledge of the **language of pediatrics** to match the statement in the left column with the correct terminology in the right column.*

_____ 5. Open-heart surgery

_____ 6. Vessel is open before birth

_____ 7. Through which fetal heart pumps blood to the placenta

_____ 8. Activity, pulse, grimace, appearance, respiration

_____ 9. "Hole in the heart"

_____ 10. Organ that allows metabolic interchange between mother and fetus

_____ 11. Blue discoloration of the skin, lips, or nail beds

_____ 12. An absence, malformation, or imperfection

A. placenta

B. umbilical arteries

C. cyanosis

D. septal defect

E. defect

F. Apgar parameters

G. ductus arteriosus

H. repairs septal defects

NEONATAL ADAPTATIONS (continued)

Brain and Neurologic Adaptations

A newborn baby's brain is a work in progress. It is one-quarter of its adult size. The brain's growth is monitored by charting increases in head circumference.

At birth, only the spinal cord and brainstem are well developed. The cortex is primitive. All of the newborn's kicking, grasping, **rooting** (searching for the nipple), and crying behaviors are functions of the brainstem, and this is why they are **involuntary** and not well coordinated.

The presence of a well-developed brainstem ensures that the **neural** circuits for the most vital bodily functions—breathing, heartbeat, sleeping, sucking, and swallowing—are in place at birth.

Three involuntary newborn reflexes that are tested are brainstem reflexes: the **Moro**, or **startle, reflex** (the baby splays out her arms and slowly closes them in response to sudden movement); the **doll's eye maneuver** (the baby's eyes stay focused forward when her head is turned to one side); and the **stepping reflex** (the baby "walks" when she is held up with her feet touching a surface). Also, babies show a **Babinski sign** or extensor response to the **plantar reflex** when stimulation of the sole of the foot extends the toes upward and fans them out instead of flexing them inward. As the cortex develops over the next 2 to 3 months, all these reflexes disappear.

Congenital neurologic abnormalities include:

- **Anencephaly**—absence of the cerebral hemispheres. This is incompatible with life.

- **Microcephaly**—small cerebral hemispheres, leading to motor and mental retardation.

- **Encephalocele**—a protrusion of nervous tissue and meninges through a defect in the skull.

- **Hydrocephalus**—enlargement of the ventricles with excessive **cerebrospinal fluid (CSF)**. This is the most common cause of a large head in the neonate *(see Chapter 10)*.

- **Spina bifida** is a failure of the vertebral column to close over the spinal cord in the lumbar and sacral regions. In **spina bifida occulta**, the vertebral arches fail to unite and there is no neurologic involvement *(see Chapter 5)*. When the vertebral defect is more open, nervous tissue can protrude through it in a sac. In **spina bifida cystica** *(Figure 16.6)*, the sac can contain meninges **(meningocele)**, part of the spinal cord **(myelocele)**, or both **(myelomeningocele)** *(see Chapter 5)*.

Neonatal seizures are a common and sometimes serious neonatal disorder. They can be:

- **Primary**—from an intracranial process such as meningitis or a cerebral hemorrhage from a difficult birth.

- **Secondary**—from a systemic or metabolic problem such as hypoxia, hypoglycemia, or hypocalcemia.

Treatment is directed to the underlying pathology. The seizure itself is treated with IV phenobarbital.

Thermoregulation and Adaptation

The infant has a larger ratio of surface area to body volume than an adult. Therefore, the infant loses heat more easily, particularly if the body surface is wet. This is why the newborn is dried, wrapped, and placed in a warmer after birth. Although growing infants accumulate subcutaneous fat to retain heat, their body temperature regulation remains more variable than that of an adult.

Hypothermia is more likely to occur in **premature** or **small-for-date (SFD)** neonates. Hypothermia is rare in the United States but is often seen in rural areas of developing countries, even in full-term babies, when informed neonatal care is lacking.

Keynote

Babies are born with more than 100 billion brain cells. In the first months and years of life, connections are made (wiring) to form complex circuits that shape their thinking, feelings, and behaviors.

Abbreviations

CSF	cerebrospinal fluid
SFD	small for date

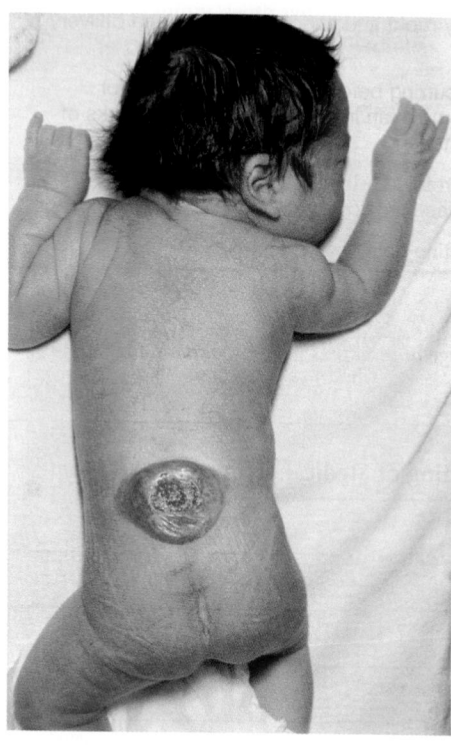

▲ **FIGURE 16.6 Child with Spina Bifida Cystica.**

WORD	PRONUNCIATION	ELEMENTS		DEFINITION
anencephaly	**AN**-en-**SEF**-ah-lee	P/ R/	**an-** *without, lack of* **-encephaly** *condition of the brain*	Born without cerebral hemispheres
Babinski sign	bah-**BIN**-skee SINE		Joseph Babinski, 1857–1932	Abnormal neurological response to plantar reflex that is normal in infants
bifid spina bifida	**BIH**-fid **SPY**-nah **BIH**-fih-dah		**bifid** Latin *split into two* **spina** Latin *backbone*	Separated into two parts Failure of one or more vertebral arches to close during fetal development
cystic cystica (adj)	**SIS**-tik		Greek *bladder*	Relating to a cyst
encephalocele	en-**SEF**-ah-loh-seal	S/ R/CF	**-cele** *hernia* **encephal/o-** *brain*	Congenital defect of the cranium with herniation of brain tissue
hydrocephalus	high-droh-**SEF**-ah-lus	P/ R/	**hydro-** *water* **-cephalus** *head*	Enlarged head due to excess CSF in the cerebral ventricles
hypothermia	high-poh-**THER**-me-ah	S/ P/ R/	**-ia** *condition* **hypo-** *below* **-therm-** *heat*	Very low core body temperature
involuntary	in-**VOL**-un-tah-ree	S/ P/ R/	**-ary** *pertaining to* **in-** *not* **-volunt-** *free will*	Not under control of the will
meningocele	meh-**NING**-oh-seal	S/ R/CF	**-cele** *hernia* **mening/o-** *meninges*	Protrusion of the meninges from the spinal cord or brain through a defect in the vertebral column or cranium
microcephaly microcephalic (adj)	**MY**-kroh-**SEF**-ah-lee	P/ R/	**micro-** *small* **-cephaly** *condition of the head*	An abnormally small head
Moro reflex (also called startle reflex)	**MOR**-oh **RE**-fleks		Ernst Moro, 1874–1951 **reflex** Latin *to bend back*	Neonatal brainstem reflex
myelocele	**MY**-eh-low-seal	S/ R/CF	**-cele** *hernia* **myel/o-** *spinal cord*	Protrusion of the spinal cord through a defect in the vertebral arch
myelomeningocele	**MY**-eh-low-meh-**NING**-oh-seal	R/CF	**-mening/o-** *meninges*	Protrusion of the spinal cord and meninges through a defect in the vertebral arch of one or more vertebrae
neural	**NYU**-ral	S/ R/	**-al** *pertaining to* **neur-** *nerve, nerve tissue*	Pertaining to nervous tissue
plantar reflex	**PLAN**-tar re-**FLEKS**		**plantar** Latin *sole of foot* **reflex** *to bend back*	Neurological response to stimulation of the sole of the foot
rooting	rue-**TING**		Latin *seek*	A neonatal reflex to turn toward the nipple and open the mouth when a nipple is placed on the cheek

EXERCISES

Build *the medical term by filling in the blanks with the correct element(s).*

1. Born without cerebral hemispheres   _____/encephaly

2. Pertaining to nervous tissue   _____/al

3. Very low core body temperature   hypo/ _____/ _____

4. Small head   _____/cephaly

5. Enlarged head due to excess CSF   hydro/ _____

6. Protrusion of the meninges   meningo/ _____

7. Congenital cranial defect with herniation of brain tissue   _____/cele

NEONATAL ADAPTATIONS (continued)

Growth Adaptations

Failure to grow fully in utero is caused by two main factors:

1. **Inadequate nutrition,** caused by poor placental function. The newborn can be delivered preterm, term, or postterm but is below the 10th percentile of babies of the same gestational age. This is called **small for gestational age (SGA).** Good nutrition after delivery will enable growth to accelerate to normal.

2. **Premature labor,** in which the infant is born before 37 weeks of gestation. The cause of premature labor is usually unknown. The premature infant weighs less than 5.5 pounds, has little subcutaneous fat or hair, and has a low level of spontaneous activity *(Figure 16.7)*. Surfactant deficiency leads to RDS. Inadequate cerebral perfusion can contribute to cerebral hemorrhage. Immature development of the CNS leads to poor sucking and swallowing. The infant may have to be fed by IV or by **gavage (stomach tube).**

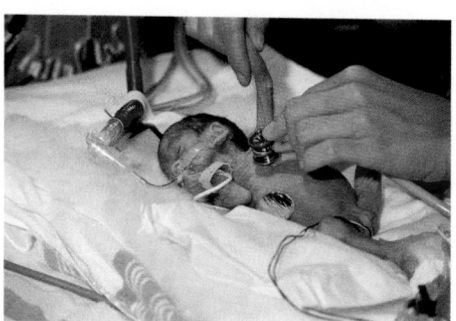

▲ **FIGURE 16.7 Premature Baby.**

Occasionally, labor does not start until after 42 weeks' of gestation and produces a **postmature infant** *(Figure 16.8)*. The problem is that past term the placenta **involutes,** and the fetus receives insufficient nutrition in the days after term. As a result, such infants have decreased subcutaneous fat and dry, peeling skin. They are prone to meconium aspiration and to neonatal hypoglycemia because their glycogen stores are depleted.

Normal full-term babies lose up to 10% of their birth weight during the first few days of life. By 1 month, they should be gaining ⅔ to 1 ounce per day. They will grow 1 to 1.5 inches per month. These changes will be plotted on **growth charts,** which indicate the size and growth patterns of individual children compared to those of other children in the United States. **Percentiles** are used. For example, a 2-year-old girl whose weight is plotted on the weight chart at the 25th percentile weighs the same or more than 25% of other 2-year-old girls. She also weighs less than 75% of other 2-year-old girls. The function of growth charts is to show how consistent the child's growth pattern is over time. You will be asked to work with growth charts at the end of this chapter.

Failure to thrive (FTT) is the term used for an infant or young child who is not growing and developing as expected. There are two main reasons for the failure:

1. **Organic disorders,** such as chronic illness (e.g., celiac disease) and genetic (e.g., Down syndrome), metabolic (e.g., **fetal alcohol syndrome [FAS]**), and hormonal disorders (e.g., pituitary dwarfism).

2. **Psychosocial disorders,** including poverty, lack of education about feeding, neglect or abuse, and parental mental illness or substance abuse.

Esophageal **atresia,** incomplete formation of the esophagus, is often associated with a fistula between the esophagus and the trachea. This leads to feeding difficulties and respiratory distress in the first few days of life.

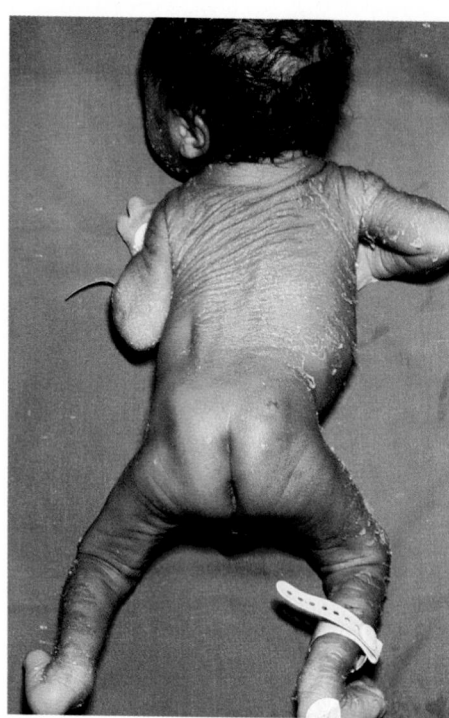

▲ **FIGURE 16.8 Postmature Infant with Skin Changes.**

Abbreviations	
FAS	fetal alcohol syndrome
FTT	failure to thrive
SGA	small for gestational age

Urinary System Adaptations

Kidneys at birth are not fully developed. Infants cannot concentrate their urine, so they have a high rate of water loss. They require more fluid intake, relative to body weight, than adults. In the first month of life, an infant will produce five to six wet diapers daily.

Congenital urinary tract disorders include renal **agenesis,** in which one or both kidneys are absent; blockage of urinary flow in utero, causing hydronephrosis of the kidneys; **polycystic kidney disease,** one of the most common genetic disorders; and **hypospadias** of the penis, in which the urethra does not extend to the end of the penis and opens along the underside of the penis. Hypospadias affects nearly 1% of baby boys *(see Chapter 11).*

WORD ANALYSIS AND DEFINITION

S = Suffix   P = Prefix   R = Root   R/CF = Combining Form

WORD	PRONUNCIATION	ELEMENTS		DEFINITION
agenesis	a-**JEN**-eh-sis	P/ R/	a- *without* -genesis *creation or production*	Failure to develop any organ or any part
atresia	a-**TREE**-zee-ah	P/ R/	a- *without* -tresia *a hole*	Congenital absence of a normal opening or lumen
gavage	guh-**VAHZH**		French *to force feed geese (to make pâté de foie gras)*	Forced feeding by stomach tube
hypospadias	high-poh-**SPAY**-dee-as	S/ P/ R/	-ias *condition* hypo- *below, under* -spad- *to tear, cut*	Urethral opening more proximal than normal on the ventral surface of the penis
involute	in-voh-**LUTE**	P/ R/	in- *in* -volute *roll up, shrink*	To return to a former condition; or decline associated with advanced age
percentile	per-**SEN**-tile	S/ P/ R/	-ile *capability* per- *through* -cent- *hundred*	One of a hundred groups in a distribution of variables
postmature	post-mah-**TYUR**	P/ R/	post- *after* -mature *fully developed*	Infant born after 42 weeks of gestation

> *Study Hint*
> **G**avage means *feeding* by a stomach (**g**astric) tube. Lavage is *washing out* a cavity, tube, or organ.

EXERCISES

Documentation: *Use the terminology and abbreviations found on these two pages to correctly fill in the following patient documentation.*

1. This infant's mother has been an alcoholic for the past year and a half. Infant was born suffering from _____ .

2. This preemie falls below the 10th percentile on a growth chart and is _____ .

3. This patient was born with a congenital absence of a normal opening in his esophagus. Diagnosis: esophageal _____

4. Patient was born with only the right kidney present. Diagnosis: renal _____

5. This infant's ventral urethral opening falls short of the tip of his penis. Diagnosis: _____

6. One of the most common urinary system genetic disorders is _____ .

7. Celiac disease has caused _____ in this patient; she is significantly below normal height and weight for her age group.

Create two sentences of patient *documentation* that demonstrate the correct usage of *gavage* and *lavage*:

8. gavage: _____

_____

_____

9. lavage: _____

_____

_____

CASE REPORT 16.2
True Story

A singer in a Master Chorale during the seventh and eighth months of pregnancy was in rehearsal for Handel's *Messiah* for a Christmas concert. At home, she frequently practiced her solo that began "I know that my redeemer liveth." When her daughter was 6 months old, the mother was changing the baby's diaper and started to sing "I know that my..." The child turned her head and chimed in "redeemer." Now, at 10 years old, the daughter has absolute pitch. She has the rare ability to replicate on the piano the note for any sound made in nature.

Keynote

Breast milk provides valuable antibodies, digestive enzymes, and hormones that infants need. It is nonallergenic.

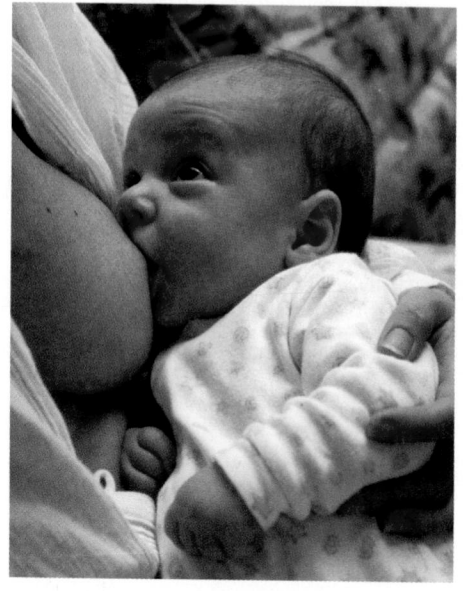

▲ **FIGURE 16.9 One-Month-Old Baby Breastfeeds and Interacts with Mother.**

Keynote

All newborn babies should receive hearing screening tests before they go home from the hospital.

NEONATAL ADAPTATIONS (continued)
Digestive System Adaptations

Until the baby is 6 months old, she needs only **breast milk** or commercially prepared **infant formula**. At 1 month of age, a breastfed baby will be feeding every 2 to 3 hours for about 10 minutes each time, and the **maternal** supply of milk will be adjusting to the baby's needs. The supply is based on the energy and frequency of the baby's sucking. Formula-fed babies will take 3 to 4 ounces every 3 to 4 hours.

Around 1 month of age, a feeding routine will be established. Breast milk can be pumped out of the breast and stored in the refrigerator for up to a week for other people to help with feeding. By 3 months, daytime feedings should be around every 4 hours, and the baby should be sleeping through the night.

An immature digestive system may be the cause of **colic,** in which the neonate cries for hours at a time until you feel like joining in. Twenty-five percent of all infants have colic. It begins between the third and sixth weeks and goes away on its own by the twelfth week. There is no known treatment.

Food intolerance, totally different from food allergy (see page 650, Immunologic Adaptations), is an adverse digestive system reaction to food. It does not involve the immune system. It can be a metabolic reaction to a digestive enzyme deficiency, such as **lactase deficiency** leading to intolerance to cows' milk. It can be an inability to deal with gluten, as in **celiac disease** *(see Chapter 6)*. The symptoms of food intolerance include feeling irritable and cranky, bloating and flatulence, nausea, vomiting, and diarrhea.

Visual Adaptations

At birth, a nonanesthetized baby is able to see and focus on an object between 8 and 12 inches away. This distance has probably **evolved** because it is the distance between mother's and baby's faces during breastfeeding *(Figure 16.9)*. For color vision, the baby will see only very brightly colored objects. Full color vision comes at between 3 and 4 months of age. Research has shown that newborns are naturally attracted to human faces, even to rough sketches of faces. This mechanism helps in **bonding,** particularly during breastfeeding.

Hearing Adaptations

The fetus begins to hear loud noises around the beginning of the third trimester (24 weeks). By the seventh month of pregnancy, the fetus can hear maternal speech and remember what is heard after she is born. Fetal experience with sounds and speech can make babies more responsive to speech after birth *(Case Report 16.2)*.

Congenital malformations of the external auditory canal and middle ear can result in a conductive hearing loss. Congenital malformations of the inner ear can result in a **sensorineural hearing loss** *(see Chapter 4)*. About 1 in 1000 newborns has a severe hearing loss.

WORD	PRONUNCIATION	ELEMENTS		DEFINITION
bonding	**BON**-ding		Latin *to hold together*	Formation of a close and lasting emotional attachment
celiac disease	**SEE**-lee-ak **DIZ**-eez	S/ R/	-ac *pertaining to* celi- *abdomen*	Disease caused by sensitivity to gluten
colic	**KOL**-ik	S/ R/	-ic *pertaining to* col- *colon*	Spasmodic, crampy pains in the abdomen; in young infants, persistent crying and irritability thought to be arising from pain in the intestines
evolve	ee-**VOLV**		Latin *to unfold*	To develop gradually
infant formula	**IN**-fant **FOR**-myu-lah	S/ R/	**infant** Latin *infans not speaking* -ula *small thing* form- *form*	Commercial product for infants manufactured from cows' milk or soy milk
intolerance	in-**TOL**-er-ance		Latin *impatient*	Inability of the small intestine to digest and dispose of a particular dietary constituent
lactase	**LAK**-tase	S/ R/	-ase *enzyme* lact- *milk*	Enzyme that breaks down lactose to glucose and galactose
maternal	mah-**TER**-nal	S/ R/	-al *pertaining to* mater- *mother*	Pertaining to or derived from the mother
sensorineural hearing loss	**SEN**-sor-ih-**NYUR**-al	S/ R/CF R/	-al *pertaining to* sensor/i- *sensation* -neur- *nerve*	Hearing loss caused by lesions of the inner ear or the auditory nerve

EXERCISES

Pediatric terminology will help you determine the correct answer for the following questions. Circle the best answer.

1. Breast milk provides:
   a. antibodies
   b. digestive enzymes
   c. hormones
   d. none of these
   e. all of these

2. Bloating, flatulence, nausea, vomiting, and diarrhea are symptoms of:
   a. food allergy
   b. immune response
   c. food intolerance
   d. urinary tract infection
   e. enzyme malabsorption

3. An immature digestive system may be the cause of:
   a. TTN
   b. colic
   c. elevated temperature
   d. FAS
   e. a rash

4. Formation of a close and lasting emotional attachment is called:
   a. independency
   b. visual adaptation
   c. bonding
   d. dependency
   e. intolerance

5. Congenital malformations of the external auditory canal can result in:
   a. FTT
   b. lactase deficiency
   c. FAS
   d. conductive hearing loss
   e. celiac disease

6. Lactase deficiency is:
   a. metabolic reaction to digestive enzyme deficiency
   b. intolerance to cow's milk
   c. food allergy
   d. a and b
   e. a and c

7. Circle the correct statement about breast milk:
   a. Breast milk is nonallergenic.
   b. Breast milk contains antibodies that babies need.
   c. Breast milk can be pumped out of the breast and put in a bottle.
   d. Breast milk can be stored in the refrigerator.
   e. All of the above.

8. The root *celi* means:
   a. stomach
   b. abdomen
   c. nerve
   d. colon
   e. bowel

NEONATAL ADAPTATIONS (continued)

Hematologic Adaptations

The newborn infant has an excess of red blood cells (RBCs). When these are broken down, bilirubin is produced *(see Chapter 7)*. In addition, the neonate's liver is immature and cannot process bilirubin quickly. The excess bilirubin is deposited in the tissues, producing jaundice. In the first 3 days after birth, neonatal jaundice affects 60% of full-term and 80% of premature infants. In most infants, no specific treatment is needed. Sunlight and **phototherapy** with a blue fluorescent light break down the bilirubin and are the mainstay of therapy *(Figure 16.10)*.

Breastfeeding is associated with hyperbilirubinemia in the first few days of life. It is related to breast milk taking a few days to come into the breast in adequate amounts to maintain hydration of the infant.

Rhesus and ABO incompatibilities that can produce neonatal jaundice and anemia are described in *Chapter 7*.

Immunologic Adaptations

Many of these adaptations occur in the first 6 months of life. The baby is born with immunoglobulin G (IgG) levels near those of an adult, having acquired them from the mother through the placenta. These levels remain high enough in the first 6 months to protect the baby against some infectious diseases but not against others, including **whooping cough (pertussis)** and **diphtheria.** This is why immunization against these diseases takes place at 2, 4, and 6 months of age. At 6 months, the IgG levels are at their lowest, and respiratory infections occur more easily.

Major failures of immunologic adaptation are discussed in *Chapter 15*.

In **food allergies,** the body's immune system reacts as though a particular food is harmful (an allergen) and creates IgE antibodies to it. This, in turn, generates chemicals such as histamine that produce symptoms of a runny nose, itchy skin rash, swelling of the lips, or wheezing. The most common allergens are **cows' milk, eggs, wheat, soy,** and **peanuts.** Between 25% and 50% of children outgrow their food allergies by age 3 years.

Social Adaptations

Identity. The building blocks of a baby's identity began in the last trimester in utero when she played with her fingers and toes and responded to sounds, music, and voices. Genes and her **inborn temperament** play their roles. At 1 month of age, her interaction with her caregiver's love, attention, and caring skills are the stimulus for how she reacts to other people. By 2 to 3 months, as she again starts to play with her fingers and toes, she will be starting the process of being aware of her own physical identity.

Communication. Crying is the baby's primary communication method. She cries in different ways to say "I'm wet, hungry, lonely, or just overwhelmed by the sights and sounds of this world around me." She'll start to "coo" and gurgle and will enjoy hearing the caregiver respond with the same sounds. When she turns away or closes her eyes, she may just need her own space.

Curiosity. A 1-month-old baby can show interest only in what is in front of her, such as a parent's face or a brightly colored toy. As her eye and neck muscles develop, she can turn her head to see any object that catches her eye. At 3 months, she'll take swipes at a mobile of shapes hanging over her crib, and she'll look into a child-safe mirror in the crib near her head.

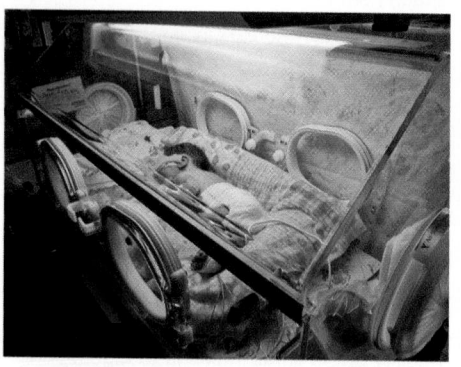

▲ **FIGURE 16.10 One-Day-Old Premature Baby Undergoing Phototherapy.**

Keynote

In the first 2 years of life, most children have 8 to 10 colds.

Six percent of children under the age of 3 have food allergies.

Abbreviation	
Ig	immunoglobulin

Keynote

By 3 months of age, the baby will smile at the sound of a known voice and turn her head to the direction of the sound.

WORD	PRONUNCIATION		ELEMENTS	DEFINITION
diphtheria	dif-**THEER**-ee-ah		Greek *leather*	Disease with a thick, membranous (leathery) coating of the pharynx
pertussis whooping cough (syn)	per-**TUSS**-is **WHO**-ping KAWF	P/ R/	per- *intense* -tussis *cough*	Infectious disease with spasmodic, intense cough ending on a whoop (stridor)
phototherapy	foh-toe-**THAIR**-ah-pee	R/CF S/	phot/o- *light* -therapy *treatment*	Treatment using light rays
temperament	**TEM**-per-ah-ment		Latin *disposition*	Predisposition to character or personality

EXERCISES

Analyze the statements and choose the correct medical term to fill in the blanks. Watch your spelling please!

1. Predisposition to character and personality is referred to as _____ .

    (parameter   temperament)

2. Treatment using light rays is called _____ .

    (fototherapy   phototherapy)

3. Excess bilirubin in tissues produces _____ .

    (jaundice   cyanosis)

4. Another name for whooping cough is _____ .

    (tonsillitis   pertussis)

5. Disease with a thick, leathery coating of the pharynx is called _____ .

    (hypospadias   diphtheria)

Utilize the *language of pediatrics* and briefly answer the following questions.

1. How is jaundice produced in the neonate? _____

   _____

2. How do the fetus's pulmonary and systemic circuits change at birth? _____

   _____

3. What key role does the development of surfactant play in a neonate's respiratory system? _____

   _____

4. What vital body functions must be in place at birth to ensure that the newborn thrives? _____

   _____

5. Why do infants have a high rate of water loss? _____

   _____

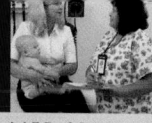

LESSON 16.2 Infant to Teenager

OBJECTIVES

To be both a pediatric medical assistant and a parent, you need to be able to use correct medical terminology to:

16.2.1 Identify the different stages of development in childhood.

16.2.2 Distinguish between acceptable and unacceptable behaviors at different stages of childhood development.

16.2.3 Describe common disorders of development in childhood.

16.2.4 Discuss common problems of childhood and adolescence.

You are

. . . a pediatric medical assistant who has been working with Sandra Mendes, MD, at Fulwood Medical Center for 7 years.

Your patients are

. . . 7-year-old Carol Hotteling and her mother.

CASE REPORT 16.3

You have watched Carol grow over the 7 years that you have worked in Dr. Mendes' well-baby clinic. Her mother, Mrs. Anna Hotteling, is telling you about her current concerns:

"As you know, she's always been a handful. The neighbors call her a tomboy. She's trashed every room in the house. The other kids' mothers have stopped inviting her to parties. Nothing holds her attention for very long. I've lost her a couple of times in the shopping mall when she's darted away. I always thought she'd grow out of it. But now she's in second grade. The teacher is complaining that Carol can't sit still, interferes with the other kids, and disrupts the class, and she's having trouble reading and staying focused. It's got to be due to something I did or didn't do?"

STAGE 1—INFANCY

Around 1 year old, your child can be taken into an optimal nutritional environment that reflects your own good eating habits *(see Chapter 17)*. This can ensure a normal growth pattern that can be disturbed only by illness or **psychosocial** disorders such as poverty or abuse as she goes through the transformation from a **dependent** infant into a **competent, independent** adult.

This dramatic transformation to adulthood has been broken down by psychologist Erik Erikson into eight stages:

Stage 1: Infancy—Age 0 to 1 year

In the first year of life, your **infant** is dependent on parents and caregivers for food, affection, and warmth. Consistently meeting these needs will result in a secure, trusting attachment to parents and their environment. If those needs are not met, your infant can develop distrust toward people and their surroundings. At the end of this year, your infant will be starting to show **independence** by pulling herself up to stand, walking by holding on to furniture, and perhaps saying her first word.

Keynote

Stage 1 issue: trust versus mistrust.

Note: Stages of development in childhood were adapted from E. H. Erikson, *Childhood and Society*, 2nd ed. New York: W. W. Norton & Co., 1963.

WORD ANALYSIS AND DEFINITION

WORD	PRONUNCIATION	ELEMENTS		DEFINITION
competent	**KOM**-peh-tent		Latin *in harmony*	Capable of performing a task or function
dependent	de-**PEN**-dent		Latin *to hang from*	Having to rely on someone else
independent	in-de-**PEN**-dent	S/ P/ R/ S/	-ent *end result* in- *not* -depend- *relying on* -ence *state of, quality of*	Able to fend for oneself
independence	in-de-**PEN**-denz			State of being independent
infant	**IN**-fant		Latin *not speaking*	Child in the first year of life
infancy	**IN**-fan-see			The first year of life
psychosocial	sigh-koh-**SOH**-shal	S/ R/CF R/	-ial *pertaining to* psych/o- *the mind* -soc- *partner*	Involving both the mind and various social and community aspects of life

EXERCISES

Lesson Objective: *Meet this lesson's objective of being able to identify stages of development in childhood by answering the following questions. Use the vocabulary on these two pages to fill in the blanks.*

1. Stage 1 of childhood development encompasses what ages? _____

2. What is the main issue in stage 1 of childhood development? _____

3. An infant must transform from a(n)_____ infant to a(n) _____ adult.

4. What can ensure a normal growth pattern for a child in stage 1? _____

5. What can disrupt a normal growth pattern for a child in stage 1? _____

6. Who is the famous psychologist who formulated the eight stages of childhood development? _____

Research the Internet for more information regarding the psychologist Erik Erikson. List below five facts you have learned about him and his theory. **Be sure you can explain and define any new terms you use here.**

7. _____

_____

8. _____

_____

9. _____

_____

10. _____

_____

11. _____

_____

STAGES 2 TO 5—TODDLER TO ADOLESCENCE

Keynote

Stage 2 issue: independence versus self-doubt.

Stage 2: Toddler—Age 1 to 2 years

Independence is the issue for your toddler, who learns to walk and talk and wants to do things for herself—like use the toilet and put on her own clothes. Out of these abilities and desires begins the development of self-confidence and self-control. If your child's initiatives are encouraged and mistakes are accepted, she will be able to make choices and achieve self-control and independence. If you are an overprotective or disapproving parent, she can have doubts about her abilities.

By the end of this year, she will run, climb on furniture, scribble artwork, say "I love you," and be able to cope with other children.

Keynote

Stage 3 issue: initiative versus impulse.

Stage 3: Early Childhood—Age 2 to 6 years

Your child finds power with **motor** skills and her ability to engage in social interaction. She wants to be the center of attention and part of an adult world for which she is not ready. Encouragement with boundaries and consistent **discipline** help her define her role in the family. *Discipline* has the same root as *disciple*, a learner of the responsible way of living. Impulse control and responsibility are learned as a key part of her independence.

Keynote

Stage 4 issue: competence versus failure.

Stage 4: Grade School Years—Age 6 to 12 years

Transition takes place from the world of home to the world of **peers.** Your parental role is to stimulate curiosity and pleasure in **intellectual** success so that your child develops a sense of competence, not feelings of inferiority and expectations of failure.

Keynote

Stage 5 issue: identity versus confusion.

Stage 5: Adolescence—Age 12 to 18 years

This is the time of identity crisis. "Who am I?"—the most powerful and critical question in anyone's lifetime. Is she able to **integrate** the trust she learned in stage 1 with the independence she learned in stage 2, with the impulse control and responsibility from stage 3, with the competence and intellectual curiosity of stage 4? If your **adolescent** can integrate these values into her being, she will have a strong identity and readiness to be an adult. If not, she will sink into confusion and fear and be unable to make choices about her roles in life.

Depression, bipolar disorder, anxiety disorders *(see Chapter 19)*, and the eating disorders of **anorexia nervosa, bulimia,** and **binge eating** and **purging** arise out of this confusion.

WORD	PRONUNCIATION	ELEMENTS		DEFINITION
adolescence	ad-oh-**LESS**-ents	S/ R/	-ence *state of, quality of* **adolesc-** *beginning of adulthood*	Stage that begins with puberty and ends with physical maturity
adolescent	ad-oh-**LESS**-ent	S/	-ent *end result*	Pertaining to adolescence or a person in that stage
anorexia	an-oh-**RECK**-see-ah	S/ P/ R/	-ia *condition* **an-** *without* **-orex-** *appetite*	Severe lack of appetite; or an aversion to food
binge eating	BINJ **EE**-ting		**binge** Old English *to soak*	Eating with periods of excessive intake
bulimia	byu-**LEEM**-ee-ah		Greek *hunger*	Episodic bouts of excessive eating with compensatory throwing up
discipline	**DIS**-ih-plin	S/ R/	-ine *pertaining to* **discipl-** *understand*	Training for proper conduct or action
integrate	**IN**-teh-grate		Latin *to make whole*	To bring together into a complete and harmonious whole
intellectual	in-teh-**LEK**-chu-al	S/ R/CF	-al *pertaining to* **intellect/u-** *perception, discernment*	Pertaining to the capacity for thinking and acquiring knowledge
motor	**MOH**-tor		Latin *to move*	Structures of the nervous system that send impulses out to cause muscles to contract or glands to secrete
peer	PEER		Latin *equal*	A person at the same level or standing
purge purging	PURJ **PURJ**-ing	S/ R/	-ing *doing, quality of* **purg-** *cleanse*	Consciously throw up, or cause bowel evacuation The act of throwing up or evacuating the bowel

EXERCISES

Lesson Objective: *Continue to meet the lesson objective of identifying Erikson's stages of childhood development. Fill in the chart.*

Stage	Ages	Major Issue in Development
2		
3		
4		
5		

Pick any one of these stages, and write a two-sentence description of what might happen to a child in this stage.

_____

_____

_____

_____

_____

Always aim for neat and legible handwriting!

Keynote

Visual acuity starts to decline very early in life. Eye exercises can be of value to prevent this.

Exercise and good nutrition help prevent osteopenia.

Exercise and good nutrition help prevent muscle degeneration.

Exercising your brain enhances the quality of life in old age.

Exercise and good nutrition extend **longevity** and enhance the quality of life.

Bronchitis and emphysema, the **chronic obstructive pulmonary diseases (COPDs)**, are the cumulative effects of cigarette smoking and are a leading cause of death in old age.

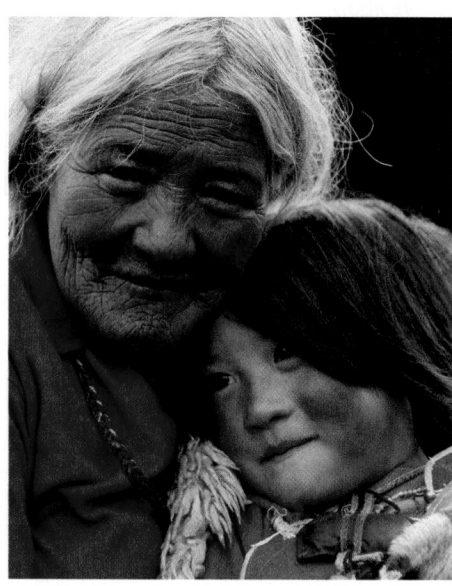

▲ **FIGURE 16.11 Senescence of the Skin.**
Elderly Tibetan woman with her granddaughter.

Keynote

The kidneys of an 80-year-old receive only half as much blood as those of a 30-year-old because of atherosclerosis.

Keynote

Because of lowered immunity, vaccinations against influenza and other seasonal infections are recommended for the elderly.

Organ systems begin to show signs of senescence at very different ages and do not degenerate at the same speed. For example, **autopsies (postmortem)** in children will often reveal atherosclerosis in the CVS. Most physiologic studies show general peak physical performance appears in the twenties. Autopsies are usually performed by a **pathologist** or a medical examiner.

Integumentary system changes begin in the forties. Melanocytes *(see Chapter 3)* die, and hair becomes gray and thinner. The skin becomes paper thin, loses elasticity, and hangs loose, and wrinkles appear *(Figure 16.11)*. Flat brown-black spots, **senile lentigines (age spots),** appear on the back of the hands and areas exposed to sunlight.

Special senses start to decline in the twenties. Visual acuity declines at that time. In the forties, presbyopia *(see Chapter 4)* begins, and many people develop cataracts in old age. Hearing loss occurs as the ossicles become stiffer and the number of cochlear hair cells *(see Chapter 4)* declines. This was the cause of Mr. Hickman's hearing loss. Taste and smell are blunted late in life as taste cells and olfactory buds decline in number.

Skeletal system changes appear in the thirties, when osteoblasts become less active than osteoclasts. The result is osteopenia, which goes on to become osteoporosis, particularly in postmenopausal women. Joints in the older age groups have less synovial fluid and thinner articular cartilage. Osteoarthritis results *(see Chapter 5)*.

Muscular system changes occur with age as muscle mass is lost **(sarcopenia)** and is replaced with fat. As muscle **atrophies,** there are fewer muscle fibers to do the work and the available blood supply is decreased. Tasks that used to be easy become difficult, such as buttoning shirts and tying shoelaces. This was one of Mr. Hickman's triumphs of the day.

Nervous system changes begin around age 30, when the brain weighs twice as much as it does by age 75. Motor coordination, intellectual function, and short-term memory decline more quickly than long-term memory and language skills.

Cardiovascular systems always show coronary artery atherosclerosis from an early age. As a result, when aging myocardial cells die, the heart wall gets thinner and weaker, and cardiac output declines. This causes the decline in physical capabilities with aging. Atherosclerotic plaques narrow arteries and trigger thrombosis, leading to strokes and heart attacks. In veins, valves become weaker, and blood flows back and pools in the legs, leading to poor venous return to the heart and heart failure.

Respiratory system changes are noticeable in the thirties when pulmonary ventilation declines, a factor in the gradual loss of stamina. The rib cage becomes less flexible; the lungs become less elastic and have fewer alveoli. Respiratory function declines. As respiratory health declines, hypoxic degenerative changes occur in all the other organ systems.

Urinary system changes begin in the twenties, when the number of nephrons starts to decline. Later in life, many of the remaining glomeruli become atherosclerotic.

Glomerular filtration rate (GFR) decreases, and the kidneys become less efficient. For example, drug doses in the elderly need to be reduced because the drugs cannot be cleared from the blood as rapidly.

Immune system function declines in the elderly as the amounts of lymphatic tissue and red bone marrow decrease with age. This leads to a reduction in both cellular and humoral (antibody) immunity *(see Chapter 15)*. This means that the elderly have less protection against infectious diseases and cancer.

The **disorders of senescence** and their terminology are described in detail in each of the body system chapters in this book.

WORD	PRONUNCIATION	ELEMENTS		DEFINITION
atrophy atrophies (verb)	**AT**-roh-fee **AT**-roh-feez	P/ R/	**a-** *without* **-trophy** *development, nourishment*	Wasting or diminished volume of a tissue or organ
autopsy postmortem (syn)	**AWE**-top-see post-**MOR**-tem	 S/ P/ R/	Greek *see with one's own eyes* **-em** *condition* **post-** *after* **-mort-** *death*	Examination of the body and organs of a dead person to determine the cause of death
lentigo lentigines (pl)	len-**TIE**-go len-**TIHJ**-ih-neez		Greek *lentil*	Age spot; small, flat, brown-black spot in the skin of older people
pathologist	pa-**THOL**-oh-jist	S/ R/CF	**-logist** *one who studies, specialist* **path/o-** *disease*	A specialist in pathology (study of disease or characteristics of a particular disease)
sarcopenia	sar-koh-**PEE**-nee-ah	S/ R/CF	**-penia** *deficiency* **sarc/o-** *muscle*	Progressive loss of muscle mass and strength in aging

Abbreviations

COPD chronic obstructive pulmonary disease
GFR glomerular filtration rate

EXERCISES

Organ systems show various signs of senescence. Provide one example of a sign of senescence in each organ system listed in the following table. Be sure to use correct medical terminology, and be able to explain every term you use. Fill in the blanks.

Organ System	Sign of Senescence
Integumentary	
Special senses (ear/eye)	
Skeletal	
Muscular	
Nervous	
Cardiovascular	
Respiratory	
Urinary	
Immune	

Have you checked your spelling?

THEORIES OF SENESCENCE, DYING, AND DEATH

The causes of senescence are unknown. **Heredity** plays a role because longevity or early death tend to run in families. Theories of senescence include:

- **Protein abnormalities.** One-quarter of the body's protein is collagen. With age, collagen and other proteins show abnormal structures in their cells and tissues and become less soluble and more rigid. The cells accumulate more of these dysfunctional proteins as they age, and their functions are impaired, leading to **senescent** changes.

- **Free radicals.** These are chemical particles with an extra electron. For example, the stable oxygen molecule has two atoms with many electrons. If it picks up an extra electron through some metabolic reaction, by radiation, or by chemicals, it becomes a free radical. The free radical's life is short because it combines quickly with other molecules that, in turn, become free radicals with the addition of the extra electron. A chain reaction occurs as more and more molecules become free radicals. Among the damage they cause are cancer, myocardial infarction, and perhaps senescence. They can be neutralized by **antioxidants** *(see Chapter 17)*.

- **Autoimmune** altered molecules *(see Chapter 15)*. These molecules may be recognized as foreign antigens, and an immune response may be generated against the body's own tissues. This theory is helped by the fact that autoimmune diseases such as rheumatoid arthritis are more common in old age.

Dying and Death

Death is inevitable. Just as fetal life in the womb is a preparation for birth, so living and aging are a preparation for death. You can prepare for death in different ways, all of which are done with your family and many of which necessitate legal assistance.

Medical issues are clearly significant in the process of dying. Your views on the types and extent of medical treatment you wish to have should be clearly stated. This is done through an **advance medical directive,** which consists of two documents:

1. **Medical (durable) power of attorney,** in which you appoint someone you know and trust as your agent and authorize that person to make medical decisions for you when you cannot.

2. **Living will,** in which you provide a set of instructions detailing what treatment you do and do not want in a terminal illness, including **hospice** treatment. If there are special instructions, such as **do not resuscitate (DNR)**, these must be stated clearly. It should also include a Health Insurance Portability and Accountability Act **(HIPAA) authorization** that enables your agent to receive the medical information about you that is necessary for making decisions about treatment. This is needed because the HIPAA of 1996 *(see Chapter 2)* imposes tough privacy-of-medical-information rules on doctors and hospitals.

Your primary care doctor should have a copy of your advance medical directive and have read the document with you.

The process of dying, rather than death itself, is of concern to most elderly people. Dying should be dignified and free from physical and emotional pain. A **hospice** provides **palliative care** and provides for the emotional and spiritual needs of terminally ill patients and their loved ones at an inpatient facility or in the patient's home. Palliative care is designed to provide pain and symptom management to maintain the highest quality of life for as long as life remains.

Just as the moment life begins is controversial, there is no universally accepted moment of biological death.

In most states in the United States, death is now defined in terms of **brain death (BD)**, when there is no cerebral or brainstem activity and the EEG is flat for a specific length of time *(Figure 16.12)*. Two other conditions involving brain damage

Abbreviations

BD	brain death
DNR	do not resuscitate
HIPAA	Health Insurance Portability and Accountability Act
MCS	minimally conscious state
PVS	persistent vegetative state

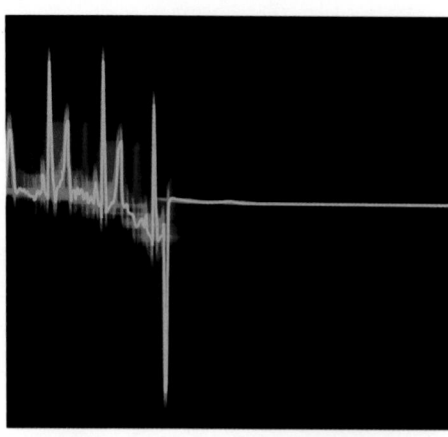

▲ **FIGURE 16.12 Electroencephalogram Shows Brain Death.**

WORD	PRONUNCIATION	ELEMENTS		DEFINITION
advance medical directive	ad-**VANTS MED**-ih-kal die-**REK**-tiv			Legal document signed by the patient dealing with issues of prolonging or ending life in the event of life-threatening illness
antioxidant	an-tee-**OKS**-ih-dant	S/ P/ R/	-ant *forming* anti- *against* -oxid- *oxidize*	Substance that can prevent cell damage by neutralizing free radicals
coma	**KOH**-mah		Greek *deep sleep*	State of deep unconsciousness
death	DETH		Old English *to die*	Total and permanent cessation of all vital functions
free radical	FREE **RAD**-ih-kal	R/ S/ R/	free *free* -al *pertaining to* radic- *root*	Short-lived product of oxidation in a cell that can be damaging to the cell
heredity	heh-**RED**-ih-tee	S/ R/	-ity *state, condition* hered- *inherited through genes*	Transmission of characteristics from parents to offspring through genes
hospice	**HOS**-pis		Latin *lodging*	Facility or program that provides care to the dying and their families
palliative care	**PAL**-ee-ah-tiv KAIR	S/ R/ R/	-ive *nature of, pertaining to* palliat- *reduce suffering* care *be responsible for*	Care that relieves symptoms and pain without curing
vegetative	**VEJ**-eh-tay-tiv	S/ R/	-ive *nature of, pertaining to* vegetat- *growth*	Functioning unconsciously as plant life is assumed to do

and loss of brain function cause medical difficulty and should be addressed in your living will:

1. **Persistent vegetative state (PVS)** occurs in people who suffer enough brain damage that they are unaware of themselves or their surroundings, even though their eyes are open. Yet they still have certain reflexes and can breathe and pump blood because the brainstem still functions. Even reflex events like crying and smiling and the sleep-wake cycle can be seen. With medical care and artificial feeding, patients can survive for decades.

2. **Minimally conscious state (MCS)** is a condition of severely altered consciousness in which minimal evidence of awareness of self or surroundings is demonstrated. There is inconsistent communication or command following. However, PET scans of MCS patients show cortical function when their loved ones speak to them. They are more likely to improve than are PVS patients.

Keynote

Both PVS and MCS differ from **coma**, in which the individual is unresponsive and keeps his eyes closed.

EXERCISES

Explain the difference among the following terms to a patient's relatives. If you understand it yourself, you can explain it to someone else. Write a brief explanation for each term.

1. Persistent vegetative state:

_____

_____

2. Minimally conscious state:

_____

_____

3. Coma:

_____

LIFE SPAN

CHALLENGE YOUR KNOWLEDGE

A. **Case Report:** Reread the following Case Report, which was presented earlier in this chapter. Use your knowledge of the *language of pediatrics* to answer the questions below. Fill in the blanks.

CASE REPORT 16.3

Your patients are

. . . 7-year-old Carol Hotteling and her mother. You have watched Carol grow over the 7 years that you have worked in Dr. Mendes' well-baby clinic. Her mother, Mrs. Anna Hotteling, is telling you about her current concerns:

"As you know, she's always been a handful. The neighbors call her a tomboy. She's trashed every room in the house. The other kids' mothers stopped inviting her to parties. Nothing holds her attention for very long. I've lost her a couple of times in the shopping mall when she's darted away. I always thought she'd grow out of it. But now she's in second grade. The teacher is complaining that Carol can't sit still, interferes with the other kids, and disrupts the class, and she's having trouble reading and staying focused. It's got to be due to something I did or didn't do?"

1. According to Erikson, what stage of development is Carol Hotteling in now, and what is the major issue in this stage of development?

   _____

2. What types of problems does Carol have?

   _____

   _____

   _____

3. Based on these symptoms and the descriptions provided by her mother, what disorders could Carol possibly have? _____

   _____

4. What type of specialist might Carol be referred to?

   _____

B. **Elements:** You need to recognize word elements in and out of context. First, match the meaning in the left column with the element in the center column. Write your answer on the blank between them. Then, fill in each blank in the right column with the type of element that is next to it.

Meaning of Element		Element	Type of Element (P, R, CF, S)
1. together	_____	A. drom	_____
2. in	_____	B. ase	_____
3. appetite	_____	C. syn	_____
4. pertaining to	_____	D. rumin	_____
5. without	_____	E. uresis	_____
6. enzyme	_____	F. an	_____
7. running	_____	G. orex	_____
8. the mind	_____	H. ine	_____
9. throat	_____	I. psycho	_____
10. to urinate	_____	J. en	_____

C. **Dictionary:** English words that are not necessarily medical terminology can still have an impact on the meaning of a medical term; for example, transient tachypnea of the newborn. Use your dictionary or go online to look up the meaning of the word **transient;** then fill in the blanks:

1. transient: _____

    Is *transient tachypnea of the newborn* a permanent condition?

    _____

2. Using your knowledge of the definition of *transient,* analyze this sentence: "Amniotic fluid remains in the infant's lungs and causes a *self-limiting* respiratory distress."

    a. What does **self-limiting** mean in this context?

    _____

    b. How will this condition resolve?

    _____

D. **Abbreviations:** Regardless of whether you are an administrative or clinical health care worker, you will be reading patient documentation with abbreviations, which can mean a diagnosis, procedure, disease, and so on. To interpret this documentation correctly and safely, you must know the meanings of the abbreviations. Challenge yourself to *define* each of the following abbreviations correctly. *Then list the specialist* connected to that medical term. Fill in the chart, and then practice your documentation.

Abbreviation	Meaning of Abbreviation	Specialist
BD		
MCS		
PVS		
PDA		
HMD		
SIDS		
SFD		
RDS		
FTT		
LD		

Choose any abbreviation from the table above, and write one sentence of patient documentation that might come from that particular specialist.

Abbreviation: _____

Specialist: _____

Patient documentation:

_____

_____

LIFE SPAN

E. Discussion: Research in the school library or on the Internet to be able to explain the statement: "Autism is a spectrum of disorders." Be sure you can define any vocabulary you use in your discussion. Briefly organize your thoughts below, or write down the words you need to look up. Use reliable medical sites on the Web—those ending with .gov, .edu, or .org.

1. Internet sites visited: _____

   _____

   _____

2. New vocabulary learned: _____

   _____

   _____

3. Useful facts (information): _____

   _____

   _____

4. Possible treatments: _____

   _____

   _____

5. Synthesize your information: Autism is a spectrum of disorders because _____

   _____

   _____

   _____

F. Education: Convert the following sentences into layman's terms to explain them to the parent of a patient.

1. "Infants with RDS are at risk for cerebral ischemia, hemorrhage, and neonatal death."

   _____

   _____

   _____

   _____

2. "Postmature infants are prone to meconium aspiration and neonatal hypoglycemia."

   _____

   _____

   _____

   _____

G. **Prefixes and suffixes are good clues to the meaning of a medical term.** Analyze each medical term for the meaning of its prefix and suffix. Then give the complete meaning of the medical term in the last column. Every term may not have both a prefix and a suffix. Fill in the table.

Medical Term	Meaning of Prefix	Meaning of Suffix	Meaning of Medical Term
agenesis			
anorexia			
colic			
encephalocele			
enuresis			
pediatric			
psychosocial			
senile			
stereotype			
syndrome			

H. **English and Medical Terminology:** Some of the terminology in this chapter is rooted in Latin or Greek and can be literally translated and used in the English language or the language of medicine. On the line below each sentence, fill in the meaning of the bold word in that particular sentence.

1. My sister is **depressed** and has been on medication for 6 years.

   _____

   Her immune system is **depressed,** and she is much more susceptible to disease.

   _____

2. Her **precipitate** labor threatened the life of her unborn child.

   _____

   In the centrifuge, the **precipitate** fell to the bottom of the tube.

   _____

   OR: A term may have more than one meaning, but only one meaning is specific to that particular context. Write the correct meaning of the bold word on the line below each of the following sentences.

3. The young child **aspirated** a peanut at the picnic and had to be rushed to the ER.

   _____

   The fluid in the patient's lungs was **aspirated** by a thoracentesis.

   _____

4. The Poison Control Center advised an emetic and **purging** of the child's stomach.

   _____

   The health information (HI) department is **purging** all the outdated patient files.

   _____

LIFE SPAN

I. Similar but Different: Terms that appear similar can have very different meanings. When you know the terms well enough, you can briefly explain the difference between the terms. Write a short answer.

1. food intolerance:

_____

_____

food allergy:

_____

_____

2. enuresis:

_____

_____

encopresis:

_____

_____

J. Elements: Even though these elements do not appear in the context of a medical term, you should be able to recognize their meaning out of context. Match the correct element in the left column with its meaning in the right column. Fill in the blanks.

_____	1. plasia	A.	to adjust
_____	2. neo	B.	old age
_____	3. faci	C.	forming
_____	4. thermo	D.	relating to medicine
_____	5. ile	E.	without
_____	6. ped	F.	formation
_____	7. adapt	G.	to roll up
_____	8. a or an	H.	capability
_____	9. iatric	I.	new
_____	10. ant	J.	face
_____	11. volute	K.	child
_____	12. geronto	L.	heat

K. **Medical Language:** Employ the *languages of pediatrics and gerontology* to answer the following multiple-choice questions. Circle the correct answer.

1. The term **sensorineural** has to do with:

    a. body weight

    b. blood pressure

    c. peripheral vision

    d. hearing loss

    e. metabolism

2. Which of the following conditions results from a "blue" baby?

    a. cleft lip

    b. cyanosis

    c. hypoglycemia

    d. OCD

    e. encopresis

3. The medical term for feeding through a stomach tube is:

    a. senescence

    b. lavage

    c. vegetative

    d. resuscitation

    e. gavage

4. This occurs most frequently in infants from C-sections and precipitate deliveries:

    a. transient tachypnea

    b. dyspnea

    c. enuresis

    d. dysplasia

    e. SIDS

5. Appointing someone you trust to make medical decisions for you is called:

    a. living will

    b. medical power of attorney

    c. DNR order

    d. consent form

    e. HIPAA authorization

LIFE SPAN

L. Medical Language: Employ the *languages of pediatrics and gerontology* to answer the following multiple-choice questions. Circle the best answer.

1. Neonatal reflex to turn toward nipple and open mouth when nipple is placed on cheek:

   a. Moro reflex

   b. rooting

   c. stepping reflex

   d. startle reflex

   e. doll's eye maneuver

2. Synthetic surfactant is instilled:

   a. intertracheally

   b. subcutaneously

   c. intratracheally

   d. subdermally

   e. by gavage

3. Free radicals can be neutralized by:

   a. T lymphocytes (T cells)

   b. organ systems

   c. antioxidants

   d. enzymes

   e. hormones

4. Hypothermia is more likely to occur in infants who are:

   a. SFD

   b. premature

   c. postmature

   d. a and b

   e. a and c

5. Eating with periods of excessive intake:

   a. bulimia

   b. anorexia nervosa

   c. binge-eating disorder

   d. dyslexia

   e. pica

6. Fetal distress can cause:

   a. Asperger syndrome

   b. meconium aspiration syndrome

   c. cleft palate

   d. Down syndrome

   e. HMD

7. The development of _____ is the key to the development of fully functioning lungs:

   a. ventilation

   b. surfactant

   c. precipitate

   d. osteoclasts

   e. protein

8. Exercise and good nutrition are helpful in preventing:

   a. cancer

   b. tumors

   c. freckles

   d. osteopenia

   e. COPD

9. Another name for whooping cough is:

   a. OCD

   b. TTN

   c. pertussis

   d. celiac disease

   e. jaundice

10. A milder form of autism is:

    a. Down syndrome

    b. hyaline membrane disease

    c. Asperger syndrome

    d. dyslexia

    e. ODD

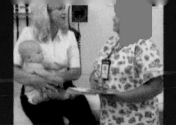
LIFE SPAN

M. Deconstruct: The language of any body system can be analyzed by its basic elements. Deconstruct each of the following medical terms into the elements, which will reveal its meaning. Fill in the chart; then use any two of the terms in patient documentation. The first entry on the chart has been done for you.

Medical Term	Prefix/Meaning	Root/CF/Meaning	Suffix/Meaning	Meaning of Term
hydrocephalus	hydro water	cephalus head		Enlarged head due to excess CSF in the cerebral ventricles
involuntary				
anencephaly				
neural				
phototherapy				
pertussis				
neonatal				
microcephaly				
hypospadias				
atrophy				
postmortem				

Patient documentation:

1. _____

_____

2. _____

_____

N. Terminology Challenge: Find the synonym for the medical term **autopsy**. Deconstruct each term, and provide a definition. Fill in the blanks.

1. The synonym for autopsy is _____ .

2. Deconstruct the synonym into elements with their meanings.

(synonym): _____

3. What is the definition of autopsy? _____

_____

4. What type of specialist is likely to perform an autopsy? _____

5. What can be learned from an autopsy? _____

_____

O. **Language of Gerontology:** The following medical terms are all applicable to the *language of gerontology.* Build your knowledge of their meanings by correctly using each term in a sentence of your choice that is *not a definition that appears in the text.* **Example:** "The life expectancy at any given age will be considerably shortened if that person smokes cigarettes."

life span	life expectancy	longevity	aging	senescence

1. _____

_____

_____

_____

2. _____

_____

_____

_____

3. _____

_____

_____

_____

4. _____

_____

_____

_____

5. _____

_____

_____

6. Meet a lesson objective by distinguishing *aging* from *senescence.* Be prepared to discuss your answer in class. Write your discussion notes here:

_____

_____

_____

_____

LIFE SPAN

P. Recall and Review: How well do you remember these word elements from the previous chapter? Try to answer without first looking back to check. Fill in the blanks.

Element	Type of Element (P, R, CF, S)	Meaning of Element
megaly	_____	_____
oid	_____	_____
ism	_____	_____
agglutin	_____	_____
macro	_____	_____

Q. Latin and Greek terms cannot be further deconstructed into prefix, root, or suffix. You must know them for what they are. Test your knowledge of these terms with this exercise. Match the meaning in the left column with the correct medical term in the right column.

_____ 1. to bend back   A. rooting

_____ 2. to hang from   B. peer

_____ 3. to grow old   C. bulimia

_____ 4. seek   D. diphtheria

_____ 5. age spots   E. senescence

_____ 6. equal   F. purge

_____ 7. excessive eating, then vomiting   G. reflex

_____ 8. disposition   H. lentil

_____ 9. to cleanse   I. dependent

_____ 10. leather   J. temperament

R. How well do you understand what you read? Briefly explain, in your own words, each of the following statements. If there is an abbreviation, rewrite it in complete medical terms.

1. "SIDS is thought to be caused by a failure of the cardiorespiratory control mechanisms to mature."

   _____

   _____

2. "Infants with RDS are at risk for cerebral ischemia, hemorrhage, and neonatal death."

   _____

   _____

3. "Treatment for secondary neonatal seizures is directed at the underlying pathology."

   _____

   _____

4. "The musculoskeletal system can develop abnormally in utero and produce congenital malformations in different parts of the newborn's body."

   _____

   _____

S. Meet a lesson objective by demonstrating your knowledge and recognition of medical terms that have appeared in Chapters 2 through 15. Circle the correct medical term that matches the brief description.

1.	Specialist in the study of cells	histologist	cytologist
2.	Invasion of a parasite on the skin	infection	infestation
3.	Complete loss of sensation	anesthesia	analgesia
4.	Forward curvature of the spine	kyphosis	lordosis
5.	Abnormal passage	fissure	fistula
6.	To ooze out from a vessel into tissue	disseminate	extravasate
7.	Constriction/stenosis of the aorta	coarctation	infarction
8.	Wheezing sounds heard on auscultation	rales	rhonchi
9.	Network of joined nerves	synapse	plexus
10.	Outside the body	extracorporeal	interstitial
11.	Neoplasm of a testis or ovary	seminoma	teratoma
12.	Opening into a canal	orifice	os
13.	Excessive body and facial hair	hirsutism	prognathism
14.	Weaken the ability of an organism to produce disease	attenuate	agglutinate

T. Identify the following medical terms and place them in the correct body system. The first one is done for you.

Medical Term	Body System
hypothenar	*musculoskeletal*
verruca	
cochlear	
diaphragm	
deglutition	
hemodialysis	
emmetropia	
thelarche	
mitral	
thyrotoxicosis	
laceration	
postictal	
balanitis	
flexion	
plaque	
ileocecal	
myelomeningocele	

LIFE SPAN

CHAPTER SUMMARY EXERCISE

1. *Listen to the pronunciation of the medical terms as given by your instructor.*
2. *Circle the correct spelling of the medical term.*
3. *Match the correctly spelled terms to the brief descriptions below.*
4. *Write a sentence for each of the 10 terms that appear in this exercise.*

A. SPELLING COMPREHENSION: CIRCLE THE CORRECT SPELLING OF THE TERM.

1. tetrailogy	tettrology	tetralogy	tedtrology	tidtrology
2. bullemia	bulimia	bulemia	buleemia	bulemea
3. jerontelogist	geronntologist	jerontologist	gerontologist	jirontologist
4. seenesence	cenescence	sinescence	ceniscence	senescence
5. purtusis	pertusis	pertussis	putussis	pertuses
6. rumination	rumenation	rummination	rimination	remination
7. hialine	hyline	hyaline	hilyne	hylene
8. innvolude	involute	involude	involede	invelute
9. deptheria	deeptheria	diphtheria	diptheria	dipteria
10. percentile	persentile	pircentile	pirsentile	persentiel

B. MATCH THE NUMBER OF THE CORRECT TERM IN PART A WITH THE BRIEF DESCRIPTION OF THE TERM BELOW.

a. Disease with leathery coating on the pharynx _____

b. Whooping cough _____

c. Decline associated with advanced age _____

d. Thin membrane in lung alveoli _____

e. To bring back food into the mouth to chew
over and over _____

f. A set of four congenital heart defects _____

g. Medical specialist for aged patient population _____

h. State of being old _____

i. Episodic bouts of eating and then throwing up _____

j. One of a hundred groups in a distribution of
variables _____

C. USING YOUR KNOWLEDGE OF TERMS 1–10 IN PART A AND THEIR CORRECT SPELLING, WRITE A BRIEF SENTENCE AS IT MIGHT APPEAR IN PATIENT DOCUMENTATION.

1. _____

2. _____

3. _____

4. _____

5. _____

6. _____

7. _____

8. _____

9. _____

10. _____

D. YOUR INSTRUCTOR WILL DIRECT YOU TO MCGRAW-HILL CONNECT. OPEN THE AUDIO GLOSSARY AND PRACTICE YOUR PRONUNCIATION OF THE TERMS IN PART A OF THIS EXERCISE.

E. EACH OF THE FOLLOWING SURGICAL PROCEDURES IS A REMOVAL OF SOME BODY PART. IDENTIFY WHAT IS REMOVED IN EACH SURGERY.

1. appendectomy _____

2. lymphadenectomy _____

3. nephrectomy _____

4. pneumonectomy _____

5. splenectomy _____

6. hysterectomy _____

7. ureterectomy _____

8. mastectomy _____

9. endarterectomy _____

10. cystectomy _____

11. myomectomy _____

12. cholecystectomy _____

13. vasectomy _____

14. prostatectomy _____

15. thymectomy _____

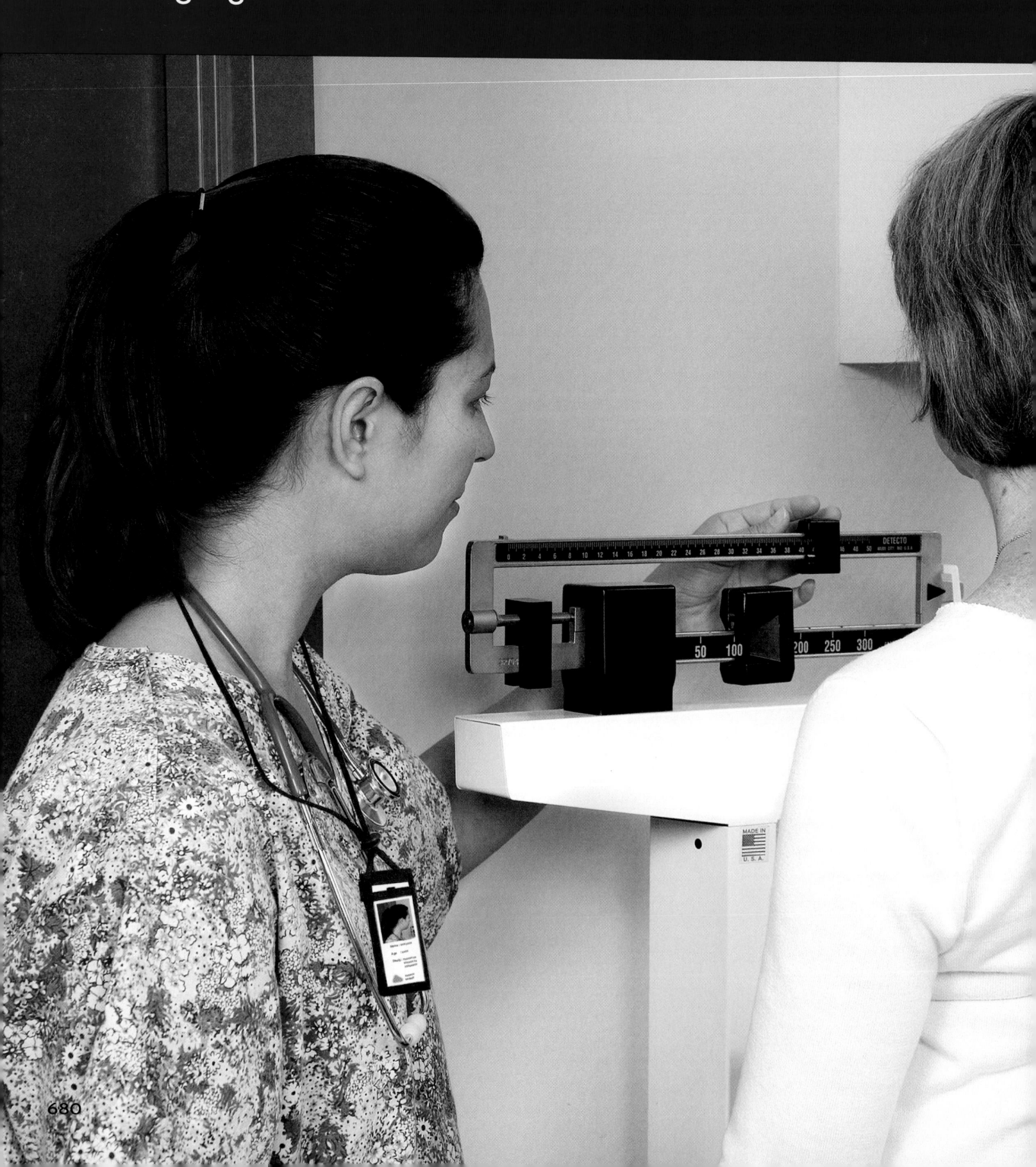

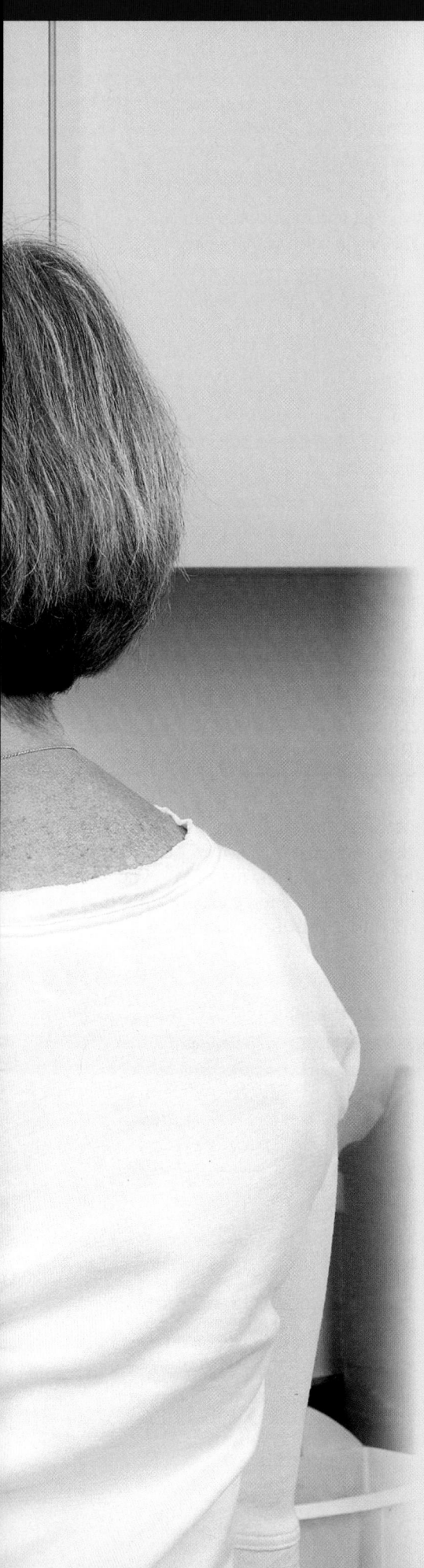

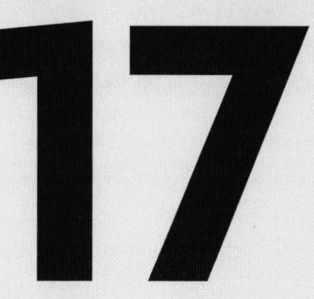
CASE REPORT 17.1

You are

. . . a **nutrition** assistant working with Karen Goodrich, MS, PhD, a **nutritionist** who provides guidance to patients referred from the different clinics at Fulwood Medical Center.

Your patient is

. . . Ms. Karen Johnson, a 20-year-old single woman, who is enrolled in a 6-month nursing assistant program. She is concerned about her weight (140 pounds, 5 feet 4 inches) and the nutritional lifestyle she should adopt. She has heard that she should be eating a high-carbohydrate **diet.** Her breakfast is a bowl of cereal with skim milk. For lunch, Ms. Johnson brown-bags a turkey sandwich with white bread, lettuce, tomato, and mustard and an 8-ounce bottle of apple juice. Dinner is either a frozen dinner entrée or pasta with a packaged marinara sauce. She snacks on fat-free yogurt and low-fat cookies. Once a week she goes out with her boyfriend and has several light beers and nachos.

Learning Outcomes

To be able to provide optimal care and communicate with your patient, other health care professionals, dieticians, and nutritionists, you need to be able to:

17.1 Apply the language of nutrition to the form, function, metabolism, and well-being of the cells, tissues, and organs of the body.

17.2 Describe in correct medical terminology the different nutrients and their roles in cell metabolism.

17.3 Comprehend, analyze, spell, and write the language of nutrition so that you can communicate in writing and document accurately and precisely in any health care setting.

17.4 Recognize and pronounce the language of nutrition so that you can communicate verbally with accuracy and precision in any health care setting.

17.5 Explain the effects of a balanced diet and improper nutrition on health.

LESSON 17.1 Nutrients

OBJECTIVES

Nutrition is the taking in and use of food and other nourishing material by the body. It is a three-part process:

1. The food or drink is consumed **(ingested)** into the digestive system *(see Chapter 6).*
2. The food or drink is **digested** and broken down into **nutrients** that are **absorbed** from the digestive tract into the bloodstream.
3. The nutrients are **transported** by the bloodstream to cells all over the body to be used for energy, cell maintenance, reproduction, growth, and repair.

In *Chapter 6* (digestive system), you learned how different foods were digested, metabolized into nutrients, and absorbed into the bloodstream. The information in this lesson will enable you to use correct medical terminology to:

17.1.1 Define the term *Calorie* **and the sources of** *dietary* **calories.**
17.1.2 Identify the major groups of *nutrients* **and their functions.**
17.1.3 Describe the food sources of the nutrients.
17.1.4 Discuss the roles of dietary fiber.
17.1.5 Explain the effects of nutrients on body functions.

Keynote

The term **Calorie** in metabolism always has an uppercase "C" and represents 1000 calories (lowercase "c").

Abbreviations

AI	adequate intake
BMR	basal metabolic rate
g	gram
RDA	recommended dietary allowance

NUTRIENTS

The energy stored by most **nutrients** is taken and used by your body in cellular metabolism. The term **Calorie** is used to express the quantities of energy supplied by foods and to measure the energy needs of your body. Each **gram (g)** of carbohydrate yields 4 Calories of energy. Each gram of protein yields 4 Calories. Each gram of fat yields 9 Calories. This daily input of energy supplied by food should equal your body's metabolic expenditure of energy *(Table 17.1)*.

Basal metabolic rate (BMR) is the energy expended by your body when at rest. Total energy expenditure depends on the BMR, the energy expended for physical activity, and the energy expended in synthesizing reserves of energy such as glycogen, fat, and protein.

Exercise increases your **metabolic rate,** the total amount of energy produced and used by the body in a unit of time. Walking briskly will use 7 Calories per minute; jogging, 13 Calories per minute. If you jog for 40 minutes each day for a week, you can lose a pound of body fat. Exercise is the only component of energy expenditure that you can control. A combination of exercise and dietary control can modify weight.

TABLE 17.1 Caloric Needs per Day

	Caloric Range	
Children	**Sedentary**	**Active**
2–3 years	1000	1400
Females		
14–18	1800	2400
19–30	1800	2400
31–50	1500	2200
50 +	1500	2000
Males		
14–18	2200	3000
19–30	2400	3200
31–50	2200	3000
50 +	2000	2800

Based on U.S. Department of Agriculture (USDA), www.mypyramid.gov, 2005.

WORD	PRONUNCIATION	ELEMENTS		DEFINITION
absorption	ab-**SORP**-shun	S/ R/	-ion *action condition* absorpt- *take in*	Uptake of nutrients and water by cells in the GI tract
basal metabolic rate (BMR)	**BAY**-sal met-ah-**BOL**-ic RATE	S/ R/ S/ R/	-al *pertaining to* bas- *base* -ic *pertaining to* metabol- *change* rate Latin *a reckoning*	Energy the body requires to function at rest
Calorie caloric (adj)	**KAL**-oh-ree kah-**LOR**-ik	S/ R/	Latin *heat* -ic *pertaining to* calor- *heat*	An expression of the energy content of food; capitalize "C" always Pertaining to Calories
diet dietary dietetics dietician (alternative spelling: dietitian)	**DIE**-et **DIE**-et-ary die-eh-**TET**-iks die-eh-**TISH**-un	 S/ R/ S/ S/	Greek *a way of life* -ary *pertaining to* diet- *a way of life* -etics *pertaining to* -ician *expert*	Specific course of eating and drinking Pertaining to a diet Application of diet to prevention and treatment of disease Licensed professional in dietetics
nutrient nutritive (adj) nutrition nutritionist	**NYU**-tree-ent **NYU**-trih-tiv nyu-**TRISH**-un nyu-**TRISH**-un-ist	 S/ R/ S/ S/ R/	Latin *to nourish* -ive *nature of, pertaining to* nutrit- *nourishment* Latin *to nourish* -ion- *action, condition* -ist *specialist in* nutrit- *nourishment*	A substance in food required for normal physiologic function Providing nourishment The study of food and liquid requirements for normal function of the human body Certified professional in nutrition science

The intake of a nutrient that is sufficient to meet the daily needs of 97% of individuals in a specific age and gender group is called the **recommended dietary allowance (RDA)**. If there is insufficient information available to calculate an RDA, the nutrient is given a recommended value called its **adequate intake (AI)**.

The six groups of nutrients are carbohydrates, lipids, proteins, vitamins, minerals, and water (see the following sections of this chapter).

EXERCISES

Language of Nutrition: *This knowledge about nutrition and its specialized vocabulary will aid you in taking better care of your patients and provide you with an awareness of how to improve and maintain your own health. Apply correct medical terminology to fill in each blank.*

1. Nutrition is a three-part process. Briefly define each part.

   a. Ingestion: _____

   b. Digestion: _____

   c. Transportation: _____

2. The term _____ is used to express the quantities of energy supplied by foods and to measure the energy needs of your body.

3. _____ is the energy expended by the body when at rest.

4. Exercise increases _____ rate—the total amount of energy produced and used by the body in a unit of time.

5. The intake of a nutrient that is sufficient to meet the daily needs of 97% of individuals in a specific age and gender group is called the _____ or _____ (abbreviation).

CARBOHYDRATES

Carbohydrates vary from the complex starch in potatoes to the simple sugars of **glucose, fructose** (fruit sugar), and **sucrose** (table sugar). The simple sugars on their own have calories but no nutrient value. They are said to have **empty calories.**

Most carbohydrates are broken down to glucose, the major source of energy in cells.

Glycogen, the storage form of carbohydrate, is found in the liver and skeletal muscles. Glycogen in muscles supplies glucose during high-intensity and endurance exercise.

The leading sources of carbohydrate intake are bread, soft drinks, cookies, cakes and doughnuts, syrups, jams, and potatoes.

Artificial Sugars

Nutritive sweeteners is a term used for all of the sugars that provide energy as well as sweetness. **High-fructose corn syrup** is manufactured from cornstarch. It is used in many processed foods such as cookies, soft drinks, jam, and jelly. It is mostly fructose and is cheaper than sucrose. **Brown sugar** is sucrose with some **molasses. Maple syrup** is made by boiling down the sap of sugar maple trees. **Honey** is plant nectar broken down by bee enzymes into fructose and glucose. It offers only the same nutritional value as that of the other sugars.

Alternative or **artificial sweeteners** provide no energy, only sweetness *(Table 17.2).* Six are currently available in the United States:

- **Saccharin,** no longer considered a potential cause of cancer, is used in diet drinks.
- **Aspartame,** sold as Nutrasweet and Equal, is used in diet beverages, gelatin desserts, chewing gum, and toppings and fillings in bakery goods and cookies. Because aspartame is made from **phenylalanine,** people with **phenylketonuria (PKU)** *(see Chapter 21)* must avoid it.
- **Neotame** is also a phenylalanine derivative that is heat-stable and can be found in cooked products, as well as soft drinks and chewing gum.
- **Acesulfame-K** is heat-stable and is found in many baked goods.
- **Sucralose** is derived from sucrose, is heat-stable, and is used in baked goods, ice creams, and juices and for tabletop use as Splenda.
- **Stevia** is a herb that is sold as a diet supplement. It is heat-stable and can be used in cooking but does not add texture to food.

TABLE 17.2 Relative Sweetness

Substance	Sweetness Compared to Sucrose
Sucrose (table sugar)	1
Saccharin	300 ×
Aspartame	180–200 ×
Neotame	7,000–13,000 ×
Acesulfame-K	200 ×
Sucralose	600 ×
Stevia	150–400 ×

Keynote

- Baked potato (without sour cream) contains 51 g of carbohydrate.
- 12-ounce cola drink contains 39 g.
- One teaspoon of sugar contains 5 g.

Keynote

The RDA of carbohydrates is 130 grams per day for an adult. Most North Americans consume 180 to 300 g/day.

Keynote

Sugar alcohols, for example, **sorbitol,** provide energy (3 Calories/g), are absorbed more slowly than sucrose, and are metabolized to glucose. They are used in sugarless gum, breath mints, and candy.

Abbreviation

PKU   phenylketonuria

WORD	PRONUNCIATION		ELEMENTS	DEFINITION
carbohydrate	kar-boh-**HIGH**-drate	S/ R/CF R/	-ate *composed of* **carb/o-** *carbon* **-hydr-** *water*	Any of a group of organic food compounds that includes sugars, starch, glycogen, and cellulose
fructose	**FRUK**-toes	S/ R/	-ose *full of* **fruct-** *fruit*	Sugar found in fruits and honey
glucose	**GLU**-kose	S/ R/	-ose *full of* **gluc-** *sugar, glucose*	The final product of carbohydrate digestion and the main sugar in the blood
glycogen	**GLYE**-koh-jen	S/ R/CF	-gen *to produce* **glyc/o-** *glycogen*	The body's principal carbohydrate reserve, stored in the liver and skeletal muscle
molasses	mo-**LASS**-iz		Latin *honeylike*	Dark-colored syrup produced during the refining of sugar
phenylalanine	fen-il-**AL**-ah-neen	R/ R/	**phenyl-** *chemical group* **-alanine** *protein synthesized in muscle*	An amino acid
phenylketonuria	**FEN**-il-**KEE**-toe-**NYU**-ree-ah	S/ R/ R/	-uria *urine* **phenyl-** *chemical group* **-keton-** *ketone*	Hereditary disease with accumulation of phenylalanine and urinary excretion of its metabolites; leads to mental retardation if not controlled
sorbitol	**SOR**-bih-tol	S/ R/	-ol *alcohol* **sorbit-** *fruit of a tree*	Alcohol derivative of glucose
sucrose	**SUE**-krose	S/ R/	-ose *full of* **sucr-** *sucrose, table sugar*	Table sugar
sugar	**SHUH**-gar		Latin *sugar*	Basic carbohydrate; term sometimes used for glucose or sucrose

EXERCISES

Deconstruct *the following medical terms into their basic elements. Write the meaning of the medical term in the last column. Remember to answer the question following the table.*

Medical Term	Root/CF	Suffix	Meaning of Medical Term
phenylketonuria			
carbohydrate			
phenylalanine			
sorbitol			

What is one important fact about carbohydrates that you did not know until you read this lesson? _____

_____

CARBOHYDRATES (continued)

Fiber

Fiber consists of complex carbohydrates that cannot be broken down by the human digestive process. These carbohydrates are dietary fiber. It is undigested as it leaves the small intestine to enter the colon, where it provides bulk and softness for the stool. Whole grains have their outer covering intact and are a good source of dietary fiber, some vitamins, and magnesium.

Water-soluble dietary fiber, including pectin and gum, slows glucose absorption from the small intestine, of value to diabetics and overweight people. It also inhibits absorption of cholesterol, reducing the risk of cardiovascular disease and gallstones. Fruits, vegetables, and beans in general are rich sources of soluble fiber.

Functional fibers are those that can be added to foods. They are plant-based compounds such as **cellulose, pectins,** and gums. Some of these fibers are soluble and are fermented by bacteria in the large intestine to produce gases such as methane.

The AI for fiber is 25 g/day for women and 38 g/day for men. In North America, the average intake is about half these figures.

Lack of fiber in the diet can lead to small, hard stools and constipation. Excessive pressure may be needed for defecation. This high pressure developed in the colon can force parts of the colon wall out between the bands of muscle, producing pouches called diverticula and the asymptomatic disorder called diverticulosis *(see page 246)*. If the diverticula stay filled with feces, they can become inflamed and painful, a condition called diverticulitis *(see page 246)*.

Choice of Carbohydrates

Simple sugars provide calories but have no nutritional value. Overcrowding the diet with sugar can mean that foods such as fruits and vegetables, which are dense in nutrients, are left out. Foods that are advertised as low-fat and fat-free usually contain lots of added sugar to produce an acceptable taste.

Simple sugars are absorbed rapidly and converted into blood glucose. This rapid blood glucose response is called a high **glycemic index (GI)** and results in a high **glycemic load (GL)** in the body. These high-glycemic-load carbohydrates generate a high insulin output from the pancreas *(see page 586)*. A persistent high insulin output produces numerous ill effects on the body:

- Increased **fat deposits** in adipose tissue.
- Increased **fat synthesis** in the liver.
- High **low-density lipoprotein (LDL)**—"bad cholesterol"—levels and high triglycerides *(see Chapter 6)*.
- Rapid return of **hunger** after a meal.

Complex carbohydrates with a **starch** structure and fiber content are absorbed much more slowly and have a lower glycemic index. Glucose is given a glycemic index of 100. Low GI foods are below 55 and should be chosen when possible. High GI foods are over 70 and should be chosen in minimal quantities, if at all. A glycemic load of 20 is high and 10 or below is low *(Table 17.3)*.

Abbreviations

GI	glycemic index
GL	glycemic load
LDL	low-density lipoprotein

Case Report 17.1 *(continued)*

Your training as a nutrition assistant tells you that, from the carbohydrate perspective, Karen Johnson's diet is lacking in fruits and vegetables, and this affects her fiber intake. Also, her bread should be changed to whole grain to increase her fiber. Her snacks of fat-free yogurt and low-fat cookies will have added simple sugars and will generate a high glycemic load. The snacks should be replaced by fresh produce, such as apples and other fruits and any raw vegetables that she enjoys.

WORD	PRONUNCIATION	ELEMENTS		DEFINITION
cellulose	**SELL**-you-lohse	S/ R/	-ose *full of* cellul- *small cell*	Major constituent of cell walls of plants
fiber	**FIE**-ber		Latin *fiber*	Carbohydrate not digested by intestinal enzymes; or a strand or filament
glycemic index	glye-**SEE**-mic **IN**-deks	S/ R/ R/	-emic *in the blood* glyc- *glycogen* index *to declare*	Measure of the rapidity in rise of blood glucose after ingestion of carbohydrates
glycemic load	glye-**SEE**-mic LOHD	R/	load *to carry*	System that takes into account the amount of sugar available in the food to cause the rise in blood sugar
pectin	**PEK**-tin		Greek *to make solid*	Plant fiber with the ability to thicken and solidify to a gel
starch	STARCH		Anglo-Saxon *stiffen*	Complex carbohydrate made of multiple units of glucose attached together

TABLE 17.3 Glycemic Index and Glycemic Load of Foods

Food	Glycemic Index	Glycemic Load
Glucose	100	50
Potato (baked)	85	26
Honey	73	10
Cheerios	74	15
White rice	72	23
Bread (white or whole grain), bagel	70	10
Coca-Cola	63	16
Carrots	49	3
Apple	38	6
Milk (skim)	32	4
Lentils	30	5
Peanuts	14	2

EXERCISES

After reading Case Report 17.1 on the opposite page, answer the following questions. Be prepared to discuss your answers in class.

1. What is the major function of fiber in the body? _____

2. What types of foods will increase Karen Johnson's fiber intake? _____

_____

3. What is *water-soluble dietary fiber,* and what is its function in the body?

_____

4. What are the results of lack of fiber in the body? _____

_____

5. Briefly explain the difference between *glycemic index* and *glycemic load.*

_____

_____

TABLE 17.4 Foods with High Saturated-Fat Content

Food Item and Amount	Fat (grams)	Saturated Fat (grams)
T-bone steak, 6 oz.	34.0	14.0
Hamburger, 4 oz.	20.0	8.0
Peanuts, oil roasted, ½ cup	35.7	5.0
Doughnut, plain, 1	13.0	3.0

Abbreviations

EFA	essential fatty acid
HDL	high-density lipoprotein
LDL	low-density lipoprotein
omega-3	alpha-linolenic acid
omega-6	linolenic acid

Keynote

Two-thirds of your body cholesterol is made by your cells, and the remaining one-third is derived from your diet. Plant foods do not contain cholesterol.

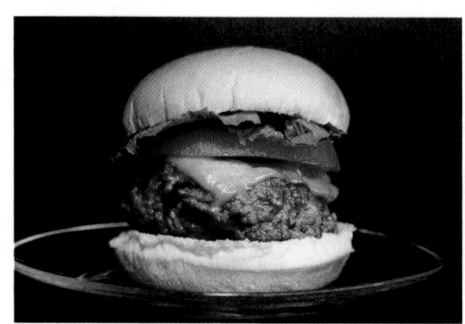

▲ **FIGURE 17.1 Tastes Great but High in Saturated Fat.**

LIPIDS

Lipids that are solid at room temperature are called **fats**; for example, the solid fat around an uncooked steak. Lipids that are liquid are called **oils.** Lipids do not dissolve in water. For example, the oil in an oil and vinegar salad dressing will not mix with the water-based vinegar.

Triglycerides account for 95% of the fat in the human diet and have three main categories:

- **Saturated fats** or **fatty acids** are found in meats, dairy products (milk, cheese, butter), and eggs. These are solid at room temperature.
- **Unsaturated fats** or **fatty acids** are found mostly in oils such as olive, peanut, safflower, and canola oil. These are liquid at room temperature.
- **Hydrogenated trans fatty acids** are formed commercially by partial hydrogenation of unsaturated vegetable oils to make them solid or semisolid. Trans fatty acids are found in margarine, shortenings, pie crusts, crackers, croissants, and French fries. The labeling of the content of trans fatty acids in food is required. They raise **LDL** levels, lower **high-density lipoprotein (HDL)** levels *(see Chapter 8)*, and have no role in maintaining body health. They should be avoided as much as possible. Some cities and states are banning their use.

Essential fatty acids (EFAs) are so-called because the body cannot synthesize them and they must be ingested. **Linolenic acid (omega-6)** and **alpha-linolenic acid (omega-3)** are essential fatty acids, which have important roles in cell structure and immune system function. The EFAs are found in plant oils or fatty fish such as salmon, tuna, and sardines.

Cholesterol is a steroid characterized as a lipid because it does not dissolve in water. Cholesterol has the following functions:

- Forms part of hormones (such as estrogen and testosterone) and active vitamin D.
- Precursor of bile acids, which are essential for fat digestion *(see Chapter 6)*.
- An essential component of cell membranes.
- An essential component of the LDL and HDL particles that transport lipids in the blood *(see Chapter 8)*.

Fat Intake

There are no RDAs for fat intake for adults. Most authorities recommend that fat intake should be between 30% and 35% of energy intake, with minimal trans-fat and saturated-fat intake *(Table 17.4)*. Omega-3 and omega-6 fatty acids should be included in the diet. For a person on a 2000-Calorie diet, this would involve 600 to 700 Calories coming from fat. At 9 Calories/g, this means eating 65 to 80 g of fat per day.

Combining these concepts with what you have learned about carbohydrates, a good diet plan could emphasize vegetables, fruits, plant oils, and whole grains; use fish, poultry, eggs, and dairy products daily but sparingly; and avoid red meats, white rice, white bread, potatoes, pasta, and sweets *(Figure 17.1)*.

Case Report 17.1 (continued)

As a nutrition assistant, you would advise Karen Johnson to avoid nachos, which contain saturated fats and lots of calories, and the processed frozen dinner, which probably contains trans fats.

WORD	PRONUNCIATION		ELEMENTS	DEFINITION
cholesterol	koh-**LESS**-ter-ol	S/ R/CF	-sterol *steroid* chol/e- *bile*	Substance formed in liver cells; it is the most abundant steroid in tissues and it circulates in the plasma attached to proteins of different densities
fat fatty acid	FAT **FAT**-ee **ASS**-id		Old English *fat*	Lipid that is solid at room temperature An acid obtained from the hydrolysis of fats
hydrogenated	**HIGH**-droh-jeh-**NAY**-ted	S/ S/ R/CF	-ated *composed of, process* -gen- *produce* hydr/o- *water*	Addition of hydrogen to unsaturated oils to solidify them and produce trans fats
lipid	**LIP**-id		Greek *fat*	General term for all types of fatty compounds; for example, cholesterol, triglycerides, and fatty acids
saturated fatty acid	satch-you-**RAY**-ted **FAT**-ee **ASS**-id	S/ R/	-ated *composed of, process* satur- *to fill*	Substance that is incapable of absorbing any more hydrogen, and is solid at room temperature
trans fatty acid	TRANZ **FAT**-ee **ASS**-id		**trans** Latin *through, across*	Solid or semisolid product of hydrogenation of unsaturated plant oils
triglyceride	tri-**GLISS**-eh-ride	S/ P/ R/	-ide *having a particular quality* tri- *three* -glycer- *glycerol, sweet*	Substance with three fatty acids
unsaturated fatty acid	un-**SATCH**-you-ray-ted **FAT**-ee **ASS**-id	S/ P/ R/	-ated *composed of, process* un- *not* -satur- *to fill*	Found mostly in oils and is liquid at room temperature

EXERCISES

Elements are the key to learning medical terminology. Build your knowledge of elements with this exercise. Match the meaning in the left column with the correct element in the right column.

_____ 1. three   A. chol/e

_____ 2. not   B. gen

_____ 3. composed of, process   C. sterol

_____ 4. water   D. glycer

_____ 5. through, across   E. satur

_____ 6. sweet   F. tri

_____ 7. produce   G. trans

_____ 8. steroid   H. hydro

_____ 9. to fill   I. un

_____ 10. bile   J. ated

Proteins are essential for health. **Amino acids** are the building blocks of proteins and help build and repair tissue. They consist of carbon linked to nitrogen. Twenty different amino acids are divided into two groups:

1. **Essential amino acids,** which the body cannot **synthesize** and therefore have to be obtained in the diet.
2. **Nonessential amino acids,** which the body can synthesize from other molecules.

A **complete protein food** contains all **nine** essential amino acids. Examples are meat, fish, poultry, cheese, and eggs. **Incomplete protein foods** do not contain all nine essential amino acids. Examples are grains, leafy green vegetables, and **legumes** (beans and peas). A variety of plant proteins have to be consumed to obtain the different essential amino acids.

Proteins perform numerous functions in the body:

- **Collagen** provides structural strength in connective tissue *(see Chapter 5)*.
- **Keratin** provides structural strength in skin *(see Chapter 3)*.
- **Hormones** regulate physiologic processes by communicating between cells *(see Chapter 14)*.
- **Enzymes** regulate the rate of chemical reactions and function as catalysts *(see Chapter 6)*.
- **Hemoglobin** transports oxygen and carbon dioxide in the blood *(see Chapter 7)*.
- **Antibodies, complement, and lymphokines** are essential components of the immune system *(see Chapter 15)*.
- **Proteins transport** other molecules outside the cell, through the cell membrane, and inside the cell.
- **Proteins bind** cells to each other to keep tissues from falling apart and enable immune cells to bind to cancer cells.

TABLE 17.5 Food Sources of Protein

Food Item and Amount	Protein (Grams)
Roast beef, 3.5 oz.	28.0
Fish, 3.5 oz.	21.0
Hamburger, 3.5 oz.	20.0
Peanut butter, 2 tablespoons	10.0
Baked potato, 8 oz.	9.0
Whole milk, 8 oz.	8.0
Peanuts, 1 oz.	7.3
Cheddar cheese, 1 oz.	7.0
Egg, 1	6.0
Oatmeal, cooked, 1 cup	6.0
Natural cereal, ½ cup	4.0
Whole-grain bread, 1 slice	2.6
Raw vegetables, ½ cup	2.6

Keynote

Proteins form the major part of lean body tissue, about 17% of body weight.

Keynote

There are nine essential amino acids.

Keynote

Proteins are a source of energy, providing 4 Calories per gram.

Keynote

Excess protein is turned into glucose or fat and used for energy or stored in adipose tissue.

WORD	PRONUNCIATION	ELEMENTS		DEFINITION
amino acid	ah-**ME**-no **ASS**-id	R/CF	**amin/o** *nitrogen compound*	The basic building block for protein
complete	kom-**PLEET**	P/ R/	**com-** *with, together* **-plete** *filled*	Whole, entire, total
essential nonessential	eh-**SEN**-shal **NON**-ee-**SEN**-shal	S/ R/ P/	**-ial** *pertaining to* **essent-** *existence* **non-** *not*	Required, amino acids that cannot be synthesized by the body Not required, as amino acids that can be synthesized by the body
incomplete (***Note:*** This word has two prefixes.)	in-kom-**PLEET**	P/ P/ R/	**in-** *not* **-com-** *with, together* **-plete** *filled*	Lacking some part
legume	**LEG**-yoom		Latin *plant with seedpods*	Family of plants including peas, beans, and lentils
protein	**PRO**-teen	S/ R/CF	**-in** *chemical compound* **prot/e-** *first*	Class of food substances based on amino acids
synthesis synthesize (verb)	**SIN**-the-sis **SIN**-the-size	P/ R/	**syn-** *together* **-thesis** *arrange, place*	The process of building a compound from different elements

Protein Intake

The RDA for protein intake is expressed as 0.8 g of protein per kilogram of body weight. This works out to about 56 g of protein per day for a person weighing 154 pounds and 46 g of protein for a person weighing 125 pounds. North American men consume about 95 g of protein daily, and women consume about 65 g daily.

Pregnant women require an extra 10 g of protein daily; lactating women, an extra 15 g.

For most North Americans, 70% of protein comes from animal sources. Vegetable sources of protein include soy, nuts, and legumes *(Table 17.5)*. They contain no cholesterol and little saturated fat, and legumes contain soluble fiber.

EXERCISES

Lesson Objective: *Meet the lesson objective and relate medical vocabulary to function by matching the correct medical terminology in the left column with the correct function in the right column.*

_____ 1. hemoglobin

_____ 2. hormones

_____ 3. enzymes

_____ 4. antibodies

_____ 5. keratin

_____ 6. collagen

_____ 7. proteins

A. enable immune cells to bind to cancer cells

B. provides structural strength in skin

C. components of the immune system

D. provides structural strength in tissue

E. regulate physiologic processes

F. transports O_2 and CO_2 in blood

G. regulate chemical reactions

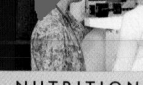

LESSON 17.2 Vitamins and Minerals

OBJECTIVES

Neither vitamins nor minerals are used as fuel to provide calories, but both are essential to our ability to use the other nutrients and are needed only in small quantities. The information in this lesson will enable you to use correct medical terminology to:

17.2.1 Identify the major vitamins and minerals needed by the body.

17.2.2 Describe the sources and functions of the major vitamins and minerals.

17.2.3 Explain the sources and functions of trace minerals.

17.2.4 Use correct medical terminology to describe the effects of vitamins and minerals on body functions.

Keynote

Only vitamin D and niacin can be synthesized by the body—but in inadequate amounts. Therefore, all vitamins have to be acquired in the diet or through supplements.

Abbreviations

IU	international unit
µg	microgram, one-millionth of a gram

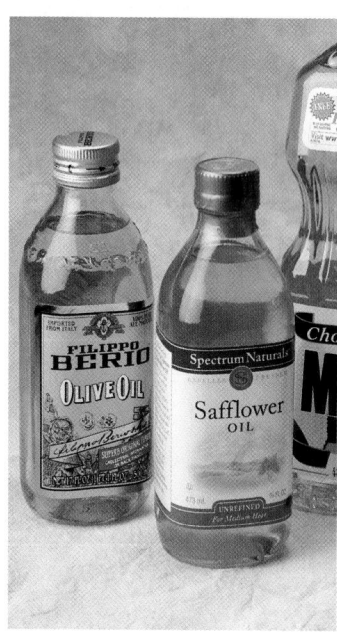

▲ **FIGURE 17.2 Plant Oils Are Rich Sources of Vitamin E.**

VITAMINS

Vitamins are **organic** (carbon-containing) substances that are essential in small amounts for the normal function of cells. Both plant and animal foods supply vitamins. Vitamins synthesized in the laboratory are no different from natural vitamins, except for vitamin E, which is twice as potent in its natural form.

Water-soluble vitamins are vitamin C and the B vitamins.

Fat-soluble vitamins do not dissolve in water and are vitamins A, D, E, and K.

Some of the vitamins in foods can be lost during transport from the field to the store, and cooking in water can remove more. The least contact with water and as short a cooking time as possible preserves more nutrients and vitamins.

Vegetables and fruits frozen soon after picking contain as many nutrients and vitamins as fresh supermarket produce.

FAT-SOLUBLE VITAMINS

Vitamin E

Vitamin E functions as an efficient **antioxidant,** preventing the propagation of cell-damaging chain reactions caused by **free radicals**. There is widespread scientific agreement that adequate quantities of fruits and vegetables help to lower the incidence of cancer and cardiovascular disease. It has not yet been proved that this effect is due to antioxidants.

Vitamin E deficiency can occur in premature newborns because only small amounts cross the placenta. Premature newborns can develop anemia and bleeding into the brain and retina. Deficiency is rare among older children and adults.

Excess vitamin E can lead to hemorrhagic stroke, particularly in people taking the anticoagulant Coumadin (warfarin) *(see Chapter 7)*.

Sources of vitamin E are plant oils (e.g., corn, safflower, soybean), asparagus, peanuts, oatmeal, nuts, and seeds (e.g., sunflower seeds) *(Figure 17.2)*. The RDA for vitamin E is 15 mg/day for men and women. This is equivalent to 22 **international units (IUs)** of a natural source and 33 IU of a **synthetic** source. Two tablespoons of chunky peanut butter contain 3.6 IU of vitamin E.

WORD	PRONUNCIATION	ELEMENTS		DEFINITION
antioxidant	an-tee-**OKS**-ih-dant	S/ P/ R/	-ant *forming* anti- *against* -oxid- *oxidize*	Substance that can prevent cell damage by neutralizing free radicals
free radical	FREE **RAD**-ih-kal	R/ S/ R/	free *free* -al *pertaining to* radic- *root*	Short-lived product of oxidation in a cell that can be damaging to the cell
mineral	**MIN**-er-al	S/ R/	-al *pertaining to* miner- *mines*	Inorganic compound usually found in earth's crust
organic	or-**GAN**-ik		Greek *organ*	Compound with carbon atoms; food produced without using chemicals
synthetic	sin-**THET**-ik	S/ P/ R/	-ic *pertaining to* syn- *together* -thet- *place, arrange*	Built up or put together from simpler compounds
vitamin	**VYE**-tah-min	R/ R/	vit- *life* -amin *nitrogen containing*	Essential organic substance necessary in small amounts for normal cell function

Vitamin K

Vitamin K is essential for blood clotting and is required for the synthesis of the clotting factors by the liver *(see Chapter 7)*. One example is the formation of prothrombin. Sources of vitamin K are liver, green leafy vegetables, salad greens *(Figure 17.3)*, broccoli, peas, green beans, and vegetable oils. The AI is 90 μg/day for women and 120 μg/day for men. One-half cup cooked green beans contains 49 μg of vitamin K.

Vitamin K deficiency can occur in newborns, and vitamin K is given routinely by injection within 6 hours of birth. Deficiency can also occur in patients taking antibiotics for a long period of time.

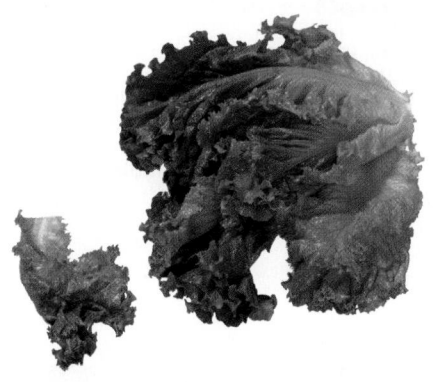

▲ **FIGURE 17.3 Salad Greens.** A salad containing dark greens (or other green vegetables) each day provides abundant vitamin K for a diet.

EXERCISES

*Build more knowledge of the **language of nutrition**. Answers to all the questions can be found on these two pages. Circle the best answer.*

1. Preventing the propagation of cell-damaging chain reactions caused by free radicals is the function of an:
   a. antibiotic
   b. antiemetic
   c. anticonvulsant
   d. antioxidant
   e. anticoagulant

2. Vitamins are supplied by:
   a. plant foods
   b. water
   c. animal foods
   d. only a and c
   e. a, b, and c

3. Which of these will help preserve more of the vitamins in food:
   a. quicker transportation from field to store
   b. shorter cooking time
   c. less contact with water
   d. all of these
   e. only a and b

4. Vitamin K is essential for:
   a. digestion
   b. higher RBC count
   c. blood clotting
   d. strong bones
   e. smoother skin

5. The water-soluble vitamins are:
   a. A
   b. B vitamins
   c. C
   d. all of these
   e. only b and c

6. Name one source of vitamin K:
   a. milk
   b. cheese
   c. liver
   d. nuts
   e. oatmeal

Vitamin A

Vitamin A is found in two forms.

1. **Carotenoids** are vitamin A precursors and produce the yellow-orange pigment in fruits and vegetables. Carotenoids are also found in green vegetables and fruits *(Figure 17.4)*. **Beta carotene** can be converted to vitamin A and provides the skin with some protection from ultraviolet light damage. **Lutein** and **zeaxanthin,** the yellow pigment in corn, appear to delay the age-related eye diseases macular degeneration and cataracts *(see Chapter 4)*. **Lycopene,** the red pigment in tomatoes, provides some protection against prostate cancer *(see Chapter 12)*. Carotenoids also act as antioxidants *(see Vitamin E)*.

2. **Retinoids** are preformed vitamin A and are found in liver, egg yolk, butter, fish oils, and fortified milk. Vitamin A is needed by the retina to change visual light into nerve signals to the brain and to maintain the cell types in the retina, cornea, and epithelium of the eye. It is also necessary for the function of epithelial cells in the lungs, trachea, gastrointestinal tract, and skin. Because of its effect on skin, forms of **retinoic acid,** such as Retin-A, are used to treat skin damage.

Vitamin A deficiency can lead to impaired dark adaptation and night blindness and to growth retardation in children.

Vitamin D

Skin cells can synthesize vitamin D with exposure to sunlight. This can provide 90% of your needs, except in winter in northern climates and in elderly people when aging decreases production. The most active form of vitamin D is called **calcitriol,** a potent hormone that raises blood calcium concentration.

Dietary sources of vitamin D include fatty fish (such as salmon and sardines), fish oils, and fortified milk. Eight ounces of fortified milk contains 99 IU of vitamin D.

The AI of vitamin D for adults is 200 IU per day; this increases to 400 IU per day for those over 50 years. Infants are born with sufficient vitamin D to last about 6 months, at which time a breastfed infant should be exposed to sunlight or given a vitamin D supplement. Breast milk does not come fortified with vitamin D.

Vitamin D's functions relate primarily to calcium and phosphorus metabolism to:

- Increase **intestinal absorption of calcium** from foods; this makes calcium available for incorporation into bones and teeth.

- **Release calcium from bone** if blood calcium levels are low.

- **Maintain the function of neuromuscular junctions.**

Vitamin D deficiency leads to inadequate calcium and phosphorus deposition in bone. In children, this causes **rickets,** in which the weakened leg bones bow under weight-bearing pressure *(Figure 17.5)* and the pelvis is deformed. In adults, this disease is called **osteomalacia.** This is different from osteoporosis, in which the rate of bone resorption exceeds the rate of bone formation and the bones are liable to fracture *(see Chapter 5)*.

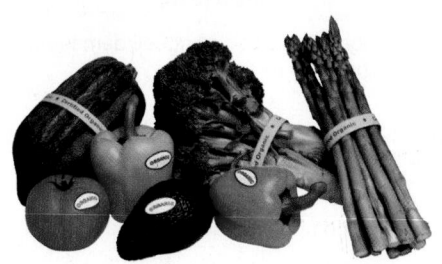

▲ **FIGURE 17.4 Carotenoids Are Vitamin A Precursors.** Many vegetables, such as asparagus and broccoli, are rich in carotenoids.

Keynote

Infants who drink too much carrot juice or eat too much winter squash can turn a yellow-orange color due to high carotenoid deposition in the skin. This **hypercarotenemia** can be mistaken for the **hyperbilirubinemia** of jaundice.

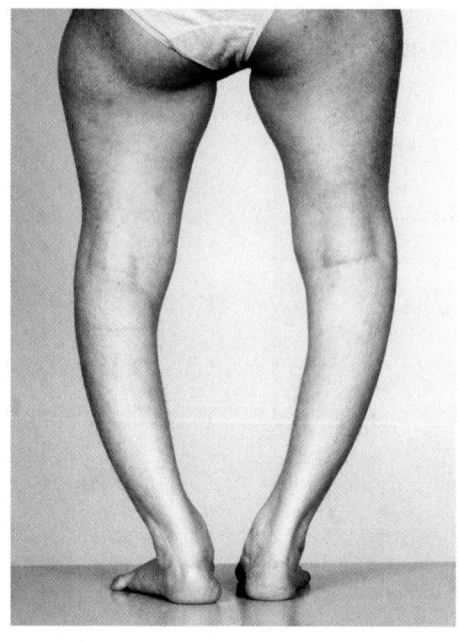

▲ **FIGURE 17.5 Bowed Legs of Rickets.**

WORD ANALYSIS AND DEFINITION

S = Suffix   P = Prefix   R = Root   R/CF = Combining Form

WORD	PRONUNCIATION	ELEMENTS		DEFINITION
beta carotene	BAY-tah KAR-oh-teen	R/ R/CF	beta *second letter of Greek alphabet* caroten/e *yellow-red pigment*	Yellow-red pigment in fruits and vegetables
calcitriol (*Note:* The prefix **tri-** relates to the chemical substance.)	KAL-sih-TRY-ol	S/ P/ R/CF	-ol *chemical substance* -tri- *three* calc/i- *calcium*	Potent form of vitamin D that acts as a hormone
carotenoid	kah-ROT-en-oyd	S/ R/	-oid *resemble* caroten- *yellow-red pigment*	Organic pigment occurring naturally in plants
hypercarotenemia (*Note:* The final "e" in -carotene is dropped for easier flow and pronunciation.)	HIGH-per-KAR-o-teh-NEE-me-ah	S/ P/ R/	-emia *blood condition* hyper- *above, excessive* -caroten- *yellow-red pigment*	Excessive level of the yellow-red pigment carotene in the blood
lutein	LOO-tee-in		Latin *saffron yellow*	Yellow pigment
lycopene	LIE-koh-peen		Latin *tomato*	Carotenoid that gives tomatoes their red color
retinoid	RET-ih-noyd	S/ R/	-oid *resembling* retin- *resin*	A class of keratolytic agents
retinoic acid	ret-ih-NO-ik ASS-id	S/ R/CF	-ic *pertaining to* retin/o- *resin*	A compound derived from vitamin A and used topically to treat acne
rickets	RICK-ets		Old English *to twist*	Disease due to vitamin D deficiency, producing soft, flexible bones
zeaxanthin	ZEE-ah-ZAN-thin	S/ P/ R/	-in *chemical compound* zea- *to live* -xanth- *yellow*	Carotenoid found in pepper, corn, and spinach

EXERCISES

Identify the correct nutritional vocabulary on the basis of the clues given. After you have identified the term, deconstruct the term into its elements; then answer the questions. Fill in the blanks.

1. Carotenoid found in pepper, corn, spinach _____ / _____ / _____

2. Organic pigment found naturally in plants _____ / _____ / _____

3. Excessive level of carotene in the blood _____ / _____ / _____

4. Yellow-red pigment in fruits and vegetables _____ / _____ / _____

5. A class of keratolytic agents _____ / _____ / _____

6. Potent form of vitamin D that acts as a hormone _____ / _____ / _____

7. List any term that could be a diagnosis: _____

8. List any term that contains elements meaning a color: _____

9. List any term with an element that means a number: _____

Vitamin C

All fruits and vegetables contain some vitamin C, but citrus fruits, green vegetables, and potatoes are very good sources *(Figure 17.8)*. Vitamin C is easily destroyed in cooking and processing.

Vitamin C **(ascorbic acid)** is involved:

- In collagen synthesis to provide strength to connective tissue and bone.
- In wound healing.
- In moving fatty acids from cell cytoplasm to mitochondria for energy production.
- In increasing iron absorption.
- As an antioxidant. Vitamin C is found in high concentrations in the eye and in white blood cells to protect against free radicals.

The RDA for vitamin C is 90 mg/day in men and 75 mg/day in women. There is no agreement on whether higher doses of vitamin C are of value in preventing and treating colds and other illnesses. One fresh orange provides 70 mg of vitamin C.

Vitamin C deficiency interferes with the formation of collagen and affects connective tissues all over the body, producing **scurvy.** Pinpoint hemorrhages around hair follicles and bleeding gums are the characteristic signs, together with bone and joint pain and impaired wound healing. The risk factors for developing scurvy today are poverty, alcoholism, drug addiction, and cigarette smoking.

Phytochemicals protect plants from external stressors such as heat, drought, and insects. For humans, they are nonnutritive chemicals that can protect against diseases. Phytochemicals in fruits and vegetables include:

- **Antioxidants** like the carotenoids and **allyl sulfides** (found in garlic, onions, leeks).
- **Polyphenols** (found in grapes and tea), which can reduce the risk of cardiovascular disease.
- **Isoflavones** (found in soy), which can imitate estrogens.
- **Indoles** (found in cabbages), which can help reduce the risk of breast cancer.
- **Saponins** (found in beans), which can reduce the multiplication of cancer cells.

Choline, while not a vitamin, is an essential nutrient as a precursor for **acetylcholine,** a neurotransmitter associated with learning, memory, and muscle control *(see Chapter 10)*. Choline is found in many foods. Milk, eggs, and peanuts are rich sources.

Water

Water has no caloric value. It constitutes about 60% of body weight (about 10 gallons). You can survive 6 to 8 weeks without food but only a few days without water. This is because water is an integral part of tissues but is not stored in a particular place from where it can be released.

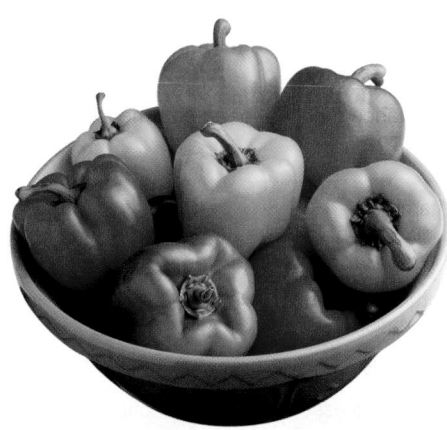

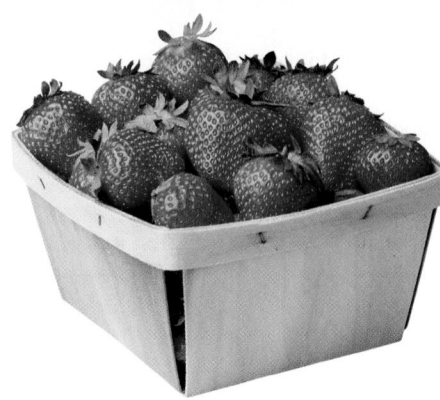

▲ **FIGURE 17.8 Sources of Vitamin C.**
Vegetables such as green peppers are a good source of vitamin C, and fruits such as strawberries are another good source.

Keynote

The Food and Nutrition Board of the **IOM** recommends an AI of water of 3.7 liters (quarts) per day for adult males and 2.7 liters (quarts) for adult females.

Abbreviation

IOM Institute of Medicine

Case Report 17.1 (continued)

As a nutrition assistant, you could advise Ms. Johnson to increase her intake of vegetables (especially greens) and fruits to supply vitamins A, K, folate, and C; to add nuts and seeds to her snacks to supply vitamin E; to add oranges and grapefruit to supply more vitamin C; and to eat salmon or other fatty fish once or twice a week to supply vitamin D.

WORD ANALYSIS AND DEFINITION

WORD	PRONUNCIATION	ELEMENTS		DEFINITION
allyl sulfides	**AL**-il **SUL**-fides	S/ R/ S/ R/	-yl *substance* all- *strange, other* -ide *having a particular quality* sulf- *sulfur*	Group of substances found in garlic and onions that can reduce blood cholesterol
ascorbic acid	as-**KOR**-bic **ASS**-id	S/ P/ R/	-ic *pertaining to* a- *without* -scorb- *scurvy*	Vitamin C, which prevents scurvy
choline	**KOH**-leen	S/ R/	-ine *pertaining to, substance* chol- *bile*	An amine found in most tissues; a precursor for acetylcholine
indole	**IN**-dole		Particular alkaloid structure	A phytochemical that makes estrogen less effective
isoflavone	I-zo-**FLAY**-vone	P/ R/	iso- *equal* -flavone *yellow*	Phytochemical that imitates estrogen
polyphenol	pol-ee-**FEE**-nol	P/ R/	poly- *many* -phenol *benzene derivative*	Antioxidant found in grapes and tea
saponin	**SAP**-oh-nin	S/ R/	-in *chemical compound* sapon- *soap*	Phytochemical that can prevent cancer cell replication
scurvy	**SKUR**-vee		Old English *scaly*	Deficiency of vitamin C

Most people consume about 1 liter of water in various liquids such as water, coffee, tea, soft drinks, and juices. Foods supply another liter of fluid, and water as a by-product of metabolism supplies another liter. *Table 17.6* outlines the functions of water.

TABLE 17.6 Functions of Water

- **Maintains** homeostasis in the body
- **Dissolves** many chemical compounds
- **Provides** a medium in which chemical reactions can occur
- **Transports** nutrients to cells
- **Regulates** temperature with its great capacity to absorb and hold heat
- **Removes** waste products of cell metabolism into the urine
- **Contributes** to lubricants in the knees and other joints
- **Forms** the base of saliva, bile, and amniotic fluid

EXERCISES

After reading Case Report 17.1 on the opposite page, answer the following questions. Be prepared to discuss your answers in class.

1. What items added to Ms. Johnson's diet will increase her vitamin C consumption? _____

2. What is another name for vitamin C? _____

3. List two functions of vitamin C. _____

_____

4. *Folate* is the generic name for _____ .

TABLE 17.7 Food Sources of Sodium
(adult minimum need for sodium: 500 mg)

Food Item and Amount	Sodium Content (mg)
Pepperoni pizza, 2 slices	2045
Slice ham, 1 oz.	1215
V8 vegetable juice, 8 oz.	620
Hamburger with bun	474
Green beans, canned, ½ cup	390
Saltine crackers, 6	234
Cheddar cheese, 1 oz.	176
Peanut butter, 2 tablespoons	156

From *Perspectives in Nutrition*, 6th ed., by Wardlaw et al. Copyright © 2004 The McGraw-Hill Companies, Inc. Reprinted with permission.

TABLE 17.8 Food Sources of Potassium
(adequate intake of potassium: 2000 mg)

Food Item and Amount	Potassium (mg)
Kidney beans, 1 cup	715
Plain yogurt, 1 cup	570
Orange juice, 1 cup	495
Banana, 1 medium	470
Tomato juice, ¾ cup	400
Baked potato, 1 small	385
Sirloin steak, 3 oz.	345

From *Perspectives in Nutrition*, 6th ed., by Wardlaw et al. Copyright © 2004 The McGraw-Hill Companies, Inc. Reprinted with permission.

TABLE 17.9 Food Sources of Calcium
(adequate intake, adults: 1000 mg)

Food Item and Amount	Calcium (mg)
Plain yogurt, 1 cup	450
Fortified orange juice, 1 cup	350
Cheddar cheese, 1.5 oz	305
Milk, 1%, 1 cup	300
Spinach, 1 cup	250
Salmon, 3 oz.	210

From *Perspectives in Nutrition*, 6th ed., by Wardlaw et al. Copyright © 2004 The McGraw-Hill Companies, Inc. Reprinted with permission.

MAJOR MINERALS

Major **minerals** are those for which you need more than 100 mg/day. The absorption of many minerals can be limited by components of fiber, particularly **phytic acid** in wheat fiber. Oxalic acid in spinach limits the absorption of calcium, which is present in large quantities, but only about 5% is **bioavailable** (i.e., not bound to oxalate). Some vitamins increase the bioavailability of minerals. For example, vitamin C improves iron absorption, and vitamin D improves calcium, phosphorus, and magnesium absorption.

Sodium (Na)

All the sodium in your diet comes from salt, whether it is added to food in cooking or at the table or is incorporated into processed food. Your body absorbs all the sodium that is consumed.

Sodium is the major electrolyte in extracellular fluid and retains fluid to maintain the extracellular volume and ensure cell function. The RDA for sodium is 500 mg/day. The Food and Nutrition Board of the IOM has set an AI of sodium as 1.5 g/day for adult males and adult females. *Table 17.7* shows how easy it is to exceed those figures.

Excess blood sodium **(hypernatremia)** is associated with hypertension and kidney stone formation.

Potassium (K)

Potassium is the major electrolyte that maintains fluid volume both inside and outside the cell, though 95% of potassium is in the intracellular fluids. Unlike sodium, it is associated with lower blood pressure values. It influences nerve impulse transmission and muscle contractility.

The AI for potassium is 2000 mg (2 grams) per day. *Table 17.8* shows the food sources of potassium. Low blood potassium **(hypokalemia)** is a life-threatening condition, causing anorexia, muscle cramps, and confusion. Eventually the heart beats irregularly and does not pump adequately, and death can occur. Some diuretics deplete potassium, and high-potassium foods—bananas, fruit juices, and vegetables—are an essential part of the diet for people taking diuretics.

Calcium (Ca)

You absorb about 25% of the calcium in the foods you eat. *Table 17.9* shows food sources of calcium. All cells need calcium, but 99% of body calcium is in bones and teeth. The functions of calcium are to:

- Form and maintain **bones and teeth** (see Chapter 5).
- Participate in **blood clotting** (see Chapter 7).
- Transmit **nerve impulses** across synapses (see Chapter 10).
- Permit **muscle contraction** (see Chapter 5).
- Regulate the activity of intracellular enzymes involved in **glucose metabolism** (see Chapter 6).

The AI for calcium in adults is between 1000 to 1200 mg/day. It is set higher for adolescents, at 1300 mg/day, because bone mass is being laid down.

Calcium deficiency is most often seen as **osteoporosis** and **osteopenia** (see Chapter 5).

Magnesium (Mg)

More than 300 enzymes require magnesium to function. It contributes to DNA and RNA synthesis, insulin action on cells, normal heart rhythm, and decreasing blood pressure by dilating arteries.

Magnesium is part of **chlorophyll** and is found in leafy green vegetables. Other good sources are beans, nuts, seeds, and chocolate. Milk and meats supply a smaller amount.

WORD	PRONUNCIATION	ELEMENTS		DEFINITION
bioavailable	**BI**-oh-ah-**VAIL**-ah-bul	S/ R/ R/	**-able** *capable of* **bio-** *life* **-avail-** *useful*	Capable of being absorbed into the bloodstream
chlorophyll	**KLOR**-oh-fil	S/ R/CF	**-phyll** *leaf* **chlor/o-** *green*	Light-absorbing pigment in plants
hyperkalemia	**HIGH**-per-kah-**LEE**-me-ah	S/ P/ R/	**-emia** *blood condition* **hyper-** *excessive, above* **-kal-** *potassium*	High level of potassium in the blood
hypokalemia	**HIGH**-poh-kah-**LEE**-me-ah	P/	**hypo-** *deficient, below*	Low level of potassium in the blood
hypernatremia	**HIGH**-per-nah-**TREE**-me-ah	S/ P/ R/	**-emia** *blood condition* **hyper-** *excessive, above* **-natr-** *sodium*	High level of sodium in the blood
hyponatremia	**HIGH**-poh-nah-**TREE**-me-ah	P/	**hypo-** *deficient, below*	Low level of sodium in the blood
mineral	**MIN**-er-al	S/ R/	**-al** *pertaining to* **miner-** *mines*	Inorganic compound usually found in earth's crust
phytic acid	**FIE**-tik **ASS**-id	S/ R/	**-ic** *pertaining to* **phyt-** *plant*	Component of fiber that can limit absorption of some minerals

The RDA for magnesium is 400 mg/day for adult men and 310 mg/day for adult women.

Magnesium deficiency causes tachycardia, muscle spasms, disorientation, and seizures. It can occur in alcoholics and patients with chronic diarrhea.

EXERCISES

Analyze the following medical terms. One element in each term is in bold—identify the type of element, and give the meaning of that element. Fill in the table; then use any two terms in sentences of your choice that are not definitions.

Medical Term	Type of Element	Meaning of Element	Meaning of Medical Term
hypo**natr**emia			
mineral			
hyperkal**emia**			
chlorophyll			
bioavailable			
hypokalemia			
phytic			

1. _____

_____

2. _____

_____

TRACE MINERALS (ELEMENTS)

Trace minerals are **dietary essentials** with a daily nutritional need of less than 100 mg/day. Their importance has been realized only since the 1960s. Food processing destroys trace minerals. For example, processing whole wheat into flour destroys most of the iron, selenium, zinc, and copper. Enriched white flour contains iron but not the other trace minerals that were removed. The trace minerals include those described below.

Iron (Fe)

Iron is found in every living cell. One-sixth of the total world population has iron-deficiency anemia. In developing nations, two-thirds of all children and women of child-bearing age have iron-deficiency anemia.

In meat, fish, and poultry, iron is mostly **hemoglobin** and **myoglobin,** which are collectively called **heme iron.** In vegetables, grains, and supplements, the iron is **nonheme,** which is less well absorbed by the body.

In hemoglobin, iron is the carrier of oxygen to all cells. In myoglobin, iron is the carrier of oxygen to skeletal and heart muscle cells. The RDA for iron is 18 mg/day for adult women and 8 mg/day for adult men. *Table 17.10* shows food sources of iron.

In iron deficiency, there is not enough iron to make all the hemoglobin needed to carry oxygen. Therefore, the red blood cells are small **(microcytic)** and pale **(hypochromic)** *(see Chapter 7).*

Too much absorption of iron can produce an inherited condition called **hemochromatosis.** The excess iron is stored in tissues, especially the liver, heart, and pancreas. It damages these organs and can cause them to fail.

Zinc (Zn)

As many as 200 **enzyme reactions** need zinc in order to function as they contribute to DNA and RNA synthesis, protein metabolism, hormone formation, antioxidant defenses, and cell membrane stabilization.

Protein-rich foods are usually good sources of zinc. Lean meats, shellfish, nuts, beans, and whole grains supply most of your zinc. The RDA for zinc is 11 mg/day for adult men, 8 mg/day for adult women.

Case Report 17.1 (continued)

Your advice to Ms. Karen Johnson about ensuring an adequate supply of minerals could be to change from fat-free yogurt to plain yogurt and to add occasional cheese to increase her calcium intake. Some lean protein or fish instead of frozen dinners would increase her intake of selenium.

Copper (Cu)

Copper is part of numerous **enzyme reactions,** including the formation of hemoglobin and norepinephrine, the protection of immune cells, and the formation of collagen and elastin in connective tissue. Good food sources include shellfish, nuts, seeds, legumes, soy, avocadoes, and dark chocolate.

Selenium (Se)

Selenium functions as part of the antioxidant defense system and as a coenzyme in the process of forming thyroid hormones. Selenium can also prevent the oxidation of HDL cholesterol and may help prevent plaque buildup in arteries.

Animal products, fish, and eggs are excellent sources of selenium.

TABLE 17.10 Food Sources of Iron
(RDA, adult men: 8 mg; RDA, adult women: 18 mg)

Food Item and Amount	Iron (mg) with Bioavailability (in parentheses)
Oat bran cereal, 1 cup	15.0 (low)
Spinach, 1 cup	6.4 (low)
Sirloin steak, 4 oz.	3.8 (high)
Shrimp, 3 oz.	2.7 (high)
Flour tortilla, 1	2.4 (low)
Baked potato, 1	1.7 (low)
Artichoke, 1	1.6 (low)
Whole-wheat bread, 1 slice	1.0 (low)

From *Perspectives in Nutrition,* 6th ed., by Wardlaw et al. Copyright © 2004 The McGraw-Hill Companies, Inc. Reprinted with permission.

Keynote

A 4-ounce sirloin steak contains 7.4 mg of zinc.

Keynote

• The RDA for copper is 1 mg/day for male and female adults.

• One ounce of semisweet chocolate supplies 110 μg of copper.

WORD	PRONUNCIATION	ELEMENTS		DEFINITION
enzyme	**EN**-zime		Greek *ferment*	Protein that induces changes in other substances
fluoride	**FLOR**-ide		Latin *to flow*	Chemical found in bones and teeth
heme	HEEM		Greek *blood*	The iron-based component of hemoglobin that carries oxygen
hemochromatosis	**HE**-mah-krom-ah-**TOE**-sis	S/ R/CF R/	-osis *condition* hem/o- *blood* -chromat- *color*	Dangerously high levels of iron in the body with deposition of iron pigments in tissues

Iodide (I)

The function of iodide is the synthesis of thyroxine (T4) *(see Chapter 14)*. People with an inadequate intake of iodide develop goiters. The RDA for iodide is 150 μg/day for adults.

Saltwater fish, shellfish, and molasses contain iodide. Many countries, including the United States, fortify table salt with iodide.

Fluoride (F)

Fluoride incorporated into developing teeth makes them resistant to acid and bacterial attack, preventing the development of caries *(Figure 17.9)*. It also helps in the remineralization of teeth after caries has begun. Most Americans obtain adequate fluoride from that added to drinking water and from toothpaste.

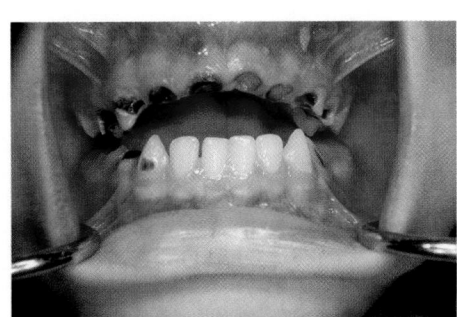

▲ **FIGURE 17.9 Dental Caries.**

Other Trace Minerals

Chromium, manganese, and **molybdenum** are other trace minerals.

EXERCISES

Test your knowledge of trace minerals with the following quiz. Check (✓) the column with the name of the mineral to which the statement applies. Fill in the table.

Statement	Iron	Zinc	Copper	Selenium	Iodide	Fluoride
Excess of this mineral can cause liver failure						
Found in every living cell						
Function of this mineral is the synthesis of thyroxine (T4)						
Part of numerous enzyme reactions						
Part of the antioxidant defense system						
Prevents the development of caries						
Protein-rich foods are a good source of this mineral						
Too much absorption of this mineral causes hemochromatosis						

The information in this lesson will enable you to use correct medical terminology to:

17.3.1 Discuss different types of diet that are recommended for different purposes.

17.3.2 Establish an eating plan in balance with different body needs.

17.3.3 Analyze the value of MyPyramid 2005 in providing individual nutrition advice.

17.3.4 Describe some common forms of metabolic and nutritional problems.

17.3.5 Explain what information is on a nutrition label and what it tells you.

You are

. . . a medical assistant working with Susan Lee, MD, a primary care physician at Fulwood Medical Center.

Your patient is

. . . Mrs. Rosa Costa, a 55-year-old medical transcriptionist working at Fulwood Medical Center.

CASE REPORT 17.2

Since menopause 4 years ago, Mrs. Costa has put on 15 pounds in weight, mostly around the lower abdomen. A recent examination by Dr. Lee in the primary care clinic showed Mrs. Costa's abdominal circumference to be 37 inches *(Figure 17.10)*. Her blood pressure was 145/90 mm Hg, and she had a triglyceride level of 150 mg/dL, a fasting blood glucose level of 100 mg/dL, and an HDL level of 40 mg/dL. Her mother died of type 2 diabetes in her midsixties. Dr. Lee made a diagnosis of metabolic syndrome, informed her of its significance, and recommended lifestyle changes.

The changes include losing 15 pounds and starting an exercise program including a brisk 30-minute walk each day. Dietary changes should be a 1600-Calorie diet, restricting carbohydrates to no more than 50% of total Calories, and eating only complex carbohydrates. She should increase fiber consumption and eat no red meats and minimal saturated and trans fats. Dr. Lee will see her again in 6 weeks.

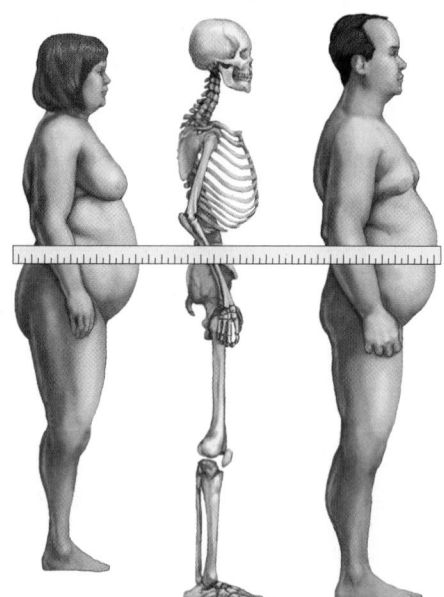

▲ **FIGURE 17.10 Waist Circumference Measurement.** Place measuring tape, holding it parallel to the floor, around abdomen at the level of the iliac crest. Hold tape snug but do not compress the skin. Measure circumference at end of normal expiration.

DIETS

There is an old saying, "Good food is good medicine." However, good food and nutrition go way beyond medicine and drugs in maintaining and treating the body as a whole. Drugs are brought in to combat a specific problem at a specific site that poor nutrition may have affected. Good nutrition could perhaps have prevented the problem, and a return to good nutrition could be a large component in correcting the problem and enabling the drug to function optimally. Good nutrition is a daily need and is an important part of any lifestyle. There is no one diet that is best for everyone.

Case Report 17.2 (continued)

The value of good, individualized nutrition, often in conjunction with exercise, is shown by Dr. Lee's recommendations for Mrs. Costa in treating her metabolic syndrome. She has prescribed no medication.

The protein, carbohydrates, and fat that you eat generate complex hormonal responses. An example of this is insulin. Insulin's role is to take excess glucose from dietary carbohydrates and excess amino acids from dietary protein, store them in adipose tissue as fat, and keep the fat locked in the adipose tissue. High-glycemic carbohydrate loads generate high levels of insulin.

Proponents of a specific type of diet often maintain that the diet is appropriate for everyone. Just as individuals respond differently to medications, so responses to different foods will vary, depending on enzyme concentrations and efficiencies during absorption, transport, and metabolism of the food. You may respond well to a high-carbohydrate diet, others to a low-carbohydrate–high-protein diet, and many to a diet balanced between carbohydrates and protein. All agree that fats in any diet should contain minimal saturated and trans fats.

WORD	PRONUNCIATION	ELEMENTS		DEFINITION
antimicrobial	**AN**-tee-my-**KROH**-bee-al	S/ P/ P/ R/	-al *pertaining to* anti- *against* -micro- *small* -bio- *life*	Agent for destroying or preventing multiplication of organisms
fertilizer	**FER**-tih-lie-zer	S/ R/	-er *agent* fertiliz- *make fruitful*	Substance used to increase the yield of crops
fungicide	**FUN**-jee-side	R/CF R/CF	-cid/e *to kill* fung/i- *fungus*	Agent for destroying fungi
herbicide	**ER**-bih-side	R/CF R/CF	-cid/e *to kill* herb/i- *plant*	Agent for destroying plants
insecticide	in-**SEK**-tih-side	R/CF R/CF	-cid/e *to kill* insect/i- *insect*	Agent for destroying insects
pesticide	**PES**-tih-side	R/CF R/CF	-cid/e *to kill* pest/i- *nuisance*	Agent for destroying flies, mosquitoes, and other pests

Good food has two other components. The food should contain appropriate levels of nutrients. Since 1950, levels of calcium and magnesium in many vegetables have dropped by one-third. Changes in the soil with the use of commercial **fertilizers** have diminished the concentration of trace minerals, including zinc and chromium. Many fruits and vegetables are picked green. Without exposure to the sun to ripen, antioxidants are not allowed to develop.

There is growing concern about different ways in which small doses of **pesticides** in food can affect people, although these are not well understood. Pesticides include **insecticides** to control insects, **herbicides** to control weeds, **fungicides** to control mold and fungus, and **antimicrobials** to control bacteria *(Figure 17.11)*. The health problems posed by pesticides include birth defects, nerve damage, and cancer, including prostate cancer. Parkinson disease, not caused by genetics or head injury, is much more common in rural areas. Researchers are now tracking farmers to document their exposure to combinations of pesticides and to determine whether there is an increased incidence of Parkinson disease in this population.

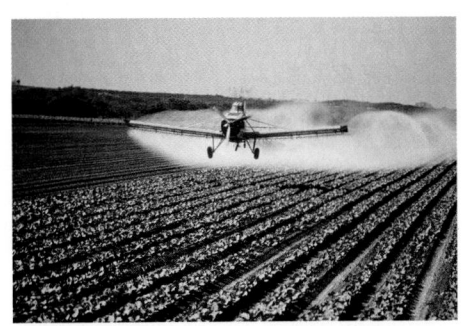

▲ **FIGURE 17.11 Spraying Insecticide on Carrots.**

EXERCISES   *"There is no one diet that is best for everyone." Use what you have learned about nutrition to briefly answer the following questions. Fill in the blanks.*

1. What exactly does the quoted statement mean?

_____

_____

_____

_____

2. Based on what you have learned about nutrition, why is this a correct statement?

_____

_____

_____

_____

DIETS (continued)

High-Carbohydrate Diet

A high-carbohydrate diet is based largely on plant foods with starch as the carbohydrate source. The only exception to plants is fruit, in which the carbohydrates are the simple sugars fructose, sucrose, and glucose, as well as pectin, a fiber. Nuts contain 20% to 30% carbohydrate in terms of energy and are part of the diet.

Most high-carbohydrate diets contain 60% to 65% of energy from carbohydrate with 15% of energy from protein and 20% to 25% from fat. *Table 17.11* shows this as grams in different Calorie diets.

The high-carbohydrate diet is rich in fiber, minerals, vitamins, and antioxidants. It is important to keep the intake of simple sugars below 10% to 15% of total energy intake and to use mostly complex, low-glycemic carbohydrates. A high-carbohydrate diet with a high percentage of high-glycemic carbohydrates is one of the reasons for the epidemic of obesity in this country.

TABLE 17.11 High-Carbohydrate Diet

Total Calories	Carbohydrate (% and grams)	Fat (% and grams)	Protein (% and grams)
1600	60% 240 g	25% 44 g	15% 30 g
2500	60% 375 g	25% 70 g	15% 40 g

High-Protein Diet

A high-protein diet usually obtains 30% of its calories from protein, 40% from carbohydrates, and 30% from fat *(Table 17.12)*. Just as in a good high-carbohydrate diet where the type of carbohydrate is important, so in a good high-protein diet the type of protein is important. In both diets, the type of fat is important.

Sources of protein to avoid are beef and red meats, cow's milk, cheese, and protein powders with artificial sweeteners. Good sources of lean protein are fish, free-range poultry (chicken and turkey), buffalo, deer, **spirulina,** the grain **quinoa,** nuts, and beans. The healthy fat intake should avoid saturated fats and trans fats.

A 2005 study showed that a diet with 25% of total calories from protein (half from vegetable protein) was more effective in reducing blood pressure and blood cholesterol than the **Dietary Approaches to Stop Hypertension (DASH)** diet (18% protein) developed by the **National Heart, Lung, and Blood Institute (NHLBI).**

TABLE 17.12 High-Protein Diet

Total Calories	Carbohydrate (% and grams)	Fat (% and grams)	Protein (% and grams)
1600	40% 160g	30% 53g	30% 60g
2500	40% 250g	30% 85g	30% 80g

Balanced Diet

A good balanced diet is what is right for you, enables you to maintain the weight you want to be, provides you with the energy you need, and has the food that you enjoy eating. In all diets, which are really a lifestyle, exercise plays an important role. One example of a balanced diet could contain 50% carbohydrate, 25% protein, and 25% fat *(Table 17.13)*. The lean protein should be from both vegetable and animal sources. Carbohydrates should be complex and high-glycemic, and fats should not be saturated or trans fats.

TABLE 17.13 Balanced Diet

Total Calories	Carbohydrate (% and grams)	Fat (% and grams)	Protein (% and grams)
1600	50% 200g	25% 44g	25% 50g
2500	50% 310g	25% 70g	25% 70g

Keynote

Consumption of refined carbohydrates—especially refined white sugar—promotes diabetes, obesity, and some forms of cancer.

Keynote

In high-protein diets, Calorie and fat intakes are carefully controlled.

Abbreviations

DASH　Dietary Approaches to Stop Hypertension

NHLBI　National Heart, Lung, and Blood Institute

Keynote

Diets are a component of a lifestyle in which exercise always plays a role.

WORD	PRONUNCIATION		ELEMENTS	DEFINITION
lactovegetarian	LAK-toe-VEJ-eh-TAR-ee-an	S/ R/CF R/	-arian *one who is* lact/o- *milk* -veget- *plants*	Person whose diet consists of only plants and dairy products
quinoa	kee-NO-ah		Inca *mother of all grains*	Plant with edible seeds high in protein
spirulina	spy-roo-LEE-nah		Genus of plant	Commercial product of blue-green algae containing 60% to 70% protein
vegan	VEE-gan		Greek *plants*	One who eats plants and no animal or dairy products

Vegetarian Diets

The two major vegetarian styles are:

- **Vegans,** who eat only plant foods.

- **Lactovegetarians,** who eat dairy products and plant foods.

A vegan diet is low in saturated fat, high in fiber, and rich in antioxidants but must find sources of vitamins D and B$_{12}$, calcium, iron, and zinc. Fortified foods or a vitamin and mineral supplement can provide these. Protein is provided by nuts, legumes, seeds and grains, and dairy products, if these are used.

The importance and the quantities of the different foods needed in a vegetarian diet is illustrated by the Vegetarian Diet Pyramid *(Figure 17.12)*.

FIGURE 17.12 The Oldways Preservation & Exchange Trust Traditional Vegetarian Diet.
The diet has the advantage of being low in saturated fat, high in fiber, and rich in antioxidants. However, it can pose a risk for an inadequate iron, vitamin D, and vitamin B$_{12}$ intake.

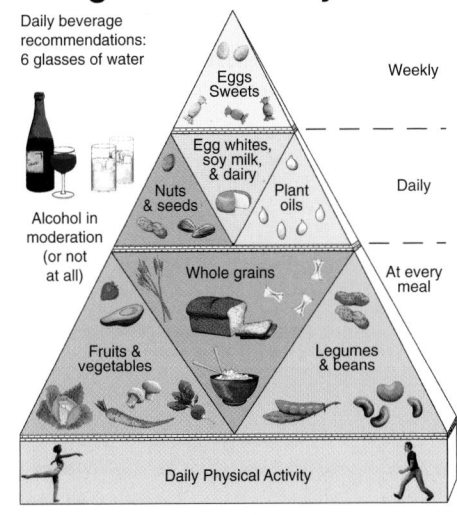

The Traditional Healthy Vegetarian Diet Pyramid

Copyright © 2000 Oldways Preservation & Exchange Trust, www.oldwayspt.org

EXERCISES

Reinforce your knowledge of various diets with this exercise. Decide whether the statements given apply to a high-carbohydrate, high-protein, or vegetarian diet. In the chart, check (✓) the appropriate boxes for each statement.

Statement	High-Carbohydrate Diet	High-Protein Diet	Vegetarian Diet
May include only dairy and plant foods			
Effective in reducing blood pressure and blood cholesterol			
Rich in fiber, minerals, vitamins, and antioxidants			
Based largely on plant foods with starch			
30% of calories from protein, 40% from carbohydrates, and 30% from fat			
May need fortified foods or vitamin supplements			

Diagnostic criteria for metabolic syndrome	
Feature	**Criterion**
Abdominal girth	Waist circumference
Men	>102 cm (40 in)
Women	>88 cm (35 in)
Fasting plasma HDL-C	
Men	<40 mg/dL (1.03mmol/L)
Women	<50 mg/dL (1.29mmol/L)
Fasting plasma triglycerides	≥150 mg/dL (1.69mmol/L)
Fasting blood glucose	≥110 m/dL (6.1 mmol/L)
Blood pressure	≥130/85 mm Hg

▲ **FIGURE 17.13 Diagnostic Criteria for Metabolic Syndrome.**

METABOLIC SYNDROME

Almost 30% (50 million) of U.S. adults and 5% of adolescents aged 12 to 19 years have metabolic syndrome. The key diagnostic components are **central adiposity, dyslipidemia, glucose intolerance,** and **hypertension.** The criteria for these are shown in *Figure 17.13.* Chronic inflammation, coagulation defects, and a genetic disposition are thought to play a role in the effects of the syndrome.

People with metabolic syndrome are at high risk for coronary heart disease and other diseases related to plaque (stroke, peripheral vascular disease), hypertension, and type 2 diabetes. The dominant underlying factors are insulin resistance and the resulting abdominal obesity.

Case Report 17.2 (continued)

Mrs. Rosa Costa has metabolic syndrome. The diagnostic criteria for this disorder are shown in *Figure 17.13.* Mrs. Costa meets four of the five criteria, and her plasma triglycerides are borderline. The diet Dr. Lee has prescribed is similar to the balanced diet shown previously. It is important for you as a medical assistant to reinforce the need for the diet and to encourage her weight loss.

MyPyramid and Diet Planning

In response to the epidemic of obesity and the recent recognition of metabolic syndrome, *The Dietary Guidelines for Americans 2005* was issued by the federal government. Based on these guidelines, MyPyramid, an interactive food guidance system, was introduced to suggest the recommended proportion and amounts of foods from different food groups needed to create a healthy diet *(Figure 17.14).* This is accessible through the website MyPyramid.gov.

Anatomy of MyPyramid

One size doesn't fit all
USDA's new MyPyramid symbolizes a personalized approach to healthy eating and physical activity. The symbol has been designed to be simple. It has been developed to remind consumers to make healthy food choices and to be active every day. The different parts of the symbol are described below.

Activity
Activity is represented by the steps and the person climbing them, as a reminder of the importance of daily physical activity.

Moderation
Moderation is represented by the narrowing of each food group from bottom to top. The wider base stands for foods with little or no solid fats or added sugars. These should be selected more often. The narrower top area stands for foods containing more added sugars and solid fats. The more active you are, the more of these foods can fit into your diet.

Personalization
Personalization is shown by the person on the steps, the slogan, and the URL. Find the kinds and amounts of food to eat each day at MyPyramid.gov.

Proportionality
Proportionality is shown by the different widths of the food group bands. The widths suggest how much food a person should choose from each group. The widths are just a general guide, not exact proportions. Check the website for how much is right for you.

Variety
Variety is symbolized by the six color bands representing the five food groups of the pyramid and oils. This illustrates that food from all groups are needed each day for good health.

Gradual Improvement
Gradual improvement is encouraged by the slogan. It suggests that individuals can benefit from taking small steps to improve their diet and lifestyle each day.

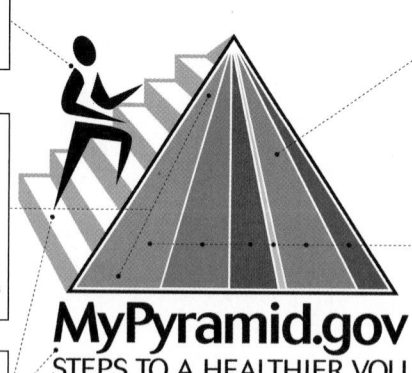

MyPyramid.gov
STEPS TO A HEALTHIER YOU

USDA U.S. Department of Agriculture Center for Nutrition Policy and Promotion April 2005 CNPP-16
USDA is an equal opportunity provider and employer.

GRAINS | VEGETABLES | FRUITS | OILS | MILK | MEAT & BEANS

▲ **FIGURE 17.14 The MyPyramid.gov Website Offers Individualized Information to the User.**

WORD	PRONUNCIATION	ELEMENTS		DEFINITION
adiposity	ad-ih-**POSS**-ih-tee	S/ R/	-ity *condition* adipos- *fat*	Excessive accumulation of fat in a site, organ, or body
dyslipidemia	**DIS**-li-pi-**DEE**-me-ah	S/ P/ R/	-emia *blood condition* dys- *bad, difficult, painful* -lipid- *fat*	Abnormal (and "bad") levels of blood lipids

In the MyPyramid guidelines, lumping together red meat, poultry, fish, and beans ignores the fact that these foods have different types of fats and ignores mounting evidence that replacing red meat with a combination of fish, poultry, beans, and nuts offers distinct health benefits. There is no advice in the guidelines about obtaining protein from plant sources.

The emphasis on milk products includes the recommendation to drink three 8-ounce glasses of low-fat milk daily. This provides 390 Calories and 4.5 grams of saturated fats, which are significant for people on a 1600-Calorie low-fat diet.

The guidelines suggest that half the grains chosen can be refined starch. This ignores the fact that refined starch behaves like sugar, providing empty calories with adverse metabolic effects.

There is no advice given about foods to avoid.

At the end of this chapter, you will be given opportunities to work with the MyPyramid website.

EXERCISES

Patient Education: *Your patient does not understand the following statements made by the doctor. Explain each statement in language a nonmedical person will understand. Fill in the blanks.*

1. "The key diagnostic components are central adiposity, dyslipidemia, glucose intolerance, and hypertension."

   Rewrite this sentence in layman's language.

   _____

   _____

   _____

   _____

   _____

   _____

2. "Chronic inflammation, coagulation defects, and a genetic disposition are thought to play a role in the effects of this syndrome."

   Rewrite this sentence in layman's language.

   _____

   _____

   _____

   _____

   _____

   _____

READING FOOD LABELS

Most foods sold in stores must be labeled with the product name, its manufacturer, the amount of product in the package, its nutritional composition, and its ingredients listed in *descending order by weight*. So, below the label in *Figure 17.15*, the two major ingredients by weight in the soup are milk and water.

Starting at the top of the label, the **serving size** is 1 cup (8 ounces), not a large serving by modern standards. With four servings per container, the **total volume** in the container is $4 \times 8 = 32$ ounces (1 quart). Knowing the total volume enables you to more easily compare prices with competing products.

In the next section, each **serving** contains 100 Calories, with 20 of them being from fat. If you consume 12 ounces (1½ servings) of the soup, you will have consumed 150 Calories, with 30 of these Calories derived from fat.

The next section shows you the quantities of the main nutrients and relates this to a percentage of the **daily value.** The daily values are set at the nutrient recommendations for a 2000-Calorie diet with 30% of the Calories derived from fat (one-third of this total from saturated fat), 60% from carbohydrates, and 10% from protein. So, if you are on a low-carbohydrate diet, the carbohydrate percentages on the label will be low.

In this soup, three-quarters of the fat is saturated, reflecting the content of butter and milk. Sixty percent of the carbohydrate (10 out of 16 g) is sugar, reflecting the use of cane syrup as the sweetener. Protein does not have a daily value because determining it would require expensive testing by the manufacturer.

The RDA for sodium for adults is 500 mg/day (0.5 g). Most adults ingest 4 to 7 g/day. This soup contains 750 mg per serving.

This soup carries the **USDA organic symbol,** which means that the product contains at least 95% organic ingredients. Organic refers to the way food is grown (or raised in the case of animals), without commercial pesticides, herbicides, or fertilizers. Irradiated or genetically engineered ingredients are not used in organic foods.

The traditional food industry lobbies the **U.S. Department of Agriculture (USDA)** continually to allow synthetic ingredients to be added. The definition of organic may well change.

The label shown in *Figure 17.16* is for a much simpler product, but if you really want to know what you are eating, you have to count the chips. Compared to the soup, the chips contain much more total fat but not much more saturated fat, and they have zero cholesterol. There is no hydrogenated oil listed in the ingredients, so there should be no trans fats. Sodium is much lower, and the chips contain small amounts of some B vitamins. There are no sugars.

At the very bottom of the label is the information about the manufacturing crossover with peanut oil. If you are allergic to peanuts, the small amount of peanut oil that might be in this food could set off your allergy.

It's always good to peruse the food label in its entirety.

Nutrition Facts

Serving Size 1 cup (8fl. oz.) 240mL
Servings Per Container 4

Amount Per Serving

Calories 100 Calories from Fat 20

	% Daily Value*
Total Fat 2g	3%
Saturated Fat 1.5g	6%
Cholesterol 10mg	3%
Sodium 750mg	31%
Total Carbohydrate 16g	5%
Dietary Fiber 1g	4%
Sugars 10g	
Protein 5g	

Vitamin A 10%	•	Vitamin C 4%
Calcium 15%	•	Iron 2%

*Percent Daily Values are based on a 2,000 calorie diet. Your daily values may be higher or lower, depending on your calorie needs.

	Calories	2,000	2,500
Total Fat	Less than	65g	80g
Sat Fat	Less than	20g	25g
Cholesterol	Less than	300mg	300mg
Sodium	Less than	2,400mg	2,400mg
Total Carbohydrate		300g	375g
Dietary Fiber		25g	30g

Ingredients: Organic Milk, Filtered Water, Organic Tomato Paste, Organic Cane Sweetener, Organic Caramelized Red Pepper Flavor (Organic Red Peppers, Sea Salt, Organic Butter), Roasted Garlic, Roasted Red Peppers, Sea Salt, Sodium Citrate, Organic Rice Flour, Organic Garlic Powder, Organic Onion Powder

▲ **FIGURE 17.15 Soup Label.**

Nutrition Facts

Serving Size 1 oz (28g/About 22 chips)
Servings Per Container 9

Amount Per Serving

Calories 150 Calories from Fat 80

	% Daily Value*
Total Fat 8g	12%
Saturated Fat 2g	10%
Cholesterol 0mg	0%
Sodium 110mg	5%
Total Carbohydrate 18g	6%
Dietary Fiber 1g	4%
Sugars 0g	
Protein 2g	

Vitamin A 0%	•	Vitamin C 10%
Calcium 15%	•	Iron 2%
Thiamin 2%	•	Niacin 4%
Vitamin B6 6%	•	Phosphorus 2%

*Percent Daily Values are based on a 2,000 calorie diet. Your daily values may be higher or lower, depending on your calorie needs.

	Calories	2,000	2,500
Total Fat	Less than	65g	80g
Sat Fat	Less than	20g	25g
Cholesterol	Less than	300mg	300mg
Sodium	Less than	2,400mg	2,400mg
Total Carbohydrate		300g	375g
Dietary Fiber		25g	30g

Ingredients: Potatoes, Vegetable Oil (Contains One or More of the Following: Corn, Cottonseed, or Sunflower Oil), and Sea Salt
Allergy Information: This product is made on equipment that also makes products containing peanut oil.

▲ **FIGURE 17.16 Potato Chip Label.**

Understand What You Read. *Reading the nutritional facts about the food you are about to consume may lead you to make wiser choices in the supermarket or at the vending machine. Refer to the food labels in Figures 17.15 and 17.16 to answer the following questions. Some answers may surprise you.*

1. Which food product contains more sodium per serving, the soup or the potato chips? _____

2. What is the serving size of potato chips? _____

3. What is the serving size of the soup? _____

4. Which product contains no sugar? _____

5. Which product contains more protein? _____

6. Which product contains less total fat? _____

7. Which product contains no cholesterol? _____

8. How many servings are in a container of chips? _____

9. How many servings are in the can of soup? _____

10. Which food product contains trace minerals? _____

11. Which product contains a warning on the label? _____

12. If you have a patient with hypertension, which component on the label should be of particular interest to him? _____

Take a moment to think about what you are eating every day and whether or not it contributes to a healthy lifestyle. Answer these questions for yourself.

13. How often in a day do you eat "junk" food? _____

14. How many potato chips do you eat at one time? _____

15. Do you drink soda more than once a day? _____

16. Do you skip meals because of limited time? _____

17. Do you eat a piece of fruit every day? _____

18. What is your "normal" breakfast? _____

19. How many glasses (or bottles) of water do you drink in any one day? _____

20. What is your main source of protein? _____

21. Can you name three things you ate today that contained sugar? _____

_____, and _____

22. Do you generally choose organic foods when you go to the supermarket?

Yes, because _____ .

No, because _____ .

23. Do you think you eat a balanced diet? _____

If not, why not? _____

_____

NUTRITION

L. **Optional Exercise:** You are almost three-quarters of the way into this text and have worked your way through numerous types of exercises at chapter ends. *Create a short exercise you will exchange with another student.* Be sure to put your answers on a separate sheet and keep that. Five questions for the exercise can be short answer, multiple choice, definitions, spelling, word elements, or fill in the blank. Be prepared to hand the sample exercise and the answers in to the instructor.

List the medical terms you want to incorporate into your questions below.

_____

_____

_____

_____

M. **Diet Plans:** Not all diet plans work for everyone who tries them. Being knowledgeable about what your body needs and what you are providing it will help you choose a healthy diet plan that will work for you. Write a short answer for each question, describing the basics of each diet plan.

1. Name the two types of vegetarian eating plans, and briefly describe what types of food they permit.

   a. _____

   Food consumed: _____

   b. _____

   Food consumed: _____

2. What are the basic elements of a balanced diet?

   _____

   _____

   _____

3. What are the basic elements of a high-carbohydrate diet?

   _____

   _____

   _____

4. What are the basic elements of a high-protein diet?

   _____

   _____

   _____

   _____

5. Generally, most diet plans will tell you to avoid:

   _____

S. Deconstruct the following term
appeared in earlier chapters. In th
previously appeared in the langua

Medical Term	Prefix
hemochromatosis	
antimicrobial	
lactovegetarian	
dyslipidemia	
phenylketonuria	
hydrogenated	

List another medical term.

1. List a medical term using a p

   Previous term: _____

2. List a medical term using a r

   Previous term: _____

3. List a medical term using a s

   Previous term: _____

T. Apply the *language of nutrition* to
the first row across the top of the f
each item in the first column and p
chart.

Nutrients (Fill in across the top row.)
Constitutes 60% of body weight
Breaks down to glucose, major source cell energy
Organic substances
Can be complex starch or simple suga
Some vitamins increase the bioavailab of this nutrient
Do not dissolve in water
Zinc
Form major part of lean body tissue
No caloric value
Cholesterol

N. **Patient Documentation:** Employ your knowledge of the *language of nutrition* to correctly complete the following patient documentation. Fill in the blanks with your correct choice—choose from the answers below the statement.

1. I am prescribing daily use of _____ for the patient's acne. She will return to see me in 2 weeks so that I can check for any improvement in her skin.

   lutein   niacin   retinoic acid   beta carotene

2. What was initially thought to be hyperbilirubinemia has proved on lab results to be _____; the patient had ingested a large amount of carrot juice in the past month (which she failed to tell me).

   hypertension   hypercalcemia   hypercarotenemia   hyperketonuria

3. I am treating this patient's osteomalacia with additional supplements of _____.

   vitamin B   vitamin K   vitamin C   vitamin D

4. Because the patient is pregnant, I have recommended an additional daily intake of _____.

   amino acids   carbohydrates   folate   lipids

5. Since this patient has been on antibiotics for an extended period of time and liver function lab results are lower than normal, I am prescribing additional _____ to boost liver function.

   vitamin B_6 vitamin B_{12} vitamin K   vitamin E

O. **Critical Thinking:** Prepare a brief answer to the following statement, and be prepared to discuss your answer in class.

   In all diets, which are really a lifestyle, exercise plays an important role.

Three important questions you must address in your answer:

1. What is a lifestyle?
2. Why is it a "lifestyle" and not a "diet"?
3. What is the value of exercise in lifestyle and diet?

_____

_____

_____

P. **Recall and Review:** How well do you remember these word elements from the previous chapter? Try to answer without first looking back to check. Fill in the blanks.

Element	Type of Element (P, R, CF, S)	Meaning of Element
1. geront/o	_____	_____
2. pulmon/o	_____	_____
3. pre	_____	_____
4. ped	_____	_____
5. an	_____	_____

Q. Build your knowledge of the *langu*
key role in body nutrition. Match t
terminology in the right column.

_____ 1. Common name for so

_____ 2. Prevents development

_____ 3. Too much absorption

_____ 4. Magnesium deficiency

_____ 5. Calcium deficiency ap

_____ 6. Iron deficiency causes

_____ 7. Excess blood sodium

_____ 8. Can be absorbed into

_____ 9. Insufficient iodine inta

_____ 10. Low blood potassium

R. Terminology Challenge: Elements yo

Example: In this chapter you have th
chapters that have the *same root.*

choline: Prefix means _____

Fill in the chart with additional medical

Medical Term	Meaning of M

---

11. What is the major electrolyte in extracellular fluid?

    a. sodium

    b. potassium

    c. vitamin E

    d. copper

    e. calcium

12. Which term represents excess blood sodium?

    a. hyperglycemia

    b. hypernatremia

    c. hypoglycemia

    d. hyperkalemia

    e. hyponatremia

V. Translate the following sentences from layman's language into medical terminology.

1. "Excess blood sodium is associated with high blood pressure and kidney stones."

   Rewrite using correct medical terminology. _____

   _____

   _____

   _____

2. "In iron deficiency, there is not enough red-pigmented protein, so the RBCs are small and pale."

   Rewrite using correct medical terminology. _____

   _____

   _____

   _____

3. "Low blood potassium is a life-threatening condition causing loss of appetite, muscle cramps, and confusion."

   Rewrite using correct medical terminology. _____

   _____

   _____

W. **True or False:** Not all of the following statements are correct. Check *true* or *false* for each statement. Rewrite any false statements correctly on the lines below.

1.	Glycogen is the storage form of carbohydrate.	T	F
2.	Calcium is found in bones and teeth.	T	F
3.	Trace minerals do not dissolve in water.	T	F
4.	Neither vitamins nor minerals are used as fuel to burn Calories.	T	F
5.	Seventy-five percent of your body weight is water.	T	F
6.	Major minerals are those for which you need > 100 mg/day.	T	F

Sentences written correctly:

_____

_____

_____

_____

_____

_____

_____

_____

_____

_____

_____

X. **Study Hint: Learn to make study hints that work for you.** Make up a good study hint to help you remember:

Water-soluble vitamins are vitamin C and the B vitamins.

Fat-soluble vitamins do not dissolve in water and are vitamins A, D, E, and K.

My study hint: _____

_____

_____

_____

_____

_____

_____

NUTRITION

CHAPTER SUMMARY EXERCISE

1. *Listen to the pronunciation of the medical terms as given by your instructor.*
2. *Circle the correct spelling of the medical term.*
3. *Match the correctly spelled terms to the brief descriptions below.*
4. *Write a sentence for each of the 10 terms that appear in this exercise.*

A. SPELLING COMPREHENSION: CIRCLE THE CORRECT SPELLING OF THE TERM.

1. rickits	rickets	ricketts	ricketes	rickettes
2. colesterol	cholestrol	cholesterol	collesterol	cholisterol
3. nutrieent	nutreint	nutreent	nurtrient	nutrient
4. vegan	vigen	vagen	vagan	vegin
5. defeciency	dificiency	deficiency	defficiency	difficiency
6. pilagra	pellagra	pelagra	pillagra	pellagria
7. scurrvey	scurve	scurvie	surrvey	scurvy
8. glycogen	glicogen	glecogen	gicogen	gilcogen
9. lipid	lippid	lipidd	liped	lepid
10. ribbofavin	riboflavin	ribboflavin	ryboflavin	ribofavin

B. MATCH THE NUMBER OF THE CORRECT TERM IN PART A WITH THE BRIEF DESCRIPTION OF THE TERM BELOW.

a. Vegetarians who eat only plant foods _____

b. Disease due to lack of dietary niacin _____

c. Vitamin B_2 _____

d. Steroid characterized as a lipid _____

e. Food compound that does not dissolve in water _____

f. Storage form of carbohydrate _____

g. Vitamin D deficiency in children _____

h. Lack of, less than normal _____

i. Food required for normal physiologic function _____

j. Lack of vitamin C _____

C. USING YOUR KNOWLEDGE OF TERMS 1–10 IN PART A AND THEIR CORRECT SPELLING, WRITE A BRIEF SENTENCE FOR EACH OF THE TERMS AS IT MIGHT APPEAR IN PATIENT DOCUMENTATION.

1. _____
2. _____
3. _____
4. _____
5. _____
6. _____
7. _____
8. _____
9. _____
10. _____

D. YOUR INSTRUCTOR WILL DIRECT YOU TO MCGRAW-HILL CONNECT. OPEN THE AUDIO GLOSSARY AND PRACTICE YOUR PRONUNCIATION OF THE TERMS IN PART A OF THIS EXERCISE.

E. CARBOHYDRATES PLAY AN IMPORTANT ROLE IN THE REGULATION OF INSULIN IN THE BODY. MEET A LESSON OBJECTIVE, AND LIST THE ILL EFFECTS OF PERSISTENT HIGH INSULIN OUTPUT ON THE BODY.

1. _____
2. _____
3. _____
4. _____
5. What organ is responsible for insulin output? _____

Rehabilitation Medicine
The Language of Rehabilitation

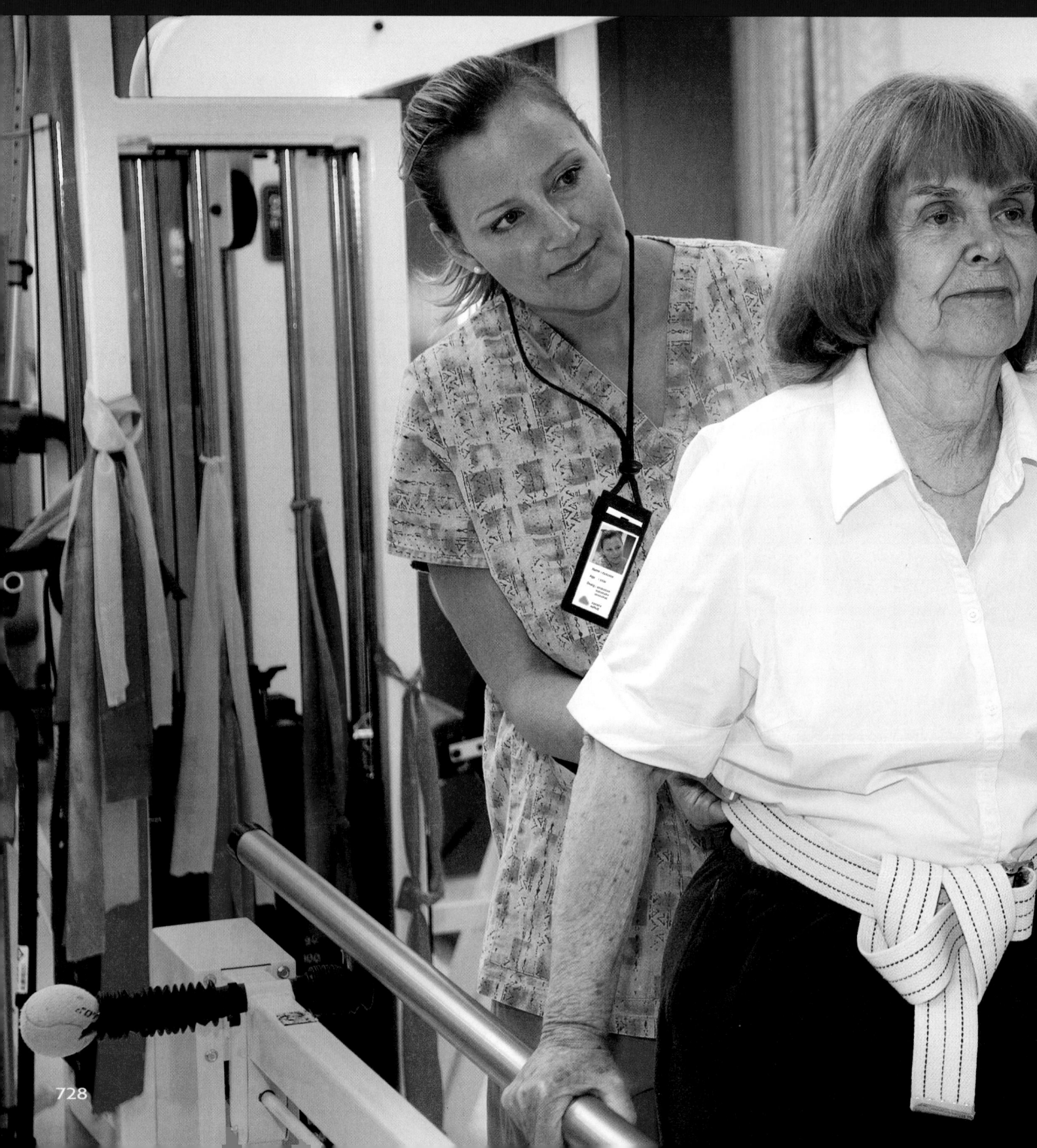

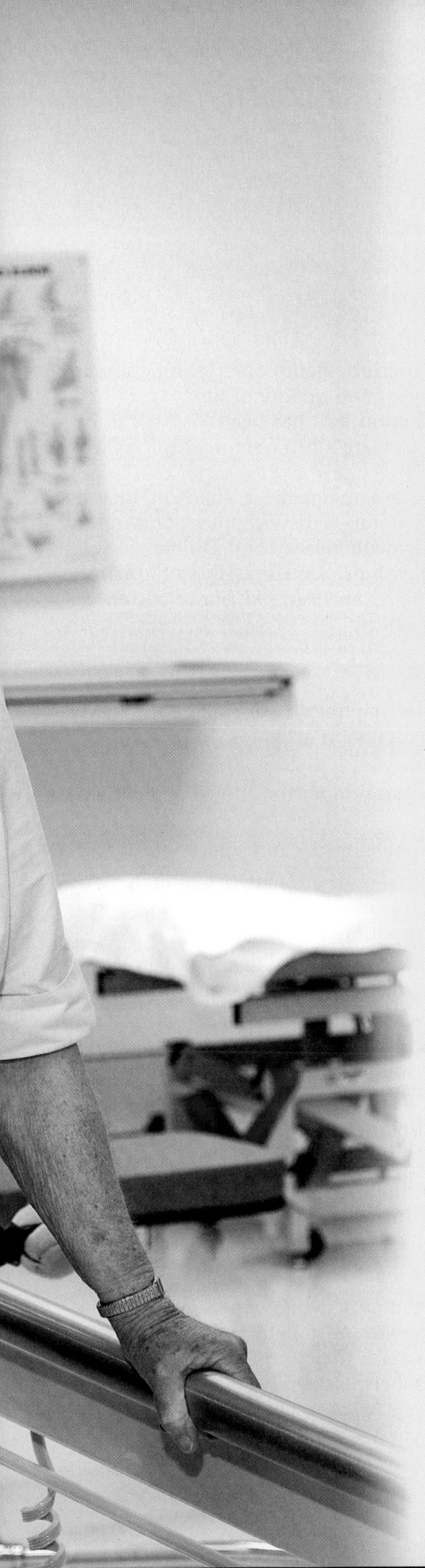

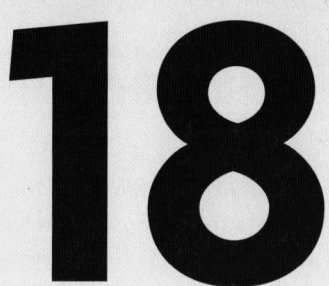

18

CASE REPORT 18.1

You are

... A **physical therapy assistant (PTA)** employed in the Rehabilitation Unit at Fulwood Medical Center.

Your patient is

... Mrs. Amy Vargas, a 70-year-old housewife, who is 2 weeks postop following an emergency hip replacement for a hip fracture. She also has osteoporosis. She is able to walk about 100 feet with a walker and is taking pain medication only at night.

Her rehabilitation treatment plan involves increasing her walking, progressing to a cane, and using exercises to increase strength and mobility in the hip joint and increase strength in her upper arms.

She is living with her daughter, whose home is on one level and has been made safe for Mrs. Vargas to move around in. Mrs. Vargas is taking alendronate (Fosamax) for her osteoporosis. Her diet is structured to give her 1500 **milligrams (mg)** of calcium daily, and she is taking a supplement of 600 **international units (IUs)** of vitamin D daily.

Learning Outcomes

Mrs. Vargas' rehabilitation will involve a team of people of different specialties. To participate fully in her care and communicate with team members, you need to be able to:

18.1 Apply the language of rehabilitation medicine to the therapeutic methods used to assist recovery from injury and disease.

18.2 Comprehend, analyze, spell, and write the medical terms of rehabilitation medicine so that you communicate and document accurately and precisely in any health care setting.

18.3 Recognize and pronounce the medical terms of rehabilitation medicine so that you communicate verbally with accuracy and precision in any health care setting.

18.4 Identify common conditions requiring restorative rehabilitation.

18.5 Specify common techniques used in rehabilitation.

OBJECTIVES

The information in this lesson will enable you to use correct medical terminology to:

18.1.1 Identify the members of the rehabilitation team.

18.1.2 Discuss the purposes of rehabilitation medicine.

18.1.3 Define the goals for a restorative rehabilitation program for specific common problems.

18.1.4 Detail common medical problems that arise during rehabilitation.

DEFINITIONS

Rehabilitation medicine focuses on **function.** Being able to function is essential for being independent and having a good quality of life.

Restorative rehabilitation restores a function that has been lost. It can be intense and short-term. Examples occur following a hip fracture, hip replacement, or stroke.

Maintenance rehabilitation strengthens and maintains a function that is gradually being lost. It is less intense and often long-term. Examples occur in the problems of senescence; for example, difficulty with balance or flexibility.

Rehabilitation medicine is also involved with **prevention** of loss of function and prevention of injury. In sports medicine, an example is prevention of shoulder and elbow injuries in baseball pitchers.

Rehabilitation Team

Rehabilitation programs involve a **multidisciplinary** team approach. Each member of the team manages different rehabilitation activities. Team members include:

- **Physiatrist**—a physician specializing in **physical medicine** and rehabilitation. This person is often the team leader.

- **Medical specialists**—manage acute or chronic illnesses and pain.

- **Occupational therapists**—improve performance of the **activities of daily living (ADLs)** that are described below and help patients adapt to visual and other perceptual deficits. They practice **occupational therapy (OT).**

- **Physical therapists**—improve strength, **range of motion (ROM)**, balance, and endurance and teach the use of assistive devices. They practice **physical therapy (PT)** assisted by **restorative aids.**

- **Rehabilitation psychologists**—specialists in helping people undergoing rehabilitation and those with resulting disabilities to reclaim their sense of belonging, contributing to, and participating in the world around them.

- **Social workers**—provide support and assistance with social issues such as health insurance, care facilities, and employment.

- **Speech therapists**—evaluate and treat communication, speech, and swallowing disorders.

- **Orthotists**—make and fit orthopedic appliances **(orthotics).**

- **Nutritionists**—evaluate and improve nutritional status.

Activities of daily living (ADLs) are the routine activities of personal care. The six basic ADLs are eating, bathing, dressing, grooming, toileting, and transferring. **Assistive devices** are designed to make ADLs easier to perform and help maintain independence. Examples are reachers and grabbers, easy-pull sock aids, long shoe-horns, jar openers, and eating aids *(Figure 18.1)*. ADLs are also a measurement to assess therapy needs and monitor its effectiveness.

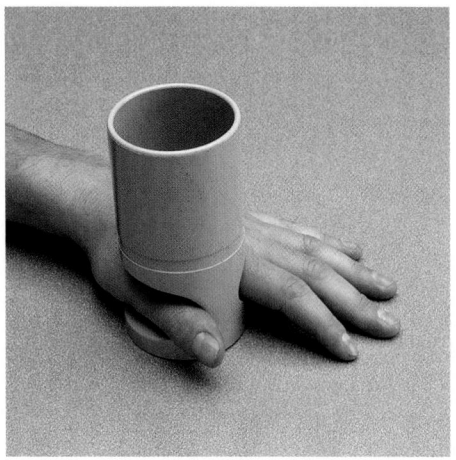

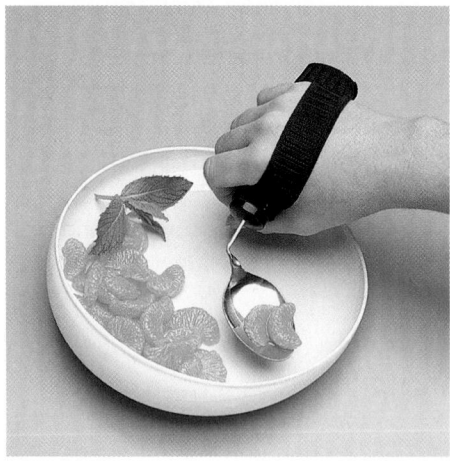

▲ **FIGURE 18.1 Assistive devices for eating.**

Abbreviations	
ADLs	activities of daily living
IADLs	instrumental activities of daily living
IU	international unit
mg	milligram
OT	occupational therapy
PT	physical therapy
PTA	physical therapy assistant
ROM	range of motion

WORD	PRONUNCIATION		ELEMENTS	DEFINITION
assistive device	ah-**SIS**-tiv de-**VICE**	S/ R/	-ive *nature of* assist- *aid, help* **device** *an appliance*	Tool, software, or hardware to assist in performing daily activities
multidisciplinary	mul-tee-**DIS**-ih-plih-**NAR**-ee	S/ P/ R/	-ary *pertaining to* multi- *many* -disciplin- *instruction*	Involving health care providers from more than one profession
occupational therapy	**OCK**-you-**PAY**-shun-al **THAIR**-ah-pee	S/ R/ R/	-al *pertaining to* occupation- *work* therapy *treatment*	Use of work and recreational activities to increase independent function
orthotic	or-**THOT**-ik	S/ R/	-ic *pertaining to* orthot- *correct*	Orthopedic appliance to correct an abnormality
orthotist	or-**THOT**-ist	S/	-ist *specialist*	Maker and fitter of orthopedic appliances
physiatry physiatrist	fih-**ZIE**-ah-tree fih-**ZIE**-ah-trist	 S/ R/ R/	Greek *science of nature* -ist *specialist* phys- *nature* -iatr- *treatment*	Physical medicine Specialist in physical medicine
physical medicine	**FIZ**-ih-cal **MED**-ih-sin	S/ R/	-al *pertaining to* physic- *body*	Diagnosis and treatment by means of remedial agents, such as exercises, manipulation, heat, etc.
physical therapy (also known as physiotherapy)	**FIZ**-ih-cal **THAIR**-ah-pee	S/ R/ R/	-al *pertaining to* physic- *body* therapy *treatment*	Use of remedial processes to overcome a physical defect
physiotherapy (syn)	**FIZ**-ee-oh-**THAIR**-ah-pee	R/CF	physi/o- *body*	Another term for physical therapy
prevention	pree-**VEN**-shun	S/ R/	-ion *action, condition* prevent- *prevent*	Process to prevent occurrence of a disease or health problem
rehabilitation	**REE**-hah-bill-ih-**TAY**-shun	S/ P/ R/	-ion *action, condition* re- *again* -habilitat- *restore*	Therapeutic restoration of an ability to function as before
restorative rehabilitation	ree-**STOR**-ah-tiv **REE**-hah-bill-ih-**TAY**-shun	S/ R/	-ative *quality of* restor- *renew*	Therapy that promotes renewal of health and strength

Instrumental activities of daily living (IADLs) relate to independent living. They include managing money, using a telephone, cooking, driving, shopping for groceries and personal items, and doing housework.

EXERCISES

Deconstruct the following medical terms into their word elements. Some terms will not have every element present. Then use any one term in a sentence of patient documentation. Fill in the blanks.

Medical Term	Prefix	Root/CF	Suffix	Meaning of Term
physiatrist				
rehabilitation				
orthotic				
multidisciplinary				
orthotist				
physiotherapy				

Sentence: _____

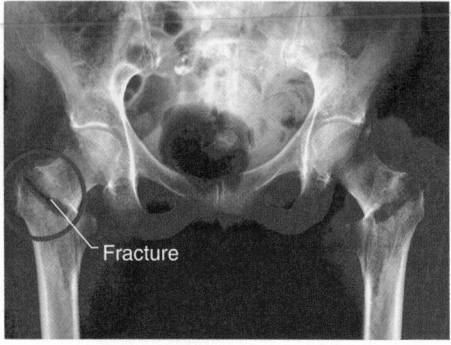

(a)

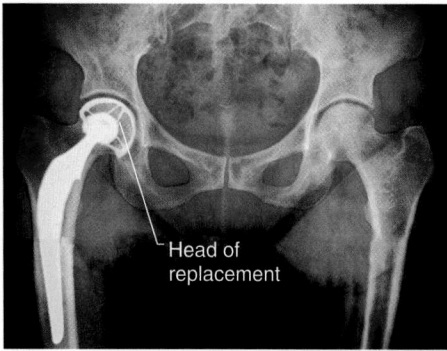

(b)

▲ **FIGURE 18.2 Hip Fracture.** (*a*) Fractured neck of femur in an osteoporotic woman. (*b*) Total hip replacement to repair the fracture.

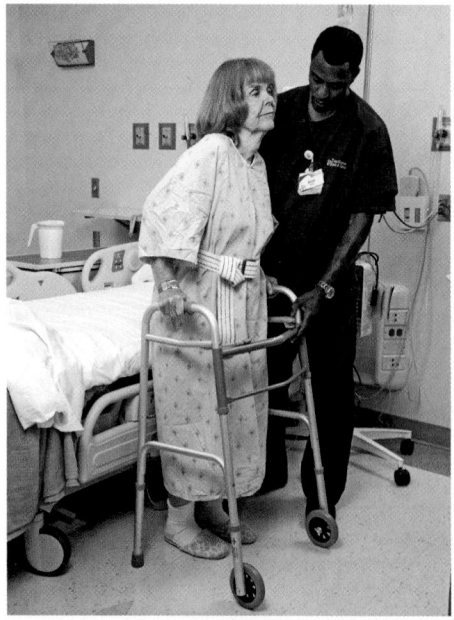

▲ **FIGURE 18.3 Postop: Starting to Bear Weight and Ambulate.**

Abbreviation	
DVT	deep vein thrombosis

Case Report 18.1 (continued)

For Mrs. Vargas the goal of hip fracture *(Figure 18.2)* rehabilitation is to regain as much pain-free function as possible. The rehabilitation focuses on:

- Strengthening the leg, buttock, and low-back muscles.
- Strengthening arm muscles to help with walking aids and with bathing and dressing.
- Improving balance.
- Progressing from walker to cane to walking without an aid.
- Treating underlying disease such as osteoporosis.
- Preventing further injury.

Mrs. Vargas was able to get out of bed the day after surgery with the physical therapist's assistance and to take a few steps in her room with a walker *(Figure 18.3)*. During her hospital stay, she progressed to walking several yards in the corridor with her walker. In her daughter's home, physical therapy has continued three times a week, and she is about to progress to using a four-prong cane (quad cane, or "quad") instead of a walker.

REHABILITATION CONSIDERATIONS

Numerous factors influence the course and outcome of rehabilitation after hip fracture:

- What physical shape the person was in before surgery, particularly in terms of muscle strength.
- The presence of underlying and other health problems.
- The type and severity of the fracture.
- The will and spirit of the patient (**motivation** and commitment).

Most people are allowed to bear weight on their leg the first day after hip surgery, depending on the surgeon's **protocol.** People who can do this early on require less physical therapy and progress quicker than the others. After hip replacement surgery, the patient should not internally rotate or adduct the leg and should not bend the trunk to below 90 degrees to the thigh. These three movements can be the cause of a very painful dislocation of the head of the hip replacement *(Figure 18.2b).*

Medical Considerations

Blood Clots Patients with hip fractures and with hip replacements are susceptible to **deep vein thrombosis (DVT)** in the affected leg. Anticoagulants, such as Heparin and Coumadin, are given, and **sequential (intermittent) pressure cuffs** on the legs are used postoperatively to prevent DVT. These **pneumatic** leg cuffs are pumped up and emptied by an electric pump to **simulate** the pressures in the veins generated by walking.

Cardiac Considerations

Most physical therapy programs do not require a high level of physical activity, such as running. Occupational therapy puts more stress on the heart than does physical therapy because exercising the arms increases blood pressure and pulse rate more than exercising the legs. However, particularly in the elderly, symptoms of shortness of breath (SOB), fatigue, and chest pain are watched for carefully.

WORD	PRONUNCIATION	ELEMENTS		DEFINITION
motivation	moh-tih-**VAY**-shun	S/ R/	-ation *process* motiv- *move*	Force that enables a person to meet a need or achieve a goal
pneumatic	new-**MAT**-ik	S/ R/	-ic *pertaining to* pneumat- *structure filled with air*	Pertaining to a structure filled with air
protocol	**PRO**-toe-kol		Latin *contents page of a book*	Detailed plan; in this case, for a regimen of therapy
sequence sequential (adj)	**SEE**-kwens see-**KWEN**-shal		Latin *to follow*	The succession of one event after another One event following another
simulate simulation	**SIM**-you-late sim-you-**LAY**-shun	S/ R/ S/	-ate *composed of, pertaining to* simul- *imitate* -ation *process*	To imitate a disease process

Joints

Arthritis that is already present can give rise to more pain during physiotherapy, as progressive weight bearing and movement stress the joints, and will influence the progression of the therapy.

Lung Rehabilitation

Again in the elderly, lung rehabilitation as part of the physical or occupational therapy program to work on breathing techniques is often essential even when there is no specific underlying lung problem present.

EXERCISE

After reading Case Report 18.1 on the opposite page, answer the following questions. Be prepared to discuss your answers in class.

1. Name two assistive devices Mrs. Vargas used to help her walk.

_____

2. What was the goal of her rehabilitation?

_____

3. What muscles are receiving specialized attention in Mrs. Vargas' rehabilitation therapy, and why?

_____

_____

4. Why will improving her balance help prevent further injury?

_____

5. What underlying disease needs continuing treatment for Mrs. Vargas?

_____

6. What role does patient motivation and commitment play in recovery and rehabilitation?

_____

Your patient is

...Mr. Hank Johnson, a 65-year-old owner of a printing shop.

CASE REPORT 18.2

One year ago, Mr. Johnson had an **elective** left total-hip replacement for osteo-arthritis. Four months later, he had a myocardial infarction. Two weeks ago, while on his exercise bicycle, he had a stroke. His right arm and leg were paralyzed, and he lost his speech and had difficulty swallowing. He was brought to the Emergency Department within 3 hours of the stroke and received thrombolytic **therapy** *(see Chapter 7)*. He is now receiving physical therapy, occupational therapy, and speech therapy in the inpatient Rehabilitation Unit. He is able to say some simple words and has begun to have voluntary movements in the arm and leg.

Your roles are to help him regain function in his arm and leg and to monitor and record his progress.

Abbreviations

BKA	below-the-knee amputation
COTA	certified occupational therapist assistant
PVD	peripheral vascular disease

Keynote

Coordinated multidisciplinary evaluation, management, and therapy add significantly to the chances of a good recovery.

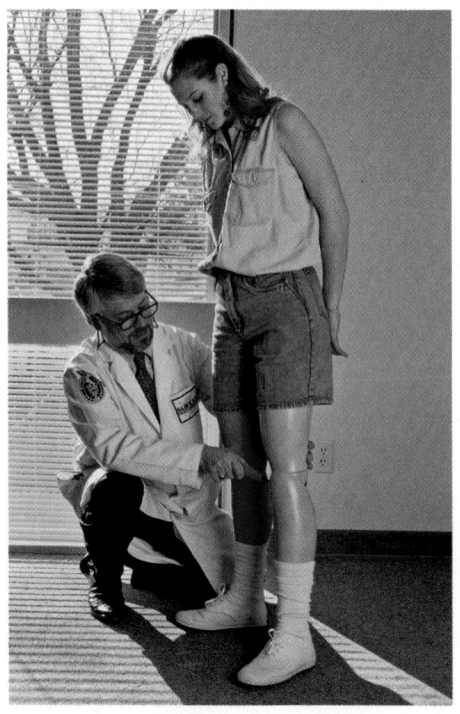

▲ **FIGURE 18.4 Sixteen-Year-Old Being Fitted with Prosthesis.**

STROKE REHABILITATION

The goals of Mr. Johnson's rehabilitation program are to enable him to:

- Walk safely using an assistive device.
- Use his hands with accuracy.
- Restore his speech abilities.
- Prevent a second stroke.

Because he received thrombolytic therapy *(see Chapter 7)* within 3 hours of the onset of his stroke, his chance of being left with little or no **residual** difficulty is around 50%, compared to 35% if he had not received the therapy.

Social workers are helping his wife to make their home safe for his return and to work with Medicare to obtain the maximum benefits allowed. They will work out the family's need for **adaptive equipment,** such as raised toilet seats, handrails in bath and shower, eating devices, and other equipment to enable Mr. Johnson to perform the activities of daily living as he recovers.

Anyone who has had one stroke is at high risk for having a second stroke. During this rehabilitative period, he will be evaluated for such risk factors as narrowing of his carotid arteries with plaque and thrombosis *(see Chapter 7)* and the presence of atrial fibrillation *(see Chapter 8)*.

AMPUTATIONS

Seventy-five percent of all **amputations** are performed on people over 65 years with **peripheral vascular disease (PVD)** with complications due to arteriosclerosis and diabetes. Most of these are **below-the-knee amputations (BKAs).** The war in Iraq has led to the loss of arms and legs in soldiers due to explosive devices. Rehabilitation after amputation is an increasingly important component in rehabilitation programs.

Immediately after surgery to perform the amputation, the objectives are to:

- Promote healing of the stump.
- Strengthen the muscles above the site of the amputation.
- Strengthen arm muscles to assist in ambulation.
- Prevent **contractures** of the joints above the amputation (knee and hip for BKAs).
- Shrink the stump with elastic cuffs or bandages to fit the socket of a temporary **prosthesis.**
- Provide emotional, psychological, and family support.

With a temporary leg prosthesis *(Figure 18.4)*, weight bearing and walking can be practiced first on parallel bars *(Figure 18.5)* and then with a walker, crutches, and cane.

WORD	PRONUNCIATION	ELEMENTS		DEFINITION
adapt	ad-**APT**		Latin *to adjust*	To adjust to different conditions
adaptive equipment	a-**DAP**-tiv ee-**KWIP**-ment	S/ R/ S/ R/	**-ive** *nature of, quality of* **adapt-** *adjust* **-ment** *action, state* **equip-** *to fit out*	Devices and supplies that enable a disabled individual to perform specific functions
amputation amputate (verb) amputee	am-pyu-**TAY**-shun am-pyu-**TATE** **AM**-pyu-tee		Latin *to prune*	Process of removing a limb, part of a limb, a breast, or other projecting part A person with an amputation
contracture	kon-**TRAK**-chur	S/ R/	**-ure** *result of* **contract-** *pull together*	Muscle shortening due to spasm or fibrosis
elective	e-**LEK**-tiv	S/ R/	**-ive** *nature of, quality of* **elect-** *choice*	Not urgent or vital, as surgery
prosthesis	**PROS**-thee-sis		Greek *an addition*	Manufactured substitute for a missing part of the body
residual	re-**ZID**-you-al	S/ R/CF	**-al** *pertaining to* **resid/u-** *left over*	Pertaining to anything left over
therapy	**THAIR**-ah-pee		Greek *medical treatment*	Systematic treatment of a disease, dysfunction, or disorder
therapeutic	**THAIR**-ah-**PYU**-tik	S/ R/	**-ic** *pertaining to* **therapeut-** *treatment*	Relating to the treatment of a disease or disorder
therapist	**THAIR**-ah-pist	S/ R/	**-ist** *specialist* **therap-** *treatment*	Professional trained in the practice of a particular therapy

A temporary prosthesis can usually be fitted 4 to 8 weeks after surgery and a permanent prosthesis 8 to 12 weeks after surgery. About 75% of older adults with a prosthesis can walk, often without a cane or walker.

For an arm and/or hand prosthesis, the decision on what type of prosthesis will be needed depends on what natural arms and hands remain, what functions the patient wants and needs to do, and which kinds of prostheses are available and affordable.

The hand or tool of the prosthesis can be a hand, hook, or some other shape to perform specific functions that are needed.

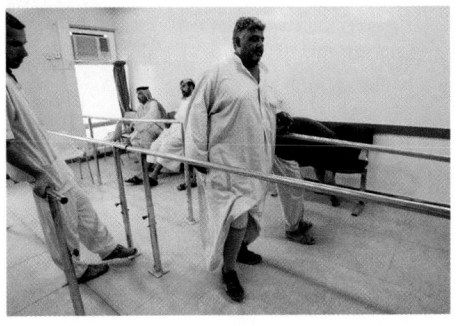

▲ **FIGURE 18.5 Trying Out a New Prosthesis in Iraq.**

EXERCISES

*Utilize the correct **language of rehabilitation** in the following paragraph. The word bank contains more terms than you need to use—some terms you may use more than once. When you have finished the exercise, proofread it again to see if it makes sense. Fill in the blanks.*

Word bank:

adapt	contracture	amputation(s)	prosthesis
amputee	adaptive equipment	elective	amputate
residual	PVD	assistive	protocol

Seventy-five percent of all _____ are performed on patients over 65 years of age with

_____ complicating arteriosclerosis and diabetes. Loss of blood flow to a limb area produces necrotic

tissue, which in time can become infected or gangrenous and makes the need for this procedure urgent, rather

than _____. A traumatic _____ can occur in an industrial accident, motor vehicle accident,

or household accident. The decision to _____ is a serious one and must be undertaken by a qualified

surgeon. The _____ will require postoperative training in how to _____ to the use of

a _____ and/or _____. Hopefully, there will be no muscle _____

or _____ pain after the surgery.

Techniques and Tools of Rehabilitation

THERAPEUTIC TECHNIQUES AND TOOLS

Physical therapists, occupational therapists, physical therapy assistants, and physical therapy aides use a wide range of therapeutic techniques and **modalities** in the rehabilitation of patients. This can range from a simple ice pack for an acute muscle injury to the stimulation of nerve and muscle by electrical currents or the use of heat to increase circulation and ease pain.

Cryotherapy

Cold has its best effects in an acute injury when it lowers the temperature in the injured area to decrease its metabolism. This enables the damaged tissue to better survive hypoxia.

When applied with **compression**, cold produces local vasoconstriction to control hemorrhage and edema and decrease pain.

After the initial acute injury, cold is used to reduce pain and reflex muscle spasm. It depresses the excitability of peripheral nerve endings and thus increases the **pain threshold,** making it less noticeable. A minimum of 15 minutes is needed to obtain analgesia. The more subcutaneous fat, the longer the cold will take to reach the underlying muscle and the longer the treatment will need to be.

The tools of **cryotherapy** include ice packs (trade-named **Hydrocollator** packs; *Figure 18.6*) containing petroleum distillate gel that are frozen in the freezer, ice massage, and cold whirlpool baths. Commercial cold sprays do not provide deep penetration and are used to reduce muscle spasm. **Cryokinetics** uses the action of cold but adds exercise and **active range of motion (AROM)** of joints when the cold has produced numbness.

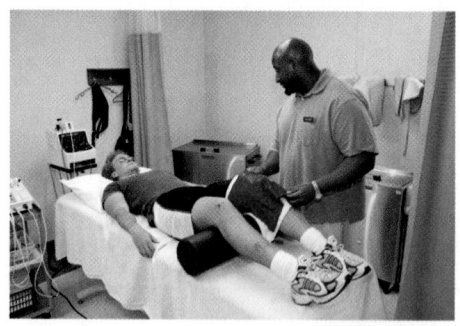

▲ **FIGURE 18.6 An Ice Pack Can Be Molded to Fit an Injured Part.**

Abbreviation	
AROM	active range of motion

Thermotherapy

Heat induces vasodilation with its hyperemia and increase in the supply of oxygen, nutrients, enzymes, and leukocytes needed in the repair process, together with an increased removal of metabolites. Heat reduces pain and increases relaxation of muscle; these are the bases for **thermotherapy.**

Techniques for applying heat include a hot whirlpool bath (98°F to 110°F), warm Hydrocollator packs that are heated to 170°F and used wrapped in towels *(Figure 18.7),* and infrared lamps that do not penetrate beyond the superficial subcutaneous layers. **Fluidized therapy** uses a dry whirlpool of suspended fine particles in a heated air stream to apply heat, massage, and sensory stimulation. It does not penetrate into deep muscles.

Thermacare wraps contain small discs of iron, charcoal, salt, and water that heat up when unwrapped and exposed to oxygen. They reach muscles at a depth of three-quarters of an inch from the skin surface.

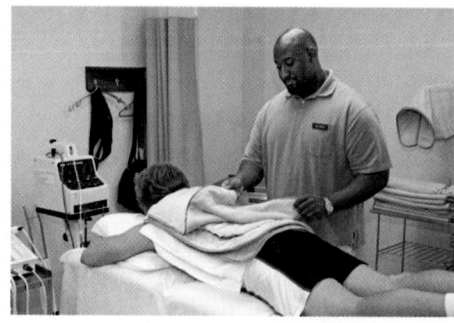

▲ **FIGURE 18.7 Warm Pack Applied to Lower Back.**

WORD	PRONUNCIATION	ELEMENTS		DEFINITION
compression	kom-**PRESH**-un	S/ R/	-ion *action, condition* compress- *press together*	Squeeze together to increase density or decrease a dimension of a structure
cryokinetics	**CRY**-oh-kih-**NET**-iks	S/ R/CF R/	-ics *knowledge of* cry/o- *cold* -kinet- *motion*	Combination of cold therapy with exercise
cryotherapy	**KRY**-oh-**THAIR**-ah-pee	S/	-therapy *treatment*	The use of cold in the treatment of injury
fluidized therapy	**FLU**-id-ized **THAIR**-ah-pee	S/ R/ R/	-ized *affected in a specific way* fluid- *to flow* therapy *medical treatment*	Use of suspended particles in hot air stream to apply heat
fluidotherapy	**FLU**-id-oh-**THAIR**-ah-pee	R/CF S/	fluid/o- *to flow* -therapy *treatment*	A form of heat therapy
Hydrocollator	high-droh-**KOLL**-ay-tor	S/ R/CF R/	-ator *that which does* hydr/o- *water* -coll- *collect*	Synthetic hot or cold gel to stimulate a rise or fall in tissue temperature
modality modalities (pl)	moh-**DAL**-ih-tee moh-**DAL**-ih-tees		Latin *a method*	A form of therapeutic agent or regimen
pain threshold	PANE **THRESH**-old		**pain** Latin *a penalty* **threshold** Anglo-Saxon *entrance*	The point at which pain is first noticed
thermotherapy	**THER**-moh-**THAIR**-ah-pee	S/ R/CF	-therapy *treatment* therm/o- *heat*	The use of heat in treatment

EXERCISES

Test your knowledge of the elements in medical terminology. Match the correct element in the left column with its meaning in the right column. Fill in the blanks.

_____ 1. therapy

_____ 2. hydr/o

_____ 3. kinet

_____ 4. cry/o

_____ 5. therm/o

_____ 6. ics

A. heat

B. cold

C. knowledge of

D. motion

E. treatment

F. water

*Define **modality**, and list several different modalities used in rehabilitation.*

7. Definition of **modality**:

_____

_____

_____

8. Types of modalities:

_____

_____

_____

_____

THERAPEUTIC TECHNIQUES AND TOOLS (continued)

Ultrasound Therapy

Therapeutic ultrasound uses its high-frequency, **acoustic** (sound) vibrations to provide deep heating (*Figure 18.8*). A **transducer** is used to convert electrical energy to sound energy that passes through tissues, generating heat.

Treatments are usually started as soon as possible after injury of muscles, tendons, and joints. Ultrasound can also be used to stimulate bone healing.

Phonophoresis uses ultrasound to facilitate delivery of some medications through the skin into tissues by increasing the permeability of the stratum corneum. Hydrocortisone or dexamethasone cream (Decadron) are commonly delivered with this technique.

Light Therapy

Laser is an acronym for **l**ight **a**mplification by **s**timulated **e**mission of **r**adiation. Low-power lasers seem to be effective in aiding wound healing and reducing pain but have not received FDA approval.

Light emission diode (LED) therapy has received FDA approval. Red LEDs help prevent the skin appearances of aging, amber LEDs trigger pain relief, and blue LEDs treat acne.

Ultraviolet therapy has a limited use for treating dermatologic conditions such as psoriasis, acne, and pressure sores.

Electrical Stimulation

Electrical stimulation is used in two forms:

1. **Functional electrical stimulation** uses an electrical current directed to a muscle. This prevents **atrophy** in muscles that are not being used. It can also help increase the function of previously paralyzed muscles.

2. **Transcutaneous electrical nerve stimulation (TENS)** stimulates peripheral nerves to improve muscle strength and mass (*Figure 18.9*). It is also used to treat pain associated with the peripheral neuropathy of diabetes and for older adults with herpes zoster (shingles).

Spinal Traction

Traction can be performed mechanically using a machine or a system of ropes and pulleys or be performed manually by a therapist. Its function is to increase the space between vertebrae, so it can be used to treat intervertebral disc herniations and lumbar and cervical muscle spasm.

Mechanical lumbar traction can be performed using a lower-body harness and a traction device to generate a force equal to half the patient's body weight. Mechanical cervical traction can use a head harness with forces of 20 to 50 pounds (*Figure 18.10*).

Hyperbaric Oxygen Therapy

Hyperbaric oxygen therapy (HBOT) chambers enable oxygen therapy to be given at pressures greater than atmospheric pressure. This promotes angiogenesis (formation of new blood vessels) and wound healing. In addition to treating decompression sickness, it is used to improve skin graft and wound healing and to treat radiation ulcers, snake bites, acute thermal burns, and foot injuries in diabetics. It also kills certain anaerobic bacteria and prevents the production of some bacterial toxins (*see Chapter 20*).

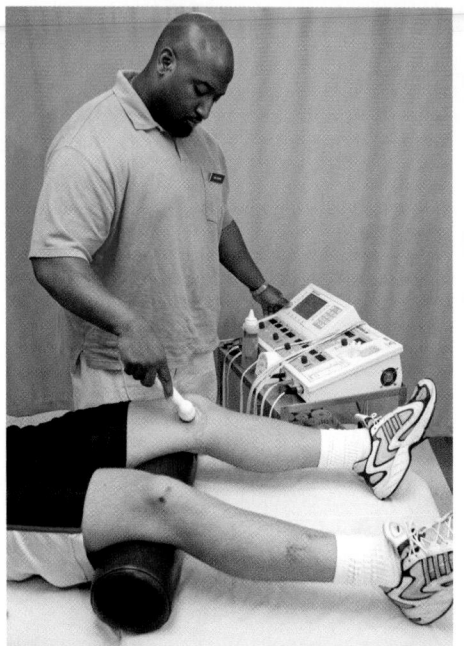

▲ **FIGURE 18.8 Ultrasound Applied Through a Gel-Like Coupling Medium.**

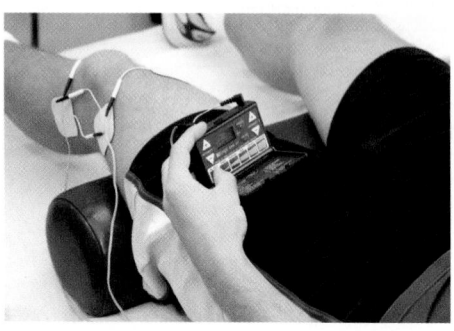

▲ **FIGURE 18.9 Application of Electrodes for TENS Stimulation.**

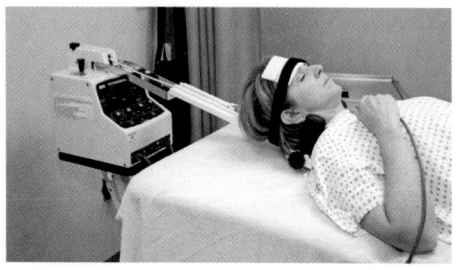

▲ **FIGURE 18.10 Mechanical Cervical Traction.**

Abbreviations

HBOT	hyperbaric oxygen therapy
LASER	light amplification by stimulated emission of radiation
LED	light emission diode
TENS	transcutaneous electrical nerve stimulation

B. **Abbreviations:** An abbreviation is a shortcut for saving time by not writing out all the words. Rewrite the following sentences in correct medical language *without* using the abbreviations. (Take the abbreviations out of these sentences, and insert the full terms.)

1. Rehabilitation for this stroke patient includes instruction in ADLs and IADLs.

   _____

   _____

   _____

2. To prevent DVT from forming, patient needs to get out of bed and walk 1 hour in the morning, afternoon, and evening.

   _____

   _____

   _____

3. The patient's ROM will be assessed by the PT tomorrow.

   _____

   _____

4. We will try to alleviate this patient's chronic pain with a TENS unit.

   _____

   _____

   _____

5. Now choose one of the sentences above and rewrite it in nonmedical language.

   _____

   _____

   _____

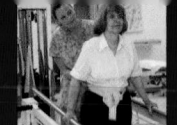

REHABILITATION MEDICINE

C. **Greek and Latin Terms:** A lot of medical terms are formed directly from Greek and Latin terms. You are given the medical term; list its meaning, and then define the term. The first one is done for you. Fill in the chart.

Medical Term	Greek/Latin	Definition
adapt	*To adjust*	*To adjust to different conditions*
amputation		
assist		
modality		
physiatry		
prosthesis		
protocol		
traction		

Some of these terms can be used in regular English sentences with no medical meaning. Choose two terms, and write a simple English sentence for each in which the word has no medical meaning. Write a second sentence for each term that illustrates how the same term is used medically.

Term: _____ .

1. English usage: _____

   _____

   _____

2. Medical usage: _____

   _____

   _____

Term: _____ .

3. English usage: _____

   _____

   _____

4. Medical usage: _____

   _____

   _____

D. **Elements:** Identifying word elements will assist you in determining the meaning of the medical term. Test your knowledge of the elements, and circle the correct choice.

1. In the term **physiatrist,** the suffix means:

   a. agent, specialist

   b. a condition

   c. an inflammation

   d. one who leads

   e. nature

2. In the term **orthotic,** the root means:

   a. many

   b. correct

   c. move

   d. action

   e. physical

3. In the term **contracture,** the suffix means:

   a. addition

   b. movement

   c. process

   d. energy

   e. pertaining to

4. In the term **transducer,** the root means:

   a. device

   b. pulling

   c. temperature

   d. leader

   e. cold

5. In the term **multidisciplinary,** the prefix means:

   a. one

   b. specialists

   c. many

   d. across

   e. less than

REHABILITATION MEDICINE

E. **Elements:** Identifying word elements will assist you in determining the meaning of the medical term. Test your knowledge of the elements, and circle the correct choice.

1. The element **ics** is a:

   a. suffix

   b. prefix

   c. root

   d. combining form

   e. combining vowel

2. The element **sis** is a:

   a. suffix

   b. prefix

   c. root

   d. combining form

   e. combining vowel

3. The element **thermo** is a:

   a. suffix

   b. prefix

   c. root

   d. combining form

   e. combining vowel

4. The element **contract** is a:

   a. suffix

   b. prefix

   c. root

   d. combining form

   e. combining vowel

5. The element **trans** is a:

   a. suffix

   b. prefix

   c. root

   d. combining form

   e. combining vowel

F. Recall and Review: How well do you remember these word elements from the previous chapter? Try to answer without first looking back to check. Fill in the blanks.

Element	Type of Element (P, R, CF, S)	Meaning of Element
ician	_____	_____
glyc	_____	_____
tri	_____	_____
gen	_____	_____
un	_____	_____

G. Identify the elements from the language of rehabilitation. Match the meaning in the left column with the correct medical term in the right column. Fill in the blanks.

_____ 1. Combining form means *left over*

_____ 2. Combining form means *cold*

_____ 3. Root means *understand*

_____ 4. Suffix means *treatment*

_____ 5. Suffix means *abnormal condition*

_____ 6. Root means *body*

_____ 7. Suffix means *that which does*

_____ 8. Root means *to move*

_____ 9. Prefix means *across*

_____ 10. Root means *correct*

A. Hydrocollator

B. transducer

C. cryokinetics

D. phonophoresis

E. physiatrist

F. orthotic

G. residual

H. multidisciplinary

I. motivation

J. hydrotherapy

Choose any *two terms* from column 2 and use them *both in a single sentence* of your choice.

Sentence:

_____

_____

_____

_____

_____

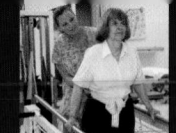
REHABILITATION MEDICINE

H. Teamwork: Being able to perform the ADLs is essential for being independent and having a good quality of life. Patients in rehabilitation often have a multidisciplinary team responsible for their care. Each member of the team contributes his or her expertise to help restore function to the patient's life. Identify the correct profession on the basis of the statement given. There are more answers than you will need. Fill in the blanks.

nutritionist	social worker	psychologist	physiatrist	restorative aide
orthopedist	physical therapist	occupational therapist	speech therapist	orthotist
pain management specialist	endocrinologist			

1. This team member works with Mrs. Vargas to improve her strength, range of motion, balance, and endurance. She is also helping Mrs. Vargas learn to use a walker. _____

2. This physician is responsible for the overall rehabilitation management of the entire team helping Mrs. Vargas. _____

3. Fitting of a brace to strengthen a patient's leg after a stroke will be done by the _____.

4. Paralysis resulting from a stroke often leaves patients unable to do even the most simple daily tasks, such as brushing their teeth or combing their hair. Working with a(n) _____ can help improve performance of these tasks.

5. Changes in diet can often improve a rehabilitation patient's health status. Consultation with a(n) _____ would be recommended.

6. The physical exertion required for rehab often exacerbates pain. This physician will be called upon for patient care. _____

7. Partial facial paralysis often follows a stroke, and this can result in slow speech or slurring of words. Mr. Johnson is able to speak only simple words. A _____ will work with him to improve his communication skills.

8. Extensive time spent in rehabilitation often takes a mental toll on patients and their families. Support can be provided by the _____.

9. The physical therapist has designed a program of treatment to help restore some of the functions the patient had before his stroke. A _____ will help her implement this program for the patient.

10. After rehab, some patients will still need skilled nursing care in a nursing home. This can be arranged with the help of the _____.

11. The _____ has performed the surgery that now requires rehabilitation for the patient.

I. **Roots/Combining Forms:** Continue building and testing your knowledge of the root/combining form elements found in this chapter. Fill in the table.

Element	Meaning of Element	Medical Term with This Element	Meaning of This Medical Term
cry/o			
ducer			
habilitat			
hydr/o			
iatri			
orthot			
phon/o			
physic			
resid/u			
therm/o			

J. **Difference Between:** Patients will often ask for an explanation of medical terms they do not understand. Your patients have been referred to the following health care professionals. Explain to your patients the difference between:

1. An orthotist and an orthopedist

    Orthotist: _____

    Orthopedist: _____

2. A physiatrist and a psychiatrist

    Physiatrist: _____

    Psychiatrist: _____

K. **In Your Own Words:** Essential to insight into the concept of rehabilitation is understanding the focus rehabilitation places on function. In your own words, briefly describe how rehabilitation can restore, maintain, or prevent loss of function. Give examples when possible. Write a brief answer.

1. Restore a function:

    _____

    _____

2. Maintain a function:

    _____

    _____

3. Prevent loss of function:

    _____

    _____

REHABILITATION MEDICINE

L. **Classroom Discussion:** What kinds of medical advances are made as a result of an influx of patients with war injuries? Can you back up your opinion with any research or recent articles on this subject? (Check reliable Internet sites: .gov, .edu, or .org.)

Outline your thoughts for the discussion or write your notes from your research here:

_____

_____

_____

_____

_____

_____

_____

_____

_____

_____

M. **Accurate documentation requires using correct terminology.** Apply the following rehabilitation terminology to the exercise. There are more answers than questions. Fill in the blanks.

modalities	TENS	traction	protocol
amputation	orthotist	orthopedist	prosthesis
orthotic	contracture	ECG	residual

1. The _____ referred the patient to an _____ for fitting of a special leg brace following his surgery. This _____ device was covered by the patient's insurance company.

2. The _____ for the clinical trial stipulated surgery and chemotherapy as the treatment of choice for this patient.

3. Arthritis caused painful _____ of the patient's fingers and toes.

4. The patient's leg was so badly crushed in the accident that it required _____.

5. The patient suffered _____ effects of her stroke and requires speech therapy for several more months.

6. Because of his hip _____, the patient will be required to take a blood thinner for the rest of his life.

7. The patient has been given a(n) _____ unit for pain relief after her spinal surgery.

8. In an effort to increase the space between the fourth and fifth vertebrae and reduce the disc herniation, I am recommending _____ for this patient.

9. This patient may be treated with any of the following _____: ice packs, ice massage, or cold whirlpool baths.

N. **Language of Rehabilitation:** Build your knowledge of the *language of rehabilitation* by filling in the correct term for the definitions given. Some terms form part of additional terms with similar meanings. Fill in the blanks.

1. Pertaining to aid or help: _____

   A tool to help you perform a daily activity: _____

   Give an example: _____

2. *That which is left over or remaining:* _____

   What could remain after a patient has had a stroke? _____

3. Surgery that *is not* urgent or vital: _____

   Surgery that *is* urgent or vital: _____

4. From the Latin *to adjust:* _____

   Devices and supplies that help a patient conduct normal activities: _____

   Give an example: _____

5. *The result of pulling together:* _____

   Give an example in an arthritic patient: _____

6. From the Latin *to prune:* _____

   The result of a radical mastectomy: _____

   A person missing a limb or body part: _____

O. **Similar but Different:** The difference of one word completely alters the meaning of an order from a physician. Can you interpret the terminology well enough to perform responsibly?

   The physiatrist has ordered the following equipment for the patient. Give an example of each type of equipment, and briefly describe the help it provides to the patient.

1. *adaptive* equipment:

   Example: _____

   Help: _____

2. *assistive* device:

   Example: _____

   Help: _____

   Mr. Johnson has received thrombolytic therapy in the past. Another one of your patients is scheduled for thermotherapy. Briefly describe each type of therapy and explain its purpose.

3. thrombolytic therapy: _____

   _____

4. thermotherapy: _____

   _____

REHABILITATION MEDICINE

P. **Research:** Use your dictionary, glossary, school library, and/or the Internet to research the medical term **pain threshold.**

    1. Write a definition for this term.

_____

_____

_____

    2. Write three facts you have learned about this medical term.

_____

_____

_____

_____

_____

_____

_____

_____

_____

_____

_____

_____

    3. Use this term in a sentence of patient documentation.

_____

_____

_____

_____

Q. **Terminology Challenge: ultrasound** versus **hyperbaric.**

Both these prefixes denote some degree of measurement. Give the exact meaning of each prefix, and explain how they are similar and how they are different. Fill in the blanks.

    ultrasound: Prefix is _____ and means _____.

    hyperbaric: Prefix is _____ and means _____.

Similar but different:

_____

_____

_____

R. Elements: Demonstrate your knowledge of word elements and definitions for each of the following rehabilitation terms. Circle the correct answer.

1. **cryotherapy:** The element **cryo** is a:

   suffix   prefix   root   combining form

2. **transducer:** The prefix means:

   beneath   beside   on top of   across

3. **modality:** The term means a:

   condition   method   disease   sound

4. **thermotherapy:** The element **thermo** is a:

   suffix   prefix   root   combining form

5. **Hydrocollator:** The element **hydro** means:

   white   water   heat   excessive

6. **cryokinetics:** The root means:

   motion   collect   being born   leader

7. **traction:** The term means:

   sleep   walk   pull   turn

8. **phonophoresis:** The suffix means:

   abnormal condition   that which does   treatment   sound

9. **acoustic:** The root means:

   seeing   walking   hearing   standing

10. **atrophy:** The root means:

    development   abnormal   without   beside

Pick one term from above, and use it to communicate a message about a patient:

Term:_____

Message: _____

_____

Study Hint
Equate the term *traction* to a certain farm machine. It serves the same purpose.

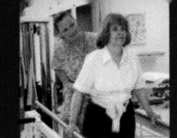
REHABILITATION MEDICINE

S. Apply the *language of rehabilitation* to the following questions. Circle the correct answer.

1. Rehabilitation medicine focuses on:

   a. prevention

   b. restoration

   c. function

   d. strength

   e. all of the above

2. A *protocol* is a:

   a. rehabilitation team

   b. treatment plan

   c. medical specialist

   d. special piece of equipment

   e. treatment modality

3. Name one tool of cryotherapy:

   a. subcutaneous injection

   b. heating pad

   c. Hydrocollator

   d. hot wax

   e. acupuncture

4. Name one example of adaptive equipment:

   a. raised toilet seat

   b. walker

   c. prosthesis

   d. orthotic

   e. quad cane

5. How many prongs does a quad cane have?

   a. one

   b. two

   c. three

   d. four

   e. five

6. Can be used to treat decompression sickness, snake bites, and radiation ulcers:

   a. ADL

   b. LED

   c. TENS

   d. ROM

   e. HBOT

7. In a rehabilitation multidisciplinary team, the _____ leads the team.

   a. social worker

   b. orthopedist

   c. physiatrist

   d. orthotist

   e. physical therapist

8. Patients with hip fractures and hip replacements are susceptible to:

   a. BKA

   b. DVT

   c. ADL

   d. ROM

   e. PVD

9. Heat reduces pain and increases:

   a. body metabolism

   b. relaxation of muscle

   c. vasoconstriction of blood vessels

   d. pulse rate

   e. tendon elasticity

10. A maker and fitter of orthopedic appliances is called a(n):

   a. orthopedist

   b. ophthalmologist

   c. histologist

   d. orthotist

   e. physiatrist

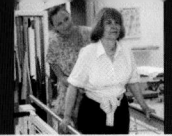

REHABILITATION MEDICINE

CHAPTER SUMMARY EXERCISE

1. *Listen to the pronunciation of the medical terms as given by your instructor.*
2. *Circle the correct spelling of the medical term.*
3. *Match the correctly spelled terms to the brief descriptions below.*
4. *Write a sentence for each of the 10 terms that appear in this exercise.*

A. SPELLING COMPREHENSION: CIRCLE THE CORRECT SPELLING OF THE TERM.

1. fonophoresis	phonophoresis	funoporesis	phonoporesis	ponophoresis
2. restoreitive	ristoritive	restorative	ristorative	ristoriteve
3. ultravilet	ultreviolet	ultreeviolet	ultraviolet	ultraviolette
4. pysiatry	phsiatry	physiatrey	phsiatrey	physiatry
5. therapeutic	teraputetic	thereputic	terapeutic	theraputic
6. kryocinetics	cryocinetics	kryokinetics	cryokinetics	criocinetics
7. trackion	tracktion	tracion	treckion	traction
8. rehabilitation	rehabillition	rehavilitation	rehabillitation	rehebiliation
9. orthotic	othotick	ortotic	orthotick	orrthotic
10. hyperberric	hypoberic	hyperbarrick	hyperbaric	hypobaric

B. MATCH THE NUMBER OF THE CORRECT TERM IN PART A WITH THE BRIEF DESCRIPTION OF THE TERM BELOW.

a. Pressure greater than atmospheric pressure _____

b. Uses ultrasound to facilitate delivery of medication _____

c. Combines cold with exercise _____

d. Limited use for dermatologic conditions _____

e. Physical medicine _____

f. Focuses on function _____

g. Corrects an orthopedic abnormality _____

h. Pertaining to treatment _____

i. To return something to what it was _____

j. Can be manual or mechanical _____

C. USING YOUR KNOWLEDGE OF TERMS 1–10 IN PART A AND THEIR CORRECT SPELLING, WRITE A BRIEF SENTENCE FOR EACH OF THE TERMS AS IT MIGHT APPEAR IN PATIENT DOCUMENTATION.

1. _____

2. _____

3. _____

4. _____

5. _____

6. _____

7. _____

8. _____

9. _____

10. _____

D. YOUR INSTRUCTOR WILL DIRECT YOU TO MCGRAW-HILL CONNECT. OPEN THE AUDIO GLOSSARY AND PRACTICE YOUR PRONUNCIATION OF THE TERMS IN PART A OF THIS EXERCISE.

Mc Graw Hill **connect**™ (plus+)

E. AFTER READING CASE REPORT 18.1, ANSWER THE FOLLOWING QUESTIONS. BE PREPARED TO DISCUSS YOUR ANSWERS IN CLASS.

CASE REPORT 18.1

You are

. . . a **physical therapy assistant (PTA)** employed in the Rehabilitation Unit at Fulwood Medical Center.

Your patient is

. . . Mrs. Amy Vargas, a 70-year-old housewife, who is 2 weeks postop following an emergency hip replacement for a hip fracture. She also has osteoporosis. She is able to walk about 100 feet with a walker and is taking pain medication only at night.

Her rehabilitation treatment plan involves increasing her walking, progressing to a cane, and using exercises to increase strength and mobility in the hip joint and increase strength in her upper arms.

She is living with her daughter, whose home is on one level and has been made safe for Mrs. Vargas to move around in. Mrs. Vargas is taking alendronate (Fosamax) for her osteoporosis. Her diet is structured to give her 1500 **milligrams (mg)** of calcium daily, and she is taking a supplement of 600 **international units (IUs)** of vitamin D daily.

1. Mrs. Vargas' hip surgery was an emergency, rather than "elective." Why?

   _____

2. Choose the correct abbreviation for her surgery. _____

   HBV   TAH   THR   TURP   HDL

3. What disease is in her past medical history? _____

4. What nutrients are now an important part of Mrs. Vargas' diet?

   _____

5. What prescribed medication is she taking for her condition?

   _____

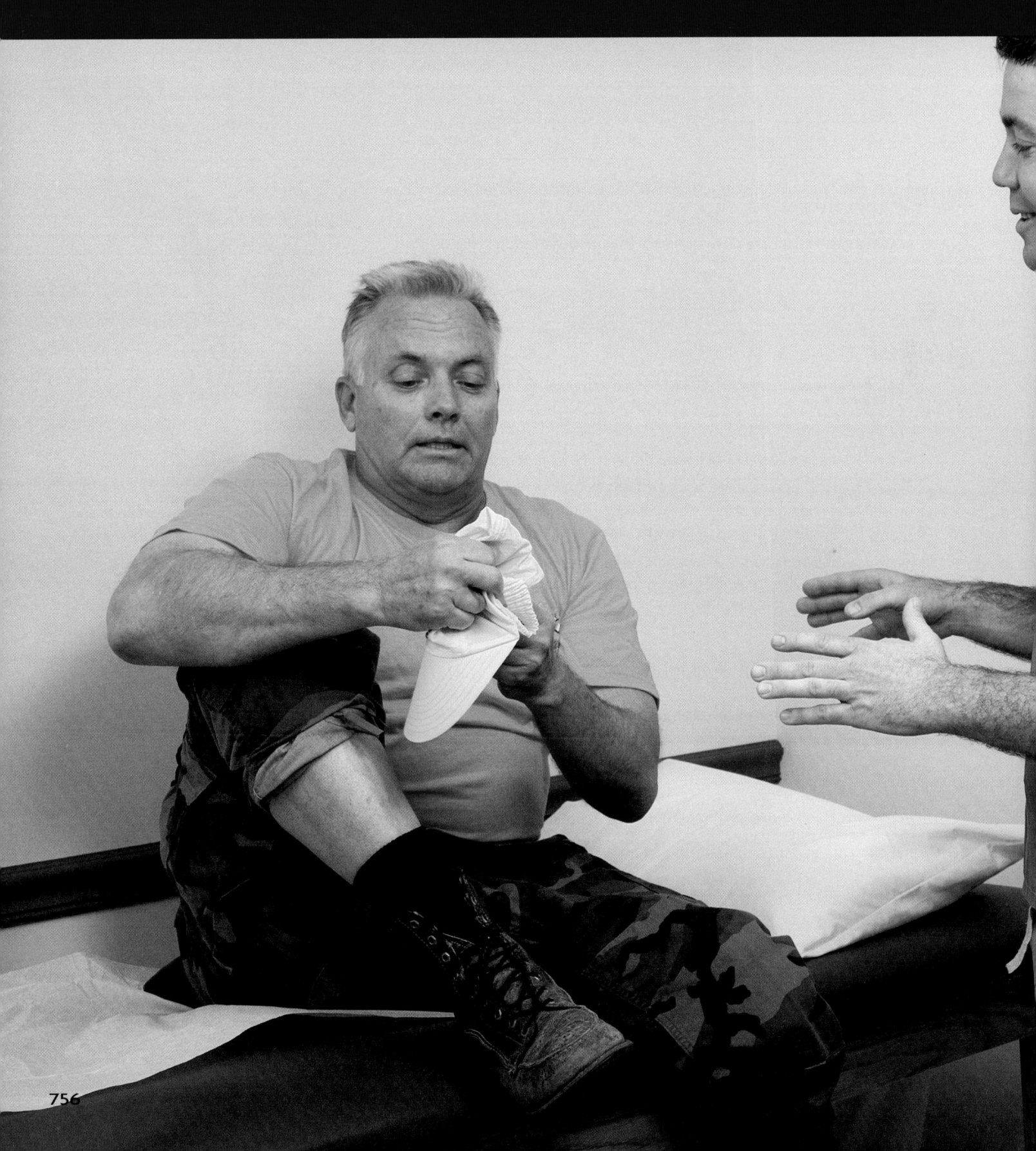

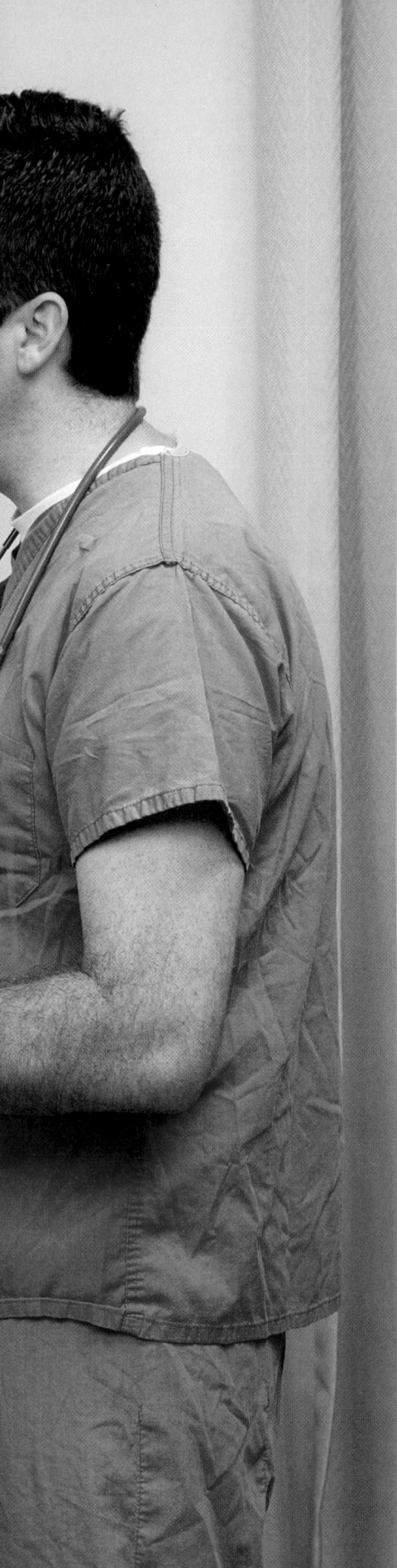

CASE REPORT 19.1

You are

. . . A **psychiatric technician** employed in the Psychiatric Department of Fulwood Medical Center. Your patient has been referred from the Emergency Department, where he was seen earlier this morning.

Your patient is

. . . Mr. Harlan Diment, a 40-year-old construction worker. He was brought to the Emergency Department by his roommate, who says that Mr. Diment has slept only a couple of hours each night for the past 3 weeks. He stays up most of the night, cleaning their apartment and drinking beer. He has bought a new home entertainment set, including a big-screen plasma TV, that he cannot afford. He is very irritable and explosive when challenged about his behavior. His roommate has seen no signs of drugs and is not aware of any medical problems. Mr. Diment is usually very quiet, thoughtful, and introverted.

A mental status examination shows Mr. Diment to be alternately irritable and excited. He is wearing a bright orange top and camouflage slacks and is carrying a soft green cap. His speech is rapid and loud, and it is difficult to interrupt him. He paces the room, claims to feel "great," and is angry with his roommate for insisting that he come to the hospital. His thought processes and verbalization go off on different **tangents (tangentiality).** He says he has no suicidal thoughts, **hallucinations,** or **delusions.**

Learning Outcomes

To be an effective member of the mental health team that will be responsible for Mr. Diment's care, you will need to be able to:

19.1 Apply the languages of psychology and psychiatry to disorders of mental health.

19.2 Comprehend, analyze, spell, and write the medical terms of psychology and psychiatry to communicate and document accurately and precisely in any health care setting.

19.3 Recognize and pronounce the medical terms of psychology and psychiatry to communicate verbally with accuracy and precision in any health care setting.

19.4 Explain the effects of common psychiatric disorders on health.

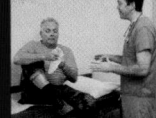

Mental Health and Affective Disorders

OBJECTIVES

Mental health is defined as emotional, behavioral, and social well-being such that an individual can cope with internal and external events. In this lesson, you will be given information about affective disorders, mood disorders, schizophrenia, anxiety disorders, and psychosomatic and somatoform disorders.

This lesson and the introduction will enable you to use correct medical terminology to:

19.1.1 **Distinguish between psychology and psychiatry.**

19.1.2 **Define** *mental disorder* **and** *insanity*.

19.1.3 **Discuss affective disorders.**

19.1.4 **Describe the differences between the two main types of mood disorder.**

Keynote

Psychologists are not licensed to prescribe medications.

As physicians, psychiatrists are licensed to prescribe medications.

Abbreviations

DSM-IV-TR	*Diagnostic and Statistical Manual of Mental Disorders,* fourth edition, text revision; referred to as "DSM-IV"
PhD	doctorate in philosophy
PsyD	doctorate in psychology

Keynote

The DSM-IV classifies and describes psychiatric disorders.

The DSM-IV contains over 200 diagnoses grouped into 17 major categories.

DSM-V is scheduled for release in 2012.

DEFINITIONS IN MENTAL HEALTH

Psychology is defined as the scientific study of behavior and mental processes. **Behavior** is anything you do—talking, sleeping, reading, interacting with others. **Mental processes** are your private, internal experiences—thinking, feeling, remembering, dreaming.

A licensed specialist in psychology is called a **psychologist.** Psychologists can have a master's degree or a doctorate in philosophy **(PhD)** or a doctorate in psychology **(PsyD).** They can practice in many different career specialties, including being a **psychotherapist** or a **psychoanalyst.**

Psychiatry is the medical specialty concerned with the origin, diagnosis, prevention, and treatment of mental, emotional, and behavioral disorders. **Psychiatrists** have an MD or DO degree and a minimum of 4 years of residency training in the specialty.

Many psychiatrists and psychologists work together in a team approach to therapy. Other health professionals in the mental health team include **clinical social workers, psychiatric nurses, mental health technicians,** and **psychiatric technicians.**

Mental disorder can be defined as any behavior or emotional state that:

- Causes a person to suffer emotional distress (e.g., depression, anxiety).

- Is harmful to the individual sufferer (impairs the individual's ability to work, take care of personal needs, or get along with others).

- Is self-destructive (e.g., substance abuse, gambling and other addictions, self-injury).

- Endangers others or the community (antisocial behaviors, **homicidal** intent, **pyromania** [setting fires]).

Insanity is a *legal* term for a severe mental illness, present at the time a crime was committed, that impaired the defendant's capacity to understand the moral wrong of the act. *It is not a medical diagnosis.*

Mental disorders are numerous and very diverse. A uniform system for classifying and describing them has been developed by the American Psychiatric Association. It is called the *Diagnostic and Statistical Manual of Mental Disorders,* fourth edition, text revision **(DSM-IV-TR).** The "IV" indicates that this is the fourth conceptual revision; "TR" indicates a text revision of the fourth edition. The manual is usually referred to as **DSM-IV** ("DSM-4").

The DSM-IV provides a detailed description of the symptoms seen in psychiatric disorders. These descriptions allow psychiatric disorders to be classified. It is the disorders that are classified, not the people who have the disorders. Modern mental health terminology does not use the term **schizophrenic** but uses the phrase "a person with **schizophrenia.**"

WORD ANALYSIS AND DEFINITION

S = Suffix   P = Prefix   R = Root   R/CF = Combining Form

WORD	PRONUNCIATION		ELEMENTS	DEFINITION
delusion	de-**LOO**-shun	S/ R/	-ion *condition, process* delus- *deceive*	Fixed, unyielding, false belief or judgment held despite strong evidence to the contrary
delusional (adj)	de-**LOO**-shun-al	S/	-al *pertaining to*	
hallucination	hah-loo-sih-**NAY**-shun	S/ R/	-ation *process* hallucin- *imagination*	Perception of an object or event when there is no such thing present
homicide	**HOM**-ih-side	R/CF R/CF	hom/i- *man* -cid/e *to kill*	Killing of one human by another
homicidal	hom-ih-**SIDE**-al	S/ R/	-al *pertaining to* -cid- *to kill*	Having a tendency to commit homicide
insanity	in-**SAN**-ih-tee	S/ P/ R/	-ity *condition* in- *not* -san- *sound, healthy*	Nonmedical term for person unable to be responsible for actions
psychiatry	sigh-**KIGH**-ah-tree	S/ R/	-iatry *treatment* psych- *mind*	Diagnosis and treatment of mental disorders
psychiatric	sigh-kee-**AH**-trik	S/	-ic *pertaining to*	Pertaining to psychiatry
psychiatrist	sigh-**KIGH**-ah-trist	S/	-iatrist *one who treats, practitioner*	Licensed medical specialist in psychiatry
psychology	sigh-**KOL**-oh-jee	S/ R/CF	-logy *study of* psych/o- *mind*	Scientific study of the human mind and behavior
psychological	sigh-koh-**LOJ**-ik-al	S/	-ical *pertaining to*	Pertaining to psychology
psychologist	sigh-**KOL**-oh-jist	S/	-logist *specialist*	Licensed specialist in psychology
psychoanalysis	sigh-koh-ah-**NAL**-ih-sis	R/	-analysis *process to define*	Method of psychotherapy
psychoanalyst	sigh-koh-**AN**-ah-list	R/	-analyst *one who defines*	Practitioner of psychoanalysis
psychotherapy	sigh-koh-**THAIR**-ah-pee	S/	-therapy *treatment*	Treatment of mental disorders through communication
psychotherapist	sigh-koh-**THAIR**-ah-pist	S/	-therapist *one who treats*	Practitioner of psychotherapy
pyromania	pie-roh-**MAY**-nee-ah	S/ R/CF	-mania *frenzy* pyr/o- *fire*	Morbid impulse to set fires
schizophrenia	skitz-oh-**FREE**-nee-ah	S/ R/CF R/	-ia *condition* schiz/o- *to split, cleave* -phren- *mind*	Disorder of perception, thought, emotion, and behavior
tangentiality	tan-jen-she-**AL**-ih-tee	S/ S/	-ity *condition, state* -al- *pertaining to*	Disturbance in thought processes, which move rapidly from one topic to another
tangent	**TAN**-jent	R/CF	tangent/i- *touch*	Sudden change of course

EXERCISES

Elements remain your best clue to the meaning of a medical term. Match the element in the left column with its correct meaning in the right column.

_____ 1. psych/o   A. pertaining to   _____ 6. pyr/o   F. mind

_____ 2. logy   B. condition   _____ 7. logist   G. to split

_____ 3. mania   C. specialist   _____ 8. in   H. frenzy

_____ 4. schiz/o   D. not   _____ 9. ic   I. treatment

_____ 5. ity   E. fire   _____ 10. iatry   J. study of

AFFECTIVE DISORDERS

Affective disorders are not a clearly delineated group of disorders. Included are the **mood disorders** of **unipolar** and **bipolar depression**, generalized anxiety disorder and more specific anxiety disorders, **phobias, obsessive-compulsive disorder (OCD)**, and posttraumatic stress disorder.

Mood Disorders

You will feel sad and blue and down in the dumps from time to time and occasionally feel the grief of the death of a loved one and the tragedy of injury or severe emotional hurt. Everyone does. But people with **major depression** are so deeply sad for at least 2 weeks that they feel despairing and hopeless, see nothing but sorrow in the future, and may not want to live anymore *(Figure 19.1)*. They see themselves as worthless and unlovable. They have difficulty getting up and going to school or work. One person's depression can hurt everyone in the entire family.

Physical symptoms occur. These may include difficulty concentrating, difficulty falling asleep, feeling tired all the time, losing weight. Violent behavior or substance abuse occurs more often in depressed men than in women, though depression is more common in women.

When depression is unipolar, the episode will ease with medication. Since the 1950s, **tricyclic antidepressant (TCA) drugs** have been used for depression, but since 1990 they are being replaced by **selective serotonin reuptake inhibitors (SSRIs)** or **serotonin and norepinephrine reuptake inhibitors (SNRIs)** *(Table 19.1)*. Moderate exercise for 3 hours weekly has been shown to reduce symptoms by 47%. It is believed to alter the serotonin chemistry in the brain.

Some people rebound to the opposite extreme of depression called **mania**, an excessive state of overexcitement and impulsive behavior. This alternation of episodes of depression with mania is called **bipolar disorder**. It used to be called **manic-depressive disorder**.

In the **manic** phase, the person is hyperactive and distractible and may not sleep for days yet shows no fatigue. Thinking and speech are rapid and disjointed and cannot be interrupted. The person may give away possessions or go on a spending spree.

Untreated pure manic episodes usually last 6 weeks. Untreated mixed (manic and depressive) episodes usually last 17 weeks. The choice of treatments for bipolar disorder is shown in *Table 19.2*.

Seasonal affective disorder (SAD) is a mood disorder associated with episodes of depression during the fall and winter months, subsiding during spring and summer. It appears to be related to a lack of sunshine causing increased melatonin production by the pineal gland *(see Chapter 14)*. It can be helped by phototherapy with bright white fluorescent lights. Antidepressant drugs can also be helpful.

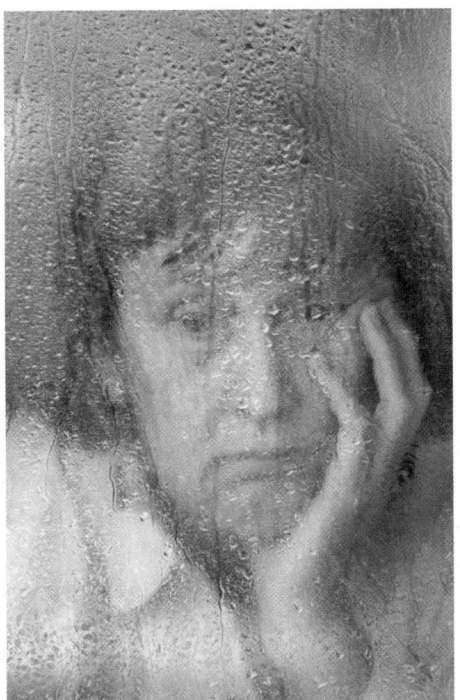

▲ **FIGURE 19.1 Depressed Woman at Window.**

Abbreviations

ECT	electroconvulsive therapy
OCD	obsessive-compulsive disorder
SAD	seasonal affective disorder
SNRI	serotonin and norepinephrine reuptake inhibitor
SSRI	selective serotonin reuptake inhibitor
TCA	tricyclic antidepressant

Case Report 19.1 (continued)

Mr. Harlan Diment is clearly in a manic phase. When Dr. Robert Nguyen, a psychiatrist, examined him in the Emergency Department, he believed the most likely diagnosis to be bipolar disorder. He has asked you to obtain a urine specimen to test for drugs of abuse and to do a blood test for his alcohol level to exclude those as causes. Dr. Nguyen has ordered that Mr. Diment be admitted to the Psychiatric Unit. He will need treatment with a mood stabilizer such as lithium. If he resists admission, he can be placed on a 72-hour hold because he is a danger to himself and to others.

TABLE 19.1 The Depression Arsenal of Drugs

Drug Type	Generic or Brand Name
tricyclic antidepressants (TCAs)	Generic names: amitriptyline, nortriptyline, protriptyline, clomipramine, imipramine, trimipramine
selective serotonin reuptake inhibitors (SSRIs)	Generic and brand names: fluoxetine (Prozac), fluvoxamine maleate (Luvox), paroxeline (Paxil), citalopram (Celexa), sertraline (Zoloft)
serotonin and norepinephrine reuptake inhibitors (SNRIs)	Generic and brand names: venlafaxine (Effexor), milnacipran (Dalcipran), duloxetine (Cymbalta)

WORD	PRONUNCIATION		ELEMENTS	DEFINITION
bipolar disorder	bi-**POH**-lar dis-**OR**-der	S/ P/ R/	-ar *pertaining to* bi- *two* -pol- *pole*	A mood disorder with alternating episodes of depression and mania
depression	de-**PRESH**-un	S/ R/	-ion *condition, process* depress- *press down*	Mental disorder with feelings of deep sadness and despair
electroconvulsive therapy	ee-**LEK**-troh-kon-**VUL**-siv **THAIR**-ah-pee	R/CF P/ R/ S/	electr/o- *electricity* -con- *with* -vuls- *tear, pull* -ive *quality of*	Passage of electric current through the brain to produce convulsions and treat persistent depression, mania, and other disorders
mania manic (adj) manic-depressive disorder	**MAY**-nee-ah **MAN**-ik **MAN**-ik de-**PRESS**-iv dis-**OR**-der	 R/ S/ R/	Greek *frenzy* manic *affected by frenzy* -ive *quality of* depress- *press down*	Mood disorder with hyperactivity, irritability, and rapid speech An outdated name for bipolar disorder
phobia	**FOH**-bee-ah		Greek *fear*	Pathologic fear or dread
unipolar disorder	you-nih-**POLE**-ar dis-**OR**-der	S/ P/ R/	-ar *pertaining to* uni- *one* -pol- *pole (at the pole of depression)*	Depression

TABLE 19.2: Treatment of Bipolar Disorder

Medications for Depression (in bipolar disorder)	Medications for Mania (in bipolar disorder)
lithium—prevention of future depression and suicide	lithium—for mania and prevention of future mania (60% success rate)
carbamazepine (Tegretol)—prevention of future depression	carbamazepine (Tegretol)—for mania and prevention of future mania
lamotrigine (Lamictal)—for depression	valproic acid (Valproate)—for mania
fluvoxamine (Luvox)—for depression	haloperidol (Haldol)—for mania
electroconvulsive therapy (ECT)	aripiprazole (Abilify)—for mania and prevention of future mania
Ancillary Treatments for Depression	**Ancillary Treatments for Mania**
cognitive therapy	lamotrigine (Lamictal)—to prevent future rapid cycling
family education	electroconvulsive therapy (ECT) as a last resort
group education	

EXERCISES

*Reinforce your learning of the **languages of psychology and psychiatry** by defining the difference between the following medical terms.*

1. psychologist: _____

2. psychiatrist: _____

3. mental disorder: _____

4. insanity: _____

5. Describe the differences between the two main types of mood disorders. _____

_____

_____

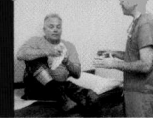

LESSON 19.2 Anxiety Disorders

MENTAL HEALTH

OBJECTIVES

To work effectively with patients with anxiety disorders, you will need to be able to use correct medical terminology to:

19.2.1 **Discuss the symptoms of the five major types of anxiety disorder.**

19.2.2 **Specify the diagnostic criteria for posttraumatic stress disorder.**

19.2.3 **List some of the drugs used to treat anxiety disorders.**

19.2.4 **Differentiate between psychosomatic and somatoform disorders.**

You are

. . . a readjustment counseling technician in a Veterans Administration Counseling Center attached to Fulwood Medical Center.

Your patient is

. . . Sergeant Mike West, an Army reservist who returned from Iraq 6 months ago after his second tour of duty.

CASE REPORT 19.2

As you interview Sergeant West, you learn that he is having difficulty coping with what he experienced in Iraq. His Humvee ran over an improvised explosive device. Two of his comrades died. Sergeant West took shrapnel in his leg and hand. Insurgents then attacked with mortars.

He plays the tape-in-his-mind of the incident over and over again. Loud noises, like thunderstorms, trigger paralysis. The smell of diesel brings back the memory of the Humvee on fire. Chicken on the barbecue smells like searing flesh. He can't sleep more than 3 or 4 hours a night, and then he wakes up in cold sweats. Sergeant West has become quick-tempered and doesn't like the way he's treating his wife. He's frightened to have children because of his outbursts of anger at seemingly minor upsets.

Abbreviations

CBT	cognitive behavioral therapy
CPT	cognitive processing therapy
EMDR	eye movement desensitization and reprocessing
GAD	generalized anxiety disorder
MAOI	monoamine oxidase inhibitor
PTSD	posttraumatic stress disorder

ANXIETY DISORDERS

Anxiety disorders are the most common category of mental disorders found in the United States. They are characterized by an **unreasonable anxiety** or **fear** that is inappropriate to the circumstances and so intense and chronic that it disrupts the person's life.

There are five major categories of anxiety disorder:

1. **Generalized anxiety disorder (GAD)** consists of persistent, excessive worrying and uncontrollable anxiety that is not focused on one particular situation and has lasted for at least 6 months. People with this disorder are frightened of something but are *unable to articulate a specific fear.* They develop physical fear reactions including palpitations, **insomnia,** difficulty concentrating, and irritability.

2. **Posttraumatic stress disorder (PTSD)** occurs when a person who has gone through a significant trauma shows stress symptoms that last for longer than a month and impair the person's ability to function. The trauma can be a life-threatening accident, a natural disaster, loss of a loved one, torture or abuse, or combat and its related incidents. Table 19.3 lists drugs used to treat PTSD and the effects of the drugs. PTSD is the diagnosis for Sergeant West.

The treatment of PTSD is **multimodal,** involving **psychopharmacotherapy, psychotherapy, social interventions,** and **patient and family education.** Forms of psychotherapy are **cognitive behavioral therapy (CBT),** in which the traumatic experiences are relived and worked through, and **cognitive processing therapy (CPT),** in which the thoughts and beliefs generated by the trauma are explored and reframed. **Eye movement desensitization and reprocessing (EMDR)** is also used. Social interventions to restore a sense of safety and security are a crucial element in therapy.

WORD	PRONUNCIATION		ELEMENTS	DEFINITION
anxiety	ang-**ZI**-eh-tee		Greek *distress, anxiety*	Distress caused by fear
cognitive	**KOG**-nih-tiv		Latin *knowledge*	Pertaining to the mental activities of thinking and learning
cognitive behavioral therapy (CBT) (***Note:*** Behavioral has two suffixes to make the word flow.)	**KOG**-nih-tiv be-**HAYV**-yur-al **THAIR**-ah-pee	S/ R/ S/ S/ R/ R/	-ive *quality of* cognit- *thinking* -al *pertaining to* -ior- *pertaining to* behav- *mental activity* therapy *medical treatment*	Psychotherapy that emphasizes thoughts and attitudes in one's behavior
cognitive processing therapy (CPT)	**KOG**-nih-tiv **PROS**-es-ing **THAIR**-ah-pee	S/ R/ S/ P/ R/	-ive *quality of* cognit- *thinking* -ing *doing* pro- *before* -cess- *going forward*	Psychotherapy to build skills to deal with effects of the trauma in other areas of life
insomnia	in-**SOM**-nee-ah	S/ P/ R/	-ia *condition* in- *not* -somn- *sleep*	Inability to sleep
multimodal	mul-tee-**MOH**-dal	S/ P/ R/	-al *pertaining to* multi- *many* -mod- *method*	Using many methods
posttraumatic	post-traw-**MAT**-ik	S/ P/ R/	-ic *pertaining to* post- *after* -traumat- *wound*	Occurring after and caused by trauma
psychopharmaco-therapy	**SIGH**-koh-**FAR**-mah-koh-**THAIR**-ah-pee	S/ R/CF R/CF	-therapy *treatment* psych/o- *mind* -pharmac/o- *drugs*	Drug treatment of mental disorders

TABLE 19.3 Pharmacotherapy of PTSD

Type of Drug	Effect
Selective serotonin reuptake inhibitors (SSRIs):	Reduce most symptom clusters and depression
sertraline (Zoloft)	Sertraline may reduce alcohol consumption
paroxetine (Paxil)	Paroxetine reduces nightmares
fluvoxamine (Luvox)	Fluvoxamine reduces insomnia
Antiadrenergic agents: clonidine (Catapres); propranolol (Inderal)	Reduce autonomic activity, including startle reactions and outbursts of rage
Monoamine oxidase inhibitors (MAOIs): phenelzine (Nardil)	Reduce reexperiencing symptoms, nightmares, and insomnia

EXERCISES

After reading Case Report 19.2 on the opposite page, answer the following questions. Be prepared to discuss your answers in class.

1. Specify the diagnostic criteria for postraumatic stress disorder. (What can the diagnosis be based on?) _____

_____

2. What aftereffects of PTSD does Sergeant West now deal with on a daily basis? _____

_____

3. Is PTSD a generalized anxiety disorder? _____

4. List some of the specific drugs used to treat PTSD. _____

_____

5. What are some of the causes of PTSD? _____

_____

3. **Panic disorder** is characterized by sudden, brief attacks of **intense fear** that cause physical symptoms. The fear rises abruptly, often for no reason, and peaks in 10 minutes or less. The frequency of the attacks varies widely over many years. The disorder runs in families, but whether it is due to genetics or a shared environment is not clear. Treatment consists of medication *(Table 19.4)* and cognitive behavioral therapy.

4. **Phobias** differ from generalized anxiety and panic attacks in that it is a *specific* situation or object that brings on the strong fear response. The danger is small and the person realizes the fear is irrational, but there is still overwhelming anxiety. There are two categories of phobia:

   - **Situational phobias** involve a fear of specific situations. Examples include **agoraphobia** (fear of crowded places, buses, and elevators), **acrophobia** (fear of heights), fear of flying or driving in tunnels, and fear of specific animals (snakes, mice). The basic fear of being trapped in a confined space is called **claustrophobia.**

   - **Social phobias** involve fear of being embarrassed in social situations. The most common are fear of public speaking (stage fright) or of eating in public. In many, the fear is so strong that it makes normal life impossible.

5. **In obsessive-compulsive disorder (OCD),** a majority of patients have both **obsessions** and **compulsions.** The obsessions are recurrent thoughts, fears, doubts, images, or impulses. The compulsions are recurrent, irresistible actions such as counting, hand washing, checking, and systematically arranging things. The recurrent actions can be violent or sexual.

   Most patients recognize the senselessness of their behaviors; but if they resist doing them, the fear and anxiety become intolerable. Treatment is with cognitive behavioral therapy and one of the SSRIs listed in *Tables 19.1 to 19.4.*

PSYCHOSOMATIC AND SOMATOFORM DISORDERS

Psychosomatic disorder is a real, physical disorder that, at least in part, has a psychological cause. Tension headaches have real pain caused by muscle spasm, but stress and anxiety play a role in causing the symptoms. **Biofeedback** *(Figure 19.2)* and relaxation techniques can be helpful in reducing the tension and spasm *(see Chapter 23).*

Somatoform disorder occurs when there is no identifiable physical cause to explain physical symptoms. The symptoms are real to the patient and are not under voluntary control. In **conversion disorder,** symptoms progress to involve loss of feeling, paralysis, deafness, or blindness.

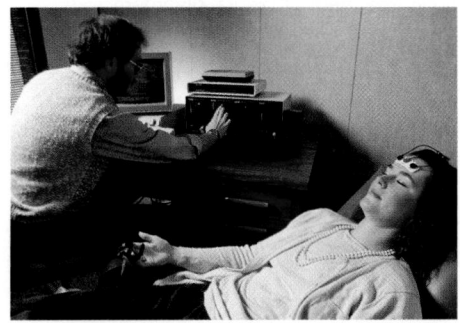

▲ **FIGURE 19.2 Person Undergoing Biofeedback.**

TABLE 19.4 Pharmacotherapy of Panic Disorder

Type of Drug	Effect
Benzodiazepines:	Effective prophylaxis
alprazolam (Xanax)	Reduce anticipatory anxiety
clonazepam (Klonopin)	Rapid onset of action
lorazepam (Ativan)	
diazepam (Valium)	
Selective serotonin reuptake inhibitors (SSRIs):	Reduce frequency of attacks
	Reduce intensity of panic
sertraline (Zoloft)	Take 2 weeks to produce effect
paroxetine (Paxil)	
fluvoxamine (Luvox)	

WORD	PRONUNCIATION	ELEMENTS		DEFINITION
acrophobia	ak-roh-**FOH**-be-ah	S/ R/CF	-phobia *fear* acr/o- *peak, highest point*	Pathologic fear of heights
agoraphobia	ah-gor-ah-**FOH**-be-ah	S/ R/CF	-phobia *fear* agor/a- *marketplace*	Pathologic fear of being trapped in a public place
biofeedback (***Note:*** This term has no prefix or suffix.)	bi-oh-**FEED**-back	R/CF R/ R/	bi/o- *life* -feed- *to give food, nourish* -back *back, return*	Training techniques to achieve voluntary control of responses to stimuli
claustrophobia	klaw-stroh-**FOH**-be-ah	S/ R/CF	-phobia *fear* claustr/o- *confined space*	Pathologic fear of being trapped in a confined space
compulsion	kom-**PULL**-shun	S/ R/	-ion *action, condition* compuls- *drive, compel*	Uncontrollable impulses to perform an act repetitively
compulsive (adj)	kom-**PULL**-siv	S/	-ive *nature of, quality of*	Possessing uncontrollable impulses to perform an act repetitively
conversion disorder	kon-**VER**-shun dis-**OR**-der		Latin *turn around or change*	An unconscious emotional conflict is expressed as physical symptoms with no organic basis
hypochondriac	high-poh-**KON**-dree-ack	S/ P/ R/	-iac *pertaining to* hypo- *below* -chondr- *cartilage, rib*	A person who exaggerates the significance of symptoms
hypochondriasis	**HIGH**-poh-kon-**DRY**-ah-sis	S/	-iasis *condition, state of*	Belief that a minor symptom indicates a severe disease
obsession	ob-**SESH**-un	S/ R/	-ion *action, condition* obsess- *besieged by thoughts*	Persistent, recurrent, uncontrollable thoughts or impulses
obsessive (adj)	ob-**SES**-iv	S/	-ive *nature of, quality of*	Possessing persistent, recurrent, uncontrollable thoughts or impulses
phobia	**FOH**-be-ah		Greek *fear*	Pathologic fear or dread
psychosomatic	sigh-koh-soh-**MAT**-ik	S/ R/CF R/	-tic *pertaining to* psych/o- *mind* -soma- *body*	Pertaining to disorders of the body usually resulting from disturbances of the mind
somatoform	so-**MAT**-oh-form	S/ R/CF	-form *appearance of* somat/o- *body*	Physical symptoms occurring without identifiable physical cause

EXERCISES

Meet lesson objectives by applying correct medical terminology to answer the following questions. Fill in the blanks.

1. What is the difference between *psychosomatic* and *somatoform* disorders?

_____

_____

2. Which disorder runs in families? _____

3. What is the correct medical term for a disorder that "runs in families"? _____

4. What is the difference between *obsession* and *compulsion*? _____

_____

_____

5. Explain what characterizes a *situational phobia* and a *social phobia*. _____

_____

_____

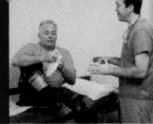

LESSON 19.3 Schizophrenia and Personality Disorders

OBJECTIVES

The information in this lesson will enable you to use correct medical terminology to:

19.3.1 Detail the symptoms of schizophrenia.

19.3.2 Discuss the use of lithium in schizophrenia.

19.3.3 Describe the different types of personality disorders.

19.3.4 Recognize classes of psychoactive drugs.

You are

. . . an EMT working in the Emergency Department at Fulwood Medical Center.

Your patient is

. . . Mr. Dante Costello, a 21-year-old homeless man, brought in by the police after he was found sitting in the middle of a main street.

CASE REPORT 19.3

Mr. Costello's explanation is "the voices told me to do it." He has heard voices telling him to do things for the past year. The voices often comment on his behavior. He has isolated himself from other people because "they are not who they say they are, and they are trying to get me." He is taking no drugs or medications and denies any **suicidal** or homicidal intent.

Mr. Costello is dirty and disheveled, with poor hygiene. He can give no home or family address. His **affect** is **congruent,** though expressionless. His speech is slow, and his thoughts are disorganized and confused.

The most probable diagnosis is **schizophrenia.** He needs to be admitted to the hospital because he is a danger to himself and other people.

SCHIZOPHRENIA

Schizophrenia is a form of **psychosis** in which there is a loss of contact with reality. People with schizophrenia do *not* have a split personality, but their words are separated from the meaning, their perceptions are separated from reality, and their behaviors are separated from their thought processes *(Figure 19.3)*.

People with schizophrenia have their sensory perceptions jumbled and distorted, have difficulty concentrating, and perceive things without a stimulation—**hallucinations.** Hallucinations can occur in any of the senses but are most often auditory. These people also suffer from **delusions,** mistaken beliefs that are contrary to facts. The delusions can be **paranoid,** with pervasive distrust and suspicion of others. People with schizophrenia can withdraw from society, become homeless, and refuse to communicate.

Their speech is disorganized and can be incoherent. Their behaviors are often totally inappropriate. Their blunted emotions and withdrawal can progress to **catatonia,** motor immobility that can last for hours. **Mutism** is the inability or refusal to speak.

Magnetic resonance imaging (MRI) and positron emission tomography (PET) scans show brain abnormalities and changes in function.

Symptoms of schizophrenia typically come on in the late teens and twenties. While there is no cure, it can be effectively treated with medications and programs of psychological rehabilitation *(see Chapter 18)*. The goals of therapy are to reduce schizophrenic symptoms, prevent their return, and enable the patient to function in society. **Antipsychotic** medications such as olanzapine, quetiapine, and risperidone are used, either singly or in combinations if necessary.

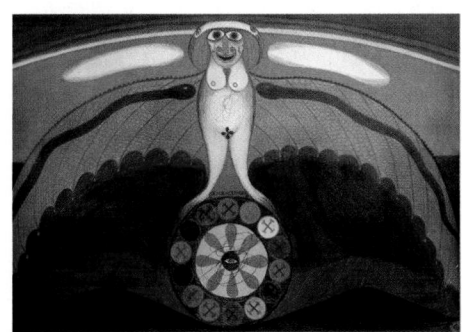

▲ **FIGURE 19.3 Artwork by Schizophrenic Patient.**

Case Report 19.3 (continued)

Mr. Costello stated he was hearing voices of people who were not there speaking to him (hallucination). Mr. Costello was also paranoid, believing that people were "out to get him." He withdrew from society and became homeless. His behavior of sitting immobile in the middle of the street for long periods is inappropriate and is catatonic.

WORD	PRONUNCIATION		ELEMENTS	DEFINITION
affect (noun)	**AF**-fekt		Latin *state of mind*	External display of feelings, thoughts, and emotions
catatonia	kat-ah-**TOE**-nee-ah	S/ P/ R/	-ia *condition* cata- *down* -ton- *pressure, tension*	Syndrome characterized by physical immobility and mental stupor
catatonic (adj)	kat-ah-**TON**-ic	S/	-ic *pertaining to*	
congruent	**KON**-gru-ent	S/ P/ R/	-ent *end result* con- *with* -gru- *to move*	Coinciding or agreeing with
mute	MYUT		Latin *silent*	Unable or unwilling to speak
mutism	**MYU**-tizm	S/ R/	-ism *condition, process* mut- *silent*	Absence of speech
paranoia	par-ah-**NOY**-ah	P/ R/	para- *abnormal, beside* -noia *to think*	Mental disorder with persecutory delusions
paranoid (adj)	**PAR**-ah-noyd	S/	-oid *resembling*	Having delusions of persecution
psychosis	sigh-**KOH**-sis	S/ R/	-osis *condition* psych- *mind*	Disorder causing mental disruption and loss of contact with reality
psychotic (adj)	sigh-**KOT**-ik	S/	-tic *pertaining to*	Pertaining to or affected by psychosis
antipsychotic	**AN**-tih-sigh-**KOT**-ik	P/ R/CF	anti- *against* psych/o- *mind*	An agent helpful in the treatment of psychosis
schizophrenia schizophrenic (adj)	skitz-oh-**FREE**-nee-ah skitz-oh-**FREN**-ik	S/ R/CF R/	-ia *condition* schiz/o- *to split, cleave* -phren- *mind*	Disorder of perception, thought, emotion, and behavior
suicide	**SOO**-ih-side	R/CF R/CF	su/i- *self* -cid/e *kill*	The act of killing oneself
suicidal (adj)	**SOO**-ih-**SIGH**-dal	S/	-al *pertaining to*	Wanting to kill oneself

Mood stabilizers such as lithium are also used. Treatment is for a minimum of a year and can be indefinite. Unfortunately, more than 50% of patients stop taking the drugs because of unpleasant side effects. These include loss of bladder control, increased thirst, nausea, trembling of hands, and an acnelike skin rash. Others stop treatment because they are feeling better. Blood levels of lithium have to be monitored, and signs of overdose include diarrhea, drowsiness, loss of appetite, muscle weakness and trembling, and slurred speech.

EXERCISES

After reading Case Report 19.3 on the opposite page, answer the following questions. Be prepared to discuss your answers in class.

1. What is the difference between *suicidal* intent and *homicidal* intent?

_____

2. What is inappropriate about Mr. Costello's behavior?

_____

_____

3. What is amiss about his appearance?

_____

4. Explain this sentence: "His affect is congruent, though expressionless." What does that mean?

_____

_____

5. Why is Mr. Costello being admitted to the hospital?

_____

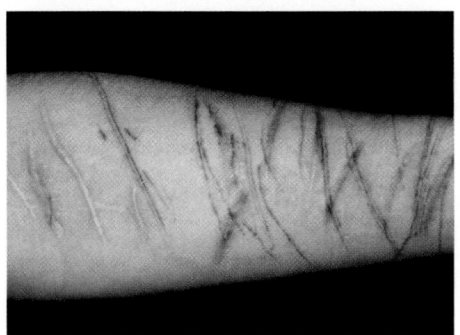

▲ FIGURE 19.4 Self-Mutilated Arm.

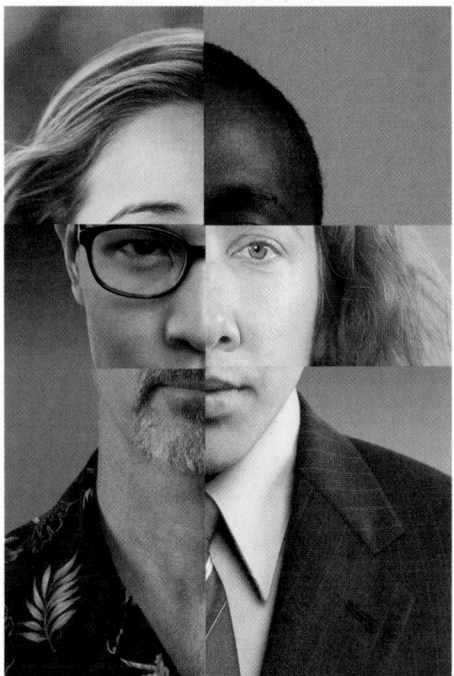

▲ FIGURE 19.5 Dissociative Identity Disorder (Multiple Personality Disorder).

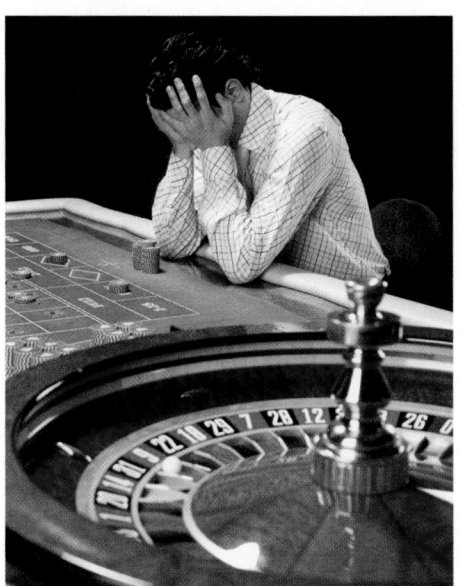

▲ FIGURE 19.6 Compulsive Gambler.

PERSONALITY DISORDERS

Personality is defined as an individual's unique and stable patterns of thoughts, feelings, and behaviors. When these patterns become rigid and inflexible in response to different situations, they can cause impairment of the individual's ability to deal with other people (i.e., to function socially).

Borderline personality disorder (BPD) is a frequent diagnosis in people who are impulsive, unstable in mood, and manipulative. They can be exciting, charming, and friendly one moment and angry, irritable, and sarcastic the next. Their identity is fragile and insecure, their self-worth low. They can be promiscuous and self-destructive; for example, with **self-mutilation (self-injury)** *(Figure 19.4)* or suicide. People with **narcissistic personality disorder** have an exaggerated sense of self-importance and seek constant attention.

Antisocial personality disorder, used interchangeably with the terms **sociopath** and **psychopath,** describes people who lie, cheat, steal, and have no sense of responsibility and no anxiety or guilt about their behavior. The psychopaths have these characteristics but tend to be more violent and anger easily.

Schizoid and **paranoid personality disorders** describe people who are absorbed with themselves, untrusting, and fearful of closeness with others.

Treatment for personality disorders is not successful.

Dissociative Disorders

Dissociative disorders involve a disassociation (splitting apart) of past experiences from present memory or consciousness. Being unable to recall identity is called dissociative **amnesia**. The development of distinctly separate personalities is called **dissociative identity disorder (DID).** It was formerly called **multiple personality disorder (MPD).**

The basic origin of all these disorders is the need to escape, usually from extreme trauma, and most often from sexual, emotional, or physical abuse in childhood.

The most severe of this group of disorders is DID. Two or more distinct personalities, each with their own memories and behaviors, inhabit the same person at the same time *(Figure 19.5)*. Treatment is with psychotherapy.

Impulse Control Disorders

Impulse control disorders are an inability to resist an impulse to perform an action that is harmful to the individual or to others. These disorders include:

- **Intermittent explosive disorder** is characterized by recurrent episodes of unrestrained aggression toward people, furniture, or property, with violent resistance to attempts to restrain. The etiology is thought to be epileptic-like activity in the brain. Medications that generate some improvement include propranolol, lithium, valproate, and phenytoin.

- **Kleptomania** is characterized by stealing—not for gain, but to satisfy an irresistible urge to steal. Behavior therapy can help, and SSRIs appear to be of value.

- **Trichotillomania (TTM)** is characterized by the repeated urge to pull out scalp, beard, pubic, and other body hair.

- **Substance abuse** and **chemical dependence** involve a person's continued use of drugs or alcohol despite having had significant problems or distress related to their use. This **addiction** affects the brain and behavior and develops an increased need for the substance and an inability to stop using it.

- **Pyromania** is repeated fire setting with no motive other than a fascination with fire and fire engines. Some pyromaniacs end up as volunteer firefighters. Treatment with behavior therapy is sometimes successful.

WORD	PRONUNCIATION	ELEMENTS		DEFINITION
addict	**ADD**-ikt	P/	ad- *toward*	Person with a psychologic or physical dependence on a substance or practice
addiction	ah-**DIK**-shun	R/ S/	-dict *surrender* -ion *condition, action*	Habitual psychologic and physiologic dependence on a substance or practice
amnesia	am-**NEE**-zee-ah		Greek *forgetfulness*	Total or partial inability to remember past experiences
antisocial personality disorder	**AN**-tee-**SOH**-shal per-son-**AL**-ih-tee dis-**OR**-der	S/ P/ R/ S/ S/ R/	-al *pertaining to* anti- *against* -soci- *partner, ally, community* -ity *condition, state* -al- *pertaining to* -person- *person*	Disorder of people who lie, cheat, steal, and have no guilt about their behavior
dissociative identity disorder	di-**SO**-see-ah-tiv eye-**DEN**-tih-tee dis-**OR**-der	P/ R/ S/	dis- *apart, away from* -soci- *partner, ally, community* -ative *quality of*	Mental disorder in which part of an individual's personality is separated from the rest, leading to multiple personalities
kleptomania	klep-toe-**MAY**-nee-ah	S/ R/CF	-mania *frenzy* klept/o- *to steal*	Uncontrollable need to steal
narcissism	**NAR**-sih-sizm		Greek mythical character, Narcissos, who was in love with his own reflection in water	Self-love; person interprets everything purely in relation to himself or herself
narcissistic (adj)	**NAR**-sih-**SIS**-tik	S/ R/ S/	-ism *a process* narciss- *self-love* -istic *pertaining to*	Relating everything to oneself
pathologic gambling	path-oh-**LOJ**-ik **GAM**-bling	S/ R/ R/	-ic *pertaining to* path/o- *disease* -log- *study of*	Morbid, constant, uncontrollable, destructive gambling
psychopath	**SIGH**-koh-path	S/ R/CF	-path *disease* psych/o- *mind*	Person with antisocial personality disorder
pyromania	pie-roh-**MAY**-nee-ah	S/ R/CF	-mania *frenzy* pyr/o- *fire*	Morbid impulse to set fires
schizoid	**SKITZ**-oyd	S/ R/	-oid *resemble* schiz- *split*	Withdrawn, socially isolated
self-mutilation	self-myu-tih-**LAY**-shun	S/ R/ R/	-ation *process* self- *own individual* -mutil- *to maim*	Injury or disfigurement made to one's own body
sociopath	**SO**-see-oh-path	S/ R/CF	-path *disease* soci/o- *partner, ally, community*	Person with antisocial personality disorder

- **Pathologic gambling** is a recurrent, compelling fascination to spend time and money on gambling, despite ever-mounting losses *(Figure 19.6)*. Gambling becomes the reason for living. Financial ruin does not stop the gambling. Fraud and theft then support it. Treatment with behavior therapy helps, in tandem with participation in Gamblers Anonymous.

Abbreviations

BPD borderline personality disorder
DID dissociative identity disorder
MPD multiple personality disorder
TTM trichotillomania

EXERCISES

Use your knowledge of medical language to answer the following question.

How are psychopaths and sociopaths the same and how are they different?

1. _____

2. _____

PSYCHOACTIVE DRUGS

Psychoactive drugs are chemicals that change consciousness, awareness, or perception *(Table 19.5)*. The most commonly used drugs are caffeine, tobacco, and alcohol.

Drug abuse refers to the use of drugs that cause emotional or physical harm to an individual as consumption becomes frequent and compulsive.

Addiction occurs when a person feels compelled to use a drug or perform a certain activity and cannot control the use.

Psychological dependence is the mental desire or **craving** for the effects produced by a drug.

Physical dependence is the changes in the body processes that make the drug necessary for daily functioning. If the drug is stopped, the withdrawal symptoms include physical pain, as well as intense cravings.

Tolerance occurs when the body adjusts to the effects of the drug, and higher and higher doses produce less and less effect. The brain, liver, heart, and other organs can be damaged.

Comorbidity is the presence of a combination of disorders. It is very common. Alcohol dependence and abuse overlap with almost all other mental disorders, including anxiety disorders, mood disorders, and personality disorders. In such cases, stopping drinking alcohol is only the first step in solving the problem.

Keynote

Dependence on drugs can be both psychological and physical.

TABLE 19.5 Psychoactive Drugs

Type/Mode of Action	Name	Common Effects	Effects of Abuse
Stimulants ("uppers") Speed up activity in the CNS	caffeine	Wakefulness, shorter reaction time, alertness	Restlessness, insomnia, heartbeat irregularities
	nicotine	Varies from alertness to calmness, appetite for carbohydrates decreases	Heart disease; high blood pressure; vasoconstriction; bronchitis; emphysema; lung, throat, mouth cancer
	amphetamines	Wakefulness, alertness, increased metabolism, decreased appetite	Nervousness, high blood pressure, delusions, psychosis, convulsions, death
	cocaine	**Euphoria**, high energy, illusions of power	Excitability, paranoia, anxiety, panic, depression, heart failure, death
Depressants ("downers") Slow down activity in the CNS	alcohol	**1–2 drinks**—reduced inhibitions and anxiety	Blackouts, mental and neurologic impairment, psychosis, cirrhosis of liver, death
		Many drinks—slow reaction time, poor coordination and memory	Impaired motor and sensory functions, amnesia, loss of consciousness, death
	barbiturates and tranquilizers	Reduced anxiety and tension, sedation	
Narcotics Mimic the actions of natural endorphins	codeine, opium, morphine, heroin	Euphoria, pleasure, relief of pain	High tolerance of pain, nausea, vomiting, constipation, convulsions, coma, death
Psychedelics Disrupt normal thought processes	marijuana	Relaxation, euphoria, increased appetite, pain relief	Sensory distortion, hallucinations, paranoia, throat and lung damage
	LSD, mescaline, MDMA (Ecstasy)	Exhilaration, euphoria, hallucinations, insightful experiences	Panic, extreme delusions, bad "trips," paranoia, psychosis

WORD	PRONUNCIATION	ELEMENTS		DEFINITION
comorbidity	koh-mor-**BID**-ih-tee	S/ P/ R/	-ity *condition, state* co- *with, together* -morbid- *disease*	Presence of two or more diseases at the same time
craving	**KRAY**-ving		Latin *desire*	Deep longing or desire
dependence	de-**PEN**-dense		Latin *to hang from*	State of needing someone or something
depressant	de-**PRESS**-ant	S/ P/ R/	-ant *agent* de- *away from* -press- *press down*	Substance that diminishes activity, sensation, or tone
endorphin	en-**DOR**-fin	P/ R/	end- *within* -orphin *morphine*	Natural substance in the brain that has same effect as opium
euphoria	yoo-**FOR**-ee-ah	S/ P/ R/	-ia *condition* eu- *normal* -phor- *bear, carry*	Exaggerated feeling of well-being
narcotic	nar-**KOT**-ik	S/ R/CF	-tic *pertaining to* narc/o- *sleep, stupor*	Drug derived from opium or a synthetic drug with similar effects
psychedelic	sigh-keh-**DEL**-ik	S/ R/CF R/	-ic *pertaining to* psych/e- *mind, soul* -del- *manifest, visible*	Agent that intensifies sensory perception
psychoactive	sigh-koh-**AK**-tiv	S/ R/CF R/	-ive *quality of, nature of* psych/o- *mind, soul* -act- *performance*	Able to alter mood, behavior, and/or cognition
stimulant	**STIM**-you-lant	S/ R/	-ant *agent* stimul- *excite*	Agent that excites or strengthens functional activity
tolerance	**TOL**-er-antz	S/ R/	-ance *condition, state of* toler- *endure*	The capacity to become accustomed to a stimulus or drug

EXERCISES

Review all the new terms you have learned on these two pages. Choose the correct medical terminology to insert into each of the following sentences. You will use some terms twice.

1. Overuse of antibiotics builds up a(n) _____ to certain drugs, and they are no longer effective.

2. A diabetic with high blood pressure has a _____.

3. Caffeine and nicotine can be *both* a(n) _____ and a(n) _____.

4. Marathon runners can experience the natural stimulatory effect from _____.

5. _____ is a state that can be physical or mental.

6. The two opposite terms in this WAD are _____ and _____.

7. An agent able to alter mood, behavior, and/or cognition is _____.

8. A natural substance in the brain that has the same effect as opium is _____.

9. A(n) _____ is an agent that excites or strengthens functional activity.

10. Deep longing or desire is a(n) _____.

MENTAL HEALTH
CHALLENGE YOUR KNOWLEDGE

A. You will be required to document certain notes concerning Mr. Diment's behavior. Your patient has been diagnosed with a manic episode of bipolar disorder. Reread this case report, and answer the following questions.

CASE REPORT 19.1

Your patient is

. . . Mr. Harlan Diment, a 40-year-old construction worker. He was brought to the Emergency Department by his roommate, who says that Mr. Diment has slept only a couple of hours each night for the past 3 weeks. He stays up most of the night, cleaning their apartment and drinking beer. He has bought a new home entertainment set, including a big-screen plasma TV, that he cannot afford. He is very irritable and explosive when challenged about his behavior. His roommate has seen no signs of drugs and is not aware of any medical problems. Mr. Diment is usually very quiet, thoughtful, and introverted.

A mental status examination shows Mr. Diment to be alternately irritable and excited. He is wearing a bright orange top and camouflage slacks and is carrying a soft green cap. His speech is rapid and loud, and it is difficult to interrupt him. He paces the room, claims to feel "great," and is angry with his roommate for insisting that he come to the hospital. His thought processes and verbalization go off on different tangents. He says he has no suicidal thoughts, hallucinations, or delusions.

Mr. Harlan Diment is clearly in a manic phase. When Dr. Robert Nguyen, a psychiatrist, examined him in the Emergency Department, he believed the most likely diagnosis to be bipolar disorder. He has asked you to obtain a urine specimen to test for drugs of abuse and to do a blood test for his alcohol level to exclude those as causes. Dr. Nguyen has ordered that Mr. Diment be admitted to the Psychiatric Unit. He will need treatment with a mood stabilizer such as lithium. If he resists admission, he can be placed on a 72-hour hold because he is a danger to himself and to others.

1. Describe the symptoms that indicate Mr. Diment is in a manic phase of this disorder.

   _____

   _____

   _____

2. If this is a *bipolar* disorder, what is the opposite type of behavior Mr. Diment could have been exhibiting?

   _____

   _____

   _____

3. What diagnostic tests have been ordered for Mr. Diment?

   _____

   _____

4. What two factors are Dr. Nguyen looking to *exclude* as possible causes of Mr. Diment's behavior?

   _____

   _____

5. What treatment was prescribed for Mr. Diment?

_____

_____

_____

6. How or why can Mr. Diment be considered a danger to himself or others?

_____

_____

B. **Deconstruct the following medical terms from this lesson into their basic elements.** Then choose any four terms, and use each of them in a sentence of patient documentation. Fill in the blanks.

Medical Term	Prefix	Root/CF	Suffix
obsessive			
psychosomatic			
hypochondriac			
antipsychotic			
sociopath			
paranoia			
schizophrenia			

1. _____

_____

2. _____

_____

3. _____

_____

4. _____

_____

MENTAL HEALTH

C. **Difference Between:** Any health care worker in the mental health field will be interacting with psychologists and psychiatrists. Write a brief answer *in layman's terms* that explains the basic differences between the two practitioners.

   1. psychologist:

      _____

      _____

      _____

   2. psychiatrist:

      _____

      _____

      _____

   Meet the lesson objective by explaining the difference between:

   3. mental disorder:

      _____

      _____

      _____

   4. insanity:

      _____

      _____

      _____

   5. There is no listing for insanity in the DSM-IV. Why not?

      _____

D. **Anxiety and Impulse Control Disorders:** Patients with various types of anxiety and impulse control disorders would be seen in the Fulwood Psychiatric Clinic. Determine the specific disorder from the description of the patient and the symptoms in the following documentation. The first one is done for you. Fill in the blanks.

   1. Patient suffers sudden bouts of intense fear that cause profuse sweating, nausea, and occasional vomiting.

      panic disorder
      _____

   2. Patient has been arrested for shoplifting but admits to stealing many more items before she was caught today. Patient states

      she steals for the "thrill of it." _____

   3. Patient's house was destroyed in the flooding following Hurricane Katrina. He barely escaped with his life and now suffers

      from almost daily stress headaches and physical aches and pains. _____

   4. Patient was locked in closets for hours at a time as a young boy. _____

5. Patient is here today by court order for psychiatric examination. Patient is suspected of setting two fires in the same neighborhood in the last 2 weeks. _____

6. Patient is so uncomfortable on buses, subways, elevators, and crowded sidewalks that she is unable to get to work.

   _____

7. Patient presents today with severe dermatitis on both hands. Patient states she washes her hands at least 50 times a day to be sure they are germ-free. _____

8. Patient's chief complaint today is palpitations and insomnia, which keep him awake most nights. He feels worried and anxious all the time but can give no specific reason for it. _____

E. **Suffixes:** Mental health practitioners can be either *psycho*logists or *psychi*atrists. The root/combining form **psych/o-** is present in all the following terms. The suffix is what makes the difference. Challenge your knowledge of the language of mental health by applying the correct term to the following statements. Fill in the blanks, using the choices below.

psychopath	**psychiatry**	**psychiatric**	**psychotherapy**
psychotic	**psychopharmacotherapy**	**psychoanalysis**	**psychology**
psychiatrist	**psychoanalyst**	**psychologist**	**psychological**
psychosomatic	**psychotherapist**	**psychosis**	**psychoactive**

1. An agent able to alter mood, behavior, or cognition: _____

2. Treatment of mental disorders through communication is called _____.

3. _____ is the science concerned with the behavior of humans.

4. A licensed specialist in psychology is known as a _____.

5. The patient's _____ state was starting to affect his physical well-being.

6. A method of psychotherapy is _____.

7. What type of technician is the health care worker in the first Case Report at the beginning of this chapter?

   _____ technician

8. Drug treatment of mental disorders: _____

9. A medical specialist in psychiatry is a _____.

10. A practitioner of psychoanalysis is called a _____.

11. Disorder causing mental disruption and loss of contact with reality: _____

12. _____ is the medical specialty dealing with the diagnosis and treatment of mental disorders.

13. A practitioner of psychotherapy is a _____.

14. Real, physical disorder that, at least in part, has a psychological cause: _____

15. Pertaining to or affected by psychosis: _____

16. A serial killer can be termed a _____.

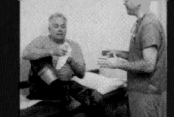

MENTAL HEALTH

F. Terminology Challenge: Once you know the meaning of an element, it always applies. First circle the prefix in each of the four terms in the left column; then write the meaning of the prefix in the middle column. Write the meaning of the term in the right column. Relate this prefix to different medical terms in other chapters.

Medical Term	Meaning of Prefix	Meaning of Medical Term
insomnia		
multimodal		
posttraumatic		
bipolar		

Terms with the same prefix from other chapters already studied:

Medical Term	Meaning of Prefix	Meaning of Medical Term
i		
m		
p		
b		

G. Abbreviations: Apply your knowledge of abbreviations to complete the patient documentation below. Choose from the following abbreviations to correctly fill in the blanks. You have more answers than questions.

ECT   CNS   PTSD   BPD   DID   CBT   SSRI   CPT   STAT

1. Patient now has developed three distinct, separate personalities. Her _____ is rapidly progressing.

2. Patient is suffering from unipolar depression, and a(n) _____ medication will be prescribed.

3. Patient's nightmares are increasing and are always the same replay of his automobile accident. I am sending him for

   _____ and _____ in the hopes this can alleviate some of his _____ and help him sleep better. Sleep

   medication is also prescribed.

4. Patient exhibits frequent mood changes and has become manipulative in her relationship with her parents.

   Her _____ is escalating her insecurity.

5. _____ will be prescribed for this patient as a last resort for treatment of his mania.

H. Recall and Review: How well do you remember these word elements from the previous chapter? Try to answer without first looking back to check. Fill in the blanks.

Element	Type of Element (P, R, CF, S)	Meaning of Element
ary	_____	_____
orthot	_____	_____
re	_____	_____
kinet	_____	_____
therm/o	_____	_____

I. **Patient Education:** As a health care worker, you should be prepared and equipped to explain any medical term to a patient, whether the patient requests it or you can see that the patient is not understanding what has been said by the physician. Explain to your patient the difference between:

1. unipolar disorder:

    _____

    _____

    _____

    bipolar disorder:

    _____

    _____

    _____

2. psychotherapy:

    _____

    _____

    _____

    psychopharmacotherapy:

    _____

    _____

    _____

3. addiction:

    _____

    _____

    _____

    abuse:

    _____

    _____

    _____

Use any one term from above in a sentence of patient documentation.

   Sentence:

    _____

    _____

    _____

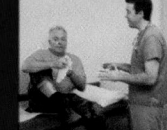

MENTAL HEALTH

J. **Prefixes:** Test your recall of word element meanings by answering the following questions about prefixes. The medical term is given; on the line beside the term, write the prefix, and then circle the meaning of the prefix.

1. **bipolar:**   Prefix is _____ and means

    a. one

    b. two

    c. three

    d. four

    e. five

2. **hypochondriasis:**   Prefix is _____ and means

    a. after

    b. around

    c. below

    d. next to

    e. excessive

3. **depressant:**   Prefix is _____ and means

    a. toward

    b. forming

    c. within

    d. away from

    e. around

4. **catatonia:**   Prefix is _____ and means

    a. up

    b. around

    c. through

    d. down

    e. beside

5. **addiction:**   Prefix is _____ and means

    a. toward

    b. from

    c. for

    d. with

    e. up

6. **euphoria:** Prefix is _____ and means

   a. marketplace

   b. mind

   c. normal

   d. madness

   e. wound

7. **paranoia:** Prefix is _____ and means

   a. above

   b. excessive

   c. abnormal

   d. condition

   e. study of

8. **unipolar:** Prefix is _____ and means

   a. one

   b. four

   c. many

   d. few

   e. none

9. **dissociative:** Prefix is _____ and means

   a. painful

   b. apart

   c. abnormal

   d. irregular

   e. together

10. **convulsive:** Prefix is _____ and means

    a. in front of

    b. with

    c. next to

    d. yellow

    e. small

MENTAL HEALTH

K. Psychoactive drugs can be prescribed (like barbiturates and tranquilizers), or they can be self-administered (like caffeine and nicotine). First, group the drugs from the word bank into their proper categories. Then list three bad effects resulting from abuse of each of the drug groups. Fill in the blanks.

Word bank:

marijuana	alcohol	nicotine
cocaine	morphine	tranquilizers
amphetamines	caffeine	heroin
barbiturates	opium	codeine
Ecstacy	LSD	mescaline

Depressants:

1. Names of drugs in this group: _____

2. Effects of abuse of these drugs: _____

Psychedelics:

3. Names of drugs in this group: _____

4. Effects of abuse of these drugs: _____

Stimulants:

5. Names of drugs in this group: _____

6. Effects of abuse of these drugs: _____

Narcotics:

7. Names of drugs in this group: _____

8. Effects of abuse of these drugs: _____

L. Language of Psychology and Psychiatry: Employ your knowledge of the language of mental health to match the statement in the left column with the correct medical vocabulary in the right column. Fill in the blanks.

_____	1. lack of contact with reality	A.	delusion
_____	2. symptoms with no physical cause	B.	mutism
_____	3. refusal or inability to speak	C.	dissociative amnesia
_____	4. legal term, not a diagnosis	D.	personality
_____	5. motor immobility for hours	E.	mental disorder
_____	6. deep sadness and despair	F.	catatonia
_____	7. mistaken belief, contrary to fact	G.	somatoform
_____	8. individual's unique pattern of thought	H.	psychosis
_____	9. unable to recall identity	I.	depression
_____	10. emotional state that is self-destructive	J.	insanity

M. Terminology in Use: Psychoactive drugs are chemicals that change consciousness, awareness, or perception. The most commonly used drugs are caffeine, tobacco, and alcohol.

Review *Table 19.5,* "Psychoactive Drugs." Then write a short paragraph using as many of the following terms as possible. *For example:* You can describe something you have observed in another person (say, a person who drinks too much coffee every day or someone you know who is trying to give up smoking). You might also comment on what effects on health these drugs have and how difficult it can be to give them up.

| drug abuse | addiction | psychological dependence | tolerance | stimulant |
| physical dependence | comorbidity | craving | depressant | |

_____

_____

_____

_____

_____

_____

_____

_____

N. Roots/combining forms are the core foundation of every medical term. Test your knowledge of roots in the *languages of psychology and psychiatry* with this exercise. Fill in the blanks; then use any one medical term in a sentence of your choice that is not a definition.

Root/CF	Meaning of Element	Medical Term Containing This Element	Meaning of Medical Term
claustr/o			
bio			
agor/a			
somn			
acr/o			
klept/o			
cide			
schiz/o			
electr/o			

Sentence:

_____

_____

_____

MENTAL HEALTH

O. **Apply your knowledge of the *language of psychology and psychiatry.*** Circle the correct answer to the following questions. *Remember:* There is only one *best* answer.

1. A mood disorder more common in women is:

   a. PTSD

   b. SAD

   c. phobias

   d. OCD

   e. depression

2. Manic depressive disorder is now known as:

   a. SAD

   b. unipolar disorder

   c. generalized anxiety disorder

   d. mania

   e. bipolar disorder

3. A TCA used to treat depression is:

   a. Prozac

   b. Paxil

   c. amitriptyline

   d. Zoloft

   e. duloxetine

4. Significant trauma can lead to:

   a. OCD

   b. TTM

   c. SAD

   d. DID

   e. PTSD

5. Circle the drug *not* prescribed for a panic disorder:

   a. nortriptyline

   b. Paxil

   c. Xanax

   d. Zoloft

   e. Klonopin

6. A combination of CBT and EMDR would be treatment for:

    a. MPD

    b. DID

    c. OCD

    d. PTSD

    e. TTM

7. No identifiable physical cause to explain physical symptoms characterizes:

    a. hypochondriasis

    b. acrophobia

    c. conversion disorder

    d. agoraphobia

    e. somatoform disorder

8. Perceiving things without a stimulation is:

    a. compulsion

    b. delusion

    c. hallucination

    d. obsession

    e. tangent

9. Higher doses of a drug produce less effect:

    a. psychological dependence

    b. addiction

    c. tolerance

    d. physical dependence

    e. comorbidity

10. Schizophrenia is a form of:

    a. delusion

    b. phobia

    c. psychosis

    d. mood disorder

    e. obsession

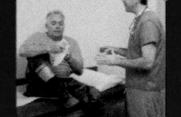
MENTAL HEALTH

P.   **Latin and Greek terms cannot be further deconstructed into prefix, root, or suffix.** You must know them for what they are. Test your knowledge of these terms with this exercise. Match the meaning in the left column with the correct medical term in the right column.

_____	1. turn around or change	A. mania
_____	2. unable to recall identity	B. affect
_____	3. knowledge	C. conversion
_____	4. frenzy	D. phobia
_____	5. desire	E. craving
_____	6. to hang from	F. anxiety
_____	7. fear	G. amnesia
_____	8. distress	H. cognitive
_____	9. state of mind	I. dependence

Q.   **Differences:** Discuss and be able to explain the basic differences among the following four terms. You should be able to describe the condition and cite an example for each. Write your notes below.

addiction:

_____

_____

_____

_____

_____

tolerance:

_____

_____

_____

_____

_____

physical dependence:

_____

_____

_____

_____

_____

_____

_____

psychological dependence:

_____

_____

_____

_____

_____

_____

R. Elements, elements, elements: Solid knowledge of elements will help increase your medical vocabulary. Identify the element as to type (P, R, CF, S), give the meaning of the element, and then provide a medical term containing the element. The first one is done for you. Fill in the table.

Element	Prefix	Root/CF	Suffix	Meaning of Element	Medical Term Containing This Element
phobia	_____	_____	✓	_fear_	_acrophobia_
iatrist	_____	_____	_____	_____	_____
phren	_____	_____	_____	_____	_____
vuls	_____	_____	_____	_____	_____
cognit	_____	_____	_____	_____	_____
somn	_____	_____	_____	_____	_____
pharmaco	_____	_____	_____	_____	_____
acro	_____	_____	_____	_____	_____
claustro	_____	_____	_____	_____	_____
agora	_____	_____	_____	_____	_____
iasis	_____	_____	_____	_____	_____
chondr	_____	_____	_____	_____	_____
mut	_____	_____	_____	_____	_____
uni	_____	_____	_____	_____	_____
sui	_____	_____	_____	_____	_____

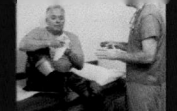

MENTAL HEALTH

CHAPTER SUMMARY EXERCISE

1. *Listen to the pronunciation of the medical terms as given by your instructor.*
2. *Circle the correct spelling of the medical term.*
3. *Match the correctly spelled terms to the brief descriptions below.*
4. *Write a sentence for each of the 10 terms that appear in this exercise.*

A. SPELLING COMPREHENSION: CIRCLE THE CORRECT SPELLING OF THE TERM.

1. lythium   lifhium   litium   lithium   lytium

2. comorrbity   comorbidity   commorbity   comorbitity   comorbity

3. paranouia   parinoia   paranoia   parenoiia   parinnoia

4. dipendance   depindince   depindance   dependence   dipendence

5. sizophrenia   schisophrenia   scizoprenia   schizophrenia   sizofrenia

6. kongruent   congruent   kongruient   congruient   congrruent

7. tolerance   tolerrence   tollerance   tolerince   tolerence

8. phobbia   pobia   fobbia   phobia   fobia

9. anesia   amisia   anmesia   amesia   amnesia

10. bipollar   bipolar   bypollar   bypolar   beipolar

B. MATCH THE NUMBER OF THE CORRECT TERM IN PART A WITH THE BRIEF DESCRIPTION OF THE TERM BELOW.

a. Pathological fear or dread   _____

b. Mood disorder with depression and mania   _____

c. Coinciding, or agreeing with   _____

d. Persecutory delusions   _____

e. Presence of two or more diseases at same time   _____

f. Inability to recall past experiences   _____

g. State of needing someone or something   _____

h. Become accustomed to a stimulus or drug   _____

i. Disorder of perception, emotion, and behavior   _____

j. Mood stabilizer   _____

C. USING YOUR KNOWLEDGE OF TERMS 1–10 IN PART A AND THEIR CORRECT SPELLING, WRITE A BRIEF SENTENCE FOR EACH OF THE TERMS AS IT MIGHT APPEAR IN PATIENT DOCUMENTATION.

1. _____

2. _____

3. _____

4. _____

8. _____

9. _____

10. _____

D. YOUR INSTRUCTOR WILL DIRECT YOU TO MCGRAW-HILL CONNECT. OPEN THE AUDIO GLOSSARY AND PRACTICE YOUR PRONUNCIATION OF THE TERMS IN PART A OF THIS EXERCISES.

E. TO MEET LESSON OBJECTIVES, BE PREPARED TO DISCUSS THE FOLLOWING QUESTIONS IN CLASS. BE SURE YOU CAN SPELL AND PRONOUNCE EACH MEDICAL TERM CORRECTLY.

1. List the symptoms of the five major types of anxiety disorders.

_____

_____

_____

_____

_____

2. Detail the symptoms of schizophrenia, and explain the use of lithium in treating this condition.

_____

_____

_____

_____

3. What are the classes of psychoactive drugs? (Refer to *Table 19.5.*)

_____

_____

_____

_____

4. Describe the different types of personality disorders.

_____

_____

_____

_____

_____

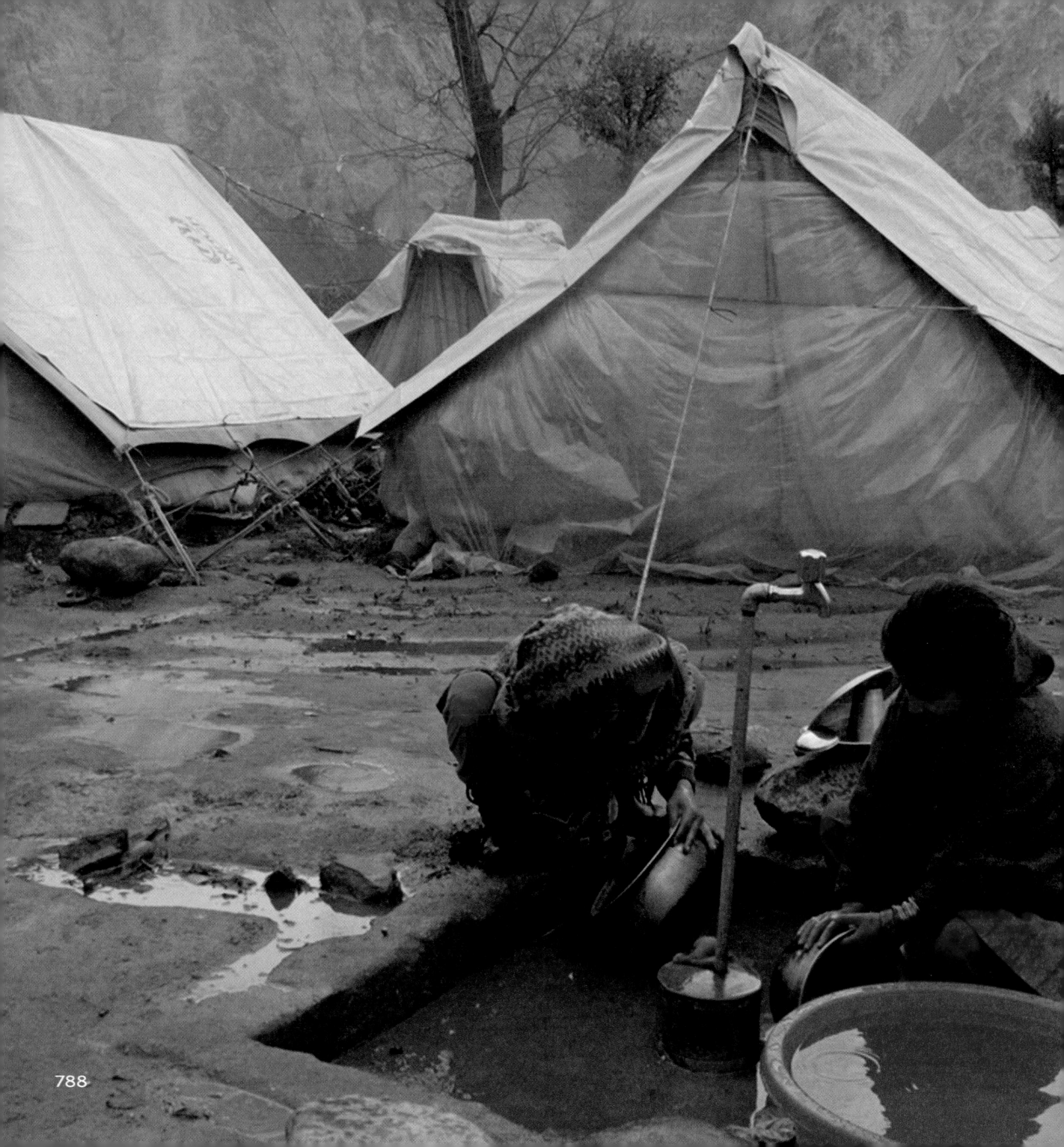

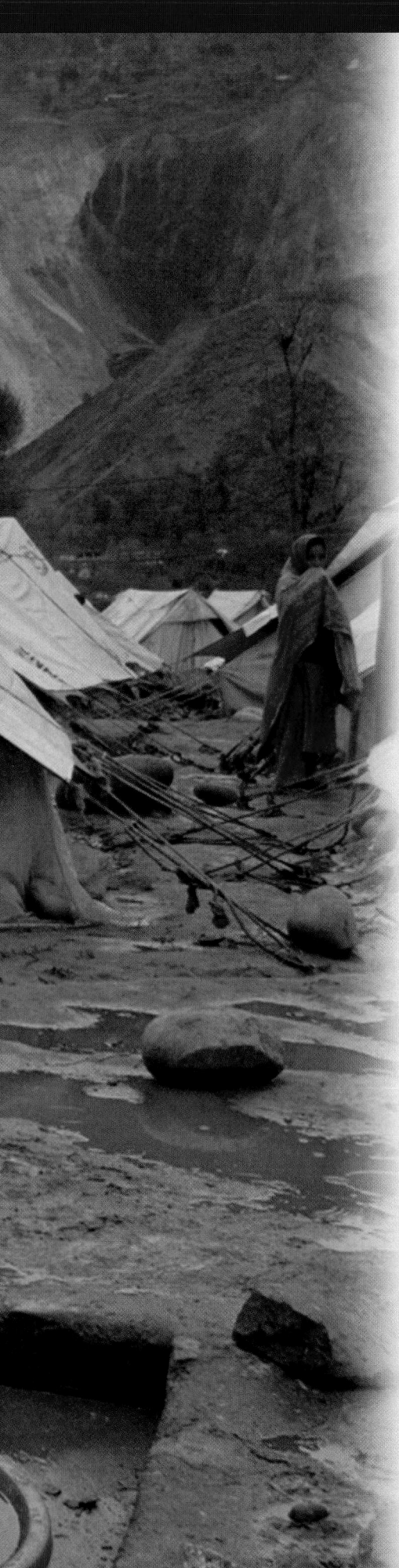

CASE REPORT 20.1

You are

. . . a physician assistant working as a volunteer with a health care team from Fulwood Medical Center in a tented camp outside Muzaffarabad, the capital of the state of Azad Kashmir in Pakistan. It is close to the epicenter of the earthquake of October 8, 2005, that killed more than 87,000 people and destroyed 70% of the buildings in Muzaffarabad. The tent city holds 1500 people whose homes have been destroyed. It is winter 2006. The temperature is around 0°C (32°F).

Your patients are

. . . Mrs. Uzma Aziz and her 2-year-old daughter Alisha, the youngest of her five children. The woman and child arrived in the tent city 2 weeks ago from a remote village high in the Himalaya mountains, where their home had been destroyed by the earthquake. The intense cold at the higher altitude made staying in their makeshift tent impossible.

Your interpreter tells you that Alisha was well until 3 days earlier, when she developed a runny nose, red eyes, and a cough. Today she has developed a rash on her forehead and neck that is spreading down onto her body.

Your examination shows T 104.2°F, P 120, R 24. A rash of red-brown macules is present on her face, neck, and shoulders. She has bilateral conjunctivitis. As you proceed with your examination, the rash continues to extend down the trunk. On the buccal mucosa (inside the mouth) are some small red spots with white centers (Koplik spots). You hear rales at the base of her right lung, and her left tympanic membrane is inflamed. She is diagnosed as having measles.

Learning Outcomes

In situations like this where the patient load is high and resources are limited, it is essential to communicate clearly with the other team members. You need to be able to:

20.1 Apply the language of infectious diseases to the causes, treatment, and prevention of infections.

20.2 Comprehend, analyze, spell, and write the medical terms of infectious diseases so that you can communicate and document accurately and precisely in any health care setting.

20.3 Recognize and pronounce the medical terms of infectious diseases so that you can communicate verbally with accuracy and precision in any health care setting.

20.4 Explain the effects of common infectious diseases on health.

Through the interpreter, you learn that none of the five children has been immunized for any disease. When they arrived at the camp, the mother refused to start a program of immunization for the children.

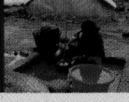

Normal Flora and Defenses Against Infections

The information in this lesson will enable you to use correct medical terminology to:

20.1.1 Describe normal flora.

20.1.2 Specify the differences between colonization and infectious disease.

20.1.3 Detail the host defense mechanisms.

20.1.4 Define the mechanisms of infection.

NORMAL FLORA AND MECHANISMS OF INFECTION

Normal Flora

Microbes (microorganisms) are everywhere—in the air, water, and soil, where they are essential for the physiology and nutrition of animals (including humans) and plants. Roughly 100 billion individual **bacteria** of 1000 different species cover your body and are called **normal flora,** while the human body is called their **host.** Their presence not only is harmless but is essential for normal functioning of the body.

These normal microorganisms are found on your skin, in your nose and respiratory tract, and in your mouth and digestive tract. This is called **colonization.** Areas like the brain and cardiovascular system remain **sterile** (microbe-free).

The host tolerates colonization by the organisms of the normal flora but restricts them to areas where they can do no harm. For example, the **bacterium** *Streptococcus pneumoniae* is found in the nasopharynx of many healthy adults. If the microbes invade the body by penetrating the nasal mucosa *(see Chapter 9)* or progressing beyond the nose into sinuses, middle ear, and the respiratory tract, they become pathogens, and an **infection** occurs *(Figure 20.1b)*. If the infection causes harm to the host, then an **infectious disease** is present. *Streptococcus pneumoniae* can invade and infect various sites in the respiratory tract and the meninges *(Figure 20.1a)*.

A healthy host defends against these pathogens through the response of the immune system *(see Chapter 15)*. These defenses may be able to prevent an infection occurring. If infection does occur, the defenses may stop the process before any harm (disease) is done *(Figure 20.1b)*. Other defenses may not come into play until the infectious disease is apparent.

Mechanisms of Infection

Toxins can be formed and released by pathogens to bind to specific adjacent or distant cells' receptors. The toxins can damage or **lyse** the cell membranes and inhibit protein synthesis and other intracellular functions.

Virulence factors in the microorganisms overcome host resistance and cause disease. **Bacterial** proteins can both facilitate local spread in tissues and penetrate intact cells, allowing the bacteria to enter the body through mucosal surfaces. Some bacteria can block antibody production, and others have developed methods to inactivate or survive phagocytosis *(see Chapter 7)*.

Microbial **adherence** to different surfaces of the host gives **pathogens** a base from which to invade cells and tissues. Some pathogens, such as *Escherichia coli*, have **fimbriae** that will attach to most human cells. Pathogens can bind to medical devices, such as IV (intravenous) catheters, shunts, stents, and vascular grafts, making them a possible source of infection.

Antimicrobial resistance involves the antibiotics used against the pathogens acting as mutagens *(see Chapter 21)* and causing mutations in the pathogens' DNA. This, in turn, enables the pathogen to become resistant to the antimicrobial agent. This resistance to antibiotics is an increasing problem, particularly in hospitals.

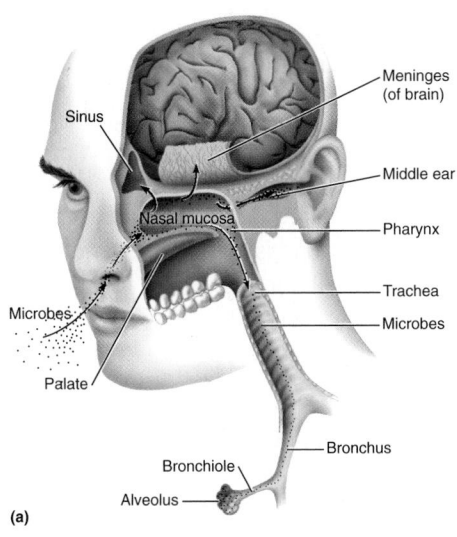

(a)

(b)

▲ **FIGURE 20.1 Associations Between Microbes and Humans.**

Keynote

Bacterial pathogens have several specific weapons to invade cells.

WORD	PRONUNCIATION		ELEMENTS	DEFINITION
adherence adhere (verb)	ad-**HERE**-ents ad-**HERE**		Latin *to stick to*	The act of sticking to something
bacterium bacteria (pl) bacterial (adj)	bak-**TEER**-ee-um bak-**TEER**-ee-ah bak-**TEER**-ee-al	S/ R/	Latin *walking stick* -ial *pertaining to* bacter- *bacterium*	A unicellular, simple, microscopic organism Pertaining to bacteria
colonization	**KOL**-on-ih-**ZAY**-shun	S/ R/	-ization *process of creating* colon- *colony*	Formation of a population of microorganisms
fimbria fimbriae (pl)	**FIM**-bree-ah **FIM**-bree-ee		Latin *fringe*	A fringelike structure on the surface of a cell or microorganism
flora	**FLO**-rah		Latin *flower*	Microorganisms covering the exterior and interior of a healthy animal
host	HOST		Latin *host*	Organism on which organisms live
infect	in-**FEKT**		Latin *invade internally*	To invade an organism with disease-producing microorganisms
infection	in-**FEK**-shun	S/ R/	-ion *condition, process* infect- *internal invasion*	Invasion of the body by disease-producing microorganisms
infectious	in-**FEK**-shus	S/	-ious *pertaining to*	Capable of being transmitted; or caused by infection by a microorganism
lysis lyse (verb)	**LIE**-sis		Greek *dissolve*	Destruction of a cell; gradual decline of a disease (as opposed to a crisis)
microbe	**MY**-krohb	P/ R/	micro- *small* -be *life*	Short for microorganism
microorganism	**MY**-kroh-**OR**-gan-izm	S/ R/	-ism *process* -organ- *instrument*	Any organism too small to be seen by the naked eye
pathogen	**PATH**-oh-jen	S/ R/CF	-gen *produce, create* path/o- *disease*	A disease-causing microorganism
pathogenic (adj)	path-oh-**JEN**-ik	S/	-ic *pertaining to*	
resistance	ree-**ZIS**-tants		Latin *to withstand*	Ability of an organism to withstand the effects of an antagonistic agent
sterile	**STER**-isle		Latin *barren*	Free from all living organisms and their spores, or unable to fertilize or reproduce
sterilize (verb) sterilization	**STER**-ih-lize **STER**-ih-lih-**ZAY**-shun			To make sterile Process of making sterile
toxin	**TOK**-sin		Greek *poison*	Poisonous substance formed by a cell or organism
toxic (adj)	**TOK**-sick	S/ R/	-ic *pertaining to* tox- *poison*	Pertaining to a toxin
toxicity (**Note:** This word contains two suffixes.)	toks-**ISS**-ih-tee	S/	-ity *state, condition*	The state of being poisonous
virulent virulence (noun)	**VIR**-you-lent **VIR**-you-lence		Latin *poisonous*	Extremely toxic or pathogenic The power of a toxin or pathogen

EXERCISES

Usage: *Employ the **language of infectious diseases** to convey the correct meaning in the following sentences. You may be asked to fill in the adjective, noun, verb, or plural form of the term. Fill in the blanks. Some terms you may use more than once.*

bacterium   **bacteria**   **bacterial**

1. Lab results showed the myco _____ tuberculosis organism to be present.

2. Her _____ infection showed major improvement after administration of antibiotics.

3. Lacerated or open skin allows _____ to invade the body.

4. A single _____ can develop into a colony of _____, producing a _____ infection.

DEFENSE MECHANISMS

Host defense mechanisms determine whether infection will occur and an infectious disease will be produced. The defense mechanisms are in four main categories:

1. **Innate resistance:**
   - **Species** have a resistance to certain **pathogens.** For example, syphilis, gonorrhea, measles, and poliomyelitis affect humans but not lower animals. The canine distemper virus does not affect humans.
   - **Individuals** within the same species have greater or lesser innate resistance to the same pathogen. Reasons for this include age, diet, malnutrition, trauma, intercurrent disease, tobacco use, immunization status, and stress.

2. **Natural barriers:**
   - **Skin** *(see Chapter 3)* effectively prevents invasion by microorganisms unless it is breached by trauma, an incision, a puncture, or any lesion. Exceptions to this rule are the **human papillomavirus (HPV)** *(see Chapter 13)* that can invade normal tissue to produce warts and cancer and some parasites that can penetrate intact skin *(see Chapter 3)*.
   - **Mucous membranes** produce secretions containing lysozyme, which has antimicrobial properties, and immunoglobulins **IgG** and **IgA** that block the attachment of microorganisms to host cells *(see Chapter 15)*. Breast milk contains IgA.
   - **Respiratory tract** has a filter system in the nose and upper airways and a **mucociliary** system to transport microorganisms away from the lung *(Figure 20.2)*. This is helped by coughing and sneezing *(see Chapter 9)*.
   - **Gastrointestinal tract** is protected by the acid pH of the stomach and the antibacterial activity of intestinal secretions. Bile and pancreatic enzymes are natural barriers to invasion by pathogens *(see Chapter 6)*.
   - **Genitourinary tract** is protected in men by the length of their urethra and in women by the acid pH of their vagina *(see Chapters 12 and 13)*.

3. **Specific immune responses:**
   The infected host produces a variety of antibodies (immunoglobulins) that bind to specific microbial antigens *(see Chapter 15)*. The antigen-antibody complexes activate the **complement** system to destroy the cell walls of the microbes *(Figure 20.3)* and stimulate the macrophage system to remove them.

4. **Nonspecific immune responses:**
   - **Cytokine production** by macrophages and lymphocytes *(see Chapter 15)* in response to an infection occurs regardless of the nature of the invading microorganism. Cytokines can generate fever and an increase in neutrophil production and activity.
   - **Inflammatory responses** *(see Chapter 15)* to infection generate an increased blood supply and increased vascular permeability at the site of the infection. The result is that neutrophils and phagocytes can leave the intravascular compartment and attack the invading microorganism.

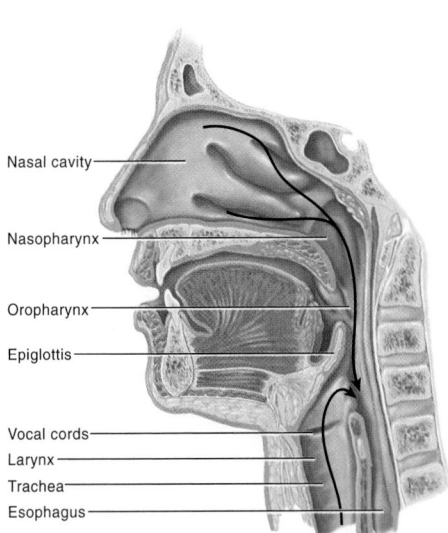

▲ FIGURE 20.2 **Filter and Transport System of Upper Respiratory Tract to Prevent Microorganisms and Pollutants from Entering the Lungs.**

Nasal cavity
Nasopharynx
Oropharynx
Epiglottis
Vocal cords
Larynx
Trachea
Esophagus

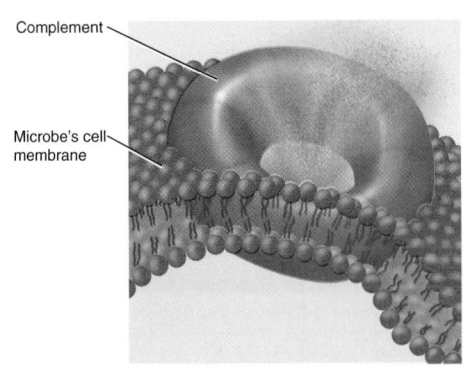

Complement
Microbe's cell membrane

▲ FIGURE 20.3 **Complement System Attacks Microbe's Cell Wall to Cause Its Death.**

Abbreviations

HPV	human papillomavirus
IgA	immunoglobulin A
IgG	immunoglobulin G

Case Report 20.1 (continued)

People, especially children, who have seen their home destroyed in the explosion of an earthquake, have tried to survive extreme cold in a simple tent, and have had to move into a foreign, primitive environment will be stressed. Their resistance to disease will be low. Add to this the lack of protection by **immunizations,** and the children will be susceptible to all the **contagious** childhood diseases, including the **measles** that Alisha has contracted.

WORD	PRONUNCIATION	ELEMENTS		DEFINITION
complement	**KOM**-pleh-ment		Latin *that which completes*	Group of proteins in serum that destroy bacteria and other cells
contagious	kon-**TAY**-jus	S/ P/ R/	-ious *pertaining to* con- *with, together* -tag- *touch*	Able to be transmitted, as infections transmitted from person to person or from person to air or surface to person
cytokine	**SIGH**-toh-kine	S/ R/CF	-kine *movement* -cyt/o- *cell*	Proteins produced by different cells that communicate with other cells in the immune system
immune	im-**YUNE**	P/ R/	im- *not* -mune *in service*	Protected from an infectious disease
immunize immunization	**IM**-you-nize im-you-nih-**ZAY**-shun	S/ S/	-ize *affect in a specific way* -ization *the process of creating*	To make resistant to an infectious disease Administration of an agent to provide immunity
innate	ih-**NATE**	P/ R/CF	in- *in* -nat/e *birth*	Present at birth; arising from the intellect
measles (also known as rubeola)	**ME**-zelz		Old English *measles*	Acute, contagious disease of childhood
mucociliary	**MYU**-koh-**SIL**-ih-ah-ree	S/ R/CF R/	-ary *pertaining to* muc/o- *mucous membrane* -cili- *hairlike structure*	Pertaining to the ciliated epithelium lining the bronchial tree
species	**SPEE**-sheez		Latin *form, kind*	A group of organisms with certain common characteristics

EXERCISES

Usage: *Continue to employ the **language of infectious diseases** to convey the correct meaning in the following sentences. Fill in the adjective, noun, verb, or plural form of the term.*

immune   immunity   immunize   immunization

1. You may be born with a natural _____ against a certain disease. In that case, there is no need for an

_____ to _____ you against the disease. You are already _____ to it.

infected   infection   infectious

2. The body can be invaded by _____ organisms with the potential to cause disease. The

_____ body part (such as a cut) may be red, swollen, and warm to the touch. Fever can also be a sign

of _____.

Use each of the following three terms in sentences that could be used for patient education. Remember to use language a nonmedical person would understand.

3. contagious: _____

_____

4. innate: _____

_____

5. rubeola: _____

_____

LESSON 20.2 Viral Diseases

The information in this lesson will enable you to use correct medical terminology to:

20.2.1 Identify the characteristics and properties of viruses.

20.2.2 Describe some of the viral diseases of children.

20.2.3 Detail some of the viral respiratory diseases.

20.2.4 Define diagnostic methods for viruses.

20.2.5 Discuss the prevention of viral infections.

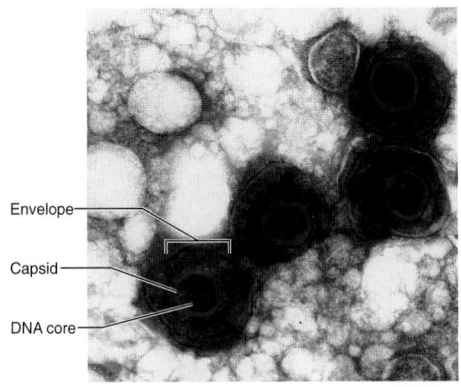

Envelope

Capsid

DNA core

300,000×

▲ **FIGURE 20.4   Electron Microscopy of Herpesvirus.**

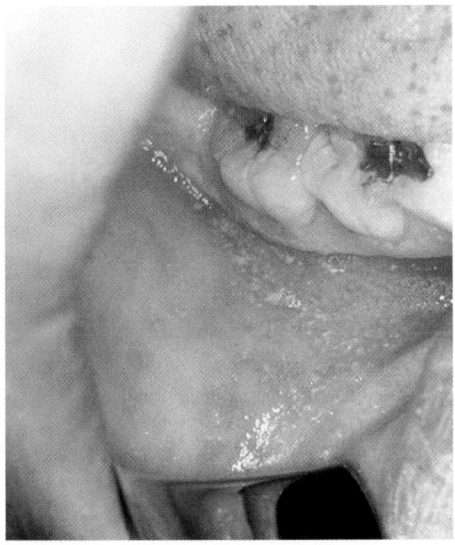

▲ **FIGURE 20.5   Koplik Spots on the Buccal Mucosa Early in Measles.**

Abbreviations	
BSE	bovine spongiform encephalopathy
CJD	Creutzfeldt-Jakob disease
EBV	Epstein-Barr virus

VIRUSES

Viruses are the smallest of microorganisms. They are too small to be seen under an ordinary light microscope but are visible using electron microscopy *(Figure 20.4)*. They are composed of an outer membrane (envelope) of protein and lipid with a nucleic acid core of RNA or DNA enclosed in a **capsid.**

Viruses are not "living" organisms, so they need living cells in order to multiply. The viruses invade cells and redirect the cells from their normal functions to replicate the virus. Viruses stimulate antibody production by the host.

Hundreds of viruses can infect humans and are spread mainly by **respiratory** (coughs, sneezes) *(see Chapter 9)* and **enteric excretions** *(see Chapter 6)* via hands when they are not properly washed. When viruses can spread from person to person, they are said to be contagious.

Some viruses are **oncogenic** (cancer-producing). For example, the **Epstein-Barr virus (EBV)** is associated with Hodgkin disease, nasopharyngeal carcinoma, and lymphomas in immunosuppressed patients *(see Chapter 15)*.

Slow viral diseases are characterized by lengthy **incubation** periods and the production of chronic degenerative diseases. An example is the JC (patient's initials) virus that is firmly associated with **progressive multifocal leukoencephalopathy,** with its destruction of brain cells, progressive dementia, and paralysis.

Bovine spongiform encephalopathy (BSE), called mad cow disease, and the associated human **spongiform encephalopathy,** called **Creutzfeldt-Jakob disease (CJD),** are not caused by a virus but by a **prion,** a small protein particle in cells capable of causing an infection.

Latency—a long period in which the virus is quiescent (dormant)—permits recurrent infection and person-to-person spread. Herpesviruses exhibit latency.

VIRAL DISEASES OF CHILDHOOD

Many viral childhood diseases have a skin rash **(exanthem)** associated with them.

Measles (rubeola), in its **prodromal** phase, produces signs similar to an upper respiratory infection (URI), but inside the mouth on the buccal mucosa are found small red spots with white centers. These are called **Koplik spots** *(Figure 20.5)*. The reddish-brown **macular** rash *(see Chapter 3)* comes out on the face and body on the third or fourth day of the illness. A safe and effective vaccine is available to prevent measles.

Case Report 20.1 (continued)

Alisha had two of the complications of measles. The rales heard at the base of her right lung indicated a right lower-lobe pneumonia, and she had an otitis media. The medical staff wanted to admit Alisha to the hospital set up on the edge of the tent city. Alisha's mother refused to let her be admitted. She was shown how to give antibiotics orally, and they went back to their tent.

WORD	PRONUNCIATION	ELEMENTS		DEFINITION
capsid	**KAP**-sid	S/	-id *having a particular quality*	Protein shell surrounding the nucleic acid in the core of a virus
		R/	caps- *cover, shell*	
enteric	en-**TEHR**-ik	S/	-ic *pertaining to*	Pertaining to the intestine
		R/	enter- *intestine*	
exanthem	ek-**ZAN**-them		Greek *an eruption*	Skin eruption or rash occurring as the outward sign of a viral or bacterial disease
incubation	in-kyu-**BAY**-shun	S/	-ation *process*	Process to develop an infection
incubate (verb)	**IN**-kyu-bate	R/	incub- *lie on, hatch*	
Koplik spots	**KOP**-lik SPOTZ		Henry Koplik, 1858–1927, American pediatrician	Small red spots with a white center on the buccal mucosa seen early in measles
latent	**LAY**-tent		Latin *lie hidden*	Dormant, not discernible
latency (noun)	**LAY**-ten-see			
leukoencephalopathy	**LOO**-koh-en-sef-ah-**LOP**-ah-thee	S/	-pathy *disease*	Disease-producing destruction of white matter of the brain
		R/CF	leuk/o- *white*	
		R/CF	-encephal/o- *brain*	
macule	**MAK**-yul		Latin *spot*	Small, flat spot or patch on the skin
macular (adj)	**MAK**-you-lahr			
multifocal	mul-tee-**FOH**-kal	S/	-al *pertaining to*	Arising from many centers
		P/	multi- *many*	
		R/	-foc- *center*	
oncogenic	**ONG**-koh-**JEN**-ik	S/	-genic *producing*	Capable of producing a neoplasm
		R/CF	onc/o- *tumor*	
prion	**PREE**-on		Derived from *proteinaceous infectious particle*	Small infectious protein particle
prodromal	pro-**DRO**-mal		Greek *running before*	Beginning of disease before signs become overt
spongiform	**SPON**-jih-form	S/	-form *resembling*	Looking like a sponge
		R/CF	spong/i- *sponge*	
virus	**VIE**-rus		Latin *poison*	Group of infectious agents that require living cells for growth and reproduction
		S/	-al *pertaining to*	
viral (adj)	**VIE**-ral	R/	vir- *virus*	Pertaining to a virus

*Meet lesson objectives and employ the **language of infectious diseases** to answer the following questions.*

1. What is the *prodromal* phase of a disease? _____

_____

2. What is the period called in which a virus is *quiescent*? _____

3. What is another medical term for the answer in question 2? _____

4. The terms in questions 2 and 3 all mean the same thing: _____

_____

5. Make your own study hint for the terms in questions 2 and 3.

_____

_____

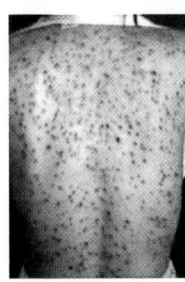

▲ FIGURE 20.6   Chickenpox.

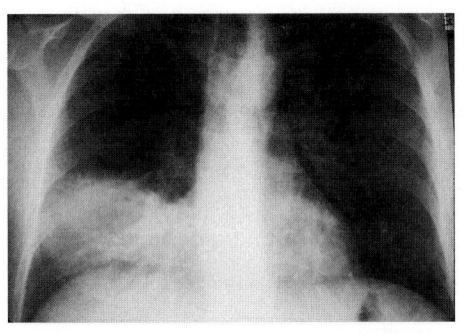

▲ FIGURE 20.7   Chest X-Ray of Patient with RML Pneumonia.

Abbreviations

H5N1 subtype of avian influenza virus
RML right middle lobe
RSV respiratory syncytial virus
SARS severe acute respiratory syndrome
WNV West Nile virus

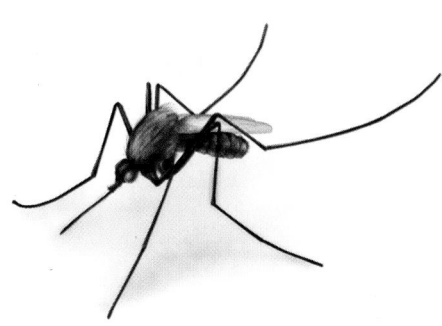

▲ FIGURE 20.8   Mosquito.

VIRAL DISEASES OF CHILDHOOD (continued)

German measles (rubella) is a much milder disease than rubeola. It can also be prevented with an effective vaccine. If a woman develops rubella early in pregnancy, the unborn child can develop serious birth defects, including hearing loss, cataracts, congenital heart disease, and mental retardation.

Chickenpox (varicella) produces an itchy, blistered **rash** that crusts *(Figure 20.6)*. The virus can remain **quiescent** (dormant) in nerve fibers for many years before producing the painful lesions of **herpes zoster (shingles)**. There is an effective **vaccine** to prevent varicella and to prevent shingles in older adults.

Other childhood viral diseases with a rash are **erythema infectiosum (fifth disease), roseola infantum, hand-foot-and-mouth disease,** and **herpangina.**

Mumps causes swelling of the parotid salivary glands and can cause **orchitis** (inflammation of the testis) in the male *(see Chapter 12)*. There is an effective vaccine to prevent the disease.

VIRAL RESPIRATORY DISEASES

The common cold, influenza, pharyngitis, laryngitis, and **laryngotracheobronchitis (croup)** *(see Chapter 9)* are all upper respiratory infections caused by viruses. Symptoms can be more severe in the very young because of the relative narrowness of their respiratory passages and in the very old because of their decreased immune response.

Viral pneumonia *(see Chapter 9)* is common in winter months, can affect small or large areas of the lungs, and is more serious in the very young and very old *(Figure 20.7)*.

Respiratory syncytial virus (RSV) is the most common cause of bronchiolitis and pneumonia in infants and children under 1 year of age.

Severe acute respiratory syndrome (SARS) is a viral respiratory tract infection that first appeared in China in 2002. Of all SARS cases, 80% to 90% are mild, but the remaining 10% to 20% develop severe respiratory distress and may require mechanical ventilation. The overall death rate is 3% to 4% of those infected.

Avian influenza (bird flu) is caused by avian influenza viruses that are **endemic** in wild birds worldwide. When domesticated birds such as chickens, turkeys, and ducks are infected, they become very sick and die. It rarely spreads to humans.

A subtype of the avian influenza viruses called **H5N1** virus caused outbreaks of the disease among poultry in Asia in late 2003 and early 2004. One hundred million birds died from the disease or were killed in attempts to control the outbreaks. More than 100 human cases were reported, mostly in poultry workers. In 2005, worries about a **pandemic** were fueled by the disease spreading to Eastern Europe.

West Nile virus (WNV) is established as a seasonal **epidemic** in North America, flaring up in the summer and fall. Mosquitoes become infected when they feed on infected birds and then spread the disease to humans when they bite *(Figure 20.8)*. The fever and aches may last for several weeks. There is no specific treatment.

The prevention of viral diseases is discussed in Lesson 20.5 of this chapter.

Most viral diseases do not respond to antibiotics. Many physicians do not prescribe antibiotics to patients with upper respiratory diseases unless a bacterial cause or complication is identified.

Swine flu is a global outbreak of a new subtype of influenza A virus named H1N1. Transmission of the virus is typically human to human, by coughing, sneezing, or touching contaminated surfaces. Eating cooked pork products does not transmit the virus. The illness is generally mild, except in people with underlying diseases and weakened immune systems.

WORD	PRONUNCIATION		ELEMENTS	DEFINITION
avian	**A**-vee-an		Latin *a bird*	Pertaining to birds
epidemic	ep-ih-**DEM**-ik	S/ P/ R/	-ic *pertaining to* epi- *above, upon* -dem- *the people*	Outbreak in a community of a disease or a health-related behavior
endemic pandemic	en-**DEM**-ik pan-**DEM**-ik	P/ P/	en- *in* pan- *all*	Disease always present in a community Disease attacking the population of a very large area
erythema infectiosum (also called **fifth disease**)	er-ih-**THEE**-mah in-fek-she-**OH**-sum	S/ R/	Greek *flushed skin* -iosum *pertaining to* infect- *internal invasion*	Mild infectious disease of childhood with a flushed-cheek appearance
herpangina	her-**PAN**-ji-nah	R/ R/	-angina *sore throat* herp- *blister*	Ulcerative disease of the throat
laryngotracheo-bronchitis (also called **croup**)	lah-**RING**-oh-**TRAY**-kee-oh- brong-**KI**-tis KROOP	S R/CF R/CF R/	-itis *inflammation* laryng/o- *larynx* -trache/o- *trachea* -bronch- *bronchus*	Inflammation of the larynx, trachea, and bronchi Infection of the upper airways in children, characterized by a barking cough
quiescent	kwi-**ESS**-ent		Latin *quiet*	Latent, dormant
rash	RASH		French *skin eruption*	Cutaneous eruption
roseola infantum	roh-**ZEE**-oh-lah in-**FAN**-tum	S/ R/ S/ R/	-ola *small* rose- *rose* -um *tissue, structure* infant- *infant*	Skin rash in infants and young children caused by a herpesvirus
syncytium syncytial (adj)	sin-**SISH**-ee-um sin-**SISH**-ee-al	S/ P/ R/CF S/	-um *tissue, structure* syn- *together* -cyt/i- *cell* -al *pertaining to*	A multinucleated mass not separated into cells Pertaining to the syncytium
vaccine vaccinate (verb) vaccination	**VAK**-seen **VAK**-sin-ate vak-sih-**NAY**-shun	S/ R/ S/	Latin *relating to a cow* -ate *process* vaccin- *giving a vaccine* -ation *process*	Preparation to generate active immunity To administer a vaccine Administration of a vaccine

EXERCISES

Circle the correct answer in the following questions on viral diseases. Remember: There is only one best answer.

1. Which of the following childhood diseases does *not* have a rash as a symptom?

    chickenpox   German measles   roseola   mumps

2. Which childhood disease, if contracted early in pregnancy, can cause serious birth defects in the fetus?

    rubella   roseola   rubeola   rosacea

3. Another name for the *chickenpox* virus is:

    verruca   vermiform   varicella   viscera

4. Many viral childhood diseases exhibit skin *rash*. Another name for this is:

    eczema   exanthem   exacerbation   excoriation

5. *Herpes zoster* is another name for:

    croup   shingles   pertussis   whooping cough

6. A multinucleated mass not separated into cells is called:

    mucociliary   fimbria   spongiform   syncytium

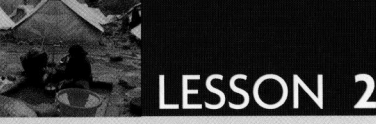

INFECTION

LESSON 20.3 Bacterial Infections

OBJECTIVES

The information in this lesson will enable you to use correct medical terminology to:

20.3.1 Classify bacteria.

20.3.2 Discuss the infections produced by different types of bacteria.

20.3.3 Define the routes of transmission of bacterial infections.

You are

. . . a licensed vocational nurse **(LVN/LPN)** working in a medical ward in Fulwood Medical Center.

Your patient is

. . . Mr. Martin Geller, a frail 70-year-old man, who has been admitted with right lower-lobe pneumonia, shortness of breath, and general weakness.

CASE REPORT 20.2

Mr. Geller is being treated with doxycycline (Vibramycin) and moxifloxacin (Avelox). He has been taking omeprazole (Prilosec) for heartburn for several months.

During the previous night, he became **febrile.** He is complaining of stomach cramps and has passed two loose stools containing blood and mucus. He is asking for the bedpan to pass another stool.

What precautions should you take before you can meet his needs?

Abbreviations

LPN	licensed practical nurse
LVN	licensed vocational nurse

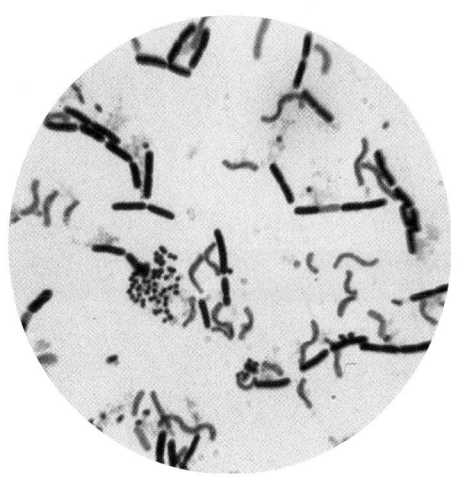

▲ **FIGURE 20.9 Gram Stain.** Blue or purple cells are Gram-positive; red or pink cells are Gram-negative.

CLASSIFICATION OF BACTERIA

Bacteria are single-celled microorganisms that reproduce by dividing. There are thousands of different bacteria, and only a few cause disease. Some bacterial infections, like strep throat, are contagious.

Bacteria are classified in several ways:

- By their **distinctive shapes.** Spherical bacteria are called **cocci.** Rodlike bacteria are called **bacilli.** Helical or spiral bacteria are called **spirochetes.**
- By their **color** after a **Gram stain** is applied to them. Bacteria that stain blue or purple are called **Gram-positive.** Bacteria that stain pink or red are called **Gram-negative** *(Figure 20.9).*
- By their **use of oxygen.** Bacteria that can grow in the presence of oxygen are called **aerobes.** Those that do not require oxygen are called **anaerobes.**

INFECTIONS CAUSED BY GRAM-POSITIVE COCCI

Pathogenic staphylococci are everywhere, including in your nose and on your skin. Transmission is most common via the hands of individuals, but airborne spread can occur; for example, if infected bedding is shaken.

The diseases produced by staphylococci include:

- Postoperative infections.
- Furuncles, carbuncles, cellulitis, impetigo *(see Chapter 3).*
- Pneumonia in newborns or immunosuppressed patients *(see Chapter 15).*
- Endocarditis in IV drug users and patients with prosthetic heart valves *(see Chapter 8).*
- Osteomyelitis, particularly in children *(see Chapter 5).*
- Bacteremia in severe burns or patients with IV catheters *(see Chapter 3).*
- Toxic shock syndrome caused by an exotoxin produced by the *Staphylococcus* bacterium and associated with tampon use *(see Chapter 13).*
- Puerperal sepsis *(see Chapter 13).*

WORD	PRONUNCIATION		ELEMENTS	DEFINITION
aerobic (adj) **aerobe (noun)**	air-**OH**-bik **AIR**-obe	S/ R/CF	**-bic** *life* **aer/o-** *air*	An organism capable of living in the presence of oxygen
anaerobic (adj) **anaerobe (noun)**	an-air-**OH**-bik **AN**-air-obe	S/ P/ R/CF	**-bic** *life* **an-** *without* **–aer/o-** *air*	An organism capable of growing in the absence of oxygen
bacillus **bacilli (pl)**	ba-**SIL**-us ba-**SIL**-ee		Latin *little rod*	A rod-shaped bacterium
coccus **cocci (pl)**	**KOK**-us **KOK**-see		Greek *berry*	Round, spheroid bacterium
fever **febrile (adj)**	**FEE**-ver **FEB**-ril or **FEB**-rile	 S/ R/	Old English *fever* **-ile** *capable of* **febr-** *fever*	Increased body temperature that is a physiologic response to disease Pertaining to or suffering from a fever
Gram stain	GRAM STAYN		Hans Christian Gram, 1853–1938, Danish bacteriologist	A method for differential staining of bacteria
spirochete	**SPY**-roh-keet	P/ R/	**spiro-** *spiral, coil* **-chete** *hair*	Spiral-shaped bacterium causing a sexually transmitted disease (syphilis)
Staphylococcus **staphylococci (pl)**	**STAF**-ih-loh-**KOK**-us **STAF**-ih-loh-**KOK**-sigh	S/ R/CF R/	**-us** *pertaining to* **staphyl/o-** *bunch of grapes* **-cocc-** *berry*	Gram-positive bacteria that divide in more than one plane to form clusters

EXERCISES

After reading Case Report 20.2 on the opposite page, answer the following questions. Be prepared to discuss your answers in class.

1. Mr. Geller is described as "frail." What does that mean?

_____

2. What two abbreviations could be inserted into this Case Report?

_____

3. What symptoms or conditions does Mr. Geller have on admission?

_____

4. What are his current medications?

_____

5. What VS indicates that Mr. Geller is *febrile?*

_____

6. What additional problems has Mr. Geller developed since he has been admitted? _____

_____

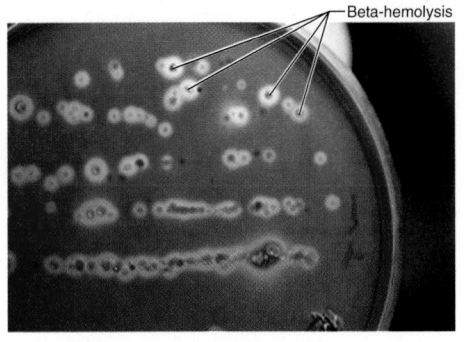

▲ **FIGURE 20.10 Blood Agar Plate Growing Bacteria from Human Throat.** Clear areas of hemolysis are shown around beta-hemolytic *streptococcal* colonies.

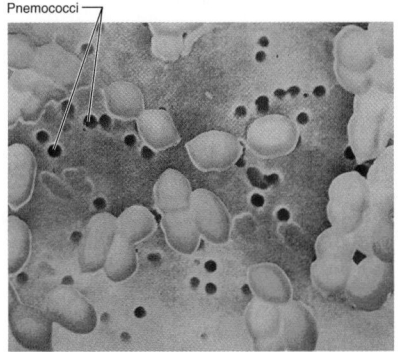

▲ **FIGURE 20.11 Spherical Bacteria of Pneumococcus.**

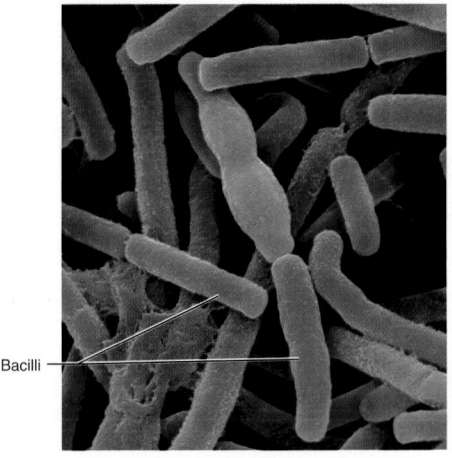

▲ **FIGURE 20.12 *Bacillus Anthracis***

INFECTIONS CAUSED BY GRAM-POSITIVE COCCI (continued)

Streptococcal Infections

Streptococci are classified according to their reaction when grown on sheep **blood agar.**

Beta-hemolytic streptococci produce an area of clear hemolysis around each colony *(Figure 20.10)*. Diseases produced by beta-hemolytic **strep,** one of which is *Streptococcus pyogenes,* include:

- Tonsillitis, pharyngitis, scarlet fever, glomerulonephritis, septicemia.
- Wound and skin infections, cellulitis, impetigo, erysipelas.
- Neonatal sepsis, puerperal sepsis, septic arthritis, endocarditis, toxic shock syndrome, necrotizing fasciitis.

Alpha-hemolytic streptococci produce a green area around each colony on the agar plate. Diseases produced by these bacteria, also called *Streptococcus viridans,* include:

- Bacterial endocarditis, localized abscesses, cellulitis, and invasive soft tissue infections.

Pneumococcal Infections

Pneumococci *(Streptococcus pneumoniae)* are found in the respiratory tract of about 50% of the population in winter and early spring. The organisms spread from person to person by droplets through coughing or sneezing or via the hands *(Figure 20.11)*. Infections caused by pneumococci include:

- **Pneumonia,** usually lobar, but occasionally bronchopneumonia *(see Chapter 9)*.
- Half of the cases of acute otitis media in infants and children *(see Chapter 4)*.
- Conjunctivitis, sinusitis, meningitis, bacteremia, endocarditis, and septic arthritis. A vaccine against **pneumococcal** disease is available.

INFECTIONS CAUSED BY GRAM-POSITIVE BACILLI

The **spores** of the **anthrax** bacillus *(Bacillus anthracis)* resist destruction by disinfectants and heat *(Figure 20.12)*. They can enter your body through broken skin or, more rarely, be inhaled. Inside the body, the spores germinate in macrophages to produce bacteria that are transported to lymph nodes, where they multiply. The bacteria produce a variety of toxins capable of causing sudden death.

The term "weapons of mass destruction" includes nuclear, chemical, radiological, and biological agents. Biological (germ) warfare is the use of microbiological agents such as anthrax, smallpox, and botulinum toxin for hostile purposes, though this is against international law. In 2001, anthrax was deliberately spread through the postal system in and around Washington, DC. Twenty-one cases of anthrax were caused.

Clostridium difficile (C. difficile) is a Gram-positive anaerobic spore-forming bacillus that is the major cause of antibiotic-associated diarrhea. The antibiotics alter the normal intestinal flora, allowing *C. difficile* to flourish. It produces two exotoxins that generate watery, bloody diarrhea and mucus and promote marked swelling of the bowel wall with edema.

Case Report 20.2 (continued)

Any patient in a hospital who is on antibiotics and is elderly and frail is suspected of having *C. difficile* disease if the patient has an onset of diarrhea. A stool sample taken for laboratory analysis from Mr. Geller is positive for the toxin of *C. difficile.* The bacterium is highly contagious, and patients require isolation. The antibiotics Mr. Geller had been taking were discontinued, and he has been started on IV metronidazole (Flagyl).

WORD	PRONUNCIATION		ELEMENTS	DEFINITION
agar	**AH**-gar		Malaysian *seaweed*	A derivative of seaweed used as a culture medium
anthrax	**AN**-thraks		Greek *carbuncle*	A severe infectious disease
Clostridium difficile	klos-**TRID**-ee-um dif-ih-**SEE**-il		***Clostridium*** Greek *a spindle* **difficile** French *difficult*	Gram-positive rod producing powerful exotoxins that cause colitis
Pneumococcus pneumococci (pl)	new-moh-**KOK**-us	S/ R/ R/CF	**-us** *pertaining to* **-cocc-** *berry* **pneum/o-** *lung, air*	Gram-positive cocci associated with respiratory infection
pneumococcal (adj)	new-moh-**KOK**-al	S/	**-al** *pertaining to*	Pertaining to the *Pneumococcus*
pneumonia	new-**MOH**-nee-ah	S/ R/	**-ia** *a condition* **pneumon-** *lung, air*	Inflammation of the lung parenchyma
pneumonic (adj)	new-**MON**-ik	S/	**-ic** *pertaining to*	Relating to pneumonia
pyogenic (adj)	**PIE**-o-**JEN**-ik	S/ R/ R/CF	**-ic** *pertaining to* **-gen-** *produce* **py/o-** *pus*	Pus-producing
spore	SPOR		Greek *seed*	Generic term for any tiny compact cells produced during reproduction by bacteria
Streptococcus streptococci (pl)	strep-toe-**KOK**-us strep-toe-**KOK**-sigh	S/ R/CF R/	**-us** *pertaining to* **strept/o-** *twisted* **-cocc-** *berry*	Gram-positive bacteria that grow in chains
streptococcal (adj)	strep-toe-**KOK**-al	S/	**-al** *pertaining to*	Pertaining to the *Streptococcus*

EXERCISES

Employ all the medical terminology you have learned thus far to answer the following questions.

1. "Infections caused by pneumococci include <u>conjunctivitis</u>, <u>sinusitis</u>, <u>meningitis</u>, <u>bacteremia</u>, <u>endocarditis</u>, and <u>septic</u> <u>arthritis</u>."

   Briefly define each of the underlined terms in this sentence, and then identify which body system is affected.

   Definition   **Body System Affected**

   _____   _____

   _____   _____

   _____   _____

   _____   _____

   _____   _____

   _____   _____

2. *Neonatal sepsis* and *puerperal sepsis* can occur in what circumstance? _____

3. On the basis of an element in the term *Streptococcus pneumoniae*, this bacterium will be found in the _____ .

4. What is the difference between *lobar pneumonia* and *bronchopneumonia*? _____

   _____

   _____

5. Drawing on your knowledge of elements, what is an *exotoxin*? _____

   _____

6. How can anthrax spores enter your body? _____

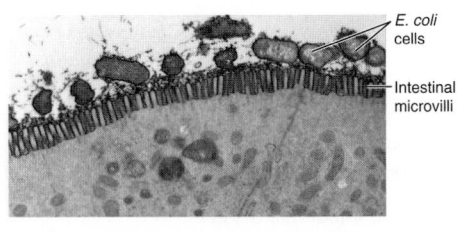

▲ **FIGURE 20.13** **A Row of *Escherichia coli* Cells Clinging to the Surface of Intestinal Cells.**

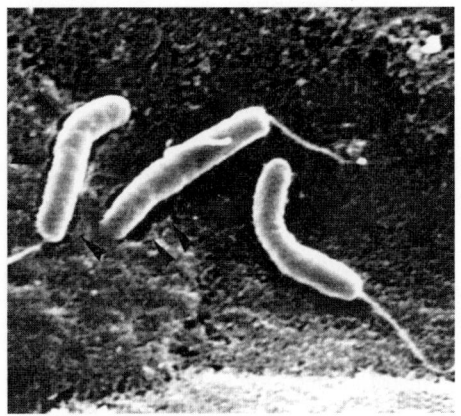

▲ **FIGURE 20.14** **Bacteria That Cause Cholera.**

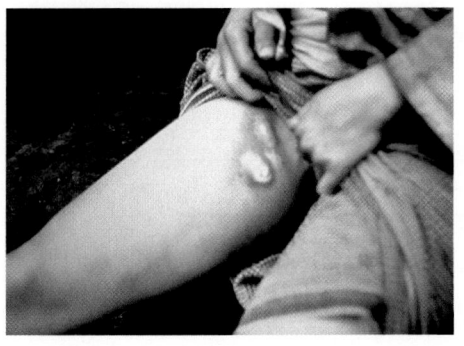

▲ **FIGURE 20.15** **Inguinal Bubo of Bubonic Plague.**

Keynote

Common side effects of antibiotics include diarrhea and, in women, vaginal yeast infections.

Abbreviation

MRSA *methicillin-resistant Staphylococcus aureus*

INFECTIONS CAUSED BY GRAM-NEGATIVE BACILLI

Escherichia coli (E. coli) inhabits the gastrointestinal tract of humans and animals *(Figure 20.13)*. Most strains are harmless, but several produce toxins that can cause diarrhea. **Contamination** of meat can occur in the animal slaughtering process. Humans acquire the infection by eating inadequately cooked meat. Person-to-person transmission can occur if infected people do not wash their hands after using the toilet.

Salmonella infections are another cause of gastroenteritis. They result from eating contaminated food, often of animal origin. Thorough cooking kills the germ. *Salmonella typhi (S. typhi)* causes **typhoid fever**, sometimes called **enteric fever.** A few people continue to shed organisms in their stool for longer than a year and are called **chronic enteric carriers.**

Shigellosis (bacillary dysentery) is a severe form of gastroenteritis, with marked diarrhea containing blood, pus, and mucus. It is transmitted in contaminated food or water.

Brucellosis (undulant fever) is an acute febrile illness acquired from infected animals or by drinking infected raw milk. Symptoms persist for 1 to 5 weeks, remit for 2 to 14 days, and then return. **Remissions (undulations)** can recur over months or years.

Cholera is an acute infection with watery diarrhea, vomiting, dehydration, and collapse *(Figure 20.14)*. It is spread by ingestion of water and foods contaminated with the **excrement** of infected persons. It is endemic in numerous parts of the world where sanitation is poor.

Plague occurs in rats and mice and is transmitted to humans by the bite of an infected flea vector. **Bubonic plague** is characterized by fever and enlarged lymph nodes (**buboes;** *Figure 20.15*). **Pneumonic plague** is characterized by acute respiratory symptoms and pneumonia. The mortality rate is high in any plague epidemic.

Pseudomonas **infections** mostly occur in hospitalized patients who are debilitated or immunosuppressed. They occur in many anatomical sites, particularly where there has been trauma, catheters, or other invasive procedures.

INFECTIONS CAUSED BY GRAM-NEGATIVE, AEROBIC COCCI

Organisms of the *Neisseria* group include:

- *N. meningitides*, which causes meningitis *(see Chapter 10)*.
- *N. gonorrhoeae*, which causes **gonorrhea** *(see Chapter 13)*.

ANTIBIOTICS

Antibiotics are drugs used to treat bacterial infections. They either kill microorganisms or stop them from reproducing; this allows the body's natural defenses to eliminate them. Antibiotics are ineffective against viral and fungal infections.

Each antibiotic is effective against only certain bacteria. If a specific infection may be caused by several types of bacteria, samples of blood, urine, or tissue are sent to a laboratory to identify the infecting bacteria. Combinations of antibiotics are used to treat life-threatening infections and infections caused by bacteria that quickly develop resistance to a single antibiotic.

Because of the widespread use and misuse of antibiotics, some bacteria develop **resistance** (see page 791) to the antibiotics, which become ineffective for those bacteria. Examples of this are methicillin-resistant *Staphylococcus aureus* (**MRSA**) and *Clostridium difficile*, which occur most frequently in hospitals and other health care facilities and cause life-threatening illnesses.

WORD	PRONUNCIATION	ELEMENTS		DEFINITION
antibiotic	**AN**-tih-bye-**OT**-ik	S/ P/ R/CF	-tic *pertaining to* anti- *against* -bi/o- *life*	A substance that has the capacity to destroy bacteria and other microorganisms
brucellosis	brew-sel-**OH**-sis	S/ R/	-osis *condition* brucell- *from pathologist David Bruce*	Undulant fever
bubo buboes (pl) bubonic (adj)	**BYU**-bo **BYU**-bose **BYU**-bon-ik		Greek *swelling in groin*	Swollen, inflamed lymph node
cholera	**KOL**-er-ah		Greek *bile*	Acute endemic infectious disease
contamination	**KON**-tam-ih-**NAY**-shun	S/ R/	-ation *process* contamin- *to corrupt, make unclean*	Presence of an infectious agent on a surface or in a substance
dysentery dysenteric (adj)	**DIS**-en-tare-ee dis-en-**TARE**-ik	P/ R/ S/ R/	dys- *bad, difficult, painful* -entery *intestine* -ic *pertaining to* -enter *intestine*	Disease with diarrhea, bowel spasms, fever, and dehydration
Escherichia coli	esh-eh-**RIK**-ee-ah **KOH**-lie		T. Escherich, 1857–1911, German pediatrician and bacteriologist	Organism in the intestine; releases an exotoxin that causes diarrhea
excrement (noun) excrete (verb)	**EKS**-kreh-ment eks-**KREET**	S/ P/ R/	-ment *resulting state* ex- *out, away from* -cre- *separation*	Waste matter such as feces To pass out of the body waste products of metabolism
gonorrhea *Neisseria gonorrhoeae*	gon-oh-**REE**-ah ni-**SEE**-ree-ah gon-oh-**REE**-ee	S/ R/CF	-rrhea *flow* gon/o- *seed* Albert Neisser, 1855–1916, German bacteriologist	Specific contagious sexually transmitted infection Bacterium that causes gonorrhea
plague	PLAYG		Latin *stroke, injury*	Infectious disease causing excessive mortality
Pseudomonas	soo-doh-**MOH**-nas	P/ R/	pseudo- *false* -monas *unit*	Gram-negative aerobic rods
remit remission	ree-**MIT** ree-**MISH**-un	S/ R/	Latin *to send back* -ion *action, process* remiss- *send back*	To diminish in intensity Period in which there is a lessening or absence of the symptoms of a disease
Salmonella	sal-moh-**NELL**-ah		Daniel Salmon, 1850–1914, U.S. pathologist	Pathogenic Gram-negative rods causing dysentery
Shigella shigellosis	she-**GEL**-ah shig-eh-**LOH**-sis	S/	Kiyoshi Shiga, 1870–1957, Japanese bacteriologist -osis *condition*	Genus of Gram-negative rods Dysentery caused by *Shigella*
typhoid	**TIE**-foyd	S/ R/	-oid *resembling* typh- *typhus*	Acute infectious disease caused by *Salmonella typhi*

EXERCISES

*Apply the **language of infectious diseases**, and match the meaning in the left column with the correct medical terminology in the right column.*

_____ 1. enteric fever

_____ 2. occur mostly in hospitalized patients

_____ 3. undulant fever

_____ 4. another name for shigellosis

_____ 5. transmitted to humans by a vector

_____ 6. endemic in some parts of the world

_____ 7. severe form of gastroenteritis

_____ 8. most strains are harmless

A. plague

B. bacillary dysentery

C. shigellosis

D. *E. coli*

E. typhoid

F. pseudomonas

G. cholera

H. brucellosis

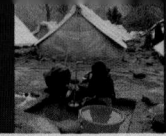

LESSON 20.4 Fungal and Parasitic Infections

INFECTION

Fungi and parasites are widespread in the **ecologic** environment of the earth, and some fungi can be parasitic. Relatively few of the 100,000 species of fungi are pathogenic for humans, but about 50 species of parasitic **helminths** (worms) can infect humans.

The information in this lesson will enable you to use correct medical terminology to:

20.4.1 Differentiate between fungi and parasites.

20.4.2 Identify different types of fungi and the diseases they cause.

20.4.3 Name different parasites and the diseases they cause.

FUNGAL INFECTIONS

Fungi are very different from bacteria in that their structure is more complex, with multiple chromosomes in a nucleus within a nuclear membrane, and cytoplasmic organelles *(see Chapter 2)*. Many fungi are "good" fungi; for example, the mushrooms you eat, and the yeasts that ferment beer and bread. Penicillin was derived from a fungal colony *(Figure 20.16)*.

Mycology is the study of fungi. **Mycologists** are the scientists who study fungi. There are two broad groups of fungi:

- **Yeasts** are solitary, small, rounded forms that reproduce by budding.
- **Molds** are a mass of filaments called **hyphae,** divided into segments by septa *(Figure 20.17b and c)* often with spores at their tips. The mass of hyphae is called a **mycelium** *(Figure 20.17a)*.

Pathogenic fungi can cause infections in healthy people. The most common of these are the dermatophyte fungi that cause skin infections. They have been discussed in *Chapter 3.*

Opportunistic fungi are normally harmless but cause disease in people with preexisting risk factors, such as those who are taking antibiotics or receiving cytotoxic or immunosuppressive therapy or who have diabetes mellitus or AIDS.

Candida albicans is an example of an opportunistic fungus. It is normally present in small numbers on the mucosa of the mouth and vagina. When it overgrows, it produces a white coating and white discharge and is called **candidiasis** *(Figure 20.18)*. It also causes diaper rash when the skin of the baby's diaper area is irritated.

Invasive fungal infections caused by *Candida albicans* or *Aspergillus* entering the bloodstream are becoming increasingly prevalent and important in hospitalized patients. They occur in those who are profoundly immunosuppressed, have central venous lines, receive **total parenteral nutrition (TPN),** or have prolonged administration of antibiotics.

Aspergillus is a mold that can colonize the lower respiratory tract and cause a hypersensitivity response similar to asthma or produce an **aspergilloma,** a ball of fungus in the cavities of areas of damaged lung. If there is a persistent neutropenia (low levels of neutrophils in the blood), the mold can invade the bloodstream and give rise to **aspergillosis.**

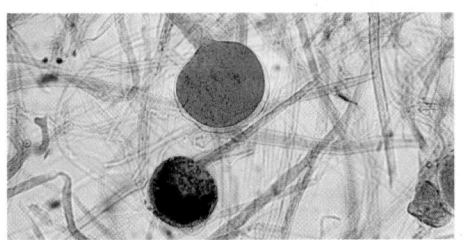

▲ **FIGURE 20.16   Structure of Penicillin.**

Keynote

- 100,000 different species of fungi have been identified, and another 1.5 million remain to be discovered.
- Fungi are everywhere—in the air, soil, sea, and on your skin and in your mucosal cavities.

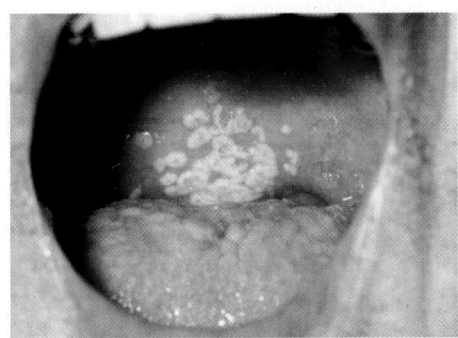

▲ **FIGURE 20.18   Oral Candidiasis.**

Abbreviation

TPN total parenteral nutrition

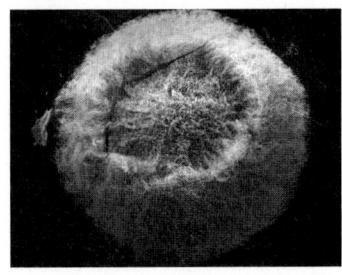

(a)

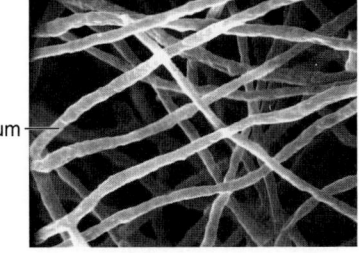

Septum ─

(b)

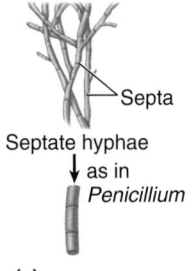

Septa

Septate hyphae
as in
Penicillium

(c)

▲ **FIGURE 20.17   Mold.** (*a*) Mycelium showing filamentous mass of hyphae. (*b*) Individual hyphae showing septa. (*c*) Septate hyphae as in *Penicillium.*

WORD ANALYSIS AND DEFINITION

WORD	PRONUNCIATION		ELEMENTS	DEFINITION
Aspergillus	as-per-**JILL**-us		Latin *to sprinkle*	A type of fungus
aspergilloma	**AS**-per-ji-**LOH**-mah	S/	-oma *tumor*	Infectious granuloma
		R/	aspergill- *Aspergillus*	
aspergillosis	**AS**-per-ji-**LOH**-sis	S/	-osis *condition*	Presence of *Aspergillus* in the body
ecology	ee-**KOL**-oh-jee	P/	eco- *environment*	Interrelationship between living organisms with each other and the environment
		R/	-logy *study of*	
ecologic (adj)	ee-koh-**LOJ**-ik	S/	-ic *pertaining to*	Pertaining to the study of the environment
		R/	-log- *study of*	
fungus	**FUN**-gus		Latin *a mushroom*	General term used to describe yeasts and molds
fungi (pl)	**FUN**-ji			
fungal (adj)	**FUN**-gal			
helminth	**HELL**-minth		Greek *worm*	Any intestinal wormlike parasite
hypha	**HIGH**-fah		Greek *a web*	Branching tubular fungal cell
hyphae (pl)	**HIGH**-fee			
mold	MOLD		Old English *dust, decay*	Filamentous fungus
mycelium	my-**SEE**-lee-um	S/	-ium *structure*	Mass of hyphae forming a colony of fungi
		R/	myc- *fungus*	
		R/	-el- *wart, nail*	
mycology	my-**KOL**-oh-jee	S/	-logy *study of*	Study of fungi
		R/CF	myc/o- *fungus*	
mycologist	my-**KOL**-oh-jist	S/	-logist *specialist*	Specialist in mycology
parenteral	pah-**REN**-ter-al	S/	-al *pertaining to*	Giving medication by any means other than the gastrointestinal tract
		P/	par- *abnormal, beside*	
		R/	-enter- *intestine*	
yeast	YEEST		Old English *ferment*	Microscopic fungus

EXERCISES

Build your knowledge of the **language of infectious diseases.** *Circle the correct answer.*

1. Parasitic worms that infect humans are called:

   molds   yeast   fungus   helminths   dermatophytes

2. Ball of fungus in a damaged lung:

   hypha   organelles   aspergilloma   mycelium   cytoplasmic

3. Because of its combining form, you can tell that *dermatophyte fungi* cause _____ infections:

   ear   kidney   skin   blood   brain

4. Causes diaper rash:

   Aspergillus   *Candida albicans*   plasmodium   stevia   salmonella

5. The study of fungi is called:

   pathology   cytology   nephrology   histology   mycology

6. Penicillin was derived from:

   Aspergillus   infection   candidiasis   fungus   tangent

7. A mass of hyphae is called:

   mycology   mycelium   aspergilloma   helminth   yeast

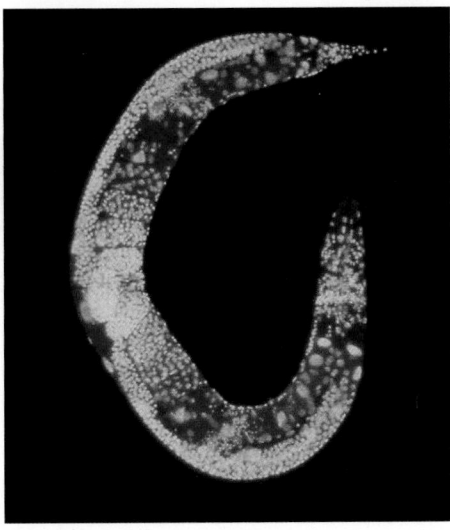

▲ FIGURE 20.19 Roundworm.

PARASITIC INFECTIONS

Parasites are organisms that live on or inside another organism (the host). The more virulent parasites for humans are endemic in rural parts of Africa, Asia, and Latin America. They may be present in food and water. They range in size from tiny single-cell organisms to large worms *(Figure 20.19)*. They are being increasingly identified as causes of food-borne illness in the United States.

Parasites that enter through the mouth are swallowed and can remain in the intestine or burrow through the wall to invade other organs. Parasites that enter through the skin can burrow through the skin or be introduced by the bite of an infected insect, the **vector**. **Malaria** is an example of a vector-borne parasitic infection. It is caused by the parasite *Plasmodium,* which is transmitted from person to person by the bite of the female *Anopheles* mosquito; the mosquito requires blood that it obtains through the bite to nurture her young.

Inside the human host, the malarial parasite takes about 10 to 14 days to mature into a form that can infect a mosquito again when it draws blood. In the mosquito, the parasite develops further and is then able to infect another human.

Malaria kills an African child every 30 seconds. Malaria kills by infecting and destroying red blood cells and by clogging the capillaries that supply the brain. The parasites are developing resistance to drugs, and many insecticides are no longer useful against mosquitoes.

Giardia lamblia is a parasite that causes a disease called **giardiasis,** an infection of the small intestine causing diarrhea, flatulence, and cramps. It is the most common intestinal parasitic infection in the United States and is mostly acquired from contaminated lakes and streams. Direct person-to-person transmission of the parasite can occur in day care centers and between homosexual men.

Pinworms are the most common parasite in children in this country. Pinworm eggs are ingested, they hatch in the intestine, and the young worms migrate to the anus, where the female deposits her eggs. The eggs can be transferred by fingers from the anus or from infected bedding **(fomites)** to the mouth of the same child or another.

Tapeworms are large, flat worms that live in the intestine and can grow 15 to 30 feet in length *(Figure 20.20)*. The parasite is acquired by eating raw or undercooked meat or fish.

Ascaris lumbricoides, an intestinal roundworm *(see Figure 20.19)*, affects people worldwide in areas of poor sanitation. Adult worms in the intestine range from 6 to 20 inches in length.

Trichinosis is a roundworm infection developed if people eat poorly cooked meat (usually pork) from an animal with the parasite. **Larvae** migrate from the intestine to muscle, where they can produce pain and swelling.

Toxoplasmosis can be acquired by eating undercooked meat from infected animals or from cats. It can infect the brain of immunosuppressed people.

Amoebiasis is another disease of poor sanitation with fecal contamination of food and water. A few people develop symptoms of an intestinal infection, and it occasionally spreads to other organs, including the liver and brain.

Food and water are often contaminated with parasites in regions of the world where there is poor sanitation and hygiene. The advice given to travelers in these areas is "Cook it, boil it, peel it, or don't eat it." Some parasites survive freezing, and ice cubes made from unpurified water can transmit disease.

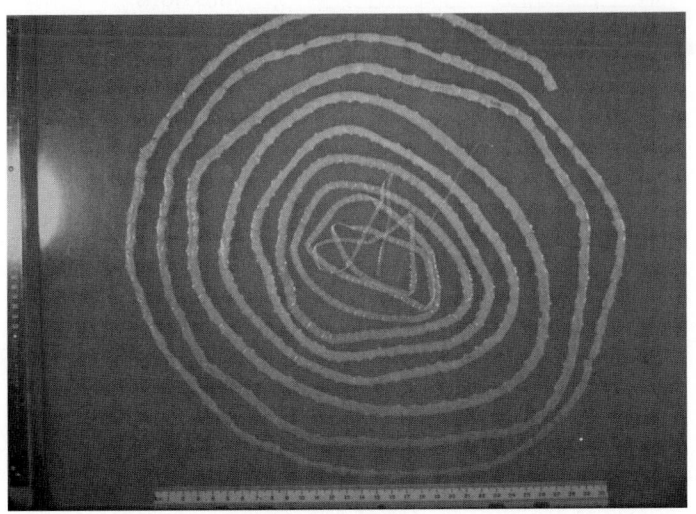

◄ FIGURE 20.20 Tapeworm.

WORD	PRONUNCIATION		ELEMENTS	DEFINITION
amoeba	ah-**ME**-bah	S/	Greek *change* -iasis *condition*	Single-celled organism that changes shape as it moves
amoebiasis	ah-me-**BY**-ah-sis	R/	amoeb- *amoeba*	Infection with *Amoeba*
Anopheles	ah-**NOF**-eh-leez	P/ R/	an- *not* -opheles *be of service*	A type of mosquito
Ascaris lumbricoides	**AS**-kah-ris lum-bri-**KOY**-deez		Greek *intestinal worm*	Large roundworm parasite
fomites	**FO**-my-teez		Latin *to keep warm*	Bedding, clothing, towels, etc., that can harbor and transmit a disease agent
Giardia	jee-**AR**-dee-ah		Alfred Giard, 1846–1908, French biologist	Parasite in the small intestine
giardiasis	jee-ar-**DIE**-ah-sis			Infection with *Giardia*, causing diarrhea
larva larvae (pl)	**LAR**-vah **LAR**-vee		Latin *a mask*	Stage in the development of an insect or intestinal parasite
malaria	mah-**LAIR**-ee-ah	P/ R/	mal- *bad* -aria *air*	Disease transmitted by the bite of a female *Anopheles* mosquito
mosquito mosquitoes (pl)	mos-**KEY**-toe		Latin *little fly*	Blood-sucking insect
parasite	**PAR**-ah-site		Greek *guest*	An organism that attaches itself to, lives on or in, and derives its nutrition from another species
parasitic (adj)	par-ah-**SIT**-ik	S/ R/	-ic *pertaining to* parasit- *parasite*	Pertaining to a parasite
pinworm	**PIN**-worm		Worm thin as a pin	Intestinal parasite
Plasmodium	plaz-**MOH**-dee-um	S/ R/CF	-dium *appearance* plasm/o- *to form*	Causal agent for malaria
tapeworm	TAPE WORM		**tape** Old English *strip* **worm** Old English *worm*	Intestinal parasitic worm
toxoplasmosis	**TOK**-soh-plaz-**MOH**-sis	S/ R/CF R/CF	-sis *abnormal condition* tox/o- *poison* -plasm/o- *to form*	Parasitic infection acquired from undercooked meat from infected animals
trichinosis	trik-ih-**NOH**-sis	S/ R/	-osis *condition* trichin- *hair*	Disease from ingestion of undercooked pork containing the roundworm
vector	**VEK**-tor		Latin *a carrier*	An animal or insect capable of transmitting an infection

EXERCISES   *Apply your knowledge of the elements and terms of infectious diseases. Circle the correct answer.*

1. Give an example of a vector-borne parasitic infection:
   a. polio
   b. osteomyelitis
   c. nephritis
   d. malaria
   e. bronchopneumonia

2. Most common parasite in children in this country:
   a. pinworm
   b. toxoplasmosis
   c. tapeworm
   d. amoebiasis
   e. trichinosis

3. Parasitic infection of the small intestine causing diarrhea, flatulence, and cramps:
   a. colic
   b. malaria
   c. giardiasis
   d. plasmodium
   e. colitis

4. This element has the same meaning as **sis** and **osis**:
   a. dium
   b. aria
   c. iasis
   d. an
   e. toxo

5. Malaria kills by infecting and destroying:
   a. WBCs
   b. platelets
   c. RBCs
   d. organelles
   e. none of these

6. Disease that can be caused by eating undercooked pork:
   a. toxoplasmosis
   b. trichinosis
   c. malaria
   d. dysentery
   e. typhoid

LESSON 20.5 Prevention of Infections

OBJECTIVES

The information in this lesson will enable you to use correct medical terminology to:

20.5.1 Define the common terms used in infection prevention and control.

20.5.2 Detail the rationale for and use of Standard Precautions and Transmission-Based Precautions.

20.5.3 Identify diseases for which there are vaccinations and immunizations.

20.5.4 Discuss the prophylactic use of antibiotics.

20.5.5 Describe methods for preventing the transmission of food-borne and water-borne diseases.

Case Report 20.2 (continued)

Preventive measures must be taken to inhibit the highly contagious *C. difficile* from spreading to caregivers, patients, and visitors. Caregivers must wash their hands before and after patient contact and wear disposable gloves and gowns. After Mr. Geller has been moved to an **isolation** setting, his room must be vigorously cleaned to remove **spores** that can spread the condition and then be disinfected with an EPA-registered hypochlorite-based disinfectant. Handwashing is done with soap and water. Alcohol-based gels are not as effective against spores.

Mr. Geller had a very difficult 10 days, with abdominal distension and circulatory failure, before he gradually improved and was able to be transferred to a skilled nursing facility.

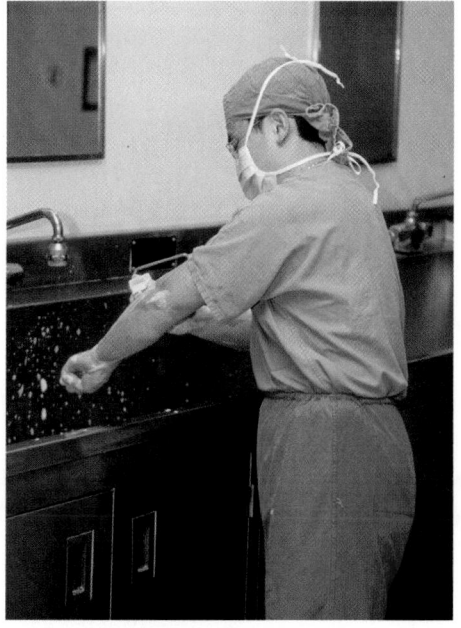

▲ **FIGURE 20.21   Surgical Scrub.**

DEFINITIONS

Cleaning is the process of removing all visible contamination from inanimate objects. It consists of thoroughly washing with soap or detergent and water, rinsing with clean water, and drying.

Sanitization is the process of removing pathogens from surfaces by chemical means, such as chlorine.

Disinfection is the destruction of pathogenic and other microorganisms on surfaces, instruments, and other man-made objects by using **disinfectants.** Commonly used disinfectants include alcohol, hydrogen peroxide, phenols, and hypochlorites.

High-level disinfection (HLD) is a process that eliminates all microorganisms, except some endospores, from inanimate objects by boiling, steaming, or using chemical disinfectants.

Sterilization eliminates all microorganisms, including **endospores,** by high-pressure steam **(autoclave),** dry heat (oven), or radiation.

Antisepsis is the process of reducing the number of microorganisms on skin, mucous membranes, or other tissue by applying an antimicrobial **(antiseptic)** agent. Preoperatively, the agents used are 70% isopropyl alcohol, 0.5% chlorhexidine, or 70% povidone-iodine. Hand antisepsis is achieved with a surgical scrub *(Figure 20.21).*

Asepsis is the process of eliminating all microorganisms on both living surfaces (skin and mucous membranes) and inanimate objects (surgical instruments and other items) to produce a state of sterility.

NOSOCOMIAL INFECTIONS

Nosocomial infections (hospital-acquired infections) are becoming increasingly common. They are estimated to occur in 5% to 10% of acute care hospital admissions. There are some 2 million cases and about 200,000 deaths per year as a result of them.

Abbreviation

HLD   high-level disinfection

WORD	PRONUNCIATION	ELEMENTS		DEFINITION
antisepsis	an-tih-**SEP**-sis	S/ P/ R/	-is *pertaining to* anti- *against* -seps- *decay*	Inhibiting the growth of infectious agents
antiseptic (adj)	an-tih-**SEP**-tic	S/	-tic *pertaining to*	Pertaining to antisepsis, or an agent capable of producing antisepsis
asepsis aseptic (adj)	a-**SEP**-sis a-**SEP**-tik	S/ P/ R/	-is *pertaining to* a- *without* -seps- *decay*	Absence of living pathogenic organisms
autoclave	**AW**-toe-klayv	P/ R/	auto- *self* -clave *lock*	Apparatus for sterilization by steam under pressure
clean	KLENE		Old English *pure*	Free from visible contamination
disinfection	dis-in-**FEK**-shun	S/ P/ R/	-ion *process, condition* dis- *apart, away from* -infect- *internal invasion*	Process of destruction of microorganisms by chemical agents
disinfectant	dis-in-**FEK**-tant	S/	-ant *agent, forming*	Agent that disinfects
isolate (verb) isolation (noun)	**I**-so-late i-so-**LAY**-shun		Latin *an island*	To separate from others
nosocomial	noh-soh-**KOH**-mee-al	S/ R/CF R/	-ial *pertaining to* nos/o- *disease* -com- *take care of*	Acquired while in the hospital
sanitization	**SAN**-ih-tih-**ZAY**-shun	S/ R/	-ation *process* sanitiz- *make healthy*	Process of using chemicals to remove pathogens from surfaces
sepsis septic (adj)	**SEP**-sis **SEP**-tik		Greek *decay*	Presence of pathogenic organisms or their toxins in blood or tissues
spore	SPOR		Greek *seed*	Generic term for any tiny compact cell produced during reproduction by bacteria
endospore	**EN**-doh-spor	P/ R/CF	endo- *within* -spor/e *spore*	Spore produced inside a cell and capable of resisting heat, freezing, radiation, and chemicals

Nosocomial infections are the result of several factors working together:

- High incidence of pathogens in a hospital.
- High incidence of immunocompromised patients.
- High incidence of invasive procedures.
- High incidence of people close together.
- High incidence of pathogens becoming resistant to antibiotics.
- Routes of transmission of pathogens from individual to individual are in place in hospital settings.

Keynote

Within hours of admission to the hospital, a patient's flora begin to acquire the characteristics of the hospital's infection pool.

EXERCISES *Meet lesson objectives by answering the following questions about prevention of infections.*

1. Where can you sterilize instruments by high-pressure steam? _____

2. How is hand *asepsis* achieved? _____

3. What is the difference between *asepsis* and *antisepsis?* _____

_____

4. What are some commonly used disinfectants? _____

_____

5. What is the only way to eliminate endospores? _____

Keynote

Standard Precautions combine Universal Precautions and Body Substance Isolation in the theoretical assumption that every patient with whom you come into contact has an HIV infection.

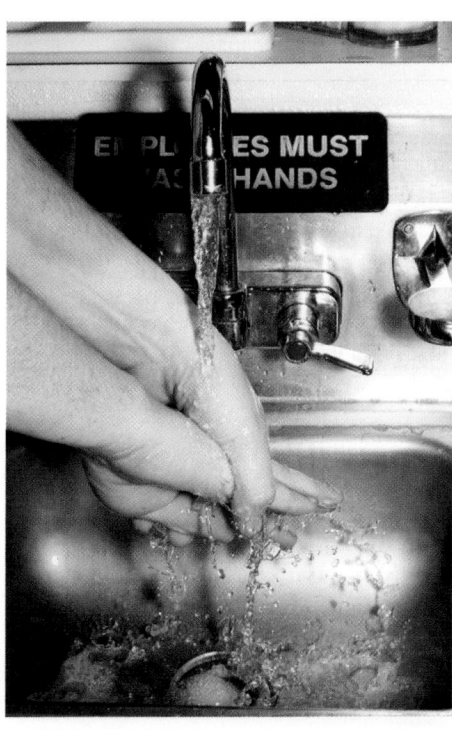

▲ **FIGURE 20.22   Employee Washes Hands in Kitchen.**

Keynote

In all cases, Transmission-Based Precautions must be used with Standard Precautions.

PRECAUTIONS TO PREVENT INFECTION

To reduce the transmission of nosocomial infections to and from patients and to protect caregivers, different systems of precautions have been introduced at different times. In the 1980s, systems called **Universal Precautions (UP)** and **Body Substance Isolation (BSI)** were put in place. As the problems of transmission of infections in a hospital continued to grow, in 1996 the **Centers for Disease Control and Prevention (CDC)** issued a new system, combining UP and BSI, called **Standard Precautions (SP)**.

Standard Precautions

Standard Precautions guidelines are designed for use in all health care facilities all the time for treating all patients, regardless of their presumed diagnosis. The key components of SP address the areas of:

- Hand washing
- Gloves
- Patient placement
- Gowns
- **Sharps**
- Masks, goggles, face masks
- Patient care equipment
- Environmental cleaning
- Linens
- Patient resuscitation

In any health care setting, hand washing is the most important factor in preventing the transmission of infections.

Details of the implementation of each component are not given here, as they do not add to your knowledge of medical terminology and are freely available elsewhere.

Transmission-Based Precautions

In addition to SP, three sets of precautions based on routes of transmission of infections (called **Transmission-Based Precautions**) apply to hospitalized patients and those in nursing homes or other types of extended care facilities. The three routes of transmission of pathogens are by:

- **Air** (tuberculosis, chickenpox, measles).
- **Droplet** (flu, mumps, rubella).
- **Contact** (hepatitis A and other enteric pathogens, including *E. coli* and *C. difficile;* staph infections; herpes simplex; skin or eye infections).

The use of Transmission-Based Precautions is designed to reduce the risk of spreading infections between hospitalized patients and health care staff.

Personal health precautions include:
- **Wash hands frequently,** particularly before and after food preparation.
- **Sanitize** food preparation areas.
- **Avoid** inadequately cooked meat.
- **Drink only purified water** in endemic areas.
- **Avoid** leafy vegetables and salads in endemic areas.
- **Avoid** ice made from nonpurified water in endemic areas.

Public health precautions include:
- **Purification** of drinking water.
- **Effective disposal** of **sewage.**
- **Pasteurization** of milk, juice, and other beverages.
- **Hand-washing laws** for food handlers *(Figure 20.22).*
- **Immunization** programs.

WORD	PRONUNCIATION	ELEMENTS		DEFINITION
droplet	**DROP**-let	S/ R/	**-let** *small* **drop-** *liquid globule*	Globule of liquid; for example, that which is ejected from the mouth during speaking, coughing, sneezing
pasteurization	**PAS**-tyur-ih-**ZAY**-shun		Louis Pasteur, 1822–1895, French chemist and bacteriologist	The heating of fluids to moderate temperatures to destroy microorganisms
purification	**PYUR**-if-ih-kay-shun	S/ R/	**-ation** *process* **purific-** *make pure*	Make free from pathogens
sewage	**SOO**-aje		Latin *drain off*	Waste matter from populated areas
sharps	SHARPS		Greek *pointed*	Any medical instrument capable of puncturing skin
sharps container	SHARPS kon-**TAY**-ner	S/ P/ R/	**-er** *agent* **con-** *with* **-tain-** *hold*	Puncture-resistant container for disposal of sharps

EXERCISES

Short Answers: *Any health care worker needs to learn the value of precautions to prevent transmission of infection in patient care. This ensures your safety and that of the patient. Employ the* **language of infectious diseases** *to briefly answer the following questions. Fill in the blanks.*

1. What exactly is a *precaution?* (*Hint:* Start with the prefix.)

   _____

   _____

2. Why are precautions necessary?

   _____

   _____

3. Give one example of what a precaution might be.

   _____

4. What can precautions achieve?

   _____

   _____

5. Detail the rationale for, and use of, Standard Precautions and Transmission-Based Precautions. What types of patients do they apply to, and what facilities require them?

   _____

   _____

   _____

6. What precautions can you take personally? _____

   _____

   _____

OTHER METHODS OF PREVENTION OF INFECTIONS

Chemoprophylaxis is the use of antimicrobial agents to prevent infection in nonimmune individuals exposed to the infection. These agents can be used against:

- **Exogenous pathogens** that are not part of the normal flora before they can invade and attach to cells or produce toxins. An example is the use of 2 grams of amoxicillin 1 hour before a dental procedure in individuals with a prosthesis such as an artificial hip. Amoxicillin is also effective in preventing Lyme disease after a tick bite. Individuals exposed to the respiratory secretions of patients with meningococcal disease should receive a fluoroquinolone antibiotic.

- **Endogenous pathogens** such as *Staphylococcus aureus*. For example, adults with recurrent infections caused by *S. aureus* have fewer infections while receiving oral clindamycin. Patients undergoing hemodialysis, intensive chemotherapy, or bone marrow transplantation leading to low neutrophil counts benefit from chemoprophylaxis.

- **Latent pathogens** that are microorganisms already residing in the human host but are not causing disease. For example, use of acyclovir significantly reduces the rate and severity of recurrences of genital herpes in infected individuals.

Immunization is one of the primary preventive measures. All health care workers providing direct patient care should be immune to rubella, measles, mumps, varicella, and hepatitis A and B. They should receive **tetanus toxoid.** Caregivers should also receive an annual influenza vaccine, as should the elderly and people with chronic diseases *(Figure 20.23)*. Children also receive immunization against poliomyelitis, pneumococcal disease, and *Haemophilus influenzae* type b. Other vaccines for yellow fever, typhoid, anthrax, and meningococcal disease are available to high-risk populations.

Passive immune prophylaxis is the transfer of immunity to prevent viral infections in exposed but nonimmune individuals. Short-lived immunity is achieved through immunoglobulins (preformed IgG antibodies) prepared from large pools of serum from blood donors. This pooled product is used as prophylaxis against hepatitis A infection and enterovirus infections in neonates and for HIV-infected neonates.

Hyperimmune globulin is immunoglobulin prepared from the serum of individuals who have a high **titer** of antibody to a specific virus. These include:

- **Zoster immune globulin** for prevention of varicella in immunocompromised children and neonates.

- **Human rabies immunoglobulin** for an individual bitten by a **rabid** animal.

- **Hepatitis B immunoglobulin** for a nonimmune individual exposed to the **hepatitis B virus** (HBV).

- **RSV immunoglobulin** for treatment of **respiratory syncytial virus (RSV)** in the neonatal period.

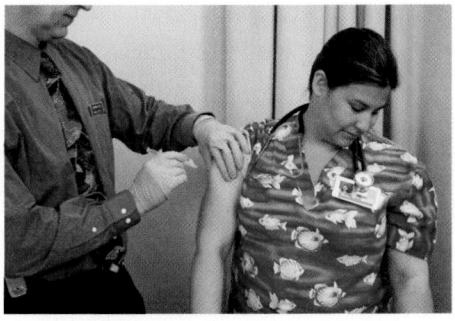

▲ **FIGURE 20.23   Caregiver Receiving Immunization.**

Abbreviations

HBV hepatitis B virus
RSV respiratory syncytial virus

WORD	PRONUNCIATION	ELEMENTS		DEFINITION
chemoprophylaxis (*Note:* The "c" in prophylac- is dropped.)	**KEEM**-oh-**PRO**-fil-ak-sis	S/ R/CF P/ R/	**-xis** *condition* **chem/o-** *chemical* **-pro-** *before* **-phylac-** *protect*	Prevent infection by use of chemicals or drugs
endogenous	en-**DOJ**-en-us	S/ P/ R/	**-ous** *pertaining to* **endo-** *within* **-gen-** *produce, create*	Produced within the organism
exogenous	ex-**OJ**-en-us	S/ P/ R/	**-ous** *pertaining to* **exo-** *outside* **-gen-** *produce, create*	Originating outside the organism
hyperimmune globulin	**HIGH**-per-im-**YUNE** **GLOB**-you-lin	P/ R/ S/ R/	**hyper-** *excessive* **-immune** *immune response* **-in** *chemical compound* **globul-** *protein*	Immunoglobulin prepared from serum of people with high antibody titer to a specific virus
prophylaxis **prophylactic** (adj)	pro-fih-**LAX**-is pro-fih-**LAK**-tik	S/ P/ R/	Greek *to take precautions* **-tic** *pertaining to* **pro-** *before* **-phylac-** *protect*	Prevention of disease The act or the agent that prevents a disease
rabies **rabid** (adj)	**RAY**-beez **RAB**-id		Latin *to be mad*	Highly fatal infectious disease transmitted by the bite of infected animals Suffering from rabies
tetanus	**TET**-ah-nuss		Greek *convulsive tension*	A disease with painful, tonic, muscular contractions caused by the toxin produced by *Clostridium tetani*
titer	**TIE**-ter		French *standard*	The strength of a substance in a solution as compared to a standard
toxoid	**TOK**-soyd	S/ R/	**-oid** *resembling* **tox-** *poison*	Toxin treated to destroy its toxic capability but retain its antigenic capability

EXERCISES

Communication: *Use the **language of infectious diseases** to communicate information to your patients, coworkers, and fellow students. Provide a brief answer to each of the following questions.*

1. A patient has asked you to explain to him the difference between *passive immune prophylaxis* and *chemoprophylaxis*.

   passive immune prophylaxis: _____

   _____

   chemoprophylaxis: _____

   _____

2. The pathologist has explained to you the difference between an *exogenous* pathogen and an *endogenous* pathogen. Can you summarize what he said for a fellow student?

   exogenous pathogen: _____

   _____

   endogenous pathogen: _____

   _____

INFECTION

CHALLENGE YOUR KNOWLEDGE

A. **Case Report Revisited:** Apply your knowledge of *all* the medical terminology you have learned up to this point to the questions asked about the following Case Report.

CASE REPORT 20.1

Your patients are

. . . Mrs. Uzma Aziz and her 2-year-old daughter Alisha, the youngest of her five children.

Your interpreter tells you that Alisha was well until 3 days earlier, when she developed a runny nose, red eyes, and a cough. Today she has developed a rash on her forehead and neck that is spreading down onto her body.

Your examination shows T 104.2°F, P 120, R 24. A rash of red-brown macules is present on her face, neck, and shoulders. She has bilateral conjunctivitis. As you proceed with your examination, the rash continues to extend down her trunk. On the buccal mucosa inside her mouth are some small red spots with white centers (Koplik spots). You hear rales at the base of her right lung, and her left tympanic membrane is inflamed. She is diagnosed as having measles.

Through the interpreter, you learn that none of the five children has been immunized for any disease. When they arrived at the camp, the mother refused to start a program of immunization for the children.

1. What are Alisha's symptoms? _____
   _____
   _____

2. What are Alisha's signs of measles? _____
   _____

3. How do you know Alisha is febrile? _____
   _____

4. What does a macule look like? _____
   _____

5. What is conjunctivitis? _____
   _____
   _____

6. Exactly where in the body is the buccal mucosa? _____
   _____

7. What would you use to hear the rales in her lung? _____

8. What might the rales signify? _____

9. What instrument did you use to discover her left tympanic membrane was inflamed?

_____

_____

10. Does Alisha have *rubella* or *rubeola?* _____

11. What could have prevented this? _____

12. What body systems that you have already studied have helped you understand this report? _____

_____

_____

B. **Prefixes:** Not every medical term will have a prefix. When they do have a prefix, it is another clue to the meaning of the entire term. Match the prefix in the left column to its correct meaning in the right column.

_____	1.	im	A.	small
_____	2.	mal	B.	false
_____	3.	ex	C.	together
_____	4.	a/an	D.	bad
_____	5.	dis	E.	within
_____	6.	micro	F.	not
_____	7.	endo	G.	away from
_____	8.	dys	H.	apart
_____	9.	pseudo	I.	difficult
_____	10.	syn	J.	without

C. **Patient Education:** Explain to your patients, in a language they can understand, the difference between the following medical terms.

1. contagious: _____

2. infectious: _____

3. pathogen: _____

4. toxin: _____

5. anaerobe: _____

6. aerobe: _____

7. pinworm: _____

8. tapeworm: _____

INFECTION

D. Elements: The following medical terms are composed of roots, combining forms, and suffixes only. Deconstruct the term into its basic elements, and write the meaning of each element in the proper column. Fill in the blanks.

Medical Term	Root/CF	Meaning of Root/CF	Suffix	Meaning of Suffix
infection				
pathogen				
vaccinate				
aerobic				
hemolysis				
enteric				
gonorrhea				
trichinosis				
toxoid				

E. Disease Process: Understanding the infectious disease process can help us all take better care of our bodies. Apply your knowledge of the **language of infectious diseases** to the following exercise. *Remember: There is only one best answer*—circle it.

1. Innate resistance, natural barriers, nonspecific immune responses, and specific immune responses are all part of:

   a. colonization

   b. host defense mechanisms

   c. mechanisms of infection

   d. virulence factors

   e. inflammatory response

2. If a *mycologist* studies fungus, what does a *toxicologist* study?

   a. viruses

   b. bacteria

   c. poisons

   d. tissues

   e. cells

3. What is the human spongiform encephalopathy associated with BSE?

   a. WNV

   b. SARS

   c. EBV

   d. CJD

   e. RSV

4. Bacteria can be classified by their shapes, use of oxygen, and:

   a. Gram stain color

   b. DNA

   c. size

   d. location

   e. infections they cause

5. What is the most common intestinal parasitic infection in the United States?

   a. toxoplasmosis

   b. giardiasis

   c. trichinosis

   d. amoebiasis

   e. malaria

6. Hand antisepsis is achieved with:

   a. lotion

   b. extremely hot water

   c. special soap

   d. surgical scrub

   e. fingernail brush

7. A nosocomial infection would be acquired from:

   a. school

   b. dormitory

   c. workplace

   d. airplane

   e. hospital

8. Which pathogen is the major cause of antibiotic-associated diarrhea?

   a. *E. coli*

   b. streptococcus

   c. staphylococcus

   d. *C. difficile*

   e. pneumococci

INFECTION

F. **Disease Process:** Understanding the infectious disease process can help us all take better care of our bodies. Apply your knowledge of the **language of infectious diseases** in this exercise. Remember: *There is only one best answer*—circle it.

1. The smallest of *microorganisms* is:

   a. bacterium

   b. prion

   c. fungus

   d. spores

   e. virus

2. The stage in development in which an insect hatches from an egg:

   a. vector

   b. parasite

   c. larva

   d. plasmodium

   e. colonization

3. The term *exanthem* means:

   a. outside the cells

   b. rash as the outward sign of disease

   c. outside the uterus

   d. bulging eyeball

   e. falling forward of an organ

4. *Rubeola,* in its prodromal phase, produces signs similar to:

   a. rubella

   b. URI

   c. pharyngitis

   d. varicella

   e. BSE

G. **Latin and Greek terms cannot be further deconstructed into prefix, root, or suffix.** You must know them for what they are. Test your knowledge of these terms with this exercise. Match the meaning in the left column with the correct medical term in the right column.

_____	1. fringe	A.	lysis
_____	2. running before	B.	bubo
_____	3. poison	C.	parasite
_____	4. berry	D.	latent

_____	5. destruction	E.	fimbria
_____	6. swelling in the groin	F.	coccus
_____	7. to take precautions	G.	prodromal
_____	8. a guest	H.	sterile
_____	9. barren	I.	prophylactic
_____	10. lie hidden	J.	toxin

H. **Test Review:** Microbes are everywhere, and they can have a good or bad effect on the body. The *language of infectious diseases* will help you understand the questions and formulate your answers to make a test review sheet for yourself on microbes. Fill in the blanks. *Refer to this exercise for test review.*

1. Give an example of five places on the body where you will find normal flora.

   a. _____

   b. _____

   c. _____

   d. _____

   e. _____

2. What two areas of the body remain microbe-free?

   a. _____   b. _____

3. What is the medical term for *microbe-free?* _____

4. At what point do normal bacteria become pathogens? _____

5. If an infection causes harm to the host, what is present? _____

6. What helps a healthy host defend itself? _____

7. **Recall question:** What is present inside the skull that contributes to the protection of the brain by preventing cross-

   contamination? _____

I. **Research and Discuss:** Pick any one of the natural barriers the body has to resisting infection (skin, mucous membranes, respiratory tract, gastrointestinal tract, genitourinary tract).

   1. Review previous chapters on those subjects.

   2. Add to that your new knowledge of the infectious disease process, and prepare a 5-minute class discussion on any one of the body's natural defense barriers, including how it prevents disease or, if it fails, how the disease process begins. Remember the role of the immune system in this as well.

   3. Use your school library and online research to supplement your text material.

   4. Make a list of 10 key terms you are going to use in your discussion.

   _____

   _____

   _____

   _____

   5. Print out your notes, and be prepared to hand them in to your instructor.

INFECTION

J. Terminology Applied to Coding: Solid comprehension of medical terminology can make you a better coder. Challenge your knowledge of the medical terms you have studied so far in this text with this exercise. Each medical code is first listed with the corresponding medical term. In the table that follows, use the *description* of the medical term to determine the appropriate code.

Medical Term	ICD-9-CM code
osteomyelitis	730.20
bacteremia	790.7
furuncle	680.9
pneumonia	486
toxic shock syndrome	040.82
endocarditis	424.90
impetigo	684
rubeola	055.9
herpangina	074.0
malaria	084.6

Description of the Medical Term	Correct ICD-9-CM Code
Infected hair follicle	
Inflammation of the lining of the heart	
Acute, contagious childhood disease	
Ulcerative disease of the throat	
Inflammation of an area of bone due to bacterial infection	
Infection of the skin producing thick, yellow crusts	
Inflammation of the lung parenchyma	
Life-threatening illness caused by toxins circulating in the blood	
Vector-borne parasitic infection	
Presence of bacteria in the blood	

K. Medical Language: A good knowledge of medical terminology will enable you to clarify, describe, and explain a term's meaning and use. Using medical language, provide short answers in this exercise.

   1. The term **parasite** comes from the Greek meaning *a guest*. Explain how a parasite becomes "a guest" of the host and what is involved in that relationship.

   _____

   _____

_____

_____

_____

2. Explain this chapter keynote: "Within hours of admission to the hospital, a patient's flora begin to acquire the characteristics of the hospital's infection pool."

_____

_____

_____

_____

_____

_____

L. **Precautions:** The best defense is often a good offense—so to prevent infections from starting, medical facilities use a variety of methods of infection prevention and control. A brief description is given of each method. Fill in the correct medical term in the blanks.

asepsis   **antisepsis**   **hand antisepsis**   **sterilization**

sanitization   **disinfection**   **HLD**   **cleaning**

1. Boiling, steaming, or using chemical disinfectants on inanimate objects: _____

2. Removing pathogens from surfaces by chemical means: _____

3. Surgical scrub: _____

4. Washing with soap and water, rinsing with clean water, and drying: _____

5. Use of autoclave: _____

6. Reducing microorganisms on skin with antimicrobial agents: _____

7. Destroying microorganisms with chlorine, alcohol, or hydrogen peroxide: _____

8. Eliminating microorganisms on living surfaces and inanimate objects: _____

M. **Terminology Challenge:** For the following three similar medical terms, analyze each prefix. This will help you understand how the terms are different. Write a brief definition that explains the difference in each term.

epidemic: _____

_____

endemic: _____

_____

pandemic: _____

_____

INFECTION

N. Word Elements: The better your knowledge of word elements, the easier you will find understanding the meaning of medical terms. Challenge your knowledge of word elements with this exercise. First, listen to the correct pronunciation of each term in the audio glossary at McGraw-Hill CONNECT. Then read each of the terms aloud *using your best pronunciation.* Don't forget to circle the correct choice.

1. In the term **endogenous,** the suffix is _____ and means:

   a. pertaining to

   b. within

   c. production

   d. action

   e. outside

2. In the term **anaerobic,** the prefix is _____ and means:

   a. within

   b. without

   c. on top of

   d. behind

   e. underneath

3. In the term **toxin,** the Greek root means:

   a. barren

   b. life

   c. poison

   d. sterile

   e. intestine

4. In the term **contamination,** the root is _____ and means:

   a. to corrupt

   b. bowels

   c. to produce

   d. separation

   e. to change

5. In the term **pyogenic,** the root/combining form is _____ and means:

   a. fever

   b. pus

   c. pain

   d. swelling

   e. rash

6. In the term **prodromal,** the Greek root means:

   a. in the middle

   b. coming before

   c. running after

   d. in between

   e. at the end of

7. In the term **syncytium,** the prefix is _____ and means:

   a. together

   b. apart

   c. beside

   d. on top of

   e. below

8. In the term **antisepsis,** the root is _____ and means:

   a. liquid

   b. decay

   c. chlorine

   d. exempt

   e. precaution

9. In the term **infection,** the suffix is _____ and means:

   a. a process

   b. an action

   c. a condition

   d. a disease

   e. a policy

10. In the term **latent,** the Latin root means:

    a. to produce something

    b. to lie hidden

    c. to come in waves

    d. to push under

    e. to burst forth

INFECTION

O. **Language of Infectious Diseases:** Apply your knowledge of the terminology of infectious diseases to match the description given in the left column with the correct medical term *or* abbreviation in the right column.

_____ 1. carried by birds

_____ 2. viral respiratory tract infection

_____ 3. german measles

_____ 4. bacillary dysentery

_____ 5. an oncogenic virus

_____ 6. undulant fever

_____ 7. cause of bronchiolitis in infants

_____ 8. also carried by mosquitoes

_____ 9. herpes zoster

_____ 10. caused by a prion

A. Epstein-Barr

B. BSE

C. shingles

D. WNV

E. SARS

F. rubella

G. avian influenza

H. shigellosis

I. RSV

J. brucellosis

P. **Deconstruct the following medical terms into elements.** Analyze the elements, and give a layman's definition of the medical term. Fill in the blanks; then use any one term in a sentence that is not directly out of the text.

Medical Term	Prefix	Root/CF	Suffix	Meaning of Term
microorganism				
anaerobic				
oncogenic				
pyogenic				
streptococcus				
exogenous				
prophylactic				
toxoid				
enteric				
herpangina				

Sentence:

_____

_____

_____

Q. Teamwork: Pair up with another student, and prepare answers to the following questions. Make your answers as complete as possible. Take turns asking other teams the questions. How do their answers compare with yours? Note any important additions to the material their answers may have contributed to what you originally wrote. Hand the answers in to the instructor.

1. What do *pneumococcus, staphylococcus,* and *streptococcus* all have in common?

   _____

   _____

2. Nosocomial infections account for approximately 200,000 deaths per year. List six factors that contribute to the spread of nosocomial infections.

   _____   _____

   _____   _____

   _____   _____

3. Give three examples of prophylactic practices to prevent the spread of nosocomial infections.

   _____

   _____

   _____

R. Prefixes: Some, but not all, of the following medical terms have a prefix. Identify each medical term that has a prefix; then write the meaning of the prefix in the last column. If there is no prefix in the term, leave the line blank. Fill in the chart.

Medical Term	Prefix	Meaning of Prefix	Meaning of Medical Term
dysentery			
malaria			
immunize			
disinfection			
prophylaxis			
antisepsis			
asepsis			
autoclave			

1. Choose any prefix from the chart, and write a medical term *from a different chapter* that has the same prefix. _____

   _____

2. Define the term you chose. _____

INFECTION

S. Apply your knowledge of the language of infectious diseases. Circle the correct answer.

1. A tell-tale sign of bubonic plague was the appearance of:

   Pseudomonas   *Shigella*   bubo   spore

2. Presence of an infectious agent on a surface is:

   mutation   immunization   contamination   vaccination

3. *E. coli* causes diarrhea by releasing:

   hormone   enzyme   endorphin   exotoxin

4. **Enteric** means pertaining to the:

   feces   intestines   anus   rectum

5. Diarrhea, spasms, fever, and dehydration are symptoms of:

   dysentery   dysentary   dsyentary   dysinteray

6. In the term *Pseudomonas,* **pseudo-** means:

   difficult   away from   false   painful

7. A fever that comes and goes is termed:

   undulant   infectious   contagious   septic

8. **Spore** is the Greek word for:

   bowel   seed   feces   carbuncle

T. Dictionary Exercise: Use your glossary or a medical dictionary (textbook or online) to define the term.

virulence: _____

Then explain this sentence in layman's terms: "Virulence factors assist pathogens to overcome host resistance and cause disease."

_____

_____

_____

_____

_____

_____

U. Brain Teasers: Leukoencephalopathy is a term presented in this chapter. Relate the elements in this term to other terms from *previous* chapters that contain the same elements. See how many terms you can enter in the chart. The first one is done for you.

Definition of elements:

1. leuk/o (*or* leuc/o): _____

2. encephal/o: _____

3. pathy: _____

Element	Another Medical Term Containing This Element	Meaning of This Medical Term
leuk/o (*or* leuc/o) (*Note:* **This element can be spelled two ways.**)	*leukoplakia*	*white plaque seen inside the mouth*
encephal/o		
pathy		

4. What other medical term in this chapter means the same as **latent** or **dormant?** _____

INFECTION

CHAPTER SUMMARY EXERCISE

1. *Listen to the pronunciation of the medical terms as given by your instructor.*
2. *Circle the correct spelling of the medical term.*
3. *Match the correctly spelled terms to the brief descriptions below.*
4. *Write a sentence for each of the 10 terms that appear in this exercise.*

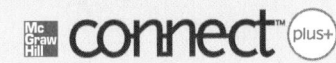

A. SPELLING COMPREHENSION: CIRCLE THE CORRECT SPELLING OF THE TERM.

1. contagius	contagious	kontagius	contajous	contajious
2. varecella	varesella	varicela	varicella	varecela
3. latency	lateincy	laytency	laytincy	lateincey
4. prodromal	prodomal	prodrumal	produmal	prodromel
5. firmbriae	fimbriae	fembriae	fimmbrie	fimbriee
6. anaerobic	anairobic	enairobic	anairobic	anerobic
7. preon	precion	prion	preion	preeon
8. xantem	exantem	xanthem	exanthem	xantum
9. orkitis	orckitus	orchitis	orchitus	orkitus
10. mycroscopy	miscroscopy	microscopy	microscopey	miccroscopy

B. MATCH THE NUMBER OF THE CORRECT TERM IN PART A WITH THE BRIEF DESCRIPTION OF THE TERM BELOW.

a. Organism can live without oxygen _____

b. Destruction of a cell _____

c. Fringelike structures on the surface of a cell _____

d. Chickenpox _____

e. Suffering from a fever _____

f. Skin rash _____

g. Spread from person to person _____

h. Beginning of disease before overt signs appear _____

i. Not currently active _____

j. Small protein particle can cause infection _____

C. USING YOUR KNOWLEDGE OF TERMS 1–10 IN PART A AND THEIR CORRECT SPELLING, WRITE A BRIEF SENTENCE FOR EACH OF THE TERMS AS IT MIGHT APPEAR IN PATIENT DOCUMENTATION.

1. _____

2. _____

3. _____

4. _____

5. _____

6. _____

7. _____

8. _____

9. _____

10. _____

D. YOUR INSTRUCTOR WILL DIRECT YOU TO MCGRAW-HILL CONNECT. OPEN THE AUDIO GLOSSARY AND PRACTICE YOUR PRONUNCIATION OF THE TERMS IN PART A OF THIS EXERCISE.

E. AFTER READING CASE REPORT 20.2, ANSWER THE FOLLOWING QUESTIONS. BE PREPARED TO DISCUSS YOUR ANSWERS IN CLASS.

CASE REPORT 20.2

Any patient in a hospital who is on antibiotics and is elderly and frail is suspected of having *C. difficile* disease if the patient has an onset of diarrhea. A stool sample taken for laboratory analysis from Mr. Geller is positive for toxin of *C. difficile*. The bacterium is highly contagious, and patients require isolation. The antibiotics Mr. Geller had been taking were discontinued, and he has been started on IV metronidazole (Flagyl).

Preventive measures must be taken to inhibit the highly contagious *C. difficile* from spreading to caregivers, patients, and visitors. Caregivers must wash their hands before and after patient contact and wear disposable gloves and gowns. After Mr. Geller has been moved to an **isolation** setting, his room must be vigorously cleaned to remove **spores** that can spread the condition and then be disinfected with an EPA-registered hypochlorite-based disinfectant. Hand washing is done with soap and water. Alcohol-based gels are not as effective against spores.

Mr. Geller had a very difficult 10 days, with abdominal distension and circulatory failure, before he gradually improved and was able to be transferred to a skilled nursing facility.

1. What diagnostic test has Mr. Geller had?

_____

2. This diagnostic test has proved positive for what bacterium?

_____

3. The results of this test have altered Mr. Geller's treatment plan—in what way?

_____

4. As a result of his diagnosis, Mr. Geller has been placed in *isolation*. What precautions must caregivers and visitors take in Mr. Geller's new room?

_____

_____

5. What must be done to the room Mr. Geller just vacated?

_____

6. It's very important that the spores of this infection do not travel through the hospital and infect other patients. If that were to happen, it would then become a _____ infection.

7. What additional problems did Mr. Geller develop after he was transferred to isolation? _____

8. What is the purpose of placing a patient in isolation? _____

_____

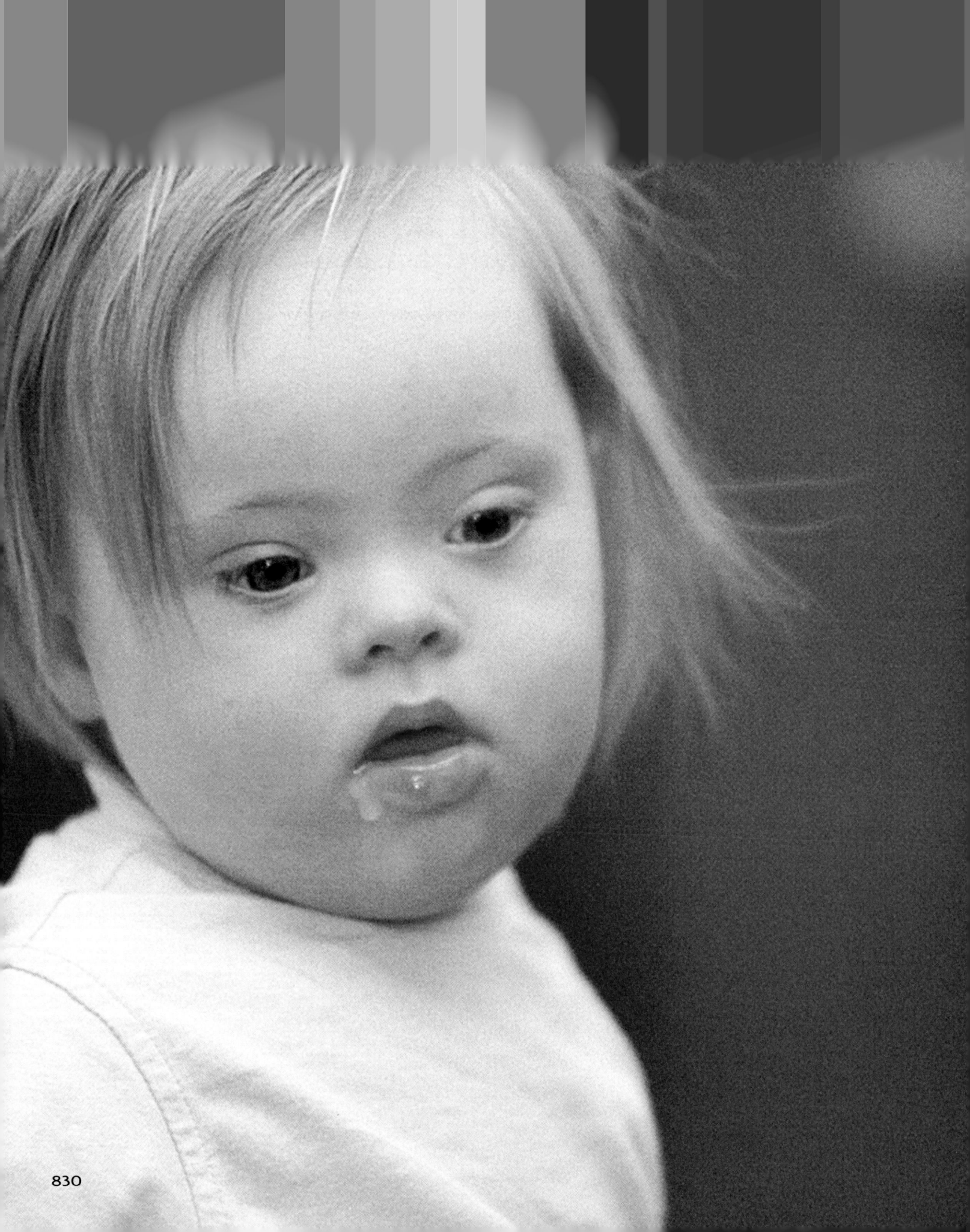

830

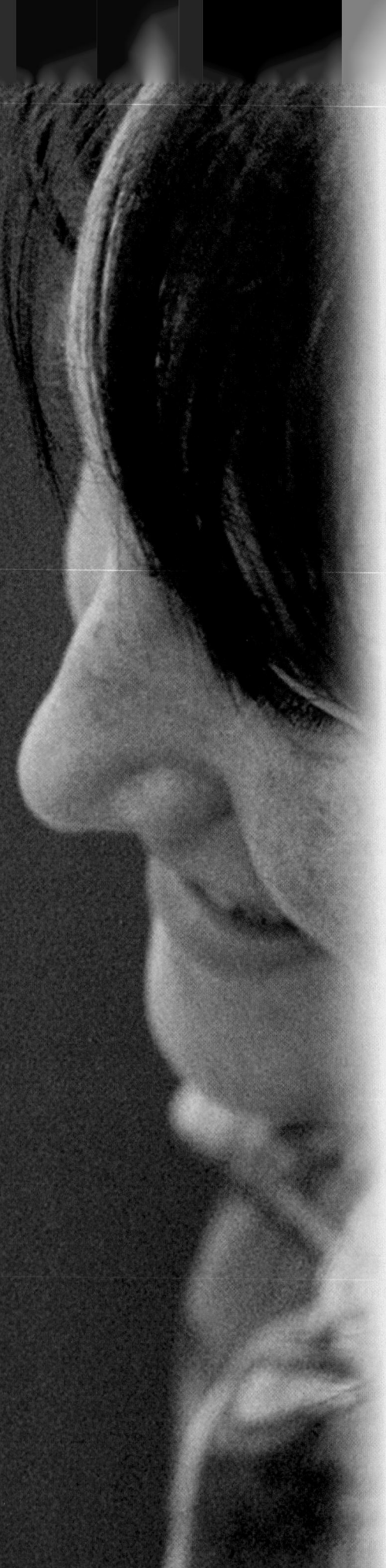

CASE REPORT 21.1

You are

. . . a **genetic** nurse working with **geneticist** Ingrid Hughes, MD, PhD, in the Genetics Department at Fulwood Medical Center.

Your patient is

. . . Mrs. Sharon Fisher, a 37-year-old administrative assistant who has been referred by Susan Lee, MD, in the primary care clinic. She is of **Ashkenazi** Jewish ancestry and has a girl aged 10 and a boy aged 7. Mrs. Fisher tries to live a healthy lifestyle. She does not smoke, drinks alcohol only occasionally, and goes to the gym two or three times a week. Physical examination and a mammogram performed a week ago were normal. Her mother, aged 62, is being treated for ovarian cancer. Her maternal grandmother is believed to have had breast cancer in her forties. Her mother's sister had breast cancer in her thirties and has recently had genetic screening at Fulwood Medical Center. She is carrying a gene mutation associated with breast cancer.

Learning Outcomes

In your role as a genetic nurse, you are a member of the genetic counseling team, and you need to be able to:

21.1 Apply the language of genetics to the anatomy and physiology of genes and chromosomes.

21.2 Comprehend, analyze, spell, and write the medical terms of genetics so that you communicate and document accurately and precisely in any health care setting.

21.3 Recognize and pronounce the medical terms of genetics so that you communicate verbally with accuracy and precision in any health care setting.

21.4 Explain the effects of common genetic modifications on health.

LESSON 21.1 DNA, RNA, and the Genetic Code

DNA, GENES, AND CHROMOSOMES

Human development depends on genetic and environmental factors. **Genetics** is the study of the transmission of information about the characteristics of our similarities and uniqueness from generation to generation, which is called **heredity.**

Your genetic composition, your **genome,** is established at conception. The genetic information is carried in **genes,** sequences of deoxyribonucleic acid **(DNA)** carried on rod-shaped structures called **chromosomes** *(see Chapter 2 and below).*

When your genes are working perfectly, your body develops and functions smoothly. But if a segment(s) of a single gene is abnormal, deformities and disease can result. Chromosomal abnormalities, including deviations from the normal number and structural defects, can also produce disorders. For example, in Down syndrome there is an extra chromosome 21 *(see page 830).*

DNA (Deoxyribonucleic acid)

Deoxyribonucleic acid (DNA) carries the instructions that enable cells to make proteins. It exists as two long, paired strands, spiraled into a **double helix** *(Figure 21.1).* Each strand is made up of millions of chemical building blocks called bases. There are only four chemical bases in DNA—**adenine, thymine, cytosine,** and **guanine**—and the order, or sequence, in which the bases appear in the strands codes the necessary information in the same way as the alphabet is used to form words and sentences.

There is DNA in the nucleus of each body cell except for mature red blood cells, which have no nucleus and cannot reproduce. Every cell in the body contains the same DNA and has 46 molecules of double-stranded DNA. Each molecule contains 50 to 250 million bases. The tightly coiled strands of DNA are packaged in paired units called **chromosomes.** Therefore, nondividing cells contain two copies of each chromosome and two copies of every gene. **Mendel's Law of Inheritance** says that during transmission from parent to offspring, the two copies of the gene separate from each other, so mature sperm and egg cells carry only a single set of 23 chromosomes.

Thus, human cells contain two pairs of chromosomes, one **inherited** from the father, one from the mother. Each set has 23 single chromosomes: 22 **autosomes** and an **X** or **Y sex chromosome,** making a total of 46 chromosomes in a cell. Males inherit an X chromosome from the mother and a Y chromosome from the father. Females inherit an X chromosome from each parent. A map of the chromosomes is called the **karyotype** *(Figure 21.2).*

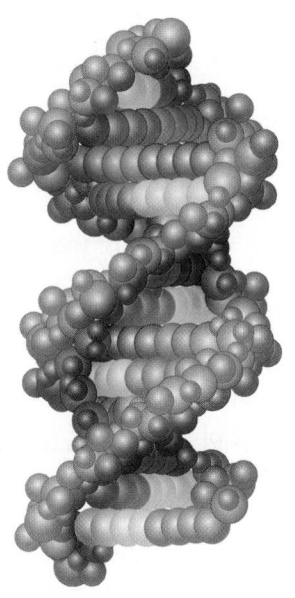

▲ **FIGURE 21.1 DNA Structure.** A molecular space-filling model of DNA giving some impression of its actual geometry.

Abbreviation	
DNA	deoxyribonucleic acid

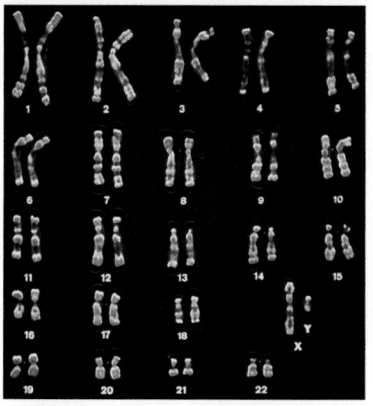

▲ **FIGURE 21.2 Karyotype Showing the Complete Set of Chromosomes of a Normal Male.**

WORD	PRONUNCIATION	ELEMENTS		DEFINITION
adenine	**AD**-eh-neen	S/ R/	-ine *pertaining to* aden- *a gland*	One of the chemical bases found in, and comprising the sequence of, both DNA and RNA
Ashkenazi	**ASH**-ke-**NAZ**-ih		Hebrew *Germany*	Jews of eastern European ancestry
autosome autosomal (adj)	**AWE**-toe-soam awe-toe-**SO**-mal	P/ R/ S/	auto- *self* -some *body* -al *pertaining to*	Any chromosome other than a sex chromosome
chromosome	**KROH**-moh-some	R/CF R/	chrom/o- *color* -some *body*	Body in the nucleus that contains DNA and genes
cytosine	**SIGH**-toh-seen	R/CF S/	cyt/o- *cell* -sine *fold, pocket*	One of the chemical bases found in, and comprising the sequence of, both DNA and RNA
deoxyribonucleic acid (DNA)	dee-**OCK**-see-**RYE**-boh-noo-**KLEE**-ik **ASS**-id	S/ P/ R/CF R/ R/ R/	-ic *pertaining to* de- *without* ox/y- *oxygen* -ribo- *pentose, a sugar* -nucle- *nucleus* acid *acid, low pH*	Source of hereditary characteristics found in chromosomes
gene genetic (adj) genetics geneticist	JEEN jeh-**NET**-ik jeh-**NET**-iks jeh-**NET**-ih-sist	 S/ S/ S/ R/	Greek *birth, origin* -ic *pertaining to* -ics *knowledge of* -ist *agent, specialist* genet- *origin*	Functional segment of DNA molecule Pertaining to a gene Science of the inheritance of characteristics A specialist in genetics
genome	**JEE**-nome	R/CF R/CF	-om/e *body* gen- *birth, to create*	Complete set of genes
guanine	**GWAH**-neen	S/ R/	-ine *pertaining to* guan- *dung*	One of the chemical bases found in, and comprising the sequence of, both DNA and RNA
helix	**HE**-liks		Greek *a coil*	A line in the shape of a coil
heredity inherited	heh-**RED**-ih-tee in-**HAIR**-it-ed	S/ R/	-ity *state, condition* hered- *inherited through genes*	Transmission of characteristics from parents to offspring through genes Acquired through genetic code
karyotype	**KAIR**-ee-oh-type	S/ R/CF	-type *model* kary/o- *nucleus*	Map of chromosomes of an individual cell
Mendelian	men-**DEE**-lee-an	S/	-ian *one who does, specialist* Gregor Johann Mendel, 1822–1884, Austrian geneticist; considered the father of genetics	Described by Gregor Mendel
thymine	**THIGH**-meen	S/ R/	-ine *pertaining to* thym- *the mind*	Chemical base found in, and comprising the sequence of, DNA but not RNA

EXERCISES

*Build your knowledge of the modern **language of genetics** by matching the following terms correctly. These are terms you will see in common usage—not just in the field of medicine but in forensics, law, and journalism as well. Fill in the blanks.*

_____ 1. study of heredity

_____ 2. prefix means *color*

_____ 3. exists in a double helix

_____ 4. complete set of genes

_____ 5. map of chromosomes

_____ 6. prefix means *self*

A. autosome

B. karyotype

C. genetics

D. chromosome

E. DNA

F. genome

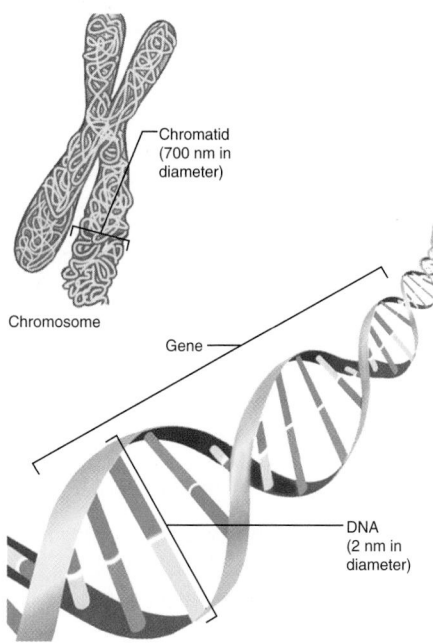

Chromatid
(700 nm in
diameter)

Chromosome

Gene

DNA
(2 nm in
diameter)

▲ **FIGURE 21.3   DNA, Gene, and Chromosome.**

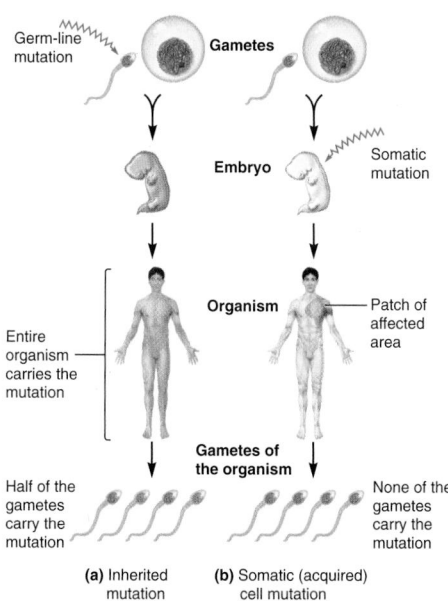

Germ-line mutation

Gametes

Embryo

Somatic mutation

Organism

Entire organism carries the mutation

Patch of affected area

Gametes of the organism

Half of the gametes carry the mutation

None of the gametes carry the mutation

(a) Inherited mutation

(b) Somatic (acquired) cell mutation

▲ **FIGURE 21.4   Genetic Mutations.**
(a) Hereditary (inherited) mutation. (b) Somatic (acquired) mutation. (Gametes are eggs and sperm.)

Abbreviations

mRNA messenger RNA
RNA ribonucleic acid

DNA, GENES, AND CHROMOSOMES (continued)

Genes

Genes are the working subunits of DNA *(Figure 21.3)*. The sum of all chromosomes (the genome) contains 25,000 to 30,000 genes, comprising some 3 billion bases. A gene is any segment along the DNA strand that **encodes** instructions to the cell to make a specific product, usually a protein such as an enzyme that initiates one specific action. Genes, through the proteins they encode, determine all body processes, including the way the body responds to challenges from the environment. A normal cell activates the genes it needs at the moment and shuts down the rest. The **genotype** is the specific genetic makeup (the specific genome) of an individual, in the form of DNA.

RNA (Ribonucleic acid)

For a cell to make a protein, the information from the gene is copied, base chemical by base chemical, from DNA into new strands of **messenger RNA (mRNA).** The newly formed mRNA travels out from the nucleus into the cell cytoplasm to organelles called ribosomes *(see Chapter 2)*. In the ribosomes, mRNA directs the assembly of amino acids into a protein molecule. The DNA stays safely behind in the nucleus, directing the operation from there.

With only 20 to 20,000 chemical bases, RNA is much smaller than DNA. RNA does not contain thymine, which is replaced by **uracil.**

Genes and Mutations

The **Human Genome Project** at the beginning of this century generated a map of specific genes linked to specific locations on chromosomes. Before this, human genetics had focused on single genes and the disorders that **malfunctions** of a single gene produced. Now, there is a new view of physiology as a complex interplay between multiple, interacting genes. This concept arises from the new science of **genomics,** the study of the structure, function, and information content of the genome. The complexity of this process is illustrated by looking at the sites where genes function at the organ level. The same genes can function at different sites.

Gene mutations occur frequently and randomly in every cell during cell division. The cells are able to recognize mistakes and correct them. However, the cells' repair ability can become less efficient with age, or it can fail because of environmental stresses such as radiation or toxins like chemotherapy or other chemicals.

When a gene mutates, the protein encoded by that gene will be abnormal. Some protein changes are insignificant; others are disabling. For example, the flawed hemoglobin in sickle cell anemia *(see Chapter 7)* is able to function but not well enough to carry oxygen normally.

Gene mutations can be inherited or **acquired.**

A hereditary mutation is a mistake that is present in virtually all the cells in the body and can be passed from generation to generation *(Figure 21.4)*.

More than 4000 disorders are thought to arise from mutated genes inherited from a parent. Common disorders, such as heart disease and cancer, arise from this complex interplay between genes and also between genes and factors in the environment.

Acquired mutations, also called **somatic mutations,** are DNA changes that develop during an individual's life. The changes arise in the DNA of individual cells and can be the result of errors during cell division or the result of environmental stresses such as radiation, chemicals, or toxins.

In the 23 pairs of chromosomes, the location of a particular gene is called its **locus.** The locus is normally the same on each chromosome, and each gene is the same. If the genes are not exactly the same, they are called **alleles,** which produce different forms of a particular **trait** or characteristic. If the trait is detectable, it is called a **phenotype,** and the allele producing the phenotype is said to be **dominant.** If the trait is not detectable, the allele is said to be **recessive.**

A phenotype is the manifestation of a trait, such as size, eye color or behavior that varies between individuals. More than one gene may contribute to a single trait.

WORD	PRONUNCIATION		ELEMENTS	DEFINITION
acquired (adj)	ah-KWIRED		Latin *to obtain*	A condition that is not inherited
allele	ah-LEEL		Greek *reciprocal*	Genetic variant found on the same locus of a pair of chromosomes
dominant gene	DOM-ih-nant JEEN		Latin *to rule*	Single allele that is expressed as a trait or characteristic
encode	en-KODE	P/ R/	en- *in* -code *information system*	Convert information
genome	JEE-nome	R/CF R/	-om/e *body* gen- *birth, to create*	Complete set of genes
genomics	jee-NOME-iks	S/ R/CF	-ics *knowledge of* gen/o- *birth, to create*	Study of the structure, function, and information content of the genome
genotype	jee-NOH-type	S/	-type *model, particular kind*	Specific genetic constitution of an individual
locus	LOW-kus		Latin, *a place*	A specific site; in this instance, the position a gene occupies on a chromosome
mutation mutate (verb)	myu-TAY-shun myu-TATE		Greek *to change*	Change in the chemistry of a gene
phenotype	FEE-noh-type	R/CF R/	phen/o- *to display* -type *model*	A visible trait
recessive gene	ree-SESS-iv JEEN		Latin *withdraw*	Allele that does not manifest as a trait or characteristic
ribonucleic acid (RNA)	RYE-boh-nyu-KLEE-ik ASS-id	S/ R/ R/ R/	-ic *pertaining to* ribo- *pentose, a sugar* -nucle- *nucleus* acid *acid, low pH*	Information carrier from DNA in the nucleus to the ribosome to produce specific protein molecules
somatic	soh-MAT-ik	S/ R/	-ic *pertaining to* somat- *body*	Relating to the body in general
trait	TRAYT		Latin *to draw out*	A discrete characteristic that has a known quality
uracil	YUR-ah-sil	S/ R/	-il *capability* urac- *urinary bladder*	Chemical found in RNA

EXERCISES

*Apply the correct **language of genetics** in this exercise. Remember: Correct spelling always counts! Fill in the blanks.*

1. A complete set of genes is called _____.

   genome   allele

2. A visible trait is _____.

   phenotype   fenotype

3. Change in the chemistry of a gene is called _____.

   recessive   mutation

4. If a gene does not manifest as a trait, it is _____.

   recessive   dominant

5. RNA stands for _____ acid.

   ribbonucelic   ribonucleic

Case Report 21.1 (continued)

Mrs. Sharon Fisher is facing two categories of risk. One is the gene mutation that she might share with her aunt and mother. The second is her family history and culture, whether or not her tests show a gene mutation. Mrs. Fisher recognized that knowing if the mutation was present had important implications for monitoring and preventing breast cancer, so she went ahead with the genetic screening.

Both Mrs. Fisher and her aunt had the *BRCA1* mutation. As her genetic nurse, you had the task of explaining to Mrs. Fisher that women with this mutation have a 50% to 85% lifetime risk of breast cancer and a 20% to 40% risk of ovarian cancer. This mutation also increases significantly the risk of developing a second case of breast or ovarian cancer within 5 years of the first case. Also, each of the Fisher children has a 50% chance of inheriting the mutation, including her son.

GENES AND THE RISK OF DISEASES

Eighty percent of the 6 million ethnic Jews in the United States are of Ashkenazi Jewish descent, with ancestors from Eastern and Central Europe. One in ten of them carries a gene mutation for **Gaucher disease.** This in itself will not cause symptoms. However, if both parents carry the gene, there is a 1-in-4 chance their children will inherit a mutated gene from both of them and develop the disease. Gaucher disease is an enzyme deficiency that leads to deposits of a fatty substance in the liver, spleen, and bone marrow. It can be treated with infusions of the defective enzyme.

Among Ashkenazi Jews, 1-in-31 carries a gene mutation for **Tay-Sachs disease,** which by itself will not cause symptoms. If both parents carry the gene mutation, their children have a 1-in-4 chance of inheriting two mutated genes and developing the disease. Tay-Sachs is a fatal lipid storage disease leading to blindness, deafness, and inability to swallow. There is no treatment.

In 1995, an alteration in the **breast cancer gene** called *BRCA1* was discovered to be present in 1% of Ashkenazi Jews, compared to 0.1% to 0.6% of the general U.S. population. In 1996, another mutation in the *BRCA1* gene and one in another breast cancer gene called *BRCA2* were identified. The risk for carrying one of these three mutations among Ashkenazi Jews is 2.3%. These mutations account for 25% of early-onset breast cancer.

The disorders became amplified in the Ashkenazi population because, until recently, Ashkenazi Jews married only other Ashkenazi Jews.

The *BRCA1* and *BRCA2* mutations can be passed on to men, where they cause a 6% risk of male breast cancer and an 8% risk of prostate cancer. They can also be passed on from the father to sons and daughters, who will benefit from screening.

In the general U.S. population of women, 1 in 8 will develop breast cancer at some point in her lifetime, and 1 in 70 will develop ovarian cancer. Of women with breast or ovarian cancer, 5% to 10% have mutations in *BRCA1* or *BRCA2*. About 1 in 800 in the general population carries a *BRCA1* mutation. The incidence of *BRCA2* is not known. The identification of close blood relatives having breast or ovarian cancer is important in genetic **counseling.**

Gene therapy is in its infancy. It can involve inserting normal copies of a gene into the cells of a person with a specific genetic disease or correcting an abnormality in egg or sperm cells. A carrier molecule, called a **vector,** delivers the therapeutic gene to the target cell. This vector is usually a virus genetically altered to carry human DNA. For this technique and others, ethical issues, lack of knowledge and experience, and expense are hurdles to be overcome. Gene therapy remains experimental and is being tried in a variety of disorders.

WORD	PRONUNCIATION	ELEMENTS		DEFINITION
congenital	kon-**JEN**-ih-tal	S/ P/ R/	-al *pertaining to* con- *with* -genit- *birth, bring forth*	Present at birth, either inherited or due to an event during gestation up to the moment of birth
counseling	**KOWN**-sel-ing		Latin *deliberation*	Professional relationship to transmit advice to direct the judgment of another
Gaucher disease	go-**SHAY DIZ**-eez		Philippe Gaucher, 1854–1918, French physician	Congenital disorder of fat metabolism
Tay-Sachs disease	TAY-SAKS **DIZ**-eez		Warren Tay, 1843–1927, British ophthalmologist; Bernard Sachs, 1858–1944, U.S. neurologist	Congenital fatal disorder of fat metabolism
vector	**VEK**-tor		Latin *a carrier*	A virus or other molecule used to carry a gene to target cells

STEM CELLS

Stem cells are distinguished from other cell types in two ways:

- They are unspecialized cells capable of replicating themselves through cell division.
- They can be induced to become organ- or tissue-specific cells with special functions.

In some organs such as the brain, gut, muscle, and bone marrow, adult stem cells regularly divide to replace worn out or damaged tissues. In 2006 some specialized adult cells were reprogrammed genetically to assume a stem cell–like state—**adult stem cells.**

In the 3- to 5-day-old embryo (blastocyst), the inner cells give rise to all the different cells in the body of the organism. These cells are called **human embryonic stem cells.**

Keynote

Although research is in its infancy, stem cells appear to offer new potentials for treating chronic diseases and injuries. This new concept is called **regenerative** or **reparative medicine.**

EXERCISES

*Analyze the Case Report on Mrs. Sharon Fisher that appears on the opposite page. Use the **language of genetics** to fill in the blanks.*

1. What is the purpose of genetic screening?

_____

2. What are Mrs. Fisher's two categories of risk?

_____

3. What medical terms can be used to describe the *BRCA1* gene?

_____

4. What can Mrs. Fisher do to help herself?

_____

See how your knowledge of medical terminology helps you understand this patient's case!

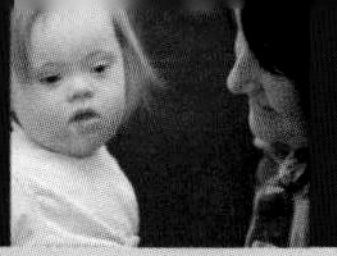

To be involved and helpful in enabling patients with abnormal genes to make informed decisions, you must be able to:

21.2.1 Explain the different types of prenatal testing.

21.2.2 Discuss the inheritance of different types of genetic disorders.

21.2.3 Describe some of the more common genetic disorders.

You are

. . . a genetic nurse working with geneticist Ingrid Hughes, MD, PhD, in the Genetics Department at Fulwood Medical Center.

Your patients are

. . . Rebecca and Paul Holyfield, a married couple in their early thirties.

CASE REPORT 21.2

The Holyfields have one daughter, Sarah (aged 5), who is doing well. Last year, they lost a son, aged 2, with **cystic fibrosis (CF)**. Rebecca is now 8 weeks pregnant, and they want to know if the new baby can also have cystic fibrosis. They did not intend to have any more children.

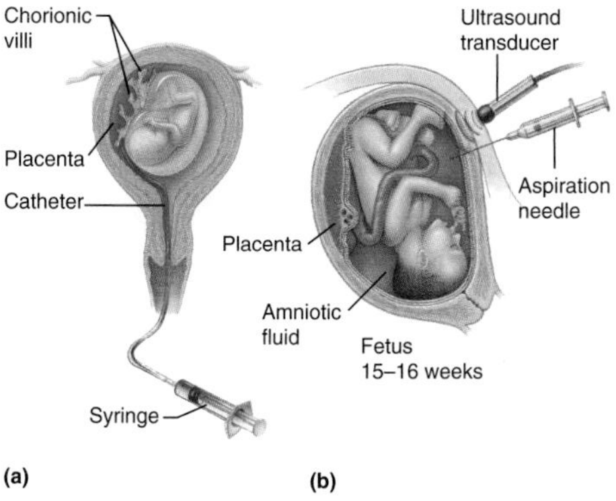

GENETIC TESTING

Genetic testing is the analysis of human DNA, RNA, chromosomes, and proteins to diagnose inheritable diseases and detect vulnerabilities to inherited diseases. In most examples, it involves examining a person's DNA from a sample of blood, hair, skin, or cells from the inside of the cheek, called a **buccal smear.**

Prenatal Genetic Diagnostic Testing

The improvement in diagnostic techniques in the past three decades has produced different options that can be used to determine whether a fetus is affected with a specific condition.

- **Chorionic villus** sampling *(Figure 21.5a)* removes placental tissue between 9 and 12 weeks of gestation. Fetal and placental positions are established by ultrasound and a transcervical biopsy is taken *(Figure 21.5b)*. The placental cells are a source of DNA and cells for cell culture and further analysis.

- **Amniocentesis** samples amniotic fluid from around the fetus using an aspiration needle. The amniotic fluid contains cells shed by the fetus that contain fetal DNA, which then can be analyzed. The fluid itself can be assayed for components such as **alpha-fetoprotein (AFP)**, the levels of which rise when neural tube defects are present *(see Chapter 10)*. Amniocentesis is a safe procedure that can be performed between 16 and 20 weeks of gestation *(Figure 21.5b)*.

- **Fetal blood** sampling takes a blood sample from the umbilical vein of the fetus using a very fine needle with ultrasound guidance. The sample provides cells for DNA or abnormal protein studies.

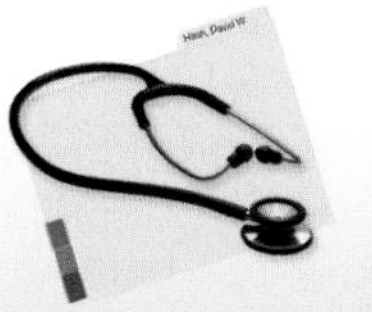

▲ **FIGURE 21.5 Prenatal Genetic Testing.**
(a) Chorionic villus biopsy.
(b) Amniocentesis, and ultrasound.

Abbreviations

AFP	alpha-fetoprotein
CF	cystic fibrosis
IVF	in vitro fertilization

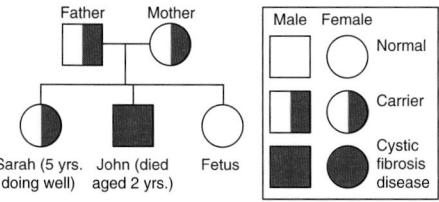

▲ **FIGURE 21.6 The Holyfield Family: Autosomal Recessive Inheritance of Cystic Fibrosis.**

Case Report 21.2 *(continued)*

When the Holyfields' son was diagnosed with cystic fibrosis, genetic testing showed that both parents carried the Mendelian autosomal recessive gene for CF *(Figure 21.6)* and that their daughter Sarah was also a **carrier,** or **heterozygote.** The child who died inherited an abnormal gene from each parent and is called a **homozygote.** Chorionic villus testing in the current pregnancy showed a fetal girl who did not carry the gene.

WORD	PRONUNCIATION	ELEMENTS		DEFINITION
alpha-fetoprotein	**AL**-fah-fee-toe-**PRO**-teen	P/ R/CF R/	**alpha-** *first letter in Greek alphabet* **fet/o-** *fetus* **-protein** *protein*	Protein normally produced only by the fetus
buccal smear	**BUCK**-al SMEER	S/ R/ R/	**-al** *pertaining to* **bucc-** *cheek* **smear** *spread*	Use of a small brush or cotton swab to collect cells from the inside surface of the cheek
carrier (also called heterozygote)	**KAH**-ree-er		Latin *vehicle*	In this setting, a person with an autosomal recessive gene for a disease
chorionic villus	koh-ree-**ON**-ik **VILL**-us		**chorion** *membrane* **villus** *fingerlike projection*	Vascular process of the embryonic chorion to form the placenta
heterozygous heterozygote (noun)	**HET**-er-oh-**ZIE**-gus **HET**-er-oh-**ZIE**-goat	S/ P/ R/	**-ous** *pertaining to* **hetero-** *different* **-zyg-** *zygote*	Carries a different version (allele) of a specific gene on each of the two corresponding chromosomes
homozygous (adj) homozygote (noun)	hoh-moh-**ZIE**-gus hoh-moh-**ZIE**-goat	S/ P/ R/	**-ous** *pertaining to* **homo-** *the same* **-zyg-** *zygote*	Having two identical copies of a specific gene on the two homologous chromosomes

- **Maternal blood** sampling provides a very small number of fetal cells that can be detected in the maternal circulation. Some chemical changes in the maternal blood can suggest the presence of a fetus with Down syndrome.

- **Preimplantation diagnosis** for **in vitro fertilization (IVF)** involves the removal of a single cell from a developing embryo for genetic study prior to implantation.

   Newborn screening is performed using a small blood sample obtained by pricking the heel of a newborn. It is taken to identify genetic disorders that can be treated early in life.

EXERCISES

*Provide brief answers to the questions, and test your knowledge of the **language of genetics.***

1. What is genetic testing?

_____

2. What samples are taken from the patient for genetic testing?

_____

3. Why is genetic testing done?

_____

4. Explain the different types of prenatal genetic testing.

_____

_____

_____

_____

5. What can the Holyfields hope to learn from this testing?

_____

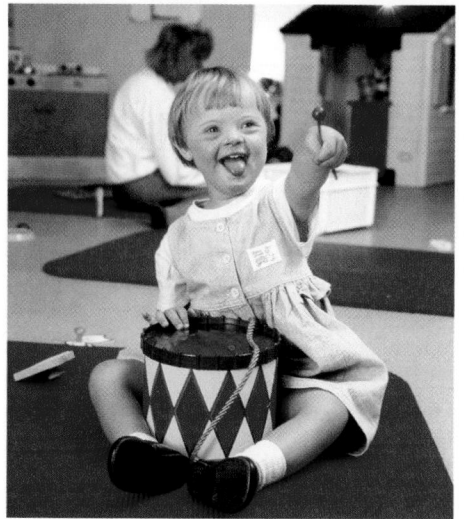

▲ FIGURE 21.7 Down Syndrome (Trisomy 21).

GENETIC DISORDERS

Changes in Chromosome Number

Down syndrome is most often associated with an extra **(trisomy)** copy of chromosome 21, and it is found in about 1 in 660 newborns *(Figure 21.7)*. People with Down syndrome are usually short, have **hypotonia,** lax joints, and soft skin. Facial features include a prominent tongue, and obliquely positioned eyes. Almost half show a single crease **(simian crease)** across the palm of the hand. About 40% have congenital heart disease, often a ventricular or atrial septal defect *(see Chapter 8)*. Mental retardation occurs in 100%, though many individuals with Down syndrome can learn basic skills and function with independence.

The most important risk factor for conceiving a child with Down syndrome is advanced maternal age. The incidence rises from an incidence of 1:1200 at maternal age 30, to 1:25 at age 45. Prenatal diagnosis uses a combination of ultrasound and the measurement of specific hormones and alpha-fetoprotein levels in maternal blood as well as a karyotype analysis of amniotic fluid for trisomy of chromosome 21.

Variations in the number of sex chromosomes in women produce **Turner syndrome.** The most common **anomaly** is the absence of one X chromosome, producing the karyotype 45,XO. The ovaries do not develop normally and do not produce adequate amounts of hormones. Treatment is to provide the hormones that are deficient.

In males, the presence of an extra X chromosome (45,XXY) produces **Klinefelter syndrome,** in which testicles are small, with few sperm developing. Treatment is with testosterone.

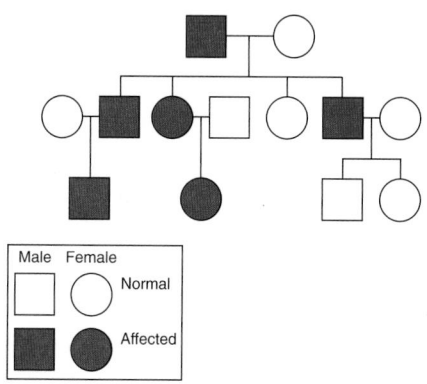

▲ FIGURE 21.8 Autosomal Dominant Family Tree.

Autosomal Dominant Conditions

In autosomal dominant inheritance, one autosome carries an abnormal gene that expresses a specific trait or characteristic, while the other autosome carries a normal copy of the same gene. This person has the disease and is called an affected heterozygote. The chance that an individual germ cell will contain the chromosome with the abnormal gene is 50%, and the chance for an affected individual to transmit the abnormal gene is 50% with each conception. Therefore, an average of 50% of the offspring of an affected individual will also be affected *(Figure 21.8)*.

Autosomal dominant disorders include:

- **Neurofibromatosis.** Neurofibromas arise from the Schwann cells that support nerve fibers *(see Chapter 10)*, and **"café-au-lait"** (coffee with cream) macules appear on the skin.

- **Achondroplasia** *(see Chapter 16)*.

- **Marfan syndrome.** This is characterized by excessive height due to growth of long bones, together with long fingers and unstable joints.

- **Huntington disease** A disorder of the **central nervous system (CNS),** this disease appears in the third and fourth decades of life, with loss of motor control, personality changes, and decreased mental capacity *(see Chapter 10)*.

Autosomal Recessive Disorders

Autosomal recessive disorders appear when there is a specific abnormality in a copy of a gene contributed by each parent. The unaffected parents are heterozygotes, and the affected offspring is a homozygote. Because each parent has only one abnormal copy of the gene, there is only a 25% likelihood of each pregnancy resulting in a homozygote.

Autosomal disorders include:

- **Sickle cell disease** *(see Chapter 7)*.

- **Gaucher disease**—reflects malfunction in a specific enzyme pathway in protein metabolism. A reliable enzyme replacement therapy is now available.

- **Phenylketonuria**—an important cause of mental retardation and tested for in newborn screening. The basis of treatment is limiting the causative amino acid phenylalanine in the serum by limiting it in the diet.

- **Albinism**—a failure to produce melanin *(see Chapter 3)*.

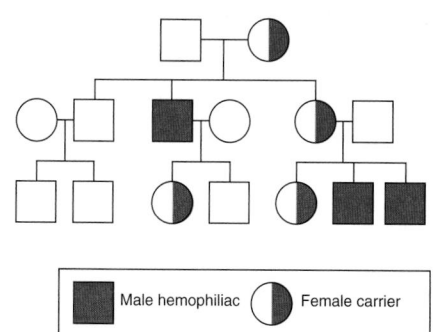

▲ FIGURE 21.9 Family History of Hemophilia.

WORD	PRONUNCIATION	ELEMENTS		DEFINITION
albinism	**AL**-bih-nizm	S/	-ism *condition*	Genetic disorder with lack of melanin
		R/	albin- *white*	
albino	al-**BY**-no	R/CF	albin/o- *white*	Person with albinism
anomaly	ah-**NOM**-ah-lee		Greek *irregularity*	A structural abnormality
café-au-lait (adj)	**KAF**-ay-oh-**LAY**		café French *coffee*	Color of skin macules in neurofibromatosis
			au French *with*	
			lait French *milk*	
Down syndrome	DOWN **SIN**-drome		John Down, 1828–1896, English physician	A syndrome with variable abnormalities associated with three chromosomes 21
Huntington disease (also called **Huntington chorea**)	**HUN**-ting-ton **DIZ**-eez		George Huntington, 1851–1916, American neurologist	Progressive, inherited, degenerative, incurable neurologic disease
hypotonia	high-poh-**TOE**-nee-ah	S/	-ia *condition*	Diminished muscle tone
		P/	hypo- *below, deficient*	
		R/	-ton- *pressure, tension*	
hypotonic (adj)	high-poh-**TON**-ik	S/	-ic *pertaining to*	Pertaining to or suffering from hypotonia
Klinefelter syndrome	**KLINE**-fel-ter **SIN**-drome		Harry Klinefelter, Jr., born 1912, Boston physician	Genetic anomaly in males with XXY chromosomes
Marfan syndrome	mahr-**FAN SIN**-drome		Antoine Marfan, 1858–1942, French pediatrician	Genetic condition with malformation of elastic connective tissue
simian crease	sih-**ME**-an KREES	S/	-an *pertaining to*	Single crease across the palm of the hand; found in monkeys
		R/	simi- *ape, monkey*	
		R/	crease *groove*	
trisomy	**TRI**-so-me	P/	tri- *three*	Presence of an extra chromosome
		R/	-somy *chromosome*	
Turner syndrome	**TER**-ner **SIN**-drome		Henry H. Turner, 1892–1970, American endocrinologist	Syndrome associated with a chromosome count of 45 and only one X chromosome

X-linked disorders occur when the altered gene is located on the X chromosome. Examples of this type of inheritance are **hemophilia A** *(Figure 21.9; see Chapter 7)*; **defective color vision** *(see Chapter 4)*; **Duchenne muscular dystrophy** *(see Chapter 5)*; **fragile-X syndrome**, the most common form of inherited mental retardation, affecting 1 in every 1000 to 2000 male individuals.

EXERCISES

*Discuss the inheritance of different types of genetic disorders; then describe some of the more common genetic disorders. Use in your discussion the **language of genetics**. Write your discussion notes below.*

1. The inheritance of genetic disorders—how does that happen?

_____

_____

2. Some of the more common genetic disorders are:

_____

_____

3. How or when would you know you need genetic counseling?

_____

_____

4. What is the ultimate goal of genetic counseling?

_____

GENETICS

CHALLENGE YOUR KNOWLEDGE

A. **Case Report:** Reread the following Case Report from this chapter, and answer the questions.

CASE REPORT 21.2

Your patients are

. . . Rebecca and Paul Holyfield, a married couple in their early thirties. They have one daughter, Sarah (aged 5), who is doing well. Last year, they lost a son, aged 2, with cystic fibrosis (CF). Rebecca is now 8 weeks pregnant, and they want to know if the new baby can also have cystic fibrosis. They did not intend to have any more children.

When the Holyfields' son was diagnosed with cystic fibrosis, genetic testing showed that both parents carried the Mendelian autosomal recessive gene for CF and that their daughter Sarah was also a carrier, or heterozygote. The child who died inherited an abnormal gene from each parent and is called a homozygote. Chorionic villus testing in the current pregnancy showed a fetal girl who did not carry the gene.

1. Explain how chorionic villus testing is done.

   _____

   _____

2. What is the purpose of this type of testing?

   _____

   _____

3. Why is the child who died termed a *homozygote,* as opposed to his sister, who is referred to as a *heterozygote?*

   _____

   _____

4. What should the Holyfields' daughter Sarah consider when she gets married and wants to have a family?

   _____

   _____

5. Define *autosomal recessive gene.*

   _____

   _____

6. What does the medical term *carrier* mean?

   _____

   _____

B. Elements: To facilitate learning medical terminology, you need to be able to recognize a word element for what it is (prefix, root, combining form, or suffix,) as well as what it means. Test your knowledge by correctly filling in the following chart with a check mark (✓) in the proper element column. Then fill in the meaning of the element and a medical term containing that element.

Element	Prefix	Root/CF	Suffix	Meaning of Element	Medical Term Using That Element
1. adeno					
2. uria					
3. ana					
4. auto					
5. bucc					
6. chromo					
7. cyst					
8. emia					
9. de					

C. Abbreviations must be interpreted correctly for safety in communication. Match the correct abbreviation from the *language of genetics* to its characteristic. Fill in the blanks.

_____ 1. Travels from nucleus to ribosome   **A.** AFP

_____ 2. Has uracil instead of thymine   **B.** DNA

_____ 3. Exists as two paired strands in a double helix   **C.** mRNA

_____ 4. Not an option for Sharon Fisher   **D.** CF

_____ 5. Protein normally produced only by the fetus   **E.** RNA

_____ 6. Can be detected in utero   **F.** HRT

D. Terminology Challenge: Medical terms can have more than one meaning, as you have seen throughout this text. The term **vector** in genetics has a different meaning than the term **vector** in infectious diseases. Compare the two terms. How are they similar, and how are they different?

Vector in genetics means _____

_____ .

Vector in infectious diseases means _____

_____

The terms are similar because _____ .

The terms are different because _____ .

GENETICS

E. Lesson Objectives: Each of the following is a lesson objective from *Chapter 21*. In your own words, provide a short answer to the question. If you are able to illustrate it with a line drawing or a photo downloaded from the Internet, so much the better.

1. Can you describe the structure of a chromosome?

   _____

   _____

   _____

2. What are the structure and functions of a gene?

   _____

   _____

   _____

F. Elements: Continue working with word elements to refine your knowledge of the *language of genetics*.

Element	Prefix	Root/CF	Suffix	Meaning of Element	Medical Term Using that Element
1. en	_____	_____	_____	_____	_____
2. feto	_____	_____	_____	_____	_____
3. hetero	_____	_____	_____	_____	_____
4. homo	_____	_____	_____	_____	_____
5. hypo	_____	_____	_____	_____	_____
6. ia	_____	_____	_____	_____	_____
7. ine	_____	_____	_____	_____	_____
8. ism	_____	_____	_____	_____	_____
9. karyo	_____	_____	_____	_____	_____

G. Pathology: The science of genetics has discovered gene mutations that account for very specific hereditary diseases. Finding the cause of a disease can eventually lead to discovering how to cure it. Use the *language of genetics* to answer the following questions. Some questions may only require a yes or no answer. Fill in the blanks.

1. Are some ethnic groups more prone to certain diseases? _____

2. If you carry a gene mutation, are there any symptoms? _____

3. If both parents carry the same mutated gene, does that increase their chances of having a child born with a hereditary disease? _____

4. Which hereditary disease is a fatal lipid storage disease? _____

5. What is the treatment for this disease? _____

6. Which hereditary disease is caused by an enzyme deficiency? _____

7. What is the treatment for this disease? _____

8. Which disease produces severe sensory and autonomic dysfunctions? _____

H. The *language of genetics* will help you understand human development. Use this terminology to provide the answers to the following questions. Circle the correct choice.

1. What factors affect human development?

    a. dietary and hereditary

    b. genetic and environmental

    c. environmental and dietary

    d. all of these

    e. none of these

2. What is the only type of body cell in which DNA does not exist?

    a. WBCs

    b. leukocyte

    c. osteoblasts

    d. mature RBCs

    e. neutrophils

3. A cell's repair ability is affected by:

    a. age

    b. environmental stress

    c. radiation

    d. chemotherapy

    e. all of these

4. The location of a particular gene is called its:

    a. vector

    b. allele

    c. phenotype

    d. locus

    e. mutation

GENETICS

I. **The *language of genetics* will help you understand human development.** Use this terminology to provide the answers to the following questions. Circle the correct choice.

1. Another name for your genetic composition is:

   a. phenotype

   b. meiosis

   c. genome

   d. autosome

   e. alleles

2. Hereditary mutations are also called:

   a. somatic mutations

   b. homozygous mutations

   c. inherited mutations

   d. statistical mutations

   e. vector mutations

3. Produce different forms of a particular trait:

   a. gamete

   b. chromosome

   c. gene

   d. ribosome

   e. allele

4. Genetic information is carried in:

   a. adenine

   b. thymine

   c. cytosine

   d. guanine

   e. all of these

5. Messenger RNA travels from the nucleus to:

   a. the bloodstream

   b. the heart

   c. an organelle

   d. a target organ

   e. another nucleus

6. A mutated gene has an abnormally encoded:

   a. nucleus

   b. protein

   c. phenotype

   d. trait

   e. locus

7. Somatic mutations are:

   a. acquired

   b. random

   c. heterozygous

   d. enzyme-related

   e. cytogenetic

8. Tightly coiled strands of DNA are packaged in units called:

   a. genes

   b. phenotypes

   c. bases

   d. chromosomes

   e. guanine

9. Delivers the therapeutic gene to the target cell:

   a. vector

   b. karyotype

   c. phenotype

   d. trait

   e. base

10. Adenine, thymine, cytosine, and guanine are:

    a. amino acids

    b. enzymes

    c. vitamins

    d. chemical bases of DNA

    e. hormones

11. *BRCA1* and *BRCA2* mutations can be passed on to men and cause:

    a. colon cancer

    b. breast cancer

    c. prostate cancer

    d. a and c

    e. b and c

J. **Recall and Review:** How well do you remember these word elements from the previous chapter? Try to answer without first looking back to check. Fill in the blanks.

Element	Type of Element (P, R, CF, S)	Meaning of Element
con		
patho		
enter		
micro		
onco		

K. **Discussion Question:** Think about what it was like before genetic counseling was available. No information and, consequently, no choices were available for certain patients. How does genetic counseling enable patients to make an informed choice and be proactive in their health care? Demonstrate your answer by using two examples of circumstances in which genetic counseling can make a difference. Write your thoughts on the lines below, and be prepared to share them with the class.

_____

_____

_____

_____

_____

_____

_____

_____

_____

_____

_____

_____

_____

GENETICS

L. **Latin and Greek terms cannot be further deconstructed into prefix, root, or suffix.** You must know them for what they are. Test your knowledge of these terms with this exercise. Match the meaning in the left column with the correct medical term in the right column.

_____ 1. withdraw   A. helix

_____ 2. to change   B. recessive

_____ 3. born with   C. vector

_____ 4. a carrier   D. heredity

_____ 5. transferred from generation to generation   E. mutation

_____ 6. a coil   F. congenital

M. **Patient Education:** You have been doing a clinical rotation in the OB (obstetrics) Clinic. Explain to your patient, in layman's terms, the difference between a congenital and a hereditary disease. Provide an example of each disease.

1. Congenital disease: _____

   _____

   Example: _____

2. Hereditary disease: _____

   _____

   Example: _____

N. Complete the following statements with the correct medical terminology.

1. _____ carries the instructions that enable your cells to make proteins.

2. What type of blood cells have no nucleus and cannot reproduce? _____

3. _____ are the working subunits of DNA.

4. Gene mutations can be _____ or acquired.

5. The location of a particular gene in the chromosome is called its _____.

6. _____ is an autosomal recessive disorder that is a failure to produce melanin.

7. Somatic mutations are also called _____ mutations.

O. **Translation:** Use your knowledge of medical terms to read and understand the following statements; then rewrite them in language your patient can understand.

1. "Hereditary traits can be dominant or recessive. If they are not hereditary, they can also be acquired."

   _____

   _____

   _____

2. "Your genetic composition is established at conception." _____

   _____

   _____

3. "A bucchal smear can be used for examination of DNA."

_____

_____

_____

4. "Chorionic villus sampling removes placental tissue between 9 and 12 weeks of gestation."

_____

_____

_____

5. "Preimplantation diagnosis for IVF involves the removal of a single cell from a developing embryo for genetic study prior to implantation."

_____

_____

_____

6. "Environmental stressors can result in acquired mutations."

_____

_____

_____

P. Test yourself on what you have learned in this chapter. Employ the new medical terms in genetics to answer the following questions.

1. Describe the structure of a chromosome.

_____

_____

2. Explain the structure and function of a gene.

_____

_____

3. Compare the structures and functions of DNA and RNA.

DNA structures: _____

_____

_____

DNA functions: _____

_____

_____

RNA structures: _____

_____

_____

RNA functions: _____

_____

_____

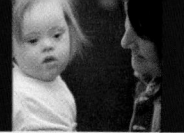

GENETICS

CHAPTER SUMMARY EXERCISE

1. *Listen to the pronunciation of the medical terms as given by your instructor.*
2. *Circle the correct spelling of the medical term.*
3. *Match the correctly spelled terms to the brief descriptions below.*
4. *Write a sentence for each of the 10 terms that appear in this exercise.*

A. SPELLING COMPREHENSION: CIRCLE THE CORRECT SPELLING OF THE TERM.

1. karytype	keriotype	karyotype	cariotype	carriotipe
2. helix	hellix	heelix	hellex	helick
3. chromosone	cromosome	chromosome	cromosom	chromosom
4. toxsin	toxin	toxsen	toxxin	toxen
5. homozygous	hommozigous	homozigous	hommozygous	homosigous
6. fenotype	penotype	phenyltype	phenotype	feenotype
7. urecell	uracil	uracell	urecil	uresell
8. congenial	congenital	congintial	congential	congeenial
9. Gaucher	Goucher	Gucher	Gowcher	Goucer
10. heridity	hereditty	herredity	heredity	herridity

B. MATCH THE NUMBER OF THE CORRECT TERM IN PART A WITH THE BRIEF DESCRIPTION OF THE TERM BELOW.

a. existing at or from birth _____

b. a line in the shape of a coil _____

c. contained in RNA _____

d. congenital disorder of fat metabolism _____

e. poison; harmful substance _____

f. similarities and uniqueness from generation to generation _____

g. having two identical copies of a specific gene on the two

homologous chromosomes _____

h. map of chromosomes _____

i. detectable trait _____

j. body in the nucleus that contains DNA and genes _____

C. USING YOUR KNOWLEDGE OF TERMS 1–10 IN PART A AND THEIR CORRECT SPELLING, WRITE A BRIEF SENTENCE FOR EACH OF THE TERMS AS IT MIGHT APPEAR IN PATIENT DOCUMENTATION.

1. _____

2. _____

3. _____

4. _____

9. _____

10. _____

D. YOUR INSTRUCTOR WILL DIRECT YOU TO MCGRAW-HILL CONNECT. OPEN THE AUDIO GLOSSARY AND PRACTICE YOUR PRONUNCIATION OF THE TERMS IN PART A OF THIS EXERCISE

E. PROOFREAD THE FOLLOWING STATEMENTS FOR ERRORS IN SPELLING AND/OR FACT. REWRITE THE SENTENCES CORRECTLY. THERE IS ONLY ONE STATEMENT WITHOUT ANY ERRORS.

1. Chromosonal abnormalities, including deviations from the normal number and structural defects, can also produce disorders.

_____

_____

_____

2. Guanine can be found only in RNA.

_____

_____

3. If a trait is not detectable, the alele is said to be dominant.

_____

_____

_____

4. In gene therapy a carrier molecule, called a vector, delivers the therapeutic gene to the target cell.

_____

_____

_____

5. A genome is any chromosome other than a sex chromosome.

_____

_____

_____

6. Fetal blood sampling takes a blood sample from the carotid artery of the fetus using a transcatheter with x-ray guidance.

_____

_____

_____

7. Gaucher disease reflects malfunction in a specific hormone pathway in protein metabolism.

_____

_____

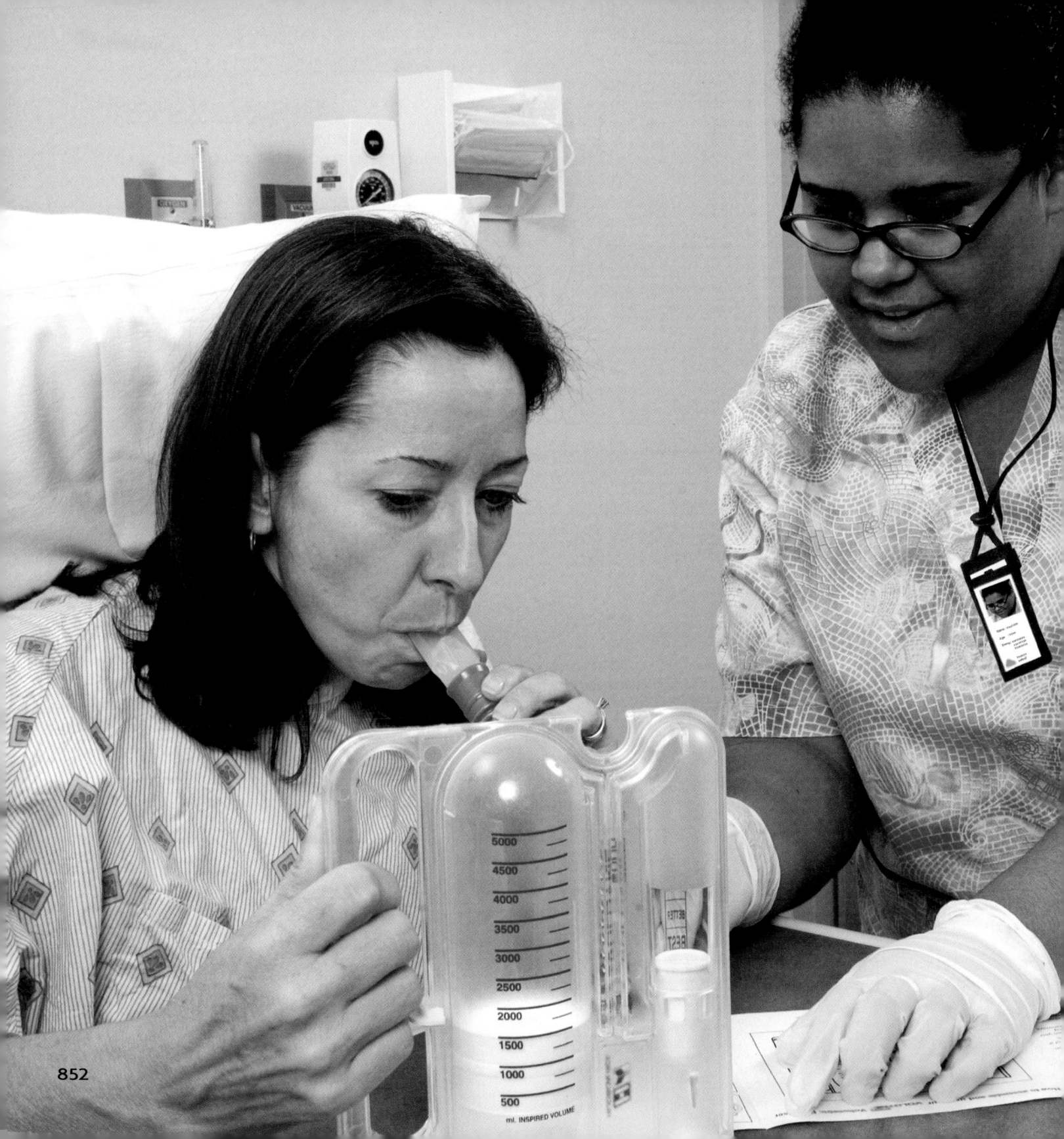

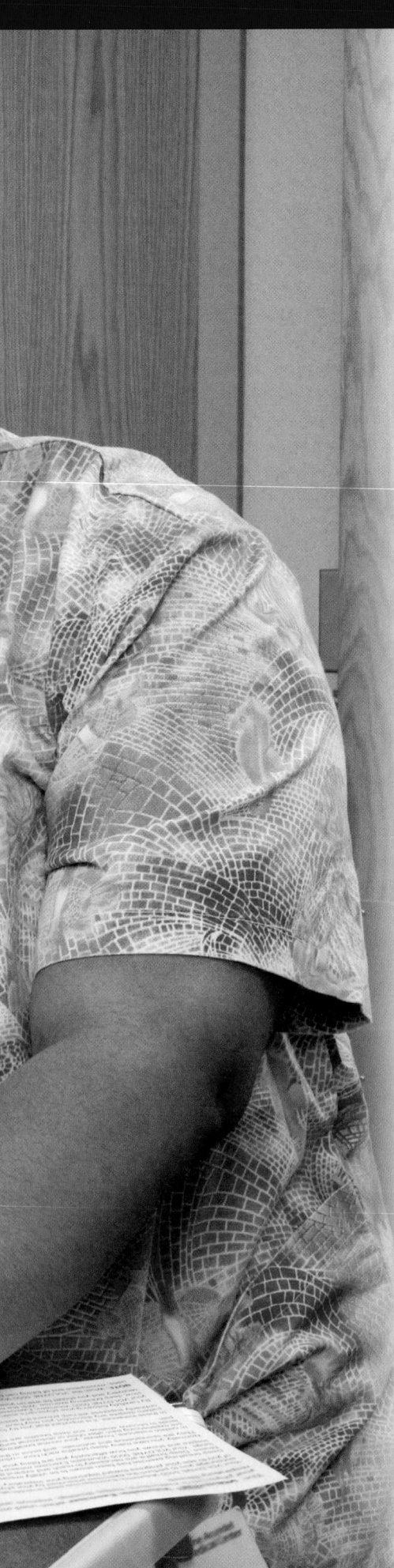

CASE REPORT 22.1

You are

. . . an advanced-level respiratory therapist employed by Fulwood Medical Center, working with Tavis Senko, MD, a pulmonologist.

Your patient is

. . . Mrs. Raquel Sacco, a 44-year-old mother of two teenage boys, who is the owner of a quilting fabrics store. She is 2 days postop from lung surgery for non-small cell lung cancer. From her records, you see that she has two secondary (2°) metastases in her brain. She has been a nonsmoker all her life. Her 70-year-old father is a two-pack-a-day smoker, as is her husband. They both show no evidence of cancer on chest x-rays. Before Mrs. Sacco is discharged, as part of her postoperative respiratory care plan you are using incentive spirometry—also called **sustained maximal inspiration (SMI)**—to increase her inspiratory volume and improve her inspiratory muscle performance. You will also be taking an arterial blood sample to check her **arterial oxygen pressure (PaO$_2$).**

Learning Outcomes

To understand the possible etiologies of cancer, its pathology and staging, and its treatment and prognosis and to communicate among the health care team as you care for Mrs. Sacco, you will need to be able to:

22.1 Apply the language of oncology to the anatomy and physiology of cancer.

22.2 Comprehend, analyze, spell, and write the medical terms of oncology so that you communicate and document accurately and precisely in any health care setting.

22.3 Recognize and pronounce the medical terms of oncology so that you communicate verbally with accuracy and precision in any health care setting.

22.4 Explain the pathophysiology, diagnosis, and therapies of common types of cancer.

Note: In previous chapters on individual body systems, the terminology of cancers specific to each body system has been detailed. In this chapter, the terminology that relates to cancer in general will be explored using lung cancer as an example.

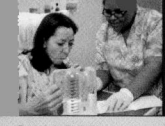

LESSON 22.1 Types of Cancer

CANCER

Normal tissue development is a balance between cell growth and cell death. If cells multiply quicker than cells die, tumors **(neoplasms)** are formed. The study of tumors is called **oncology,** and medical specialists in this field are called **oncologists.** Neoplasms whose cells **proliferate** rapidly and spread to distant sites **(metastasize)** are called **malignant.** Neoplasms that grow slowly, stay localized, do not invade surrounding tissues, and do not metastasize are called **benign.**

The information in this lesson will enable you to use correct medical terminology to:

22.1.1 Distinguish between benign and malignant neoplasms.

22.1.2 Classify the types of cancer by the type of cell from which it originates.

22.1.3 Explain the process of carcinogenesis.

22.1.4 Discuss the roles of environmental factors in carcinogenesis.

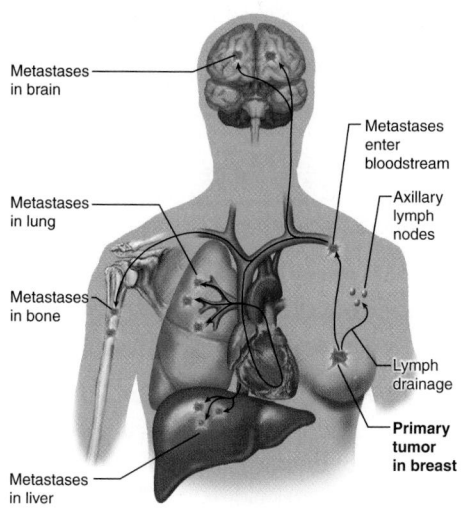

Metastases in brain

Metastases enter bloodstream

Metastases in lung

Axillary lymph nodes

Metastases in bone

Lymph drainage

Primary tumor in breast

Metastases in liver

▲ **FIGURE 22.1 Metastases from Primary Breast Cancer.** Metastasis may be via lymph drainage to the axillary lymph nodes or via the bloodstream to the brain, lung, liver, and bone.

Keynote

• Cancer death rates in the United States have declined by 1.1% a year from 1993 through 2002.

• From 2002 to 2004 the decline in cancer death rates increased to 2.1%.

• The decline in cancer death rates is due to better prevention efforts, new screening methods, and more effective treatments.

TYPES OF CANCER

Cancer (CA) is a class of malignant diseases characterized by uncontrolled cell division. The basic cause of this uncontrolled growth is damage to the cells' DNA. This damage produces mutations to the genes that control cell division. These mutations, which can be inherited or acquired, lead to the uncontrolled cell division and malignant tumor formation.

Thus all cancer is genetic; that is, it develops because something in a cell's genes has changed (mutated). Less than 10% of all cancers are inherited; that is, the genetic change is passed from parent to child. Almost 90% of cancers are acquired—something has caused the gene mutation in specific cells in a particular individual. A few genes mutated within a cell nucleus are enough to cause cancer. These gene mutations give the cells a superpower to proliferate in an uncontrolled way.

The Cells of Malignant Tumors

• Have unlimited, unregulated growth potential.

• Grow directly into adjacent tissues (invasion or **infiltration**).

• Invade the lymphatic system and are carried to local and distant lymph nodes *(Figure 22.1)*.

• Invade the bloodstream and are carried to other distant organs and tissues **(metastasis;** *Figure 22.1)*.

In contrast, benign tumors do not show such unregulated, invasive growth.

The Cells of Benign Tumors

• Grow slowly.

• Are surrounded by a connective tissue capsule.

• Do not invade or infiltrate adjacent tissues.

• Do not spread to other organs (metastasize) or to lymph nodes.

• Can compress surrounding tissues, causing functional problems.

In the United States, the three most common causes of death are:

• Cardiovascular disease (28.5% of all deaths).

• Cancer (22.8% of all deaths).

• Cerebrovascular disease, primarily stroke (6.7% of all deaths).

The leading causes of cancer death in the United States, with lung cancer by far the most common, are shown in *Table 22.1*.

Environmental factors, particularly cigarette smoke, are associated with many forms of cancer. In this chapter, we will use a case of lung cancer to illustrate the characteristics of an acquired cancer and to discuss methods of detection and treatment.

WORD	PRONUNCIATION	ELEMENTS		DEFINITION
benign (adj)	bee-**NINE**		Latin *kind*	Denoting the nonmalignant character of a neoplasm or illness
cancer cancerous (adj)	**KAN**-ser **KAN**-ser-ous	S/ R/	-ous *pertaining to* cancer- *cancer*	General term for a malignant neoplasm Pertaining to a malignant neoplasm
infiltrate infiltration	**IN**-fil-trate in-fil-**TRAY**-shun	S/ P/ R/ S/	-ate *composed of, pertaining to* in- *in* -filtr- *strain through* -ation *process*	To penetrate and invade into a tissue or cell The invasion into a tissue or cell
malignant (adj) malignancy (noun)	mah-**LIG**-nant mah-**LIG**-nan-see	 S/ R/	Latin *hurtful* -ancy *state of* malign- *cancer*	Capable of invading surrounding tissues and metastasizing to distant organs Tumor that invades surrounding tissues and metastasizes to distant organs
metastasis (noun) metastatic (adj) metastases (pl)	meh-**TAS**-tah-sis meh-tah-**STAT**-ik meh-**TAS**-tah-sez	P/ R/ S/ R/	meta- *after, beyond* -stasis *stay in one place* -ic *pertaining to* -stat- *stand still*	Spread of disease from one part of the body to another Able to metastasize
neoplasm (noun) neoplastic (adj) neoplasia (*Note:* The "m" in -plasm is removed to allow the elements to flow.)	**NEE**-oh-plazm **NEE**-oh-**PLAS**-tic **NEE**-oh-**PLAY**-zee-ah	P/ R/ S/ S/	neo- *new* -plasm- *to form* -tic *pertaining to* -ia *condition*	A new growth, either a benign or malignant tumor Pertaining to a neoplasm Process that results in formation of a tumor
oncology oncologist	on-**KOL**-oh-jee on-**KOL**-oh-jist	S/ R/CF S/	-logy *study of* onc/o- *tumor* -logist *one who studies, specialist*	The science dealing with cancer Medical specialist in oncology
proliferate	pro-**LIF**-eh-rate	S/ R/CF R/	-ate *composed of, pertaining to* prol/i- *bear offspring* -fer- *to bear*	To increase in number through reproduction
tumor	**TOO**-mor		Latin *swelling*	Any abnormal swelling

TABLE 22.1 Leading Causes of Cancer Death in the United States

Cause	Percent of Total Cancer Cases	Number per Year
Lung	30.9	154,900
Colon	9.6	48,100
Breast	8.0	40,000
Prostate	6.0	30,200

From National Vital Statistics Report, October 2004.

Abbreviations

CA	cancer
PaO₂	partial pressure of arterial oxygen
2°	secondary
SMI	sustained maximal inspiration

EXERCISES   *Demonstrate that you can use various forms of the same term in correct usage. Insert the appropriate medical term in the following blanks.*

neoplasm   neoplastic   neoplasia

1. _____ is a process that results in the formation of a tumor, which can be either malignant or benign.

2. Another name for a tumor is a _____ .

3. The tumor exhibited _____ behavior and was immediately biopsied.

metastases   metastatic   metastasis

4. A _____ carcinoma is cancer that has spread to a different site than the primary tumor.

5. The patient has _____ in his brain and kidneys.

6. Finding a primary tumor before _____ has occurred increases the chances for a cure.

The term **carcinoma in situ (CIS)**
describes an early form of carcinoma in
which there is no invasion of surrounding
tissues. In many instances, it is a precursor
that will transform into an invasive or
malignant cancer.

TYPES OF CANCER (continued)

Within the broad classes of cancer *(Table 22.2)* are many subgroups, depending on the type of cells in the cancer.

TABLE 22.2 Types of Cancer

Class of Cancer	Cells of Origin	Examples
Carcinoma	Epithelial	Cervical cancer, stomach cancer, squamous cell skin cancer, lung cancer
Sarcoma	Connective tissue, bone cartilage, muscle	**Osteosarcoma, chondrosarcoma, rhabdomyosarcoma**
Leukemia	Blood-forming tissues	Acute lymphocytic leukemia, chronic myelogenous leukemia
Lymphoma	Lymph nodes	Hodgkin disease, non-Hodgkin lymphoma
Melanoma	Melanocytes (pigment-producing skin cells)	Malignant melanoma

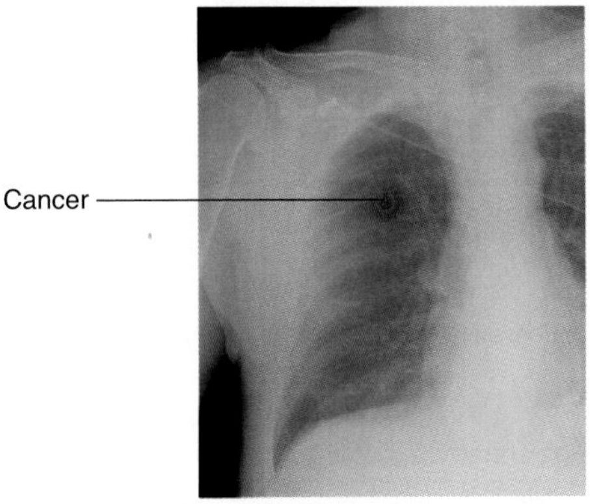

Cancer ——

▲ FIGURE 22.2 Small Cell Cancer of Right Upper Lung.

Lung cancer

Lung cancer has three main subgroups:

1. **Non-small cell lung cancer** accounts for 75% of cases, and 80% of patients die within 5 years of diagnosis. Included in this type are:

   a. **Squamous cell carcinoma,** arising from *round cells* that have replaced damaged cells in the epithelial lining cells of a major bronchus. It accounts for 25% to 40% of lung cancers.

   b. **Adenocarcinoma,** arising from the *mucus-producing cells* in the bronchi. It accounts for between 30% and 50% of lung cancers. It is the most common lung cancer in women, and its incidence is increasing.

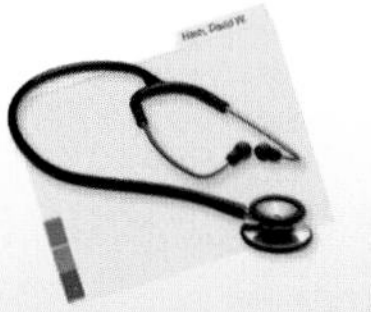

Case Report 22.1 (continued)

Adenocarcinoma was found in Raquel Sacco. It was diagnosed because she had a seizure, and neurologic tests revealed the presence of two metastases in her brain. This led to a search for the primary (1°) tumor that was found in her lung *(Figure 22.2)*.

   c. **Large cell carcinoma,** which includes cancers that cannot be identified under the microscope as squamous cell or adenocarcinoma. It accounts for 10% to 20% of lung cancers.

2. **Small cell lung cancer,** like squamous cell carcinoma, is derived from the epithelial cells of the bronchi but replicates at a faster rate, producing smaller cells. It accounts for 15% to 25% of all lung cancers; most patients die within 18 months of diagnosis.

3. **Mesothelioma** is a rare tumor of the cells lining the pleura. It is associated with **asbestosis** and accounts for 5% of lung cancers.

WORD	PRONUNCIATION	ELEMENTS		DEFINITION
adenocarcinoma	**AD**-eh-noh-kar-sih-**NOH**-mah	S/ R/CF R/	-oma *tumor* aden/o- *gland* -carcin- *cancer*	A cancer arising from glandular epithelial cells
asbestosis	as-bes-**TOE**-sis	S/ R/	-osis *condition* asbest- *asbestos*	Lung disease caused by the inhalation of asbestos particles
carcinoma	kar-sih-**NOH**-mah	S/ R/	-oma *tumor* carcin- *cancer*	A malignant and invasive epithelial tumor
carcinoma in situ (CIS)	kar-sih-**NOH**-mah in **SIGH**-tyu		in situ *Latin in its place*	Carcinoma that has not invaded surrounding tissues
chondrosarcoma	**KON**-dro-sar-**KOH**-mah	S/ R/CF R/	-oma *tumor* chondr/o- *cartilage* -sarc- *flesh*	Cancer arising from cartilage cells
mesothelioma	**MEEZ**-oh-thee-lee-**OH**-mah	S/ P/ R/	-oma *tumor* meso- *middle* -theli- *epithelium*	Cancer arising from the cells lining the pleura or peritoneum
osteosarcoma	**OS**-tee-oh-sar-**KOH**-mah	S/ R/CF R/	-oma *tumor* oste/o- *bone* -sarc- *flesh*	Cancer arising in bone-forming cells
rhabdomyosarcoma	**RAB**-doh-**MY**-oh-sar-**KOH**-mah	S/ R/CF R/CF R/	-oma *tumor* rhabd/o- *rod-shaped, striated* -my/o- *muscle* -sarc- *flesh*	Cancer derived from skeletal muscle
sarcoma	sar-**KOH**-mah	S/ R/	-oma *tumor* sarc- *flesh*	A malignant tumor originating in connective tissue

EXERCISES

Deconstruct the following **language of oncology** *into elements. These elements will form the basis for many additional oncologic terms. Fill in the chart.*

Medical Term	Meaning of Prefix	Meaning of Root/CF	Meaning of Suffix	Meaning of Medical Term
sarcoma				
adenocarcinoma				
chondrosarcoma				
osteosarcoma				
mesothelioma				
rhabdomyosarcoma				

Which of the following best describes *all* of the terms in the table above?

a. They are all malignant tumors.

b. They are all cancerous neoplasms.

c. They are all invasive.

d. a, b, and c

e. only a and b

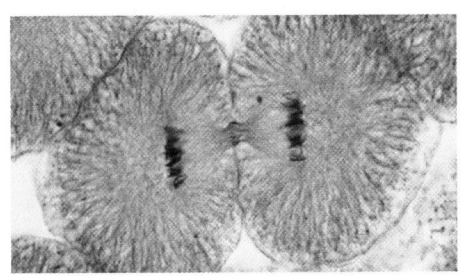

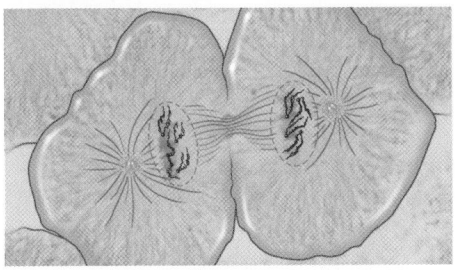

▲ FIGURE 22.3 End Stage of Mitosis. For simplicity, the schematic drawing of the cell *(bottom)* is shown with only two chromosome pairs.

Abbreviations

ETS	environmental tobacco smoke
PCD	programmed cell death
TS	tumor suppressor

Keynote

- A pack-year equals the number of packs of cigarettes smoked per day multiplied by the number of years the person has smoked.
- Cigarette smoke contains over 60 known carcinogens.

CARCINOGENESIS

Carcinogenesis, literally the creation of cancer, is the abnormal rate of cell division as a result of damaged DNA causing gene mutation. Normally, the balance between cell division and proliferation and cell death **(apoptosis,** or **programmed cell death [PCD])** is tightly controlled to maintain the integrity of organs and tissues. Gene mutations that cause cancer disrupt this orderly process. Mutation in a single gene is usually not enough to cause cancer, and carcinogenesis requires multiple mutations in many genes.

Most normal cells cannot divide unless a **growth factor** binds to a receptor on the cell's surface. This growth factor then stimulates the cell to undergo mitosis *(see Chapter 2)* and **differentiate** into mature, functional cells *(Figure 22.3).*

Two types of genes have been identified that play a part in the abnormal cell division and proliferation of cancer cells:

1. **Protooncogenes** are healthy genes that promote normal cell growth. Mutated **oncogenes** cause malfunctions in the normal growth mechanisms. For example, an oncogene called *SIS* stimulates blood vessels to grow into a tumor and provide the rich blood supply it needs to proliferate rapidly. An oncogene called *RAS* generates abnormal growth-factor receptors that switch on constant cell division signals. An oncogene called *HER-2* causes many cases of breast and ovarian cancer. The drug Herceptin is an antibody that targets the HER-2 receptors on the cancer cells. This cuts off the chemical signals that the cell needs to keep proliferating. It also marks the abnormal cells for destruction by the immune system.

2. **Tumor suppressor (TS) genes** normally suppress mitosis and are activated by DNA damage. Their function is to stop cell division so that the abnormal genetic structure cannot be passed on to daughter cells. **Mutated TS genes** cannot do this, so the abnormal cells can divide and proliferate. A mutated TS gene called *p53* is present in half of all cancers and is associated with a poor prognosis and resistance to chemotherapy.

Mutations in both types of genes are usually required for cancer to develop. The oncogenes turn on the abnormal cell growth, and the mutated TS genes cannot stop it.

Cancer is due to the accumulation of genetic injury and mutations. Agents that cause these mutations are called **mutagens,** and mutagens that cause cancer are called **carcinogens.** Particular carcinogens are linked to specific types of cancer. Examples are inhalation of asbestos fibers with mesothelioma, prolonged exposure to radiation and ultraviolet radiation with melanoma and other skin malignancies, and tobacco smoking with lung cancer. Although the link between cigarette smoking and lung cancer is well established, only 15% to 20% of smokers develop lung cancer. In addition, about 10% of the population carries a gene that protects against lung cancer.

Studies in 2004 and 2005 of the epithelial cells in the large bronchi found a large number of genes altered by cigarette smoking. The studies defined genes whose alteration correlated with cumulative pack-years of smoking, and they identified 13 genes whose alterations do not return to normal after smoking is stopped. This could explain the persistent risk of lung cancer in former smokers. In addition, a subset of smokers was identified whose gene alterations have a different profile from that of other smokers. It is possible that this subset is the group who develop lung cancer.

Secondhand smoke, called **environmental tobacco smoke (ETS),** contains the same chemicals and carcinogens as those inhaled by smokers. It is responsible for 3000 lung cancer cases each year in America. The genetic mutations caused by the carcinogens are probably similar to those in the subset of smokers discussed above, even though exposure to the carcinogens is much less than that for smokers.

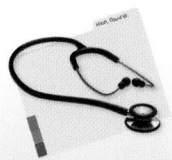

Case Report 22.1 (continued)

Raquel Sacco probably developed her lung cancer as a result of inhaling secondhand smoke all her life (from her father and husband).

WORD	PRONUNCIATION		ELEMENTS	DEFINITION
apoptosis (**Note:** The second "p" is silent.)	**AP**-op-**TOE**-sis	P/ R/	**apo-** *separation from* **-ptosis** *falling*	Programmed normal cell death
carcinogen **carcinogenic (adj)** **carcinogenesis**	kar-**SIN**-oh-jen kar-**SIN**-oh-**JEN**-ik kar-**SIN**-oh-**JEN**-eh-sis	S/ R/CF S/	**-gen** *produce* **carcin/o-** *cancer* **-genesis** *source*	Cancer-producing agent Origin and development of cancer
mutagen	**MYU**-tah-jen	S/ R/	**-gen** *produce* **muta-** *genetic change*	Agent that produces a mutation in a gene
oncogene **oncogenic (adj)**	**ONG**-koh-jeen **ONG**-koh-**JEN**-ik	S/ R/CF	**-gene** *producer, give birth* **onc/o-** *tumor*	One of a family of genes involved in cell growth that work in concert to cause cancer Capable of producing a neoplasm
protooncogene	pro-toe-**ON**-koh-jeen	S/ P/ R/CF	**-gene** *producer, give birth* **proto-** *first* **-onc/o-** *tumor*	A normal gene involved in normal cell growth

No patient with a cancer of any type passes through a hospital without it being recorded by the Tumor Registry. This enables cancer statistics to be maintained at a local level to facilitate such decisions as buying expensive equipment needed for treating certain types of cancer.

EXERCISES

Build your knowledge of elements with this exercise in the **language of oncology**. The element is given to you in the left column; fill in the meaning of the element in the middle column, and identify the type of element (prefix, root, combining form, or suffix) in the right column. The first one is done for you. Then combine the correct elements to form one medical term from this WAD, and write a definition for that term. Fill in the blanks.

> **Study Hint**
> **Ptosis** is a medical term in its own right. Another example is the term **hemolysis**, in which **lysis** is also a medical term in and of itself.

Element	Meaning of Element	Type of Element (P, R, CF, S)
proto	*first*	P
apo		
muta		
genesis		
gen		
onco		
carcino		
ptosis		
gene		

1. Term: _____

2. Definition: _____

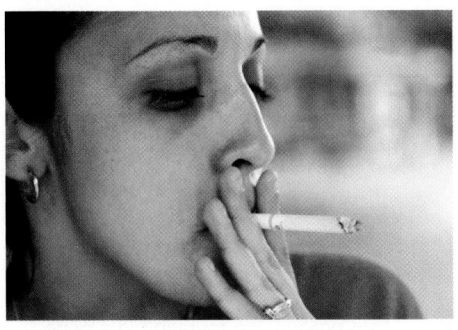

▲ **FIGURE 22.4 Woman Smoking.**

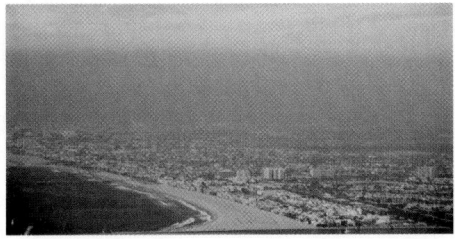

▲ **FIGURE 22.5 Air Pollution over a Large City.**

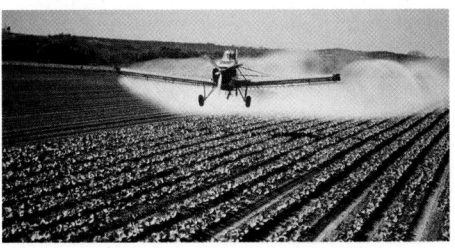

▲ **FIGURE 22.6 Pesticide Spraying of Field of Vegetables.**

Abbreviations	
EPA	Environmental Protection Agency
OSHA	Occupational Safety and Health Administration
PCBs	polychlorinated biphenyls

▲ **FIGURE 22.7 No Smoking Sign.**

ENVIRONMENTAL POLLUTION

Pollution is a trigger of many cancers. For example, cigarette smoke *(Figure 22.4)* causes 87% of all lung cancers and acts in the following way: In the smoke are approximately 4000 chemicals, some 60 of which are known to be carcinogenic and trigger genetic mutations that lead to cancer. Among the inhaled chemicals are cyanide, benzene, formaldehyde, acetylene, tar, arsenic, and ammonia, all of which can increase the risk for cancer.

Radon, a radioactive gas that you cannot see or smell, is the second leading cause of lung cancer (after smoking). It is produced by decaying **uranium** and is found in nearly all soils. In underground miners, it increases the risk of cancer to 40%. It gets into homes through cracks in the foundations or construction joints and is a problem in 1 out of 15 homes. Cigarette smoking on top of radon significantly increases the risk of lung cancer. Testing for radon is cheap and easy.

Air pollution may be the cause of the 10% to 40% increase in lung cancer mortality between urban and rural areas *(Figure 22.5)*. **Particulate matter,** especially very small particles, includes soot, organic material such as hydrocarbons, and metals such as arsenic, chromium, and nickel—all of which are known mutagens and carcinogens. A new analysis shows that premature death from cardiovascular ailments is increased by 24% among people exposed to tiny soot particles.

Chemical toxins are estimated to cause more than 75% of all cancers. Some 77,000 chemicals are used in this country. Over 3000 are added to our food, and most Americans have between 400 and 800 chemicals stored in their bodies, mostly in fat cells. The toxins known to cause cancer include:

- **Chlorine.** Used in drinking water, chlorine produces carcinogenic compounds. Cancer risk among people drinking chlorinated water is 93% higher than that of people not drinking chlorinated water.

- **PCBs (polychlorinated biphenyls).** These were banned years ago but still persist in the environment and are found in farmed salmon.

- **Pesticides.** According to the **Environmental Protection Agency (EPA),** 60% of herbicides, 90% of fungicides, and 30% of insecticides are known to be carcinogenic *(Figure 22.6)*. Farmers using pesticides have a 14% greater risk for developing prostate cancer than do organic farmers.

- **Dioxins.** These are chemical compounds produced by combustion processes from waste incineration and from burning fuels like wood, coal, and oil.

- **Asbestos.** This insulating material was used in the 1950s to 1970s on floors, ceilings, water pipes, and heating ducts. When the material becomes old and crumbly, it releases fibers into the air. Inhalation of the fibers is the cause of mesothelioma.

- **Arsenic.** This is used by insecticide and herbicide sprayers and oil refinery workers.

Occupational Safety and Health Administration **(OSHA)** regulations are designed to protect workers from these environmental hazards.

Prevention of Cancer

More than 50% of cancers could be prevented by **changes in lifestyle and environment.** The same carcinogens that affect the lining of the respiratory tract cause cancer of the oral cavity, pharynx, larynx, and esophagus. They are also absorbed into the bloodstream and disseminated, thereby becoming factors that can cause cancer in the pancreas, stomach, kidney, bladder, prostate, and cervix. **Stopping smoking** alone would reduce the 30% of all cancer deaths due to lung cancer and reduce the incidence of many of the other cancers related to smoking *(Figure 22.7)*.

Clean air measures that are being implemented to reduce the more than 2 billion pounds of toxic air pollutants emitted into the atmosphere annually in this country can reduce the incidence of cancer.

Obesity is said to be linked to about 10% of breast and colorectal cancers and up to 40% of kidney, esophageal, and endometrial cancers. The mechanisms of obesity being linked to these cancers are not understood.

WORD ANALYSIS AND DEFINITION

S = Suffix   P = Prefix   R = Root   R/CF = Combining Form

WORD	PRONUNCIATION	ELEMENTS		DEFINITION
chlorine	**KLOR**-een		Greek *greenish-yellow*	A toxic agent used as a disinfectant and bleaching agent
dioxin	die-**OK**-sin	P/ R/	**di-** *two* **-oxin** *oxygen atom*	Carcinogenic contaminant in pesticides
environment	en-**VI**-ron-ment	S/ R/	**-ment** *resulting state* **environ-** *surroundings*	All the external conditions affecting the life of an organism
environmental (adj)	en-**VI**-ron-ment-al	S/	**-al** *pertaining to*	Pertaining to the environment
flavonoid (alternative spelling: flavinoid)	**FLAY**-vih-noid	S/ R/	**-oid** *resembling* **flavon-** *yellow*	A pigment found in fruit, wine, and tea
genistein	**JEN**-is-tine	R/CF R/	**gen/i-** *produce, create* **-stein** *stone*	Flavonoid found in soy
particle particulate (adj)	**PAR**-tih-kul par-**TIK**-you-late	 S/ R/	Latin *little piece* **-ate** *composed of, pertaining to* **particul-** *little piece*	A small piece of matter Relating to a fine particle
pesticide	**PES**-tih-side	R/CF R/CF	**-cid/e** *to kill* **pest/i-** *pest*	Agent for destroying flies, mosquitoes, and other pests
phytochemical	fie-toe-**KEM**-ih-kal	S/ R/ R/CF	**-al** *pertaining to* **-chemic-** *chemical* **phyt/o-** *plant*	Biologically active, nonnutrient plant chemical
pollution	poh-**LOO**-shun		Latin *dirty*	Condition that is unclean, impure, and a danger to health
uranium	you-**RAY**-nee-um		Greek mythological character, Uranus	Radioactive metallic element

Some **phytochemicals** may offer protection against cancer *(see Chapter 17)*. These include **isothiocyanates** (found in cruciferous vegetables like broccoli and cauliflower), **flavonoids** (found in apples and tea), **resveratrol** (found in the skins of certain red grapes), **lycopene** (found in tomatoes; *Figure 22.8*), and soy protein, which contains the flavonoid **genistein**.

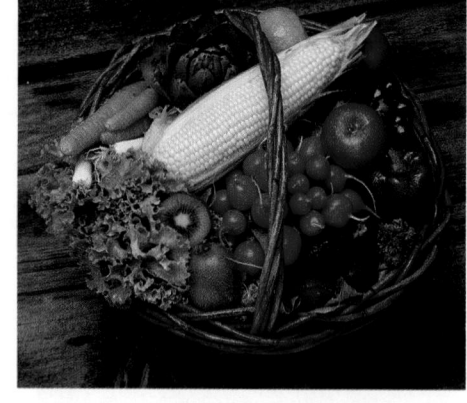

FIGURE 22.8 Foods Containing Phytochemicals That May Offer Protection Against Cancer. ▶

EXERCISES

Demonstrate your knowledge of the following terminology by deconstructing the terms into their elements and then using any one term in a sentence of your own choice (not directly from the text). Fill in the blanks.

1. phytochemical _____ / _____ / _____
           P   R/CF   S

4. pesticide _____ / _____ / _____
           P   R/CF   S

2. environment _____ / _____ / _____
           P   R/CF   S

5. genistein _____ / _____ / _____
           P   R/CF   S

3. flavonoid _____ / _____ / _____
           P   R/CF   S

6. dioxin _____ / _____ / _____
           P   R/CF   S

7. *Pick any one of these terms, and use it in a sentence.*

_____

_____

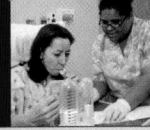

LESSON 22.2 Detecting and Treating Cancer

OBJECTIVES

All that is required for cancer to develop are genetic mutations in one cell, the mother or **progenitor** cell. The daughter cells can reproduce rapidly, but clinical detection by physical or radiographic means is rare for a tumor mass lower than 1 billion cancer cells (about 1 cm in diameter). The earlier the tumor is detected, the better the chance of cure.

The information in this lesson will enable you to use correct medical terminology to:

22.2.1 List methods of cancer prevention.

22.2.2 Discuss methods of self-examination to detect cancer.

22.2.3 Describe methods of screening for cancer.

22.2.4 Explain therapies for treating cancer.

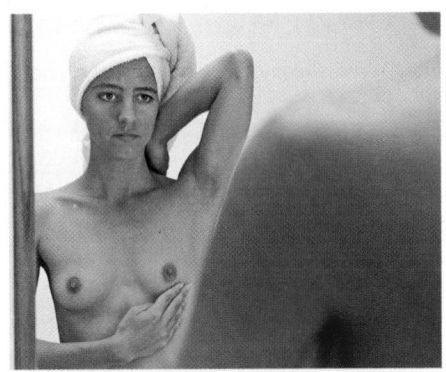

▲ **FIGURE 22.9 Breast Self-Examination.**

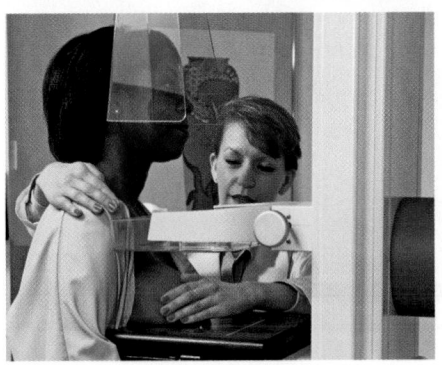

▲ **FIGURE 22.10 Mammography.**

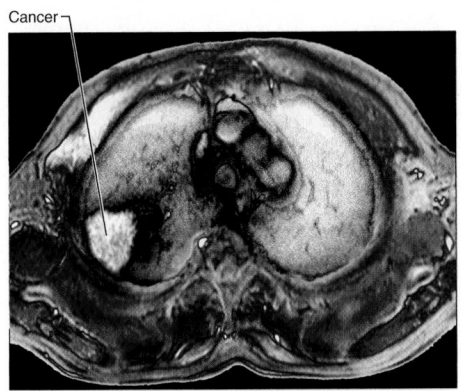

▲ **FIGURE 22.11 PET Scan Showing Cancer in Right Lung.**

DETECTING CANCER

Breast, testicular, and prostate cancers are often detected by **palpation.** This is why some advocacy organizations recommend monthly breast and testicular **self-examination** *(Figure 22.9)*. For prostate cancer, men aged 50 and over should be offered an annual **digital rectal examination (DRE)** and **prostate-specific antigen (PSA)** blood test periodically, although the value of the PSA test is controversial.

Melanoma of the skin is a visible cancer and **self-examination of the skin** in front of a full-length mirror should also be performed monthly by adults.

All self-examinations should be performed in conjunction with health care provider examinations. For example, a **cancer-related clinical examination** should be performed every year for those over age 40. Beginning at age 50, men and women should have a digital rectal examination annually, together with a **fecal occult blood test (FOBT)** as a screening for colon and rectal cancer. Every 10 years a colonoscopy (see page 248) should be performed. For women, a **Pap test** should be performed periodically to detect precancerous cells in the cervix *(see Chapter 13)*.

Screening for Breast Cancer

Mammograms should be performed every 1 to 2 years starting at age 40 *(Figure 22.10)*, and as directed by your health care provider.

Digital mammography records x-ray images in computer code instead of on x-ray film. This technique allows the images to be manipulated to enhance subtle changes in tissue density. Studies are being performed to see if digital mammography is more effective than conventional mammography at finding cancer.

Computer-aided detection scans a mammogram with a laser beam and converts it into a digital signal that can be processed by a computer to highlight suspicious areas. The effectiveness of this technique is also being evaluated.

Magnetic resonance imaging (MRI) creates detailed images of the breast in different planes. This technique is being evaluated for screening women at high risk for breast cancer. MRI is also being used to screen for lung cancer in high-risk patients.

Positron emission tomography (PET) scan uses an injection of **radioactive sugar** to locate cancer *(Figure 22.11)*. Because of their rapid cell division and higher metabolism, cancer cells absorb sugar faster than do normal cells. The areas of increased sugar uptake can be seen on the scans. The scans are good at locating large (bigger than 8 mm), aggressive tumors and sites to which the tumor has metastasized. They are also useful in evaluating and staging recurrent cancer and tracking the response of a tumor to treatment.

Electrical impedance scanning is a technique based on the fact that electricity travels at different speeds through different tissues. Electricity travels rapidly through cancer tissue and appears as white spots on the computer screen of the

WORD	PRONUNCIATION	ELEMENTS		DEFINITION
digital	DIJ-ih-tal	S/ R/	-al *pertaining to* digit- *finger or toe*	Pertaining to a finger or toe
impedance	im-PEE-dahns	S/ R/	-ance *condition, state of* imped- *obstruct*	Resistance to the flow of an electric current
lavage	lah-VAHZH		Latin *to wash*	Washing out of a hollow cavity, tube, or organ
mammogram	MAM-oh-gram	S/ R/CF	-gram *a record* mamm/o- *breast*	The record produced by x-ray imaging of the breast
mammography	mah-MOG-rah-fee	S/	-graphy *process of recording*	Process of x-ray examination of the breast
progenitor	pro-JEN-it-or	P/ R/	pro- *before* -genitor *offspring*	Founder; beginning of an ancestry
radioactive	RAY-dee-oh-AK-tiv	R/CF R/CF	radi/o- *radiation* -activ/e *movement*	Spontaneously emitting alpha, beta, or gamma rays
self-examination	SELF-ek-zam-ih-NAY-shun	S/ R/ R/	-ation *process* examin- *test, examine* self- *me*	The examination of part of one's own body
stereotactic (adj)	STER-ee-oh-TAK-tic	S/ R/CF R/	-ic *pertaining to* stere/o- *three-dimensional* -tact- *orderly arrangement*	A precise three-dimensional method to locate a lesion

scanning system. The device allows an abnormal area found on a mammogram to be viewed from different angles, and it is being studied to see if its use can reduce the need for biopsy.

Image-guided breast biopsy techniques are important in helping doctors obtain biopsies from tumors that cannot be felt but are seen on conventional mammogram. **Stereotactic-guided biopsy** is the use of a computer and scanning devices to create three-dimensional images of lesions seen on a mammogram so that a needle can be inserted accurately into the lesion. Another type of needle biopsy uses a device called a mammatome to gently vacuum out suspicious tissue through a needle.

Ductal lavage collects samples of cells from breast ducts for microscopic analysis. Saline solution is introduced into a milk duct through a fine catheter inserted into the opening of the duct on the surface of the nipple. The solution is then aspirated out through the catheter, and cells in it are analyzed under the microscope to check for evidence of abnormal cells.

Abbreviations

DRE	digital rectal examination
FOBT	fecal occult blood test
MRI	magnetic resonance imaging
Pap	Papanicolaou cervical smear test
PET	positron emission tomography
PSA	prostate-specific antigen

EXERCISES

Patient Documentation: *Insert the correct abbreviations in the following patient documentation. Fill in the blanks.*

1. The patient has been scheduled for a _____ test in the OB/GYN Clinic at noon tomorrow.

2. This patient has an appointment in the Radiology Department at 3:15 p.m. for a _____ scan and

   an _____.

3. Screening for colon and rectal cancer should include a _____ and a _____.

4. Screening for prostate cancer can be done with a _____ blood test.

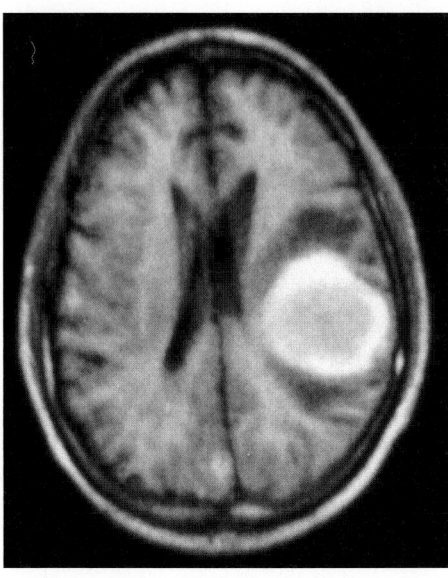

▲ **FIGURE 22.12 MRI Showing Brain Metastasis from a Lung Cancer.**

Abbreviations

AMAS	anti-malignin antibody screen
BAL	bronchoalveolar lavage
CEA	carcinoembryonic antigen
^{99m}Tc	technetium 99m, a radionuclide
TNM	tumor-node-metastasis

Case Report 22.1
(continued)

Because Mrs. Raquel Sacco's cancer has metastasized to her brain, she is placed in stage IV, which has only a 2% 5-year survival rate.

DETECTING LUNG CANCER

Chest x-rays, as a screening tool, rarely provide the first indication of lung cancer. By the time lung cancer is diagnosed by chest x-ray, it often has spread beyond the lungs.

Computed tomography (CT) scans are more effective at identifying early tumors than are chest x-rays.

Positron emission tomography (PET) scans are expensive and not widely available, but they are the most accurate noninvasive test for identifying if the cancer has spread outside lung tissue. PET use may prevent unnecessary surgeries by identifying patients whose cancer has progressed beyond the stage at which surgery is beneficial.

Magnetic resonance imaging (MRI) can locate brain and bone metastases from lung cancer *(Figure 22.12)*.

Scintigraphy utilizes low-level radioactive agents that bind to cancer cells and can be tracked by special cameras to reveal the locations of cancer cells.

Bronchoscopy can locate cancers in the major airways of the lung. Specimens are obtained for biopsy by cutting tissue, using brushings, and using a washing process called **bronchoalveolar lavage (BAL).**

Needle biopsy of tumors in the **periphery** of the lungs is performed by inserting a needle between the ribs and guiding it to the tumor by **fluoroscopy** or CT scan. The biopsy can also be performed using **thoracoscopy,** in which a fiber-optic tube with a camera is inserted between the ribs into the pleural space to view the lungs and take a biopsy.

Mediastinoscopy uses a fiber-optic tube with a camera inserted into the mediastinum via the suprasternal notch to locate appropriate areas for biopsy if the cancer has spread to mediastinal lymph nodes.

Sputum analysis of coughed-up sputum can be a useful and cost-effective method of identifying cancer cells arising from the lining of the airways.

Biomarkers are substances that are released by specific cancers. They can be found in blood, sputum, and tissue samples. Biomarkers under investigation include **carcinoembryonic antigen (CEA),** which is found in 50% of cases of non-small cell lung cancer but is also found in colorectal, pancreatic, and breast cancer.

The blood test **anti-malignin antibody screen (AMAS)** is a general test for detecting any kind of cancer. Most cancers in their early stages secrete the antigen malignin; by using an antibody against malignin, the presence of the biomarker can be detected in the laboratory.

Alpha-fetoprotein levels may be elevated as a biomarker in cancer patients because cancer cells tend to revert to fetal characteristics.

Staging Lung Cancer

Staging defines how localized or how widespread the cancer is. Treatment and prognosis depend on the cancer's stage. The diagnostic tests described above are used to stage the cancer. In addition, brain metastases are identified by MRI and bone metastases by **technetium-99m (^{99m}Tc) radionuclide** bone scans.

The **TNM (tumor-node-metastasis) staging system** is used:

- "T" stands for *tumor* and describes its size and how far it has spread within the lung and to nearby tissues such as the pleura, diaphragm, and pericardium.

- "N" stands for spread to lymph *nodes* around the affected lung or around the other lung.

- "M" stands for *metastasis* to distant sites such as brain, liver, and bones.

Once the T, N, and M categories have been assigned, the information is combined (stage grouping) and given an overall stage of 0, I, II, III, or IV.

In many cancers, another measure of staging, called **grade,** is used. This depends on an assessment by a **pathologist** of the rate of growth of the cancer cells and how likely the cancer is to spread. The most **virulent** cancers are given a grade of 4.

WORD	PRONUNCIATION	ELEMENTS		DEFINITION
biomarker	**BI**-oh-**MARK**-er	P/ R/	bio- *life* -marker *sign*	A biological marker or product by which a cell can be identified
bronchoalveolar	**BRONG**-koh-al-**VEE**-oh-lar	S/ R/CF R/	-ar *pertaining to* bronch/o- *bronchus* -alveol- *alveolus*	Pertaining to the bronchi and alveoli
fluoroscopy	flor-**OS**-koh-pee	S/ R/CF	-scopy *to examine* fluor/o- *x-ray beam*	Examination of the structures of the body by x-rays
grade	GRAYD		Latin *step*	In cancer pathology, a classification of the rate of growth of cancer cells
mediastinoscopy	**ME**-dee-ass-tih-**NOS**-koh-pee	S/ R/CF	-scopy *to examine* mediastin/o- *mediastinum*	Examination of the mediastinum using an endoscope
pathology pathologist	pa-**THOL**-oh-jee pa-**THOL**-oh-jist	S/ R/CF S/	-logy *study of* path/o- *disease* -logist *one who studies, specialist*	Medical specialty dealing with the structural and functional changes of a disease process A specialist in pathology
periphery peripheral (adj)	peh-**RIF**-eh-ree peh-**RIF**-eh-ral	P/ R/	peri- *around* -phery *outer edge*	Outer part of a structure away from the center
radionuclide	**RAY**-dee-oh-**NYU**-klide	S/ R/CF R/	-ide *having a particular quality* radi/o- *radiation* -nucl- *nucleus*	Radioactive agent used in diagnostic imaging
scintigraphy	sin-**TIG**-rah-fee	S/ R/	-graphy *process of recording* scinti- *spark*	Recording of radioactivity with a special camera
stage staging	STAYJ **STAY**-jing		Latin *to stand*	Definition of extent and dissemination of a malignant neoplasm Process of determination of the extent of the distribution of a neoplasm
thoracoscopy	thor-ah-**KOS**-koh-pee	S/ R/CF	-scopy *to examine* thorac/o- *chest*	Examination of the pleural cavity with an endoscope
virulent	**VIR**-you-lent		Latin *poisonous*	Extremely toxic or pathogenic

---

EXERCISES   **Language of Oncology:** *Test your knowledge of the* **language of oncology** *with this exercise. Circle the best answer(s). Some questions may have more than one correct answer.*

1. Which of the following terms contains a prefix?

   periphery   thoracoscopy   virulent   pathology

2. Which term means *specialist?*

   nephrology   pathologist   pathology   fluoroscopy

3. Which term would mean a recording with a special camera?

   biomarker   thoracoscopy   scintigraphy   mediastinoscopy

4. Which is the term for something extremely toxic or poisonous?

   virulent   scintigraphy   bronchoalveolar   peripheral

5. Which of the following terms does *not* mean *to examine?*

   thoracoscopy   scintigraphy   mediastinoscopy   cystoscopy

6. Which of the following terms is a procedure on the chest?

   pathology   bronchoalveolar   biomarker   thoracoscopy

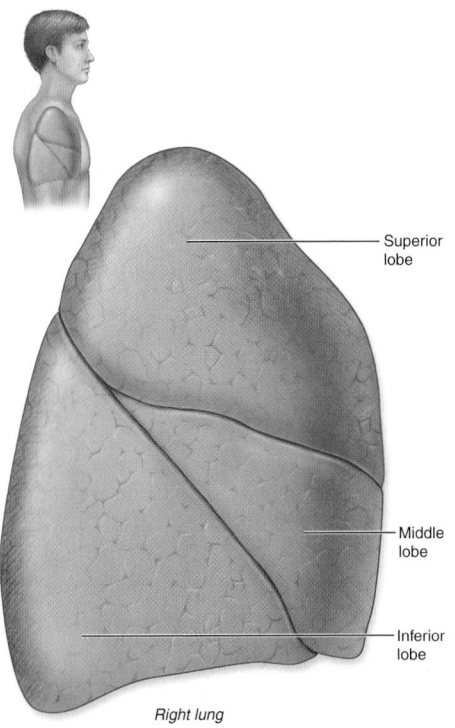

▲ **FIGURE 22.13 Lateral View of Right Lung Showing Lobes That Could Be Removed Surgically.**

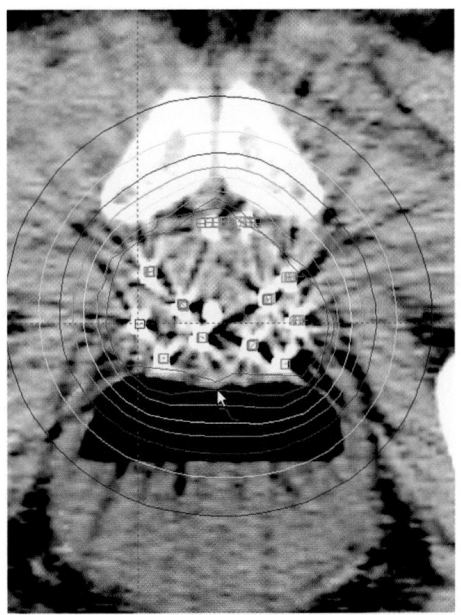

▲ **FIGURE 22.14 Radioactive Seeds Implanted in a Tumor.**

Abbreviations

CHART	continuous hyperfractionated accelerated radiotherapy
SRS	stereotactic radiosurgery

TREATING CANCER

Treatment of any cancer depends on its location, its size, its localization or spread to surrounding tissues and lymph nodes, the presence of metastases, and the cancer's aggressiveness (as determined by pathologic findings on biopsy or surgical removal).

If the cancer is still localized, it can be removed and cure is possible. Unfortunately, few patients are diagnosed at such an early stage, particularly with lung cancer. Even if the original tumor is removed, cancer recurrence rates are high. Additional treatments with **radiation** and **chemotherapy** are used and can produce unpleasant side effects. A patient will have to balance a diminished quality of life against a chance for a modestly prolonged survival.

In the elderly, studies have shown that survival rates are the same for therapies aimed at relieving pain as they are for aggressive, unpleasant treatment **regimens** with their diminished quality of life.

Surgical Procedures

Surgical procedures for specific body system cancers are discussed in the relevant chapters. For example, surgery for breast cancer is covered in *Chapter 13* and for prostate cancer in *Chapter 12*.

The type of surgery for lung cancer depends on the amount of lung tissue that has to be removed.

Wedge resection (segmentectomy) removes only a small part of the lung. It is used for carcinoma in situ, small tumors, frailer patients who cannot tolerate lobectomy, or patients with lung disease.

Lobectomy is removal of one lobe of the lung and is used if the cancer has not spread beyond the lobe or into lymph nodes *(Figure 22.13)*.

Pneumonectomy removes an entire lung and has a mortality of 5% to 8%.

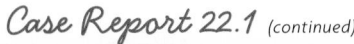

Case Report 22.1 (continued)

Lobectomy was the procedure performed on Mrs. Raquel Sacco. The respiratory therapy she is having is designed to enhance the function of her residual lung tissue.

Laser surgery enables small amounts of lung tissue to be removed and is used for improving symptoms in patients in whom more major surgery is not indicated.

Photodynamic therapy uses bronchoscopy and laser light beams combined with a photosensitive drug called porfimer sodium (Photofrin) to kill cancer cells in the lining of the bronchi in early-stage disease.

Cryosurgery uses a probe chilled to below freezing to destroy early-stage cancer cells.

Radiation Procedures (Radiotherapy)

Radiotherapy does not remove the lesion but distorts the DNA of the cancer cells so that they lose their ability to reproduce and to retain fluids; the cells shrink over time. Side effects of radiotherapy depend on the type of therapy used and occur when healthy cells are damaged during the treatment. Tiredness, nausea and loss of appetite, and sore skin in the treatment area can be short-term effects.

External-beam radiation focuses a beam of radiation directly on the tumor. It is generally used for metastasized cancer.

Brachytherapy implants radioactive seeds through thin tubes directly into the tumor to give high doses of radiation to the tumor while reducing radiation exposure to the surrounding tissues *(Figure 22.14)*. It can be used for inoperable cancers.

Continuous hyperfractionated accelerated radiotherapy (CHART) administers standard doses of radiation multiple times per day. It allows the total dose of radiation to be administered in a shorter period of time than the standard 6 weeks.

WORD	PRONUNCIATION	ELEMENTS		DEFINITION
brachytherapy	brah-kee-**THAIR**-ah-pee	R/ P/	-therapy *medical treatment* brachy- *short*	Radiation therapy in which the source of irradiation is implanted in the tissue to be treated
chemotherapy	**KEY**-moh-**THAIR**-ah-pee	R/ R/CF	-therapy *medical treatment* chem/o- *chemical*	Treatment using chemical agents
hyperfractionated (adj)	high-per-**FRAK**-shun-ay-ted	S/ P/ R/	-ated *process* hyper- *excessive* -fraction- *small amount*	Given in smaller amounts and more frequently
lobectomy	low-**BECK**-toe-me	S/ R/	-ectomy *surgical excision* lob- *lobe*	Surgical removal of a lobe of the lungs
photodynamic	foh-toe-die-**NAM**-ik	S/ R/CF R/	-ic *pertaining to* phot/o- *light* -dynam- *power*	Use of a light-sensitive drug with a laser beam to destroy cells
pneumonectomy	**NEW**-moh-**NEK**-toe-me	S/ R/	-ectomy *surgical excision* pneumon- *lung*	Surgical removal of a whole lung
radiation	ray-dee-**AY**-shun	S/ R/	-ation *process* radi- *x-ray, radiation*	Treatment with x-rays
radiotherapy	**RAY**-dee-oh-**THAIR**-ah-pee	R/CF R/	radi/o- *x-ray, radiation* -therapy *medical treatment*	Treatment using radiation
regimen	**REJ**-ih-men		Latin *direction*	Program of treatment
segmentectomy	seg-men-**TEK**-toe-me	S/ R/	-ectomy *surgical excision* segment- *section*	Surgical excision of a segment of a tissue or organ

Stereotactic radiosurgery (SRS) uses three-dimensional computer programming to deliver a precise, single high dose of radiation in a 1-day session. The most common form of SRS used in the United States is a cobalt-60–based machine called the gamma knife. Though this technique is labeled and implied as "surgery," there is no actual surgery involved.

EXERCISES

Match the element in the left column with its correct meaning in the right column. Some of these elements have appeared in earlier chapters as well.

_____ 1. phot/o

_____ 2. pneumon

_____ 3. brachy

_____ 4. hyper

_____ 5. ectomy

_____ 6. lob

_____ 7. therapy

_____ 8. osis

_____ 9. chemo

_____ 10. otomy

A. condition

B. lobe

C. excessive

D. incision

E. lung

F. light

G. chemical

H. surgical excision

I. treatment

J. short

Abbreviations

MOAB	monoclonal antibody
NCI	National Cancer Institute
NHGRI	National Human Genome Research Institute

TREATING CANCER (continued)

Chemotherapy

Chemotherapy is the use of chemical agents, the majority of which exert their effect by DNA damage that causes the cancer cells to be unable to reproduce and function, and thus they die. Unfortunately, these agents can also harm healthy cells, and that is what causes side effects. The kinds of side effects and their severity depend on the type and dose of chemotherapy. Fatigue, nausea, vomiting, and hair loss are common. Anemia and blood clotting problems can arise from the effects of the chemotherapy on the bone marrow.

Chemotherapy is usually given in regular cycles over several months. Platinum compounds, either cisplatin (Platinol) or carboplatin (Paraplatin) are used in many treatment regimens. They are mostly used with other types of **cytotoxic** drugs in two-drug or three-drug combinations. Side effects are common and vary in severity.

For some cases, chemotherapy alone can be the treatment of choice; for others, a combination of chemotherapy and radiation is used. In many cases, surgery is performed prior to or following these forms of treatment.

Biologic Therapies

Biologic therapies use the body's immune system, directly or indirectly, to attack cancer cells or to lessen the side effects that can be caused by radiation and chemotherapy. **Biologic response modifiers** alter the immune system's response to cancer cells and include interferons, interleukins, monoclonal antibodies, vaccines, and gene therapy.

Monoclonal antibodies (MOABs) are antibodies produced by a single type of cell and are specific for a single antigen. Examples of MOABs are rituximab (Rituxan), used for non-Hodgkin lymphoma, and trastuzumab (Herceptin), used in breast cancer for tumors that produce a protein called HER-2.

Antiangiogenesis therapy interferes with the genetic mechanisms that increase blood supply for the active growth of cancer cells. The drug Avastin has led to a great increase in the survival of patients with colon cancer and is also being used in lung and breast cancer.

Gene therapy is now a focus of cancer therapy. In 2005, the **National Cancer Institute (NCI)** and the **National Human Genome Research Institute (NHGRI)** announced a 3-year pilot project to map the genetic alterations in cancer cells. New technologies called **microarrays** or **gene chips** (small slivers of glass or nylon that can be coated with genes) enable every gene that is active in a cancer cell to be identified.

Gene therapy involves introducing a normal gene into a person's cells to replace an abnormal disease-producing gene *(see Chapter 21)*. Numerous trials are under way to define gene therapy's applications in the biologic treatment of cancer.

Immune therapy is a recent focus of cancer therapy research. Vaccines against lymphoma, prostate cancer, and neuroblastoma have shown promise in extending survival rates.

WORD ANALYSIS AND DEFINITION

S = Suffix   P = Prefix   R = Root   R/CF = Combining Form

WORD	PRONUNCIATION		ELEMENTS	DEFINITION
angiogenesis	**AN**-jee-oh-**JEN**-eh-sis	S/ R/CF	**-genesis** *formation* **angi/o-** *blood vessel*	New formation of blood vessels
antiangiogenesis	anti-**AN**-jee-oh-**JEN**-eh-sis	P/	**anti-** *against*	The prevention of growth of new blood vessels
biology **biologic (adj)**	bi-**OL**-oh-jee **BI**-oh-**LOJ**-ik	S/ R/CF	**-logy** *study of* **bi/o-** *life*	Science concerned with life and living organisms
clone	KLOHN		Greek *cutting used for propagation*	A colony of organisms or cells all having identical genetic constitutions
cytotoxic (adj)	sigh-toh-**TOX**-ik	S/ R/CF	**-toxic** *able to kill* **cyt/o-** *cell*	Destructive to cells
microarray (also called gene chips)	**MY**-kroh-ah-**RAY**	P/ R/	**micro-** *small* **-array** *place in order*	Technique for studying one gene in one experiment
monoclonal (adj)	**MON**-oh-**KLO**-nal	S/ P/ R/	**-al** *pertaining to* **mono-** *one* **-clon-** *cutting used for propagation*	Derived from a protein from a single clone of cells, all molecules of which are the same

EXERCISES

Review the Word Analysis and Definition box on this page to find the answers to the following questions. Circle the best answer, and then fill in the blanks.

1. The term containing a combining form that means *blood vessel* is:

   hemolysis   angiogenesis   environmental

2. The prefix in this term means *one*:

   biologic   dioxin   monoclonal

3. The suffix in this term means *study of:*

   microarray   biology   brachytherapy

4. The suffix in this term means *able to kill:*

   cytotoxic   pnemonectomy   biologic

5. The term containing a word element that means *small* is:

   lobectomy   stereotactic   microarray

6. The term that does *not* contain a prefix is:

   biology   monoclonal   microarray

Test your recall of terms from previous chapters.

7. List as many terms as you can that have the suffix **-logy**, and give a brief definition of each term.

   _____ means _____ .

   _____ means _____ .

   _____ means _____ .

   _____ means _____ .

   _____ means _____ .

CANCER

CHALLENGE YOUR KNOWLEDGE

A. Case Report: The following exercise is based entirely on the Case Report of Raquel Sacco, which was presented in this chapter.

1. Read this entire Case Report out loud to yourself for pronunciation practice. The medical terms you should pay particular attention to have been underlined.

2. Utilize your knowledge of the *language of oncology* (and previous chapters) to answer the following questions based on the Case Report. Fill in the blanks.

CASE REPORT 22.1

You are

. . . an advanced-level <u>respiratory</u> <u>therapist</u> employed by Fulwood Medical Center, working with Tavis Senko, MD, a <u>pulmonologist.</u>

Your patient is

. . . Raquel Sacco, a 44-year-old mother of two teenage boys, who is the owner of a quilting fabrics store. She is 2 days postop from a lung surgery for non-small cell lung cancer. From her records, you see that she has two <u>secondary</u> <u>metastases</u> in her brain. She has been a nonsmoker all her life. Her 70-year-old father is a two-pack-a-day smoker, as is her husband. They both show no evidence of cancer on chest x-rays. Before Raquel is discharged, as part of her <u>postoperative</u> respiratory care plan you are using <u>incentive spirometry</u>—also called <u>sustained maximal inspiration</u> (SMI)—to increase her <u>inspiratory</u> volume and improve her inspiratory muscle performance. You will also be taking an <u>arterial</u> blood sample to check her arterial oxygen pressure (PaO_2).

<u>Adenocarcinoma</u> was found in Raquel Sacco. It was <u>diagnosed</u> because she had a <u>seizure,</u> and <u>neurologic</u> tests revealed the presence of two metastases in her brain, leading to a search for the primary tumor that was found in her lung. Raquel Sacco probably developed her lung cancer as a result of inhaling secondhand smoke all her life (from her father and husband). Because Raquel Sacco's cancer has metastasized to her brain, she is placed in stage IV. The outlook for Mrs. Sacco is bleak.

Non-Small Cell Lung Cancer Survival

Stage	5-Year Relative Survival Rate
I	47%
II	26%
III	8%
IV	2%

1. What is the meaning of the term **postoperative?** _____

   _____

2. Does Mrs. Sacco have a personal history of smoking? _____

3. Is there anyone in her immediate family with a history of cancer? _____

   _____

4. Define **metastases.** _____

5. Where did the metastases appear?

    _____

6. Are the metastases the 1° or 2° cancer? _____

7. Where does her 1° cancer originate? _____

8. What specific type of cancer is the 1° cancer? _____

9. What problem first brought Mrs. Sacco to the doctor? _____

10. What stage of cancer has Mrs. Sacco been diagnosed with? _____

11. Why is her prognosis bleak? _____

B. **Short answers based on the Case Report:**

1. What is the purpose of the SMI spirometry?

    _____

    _____

    _____

2. Explain the phrase "secondhand smoke."

    _____

    _____

    _____

3. Explain the phrase "two-pack-a-day smoker."

    _____

    _____

    _____

4. How can a nonsmoker get lung cancer?

    _____

    _____

    _____

5. Record your thoughts or comments about this patient's case.

    _____

    _____

    _____

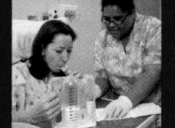

CANCER

C. **Correct Usage:** Demonstrate your knowledge of the *language of oncology.* These are similar medical terms, but each has only one correct use in the paragraph. Fill in the blanks.

carcinogen   **carcinoma**   **carcinogenic**   **carcinogenesis**

1. Raquel Sacco was unknowingly exposed to a _____ in the form of secondhand smoke. This

_____ substance brought about the _____ of her tumors. Her primary

_____ has already metastasized; her prognosis is poor.

metastasis   **metastasized**   **metastases**   **metastatic**

2. The _____ of Raquel's primary cancer to a secondary site was discovered after diagnostic study.

The _____ in her brain were not the site of her current surgery. Her _____

lesions may require radiation therapy if they are inoperable. Since her cancer has already _____, her chances of survival are poor.

D. **Prefixes:** Not every medical term will have a prefix; but when they do, it is an extra clue for you in determining the meaning of the term. Fill in the meaning of the prefix; then give an example of a medical term with that prefix and write the meaning of the term. (You may also use terms from previous chapters, but be prepared to define them.)

Prefix	Meaning of Prefix	Medical Term with This Prefix	Meaning of Term
apo			
di			
hyper			
meso			
meta			
micro			
mono			
neo			
peri			
pro			
proto			

E. Terminology Challenge: All of the following medical terms have the same ending, but one term is slightly different in meaning from the others. Find the term, and explain why it is different, even though it appears the same.

lymphoma   melanoma   hematoma   carcinoma   sarcoma

The term is _____ .

It is different because:

_____

_____ .

F. Roots: Deconstruct the following medical terms by slashing (/) the elements. Define only the roots/combining forms in every term. The first one is done for you. Fill in the blanks.

Medical Term	Root(s)/Combining Form	Meaning of Root(s)/Combining Form
adeno/carcin/oma	*aden/o; carcin*	*gland; cancer*
stereotactic		
mediastinoscopy		
neoplastic		
cytotoxic		
bronchoalveolar		
chondrosarcoma		
digital		
monoclonal		
apoptosis		
lobectomy		
progenitor		

G. Study Review: Cancer is a class of diseases characterized by uncontrolled cell division. Using the *language of oncology*, fill in this mini-outline and use it *for study review*. Fill in the blanks.

1. Uncontrolled cell division is caused by damage to a cell's _____ .

2. This damage produces _____ to the genes that cause cell division.

3. Damaged genes can be either _____ or _____ .

4. Proliferation of damaged cells leads to _____ formation.

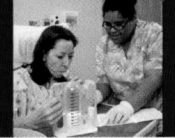

CHAPTER 22 REVIEW

CANCER

H. **Compare and contrast benign and malignant tumors to meet a lesson objective.** You are given a statement about a tumor. Indicate whether it refers to a benign or malignant tumor by placing a check mark (✓) in the appropriate column. When you have finished the chart, highlight all the statements that pertain to malignant tumors *only*.

Description of Tumor	Benign	Malignant
Grows slowly		
Invades the lymph system		
Does not metastasize to other organs		
Invades the bloodstream and travels to other organs		
Lipoma		
Surrounded by connective tissue capsule		
Can compress surrounding tissues and cause functional problems		
Does not invade or infiltrate adjacent tissues		
Unlimited, unregulated growth potential		
Invades or infiltrates adjacent tissues		
Does not spread to lymph nodes		
Mesothelioma		

I. **Elements can provide a clue to the origin of a tumor.** Analyze the medical terms in the left column, and match them to the cancer source in the right column.

Medical Term:

_____ 1. mesothelioma

_____ 2. sarcoma

_____ 3. adenocarcinoma

_____ 4. osteosarcoma

_____ 5. melanoma

_____ 6. chondrosarcoma

_____ 7. carcinoma

_____ 8. lymphoma

_____ 9. rhabdomyosarcoma

Cancer Arises From:

A. epithelial cells

B. lymph nodes

C. cells lining pleural cavity

D. connective tissue cells

E. glandular epithelial cells

F. skeletal muscle

G. bone-forming cells

H. pigment-producing skin cells

I. cartilage cells

J. **Deconstruct the following medical terms into basic elements.** These elements will be the basis for multiple terms in medical vocabulary. Fill in the chart. Complete the exercise by using any two terms from the chart in sentences of patient documentation.

Medical Term	Meaning of Prefix	Meaning of Root/CF	Meaning of Suffix	Meaning of Medical Term
pathology				
neoplasm				
infiltrate				
carcinogen				
metastasis				
pneumonectomy				
digital				
fluoroscopy				
oncology				

1. Sentence: _____

_____

_____

2. Sentence: _____

_____

_____

K. **Abbreviations must be used with care to ensure you are conveying precise information.** Demonstrate your knowledge of this chapter's abbreviations by matching them correctly.

_____ 1. genes normally suppress mitosis   A. PCD

_____ 2. injection of radioactive sugar   B. PSA

_____ 3. chemical toxin banned years ago   C. FOBT

_____ 4. general test for detecting cancer   D. PET

_____ 5. performed by respiratory therapist   E. AMAS

_____ 6. blood in stool   F. MRI

_____ 7. washing process with a scope   G. TS

_____ 8. apoptosis   H. PCB

_____ 9. detailed images in planes   I. BAL

_____ 10. blood test for men   J. SMI

CANCER

L. Procedures: There are many different procedures associated with cancer diagnosis and treatment. Can you correctly identify these procedures used for cancer patients? Circle the best choice.

1. Mrs. Sacco had this surgery at the site of her primary cancer:

   pneumonectomy   bronchoscopy   lobectomy

2. Examination of the pleural cavity with an endoscope:

   thoracoscopy   cystoscopy   bronchoscopy

3. Uses a chilled probe to destroy early cancer cells:

   brachytherapy   chemotherapy   cryosurgery

4. Fiber-optic tube with a camera is inserted into the chest:

   computed tomography   mediastinoscopy   fluoroscopy

5. Implants radioactive seeds into the tumor for direct radiation:

   brachytherapy   CHART   photodynamic therapy

6. Removes only a small part of the lung and is used for carcinoma in situ:

   SRS   segmentectomy   pneumonectomy

7. Creates three-dimensional images of a lesion for accurate insertion of a needle:

   PET scan   stereotactic guided biopsy   ductal lavage

8. Removal of an entire lung:

   lobectomy   segmentectomy   pneumonectomy

9. Employed for cutting tissue, collecting brushings, and washings in the lung:

   bronchoscopy   scintigraphy   chest x-ray

10. More effective than chest x-rays at identifying early tumors:

    CT   PET   MRI

M. Suffixes can provide additional information about a medical term. Analyze the suffix in each of the following terms, and use it to provide a clue about the term. Fill in the blanks.

1. angiogenesis: The suffix is _____ and means _____.

2. neoplasia: The suffix is _____ and means _____.

3. neoplastic: The suffix is _____ and means _____.

4. oncology: The suffix is _____ and means _____.

5. oncologist: The suffix is _____ and means _____.

6. pneumonectomy: The suffix is _____ and means _____.

7. chondrosarcoma: The suffix is _____ and means _____.

8. mediastinoscopy: The suffix is _____ and means _____.

9. scintigraphy: The suffix is _____ and means _____.

N. Recall and Review: How well do you remember these word elements from the previous chapter? Try to answer without first looking back to check. Fill in the blanks.

Element	Type of Element (P, R, CF, S)	Meaning of Element
1. auto		
2. chromo		
3. ist		
4. hetero		
5. dys		

O. Commonalities: Analyze the following medical terms, and discover what they all have in common. Circle the correct answer.

1. Lobectomy, segmentectomy, and mastectomy are all:

   diagnoses   procedures   diagnostic tests

2. Chondrosarcoma, adenocarcinoma, and osteosarcoma are all:

   neoplasms   tumors   both of these

3. PET, MRI, and CT are all:

   blood tests   diagnostic tests   surgeries

4. Thoracoscopy, bronchoscopy, and mediastinoscopy are all:

   chest procedures   pelvic procedures   abdominal procedures

5. Pathologist, oncologist, and histologist are all:

   diseases   specialists   conditions

P. Procedures: An important distinction to learn about procedures is understanding which ones are diagnostic (used to determine a diagnosis) and which ones are therapeutic (carry out treatment). Analyze the following list of medical terms and abbreviations to determine whether they are diagnostic or therapeutic procedures. Place a checkmark (✓) in the appropriate column of the chart.

Procedure	Diagnostic	Therapeutic
segmentectomy		
BAL		
brachytherapy		
DRE		
stereotactic biopsy		
pneumonectomy		
ductal lavage		
mediastinoscopy		
CHART		

CANCER

Q. Cancer Quiz: Assess your knowledge of this chapter by correctly answering the following questions on cancer. The *language of oncology* will aid your understanding of the questions and possible answers. Circle the correct choice, and remember there is only one *best* answer.

1. Second leading cause of lung cancer (after smoking):

   a. air pollution

   b. radon

   c. chemical toxins

   d. PCBs

   e. particulate matter

2. Used to vacuum out suspicious breast tissue through a needle:

   a. gamma knife

   b. lavage

   c. bronchoscopy

   d. mammatome

   e. mammogram

3. In the TNM staging system for cancer, the "N" stands for:

   a. nothing

   b. normal

   c. neoplasm

   d. node

   e. noninvasive

4. A screening test for female breast cancer is:

   a. mammogram

   b. colonoscopy

   c. Pap smear

   d. PSA blood test

   e. sigmoidoscopy

5. Tumor that has invaded or infiltrated has:

   a. grown into adjacent tissue

   b. died

   c. become weaker

   d. mutated

   e. necrotized

6. Healthy genes that promote normal cell growth are called:

   a. TS genes

   b. mutated TS genes

   c. protooncogenes

   d. mutated genes

   e. receptor genes

7. A benign tumor is:

   a. not harmful

   b. very weak

   c. metastatic

   d. necrotic

   e. harmful

8. An early form of carcinoma in which there is no invasion of surrounding tissues is:

   a. large cell carcinoma

   b. small cell carcinoma

   c. adenocarcinoma

   d. carcinoma in situ

   e. squamous cell carcinoma

9. The abbreviation PCD means the same as:

   a. protooncogene

   b. apoptosis

   c. oncogene

   d. polychlorinated biphenyls

   e. phytochemicals

10. Washing out of a hollow duct or cavity is:

    a. stereotactic biopsy

    b. lavage

    c. curettage

    d. aspiration

    e. gavage

CANCER

R. **Elements:** You are given the meaning of the element. Circle the correct term in which it appears.

1. The root meaning *surroundings* is in the term:

   environment   dioxin   pollution

2. The combining form meaning *producing* is in the term:

   genistein   pesticide   particle

3. The combining form meaning *plant* is in the term:

   phytochemical   particle   environment

4. The suffix meaning *to kill* is in the term:

   aminoketone   pollution   pesticide

5. The suffix meaning *pertaining to* is in the term:

   pollution   environmental   hemostasis

6. The prefix meaning *two* is in the term:

   pesticide   dioxin   genistein

7. The combining form meaning *chest* is in the term:

   fluoroscopy   thoracoscopy   endoscopy

8. The root meaning *flesh* is in the term:

   sarcoma   hematoma   carcinoma

S. **Patient Education:** Explain to your patient the difference between a benign and a malignant neoplasm.

benign:

_____

_____

malignant:

_____

_____

Write a sentence of patient documentation using either the term benign *or the term* malignant.

Sentence: _____

_____

_____

T. **Abbreviations:** Transcribe into plain English the following physician orders with abbreviations. Patient safety depends on your precise interpretation of these orders. Fill in the blanks.

1. Patient's next yearly physical should include PSA, DRE, and FOBT.

   _____

   _____

   _____

   _____

2. Schedule this patient for a bronchoscopy with BAL.

   _____

   _____

   _____

   _____

3. Patient's blood work should include PSA, CEA, and AMAS analysis.

   _____

   _____

   _____

   _____

4. Treatment plan includes eventual CHART or SRS after conclusion of chemotherapy.

   _____

   _____

   _____

   _____

5. I am referring this patient to the NCI for a clinical trial using MOABs for her CA.

   _____

   _____

   _____

   _____

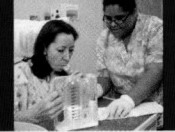

CANCER

CHAPTER SUMMARY EXERCISE

1. *Listen to the pronunciation of the medical terms as given by your instructor.*
2. *Circle the correct spelling of the medical term.*
3. *Match the correctly spelled terms to the brief descriptions below.*
4. *Write a sentence for each of the 10 terms that appear in this exercise.*

A. SPELLING COMPREHENSION: CIRCLE THE CORRECT SPELLING OF THE TERM.

1. fluoroscopy	flueroscopy	fluorroscopy	foroscopy	floroscopy
2. apotosis	apoptosis	apoptossis	apotosus	apoptossus
3. regiment	regimen	regeemen	regimin	regimine
4. radionuclede	radionuklide	radeonuclide	rodeonuclide	radionuclide
5. levage	leevage	lavage	levege	laevage
6. porliferate	porlifferate	proliferate	proleferate	porleferate
7. metastasis	metassasis	mettasasis	meatus	metasasis
8. neoplasea	nioplasia	neoplasis	neoplasia	nioplassia
9. cytotoxic	sytotoxic	cyttotoxic	cytotoxsic	cytoxic
10. steeriotactic	stereotactic	steeriotaxic	steriotaxic	stereotaxic

B. MATCH THE NUMBER OF THE CORRECT TERM IN PART A WITH THE BRIEF DESCRIPTION OF THE TERM BELOW.

a. Radioactive agent used in diagnostic imaging _____

b. Examination of the body with x-rays _____

c. Destructive to cells _____

d. Program of treatment _____

e. Process and growth of a tumor _____

f. To wash _____

g. Spread of cancer cells _____

h. Increase in number by reproducing _____

i. PCD _____

j. Three-dimensional method of locating lesions _____

C. USING YOUR KNOWLEDGE OF TERMS 1–10 IN PART A AND THEIR CORRECT SPELLING, WRITE A BRIEF SENTENCE FOR EACH OF THE TERMS AS IT MIGHT APPEAR IN PATIENT DOCUMENTATION.

1. _____

2. _____

3. _____

4. _____

5. _____

6. _____

7. _____

8. _____

9. _____

10. _____

D. YOUR INSTRUCTOR WILL DIRECT YOU TO MCGRAW-HILL CONNECT. OPEN THE AUDIO GLOSSARY AND PRACTICE YOUR PRONUNCIATION OF THE TERMS IN PART A OF THIS EXERCISE.

E. MEET LESSON OBJECTIVES: APPLY YOUR KNOWLEDGE OF MEDICAL LANGUAGE, AND BRIEFLY ANSWER THE FOLLOWING QUESTIONS.

1. Explain the role of environmental factors in carcinogenesis.

   _____

   _____

2. Classify the type of cancer by the type of cell from which it originates.

   _____

   _____

   _____

3. List methods of cancer prevention.

   _____

   _____

4. What types of self-examination should be employed to detect cancer?

   _____

5. Describe some methods of screening for cancer. _____

   _____

6. What therapies are currently available for treating cancer?

   _____

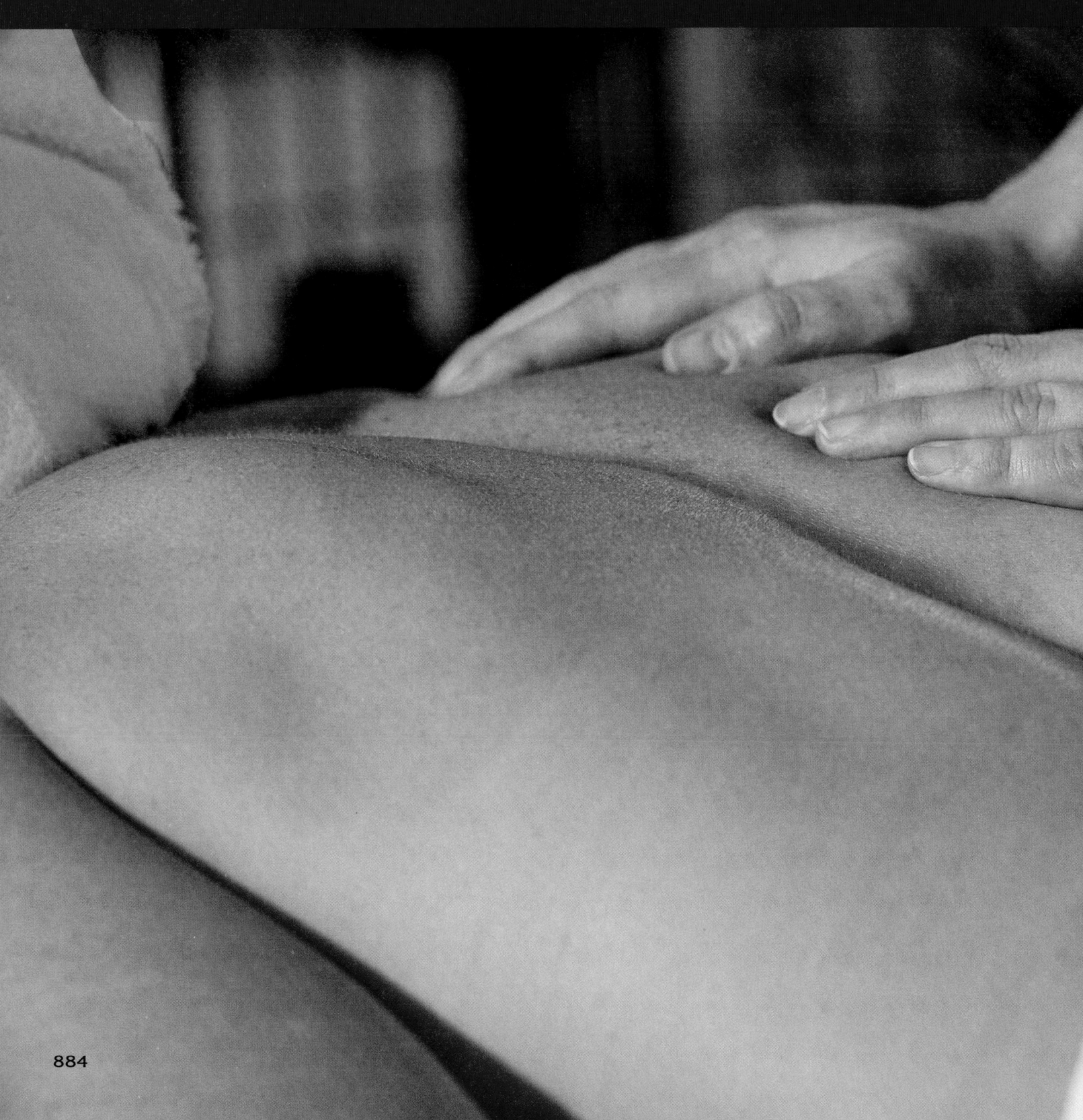

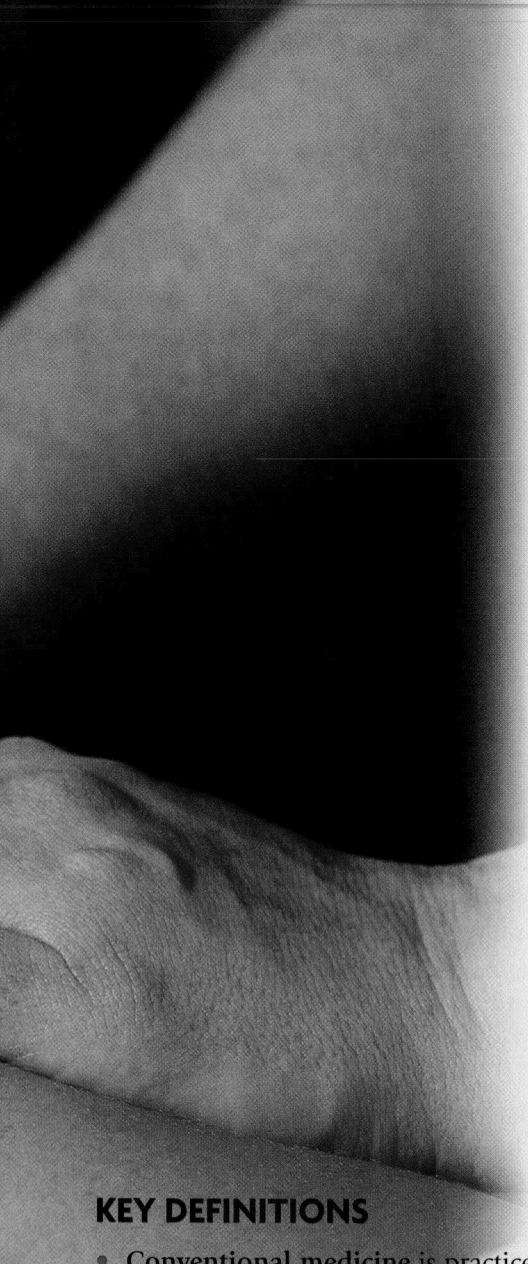

CASE REPORT 23.1

You are

...a **massage** therapist employed in the Pain Management Clinic at Fulwood Medical Center.

Your patient is

...Mrs. Mary Carr, a 65-year-old retired librarian who had been in good health until 6 months ago, when she had a sudden onset of severe pain in the muscles of her shoulders, upper arms, hips, and thighs. She was diagnosed as having polymyalgia rheumatica. Prednisone, 5 mg **t.i.d.**, has produced significant relief in the pain, but she is still having difficulty with such movements as turning over in bed and getting in and out of her car. Twice weekly, she is receiving massage therapy to the muscles of her shoulder and pelvic girdles. Once weekly, she is receiving acupuncture.

KEY DEFINITIONS

- **Conventional medicine** is practiced by holders of MD or DO degrees and their health professionals such as registered nurses and therapists. Other terms for conventional medicine include **allopathic,** Western, traditional, mainstream, or orthodox medicine.
- **Complementary and alternative medicine (CAM)** is any medical practice, system, or product that is considered not to be part of conventional medicine and standard care.
- **Complementary medicine** is used together with standard or conventional medical treatments. An example is the use of **acupuncture** to help lessen the side effects of cancer treatment.
- **Alternative medicine** is used instead of standard or conventional medical treatments. An example is the use of a special diet to treat cancer instead of conventional surgery, radiation, or chemotherapy.
- **Integrative medicine,** a total approach to care, combines conventional medicine with CAM practices that involve the patient's body, mind, and spirit in the therapeutic process. An example is the use of meditation and relaxation techniques to reduce stress during treatment for hypertension and cardiovascular disease.

Learning Outcomes

CAM practices involve new terminology, not in anatomy and physiology but in systems, techniques, and therapies. The information in this chapter will enable you to:

23.1 Apply the language of complementary and alternative medicine to its different therapies, techniques, functions, and effects.

23.2 Comprehend, analyze, spell, and write the medical terms of complementary and alternative medicine so that you communicate and document accurately and precisely in any health care setting.

23.3 Recognize and pronounce the medical terms of complementary and alternative medicine so that you communicate verbally with accuracy and precision in any health care setting.

23.4 Identify the known effects of complementary and alternative medicine on common disorders.

Complementary and Alternative Medicine Practices

The **National Center for Complementary and Alternative Medicine (NCCAM)** was established by Congress in 1998 and is one of the 27 institutes and centers that make up the **National Institutes of Health (NIH).** Its missions are to explore CAM practices in the context of rigorous science, to integrate scientifically proven CAM practices into conventional medicine, and to disseminate authoritative information about CAM practices to the public and health professionals.

The information in this lesson will enable you to use correct medical terminology to:

23.1.1 **Identify the five major groups of CAM practices.**

23.1.2 **Detail the use of complementary and alternative medicine in the United States.**

23.1.3 **Describe frequently used manipulative and body-based techniques.**

23.1.4 **Explain theories of energy fields in the body and therapeutic practices involving their use.**

23.1.5 **Recognize the benefits of certain biologic-based products.**

23.1.6 **Detail mind-body practices and their known effects.**

23.1.7 **Recognize the philosophies and uses of certain whole medical systems.**

Abbreviations	
CAM	complementary and alternative medicine
NCCAM	National Center for Complementary and Alternative Medicine
NIH	National Institutes of Health
t.i.d.	Latin *ter in die*, or three times a day

CAM PRACTICES

The NCCAM divides **CAM practices** into five major groups:

1. **Manipulative and body-based practices** are based on **manipulation** or movement of one or more body parts. Examples are:

   * **Massage**—manipulation of tissues with hands or special tools.
   * **Reflexology**—use of pressure points in the hands and feet to affect other parts of the body.

2. **Energy medicine practices** are based on the body being a web of energy fields that affect health and well-being. Examples are:

   * **Reiki**—the balance of energy by placing hands on or near the patient and the transfer of energy from one person to another.
   * **Therapeutic touch**—manipulation of a person's energy by a practitioner's hands.
   * **Acupuncture**—stimulation of specific energy points on the body to change or unblock energy fields and promote health.

3. **Biologic-based practices** use substances found in nature. These include dietary supplements, herbal products, and special diets. Examples are:

   * **Vitamins** such as vitamins C and E used with beta carotene to reduce the risk for age-related macular degeneration *(see Chapter 4).*
   * **Herbs** such as St. John's wort, used to treat depression.
   * **Special diets** such as a diet low in purine-rich foods to lower blood uric acid levels and reduce the risk of a gout attack.

4. **Mind-body practices** use a variety of techniques to enhance the mind's ability to affect body functions. Examples are:

   * **Biofeedback**—a technique in which the patient learns how to affect certain body functions, such as heart rate and blood pressure, that are normally out of the person's awareness.
   * **Hypnosis**—an altered state of consciousness in which suggestions can lead to changes in a person's behavior.
   * **Prayer and meditation**—practices that, for example, can slow the progression of cognitive impairment in Alzheimer disease.

WORD	PRONUNCIATION	ELEMENTS		DEFINITION
acupuncture	ak-you-**PUNK**-chur	S/ R/ R/	**-ure** *process, result of* **acu-** *needle, sharp* **-punct-** *puncture*	Use of sterile, hair-thin needles to stimulate the energy pathways known as meridians
allopathic medicine	al-oh-**PATH**-ik **MED**-ih-sin	S/ P/ R/ S/ R/	**-ic** *pertaining to* **allo-** *different from normal* **-path-** *disease* **-ine** *pertaining to* **medic-** *medicine*	Conventional medical practice
homeopathy homeopathic (adj)	ho-mee-**OP**-ah-thee **HO**-mee-oh-**PATH**-ik	S/ R/CF S/	**-pathy** *disease* **home/o-** *the same* **-ic** *pertaining to*	Treatment of disease with minute doses of substances
hypnosis hypnotic (adj) hypnotherapy	hip-**NOH**-sis hip-**NOT**-ic hip-noh-**THAIR**-ah-pee	S/ R/CF S/ S/	**-osis** *condition* **hypn/o-** *sleep* **-tic** *pertaining to* **-therapy** *treatment*	Changed state of consciousness Use of hypnosis in treatment of disorders
manipulation manipulative (adj)	mah-**NIP**-you-lay-shun mah-**NIP**-you-lay-tiv	S/ R/ S/	**-ation** *process* **manipul-** *handful* **-ative** *quality of, pertaining to*	Hands-on adjustment of joints, particularly of the spine Pertaining to manipulation
massage	mah-**SAHZH**		Greek *to knead, handle*	Application of pressure or vibration to soft body tissues
meditation	med-ih-**TAY**-shun		Latin *think over, contemplate*	The focusing of attention or freeing the mind of thoughts as part of a formalized spiritual practice
naturopathic medicine	**NAH**-chur-oh-**PATH**-ik **MED**-ih-sin	S/ R/CF R/	**-ic** *pertaining to* **natur/o-** *nature* **-path-** *disease*	A system of healing based on the healing power of nature
reflexology	ree-flek-**SOL**-oh-jee	S/ R/CF	**-logy** *study of* **reflex/o-** *to reflect, bend back*	Stimulation of reflexes in feet and hands, which correspond to other parts of the body
Reiki	**RAY**-kee		Japan *universal life force*	A healing method using the transfer of energy by placing hands on or near a patient

5. **Whole medical systems** are healing systems that have evolved in different cultures and parts of the world. Examples are:

- **Homeopathic** treatment is given with extremely small doses of substances that produce characteristic symptoms of illness in healthy people when given in larger doses.

- **Naturopathic medicine** emphasizes the treatment of disease through the stimulation of the inherent healing capabilities of the person's own vital force.

- **Oriental medicine** views health as a balance between yin and yang energies and views disease as the physical expressions of an imbalance.

EXERCISES

*Elements will help you understand the **language of complementary and alternative medicine** (CAM). Identify the type of element; then give its meaning. Fill in the blanks.*

Element	Type of Element (P, R/CF, S)	Meaning of Element
acu	_____	_____
allo	_____	_____
naturo	_____	_____
homeo	_____	_____
hypno	_____	_____

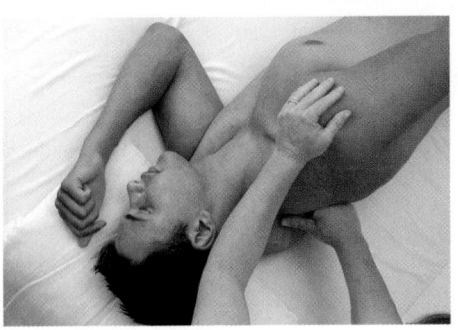

▲ **FIGURE 23.1 Rolfing.**

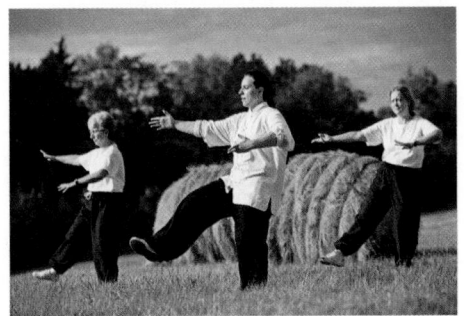

▲ **FIGURE 23.2 Tai Chi.**

Keynote

Thirty-four states require the NCTMB certification for licensure as a massage therapist.

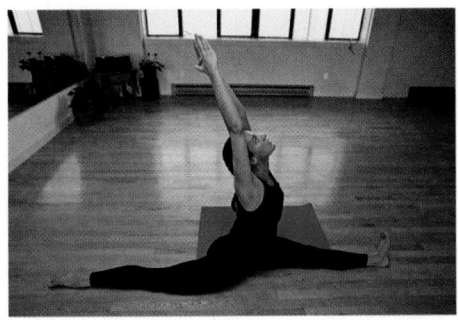

▲ **FIGURE 23.3 Yoga.**

CAM IN THE UNITED STATES

A survey released by NCCAM indicates that, in a year, 48% of adults use at least one CAM therapy. If prayer specifically for health reasons is added, the figure increases to more than 60%. If **megavitamin** therapy is included, the figure increases to more than 70%. According to government estimates, at least $27 billion is being spent annually on CAM.

The majority of people (39%) used CAM to relieve pain; 16.8% used it to relieve back pain, 10% for joint pain and arthritis, 6.6% for neck pain, 3.1% for headache, and 2.4% for recurring pain elsewhere.

Many physicians are reluctant to accept CAM practices because they have not been shown to be effective in clinical trials. Once a CAM practice has been conclusively shown to be effective in a disorder, it will no longer be a CAM practice but will be incorporated into standard medical practice.

New procedures and drugs can be approved only after tests establish that their effect is significantly greater than that of a **placebo,** any treatment or intervention with no intrinsic therapeutic effect.

Manipulative and Body-Based Practices

Massage is not just a luxury found in spas and health clubs. As a complementary treatment, it can promote healing in muscles, tendons, and connective tissues; reduce stress, tension, and anxiety; and improve blood circulation.

The **National Certification Board for Therapeutic Massage and Bodywork (NCBTMB)** is a certifying group for massage therapists in the United States and awards the **NCTMB certification.** Many states do not recognize this, and there is no universally accepted licensure or certification.

There are more than 150 types of massage. The most commonly used are:

- **Swedish massage**—concentrates on increasing circulation to superficial soft tissues.
- **Deep massage**—focuses on increasing circulation to deep muscle tissues.
- **Sports massage**—aids in the recovery of injuries related to sports trauma.
- **Craniosacral therapy**—focuses on the bones of the cranium and sacrum.
- **Neuromuscular therapy**—an umbrella term that includes **trigger point therapy, myotherapy,** and other release techniques. These all focus on the normalization of muscles and the resting length of muscle through neural and muscular interventions.
- **Myofascial release**—uses manual techniques to stretch fascia with the aim of eliminating pain and balancing the body. One form of myofascial release is called **Rolfing,** a system of soft tissue manipulation and movement education *(Figure 23.1).*
- **Thai massage**—emphasizes practitioner-assisted stretching and breathing.

Tai chi is a defined series of movements and postures that flow into each other without pause *(Figure 23.2).* They are performed in a slow, graceful manner. Its physical and mental benefits include stress reduction, improved balance and coordination, and increased muscle strength and agility.

Progressive muscle relaxation is a mental technique used to achieve total muscle relaxation, beginning at the toes and moving up the body to the head.

Relaxation breathing techniques that focus on breathing are used to relax tense muscles and break cycles of negative thoughts about one's health.

Yoga (unity) is a system of lifestyle measures used to improve flexibility and muscle tone, develop breathing and relaxation techniques, and reduce stress *(Figure 23.3).* It entails physical postures, called **asanas,** and controlled breathing exercises.

There are many different styles of yoga being practiced and taught today, including Hatha and Vinyasa.

Applied kinesiology involves testing muscle strength in response to a "question" that is presented to the body. It is used to identify substances and products that can produce benefits or harm to the body.

WORD	PRONUNCIATION	ELEMENTS		DEFINITION
Alexander technique	al-eg-**ZAN**-der tek-**NEEK**		Frederick Mathias Alexander, 1869–1955, Australian actor	The use of awareness and exercises to improve posture, breathing, and movement
asana	ah-**SAH**-nah		Hindu *posture*	Yoga posture or steady position of the body to open energy channels
craniosacral (adj)	**KRAY**-nee-oh-**SAY**-kral	S/ R/CF R/	-al *pertaining to* crani/o- *skull* -sacr- *sacrum*	Referring to the cranium and sacrum
Feldenkrais method	**FEL**-den-kries **METH**-od		Moshe Feldenkrais, 1904–1984, Russian engineer	Series of exercises to discover new ways of pain-free movement
kinesiology	ki-**NEE**-see-**OL**-oh-jee	S/ R/CF	-logy *study of* kinesi/o- *movement*	Study of muscles and body parts involved in movement
megavitamin	meg-ah-**VIE**-tah-min	P/ R/CF R/	mega- *enormous* -vit/a- *life* -min *amine*	Large dose of a vitamin
myofascial (adj)	**MY**-oh-**FASH**-ee-al	S/ R/CF R/	-al *pertaining to* my/o- *muscle* -fasci- *fascia*	Relating to the fascia surrounding and separating muscle tissue
myotherapy	**MY**-oh-**THAIR**-ah-pee	S/ R/CF	-therapy *treatment* my/o- *muscle*	Treatment of muscles by massage
placebo	plah-**SEE**-boh		Latin *I shall please*	An inert compound with no innate therapeutic value
Rolfing	**ROLF**-ing		Ida Rolf, PhD, 1896–1979	Manipulation of connective tissue to realign and balance the whole body
tai chi	tie-**CHEE**		Chinese *supreme ultimate force*	Defined series of postures performed in fluid movement
yoga	**YOH**-gah		Hindu *unity*	A system of lifestyle measures

Case Report 23.1 (continued)

For Mrs. Mary Carr, with her diagnosis of polymyalgia rheumatica, prednisone had produced marked pain relief, and massage therapy is being used to provide further pain relief and reduce associated muscle and joint stiffness.

Abbreviations

NCBTMB	National Certification Board for Therapeutic Massage and Bodywork
NCTMB	National Certificate for Therapeutic Massage and Bodywork

The **Alexander technique** reviews the body's whole movement pattern to increase self-awareness about posture and movements. It is particularly concerned with the relationship of the head to the spine. A 2009 U.K. study found that it may aid in the treatment of back pain.

The **Feldenkrais method** also works with awareness to identify and adjust ineffective, painful movements and to help regain flexibility, coordination, and comfort in movement.

EXERCISES

Complete the term with the correct missing element found in the Word Analysis and Definition (WAD) box on this page. Fill in the blanks.

1. Treatment of muscles by massage _____ /therapy

2. Study of body parts involved in movement _____ /ology

3. Large doses of vitamins, minerals, aminoacids _____ /vitamin

4. Pertaining to the total length of the spine cranio/_____ /_____

5. Relating to the fascia separating muscle tissue myo/_____ /_____

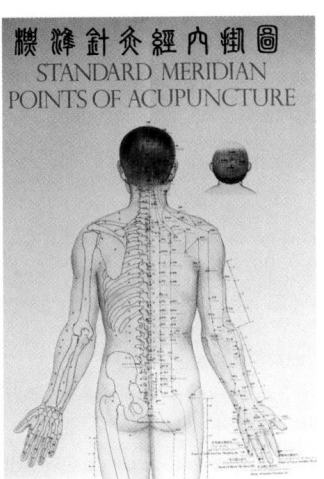

FIGURE 23.4 Chinese Energy Pathways.

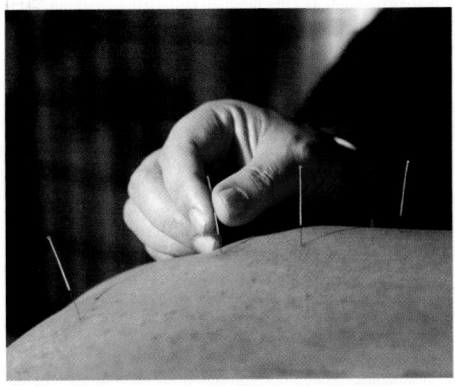

FIGURE 23.5 Acupuncture Needles.

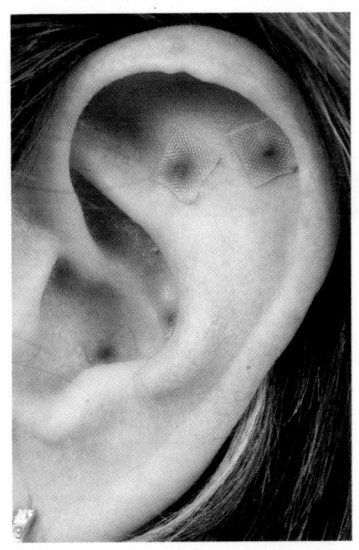

FIGURE 23.6 Use of Magnets for Sleep Therapy.

CAM IN THE UNITED STATES (continued)

Energy Medicine

Modern science, particularly **quantum physics,** has shown that we are a web of energies that exists beneath our physical characteristics, connects our body-mind-spirit system, and gives life to our bodies. This concept is not new. It has been present in other cultures for thousands of years. The energy is called **qi** or **chi** in China, **prana** in India, **ki** in Japan and Korea, and **spirit** in many modern Western healing teachings.

The term **subtle energy** is being used today by scientists to describe these energy forces in the body and environment. **Meridians** are energy pathways that carry energy into, through, and out of the body *(Figure 23.4)*. **Chakras** are seven energy centers that relate to specific organs.

Homeostasis *(see Chapter 2)* is the stable essential in body chemistry. In energy medicine, balance and stability of the body's energy systems are the main essential. When the internal energy balance is disturbed, the body does not work well.

Energy psychology consists of mind-body interventions that involve the human energy matrix. This matrix includes the **biofield** of energy that envelops the body, the energy centers (chakras), and the energy pathways (meridians). Since 2006, the **Association for Comprehensive Energy Psychology (ACEP)** has offered certification programs for both licensed mental health professionals and other energy psychology practitioners.

Acupuncture originated in China more than 2000 years ago and is based on the meridians. **Acupuncture points (acupoints)** on the skin lead into the meridians and can be stimulated with needles (acupuncture) or pressure **(acupressure)** to release or redistribute energy *(Figure 23.5)*.

In 1996, the FDA approved the use of sterile, nontoxic needles by licensed practitioners. It is frequently used as an **adjunct** or **ancillary treatment** in a comprehensive disease management program. It has been shown to be effective in treating postoperative dental pain, fibromyalgia, myofascial pain, osteoarthritis, lower-back pain, carpal tunnel syndrome, and tennis elbow. It has also been effective in treating the nausea and vomiting related to chemotherapy or following anesthesia.

Biochemical and imaging studies have shown that acupuncture triggers the release of opioids in the same areas of the brain that are responsible for the beneficial effects of narcotic analgesics.

Bioelectrical acupuncture, in which the placed needles are attached to a low-voltage electrical stimulation system, is used by many practitioners to enhance the effect of acupuncture.

Therapeutic touch is being used extensively by nurses and other health practitioners for the relief of pain. The most common technique is to keep the hands a couple of inches from the patient's body to release energy into it. Its value is being keenly debated.

Reiki is a Japanese form of healing. The practitioner places hands on specific areas of the body, some of which can relate to the chakras, channeling energy for the body to use. Using its own innate intelligence, the body takes the energy it needs and directs it to where it is needed. It is a three-way partnership among the practitioner, client, and universal energy.

Electromagnetic fields (EMFs) are invisible lines of energy that are produced by the earth, sun, and all electrical devices. We have learned to generate electromagnetic forces and saturate our environment with them. These forces influence our meridians, chakras, and subtle energy systems.

Electromagnetic therapy uses different devices to generate and open magnetic fields. They vary from strapping magnets to the skin *(Figure 23.6)*, to magnetic blankets, to machines used to stimulate the healing of bone fractures. Electromagnetic therapy has been used for numerous disorders. Scientific studies need to be done to define its efficacy.

Polarity therapy is based on the concept that the life-giving energy in the body is governed by opposite poles of positive and negative electromagnetic energy. When the flow of energy is blocked, disease results. Polarity therapy uses the practitioner's hands and fingers to balance the energy field.

WORD	PRONUNCIATION		ELEMENTS	DEFINITION
acupoint	**AK**-you-point	R/ R/	acu- *needle, sharp* -point *to pierce*	Point of entry in the skin to a meridian
acupressure	**AK**-you-presh-ur	S/ R/ R/	-ure *process, result of* acu- *needle, sharp* -press- *press down*	Application of pressure to acupoints
adjunct	**AJ**-ungkt		Latin *joined to*	Something joined to another but is not an essential part
ancillary	**AN**-sil-air-ree		Latin *relating to a servant*	Accessory, adjunct
biofield	bi-oh-**FIELD**	R/CF R/	bi/o- *life* -field *definite area*	Area of energy in and surrounding the body
chakra	**CHAK**-rah		Hindu *center of energy*	One of seven centers of energy in the body
chi (also spelled **qi**)	CHEE		Chinese *force of energy*	Universal life force
electromagnetic	ee-**LEK**-troh-mag-**NET**-ik	S/ R/CF R/	-ic *pertaining to* electr/o- *electricity* -magnet- *magnet*	Pertaining to energy propagated through matter and space
ki	KEY		Japanese *universal life force*	Universal energy of life
meridian	meh-**RID**-ee-an		Latin *midday*	Energy line connecting different anatomical sites
polarity	po-**LAR**-ih-tee		Latin *as the pole of the earth or a magnet*	Possession of opposite characteristics
prana	**PRAH**-nah		Hindu *universal life force*	Vital power
quantum physics	**KWAHN**-tum **FIZ**-iks		**quantum** Latin *how much*	The study of subatomic particles

Light therapy is the use of natural or artificial light to treat depressive and sleep disorders. A bright-light box generates full-spectrum or white light and is used for treating the "winter blues" or **seasonal affective disorder (SAD)**.

Colored light therapy uses floodlights of different colors to treat migraines, and **cold laser therapy** uses low-intensity laser light to reduce inflammation and heal wounds.

Abbreviations

ACEP	Association for Comprehensive Energy Psychology
EMF	electromagnetic field
SAD	seasonal affective disorder

EXERCISES

*Match the definitions in the left column with the correct medical **language of CAM** in the right column. Check this page spread if you are unsure of your answers to the questions.*

_____ 1. point of entry in the skin to a meridian

_____ 2. area of energy in and around the body

_____ 3. means the same as ancillary

_____ 4. transcutaneous insertion of needles

_____ 5. energy line connecting anatomical sites

_____ 6. one of seven centers of energy in the body

_____ 7. energy sent through matter and space

_____ 8. application of pressure to acupoints

_____ 9. main essential in body chemistry

_____ 10. surrounding substance

A. electromagnetic

B. acupuncture

C. matrix

D. acupressure

E. biofield

F. homeostasis

G. adjunct

H. chakra

I. meridian

J. acupoint

CASE REPORT 23.2

Fulwood Medical Center

Mr. Mathew Hickman is a 74-year-old man recently diagnosed with prostate cancer. On a routine annual physical examination, a rectal examination revealed a slightly enlarged prostate with a small central nodule, and his **prostate-specific antigen (PSA)** was elevated. The only urinary symptom he has is occasional urgency.

In consultation with urologist Phillip Johnson, MD, Mr. Hickman learned that most prostate cancers are slow-growing. With minimal symptoms and because of his age, he decided on "watchful waiting" with clinical examinations and PSA tests every 6 months. Dr. Johnson also recommended that a good nutrition program could reduce the progression of prostate cancer.

With the guidance of nutritionist Karen Goodrich, PhD, Mr. Hickman made a commitment to increase organic colorful vegetables and whole grains in his diet. This will provide vitamins, antioxidants, minerals, phytochemicals, and fiber. His supplements include an additional multivitamin, selenium, zinc, and fish oil (with omega-3). He also plans to drink green tea and to take the herb saw palmetto berry extract.

At his last examination by Dr. Johnson, Mr. Hickman's prostate had not enlarged, and his PSA was unchanged. He is continuing with his healthy lifestyle.

Keynote

The 1994 federal **Dietary Supplements Health and Education Act (DSHEA)** permits the sale of dietary supplements over the counter without requiring that the products be proved safe and effective—as is required for prescription or classic over-the-counter drugs licensed by the **U.S. Food and Drug Administration (FDA)**.

Abbreviations

DSHEA	Dietary Supplements Health and Education Act
FDA	U.S. Food and Drug Administration
GMP	good manufacturing practice

Keynote

People who are allergic to the daisy family, which includes ragweed, are more likely to have allergic reactions to *Echinacea*.

CAM IN THE UNITED STATES (continued)

Biologic-Based Practices

Dietary supplements are also called **nutritional supplements** or just **supplements**. They include:

- **Vitamins** *(see Chapter 22)*.

- **Minerals** *(see Chapter 22)*.

- **Herbs**—either as a single herb or mixtures.

- **Botanicals**—another term for herbs.

- **Spices**—such as garlic and turmeric.

- **Amino acids**—such as arginine (a vasodilator) and lysine (helps form collagen).

- **Enzymes**—proteins that speed up chemical reactions in the body. For example, digestive enzymes such as lactaid (for lactose intolerance; *see Chapter 6*), bromelain, and papain.

- **Glandular products**—ingredients made from the glands of animals; for example, extracts from animal thyroid and thymus glands. Many CAM practitioners consider these products ineffective and even dangerous.

Dietary supplements cannot claim to prevent or treat any disease but can claim to maintain "normal structure and function" of body systems. Some dietary supplements have become part of conventional medicine because of their proven efficacy. For example, the vitamin folic acid taken early in pregnancy prevents certain **neural tube** birth defects in newborns; the use of the carotenoid lutein with vitamins C and E and the mineral zinc can slow the progression of the age-related eye disease macular degeneration *(see Chapter 4)*.

Herbal medicines are derived from natural sources. However, natural does not always mean safe. Some mushrooms that grow naturally in the wild are safe, while others are poisonous.

Many herbal medicines can interact with prescription drugs. *Table 23.1* shows some of these interactions.

Supplement manufacturers must meet the requirements of the FDA's **good manufacturing practices (GMPs)** to guarantee product quality and consistency. Unfortunately, what's in the bottle does not always match what's on the label. **Echinacea** is one of the most frequently used herbs to prevent or treat colds and to stimulate the immune system. One study analyzed 59 preparations of *Echinacea* and found half did not provide accurate information about the product. A study of **ginseng** products found that most contained less than half the amount of ginseng listed on the labels.

WORD	PRONUNCIATION	ELEMENTS		DEFINITION
echinacea (common name) **Echinacea** (genus)	ek-ih-**NAY**-sha	S/ R/	**-acea** *condition, remedy* **echin-** *hedgehog*	Spiky North American herb
Ginkgo biloba	**GING**-koh **BIL**-oh-bah		Chinese tree with bilobed leaves	Extract of leaves used as a vasodilator
ginseng	**JIN**-seng		Chinese *man root or image*	Extract made from the root of a Chinese plant
neural tube	**NYU**-ral TYUB	S/ R/	**-al** *pertaining to* **neur-** *nerve, nerve tissue*	Embryologic tubelike structure that forms the brain and spinal cord
supplement	**SUH**-pleh-ment	R/	**supplement** *supply to remedy a deficiency*	Substance taken to remedy or prevent a deficiency

TABLE 23.1 Herbal Interactions with Prescription Drugs

Herb	Prescription Drug	Effect of Interaction
Ginkgo biloba	Anticoagulants (e.g., coumadin)	Increased risk of bleeding
Ginseng	Diabetes medications (e.g., insulin, tolbutamide)	Lower blood sugar levels
St. John's wort	a. Antidepressives b. Anticancer drugs c. Birth control drugs d. HIV protease inhibitor	a. Increases effects b. Reduces effects c. Reduces effects d. Reduces effects
Echinacea	Immunosuppressant drugs	Decreases effectiveness
Garlic	Anticoagulants (e.g., coumadin)	Increased risk of bleeding

EXERCISES

After reading Case Report 23.2 on the opposite page, answer the following questions. Be prepared to discuss your answers in class.

1. What findings were present on this examination that indicated Mr. Hickman has prostate cancer? _____
   _____

2. What was his only urinary symptom? _____

3. Why has Mr. Hickman elected to do "watchful waiting" for his cancer? _____
   _____

4. Do you think his age played a part in his decision to do that? Why?
   _____
   _____

5. What can Mr. Hickman do to help himself? _____
   _____

6. Name one benefit to Mr. Hickman from each of the following: "vitamins, antioxidants, minerals, phytochemicals, and fiber."
   _____
   _____
   _____
   _____

CAM IN THE UNITED STATES (continued)

Mind-Body Medicine

Mind-body medicine is based on the interactions between the mind (as expressed by the brain), body, and behavior. It shows the powerful ways in which mental, emotional, and spiritual interventions can affect behavior and health. It also emphasizes each person's individual responsibility for self-care and health.

Biofeedback is a method of taking information through a variety of monitoring procedures and equipment to learn how to control certain involuntary body responses. These responses include:

- Muscle tension
- Blood pressure
- Heart rate
- Brain activity

The machines and techniques used in biofeedback include:

- **Electromyogram (EMG)** uses electrodes to measure muscle tension. Early recognition of the tension enables relaxation of the muscles to be actively generated. It is used for headaches, neck pain, back pain, and **bruxism** (grinding the teeth).

- **Temperature biofeedback** uses sensors attached to fingers to measure skin temperature *(Figure 23.7)*. Stress often drops skin temperature due to vasoconstriction, and this technique prompts relaxation and vasodilation. It is used in peripheral vascular disease and to reduce the frequency of migraine attacks.

- **Galvanic skin response (GSR) training** uses sensors to measure the amount of perspiration on the skin, thus alerting the person to anxiety. It is used in treating emotional disorders such as anxiety and phobias.

The **Biofeedback Certification Institute of America (BCIA)** certifies biofeedback therapists, who must be licensed in another area of health care or be working under the guidance of a health care professional.

Meditation has been practiced for thousands of years, mostly in the Eastern cultures in spiritual and mystical contexts. Its technique is to concentrate on the moment and clear the mind of chattering thoughts and worries. It is used to prevent or reduce stress and for anxiety, depression, hypertension, and coronary artery disease.

Recent studies have shown that meditation increases brain activity and size in areas associated with positive emotional states and areas involved in control of the autonomic nervous system.

Prayer can be defined as an active process of appealing to a higher power. It is frequently used for health reasons on behalf of oneself or for others.

Spirituality can be defined as a person's sense of purpose or meaning to life, beyond material values. Spirituality can be practiced in many ways, including through religion.

The effects of prayer and spirituality on health outcomes are being studied extensively, particularly for their effect on the quality of life for patients with HIV/AIDS and cancer.

Hypnosis (hypnotherapy) aims to reach an altered state of consciousness in which the mind is relaxed and susceptible to suggestions to change behavior or to explore unconscious memories.

Studies of hypnotherapy have suggested a benefit for different types of chronic pain and for postprocedural pain. It is sometimes used with cognitive behavioral therapy *(see Chapter 19)* to treat anxiety, insomnia, smoking cessation, **irritable bowel syndrome (IBS)**, and **posttraumatic stress disorder (PTSD)**.

Visualization (imagery) is based on the theory that the controlled use of mental images to evoke strong emotions or fantasy can help a number of health conditions. The person clearly imagines what she wants to occur or heal and focuses on it frequently to make it part of her life. The results of using this self-help technique are very personal and inconsistent.

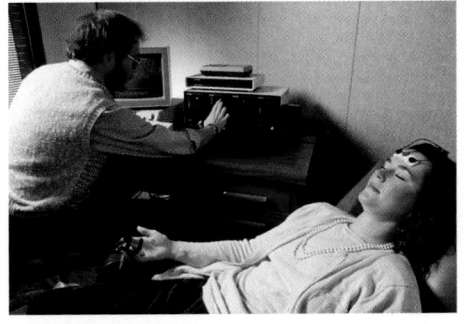

▲ **FIGURE 23.7   Patient Undergoing Biofeedback.**

Keynote

A study in 1986 by insurance companies looked at 2000 meditators in Iowa and found them to be much healthier than the rest of the population in 17 major areas of disease.

A study of AIDS patients found that frequency of prayer was related to longer survival.

A study in Iowa linked church attendance with living longer.

Abbreviations

BCIA	Biofeedback Certification Institute of America
EMG	electromyogram
GSR	galvanic skin response
IBS	irritable bowel syndrome
PTSD	posttraumatic stress disorder

Keynote

Of all adults, 10% to 15% are highly hypnotizable, and 20% are highly resistant. The rest are between these extremes.

Creative therapists are usually part of a team that includes doctors, physical therapists, speech therapists, and occupational therapists.

WORD	PRONUNCIATION	ELEMENTS		DEFINITION
bruxism	**BRUK**-sizm		Greek *to grind the teeth*	Gritting or grinding together of the teeth, often during sleep
electromyogram	ee-lek-troh-**MY**-oh-gram	S/ R/CF R/CF	**-gram** *record* **electr/o-** *electric* **-my/o-** *muscle*	Recording of electric currents associated with muscle action
galvanic	gal-**VAN**-ik	S/ R/	**-ic** *pertaining to* **galvan-** *low-voltage current*	Pertaining to electric current
imagery	**IM**-aj-ree	S/ R/	**-ery** *condition, process of* **imag-** *likeness*	Visualization of pleasant fantasies
spirituality	**SPEAR**-ih-choo-**AL**-ity	S/ S/ R/CF	**-ity** *condition* **-al-** *pertaining to* **spirit/u-** *spirit*	Meaning to life that comes from the spirit or soul rather than the physical body
visualization	**VIH**-zhoo-wah-lih-**ZAY**-shun	S/ S/ S/ R/	**-ation** *process* **-iz-** *subject to* **-al-** *pertaining to* **visu-** *sight*	The forming of mental images or pictures

Note: Not a single term in this WAD has a prefix. Roots or combining forms can appear at the beginning of a term.

Creative therapies, such as dance, music, drama, or art, allow patients to express difficult emotions such as anger or grief and to express what cannot be said. Originally designed for people with physical and mental disabilities, they are also being used in the rehabilitation phase of many illnesses and in dealing with stress and bereavement.

EXERCISES

Meet lesson objectives by briefly answering the following questions about mind-body medicine.

1. There are three types of diagnostic *biofeedback* that all involve the use of sensors. List what they are and what they measure.

_____

_____

_____

2. What is the purpose of *biofeedback?*

_____

_____

3. What body responses can *biofeedback* help control?

_____

_____

_____

_____

4. What conditions can *hypnotherapy* benefit?

_____

_____

_____

_____

5. Define *bruxism.* _____

Mrs. Andrea Turpin is a 39-year-old civil servant, married with three children between 12 and 7 years. Since adolescence, she has had a moderate scoliosis of her spine, producing recurrent back pain *(Figure 23.8)*. Her orthopedic surgeon prescribed Vioxx and suggested spinal surgery with the placement of rods.

Her Web research showed that Vioxx had significant side effects, with an increased risk of heart attacks and strokes, and that the surgery did not guarantee relief of pain and had a long and difficult rehabilitation.

She explored CAM alternatives, visited a chiropractor, and now also has acupuncture and neuromuscular massage. She has minimal pain and is able to manage her life and enjoy skiing.

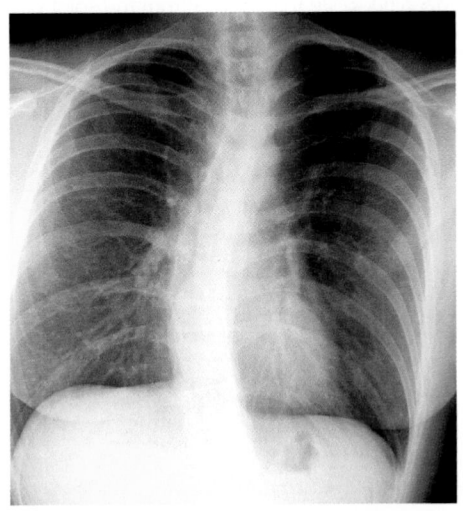

▲ **FIGURE 23.8 X-Ray of Scoliosis of the Spine.**

Keynote

The results of controlled trials of homeopathy are contradictory. In some trials, homeopathy is no more effective than a placebo. In others, the results were greater than those from a placebo.

Licensed naturopathic physicians have completed 4 years of education in basic and clinical sciences.

There is no national standard for licensing Ayurvedic practitioners in the United States.

Abbreviation

NCCAOM National Certification Commission for Acupuncture and Oriental Medicine

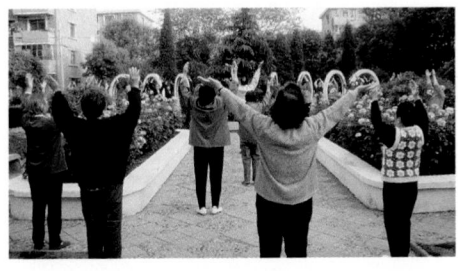

▲ **FIGURE 23.9 Qigong.**

WHOLE-MEDICINE SYSTEMS

Chiropractic medicine has its primary focus on the detection, reduction, and correction of spinal misalignments and resulting pain and nervous system dysfunction, as in Andrea Turpin's case. **Chiropractors** frequently use manipulation to move tissue. Gentle manipulations are referred to as mobilization or **adjustment.** Chiropractors in training spend 5 years in basic and clinical sciences and most complete postgraduate training in radiology and musculoskeletal therapeutics.

Osteopathic medicine began in 1892 in a similar belief to chiropractic medicine. However, it has evolved progressively toward allopathic medicine. Today, the training, practice, and licensure of osteopathic physicians **(osteopaths)** are identical to those of allopathic physicians.

Homeopathic medicine practitioners are frequently called **homeopaths.** Most **homeopathy** in the United States is practiced as part of another health care practice, such as allopathic medicine, naturopathy, or chiropractic medicine.

Homeopathy is based on the belief that every person has energy called a vital force that, when out of balance, produces health problems. Homeopathic treatment uses minuscule (extremely small) doses of substances (called remedies) that produce the characteristic symptoms of an illness in healthy people when given in larger doses. The intent is to stimulate the body's own defense mechanisms and healing responses.

The remedies used are derived from natural substances that come from plants, minerals, or animals. Because they are so diluted, they do not require FDA approval and testing for safety and efficacy.

Naturopathic medicine is a **holistic** approach to health and healing to recognize the integrity of the whole person. The **naturopath's** role is to facilitate the **inherent** capacity of the body to establish, maintain, and restore health. Symptoms are expressions of the body's attempts to heal, and the root causes of illness at the physical, genetic, mental, emotional, and spiritual level must be sought.

Naturopathic practices include nutrition, herbal medicine, homeopathic medicine, physical medicine, and acupuncture.

Oriental medicine or **Chinese medicine** is based on the concept that the body's vital energy (chi, or qi) circulates through channels called meridians that have branches to organs. Illness is a blockage or imbalance of chi. Acupuncture, herbal remedies, massage, and **Qigong** are used to restore balance. Qigong consists of numerous exercises and breathing routines performed daily to improve the function of the qi *(Figure 23.9)*. Acupuncture is discussed in the energy medicine section of this chapter.

The **National Certification Commission for Acupuncture and Oriental Medicine (NCCAOM)** has licensed more than 15,000 practitioners.

Ayurvedic medicine is based on ideas from Hinduism and aims to integrate the body, mind, and spirit into a holistic unit. Disease arises when the person is out of harmony with the universe.

Three qualities, called **doshas,** control the body's activities and are associated with different body and personality types. Ayurvedic treatments require changes in lifestyle, diet, and habits. Herbs, spices, and oils are used frequently. For example, the spice **turmeric** is used to treat rheumatoid arthritis and Alzheimer disease and to heal wounds. **Aromatherapy,** in which the essential oils extracted from plants are inhaled or applied to the skin, is also used. For example, frankincense is used to enhance meditation, and myrrh is used for positive thinking.

WORD ANALYSIS AND DEFINITION

WORD	PRONUNCIATION	ELEMENTS		DEFINITION
adjustment (also called manipulation)	ah-**JUST**-ment	S/ R/	-ment *resulting state* adjust- *alter*	The action of bringing a body part into alignment with the others
aromatherapy	ah-**ROH**-mah-**THAIR**-ah-pee	S/ R/	-therapy *treatment* aroma- *smell, sweet herb*	Use of essential oils to promote well-being
aromatic (adj)	ah-roh-**MAT**-ik	S/	-tic *pertaining to*	Having an agreeable spicy odor, or one of a group of vegetable drugs
Ayurvedic (adj) Ayurveda (noun)	ah-yur-**VED**-ik ah-yur-**VAY**-duh	S/ P/ R/	-ic *pertaining to* ayur- *life* -ved- *knowledge*	A system of medicine arising from Hindu culture
chiropractic	kye-roh-**PRAK**-tik	S/ R/CF R/	-ic *pertaining to* chir/o- *hand* -pract- *practical*	Diagnosis, treatment, and prevention of mechanical disorders of the musculoskeletal system
chiropractor	kye-roh-**PRAK**-tor	S/	-or *one who does*	Practitioner of chiropractic
dosha	**DOH**-sha		Sanskrit *fault*	Psychophysical constitution of the body in Ayurvedic medicine
holistic	ho-**LIS**-tik	S/ R/	-ic *pertaining to* holist- *entire, whole*	Pertaining to the care of the whole person in physical, mental, emotional, and spiritual dimensions
homeopathy	ho-mee-**OP**-ah-thee	S/ R/CF	-pathy *disease* home/o- *the same*	Treatment of disease with minute doses of substances
homeopath homeopathic (adj)	**HO**-mee-oh-path **HO**-mee-oh-**PATH**-ik	R/ S/	-path *disease* -ic *pertaining to*	Practitioner of homeopathy Pertaining to homeopathy
inherent	in-**HAIR**-ent		Latin *innate, inbred*	Occurring as a natural part of something
naturopathy	nah-chur-**OP**-ah-thee	S/ R/CF	-pathy *disease* natur/o- *nature*	Holistic system of medicine with a natural approach to healing
naturopath naturopathic (adj)	**NAH**-chur-oh-path **NAH**-chur-oh-**PATH**-ik	R/	-path *disease*	Practitioner of naturopathy
osteopathy	**OS**-tee-**OP**-ah-thee	S/ R/CF	-pathy *disease* oste/o- *bone*	Medical practice based on maintaining the structural integrity of the musculoskeletal system
osteopath	**OS**-tee-oh-path	R/	-path *disease*	Practitioner of osteopathy
Qigong	**CHEE**-gong	R/ R/	qi- *vital force* -gong *daily practice*	Exercises and breathing routines performed daily
turmeric	ter-**MER**-ik		Hindu *yellow root*	Spice used in Ayurvedic medicine

EXERCISES

Suffixes: *The suffix will tell you the difference between a practitioner and a practice. Choose the correct answers from among the following terms to fill in the blanks. There are more answers than questions.*

holistic	naturopathy	homeopathy	osteopath	naturopath
chiropractor	homeopath	osteopathy	aromatherapy	chiropractic

1. Holistic system of medicine with a natural approach to healing: _____

   One who practices this type of medicine: _____

2. Diagnosis, treatment, and prevention of mechanical disorders of the musculoskeletal system: _____

   One who practices this type of medicine: _____

3. Treatment of disease with small doses of substances: _____

   One who practices this type of medicine: _____

4. Medical science close to conventional medicine: _____

   One who practices this type of medicine: _____

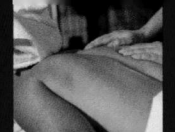

COMPLEMENTARY AND ALTERNATIVE MEDICINE

CHALLENGE YOUR KNOWLEDGE

A. **Case Report:** This exercise is based entirely on the Case Report of Andrea Turpin, which was presented in this chapter.

1. Read this report out loud to yourself for pronunciation practice.

2. Read it to yourself again and *underline* the medical terms.

3. Utilize your knowledge of the *language of complementary and alternative medicine* (and previous chapters) to answer the following questions based on the Case Report.

CASE REPORT 23.3

Mrs. Andrea Turpin is a 39-year-old civil servant, married with three children between 12 and 7 years. Since adolescence, she has had a moderate scoliosis of her spine, producing recurrent back pain. Her orthopedic surgeon prescribed Vioxx and suggested spinal surgery with the placement of rods. Her Web research showed that Vioxx had significant side effects, with an increased risk of heart attacks and strokes, and that the surgery did not guarantee relief of pain and had a long and difficult rehabilitation. She explored CAM alternatives, visited a chiropractor, and now also has acupuncture and neuromuscular massage. She has minimal pain and is able to manage her life and enjoy skiing.

1. Describe "scoliosis of the spine."

   _____

   _____

2. What is *recurrent* back pain?

   _____

3. What does an orthopedic surgeon treat?

   _____

   _____

4. What type of surgical hardware did he want to place in Mrs. Turpin's back?

   _____

5. What abbreviation can be used for heart attack? _____

6. What is another term for a stroke? _____

7. What is the purpose of rehabilitation?

   _____

   _____

8. What type of therapy would be involved in Mrs. Turpin's rehabilitation if she had this surgery performed? _____

9. What types of complementary and alternative medicine options is Mrs. Turpin now using?

   _____

10. Is a chiropractor a medical doctor? _____

   _____

J. **Abbreviations:** Some, but not all, of the sentences in this exercise contain medical t[...] sentence, substituting the correct abbreviation where applicable. Fill in the blanks.

1. Light therapy was prescribed for her seasonal affective disorder.

    _____

    _____

2. The National Certification Board for Therapeutic Massage and Bodywork is the [...] Certificate for Therapeutic Massage and Bodywork.

    _____

    _____

3. Creative therapists are usually part of a team that includes medical doctors, phy[...] pational therapists.

    _____

    _____

4. Reiki, therapeutic touch, and acupuncture are all examples of energy medicine.

    _____

    _____

5. Dietary supplements must meet the requirements of the Food and Drug Admi[...] product quality and consistency.

    _____

    _____

6. The patient was referred to the National Institutes of Health special center for [...] known as the National Center for Complementary and Alternative Medicine.

    _____

    _____

7. Both her electrocardiogram and her electromyogram were reported as normal[...] magnetic resonance imaging were rescheduled because of equipment problem[...]

    _____

    _____

8. The medication for irritable bowel syndrome just passed U.S. Food and Drug [...] prescribed three times a day.

    _____

6. Homeopathic treatment uses minuscule doses of substances called:

    a. hormones

    b. vitamins

    c. enzymes

    d. minerals

    e. remedies

7. In addition to treating SAD, light therapy is also used for:

    a. depression

    b. pain relief

    c. stress relief

    d. muscle injury

    e. cancer

8. Therapeutic touch is an example of:

    a. energy medicine

    b. manipulative practice

    c. biologic-based practice

    d. mind-body practice

    e. whole-medicine system

9. What term comes from the Greek for *to knead, to handle:*

    a. matrix

    b. massage

    c. meditate

    d. manipulate

    e. myofascial

10. Which of these responses can be controlled by biofeedback?

    a. muscle tension

    b. blood pressure

    c. sweating

    d. a and b

    e. all of the above

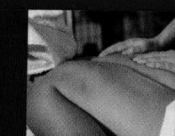

COMPLEMENTARY AND ALTERNATI[VE]

I. **The Language of CAM:** Test what you have learned about *complementary and alternative* [medi]tions correctly. Circle the best answer.

1. Trigger point therapy is also known as:

    a. neuromuscular therapy

    b. sleep therapy

    c. myotherapy

    d. a and c

    e. a and b

2. Essential oils extracted from plants are inhaled or applied to the skin in:

    a. Reiki

    b. hypnotherapy

    c. sleep therapy

    d. Ayurvedic medicine

    e. aromatherapy

3. Which product is *not* a dietary supplement?

    a. vitamins

    b. minerals

    c. hormones

    d. botanicals

    e. herbs

4. **Mobilization** and **adjustment** are two terms used by a(n):

    a. homeopath

    b. pediatrician

    c. chiropractor

    d. naturopath

    e. otolaryngologist

5. **Qi, chi, prana,** and **ki** all refer to:

    a. diseases

    b. yoga postures

    c. energy

    d. herbs

    e. tai chi

COMPLEMENTARY AND ALTERNATIVE MEDICINE

K. **Key Words:** Key definitions can contain key words that are the basic core of the statement. Understanding the essential difference in the statements will help you make a distinction in their meanings. The following definitions are taken from the first page of this chapter. Underline the key word or words in each definition, and then fill in the blanks.

Definitions:

1. Complementary medicine is used together with standard or conventional medical treatments.
2. Alternative medicine is used instead of conventional medical treatments.
3. Integrative medicine is a total approach to care that combines conventional medicine with CAM practices that involve the patient's body, mind, and spirit in the therapeutic process.

Now, utilizing the key words in the definitions, write yourself a shortcut for remembering how to tell the different systems apart.

Complementary medicine: _____

Alternative medicine: _____

Integrative medicine: _____

L. **The terminology of CAM contains Latin, Greek, and Eastern terms.** They cannot be further deconstructed into prefix, root, or suffix. You must know them for what they are. Test your knowledge of these terms with this exercise. Match the meaning in the left column with the correct medical term in the right column.

_____	1. to knead, handle	A.	Reiki
_____	2. joined to another, but not an essential part	B.	meditation
_____	3. a system of lifestyle measures	C.	yoga
_____	4. transfer of energy	D.	ancillary
_____	5. vital power	E.	tai chi
_____	6. contemplation as a formalized spiritual practice	F.	prana
_____	7. series of postures performed in fluid movement	G.	massage
_____	8. yoga posture	H.	chi or qi
_____	9. accessory, adjunct	I.	adjunct
_____	10. universal life force	J.	asana

M. **Recall and Review:** How well do you remember these word elements from the previous chapter? Try to answer without first looking back to check. Fill in the blanks.

Element	Type of Element (P, R, CF, S)	Meaning of Element
adeno	_____	_____
ectomy	_____	_____
meso	_____	_____
stasis	_____	_____
ptosis	_____	_____

N. Short Answer: Recap what you have learned in this chapter by employing medical language to give some examples of dietary or herbal supplements, and explain why it is important to tell your doctor about any dietary or herbal supplements you are taking.

Give at least one example of an interaction between drugs and supplements that could be dangerous to the patient.

_____

_____

_____

_____

O. Research and Discuss: Clinical trials and research studies often make use of placebos with their patient groups. Visit the school library or go online to research the role of _placebos_ in clinical trials, and be prepared to discuss your findings in class. You should be able to answer the following questions:

- What is a clinical trial?
- How and where do you find a clinical trial?
- What is the purpose of a clinical trial?
- How are patients picked for a clinical trial?
- What is a placebo?
- What is a placebo-controlled study?
- What is a control group?
- What is the "placebo effect"?

P. Meet lesson objectives by employing medical language to briefly answer the following questions.

1. Detail the use of complementary and alternative medicine in the United States.

_____

_____

_____

2. Describe frequently used manipulative and body-based techniques of CAM.

_____

_____

_____

3. Explain mind-body practices and their known effects.

_____

_____

_____

4. What are the benefits of biologic-based products?

_____

_____

_____

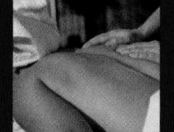
COMPLEMENTARY AND ALTERNATIVE MEDICINE

CHAPTER SUMMARY EXERCISE

1. *Listen to the pronunciation of the medical terms as given by your instructor.*
2. *Circle the correct spelling of the medical term.*
3. *Match the correctly spelled terms to the brief descriptions below.*
4. *Write a sentence for each of the 10 terms that appear in this exercise.*

A. SPELLING COMPREHENSION: CIRCLE THE CORRECT SPELLING OF THE TERM.

1. mannipulation	manipalation	manipeulation	manipulation	manipullation
2. polearity	polarity	pollarity	polarrity	polaritty
3. myofacial	myofascial	miofascial	miofacial	myofassial
4. vizulation	visualization	vizulliation	visualation	visuelation
5. creniosacral	craniosaccral	craniosacral	craniosacrul	creniosackrul
6. meridian	merridian	maridean	meridean	maridian
7. hipnossis	hypnosis	hypnossis	hipnosis	hypnoses
8. adjunct	addjunckt	adjunkt	addjunkt	adjunckt
9. Rulfing	Rolffing	Rollfing	Rolfling	Rolfing
10. placebbo	placibo	placeboo	plasebo	placebo

B. MATCH THE NUMBER OF THE CORRECT TERM IN PART A WITH THE BRIEF DESCRIPTION OF THE TERM BELOW.

a. referring to the cranium and sacrum _____

b. action performed by a chiropractor _____

c. energy line connecting anatomical sites _____

d. concentrates on connective tissue _____

e. possession of opposite characteristics _____

f. suggestions can change behavior _____

g. no therapeutic value _____

h. not an essential part _____

i. surrounds and separates muscle tissue _____

j. the forming of mental images _____

C. USING YOUR KNOWLEDGE OF TERMS 1–10 IN PART A AND THEIR CORRECT SPELLING, WRITE A BRIEF SENTENCE FOR EACH OF THE TERMS AS IT MIGHT APPEAR IN PATIENT DOCUMENTATION.

1. _____

2. _____

3. _____

4. _____

5. _____

6. _____

7. _____

8. _____

9. _____

10. _____

D. YOUR INSTRUCTOR WILL DIRECT YOU TO MCGRAW-HILL CONNECT. OPEN THE AUDIO GLOSSARY AND PRACTICE YOUR PRONUNCIATION OF THE TERMS IN PART A OF THIS EXERCISE.

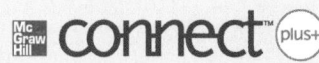

This chapter marks the end of the text. You have applied yourself to learning medical terminology, and what you take away from this course is commensurate with what you have put into learning this subject.

The authors encourage you to make use of Appendix A, both as a self-assessment tool and a comprehensive review of medical terminology for national certification examinations (coding, medical assisting, etc.). Answers are available online in McGraw-Hill Connect.

Remember: Every day on the job is a test of another kind—a test of your communication skills and professionalism. It is also an opportunity to continue your learning—which is a hallmark of a professional.

Appendices

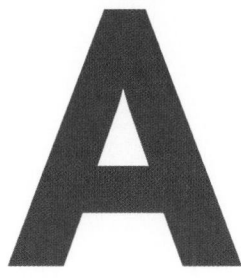

End-of-Book Exercises

The following additional exercises draw from all the previous chapters in the text and will help you review some of the basic elements of medical terminology. Fill in the blanks.

Use these exercises to prepare for cumulative exams.

A. Elements Associated with Body Systems: The body systems are listed for you in the left column. Write five different roots/combining forms for each body system, with the meaning of the element, and an example of a medical term using that element. Fill in the table.

	Body System	Root/Combining Form	Meaning of Element	Medical Term Using This Element
	Integumentary			
1.				
2.				
3.				
4.				
5.				
	Musculoskeletal			
6.				
7.				
8.				
9.				
10.				
	Nervous			
11.				
12.				
13.				
14.				
15.				
	Endocrine			
16.				
17.				
18.				
19.				
20.				

	Body System	Root/Combining Form	Meaning of Element	Medical Term Using This Element
	Cardiovascular			
21.				
22.				
23.				
24.				
25.				
	Lymphatic			
26.				
27.				
28.				
29.				
30.				
	Digestive			
31.				
32.				
33.				
34.				
35.				
	Respiratory			
36.				
37.				
38.				
39.				
40.				
	Urinary			
41.				
42.				
43.				
44.				
45.				
	Reproductive			
46.				
47.				
48.				
49.				
50.				

ELEMENTS BY GROUPING

B. List all the elements that denote a color.

	Element	Color
1.	leuk/o	white
2.		
3.		
4.		
5.		
6.		
7.		
8.		

C. List all the elements that denote a location or direction (above, below, etc.).

	Element	Location
1.	epi	above
2.		
3.		
4.		
5.		
6.		
7.		
8.		
9.		
10.		
11.		
12.		

D. List all the elements that denote a number.

	Element	Number
1.	mono	one
2.		
3.		
4.		
5.		
6.		
7.		
8.		

E. Difference Between Elements: Many elements sound and look similar but have very different meanings. Be precise in your communication—patient safety depends on you!

	Element	Type of Element (P/R/CF/S)	Meaning of Element	Medical Term from Any Chapter Containing This Element
1.	pheresis			
2.	phoresis			
3.	uretero			
4.	urethro			
5.	acro			
6.	acromio			
7.	homeo			
8.	hemo			
9.	bi			
10.	bio			
11.	inter			
12.	intra			
13.	colo			
14.	colpo			
15.	echo			
16.	ecto			
17.	radiculo			
18.	reticulo			
19.	metacarpo			
20.	metatarso			
21.	vaso			
22.	veno			
23.	thymo			
24.	thyro			
25.	diplo			
26.	dipso			
27.	necro			
28.	narco			
29.	lipo			
30.	litho			
31.	sacro			
32.	sarco			
33.	oro			
34.	orcho			
35.	brady			
36.	brachy			

F. **Elements:** Reinforce your knowledge of elements with this comprehensive list. Identify the element as to type, give its meaning, and then use it in an appropriate medical term. Fill in the chart. The first one is done for you.

	Element	Type of Element (P/R/CF/S)	Meaning of Element	Medical Term Containing This Element
1.	*a, an*	*P*	*without*	*anencephaly*
2.	adeno			
3.	alges			
4.	angio			
5.	brachio			
6.	broncho			
7.	bucc			
8.	cervic			
9.	chole			
10.	coagulo			
11.	de			
12.	dent			
13.	dia			
14.	echo			
15.	ectasis			
16.	emesis			
17.	flex			
18.	fluoro			
19.	flux			
20.	gen			
21.	gingiv			
22.	glosso			
23.	hepato			
24.	histo			
25.	hydro			
26.	iasis			
27.	ion			
28.	isch			
29.	jugul			
30.	jejun			

	Element	Type of Element (P/R/CF/S)	Meaning of Element	Medical Term Containing This Element
31.	karyo			
32.	kerato			
33.	kinesio			
34.	laparo			
35.	litho			
36.	lysis			
37.	mania			
38.	morpho			
39.	myelo			
40.	naso			
41.	necrot			
42.	neo			
43.	olfact			
44.	oligo			
45.	os			
46.	penia			
47.	procto			
48.	psycho			
49.	rrhaphy			
50.	rrhea			
51.	rrhoid			
52.	stasis			
53.	stetho			
54.	stomy			
55.	terato			
56.	thrombo			
57.	tripsy			
58.	ule			
59.	um			
60.	uria			
61.	vascul			
62.	viscer			
63.	xeno			

G. Spelling Demons: Precision in communication and professionalism require correct spelling of all medical terms. Circle the correct spelling of each term; then on the line below, deconstruct the correct spelling of the term with slashes, and write a brief explanation of the medical term.

1. acondroplasia   achondroplasia   acondroplesia

_____

2. hemorrhage   hemmorrhage   hemorhage

_____

3. escultation   auscaltation   auscultation

_____

4. cirrosis   sirosis   cirrhosis

_____

5. aneurism   aneurysm   anerysm

_____

6. antiarrythmics   antiarrhthmics   antiarrhythmics

_____

7. hysterectomy   histerectomy   hystirectomy

_____

8. systocele   cystocele   cystosele

_____

9. osteomyelitis   osteomylitis   osteomyeletis

_____

10. hernioraphy   herniorraphy   herniorrhaphy

_____

11. preeclampsia   preclampsia   preklampsia

_____

12. bronchopneumonia   broncopneumonia   bronchopeumonia

_____

13. jundice   jaundice   jaunndice

_____

14. diverticulosis   deverticulosis   diverticculosis

_____

15. cholesterol   colesterol   cholesteral

_____

16. cholecystectomy   colecystectomy   collecystectomy

___

17. ketoacidosis   ketoneacidosis   kettoacidosis

___

18. epididimis   epididymus   epididymis

___

19. immunosuppression   imunosupresion   immunosupression

___

20. laryngapharnix   laryngopharynx   laryngopharnix

___

21. exophthalmos   exopthalamos   exophtalamos

___

22. galactorhea   gallactorea   galactorrhea

___

23. rhabdomyosarcoma   rabdomyosarcoma   rhabomyosarcoma

___

24. paresthesia   parasthesia   parresthesia

___

25. fallopian   falopian   faalopian

___

26. nosocomial   nosoccomial   nossocomial

___

27. proptosis   protosis   proptossis

___

28. thrombophlebitis   thembophlebitis   thrombopelpitis

___

29. percutaneous   purcutaneous   perkutaneous

___

30. gastroesophageal   gastroesopageal   gastroesophagial

___

31. pneumonitis   penummonitis   pneumonnitis

___

32. oophorectomy   ophorectomy   ooporectomy

___

33.	uvula	uuvla	uvulla

34.	tonsillectomy	tonsilectomy	tonssilectomy

35.	streptococcus	striptococcus	streptococus

36.	vasovasostomy	vasovesostomy	vesovasostomy

37.	thyrotoxicosis	thyroidtoxicosis	thyrotoxicossis

H. Review of Latin/Greek Terms That Do Not Deconstruct into Elements: You must know these terms for what they are. Fill in the table. A sample is shown on the first line.

	Medical Term	Meaning of Term in Latin/Greek	Application to Medical Terminology
	cruciate	*cross*	*anterior cruciate ligament*
1.	integument		
2.	viscous		
3.	hirsutism		
4.	calculus		
5.	patent		
6.	zygote		
7.	Calorie		
8.	cognitive		
9.	lymph		
10.	vector		
11.	lavage		
12.	ptosis		
13.	gonad		
14.	matrix		
15.	apex		
16.	modality		
17.	ganglion		
18.	benign		
19.	cartilage		
20.	toxin		
21.	labium		
22.	node		
23.	bronchus		

I. Body Systems: Use your knowledge of medical terminology to fill in the following chart with terms applicable to each specific body system. There may not be an appropriate answer for every blank. The first one is done for you.

	Body System	Study Of (practice)	One Who Studies (practitioner)	Disease	Procedure
1.	*Integumentary*	*dermatology*	*dermatologist*	*eczema*	*excisional biopsy*
2.	Musculoskeletal				
3.	Nervous				
4.	Endocrine				
5.	Cardiovascular				
6.	Special senses/eye				
7.	Digestive				
8.	Respiratory				
9.	Urinary				
10.	Reproductive				

J. Symptoms/Chief Complaint: The patients of Fulwood Medical Center have come into the various clinics with the following complaints. Use the correct medical terminology to enter the chief complaint in the patient's chart.

	Patient Complaint	Correct Medical Terminology for Chart
1.	Double vision	
2.	Blood in urine	
3.	Ringing in ears	
4.	Painful breathing	
5.	Pus in gums	
6.	Sore throat	
7.	Earache	
8.	Pink eye	
9.	Fear of heights	
10.	Low blood pressure	
11.	Hair loss	
12.	Inability to urinate	
13.	Fainting	
14.	Lack of bowel movements	
15.	Broken wrist	
16.	Nosebleeds	
17.	Impacted earwax	
18.	Bed-wetting	
19.	Heavy menstrual bleeding	
20.	Stomachache	

K. Transcription Exercise: The following paragraphs from patient documentation and office forms contain errors. Circle the errors in the paragraph; then rewrite the correct medical terminology on the lines below.

1. This 65-year-old male with a prior history of an appendectomy awoke on the day of admission with crampy addominal pain which was accompanied by destention, nausea, and vomitting.

   _____

2. Sections show an increased number of cysstically dilated glands with the lining epithelium composed primarily of muccous secreting glands. Diagnosis: Low-grade mucoepidimoid carcinomma.

   _____

3. Hemmostasis was accomplished using electrocogulation. The patient had a slight commuted fracture of the medial maleolus. The wound was irrigated and debris was removed.

   _____

4. The patient is a 58-year-old black female with an osteosarcoma of the pelvis who underwent successful wide resuction and reconstruction; however, 2 weeks later her wound became infected and perforated the rectim, which resulted in gross contammination.

   _____

5. Under general anesthesia it was clear that the patient had a grade II tear of the latteral colateral ligament as well as an anterior and posterior cruxiate ligament tear.

   _____

6. PA/lateral CXR: The heart size is normal. There is bilateral atellectasis noted. There is density within the overlying soft tissues of the right chest consistent with recent right-sided breast biopsie. There is no evidence of plural efusion or pneumothorax.

   _____

7. Numerous enlarged, abnormal-appearing limph nodes in the right axila, with markedly thickened cortices and hillar effacement. Concerning for lympoma or metastaic disease. Further follow-up is recommended.

   _____

8. There is diffuse fatty infiltration of the liver. The spleen is unremarkable as well as kidneys and adrennal glands. There is no retroperitonial adenopathy or abdominal aortic aneursm. There are multiple calcifications within the galbladder consistent with choleithiasis.

   _____

9. Increased activity at the ankles and feet is seen bilateraly, likely related to degenerative/hypertopic changes. There is minimal increase activity at both shoulders and at the right sternocavicular joint, likely related to arthritic changes. No other significant abnormality is identified.

   _____

10. Past Medical History of childhood diseases:

diphtheria	smallpox	scarlet fever	rhumatic fever
chorea	tyhphoid	whoping cough	chickenbox
mumps	meseles	tonsilitis	rubela

   _____

11. Past Medical Illness occurring within the last 2 years:

punmonia	plurisy	arthralgia	migrain headaches
malaria	sleep apnia	broncitis	cardiomyopathy
conjunctivetis	gout	otitus media	anemmia

_____

12. The gastriscope was advanced into the distal esopagus, which was essentially normal. Advancement of the scope into the stomach showed evidence of erytema and gasritis. The pylorus was intubated and the duodenal bulb was visualized.

_____

L. Coding Exercise: Solid knowledge of medical terminology will make you better understand the coding system.

Volumes I and II of ICD-9-CM contain diagnosis codes. CPT codes are used to bill physician fees for procedures and services. In the following chart, choose whether each medical term requires an ICD-9-CM code or a CPT code (put a √ in the appropriate column), and identify the specialist associated with the medical term.

	Medical Term	Diagnosis	Procedures/Services	Specialist Consulted
1.	otitis media			
2.	CVA			
3.	carditis			
4.	blepharoplasty			
5.	thoracotomy			
6.	neuralgia			
7.	nephrosis			
8.	herniorrhaphy			
9.	uveitis			
10.	osteoporosis			
11.	lithotripsy			
12.	LEEP			
13.	osteotomy			
14.	amniocentesis			
15.	jejunostomy			
16.	hemoptysis			
17.	IVF			
18.	rhinitis			
19.	fluoroscopy			
20.	anorexia			
21.	anal fistula			
22.	MI			

	Medical Term	Diagnosis	Procedure	Specialist Consulted
23.	hematuria			
24.	hysteroscopy			
25.	neoplasm			
26.	acrophobia			
27.	dementia			
28.	CF			
29.	leiomyoma			
30.	hemogram			

M. Definitions: Write a brief definition for each of the following signs and symptoms a patient may experience.

1. gynecomastia _____
2. pallor _____
3. stridor _____
4. tic _____
5. cyanosis _____
6. colic _____
7. edema _____
8. epistaxis _____
9. alopecia _____
10. febrile _____
11. hirsutism _____
12. jaundice _____
13. hypertension _____
14. hypernatremia _____
15. albinism _____
16. hyperpnea _____
17. polydipsia _____
18. petechia _____
19. amenorrhea _____
20. pes planus _____
21. obesity _____
22. palpitation _____
23. atelectasis _____
24. effusion _____
25. malunion _____
26. tetany _____
27. hemiplegia _____
28. contracture _____
29. frequency _____
30. wheals _____

N. Surgical Suffixes: The following suffixes are all associated with surgical procedures. CPT codes are specific as to type of procedure—you can't code and bill a nephrotomy if the patient actually had a nephrectomy. You must code what is documented in the medical record. Know your suffixes!

This chart contains surgical suffixes. Give the meaning of the suffix, an example of the suffix in a term, and the definition of the term. The first one is done for you.

	Suffix	Suffix Meaning	Example of Term	Meaning of the Term
1.	ectomy	removal of	nephrectomy	removal of the kidney
2.	centesis			
3.	cision			
4.	desis			
5.	ostomy			
6.	pexy			
7.	plasty			
8.	rrhaphy			
9.	tomy			
10.	tripsy			

O. Work with more surgical terms. Write a brief description of the procedure each term represents. Fill in the blanks.

1. abdominocentesis: _____

_____

2. catheterization: _____

_____

3. ligation: _____

_____

4. amputation: _____

_____

5. incision: _____

_____

6. curettage: _____

_____

7. aspiration: _____

_____

8. debridement: _____

_____

9. cauterization: _____

_____

10. ablation: _____

_____

11. resection: _____

_____

12. dilation: _____

_____

13. manipulation: _____

_____

14. allograft: _____

_____

15. excision: _____

_____

16. suture: _____

_____

P. Abbreviations: Reading patient documentation to extract/abstract information for coding purposes requires that you understand what you are reading. Identify the abbreviations in the following chart. Check (√) whether the abbreviation is a diagnosis, a procedure, or something else. In the right column, write the meaning of the abbreviation.

	Abbreviation	Diagnosis	Procedure	Other	Meaning of Abbreviation
1.	EBV				
2.	q.i.d.				
3.	BOM				
4.	SOB				
5.	CPR				
6.	PDA				
7.	UTI				
8.	O.D.				
9.	CSF				
10.	ABG				
11.	PT				
12.	DJD				
13.	NSAID				
14.	p.r.n.				
15.	MI				
16.	CMA				
17.	CBC				
18.	ARDS				
19.	C5				
20.	AKA				
21.	WNV				
22.	CAD				

	Abbreviation	Disease	Procedure	Other	Meaning of Abbreviation
23.	AU				
24.	COPD				
25.	DEXA				
26.	WBC				
27.	EEG				
28.	ROM				
29.	STAT				
30.	CXR				
31.	AP				
32.	MRI				
33.	GYN				
34.	PVC				
35.	Pap				

Q. Use your knowledge of medical language and abbreviations to analyze the following groups of terms and determine what they have in common.

1. *comminuted, pathologic, displaced*

   All relate to _____ .

2. *onychomycosis, matrix, paronychia*

   All relate to _____ .

3. *erythrocyte, thrombocyte, leukocyte*

   All relate to _____ .

4. *canthus, orbit, tarsus*

   All relate to _____ .

5. *biceps, deltoid, brachioradialis*

   All relate to _____ .

6. *plexus, synapse, ganglia*

   All relate to _____ .

7. *enteric, flexure, ileum*

   All relate to _____ .

8. *zygote, embryo, fetus*

   All relate to _____ .

9. *vomer, occipital, zygoma*

   All relate to _____ .

10. *thelarche, pubarche, menarche*

    All relate to _____ .

11. *phobia, mania, psychosis*

    All relate to _____.

12. *cholesteatoma, tympanostomy, auricle*

    All relate to _____.

13. *typhoid, plague, cholera*

    All relate to _____.

14. *CVA, TIA, embolus*

    All relate to _____.

15. *surfactant, inflate, hilum*

    All relate to _____.

16. *crowning, effacement, dilation*

    All relate to _____.

17. *enuresis, polyuria, glycosuria*

    All relate to _____.

18. *lymphadenectomy, lymphadenitis, lymphadenopathy*

    All relate to _____.

19. *aorta, carotid, arteriole*

    All relate to _____.

20. *trimester, gravida, para*

    All relate to _____.

Congratulations on a job well done!

Word Parts

B

Note: For easy identification, the word parts in this appendix appear in the same colors as they do in the Word Analysis and Definition boxes: suffix, prefix, root, root/combining form. Any term that is used in the text in both root and combining form is shown in this appendix only as a combining form. Sometimes the same element (for example, "ac") can function in different parts of the medical term.

WORD PART	DEFINITION
-ac	pertaining to
-al	pertaining to
-ar	pertaining to
-ary	pertaining to
a-	not, without, into
ab-	away from
abdomin/o	abdomen
ability	competence
ablat	take away
-able	capable of
abort	fail at onset, expel nonviable fetus
absorpt	to swallow, take in
ac-	toward
-acea	condition, remedy
acetyl	acetyl
acid/o	acid, low pH
acin	grape
acous	hearing
acr/o	peak, extremity, highest point
acro-	peak, highest point, extremity
acromi/o	acromion
act	to do, perform, performance

WORD PART	DEFINITION
activ/e	movement
acu-	sharp
acu	needle, sharp
acumin	to sharpen
ad-	to, toward, near, into
adapt	to adjust
-ade	process
aden/o	gland
adenoid	adenoid
adipos/e	fat
adjust	alter
adjuv	give help
adnex	connected parts
adolesc	beginning of adulthood
adren/o	adrenal gland
aer/o	air, gas
ag-	to
-age	related to
agglutin	sticking together, clumping
-ago	disease
agon	contest against, fight against
-agon	contest

WORD PART	DEFINITION
agor/a	marketplace
-agra	rough
-al	pertaining to
alanine	an amino acid, protein synthesized in muscle
albin/o	white
albumin	albumin
ald/o	organic compound
-ale	pertaining to
alges	sensation of pain
-algia	pain, painful condition
aliment	nourishment
-alis	pertaining to
alkal	base
all/o	strange, other, different
aller	allergy
allo-	other, different, strange
alopec-	baldness, mange
alpha-	first letter in Greek alphabet
alveol	alveolus, air sac
-aly	condition
ambly-	dull
ambulat	to walk, walking
amin/o	nitrogen compound
-amine	nitrogen-containing
ammon	ammonia
amni/o	amnion, fetal membrane
amnios	amnion, fetal membrane
amoeb	amoeba
amph-	around
ampull	bottle-shaped
amput	to prune, lop off
amyl	starch
an-	not, lack of, without
-an	pertaining to
an/o	anus
ana-	away from, excessive

WORD PART	DEFINITION
ana	apart from
anabol	build up
analysis	process to define
analyst	one who defines
anastom	join together
-ance	condition, state of
-ancy	state of
andr/o	male, masculine
aneurysm	dilation
angi/o	blood vessel, lymph vessel
angina	sore throat, chest pain radiating to throat
ankyl	stiff
ant-	against
-ant	forming, pertaining to, agent
ante-	before, forward
anter	before, front part
anthrac	coal
anti-	against
aort	aorta
apo-	different from, separation from, off
append	appendix
apse	clasp
aqu-	water
aqu/e	watery
-ar	pertaining to
arachn	cobweb, spider
-arche	beginning
aria	air
-arian	one who is
-aris	pertaining to
aroma	smell, sweet herb
array	place in order
arteri/o	artery
arteriosus	like an artery
arthr/o	joint
articul	joint

WORD PART	DEFINITION
-ary	pertaining to
asbest	asbestos
asc	belly
ascit	fluid in the belly
-ase	enzyme
aspartate	an amino acid
aspergill	*Aspergillus*
aspirat	to breathe in, remove by suction
assay	evaluate
assist	aid, help
astr/o	star
-ata	action, place, use
-ate	composed of, pertaining to, process
-ated	process, composed of
atel	incomplete
ather/o	porridge, gruel, fatty substance
athet	without position, uncontrolled
-atic	pertaining to
-ation	process
-ative	pertaining to, quality of
-ator	agent, instrument, person or thing that does something
atri/o	entrance, atrium
-atric	treatment
attent	awareness
attenu	to weaken
audi/o	hearing
audit	hearing
aur-	ear
auscult	listen to
auto-	self, same
avail	useful
axill	armpit
ayur-	life
azot	nitrogen
back	back, return

WORD PART	DEFINITION
-back	back, toward the starting point
bacter	bacterium
bacteri/o	bacteria
balan	glans penis
bar	pressure
bari	weight
bas/o	base, opposite of acid
basal/e	deepest part
basil	base, support
be	life
behav	mental activity
beta	second letter of Greek alphabet
bi-	two, twice, double
bi/o	life
-bic	life
-bil	able
bil/i	bile
bio-	life
bio	life
biot	life
-blast	embryo, germ cell, immature cell
blast/o	immature cell, germ cell
blephar/o	eyelid
body	body, mass, substance
bov	cattle
brachi/o	arm
brachii	of the arm
brachy-	short
brady-	slow
bride	rubbish, rubble
bronch/o	bronchus
brucell	from pathologist David Bruce
bucc	cheek
buccin	cheek

WORD PART	DEFINITION
bulb/o	bulb
burs	bursa
calc/i	calcium
calcul	stone, little stone
callos	thickening
calor	heat
cancer	cancer
candid	*Candida,* a yeast
capill	hairlike structure, capillary
capit	head
capn	carbon dioxide
caps	box, cover, shell
capsul	little box
carb/o	carbon
carboxy	group of organic compounds
carcin/o	cancerous, cancer
card	heart
cardi/o	heart
cardia	heart
care	be responsible for
caroten/e	yellow-red pigment
carotid	large neck artery
carp/o	bones of the wrist
cartilag/e	cartilage
cata-	down
catabol	break down
catechol	benzene derivative
cathet	insert, catheter
caud/a	tail
cava	cave
cavern	cave
cec	cecum
-cele	cave, hernia, swelling
celi	abdomen
cellul	small cell
cent-	hundred

WORD PART	DEFINITION
cent	hundred
-centesis	to puncture
centr/o	central
cephal/o	head
cephalus	head
-cephalus	head
cephaly	condition of the head
ceps	head
-ceps	head
cept	to receive
cerebell	little brain, cerebellum
cerebr/o	brain
cervic	neck, cervix
cess	going forward
chancr	chancre
chem/o	chemical
chemic	chemical
chete	hair
-chezia	pass a stool
chir/o	hand
chlor/o	green
chol/e	bile
cholangi	bile duct
cholecyst	gallbladder
choledoch/o	common bile duct
choline	choline
chondr/o	cartilage, rib
chori/o	chorion, membrane
chorion	chorion
chrom/o	color
chromat	color
chron/o	time
chym/o	chyme
cid/e	to kill
-cidal	pertaining to killing
-cide	to kill

WORD PART	DEFINITION
cili	hairlike structure, eyelid
circum-	around
cirrh	yellow
cis	to cut
cit/i	cell
-clast	break, break down
claudic	limp
claustr/o	confined space
clav	clavicle
clave	lock
clavicul	clavicle
-cle	small
clitor	clitoris
clon	cutting used for propagation, violent action
-clonus	violent action
co-	with, together
coagul/o	clotting, clump
coarct	press together, narrow
cobal	cobalt
cocc	spherical bacterium, berry
cochle	cochlea
code	information system
cognit	thinking
coit	sexual intercourse
col-	before
col	colon
coll	collect, glue
coll/a	glue
colon	colony
colon/o	colon
coloniz	form a colony
colp/o	vagina
com-	with, together
com	take care of
combin	combine
comminut	break into small pieces

WORD PART	DEFINITION
commodat	adjust
compat	tolerate
compet	strive together
complete	fill in
complex	woven together
compli	fulfill
compress	press together
compuls	drive, compel
con-	with, together
concav	arched, hollow
concept	become pregnant
concuss	shake violently
condyl	knuckle
confus	bewildered
congest	accumulation of fluid
coni	dust
coniz	cone
conjunctiv	conjunctiva
conscious	aware
constip	press together
constrict	narrow, to narrow
contagi/o	transmissible by contact
contamin	to corrupt, make unclean
contin	hold together
contra-	against
contract	draw together, pull together
contus	bruise
convalesc	recover
cor	heart, pupil
cori	skin
corne/o	cornea
coron	crown, coronary
corpor/e	body
corpus	body
cort	cortex
cortic/o	cortex, cortisone

S = Suffix   P = Prefix   R = Root   R/CF = Combining Form

WORD PART	DEFINITION
cortis	cortisone
cost	rib
crani/o	cranium, skull
cre	separation
crease	groove
creat	flesh
creatin	creatine
cret	to separate
cretin	cretin
crimin	distinguish
crine	secrete
-crine	secrete
crista	crest
-crit	to separate
crown	crown
cry/o	icy cold
crypt-	hidden
cub	cube
cubit	elbow
cubitus	lying down
cune/i	wedge
cur	cleanse, cure
curat	to care for
curett	to cleanse
curr	to run
cursor	run
cusp	point
cutan/e	skin
cyan/o	dark blue
-cyst	cyst, sac, bladder
cyst/o	bladder, sac, cyst
cysteine	an amino acid
cyt/o	cell
-cyte	cell
cyth	cell
dacry/o	tears, lacrimal duct

WORD PART	DEFINITION
dai	day
de-	from, take away, out of, without, change of
defec	clear out waste
deferens	carry away
defici	failure, lacking, inadequate
degenerat	deteriorate
deglutit	to swallow
del	visible, manifest
deliri	confusion, disorientation
delt	Greek letter delta
delus	deceive
dem	the people
demi-	half
dendr/o	treelike, branching structure
dent	tooth
depend	relying on
depress	press down
derm/a	skin
-derma	skin
dermat/o	skin
dermis	skin
-desis	bind together, fixation of bone or joint
di-	two, complete
dia-	complete, through
diabet	diabetes
diagnost	decision
dialectic	argument
dialy	separate
diaphor	sweat
diaphragm/a	diaphragm
dict	consent, surrender
didym/o	testis
didymis	testis
diet	a way of life
different	not identical
digest	to break down, break up

WORD PART	DEFINITION
digit	finger or toe
dilat	open up, expand, open out
dips	thirst
dis-	apart, away from
discipl	understand
disciplin	disciple, instruction
dist	away from the center
-dium	appearance
diuret	increase urine output
diverticul	by-road
dorm	sleep
dors	back
dors/i	back
drome	running
drop	liquid globule
duce	to lead
ducer	to lead, leader
duct	to lead
ductus	leading
duoden	twelve, duodenum
dur/a	hard, dura mater
dwarf	miniature
dynam/o	power
-dynia	pain
dys-	bad, difficult, painful
e-	out of, from
-eal	pertaining to
ease	normal function, freedom from pain
ec-	out, outside
ech/o	sound wave
echin	hedgehog
eclamps	shining forth
eco-	environment
-ectasis	dilation
-ectomy	excision, surgical excision
ectop	on the outside, displaced

WORD PART	DEFINITION
eczema	eczema
-ed	pertaining to
edema	edema, swelling
efface	wipe out
effus	pour out
ejacul	shoot out
el	wart, nail
elasma	plate
elect	choice
electr/o	electric, electricity
elimin	throw away, expel
-elle	small
em-	in, into
-em	condition
-ema	result
emac/i	make thin
embol	plug
embry/o	embryo, fertilized egg
eme	to vomit
emesis	vomiting
-emesis	to vomit, vomiting
emia	blood
-emia	blood, blood condition
-emic	in the blood
emmetr-	measure
emuls	suspend in a liquid
emulsific	to milk out, to drain out
en-	in
-ence	forming, quality of, state of
encephal/o	brain
encephaly	condition of the brain
-ency	condition, state of, quality, quality of
end-	inside, within
endo-	inner, inside, within
-ent	end result, pertaining to, state of, end, forming
enter/o	intestine

WORD PART	DEFINITION
entery	intestine
enur	urinate
environ	surroundings
-eon	one who does
eosin/o	dawn
ependym	lining membrane
epi-	above, upon, over
epilep	seizure
epiphys/e	growth
episi/o	vulva
equi-	equal
equin/a	horse
equip	to fit out
-er	agent, one who does, work, activity
erect	straight, to set up
erg/o	work
-ergy	process of working
-ery	condition, process of
erysi-	red
erythemat	redness
erythr/o	red
-escent	process
-esis	abnormal condition
eso-	inward
esophag/e	esophagus
essent	existence
esthes	sensation
esthet	sensation, perception
estr/o	woman
ethm	sieve
eti/o	cause
-etic	pertaining to
-etics	pertaining to
-ette	little
eu-	good, normal
ex-	away from, out, out of

WORD PART	DEFINITION
exacerb	increase, aggravate
examin	test, examine
excret	separate, discharge
exo-	outside, outward
expect	await
expir	breathe out
extra-	out of, outside
fac/i	face
factor	maker
farct	stuff
fasc/i	fascia
febr	fever
fec	feces
feed	to give food, nourish
femor	femur
fer	to bear, carry
ferrit	iron
fertil	able to conceive
fertiliz	to bear, make fruitful
fet/o	fetus
fibr/o	fiber, fibrous
fibril	small fiber
fibrin/o	fibrin
-fication	remove
fida	split
field	definite area
filar	roundworm
filtr	strain through
fiss	split
fistul	tube, pipe
flat	flatus
flate	blow into
flatul	excessive gas
flavon	yellow
flavon	yellow
flex	bend

WORD PART	DEFINITION
fluid/o	to flow
fluo-	fluorine
fluor/o	flux, flow, x-ray beam
flux	flow
foc	center, focus
follicul	follicle
foramin	opening, foramen
fore-	in front
-form	appearance of, resembling
form	shape, appearance of
format	to form
fract	break
fraction	small amount
free	free
frequ	repeated, often
front	front, forehead
fruct	fruit
funct	perform
fund/o	fundus
fung/i	fungus
fusion	to pour
galact/o	milk
gall	bile
galvan	low-voltage current
gastr/o	stomach
gastrin	stomach hormone
gastrocnem	calf of leg
gemin	twin, double
gen-	birth, origin
-gen	create, produce, form
gen/o	to create, to produce
-gene	producer, give birth
gener	produce
-genes	producing
genesis	origin, creation, production
-genesis	creation, origin, formation, source

WORD PART	DEFINITION
genet	origin
-genic	creation, producing
genit	bring forth, birth, primary male or female sex organ, androgen
genitor	offspring
ger	old age
geront/o	process of aging
gest	gestation, pregnancy, produce
gestat	gestation, pregnancy, to bear
gigant	giant
gingiv	gums
gland	gland
glauc	lens opacity, gray
gli/o	glue, supportive tissue of nervous system
glia	glue, supportive tissue of nervous system
-glia	glue, supportive tissue of nervous system
glio-	glue
glob	globe
globin/o	protein
globul	globular, protein
glomerul/o	glomerulus
gloss/o	tongue
glott	mouth of windpipe
glottis	windpipe
gluc/o	glucose, sugar
glut/e	buttocks
glutin	glue, stick together
glyc/o	glycogen, glucose, sugar
glycer	glycerol, sweet
gnath	jaw
gnose	recognize an abnormal condition
gnosis	knowledge
gomph	bolt, nail
gon/o	seed
gonad/o	gonads, testes or ovaries
gong	daily practice

S = Suffix   P = Prefix   R = Root   R/CF = Combining Form

WORD PART	DEFINITION
-grade	going
graft	splice, transplant
-graft	tissue for transplant
graine	head pain
-gram	a record, drawing, recording
grand-	big
granul/o	granule, small grain
-graph	to record, write
-grapher	one who records
-graphy	process of recording
gravid	pregnant
gravida	pregnant woman
gravis	serious
green	green
gru	to move
guan	dung
gurgit	flood
gynec/o	woman, female
habilitat	restore
hale	breathe
halit	breath
hallucin	imagination
hallux	big toe
hem/o	blood
hemangi/o	blood vessel
hemat/o	blood
heme	red iron-containing pigment
hemi-	half
hepar	liver
hepat/o	liver
herb/i	plant
hered	inherited through genes
herni/o	hernia, rupture
herp	blister
heter/o	different
hetero-	different

WORD PART	DEFINITION
hist	derived from histidine
hist/o	tissue
holist	entire, whole
hom/i	man
home/o	the same
homo-	same, alike
hormon/e	chemical messenger
humor	fluid
hyal	glass
hydr/o	water
hyp-	below
hyper-	above, beyond, excess, excessive
hypn/o	sleep
hypo-	below, deficient, smaller, low, under
hyster/o	uterus
-ia	condition
-iac	pertaining to
-ial	pertaining to
-ian	one who does, specialist
-ias	condition
-iasis	condition, state of
iatr	medical treatment, treatment
-iatric	relating to medicine, medical knowledge
iatrics	field of medicine, healing
-iatrist	practitioner, one who treats
-iatry	treatment, field of medicine
-ible	can do, able to
-ic	pertaining to
-ica	pertaining to
-ical	pertaining to
-ician	expert, specialist
-ics	knowledge of
ict	seizure
icterus	jaundice
-id	having a particular quality, pertaining to
-ide	having a particular quality

S = Suffix   P = Prefix   R = Root   R/CF = Combining Form

WORD PART	DEFINITION
idi/o	personal, distinct
ifer	to bear, carry
-ify	to become
-il	capability
-ile	capable, capability, pertaining to
ile/o	ileum
ili	ilium
-ility	having the quality of, state of
im-	not, in
imag	likeness
immun/o	immune, immune response, immunity
immuniz	make immune
impair	worsen
imped/e	obstruct
imperfecta	unfinished
-imus	most
in-	not, into, in, without
-in	chemical, chemical compound, substance
incis	cut into
incub	sit on, lie on, hatch
index	to declare
-ine	pertaining to, substance
infant	infant
infect/i	tainted, internal invasion
infer	below, beneath
infest	invade, attack
inflammat	set on fire
inflat	blow up
infra-	below, beneath
-ing	quality of, doing
ingest	carry in
inguin	groin
inhal	breathe in
inhibit	repress
inject	force in

WORD PART	DEFINITION
ino	sinew
insect/i	insect
insert	put together
inspir	breathe in
insul	island
integr	whole
integument	covering of the body
intellect/u	perception, discernment
inter-	between
interstit	spaces within tissues
intestin	gut, intestine
intra-	inside, within
intrins	on the inside
intus-	within
iod/o	violet, iodine
-ion	action, condition, process
-ior	pertaining to, suffix for comparatives
-iosum	pertaining to
-ious	pertaining to
ir-	in
-is	belonging to, pertaining to, condition
isch	to keep back
-ism	action, condition, process
-ismus	take action
iso-	equal
-isone	cortisone
-ist	agent, specialist
-istic	pertaining to
-isy	inflammation
-ites	associated with
-itic	pertaining to
-ition	process
-itis	inflammation, infection
-ity	condition, state
-ium	structure
-ius	pertaining to

WORD PART	DEFINITION
-ive	nature of, quality of, pertaining to
-iz	subject to
-ization	process of creating, process of affecting in a specific way
-ize	action, affect in a specific way, policy
-ized	affected in a specific way
-izer	affects in a particular way, line of action
jejun	jejunum
jugul	throat
junct	joining together
juxta-	beside, near, close to
kal	potassium
kary/o	nucleus
kel/o	tumor
kerat/o	cornea
keratin/o	keratin
kern	nucleus
ket/o	ketone
keton	ketone
ketone	organic compound, ketone
kin	motion
kinase	enzyme
-kine	movement
kines/i	movement
kinet	motion
-kinin	move in
klept/o	to steal
kyph/o	bent
labi	lip
labyrinth	inner ear
lacer	to tear
lacrim	tears, tear duct
lact/e	milk
lactat	secrete milk
lapar/o	abdomen in general
lapse	clasp, fall together

WORD PART	DEFINITION
-lapse	fall together, slide
laryng/o	larynx
laser	acronym for *l*ight *a*mplification by *s*timulated *e*mission of *r*adiation
lash	end of whip
lat	to take
later	side, at the side
latiss	wide
-le	small
lei/o	smooth
-lemma	covering
-lepsy	seizure
lept	thin, small
-let	small
leuk/o	white
lex	word
librium	balance
ligament	ligament
ligat	tie up, tie off
lign	line
line	a mark
-ling	small
lingu	tongue
lip/o	fat, fatty tissue
lipid	fat
-lith	stone
lith/o	stone
liv	life
load	to carry
lob	lobe
locat	a place
log	to study, study of
-logist	one who studies, specialist
logous	relation
logy	study of
-logy	to study, study of

S = Suffix   P = Prefix   R = Root   R/CF = Combining Form

WORD PART	DEFINITION
longev	long life
lord	curve, swayback
lubric	make slippery
lucid	bright, clear
lumb	lower back, loin
lump	piece
lun	moon
-lus	small
lute	yellow
luxat	dislocate
ly	break down, separate
-ly	going toward, every
lymph/o	lymph
lymphaden/o	lymph node
lymphangi/o	lymphatic vessels
lys/o	decompose, decomposition, dissolve
lysis	destruction, to separate
-lysis	destroy, destruction, dissolve, separate, break down
lyt	dissolve
-lyte	soluble
-lytic	relating to destruction
lyze	destruct, dissolve, destroy
macro-	large
macul	spot
magnet	magnet
mak	makes
-maker	one who makes
mal-	bad, inadequate
mal	bad
-malacia	abnormal softness
malign	harmful, bad, cancer
malleol	small hammer, malleolus
mamm/o	breast
man/o	pressure
mandibul	the jaw

WORD PART	DEFINITION
mania	frenzy
-mania	frenzy, madness
manic	affected by frenzy
manipul	handful, use of hands
marker	sign
mast	breast
mastic	chew
mastoid	mastoid process
mater	mother
matern	mother
matur	ripe, ready
mature	ripe, ready, fully developed
medi	middle
media-	middle
media	middle
mediastin/o	mediastinum, middle septum
medic	medicine
medulla	middle
mega-	enormous
megaly	enlargement
-megaly	enlargement
mei	lessening
mela	black
melan/o	melanin, black pigment, black
mellit	sweetened with honey
membran/o	cover, skin
men/o	menses, monthly, month
mening/o	meninges, membranes
menisc	crescent, meniscus
menstru	menses, occurring monthly
ment	mind, chin
-ment	action, state, resulting state
mere	part
mero-	partial
mes-	middle
meso-	middle

S = Suffix   P = Prefix   R = Root   R/CF = Combining Form

WORD PART	DEFINITION
meta-	after, subsequent to, beyond
metabol	change
metacarp	bones of the hand
metatars	bones of the foot
meter	measure
-meter	measure, instrument to measure
metr/o	uterus
-metrist	skilled in measurement
-metry	process of measuring
mi-	derived from hemi, half
micr/o	small
micro-	small
mictur	make urine, pass urine
mid-	middle
mileusis	lathe
milli	one-thousandth
min	amine
miner	mines
mineral/o	inorganic materials
miss	send
mit/o-	thread, threadlike structure
mitr-	having two points
mitt	to send
mod	nature, form, method
molec	mass
mollusc	soft
mon	single
monas	unit
monil	type of fungus
mono-	one, single
morbid	disease
morph/o	shape
morphin	morphine
mort	death
mot	move

WORD PART	DEFINITION
motiv	move
muc/o	mucous membrane, mucus
mucos/a	lining of a cavity
multi-	many
mune	in service
muscul/o	muscle
mut	silent
muta	genetic change
mutil	to maim
my/o	muscle
myc/o	fungus
myel/o	spinal cord, bone marrow
myelin	in the spinal cord, myelin
myo-	to blink
myo	muscle
myos	muscle
myring/o	tympanic membrane, eardrum
myx-	mucus
narc/o	stupor, sleep
narciss	self-love
nas/o	nose
nat/e	birth, born
natr/i	sodium
natur/o	nature
nebul	cloud
necr/o	death
neo-	new
nephr/o	kidney
nerv	nerve
-ness	quality, state
neur/o	nerve, nervous tissue, nerve tissue
neutr/o	neutral
-nic	pertaining to
nitr/o	nitrogen
noct-	night

S = Suffix   P = Prefix   R = Root   R/CF = Combining Form

WORD PART	DEFINITION
noia	to think
nom	law
non-	no
nor-	normal
norm-	normal
nos/o	disease
nucl	nucleus
nucle/o	nucleus
nucleol	small nucleus
nutri	nourish
nutrit	nourishment
o/o	egg
oblong	elongated
obsess	besieged by thoughts
obstetr	midwifery
occipit	back of head
occult/a	hidden
occupation	work
ocul/o	eye
ode	way, road, path
odont	tooth
odyn/o	pain
-oid	appearance of, resemble, resembling
-ol	alcohol, chemical substance
-ola	small
-ole	small
olfact	smell
olig-	too little, scanty
olig/o-	scanty, too little
oligo-	too little, scanty
om/o	body, tumor
-oma	tumor, mass
omone	excite, stimulate
onc/o	tumor
-one	chemical substance, hormone

WORD PART	DEFINITION
onych/o	nail
opheles	be of service
ophthalm/o	eye
opia	sight
opportun	take advantage of
-opsis	vision
-opsy	to view
opt/o	vision
-or	a doer, one who does, that which does something
or/o	mouth
orbit	orbit
orch/o	testicle
ordin	arrange
orex	appetite
organ	organ, tool, instrument, organic
orth/o	straight
orthot	correct
-orum	function of
-ory	having the function of
os	mouth
-osa	like
-ose	full of, condition
-osis	condition
osmo	push
osmol	concentration
oss/i	bone
oste/o	bone
-osus	condition
ot/o	ear
-otomy	incision
-ous	pertaining to
ov/i	egg
ovari	ovary
ovul	ovum, egg

S = Suffix   P = Prefix   R = Root   R/CF = Combining Form

WORD PART	DEFINITION
ox/y	oxygen
-oxia	oxygen condition
oxid	oxidize
oxin	oxygen atom
oxytoc	swift birth
pace	step, pace
pact	driven in
palat	palate
palliat	reduce suffering
palpat	touch, stroke
palpit	throb
pan-	all
pancreat	pancreas
pant/o	entire
panto-	entire
papill/o	pimple
par-	abnormal, beside
para-	adjacent to, alongside, beside, abnormal
para	to bring forth
parasit	parasite
paresis	weakness
pareun	lying beside, sexual intercourse
pariet	wall
paroxysm	irritation
particul	little piece
partum	childbirth, to bring forth
pat	lie open
patell	patella
patent	lie open
-path	disease
path/o	disease
pathet	suffering
-pathic	pertaining to a disease
pathy	emotion, disease
-pathy	disease
paus/e	cessation

WORD PART	DEFINITION
-pause	cessation
pector	chest
ped	child, foot
pedicul	louse
pelas	skin
pell	skin
pelv	pelvis
pen	penis
-penia	deficient, deficiency
peps	digestion
pepsin/o	pepsin
pept/i	digest, digestion, amino acid
per-	intense, through
perforat	bore through
perfus/e	to pour
peri-	around
perin/e	perineum
peripher	external boundary, outer part, outer edge
periton/e	stretch over, peritoneum
perium	bringing forth
perm/e	pass through
person	person
pes	foot
pest/i	pest, nuisance
petit-	small
-pexy	fixation, surgical fixation
phaco-	lens
phag/e	to eat
-phage	to eat
-phagia	swallowing, eating
phalang/e	phalanx
pharmac/o	drug
pharyng/e	pharynx
pharynx	throat, pharynx
phen/o	to display

WORD PART	DEFINITION
phenol	benzene derivative
phenyl	chemical group
pheo-	gray
pher-	carrying
pher/o	to carry
-pheresis	removal
phery	outer edge
-phil	attraction
-phile	attraction
-philia	attraction
phim	muzzle
phleb/o	vein
phob	fear
-phobia	fear
phon/o	sound, voice
phor/e	bear, carry
phosph	phosphorus
phot/o	light
phren	mind
phylac	protect
phylaxis	protection
-phyll	leaf
phys	nature
physema	blowing
physi/o	body
physic	body
physis	growth
phyt/o	plant
pia	delicate
pituit	pituitary
placed	in an area
plak	plate, plaque
plant	insert, plant
planus	flat surface
plas	molding, formation

WORD PART	DEFINITION
-plasia	formation
-plasm	something formed
plasm/o	to form
-plasty	formation, repair, surgical repair
plate	flat
pleg	paralysis
plete	filled
pleur	pleura
plexy	stroke
pnea	to breathe
pneum/o	air, lung
pneumat	structure filled with air
pneumon	air, lung
pod	foot
-poiesis	to make
-poiet	the making
-poietin	the maker
poikilo-	irregular
point	to pierce
pol	pole
polio-	gray matter
pollut	to defile
poly-	excessive, many, much
polyp	polyp
poplit/e	ham, back of knee
por/o	opening
post-	after
poster	coming behind
pract	efficient, practical
prand/i	breakfast
pre-	before, in front of
precis	accurate
predn	a derivative of cholesterol
pregn	with child, pregnant
presby	old man

WORD PART	DEFINITION
press	press close, press down, squeeze
prevent	prevent
primi-	first
pro-	before, in front, projecting forward
proct/o	anus and rectum
product	lead forth
prol/i	bear offspring
prolifer	bear offspring
pronat	bend down
prost/a	prostate
prot/e	first, protein
protein	protein
proto-	first
proton	first
provis	provide
proxim	nearest
prurit	itch
pseudo-	false
psych/e	mind, soul
psych/o	mind, soul
pteryg	wing
ptosis	drooping, falling
-ptosis	drooping
ptysis	spit
pub	pubis
puber	growing up
pubesc	to reach puberty
puer	child
pulmon/o	lung
puls	to drive
pump	pump
punct	puncture
pur	pus
purg	cleanse, evacuate, throw up
purif	make pure
purul	pus

WORD PART	DEFINITION
py/o	pus
pyel/o	renal pelvis
pylor	gate, pylorus
pyr/o	fire, heat, fever
pyret	fever
pyrex	fever, heat
pyrid	heat
qi	vital force
quadr	four
quadrant	quarter
quadri-	four
radi/o	x-ray, radiation, radius
radial	radius
radic	root
re-	again, back, backward
recept	receive
rect/o	rectum
reflex/o	to reflect, bend back
regul	to rule
remiss	send back, give up
ren	kidney
replic	reply
rescein	resin
resect/o	cut off
resid/u	left over, what is left over
resist	to withstand
restor	renew
resuscit	revival from apparent death
reticul	fine net, network
retin/o	retina
retinacul	hold back
retro-	backward
rhabd/o	rod-shaped, striated
rheumat	a flow, rheumatism
rhin/o	nose
rhythm	rhythm

WORD PART	DEFINITION
rib/o	like a rib
ribo-	from gum Arabic
ribo	pentose, a sugar
rig	water
rigid	stiff
rit/u	right
rose	rose
rotat	rotate
-rrhage	to flow profusely
-rrhagia	excessive flow, discharge
-rrhaphy	suture
rrhea	flow, discharge
-rrhea	flow, discharge
-rrhoid	flow
rrythm	rhythm
-rubin	rust colored
rumin	throat
-ry	occupation
sacchar	sugar
sacr/o	sacrum
sagitt	arrow
saliv	saliva
salping/o	fallopian tube, uterine tube
salpinx	trumpet
san	sound, healthy
sanit	health
sanitiz	make healthy
sapon	soap
sarc/o	flesh, sarcoma, muscle
satur	to fill
scapul	scapula
schiz/o	to split, cleave
scinti	spark
scintill	spark
scler/o	hard, white of eye, hardness
scope	instrument for viewing

WORD PART	DEFINITION
-scope	instrument for viewing, instrument
-scopy	to examine, to view, visual examination
scorb	scurvy
script	writing, thing copied
scrot	scrotum
seb/o	sebum
sebac/e	wax
secret	secrete, produce, separate
sect	cut off
sedat	to calm
sedent	sitting
segment	section
seiz	to grab, convulse
self	me, own individual
semi-	half
semin	scatter seed
semin/i	semen
sen	old age
senesc	growing old
senil	characteristic of old age
sens	feel
sensitiv	sensitive, feeling, sensitivity
sensor/i	sensation, sensory
separat	move apart
seps	decay, infection
sept/o	septum, partition
septic	infected
ser/o	serum, serous
sib	relative
-side	glycoside
sigm	Greek letter "S"
sigmoid/o	sigmoid colon
silic	silicon, glass
simi	ape, monkey
simul	imitate
sin/o	sinus

WORD PART	DEFINITION
-sine	fold, pocket
sinus	sinus
sipid	flavor
-sis	abnormal condition, process
sit/u	place
skelet	skeleton
skin	skin
smear	spread
soc	partner
soci/o	partner, ally, community
soma	body
somat/o	body
some	body
somn/o	sleep
somy	chromosome
son/o	sound
sorbit	fruit of a tree
sorpt	swallow
sound	noise
spad	tear or cut
spasm	spasm, sudden involuntary tightening
spast	tight
specif	species
sperm/i	sperm
spermat/o	sperm
sphen	wedge
spher/o	sphere
sphygm/o	pulse
spin/o	spine, spinal cord
spir/o	spiral, coil
spirat	breathe
spirit/u	spirit
spiro-	spiral, coil
splen/o	spleen
spondyl	vertebra
spong/i	sponge

WORD PART	DEFINITION
spongios	sponge
spor/e	spore
stabil	stand firm
stable	steady
stag	standing place
stalsis	to constrict
-stalsis	constrict, constriction
staphyl/o	bunch of grapes
stasis	stagnate, stay in one place, placement
-stasis	control, stop, stand still
stat	stand still
-static	to make stand, stop
-statin	inhibit
stax	fall in drops
steat	fat
stein	stone
sten/o	narrow, contract
ster	solid, steroid
stere/o	three-dimensional
steril	barren
stern	chest, breastbone
-steroid	steroid
-sterol	steroid
steron	steroid
-sterone	sterol
steth/o	chest
sthen	strength
stick	branch, twig
stigmat	focus
stimul	excite, strengthen
stin	partition
stip	press
stit/i	space
stoma	mouth
-stomy	new opening
stone	stone, pebble

WORD PART	DEFINITION
storm	crisis
strab	squint
strat	layer
strept/o	twisted
strepto-	curved
study	inquiry
su/i	self
sub-	below, under, slightly, underneath
sucr	sucrose, table sugar
suffic/i	enough
sulf	sulfur
super-	above, excessive
super	above
supinat	bend backward
supplement	supply to remedy a deficiency
suppress	pressed under, push under
supra-	above, excessive
surf	surface
surfact	surface
surg	operate
suscept	to take up
-sylated	linked
sym-	together
symptomat	symptom
syn-	together
syn/o	synovial membrane
syndesm	bind together
synov	synovial membrane
syring/o	tube, pipe
system	body system
systol/e	contraction
tachy-	rapid
tact	orderly arrangement
tag	touch
tain	hold
tali	ankle bone

WORD PART	DEFINITION
tamin	touch
tampon	plug
tangent/i	touch
tarsus	flat surface
tax	coordination
tect/o	to shelter
tempor/o	time, temple, side of head
ten/o	tendon
tendin	tendon
tens	pressure
-tensin	tense, taut
terat/o	monster, malformed fetus
term	normal gestation
test/o	testis, testicle
testicul	testicle, testis
tetra-	four
thalam	thalamus
thalass	sea
thec	sheath
thel	breast, nipple
thel/i	lining
then	motion
thenar	palm
therap/o	healing, treatment
therapeut	healing, treatment
therapy	medical treatment
-therapy	treatment
therm/o	heat
thesis	to arrange, place
thet	place, arrange
thi	sulfur
thora	chest
thorac/o	chest
thorax	chest
thromb/o	blood clot, clot
thrombin	clot

WORD PART	DEFINITION
thym	thymus gland, the mind
thyr/o	thyroid
thyroid	thyroid
-tic	pertaining to
-tion	process, being
-tiz	pertaining to
toc	labor, birth
toler	endure
tom/o	section, incise, cut
-tome	instrument to cut
-tomy	surgical incision
ton/o	pressure, tension
tonsil	tonsil
tonsill/o	tonsil
tope	part, location
topic	local
-tous	pertaining to
tox/o	poison
-toxic	able to kill
toxic/o	poison
toxin	poison
trache/o	trachea, windpipe
tract	draw, pull
tranquil	calm
trans-	across, through
trauma	wound, injury
tresia	a hole
tri-	three
trich/o	hair, flagellum
trichin/o	hair
-tripsy	to crush
-tripter	crusher
trochle	pulley
trop	turn, turning
troph	development, nourishment
trophy	development, nourishment

WORD PART	DEFINITION
-tropic	stimulator, change
-tropin	nourishing, stimulation
tryps	friction
tub/a	tube
tubercul	swelling, tuberculosis, nodule
tubul	small tube
tuss/i	cough
tussis	cough
-ty	quality, state
tympan/o	eardrum, tympanic membrane
-type	model, particular kind, group
typh	typhus
-ula	small thing
ulcer	a sore
-ule	little, small
-ulent	abounding in
uln/a	forearm bone
ultra-	higher, beyond
-um	tissue, structure
umbilic	belly button, navel, umbilicus
un-	not
un	one
uni-	one
ur/o	urinary system
urac	urinary bladder
-ure	process, result of
uresis	to urinate
uret	ureter, urine, urination
ureter/o	ureter
urethr/o	urethra
uria	urine
-uria	urine
urin/a	urine
-us	pertaining to
uter/o	uterus
uve	uvea

WORD PART	DEFINITION
uvul	uvula
vaccin	vaccine, giving a vaccine
vag	vagus nerve
vagin	sheath, vagina
valgus	turn out
valv	valve
varic/o	varicosity; dilated, tortuous vein
vas/o	blood vessel, duct
vascul	blood vessel
ved	knowledge
veget	plants
vegetat	growth
ven/o	vein
ventil	wind
ventr	belly
ventricul	ventricle
vers	turned
verse	travel
-version	change
vert	to turn
vertebr/a	vertebra
vesic	sac containing fluid
vestibul/o	vestibule of inner ear
via	the way
violet	bluish purple
vir	virus

WORD PART	DEFINITION
viril	masculine
virus	poison
visc/o	sticky
viscer	an internal organ
visu	sight
vit/a	life
voc	voice
vol	volume
volunt	free will
volut	shrink, roll up
-volut	rolled up
volute	shrink, roll up
vuls	tear, pull
vulv/o	vulva
whip	to swing
xanth	yellow
xen/o	foreign material
xeno-	foreign
-xis	condition
-yl	substance
zea-	to live
-zoa	animal
zyg	zygote
zygot	yoked together
zyme	fermenting, enzyme, transform
-zyme	enzyme

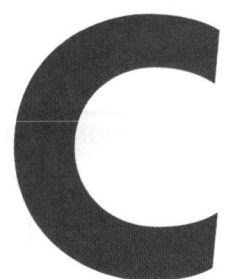

Abbreviations

ABBREVIATION	DEFINITION
μg	microgram; one-millionth of a gram
↑	increase/ above
↓	decrease/ below
1°	primary
2°	secondary
99mTc	technetium 99m, a radionuclide
ABG	arterial blood gas
ABI	ankle/brachial index
ABO	a blood group system
AC	acromioclavicular
ACE	angiotensin-converting enzyme
ACEP	Association for Comprehensive Energy Psychology; American College of Emergency Physicians
ACL	anterior cruciate ligament
ACTH	adrenocorticotropic hormone
AD	right ear
ADD	attention deficit disorder
ADH	antidiuretic hormone
ADHD	attention deficit hyperactivity disorder
ADLs	activities of daily living
AED	automatic external defibrillator
AFP	alpha-fetoprotein
AI	adequate intake
AIDS	acquired immunodeficiency syndrome
ALL	acute lymphoblastic leukemia
ALP	alkaline phosphatase
ALS	amyotrophic lateral sclerosis
ALT	alanine aminotransferase

ABBREVIATION	DEFINITION
AMAS	anti-malignin antibody screen
ANS	autonomic nervous system
AOM	acute otitis media
AP	anteroposterior
aPTT	activated partial thromboplastin time
ARDS	acute respiratory distress syndrome
ARF	acute respiratory failure
ARF	acute renal failure
AROM	active range of motion
AS	left ear
ASD	atrial septal defect
ASD	autism spectrum disorder
ASHD	arteriosclerotic heart disease
AST	aspartate aminotransferase
AU	both ears
AV	atrioventricular
AVM	arteriovenous malformation
BAL	bronchoalveolar lavage
BBB	blood-brain barrier
BCIA	Biofeedback Certification Institute of America
BD	brain death
BKA	below-the-knee amputation
BM	bowel movement
BMD	bone mineral density
BMR	basal metabolic rate
BNP	B-type natriuretic peptide
BOM	bilateral otitis media

ABBREVIATION	DEFINITION
PFT	pulmonary function test
pg	picogram; one-trillionth of a gram
PGY	pregnancy
pH	hydrogen ion concentration
PhD	doctor of philosophy
PID	pelvic inflammatory disease
PIP	proximal interphalangeal
PKD	polycystic kidney disease
PKU	phenylketonuria
PMDD	premenstrual dysphoric disorder
PMNL	polymorphonuclear leukocyte
PMS	premenstrual syndrome
PNS	peripheral nervous system
PO	by mouth
polio	poliomyelitis
PPH	postpartum hemorrhage
PPI	proton pump inhibitor
PPS	postpolio syndrome
PRL	prolactin
p.r.n.	when necessary
PSA	prostate-specific antigen
PsyD	doctor of psychology
PT	physiotherapy
PT	prothrombin time
PT	physical therapy, physical therapist
PTA	physical therapy assistant
PTCA	percutaneous transluminal coronary angioplasty
PTH	parathyroid hormone
PTSD	posttraumatic stress disorder
PVC	premature ventricular contraction
PVD	peripheral vascular disease
PVS	persistent vegetative state
q.4.h.	every 4 hours
q.i.d.	four times a day
R	respiration (rate)

ABBREVIATION	DEFINITION
RA	rheumatoid arthritis
RBC	red blood cell
RDA	recommended dietary allowance
RDS	respiratory distress syndrome
RF	radiofrequency
Rh	Rhesus
RhoGAM	Rhesus immune globulin
RICE	rest, ice, compression, elevation
RLQ	right lower quadrant
RN	registered nurse
RNA	ribonucleic acid
ROM	range of motion
RSV	respiratory syncytial virus
RT	radiology technician
RU-486	mifepristone
RUQ	right upper quadrant
S1–S5	sacral nerves or vertebrae
SA	sinoatrial
SAD	seasonal affective disorder
SARS	severe acute respiratory syndrome
SBS	shaken baby syndrome
SC	subcutaneous
SCI	spinal cord injury
SET	self-examination of the testes
SFD	small for date
SG	specific gravity
SGA	small for gestational age
SGOT	serum glutamic-oxaloacetic acid transaminase (AST)
SGPT	serum glutamic-pyruvic transaminase (ALT)
SI	sacroiliac
SIDS	sudden infant death syndrome
SLE	systemic lupus erythematosus
SMI	sustained maximal inspiration
SNRI	serotonin and norepinephrine reuptake inhibitor
SOB	short(ness) of breath

ABBREVIATION	DEFINITION
SP	Standard Precautions
SRS	stereotactic radiosurgery
SSA	Sjögren syndrome antibodies A
SSB	Sjögren syndrome antibodies B
SSRI	selective serotonin reuptake inhibitor
STAT	immediately
STD	sexually transmitted disease
SVC	superior vena cava
T	temperature
T1	first thoracic vertebra or nerve
T1–T12	thoracic spinal nerves or vertebrae
T_3	triiodothyronine
T_4	tetraiodothyronine (thyroxine)
TB	tuberculosis
TBI	traumatic brain injury
TCA	tricyclic antidepressant
TED	thromboembolic deterrent
TEE	transesophageal echocardiography
TENS	transcutaneous electrical nerve stimulation
THC	tetrahydrocannabinol (marijuana)
THR	total hip replacement
TIA	transient ischemic attack
TIBC	total iron-binding capacity
t.i.d.	(Latin *ter in die*) three times a day
TMJ	temporomandibular joint
TNM	tumor-node-metastasis (staging system for cancer)
TOF	tetralogy of Fallot

ABBREVIATION	DEFINITION
tPA	tissue plasminogen activator
TPN	total parenteral nutrition
TS	tumor suppressor
TSH	thyroid-stimulating hormone
TTM	trichotillomania
TTN	transient tachypnea of the newborn
TTP	thrombotic thrombocytopenic purpura
TURP	transurethral resection of the prostate
U	unit
UA	urinalysis
μg	microgram; one-millionth of a gram
UP	Universal Precautions
URI	upper respiratory infection
USDA	U.S. Department of Agriculture
UTI	urinary tract infection
UV	ultraviolet
VCUG	voiding cystourethrogram
VEP	visual evoked potential
V-fib	ventricular fibrillation
VS	vital signs
VSD	ventricular septal defect
vWD	von Willebrand disease
vWF	von Willebrand factor
WAD	Word Analysis and Definition (box)
WBC	white blood cell; white blood (cell) count
WNL	within normal limits
WNV	West Nile virus

Pharmacology

D

This compilation presents pharmacologic terms and classes of drugs used in this book.

A

acetaminophen Medication that is an analgesic (reduces response to pain) and antipyretic (reduces fever). (Brand name: Tylenol.) Also called *paracetamol.*

adrenaline Main catecholamine produced by the adrenal medulla. Also called *epinephrine.*

adrenocorticotropic hormone (ACTH) Hormone produced and secreted by the anterior pituitary gland. Its principal effect is stimulation of the production of androgens and cortisol from the adrenal cortex.

aldosterone The principal mineralocorticoid produced by the adrenal cortex. It promotes sodium retention and potassium excretion by the kidneys.

allergen A substance producing a hypersensitivity (allergic) reaction. Examples are animal fur and dander, penicillins, and foods such as eggs, milk, and wheat.

amphetamines A class of psychostimulants that increase levels of norepinephrine, serotonin, and dopamine in the brain. They are used to treat attention deficit hyperactivity disorder (ADHD) and narcolepsy.

anabolic steroids A class of steroid hormones related to testosterone. They increase protein synthesis in cells, particularly in muscle. They are used therapeutically to stimulate bone and muscle growth, appetite, induce male puberty, and treat chronic wasting conditions, such as cancer. Their use in sports to increase muscle power is considered doping by all major sporting bodies.

analgesic A substance that reduces or relieves the response to pain without producing loss of consciousness. Examples are aspirin and other NSAIDs, acetaminophen, and codeine.

androgen Hormone that promotes masculine characteristics. An example is testosterone.

anesthetic An agent that causes absence of feeling or sensation. Examples of a local anesthetic are lidocaine and novocaine; examples of a general anesthetic are nitrous oxide, thiopental, and ketamine.

antacid An agent that neutralizes the acidity of stomach contents. Examples are aluminum hydroxide, magnesium hydroxide, and calcium carbonate.

antiarrhythmics Drugs that change the electrical properties of myocardial cells to restore normal cardiac rate and rhythm. An example is beta-blockers.

antibiotic A substance that has the capacity to inhibit the growth of or destroy bacteria and other microorganisms. Examples are penicillin, erythromycin, cefotaxime, and flucloxacillin.

anticoagulant A substance that prevents clotting. Examples are heparin and Coumadin (warfarin).

antidepressant An agent used to treat depression and increase the amount of serotonin at synapses where it is a neurotransmitter. Examples are Prozac and Zoloft.

antidiabetic drugs Drugs used in the treatment of diabetes. Given orally, these drugs include metformin, sulfonylureas, and thiazolidinediones, such as pioglitazone. Insulin is given by injection.

antidiuretic An agent that decreases urine production. Examples are vasopressin, amiloride, and chlorpropamide.

antiepileptic An agent capable of preventing or arresting epilepsy. Examples are phenobarbital, phenytoin, and valproate.

antifungal A topical agent that eliminates or inhibits the growth of fungi. An example is Lamisil, used as a cream, gel, or spray.

antihistamine An agent used to treat allergic symptoms because of its action antagonistic to histamine. Examples are Benadryl and cimetidine.

anti-inflammatory An agent which reduces inflammation by acting on the body's responses, without affecting the causative agent; examples are corticosteroids and aspirin.

antimicrobial An agent used to destroy or prevent multiplication of organisms. (See also **antibiotic.**)

antineoplastic An agent that prevents the growth and spread of cancer cells. Examples are methotrexate, fluorouracil, and cyclophosphamide.

antioxidants Substances that can help prevent cell damage by neutralizing free radicals produced during cell metabolism. Examples are vitamins C and E.

antipruritic Medication used against itching. Examples are calamine lotion, hydrocortisone cream applied topically, and diphenhydramine (Benadryl) taken orally.

antipsychotic An agent used in the treatment of psychosis. An example is chlorpromazine (Thorazine).

antipyretic An agent that reduces fever. Examples are aspirin and acetaminophen.

antiseptic An agent that reduces the number of microorganisms on the skin and mucous membranes. Examples are alcohol, chlorhexidine, and povidone-iodine.

aseptic An agent that enables all living pathogenic organisms to be absent from a surface and produces a state of sterility.

aspirin A drug used as an analgesic to relieve minor aches and pains, as an antipyretic to reduce fever, and as an anti-inflammatory medication. It also reduces platelet adherence and aggregation and is used in long-term low doses (81 mg) to reduce the incidence of heart attacks, strokes, and blood clots. Also called *acetylsalicylic acid (ASA)*.

atropine An agent used to dilate pupils.

B

beta blocker An agent used in the treatment of cardiac arrhythmias. Examples are propranolol and acebutolol.

bronchodilator An agent that relaxes the smooth muscles of the bronchioles. Examples are theophylline; beta$_2$-agonists, such as salbutamol and terbutaline; and anticholinergics, such as ipratropium bromide.

C

calcium channel blocker An agent that decreases the force of contraction of the myocardium, dilates coronary arteries, and reduces blood pressure. Examples are amlodipine and verapamil.

chemoprophylactic A chemical or drug that prevents infection or disease. An example is the use of mefloquine or chloroquine for the prevention of malaria in tourists traveling to East Africa.

chemotherapy Treatment, often against cancer, using chemical agents. Examples are platinum compounds such as Cisplatin or Paraplatin.

chlorpromazine A tranquilizer; it was invented in 1950 and was the first drug with specific antipsychotic effects. (Brand name: Thorazine.)

coagulant A substance that causes clotting. Thrombin and fibrin glue are used surgically to treat bleeding.

cocaine An alkaloid obtained from the leaves of the coca plant that is a potent central nervous system stimulant. It is widely abused for its euphoric effects, with the risks of severe mental and physical adverse reactions.

codeine An opiate that depresses nerve transmission in the synapses of the brain and spinal cord. It is used to relieve pain and also is used in cough medicines.

contraceptive An agent that prevents conception. Examples are condoms, diaphragms, and birth control pills using a mixture of estrogen and progesterone.

corticosteroids Hormones produced by the adrenal cortex. Examples are cortisol and aldosterone.

cortisol One of the glucocorticoids produced by the adrenal cortex; has anti-inflammatory effects. Also called *hydrocortisone*.

cyanocobalamin Vitamin B$_{12}$; given by injection for the treatment of pernicious anemia (PA). PA is caused by a deficiency of B$_{12}$ when its absorption is decreased because of an absence of intrinsic factor in gastric juices.

D

decongestant An agent that reduces the swelling and fluid in the nose and sinuses. Examples are pseudoephedrine and phenylephrine.

depressant A substance that diminishes activity, sensation, or tone. Examples are alcohol, barbiturates, and benzodiazepines.

digoxin An extract from the foxglove plant that is used to treat heart conditions such as atrial fibrillation and heart failure. (Brand names include Lanoxin and Digitek.) Also called *digitalis*.

disease-modifying Term applied to agents that have partial success in slowing down the accumulation of disabilities in a specific disease process. Examples for multiple sclerosis (MS) include interferons and mitoxantrone.

disinfectant An agent used to destroy pathogenic and other microorganisms on nonliving surfaces. Examples are alcohol, hydrogen peroxide, and hypochlorites.

diuretic An agent that increases urine output. Examples are furosemide, hydrochlorothiazide, spironolactone, and mannitol.

dopamine A neurotransmitter in some specific small areas of the brain. Its absence is associated with Parkinson disease.

E

emetic An agent that induces vomiting. An example is syrup of ipecac.

epinephrine Main catecholamine produced by the adrenal medulla. Also called *adrenaline*.

estrogen Generic term for hormones that stimulate female secondary sex characteristics.

F

fertility drugs Drugs that cause the release of hormones that either trigger ovulation or regulate it. They are used for in vitro fertilization (IVF) to stimulate the ovaries to produce eggs. Clomiphene is the first choice for infertility. If this is unsuccessful, injectable hormones such as human chorionic gonadotropin or follicle-stimulating hormone can be used.

fluorescein Dye that produces a vivid green color under a blue light; used to diagnose corneal abrasions and foreign bodies in the eye.

fungicides Chemical compounds or biologic organisms that kill or inhibit the growth of fungi and molds. The most commonly used fungicide is sulfur. Other active ingredients include rosemary oil and the bacterium *Bacillus subtilis*.

H

heparin A polysaccharide widely used as an injectable anticoagulant. It also has a role as a defense mechanism against bacteria and other foreign agents at sites of tissue injury.

heroin An agent synthesized from morphine, a derivative of the opium poppy. It is used as a painkiller; as a recreational drug it has a high potential for addiction. Also called *diamorphine.*

histamine A compound liberated in tissues as a result of injury or an immune response.

hydrocortisone Potent glucocorticoid with anti-inflammatory properties. Also called *cortisol.*

hyperbaric oxygen therapy (HBOT) The medical use of oxygen in a pressure chamber at a pressure higher than atmospheric pressure. It is used to treat decompression sickness, air embolism, carbon monoxide poisoning, and severe bacterial wound infections.

I

ibuprofen A nonsteroidal anti-inflammatory drug (NSAID) used to treat minor aches and pains and fever. It is available over the counter in low dosages (Advil, Motrin).

immunization An agent to protect susceptible people from a communicable disease; used, for example, to protect against childhood diseases such as measles, rubella, and pertussis.

insecticide A pesticide used against insects to kill their eggs and larvae. Natural insecticides include nicotine and pyrethrum; in Tuscany, Italy, tobacco leaves are laid to protect grape vines and produce. Synthetic insecticides, such as DDT (dichlorodiphenyltrichloroethane), organophosphates, and related chemical warfare agents, are banned worldwide because they cause severe reductions in bird populations and are harmful to humans.

insulin Hormone produced by the islet cells of the pancreas that promotes glucose use. Injectable insulin preparations are classified by their speed of action.

iron An essential element. Supplementation tablets, such as ferrous sulfate, are used in the treatment of iron-deficiency anemias and in the prevention of anemia during pregnancy.

L

lactase An enzyme that breaks down the milk sugar lactose into glucose and galactose. It is used in the treatment of lactose intolerance.

light therapy Therapy that mimics natural outdoor light and is used in the treatment of seasonal affective disorder (SAD), shift-work problems, depression and in healthy newborns with jaundice. Also called *phototherapy.*

M

melatonin Hormone formed and secreted by the pineal gland during darkness. Serotonin is a precursor. It assists in the control of daily body rhythms, stimulates the immune system, and is an antioxidant. It has been used in the treatment of SAD and some sleep disorders.

meprobamate Available since 1955, a sedative that is listed as a controlled substance because it can cause physical and psychological dependence. (Brand names: Miltown and Equanil.)

mifepristone A synthetic steroid (RU-486) used as an abortifacient in the first 2 months of pregnancy and used in smaller doses as an emergency contraceptive. In the United States, it is a prescription drug, Mifeprex.

morphine A derivative of opium used as an analgesic or sedative.

mucolytic An agent that attempts to break up mucus to allow it to be cleared more effectively from the airways. Examples are guaifenesin (common in over-the-counter cough medications), potassium iodide, and *N*-acetylcysteine taken through a nebulizer.

N

naloxone A drug used in emergencies to counter the life-threatening CNS and respiratory depression of opiate overdose from, for example, heroin or morphine. Given intramuscularly it acts within 1 minute. (Brand names: Narcan and Nalone; also available generically.)

narcotic A drug derived from opium. Examples are heroin, morphine, codeine, and Demerol.

neurotransmitter A chemical that crosses a synapse to stimulate or inhibit another neuron or the cell of a muscle or gland. Examples are norepinephrine, serotonin, and dopamine.

O

opiate A drug derived from opium. Examples are morphine, codeine, heroin, and Demerol.

oxycodone An opiate medication used orally to combat moderate to severe pain (brand name: Oxycontin). It is also prescribed in combination with acetaminophen (Percocet), aspirin (Percodan), and ibuprofen (Combunox). It is associated with dependence and hazardous use.

oxygen A gas used in hypoxia given by nasal cannula or by mask and intubation. Patients with severe, chronic COPD can be attached to a portable cylinder of oxygen. (See also **hyperbaric oxygen therapy.**)

P

parenteral Medication taken into the body or administered other than through the digestive tract; for example, by intravenous, intramuscular, or subcutaneous injection, by transdermal patches, or by inhalation.

pesticide An agent for destroying flies, mosquitoes, and other pests.

pharmacist A person licensed by a state to prepare and dispense drugs.

pharmacology The science of the preparation, uses, and effects of drugs.

pharmacy A facility licensed to prepare and dispense drugs.

phototherapy Therapy that mimics natural outdoor light and is used in the treatment of seasonal affective disorder (SAD), shift-work problems, depression, and in healthy newborns with jaundice.

placebo An inert compound with no innate therapeutic value.

prednisone A synthetic corticosteroid that decreases the immune system's response to various diseases. It is used in the treatment of diseases such as severe asthma, severe allergies, systemic lupus erythematosus, ulcerative colitis, and rheumatoid arthritis, as well as to prevent and treat rejection in organ transplantation. The drug has significant side effects, such as adrenal suppression, increased blood glucose levels, and osteoporosis.

progesterone Hormone that prepares the uterus for pregnancy.

prophylactic A medication, treatment, public health measure, or device used to prevent a disease or an infection from occurring. Examples are vaccines, specific antibiotics, antimalarials, and condoms.

proton pump inhibitor An agent that blocks the production of gastric acid by blocking the enzyme system that produces acid in the gastric cells. Examples include Prilosec and Prevacid.

psychoactive An agent able to alter mood, behavior, and/or cognition. Examples include narcotics, stimulants, antidepressants, and hallucinogens.

S

saline Salt solution, usually sodium chloride.

sedative An agent that calms nervous excitement by decreasing the sensitivity of the postsynaptic neurons. Examples are ethanol (beverage alcohol), barbiturates, and meprobamate.

somatotropin Hormone of the anterior pituitary gland that stimulates the growth of body tissues. Also called *growth hormone (GH)*.

spermicide An agent that destroys sperm. Examples are nonoxynol-9 and benzalkonium chloride.

sterilization A method of eliminating all microorganisms by high-pressure steam (autoclave), dry heat (oven), or radiation.

steroid Large family of chemical substances found in many drugs, hormones, and body components.

stimulant An agent that excites or strengthens. Examples include caffeine, nicotine, and cocaine.

surfactant A protein and fat compound that creates surface tension to hold the lung alveolar walls apart.

T

teratogen An agent that produces fetal abnormalities—congenital malformations—while organs and structures are being formed. All medications readily cross the placenta. Examples include alcohol, valproic acid (anticonvulsant), and the rubella virus.

testosterone The major androgen that promotes development of male sex characteristics.

thrombolytic A drug injected within a few hours of a myocardial infarction (MI) or stroke to dissolve the thrombus causing the arterial blockage. Examples are streptokinase and tissue plasminogen activator (tPA). Also called *clot-busting drug.*

thyroxine Thyroid hormone T4, tetraiodothyronine.

topical Medication applied to the skin to obtain a local effect. Examples are ointments, creams, gels, lotions, patches, and sprays.

toxin A poisonous substance formed by a living cell or organism. Examples are bee stings, snake venom, and jellyfish stings.

tranquilizer An agent that acts like a sedative but without a sedative's sleep-inducing effect. Examples are chlorpromazine, haloperidol, and the benzodiazapines such as Librium and Valium.

V

vaccine An agent that is used to generate immunity and is composed of the antigenic components of a killed or attenuated microorganism or its inactivated toxins. (See also **immunization.**)

vitamin An essential organic substance necessary in small amounts for normal cell function.

vitamin D An essential compound for the formation and maintenance of bone. Men and women over 50 are often advised to take 1200 mg of calcium daily and 400 to 600 international units (IU) of vitamin D and to expose their bodies to the sun for 15 minutes daily.

W

warfarin An anticoagulant; also used as rat poison. (Brand name: Coumadin.)

A

abdomen (**AB**-doh-men) Part of the trunk between the thorax and the pelvis.

abdominal (ab-**DOM**-in-al) Pertaining to the abdomen.

abdominopelvic (ab-**DOM**-ih-no-**PEL**-vik) Pertaining to the abdomen and pelvis.

abducens (ab-**DYU**-senz) Sixth (VI) cranial nerve; responsible for eye movement.

abduction (ab-**DUCK**-shun) Action of moving away from the midline.

ablation (ab-**LAY**-shun) Removal of tissue to destroy its function.

abortion (ah-**BOR**-shun) Spontaneous or induced expulsion of an embryo or fetus from the uterus.

abortus (ah-**BOR**-tus) Product of abortion.

abrasion (ah-**BRAY**-shun) Area of skin or mucous membrane that has been scraped off.

abruptio (ab-**RUP**-she-oh) Placenta abruptio is the premature detachment of the placenta.

absorption (ab-**SORP**-shun) Uptake of nutrients and water by cells in the GI tract.

accessory (ack-**SESS**-oh-ree) Eleventh (XI) cranial nerve; supplying neck muscles, pharynx, and larynx.

accommodation (ah-kom-oh-**DAY**-shun) The act of adjusting something to make it fit the needs; in the case of the eye, the lens adjusts itself.

acetabulum (as-eh-**TAB**-you-lum) The cup-shaped cavity of the hip bone that receives the head of the femur to form the hip joint.

acetaminophen (ah-seat-ah-**MIN**-oh-fen) Medication that is an analgesic and an antipyretic.

acetone (**ASS**-eh-tone) Ketone that is found in blood, urine, and breath when diabetes mellitus is out of control.

acetylcholine (**AS**-eh-til-**KOH**-leen) Parasympathetic neurotransmitter.

Achilles tendon (ah-**KILL**-eeze) A tendon formed from the gastrocnemius and soleus muscles and inserted into the calcaneus. Also called *calcaneal tendon*.

achondroplasia (a-kon-droh-**PLAY**-ze-ah) Condition with abnormal conversion of cartilage into bone, leading to dwarfism.

acid (**ASS**-id) Substance with a pH below 7.0.

acinar cells (**ASS**-in-ar SELLS) Enzyme-secreting cells of the pancreas.

acne (**AK**-nee) Inflammatory disease of sebaceous glands and hair follicles.

acoustic (ah-**KOOS**-tik) Pertaining to hearing.

acquired (ah-**KWIRED**) A condition that is not inherited.

acquired immunodeficiency syndrome (AIDS) (ah-**KWIRED** **IM**-you-noh-de-**FISH**-en-see **SIN**-drome) Infection with the HIV virus.

acromegaly (ak-roe-**MEG**-ah-lee) Enlargement of the head, face, hands, and feet due to excess growth hormone in an adult.

acromioclavicular (AC) (ah-**CROW**-mee-oh-klah-**VICK**-you-lar) The joint between the acromion and the clavicle.

acromion (ah-**CROW**-mee-on) Lateral end of the scapula, extending over the shoulder joint.

acrophobia (ak-roh-**FOH**-be-ah) Pathologic fear of heights.

activities of daily living (ADLs) (ak-**TIV**-ih-tees of **DAY**-lee **LIV**-ing) Daily routines for mobility and personal care: bathing, dressing, eating, and moving.

acuminata (a-**KYU**-min-ah-ta) Tapering to a point.

acupoint (**AK**-you-point) Point of entry in the skin to a meridian.

acupressure (**AK**-you-presh-ur) Application of pressure to acupoints.

acupuncture (ak-you-**PUNK**-chur) Use of sterile, hair-thin needles to stimulate the energy pathways known as meridians.

acute (ah-**KYUT**) Describes a disease of sudden onset that is usually severe and of short duration.

adapt (ad-**APT**) To adjust to different conditions.

adaptation (ad-ap-**TAY**-shun) Change in function or structure of an organ to meet new conditions.

adaptive equipment (a-**DAP**-tiv ee-**KWIP**-ment) Devices and supplies that enable a disabled individual to perform specific functions.

addict (**ADD**-ikt) Person with a psychologic or physical dependence on a substance or practice.

addiction (ah-**DIK**-shun) Habitual psychological and physiologic dependence on a substance or practice.

addictive (ah-**DIK**-tiv) Pertaining to or causing addiction.

Addison disease (**ADD**-ih-son **DIZ**-eez) An autoimmune disease leading to decreased production of adrenocortical steroids.

adduction (ah-**DUCK**-shun) Action of moving toward the midline.

adenine (**AD**-eh-neen) One of the chemical bases found in, and comprising the sequence of, both DNA and RNA.

adenocarcinoma (**AD**-eh-noh-kar-sih-**NOH**-mah) A cancer arising from glandular epithelial cells.

adenohypophysis (**AD**-en-oh-hi-**POF**-ih-sis) Anterior lobe of the pituitary gland.

adenoid (**ADD**-eh-noyd) Single mass of lymphoid tissue in the midline at the back of the throat.

adenomyosis (**AD**-en-oh-my-**OH**-sis) The implantation of endometrial glandular tissue in the myometrium.

adherence (ad-**HERE**-ents) The act of sticking to something.

adipose (**ADD**-i-pose) Containing fat.

adiposity (ad-ih-**POSS**-ih-tee) Excessive accumulation of fat in a site, organ, or body.

adjunct (**AJ**-ungkt) Something that is joined to another but is not an essential part.

adjustment (ah-**JUST**-ment) The action of bringing a body part into alignment with the others. Also called *manipulation*.

adjuvant (**AD**-joo-vant) Additional treatment after a primary treatment has been used.

adnexa (ad-**NEK**-sa) Parts accessory to an organ or structure. Singular *adnexum*.

adnexal (ad-**NEK**-sal) Pertaining to accessory structures; for example, structures alongside the uterus.

adolescence (ad-oh-**LESS**-ents) Stage that begins with puberty and ends with physical maturity.

adolescent (ad-oh-**LESS**-ent) Pertaining to adolescence or a person in that stage.

adrenal gland (ah-**DREE**-nal GLAND) The suprarenal, or adrenal, gland on the upper pole of each kidney.

adrenalectomy (ah-dree-nal-**ECK**-to-me) Removal of part or all of an adrenal gland.

adrenaline (ah-**DREN**-ah-lin) One of the catecholamines. Also called *epinephrine.*

adrenergic (ad-re-**NER**-jik) Relating to the autonomic nervous system.

adrenocortical (ah-dree-noh-**KOR**-tih-kal) Pertaining to the cortex of the adrenal gland.

adrenocorticotropic hormone (ah-**DREE**-noh-**KOR**-tih-koh-**TROH**-pik HOR-mohn) Hormone of the anterior pituitary that stimulates the cortex of the adrenal gland to produce its own hormones.

adrenogenital syndrome (ah-**DREE**-no-**JEN**-it-al SIN-drome) Hypersecretion of androgens from the adrenal gland.

advance medical directive (ad-**VANTS MED**-ih-kal die-**REK**-tiv) Legal document signed by the patient dealing with issues of prolonging or ending life in the event of life-threatening illness.

adventitia (ad-ven-**TISH**-ah) Outer layer of connective tissue covering blood vessels or organs.

aerobic (air-**OH**-bik) An organism capable of living in the presence of oxygen.

affect (**AF**-fekt) External display of feelings, thoughts, and emotions.

afferent (**AF**-eh-rent) Conducting impulses inward *toward* the spinal cord or brain.

agar (**AH**-gar) A derivative of seaweed used as a culture medium.

aged (**A**-jid) Having lived to an advanced age.

agenesis (a-**JEN**-eh-sis) Failure to develop any organ or any part.

agglutinate (ah-**GLUE**-tin-ate) Stick together to form clumps.

agglutination (ah-glue-tih-**NAY**-shun) Process by which cells or other particles adhere to each other to form clumps.

aging (**A**-jing) The process of human maturation and decline.

agonist (**AG**-on-ist) Agent combines with receptors to initiate drug actions.

agoraphobia (ah-gor-ah-**FOH**-be-ah) Pathologic fear of being trapped in a public place.

agranulocyte (a-**GRAN**-you-lo-site) A white blood cell without any granules in its cytoplasm.

alanine aminotransferase (ALT) (**AL**-ah-neen ah-**ME**-no-**TRANS**-fer-aze) Enzyme that is found in liver cells and leaks out into the bloodstream when the cells are damaged, enabling liver damage to be diagnosed.

albinism (**AL**-bih-nizm) Genetic disorder with lack of melanin.

albino (al-**BY**-no) Person with albinism.

albumin (al-**BYU**-min) Simple, soluble protein.

aldosterone (al-**DOS**-ter-own) Mineralocorticoid hormone of the adrenal cortex.

aldosteronism (al-**DOS**-ter-on-izm) Condition caused by excessive secretion of aldosterone. Also called *Conn syndrome.*

aldosteronoma (al-**DOS**-ter-on-oma) Benign adenoma of the adrenal cortex.

Alexander technique (al-eg-**ZAN**-der tek-**NEEK**) The use of awareness and exercises to improve posture, breathing, and movement.

alignment (a-**LINE**-ment) A state of being in the correct position in relation to other structures.

alimentary (al-ih-**MEN**-tar-ee) Pertaining to the digestive tract.

alkaline (**AL**-kah-line) Substance with a pH above 7.0. Also called *basic.*

alkaloid (**AL**-ka-loyd) Alkaline substances with pharmacologic activity synthesized from plants.

allele (ah-**LEEL**) Genetic variant found on the same locus of a pair of chromosomes.

allergen (**AL**-er-jen) Substance producing a hypersensitivity (allergic) reaction.

allergic (ah-**LER**-jik) Pertaining to being hypersensitive.

allergy (**AL**-er-jee) Hypersensitivity to an allergen.

allogen (**AL**-oh-jen) Antigen from someone else in the same species.

allograft (**AL**-oh-graft) Tissue graft from another person or cadaver.

alloimmune (**AL**-oh-im-**YUNE**) Reaction directed against foreign tissue.

allopathic medicine (al-oh-**PATH**-ic MED-ih-sin) Conventional medical practice.

allyl sulfides (**AL**-il SUL-fides) Group of substances found in garlic and onions that can reduce blood cholesterol.

alopecia (al-oh-**PEE**-shah) Partial or complete loss of hair, naturally or from medication.

alpha-fetoprotein (**AL**-fah-fee-toe-**PRO**-teen) Protein normally produced only by the fetus.

alveolus (al-**VEE**-oh-lus) Terminal element of the respiratory tract. Plural *alveoli.*

Alzheimer disease (**AWLZ**-high-mer DIZ-eez) Common form of dementia.

amblyopia (am-blee-**OH**-pee-ah) Failure or incomplete development of the pathways of vision to the brain.

amenorrhea (a-men-oh-**REE**-ah) Absence or abnormal cessation of menstrual flow.

amino acid (ah-**ME**-no ASS-id) The basic building block of protein.

aminoketone (ah-**ME**-no-**KEY**-tone) By-product of nicotine.

ammonia (ah-**MOAN**-ih-ah) Toxic breakdown product of amino acids.

amnesia (am-**NEE**-zee-ah) Total or partial inability to remember past experiences.

amniocentesis (**AM**-nee-oh-sen-tee-sis) Removal of amniotic fluid for diagnostic purposes.

amnion (AM-nee-on) Membrane around the fetus that contains amniotic fluid.

amniotic (am-nee-OT-ic) Pertaining to the amnion.

amoeba (ah-ME-bah) Single-celled organism that changes shape as it moves.

amoebiasis (ah-me-BY-ah-sis) Infection with *Amoeba*.

ampulla (am-PULL-ah) Dilated portion of a canal or duct.

amputation (am-pyu-TAY-shun) Process of removing a limb, a part of a limb, a breast, or some other projecting part.

amputee (AM-pyu-tee) A person with an amputation.

amylase (AM-il-aze) One of a group of enzymes that break down starch.

amyotrophic (a-my-oh-TROH-fik) Pertaining to muscular atrophy.

anabolism (an-AB-oh-lizm) The buildup of complex substances in the cell from simpler ones as a part of metabolism.

anaerobic (an-air-OH-bik) An organism capable of growing in the absence of oxygen.

analgesia (an-al-JEE-ze-ah) State in which pain is reduced.

analgesic (an-al-JEE-zic) Substance that reduces the response to pain.

anaphylactic (AN-ah-fih-LAK-tik) Pertaining to anaphylaxis.

anaphylaxis (AN-ah-fih-LAK-sis) Immediate severe allergic response.

anastomosis (ah-NAS-to-MO-sis) A surgically made union between two tubular structures. Plural *anastomoses*.

anatomical (an-ah-TOM-ik-al) Pertaining to anatomy.

anatomy (ah-NAT-oh-mee) Study of the structures of the human body.

ancillary (AN-sil-air-ree) Accessory, adjunct.

androgen (AN-droh-jen) Hormone that promotes masculine characteristics.

anemia (ah-NEE-me-ah) Decreased number of red blood cells.

anemic (ah-NEE-mik) Pertaining to or suffering from anemia.

anencephaly (AN-en-SEF-ah-lee) Born without cerebral hemispheres.

anesthesia (an-es-THEE-zee-ah) Complete loss of sensation.

anesthesiologist (AN-es-thee-zee-OL-oh-jist) Medical specialist in anesthesia.

anesthesiology (AN-es-thee-zee-OL-oh-jee) Medical specialty related to anesthesia.

anesthetic (an-es-THET-ic) Substance that takes away feeling and pain.

aneurysm (AN-yur-izm) Circumscribed dilation of an artery or cardiac chamber.

angiogenesis (AN-jee-oh-JEN-eh-sis) New formation of blood vessels.

angiogram (AN-jee-oh-gram) Radiograph obtained after injection of radiopaque contrast material into blood vessels.

angiography (an-jee-OG-rah-fee) Radiography of vessels after injection of contrast material.

angioplasty (AN-jee-oh-PLAS-tee) Recanalization of a blood vessel by surgery.

angiotensin (an-jee-oh-TEN-sin) An agent that constricts blood vessels.

anomaly (ah-NOM-ah-lee) A structural abnormality.

Anopheles (ah-NOF-eh-leez) A type of mosquito.

anorchism (an-OR-kizm) Absence of testes.

anorexia (an-oh-RECK-see-ah) Severe lack of appetite; *or* an aversion to food.

anoscopy (A-nos-koh-pee) Endoscopic examination of the anus.

anoxia (an-OCK-see-ah) Without oxygen.

anoxic (an-OCK-sik) Pertaining to or suffering from a lack of oxygen.

antacid (ant-ASS-id) Agent that neutralizes acidity.

antagonism (an-TAG-oh-nizm) Situation of opposing.

antagonist (an-TAG-oh-nist) An opposing structure, agent, disease, or process.

antagonistic (an-TAG-oh-nist-ik) Having an opposite function.

anterior (an-TER-ee-or) Front surface of body; situated in front.

anteversion (an-teh-VER-shun) Forward tilting of the uterus.

antevert (an-teh-VERT) Tilted forward.

anthracosis (an-thra-KOH-sis) Lung disease caused by the inhalation of coal dust.

anthrax (AN-thraks) A severe infectious disease.

antiangiogenesis (anti-AN-jee-oh-JEN-eh-sis) The prevention of growth of new blood vessels.

antibiotic (AN-tih-bye-OT-ik) A substance that has the capacity to destroy bacteria and other microorganisms.

antibody (AN-tih-body) Protein produced in response to an antigen. Plural *antibodies*.

anticoagulant (AN-tee-ko-AG-you-lant) Substance that prevents clotting.

antidiuretic (AN-tih-die-you-RET-ik) An agent that decreases urine production.

antidiuretic hormone (ADH) (AN-tih-die-you-RET-ik HOR-mohn) Posterior pituitary hormone that decreases urine output by acting on the kidney. Also called *vasopressin*.

antiepileptic (AN-tee-epih-LEP-tik) A pharmacologic agent capable of preventing or arresting epilepsy.

antigen (AN-tee-jen) Substance capable of triggering an immune response.

antihistamine (an-tee-HISS-tah-mean) Drug used to treat allergic symptoms because of its action antagonistic to histamine.

anti-inflammatory (AN-tee-in-FLAM-ah-tor-ee) Agent that reduces inflammation by acting on the body's response mechanisms without affecting the causative agent.

antimicrobial (AN-tee-my-KROH-bee-al) Agent for destroying or preventing multiplication of organisms.

antioxidant (an-tee-OKS-ih-dant) Substance that can prevent cell damage by neutralizing free radicals.

antipruritic (AN-tee-pru-RIT-ik) Medication against itching.

antipsychotic (AN-tih-sigh-KOT-ik) An agent helpful in the treatment of psychosis.

antipyretic (AN-tee-pie-RET-ik) Agent that reduces fever.

antisepsis (an-tih-SEP-sis) Inhibiting the growth of infectious agents.

antiseptic (an-tih-SEP-tic) Pertaining to antisepsis, *or* an agent capable of producing antisepsis.

antisocial personality disorder (AN-tee-SOH-shal per-son-AL-ih-tee dis-OR-der) Disorder of people who lie, cheat, and steal and have no guilt about their behavior.

antithyroid (an-tee-THIGH-royd) A substance that inhibits production of thyroid hormones.

antrum (AN-trum) A nearly closed cavity or chamber.

anuria (an-YOU-ree-ah) Absence of urine production.

anus (A-nuss) Terminal opening of the digestive tract through which feces are discharged.

anxiety (ang-ZI-eh-tee) Distress caused by fear

aorta (a-OR-tuh) Main trunk of the systemic arterial system.

apex (A-peks) Tip or end of cone-shaped structure, such as the heart.

Apgar score (AP-gar SKOR) Evaluation of newborn status.

apheresis (a-fer-EE-sis) Extraction of one element from donated blood.

aphonia (a-FO-nee-ah) Loss of voice.

aphthous ulcer (AF-thus UL-ser) Painful small oral ulcer (canker sore).

aplastic anemia (a-PLAS-tik ah-NEE-me-ah) Condition in which the bone marrow is unable to produce sufficient red cells, white cells, and platelets.

apnea (AP-nee-ah) Absence of spontaneous respiration.

apocrine (AP-oh-krin) Apocrine sweat glands that open into the hair follicle.

apoptosis (AP-op-TOE-sis) Programmed normal cell death.

appendectomy (ah-pen-DEK-toe-me) Surgical removal of the appendix.

appendicitis (ah-pen-dih-SIGH-tis) Inflammation of the appendix.

appendix (ah-PEN-dicks) Small blind projection from the pouch of the cecum.

aqueous humor (ACHE-we-us HEW-mor) Watery liquid in the anterior and posterior chambers of the eye.

arachnoid mater (ah-RACK-noyd MAY-ter) Weblike middle layer of the three meninges.

areola (ah-REE-oh-luh) Circular reddish area surrounding the nipple.

aromatherapy (ah-ROH-mah-THAIR-ah-pee) Use of essential oils to promote well-being.

aromatic (ah-roh-MAT-ik) Having an agreeable spicy odor; *or* one of a group of vegetable drugs.

arrhythmia (a-RITH-me-ah) An abnormal heart rhythm.

arteriography (ar-teer-ee-OG-rah-fee) X-ray visualization of an artery after injection of contrast material.

arteriole (ar-TER-ee-ole) Small terminal artery leading into the capillary network

arteriosclerosis (ar-TIER-ee-oh-skler-OH-sis) Hardening of the arteries.

arteriosclerotic (ar-TIER-ee-oh-skler-OT-ik) Pertaining to or suffering from arteriosclerosis.

arteriovenous malformation (ar-TEER-e-o-VE-nus mal-for-MAY-shun) An abnormal communication between an artery and a vein.

artery (AR-ter-ee) Thick-walled blood vessel carrying blood away from the heart.

arthritis (ar-THRY-tis) Inflammation of a joint or joints.

arthrocentesis (AR-throw-sen-TEE-sis) Withdrawal of fluid from a joint through a needle.

arthrodesis (ar-THROW-dee-sis) Fixation or stiffening of a joint by surgery.

arthrography (ar-THROG-ra-fee) X-ray of a joint taken after the injection of a contrast medium into the joint.

arthroplasty (AR-throw-plas-tee) Surgery to restore as far as possible the function of a joint.

arthroscope (AR-thro-skope) Endoscope used to examine the interior of a joint.

arthroscopy (ar-THROS-koh-pee) Visual examination of the interior of a joint.

articulate (ar-TIK-you-late) To form a joint so as to allow movement.

articulation (ar-tik-you-LAY-shun) Joint formed to allow movement.

asana (ah-SAH-nah) Yoga posture or steady position of the body to open energy channels.

asbestosis (as-bes-TOE-sis) Lung disease caused by the inhalation of asbestos particles.

Ascaris lumbricoides (AS-kah-ris lum-bri-KOY-deez) Large round-worm parasite.

ascites (ah-SIGH-teez) Accumulation of fluid in the abdominal cavity.

ascorbic acid (as-KOR-bic ASS-id) Vitamin C, which prevents scurvy.

asepsis (a-SEP-sis) Absence of living pathogenic organisms.

Ashkenazi (ASH-ke-NAZ-ih) Jews of eastern European ancestry.

aspartate aminotransferase (AST) (as-PAR-tate ah-me-no-TRANS-fer-aze) Enzyme that is found in liver cells and leaks out into the bloodstream when the cells are damaged, enabling liver damage to be diagnosed.

Asperger syndrome (AHS-per-ger SIN-drome) Developmental disorder of children.

aspergilloma (AS-per-ji-LOH-mah) Infectious granuloma.

aspergillosis (AS-per-ji-LOH-sis) Presence of *Aspergillus* in the body.

Aspergillus (as-per-JILL-us) A type of fungus.

aspiration (AS-pih-RAY-shun) Removal by suction of fluid or gas from a body cavity.

assistive device (ah-SIS-tiv de-VICE) Tool, software, or hardware to assist in performing daily activities.

assistive therapy (ah-SIS-tiv THAIR-ah-pee) Use of methods, technology, and devices to help people with disabilities achieve specific functions.

asthma (AZ-mah) Episodes of breathing difficulty due to narrowed or obstructed airways.

astigmatism (ah-STIG-mah-tism) Inability to focus light rays that enter the eye in different planes.

astrocyte (ASS-troh-site) Star-shaped connective tissue cell in the nervous system.

astrocytoma (ASS-troh-sigh-TOE-mah) Brain tumor derived from astrocytes.

asystole (a-SIS-toe-lee) Absence of contractions of the heart.

ataxia (a-TAK-see-ah) Inability to coordinate muscle activity, leading to jerky movements.

atelectasis (at-el-ECK-tah-sis) Collapse of part of a lung.

atherectomy (ath-er-EK-toe-me) Surgical removal of the atheroma.

atheroma (ath-er-ROE-mah) Lipid deposit in the lining of an artery.

atherosclerosis (ATH-er-oh-skler-OH-sis) Atheroma in arteries.

athetosis (ath-eh-TOE-sis) Slow, writhing involuntary movements.

atom (AT-om) A small unit of matter.

atonic (a-TOHN-ik) Without normal muscular tone.

atopy (AY-toh-pee) State of hypersensitivity to an allergen—allergic.

atresia (a-TREE-zee-ah) Congenital absence of a normal opening or lumen.

atrioventricular (AV) (A-tree-oh-ven-TRICK-you-lar) Pertaining to both the atrium and the ventricle.

atrium (A-tree-um) Chamber where blood enters the heart on both right and left sides. Plural *atria*.

atrophy (AT-roh-fee) The wasting away or diminished volume of tissue, an organ, or a body part.

atropine (AT-ro-peen) Pharmacologic agent used to dilate pupils.

attenuate (ah-TEN-you-ate) Weaken the ability of an organism to produce disease.

attenuated (ah-TEN-you-a-ted) Weakened.

atypical (a-TIP-ih-kal) Something that does not conform to the normal type.

audiologist (aw-dee-OL-oh-jist) Specialist in evaluation of hearing function.

audiology (aw-dee-OL-oh-jee) Study of hearing disorders.

audiometer (aw-dee-OM-ee-ter) Instrument to measure hearing.

audiometric (AW-dee-oh-MET-rik) Pertaining to the measurement of hearing.

auditory (AW-dih-tor-ee) Pertaining to the sense or the organs of hearing.

aura (AWE-rah) Sensory experience preceding an epileptic seizure or a migraine headache.

auricle (AW-ri-kul) The shell-like external ear.

auscultation (aws-kul-TAY-shun) Diagnostic method of listening to body sounds with a stethoscope.

autism (AWE-tizm) Developmental disorder of children.

autoantibody (aw-toe-AN-tee-bod-ee) Antibody produced in response to an antigen from the host's own tissue.

autoclave (AW-toe-klayv) Apparatus for sterilization by steam under pressure.

autograft (AWE-toe-graft) A graft using tissue taken from the individual who is receiving the graft.

autoimmune (aw-toe-im-YUNE) Immune reaction directed against a person's own tissue.

autologous (awe-TOL-oh-gus) Blood transfusion with the same person as donor and recipient.

autolysis (awe-TOL-ih-sis) Self-destruction of cells by enzymes within the cells.

autonomic (awe-toh-NOM-ik) Not voluntary; pertaining to the self-governing visceral motor division of the peripheral nervous system.

autopsy (AWE-top-see) Examination of the body and organs of a dead person to determine the cause of death.

autosome (AWE-toe-soam) Any chromosome other than a sex chromosome.

avascular (a-VAS-cue-lar) Without a blood supply.

avian (A-vee-an) Pertaining to birds.

avulsion (a-VUL-shun) Forcible separation or tearing away, often of a tendon from bone.

axilla (AK-sill-ah) Medical name for the armpit. Plural *axillae*.

axon (ACK-son) Single process of a nerve cell carrying nervous impulses away from the cell body.

Ayurvedic (ah-yur-VED-ik) A system of medicine arising from Hindu culture.

azotemia (azo-TEE-me-ah) Excess nitrogenous waste products in the blood.

B

Babinski sign (bah-BIN-skee SINE) Abnormal neurologic response to plantar reflex that is normal in infants.

bacillus (ba-SIL-us) A rod-shaped bacterium. Plural *bacilli*.

bacterial (bak-TEER-ee-al) Pertaining to bacteria.

bacterium (bak-TEER-ee-um) A unicellular, simple, microscopic organism. Plural *bacteria*.

balanitis (bal-ah-NIE-tis) Inflammation of the glans and prepuce of the penis.

bariatric (bar-ee-AT-rik) Treatment of obesity.

basal metabolic rate (BAY-sal met-ah-BOL-ic RATE) Energy the body requires to function at rest.

basilar (BAS-ih-lar) Pertaining to the base of a structure.

basophil (BAY-so-fill) A basophil's granules attract a basic blue stain in the laboratory.

Bell palsy (BELL PAWL-ze) Paresis or paralysis of one side of the face.

benign (bee-**NINE**) Denoting the nonmalignant character of a neoplasm or illness

beriberi (**BER**-ee-**BER**-ee) Disease produced by thiamine deficiency.

beta (**BAY**-tah) Second letter in the Greek alphabet.

beta carotene (**BAY**-tah **KAR**-oh-teen) Yellow-red pigment in fruits and vegetables.

biceps brachii (**BYE**-sepz **BRAY**-key-eye) A muscle of the upper arm that has two heads or points of origin on the scapula.

biconcave (bi-**KON**-cave) Having a hollowed surface on both sides of a structure.

bicuspid (by-**KUSS**-pid) Having two points; a bicuspid heart valve has two flaps, and a bicuspid (premolar) tooth has two points.

bifid (**BIH**-fid) Separated into two parts.

bilateral (by-**LAT**-er-al) On two sides; for example, in both ears.

bile (BILE) Fluid secreted by the liver into the duodenum.

bile acids (BILE **ASS**-ids) Steroids synthesized from cholesterol.

biliary (**BILL**-ee-air-ee) Pertaining to bile or the biliary tract.

bilirubin (bill-ee-**RU**-bin) Bile pigment formed in the liver from hemoglobin.

binge eating (BINJ EE-ting) Eating with periods of excessive intake.

bioavailable (BI-oh-ah-**VAIL**-ah-bul) Capable of being absorbed into the bloodstream.

biofeedback (bi-oh-**FEED**-back) Training techniques to achieve voluntary control of responses to stimuli.

biofield (bi-oh-**FIELD**) Area of energy in and surrounding the body.

biology (bi-**OL**-oh-jee) Science concerned with life and living organisms.

biomarker (bi-oh-**MARK**-er) A biological marker or product by which a cell can be identified.

biopsy (**BI**-op-see) Removing tissue from a living person for laboratory examination.

biopsy removal (**BI**-op-see re-**MUV**-al) Used for small tumors when complete removal provides tissue for a biopsy and cures the lesion. Also called *excisional biopsy*.

biotin (**BI**-oh-tin) Vitamin B_2.

bipolar disorder (bi-**POH**-lar dis-**OR**-der) A mood disorder with alternating episodes of depression and mania

bladder (**BLAD**-er) Hollow sac that holds fluid; for example, urine or bile.

blastocyst (**BLAS**-toe-sist) The developing embryo during the first 2 weeks.

blepharitis (blef-ah-**RYE**-tis) Inflammation of the eyelid.

blepharoplasty (**BLEF**-ah-ro-plas-tee) Surgical repair of the eyelid.

blepharoptosis (**BLEF**-ah-**ROP**-toe-sis) Drooping of the upper eyelid.

blood-brain barrier (BBB) (BLUD BRAYN **BAIR**-ee-er) A selective mechanism that protects the brain from toxins and infections.

bolus (**BOH**-lus) Single mass of a substance.

bonding (**BON**-ding) Formation of a close and lasting emotional attachment.

Botox (**BO**-tox) Neurotoxin injected into the muscles of the face to prevent the muscles from contracting and causing wrinkles.

botulism (**BOT**-you-lizm) Food poisoning caused by the neurotoxin produced by *Clostridium botulinum*.

bovine spongiform encephalopathy (**BO**-vine **SPON**-jee-form en-sef-ah-**LOP**-ah-thee) Disease of cattle (mad cow disease) that can be transmitted to humans, causing Creutzfeldt-Jakob disease.

bowel (**BOUGH**-el) Another name for intestine.

brace (BRACE) Appliance to support a part of the body in its correct position.

brachial (**BRAY**-kee-al) Pertaining to the arm.

brachialis (**BRAY**-kee-al-is) Muscle that lies underneath the biceps and is the strongest flexor of the forearm.

brachiocephalic (**BRAY**-kee-oh-seh-**FAL**-ik) Pertaining to the head and arm, as an artery supplying blood to both.

brachioradialis (**BRAY**-kee-oh-**RAY**-dee-al-is) Muscle that helps flex the forearm.

brachytherapy (brah-kee-**THAIR**-ah-pee) Radiation therapy in which the source of irradiation is implanted in the tissue to be treated.

bradycardia (brad-ee-**KAR**-dee-ah) Slow heart rate (below 60 beats per minute).

bradypnea (brad-ip-**NEE**-ah) Slow breathing.

brainstem (BRAYNSTEM) Region of the brain that includes the thalamus, pineal gland, pons, fourth ventricle, and medulla oblongata.

breech (BREECH) Buttocks-first presentation of the fetus at delivery.

bronchiectasis (brong-kee-**ECK**-tah-sis) Chronic dilation of the bronchi following inflammatory disease and obstruction.

bronchiole (**BRONG**-key-ole) Increasingly smaller subdivisions of bronchi.

bronchiolitis (brong-kee-oh-**LYE**-tis) Inflammation of the small bronchioles.

bronchoalveolar (**BRONG**-koh-al-**VEE**-oh-lar) Pertaining to the bronchi and alveoli.

bronchoconstriction (**BRONG**-koh-kon-**STRIK**-shun) Reduction in diameter of a bronchus.

bronchodilator (**BRONG**-koh-die-**LAY**-tor) Agent that increases the diameter of a bronchus.

bronchogenic (brong-koh-**JEN**-ik) Arising from a bronchus.

bronchopneumonia (**BRONG**-koh-new-**MOH**-nee-ah) Acute inflammation of the walls of smaller bronchioles with spread to lung parenchyma.

bronchopulmonary dysplasia (**BRONG**-koh-**PUL**-moh-nair-ee dis-**PLAY**-zee-ah) Chronic lung disorder in premature infants after prolonged mechanical ventilation.

bronchoscope (**BRONG**-koh-skope) Endoscope used for bronchoscopy.

bronchoscopy (brong-**KOS**-koh-pee) Examination of the interior of the tracheobronchial tree with an endoscope.

bronchus (**BRONG**-kuss) One of two subdivisions of the trachea. Plural *bronchi*.

brucellosis (brew-sel-**OH**-sis) Undulant fever.

bruxism (**BRUK**-sizm) Gritting or grinding together of the teeth, often during sleep.

bubo (**BYU**-bo) Swollen, inflamed lymph node. Plural *buboes*.

buccal smear (**BUCK**-al SMEER) Use of a small brush or cotton swab to collect cells from the inside surface of the cheek.

buccinator (**BUCK**-sin-a-tor) Buccinator muscle is the muscle in the cheek.

buffer (**BUFF**-er) Substance that resists a change in pH.

bulbourethral (**BUL**-boh-you-**REE**-thral) Pertaining to the bulbous penis and urethra.

bulimia (byu-**LEEM**-ee-ah) Episodic bouts of excessive eating with compensatory throwing up.

bulla (**BULL**-ah) Bubblelike dilated structure. Plural *bullae*.

bundle of His (HISS) Pathway for electrical signals to be transmitted to the ventricles.

bunion (**BUN**-yun) A swelling at the base of the big toe.

bursa (**BURR**-sah) A closed sac containing synovial fluid.

bursitis (burr-**SIGH**-tis) Inflammation of a bursa.

C

café-au-lait (**KAF**-ay-oh-**LAY**) Color of skin macules in neurofibromatosis.

calcaneus (kal-**KAY**-knee-us) Bone of the tarsus that forms the heel.

calcitonin (kal-sih-**TONE**-in) Thyroid hormone that moves calcium from blood to bones.

calcitriol (**KAL**-sih-**TRY**-ol) Potent form of vitamin D that acts as a hormone.

calculus (**KAL**-kyu-lus) Small stone. Plural *calculi*.

callus (**KAL**-us) The mass of fibrous connective tissue that forms at a fracture site and becomes the foundation for the formation of new bone.

caloric (kah-**LOR**-ik) Pertaining to calories.

Calorie (**KAL**-oh-ree) An expression of the energy content of food; capitalize "C" always.

calyx (**KAY**-licks) Funnel-shaped structure. Plural *calyces*.

cancellous (**KAN**-sell-us) Bone that has a spongy or latticelike structure.

cancer (**KAN**-ser) General term for a malignant neoplasm.

cancerous (**KAN**-ser-ous) Pertaining to a malignant neoplasm.

Candida (**KAN**-did-ah) A yeastlike fungus.

candidiasis (can-dih-**DIE**-ah-sis) Infection with the yeastlike fungus *Candida*. Also called *thrush*.

canker; canker sore (**KANG**-ker SOAR) Nonmedical term for aphthous ulcer. Also called *mouth ulcer*.

cannula (**KAN**-you-lah) Tube inserted into a blood vessel or cavity as a channel for fluid.

canthus (**KAN**-thus) Corner of the eye where the upper and lower lids meet. Plural *canthi*.

capillary (**KAP**-ih-lair-ee) Minute blood vessel between the arterial and venous systems.

capsid (**KAP**-sid) Protein shell surrounding the nucleic acid in the core of a virus.

capsule (**KAP**-syul) Fibrous tissue layer surrounding a joint or some other structure.

carbohydrate (kar-boh-**HIGH**-drate) Group of organic food compounds that includes sugars, starch, glycogen, and cellulose.

carboxypeptidase (kar-box-ee-**PEP**-tide-ase) Enzyme that breaks down protein.

carbuncle (**KAR**-bunk-ul) Infection of many furuncles in a small area, often on the back of the neck.

carcinogen (kar-**SIN**-oh-jen) Cancer-producing agent.

carcinogenesis (kar-**SIN**-oh-**JEN**-eh-sis) Origin and development of cancer.

carcinoma (kar-sih-**NOH**-mah) A malignant and invasive epithelial tumor.

carcinoma in situ (kar-sih-**NOH**-mah IN **SIGH**-tyu) Carcinoma that has not invaded surrounding tissues.

cardiac (**KAR**-dee-ak) Pertaining to the heart.

cardiogenic (**KAR**-dee-oh-**JEN**-ik) Of cardiac origin.

cardiologist (kar-dee-**OL**-oh-jist) A medical specialist in diagnosis and treatment of the heart (cardiology).

cardiology (kar-dee-**OL**-oh-jee) Medical specialty of diseases of the heart.

cardiomegaly (**KAR**-dee-oh-**MEG**-ah-lee) Enlargement of the heart.

cardiomyopathy (**KAR**-dee-oh-my-**OP**-ah-thee) Disease of heart muscle, the myocardium.

cardiopulmonary resuscitation (**KAR**-dee-oh-**PUL**-mo-nary ree-sus-ih-**TAY**-shun) The attempt to restore cardiac and pulmonary function.

cardiovascular (**KAR**-dee-oh-**VAS**-kyu-lar) Pertaining to the heart and blood vessels.

cardioversion (**KAR**-dee-oh-**VER**-shun) Restoration of a normal heart rhythm by electrical shock. Also called *defibrillation*.

cardioverter (**KAR**-dee-oh-**VER**-ter) Device used to generate electrical shock for cardioversion.

caries (**KARE**-eez) Bacterial destruction of teeth.

carotenoid (kah-**ROT**-en-oyd) Organic pigment occurring naturally in plants.

carotid (kah-**ROT**-id) Main artery of the neck.

carotid endarterectomy (kah-**ROT**-id **END**-ar-ter-**EK**-toe-me) Surgical removal of diseased lining from the carotid artery to leave a smooth lining.

carpal (**KAR**-pal) Pertaining to the wrist.

carpus (**KAR**-pus) Collective term for the eight carpal bones of the wrist.

carrier (KAH-ree-er) A person with an autosomal recessive gene for a disease. Also called *heterozygote.*

cartilage (KAR-tih-lage) Nonvascular, firm connective tissue found mostly in joints.

cast (KAST) A cylindrical mold formed by materials in kidney tubules.

catabolism (kah-TAB-oh-lizm) Breakdown of complex substances into simpler ones as a part of metabolism.

cataplexy (KAT-ah-plek-see) Sudden loss of muscle tone with brief paralysis.

cataract (KAT-ah-ract) Complete or partial opacity of the lens.

catatonia (kat-ah-TOE-nee-ah) Syndrome characterized by physical immobility and mental stupor.

catecholamine (kat-eh-COAL-ah-meen) Any major hormones in stress response; includes epinephrine and norepinephrine.

catheter (KATH-eh-ter) Hollow tube that allows passage of fluid into or out of a body cavity, organ, or vessel.

catheterization (KATH-eh-ter-ih-ZAY-shun) Introduction of a catheter.

catheterize (KATH-eh-teh-RIZE) To introduce a catheter.

cauda equina (KAW-dah eh-KWY-nah) Bundle of spinal nerves in the vertebral canal below the ending of the spinal cord.

caudal (KAW-dal) Pertaining to or nearer to the tail.

cautery (KAW-ter-ee) Agent or device used to burn or scar a tissue.

cavernosa (kav-er-NOH-sah) Resembling a cave.

cavity (KAV-ih-tee) Hollow space or body compartment. Plural *cavities.*

cecum (SEE-kum) Blind pouch that is the first part of the large intestine.

celiac (SEE-lee-ack) Relating to the abdominal cavity.

celiac disease (SEE-lee-ak diz-eez) Disease caused by sensitivity to gluten.

cell (SELL) The smallest unit capable of independent existence.

cellular (SELL-you-lar) Pertaining to a cell.

cellulitis (sell-you-LIE-tis) Infection of subcutaneous connective tissue.

cellulose (SELL-you-lohse) Major constituent of cell walls of plants.

centromere (SEN-troh-mere) Junction that holds two chromatids together to form a chromosome.

cephalic (se-FAL-ik) Pertaining to or nearer to the head.

cerebellum (ser-eh-BELL-um) The most posterior area of the brain.

cerebrospinal (SER-eh-broh-SPY-nal) Pertaining to the brain and spinal cord.

cerebrospinal fluid (CSF) (SER-eh-broh-SPY-nal FLU-id) Fluid formed in the ventricles of the brain; surrounds the brain and spinal cord.

cerebrum (SER-ee-brum) The major portion of the brain divided into two hemispheres (cerebral hemispheres) separated by a fissure.

cerumen (seh-ROO-men) Waxy secretion of the ceruminous glands of the external ear.

cervical (SER-vih-kal) Pertaining to the cervix or to the neck region.

cervix (SER-viks) The lower part of the uterus.

cesarean section (seh-ZAH-ree-an SEK-shun) Extraction of the fetus through an incision in the abdomen and uterine wall. Also called *C-section.*

chakra (CHAK-rah) One of seven centers of energy in the body.

chalazion (kah-LAY-zee-on) Cyst on the outer edge of an eyelid.

chancre (SHAN-ker) Primary lesion of syphilis.

chancroid (SHAN-kroyd) Infectious, painful, ulcerative STD not related to syphilis.

Charcot joint (SHAR-koh JOYNT) Bone and joint destruction secondary to a neuropathy and loss of sensation.

chemoprophylaxis (KEEM-oh-PRO-fil-ak-sis) Prevent infection by use of chemicals or drugs.

chemotherapy (KEY-moh-THAIR-ah-pee) Treatment using chemical agents.

chi (CHEE) Universal life force. Also spelled *qi.*

chiasm (KYE-asm) X-shaped crossing of the two optic nerves at the base of the brain. Alternative term *chiasma.*

chickenpox (CHICK-en-pocks) Acute, contagious viral disease. Also called *varicella.*

chiropractic (kye-roh-PRAK-tik) Diagnosis, treatment, and prevention of mechanical disorders of the musculoskeletal system.

chiropractor (kye-roh-PRAK-tor) Practitioner of chiropractic.

chlamydia (klah-MID-ee-ah) A species of bacteria causing a sexually transmitted disease.

chlorine (KLOR-een) A toxic agent used as a disinfectant and bleaching agent.

chlorophyll (KLOR-oh-fil) Light-absorbing pigment in plants.

cholangiography (KOH-lan-jee-OG-rah-fee) X-ray of the bile ducts after injection or ingestion of a contrast medium.

cholecystectomy (KOH-leh-sis-TECK-toe-me) Surgical removal of the gallbladder.

cholecystitis (KOH-leh-sis-TIE-tis) Inflammation of the gallbladder.

cholecystokinin (KOH-leh-sis-toe-KIE-nin) Hormone secreted by the lining of the intestine that stimulates secretion of pancreatic enzymes and contraction of the gallbladder.

choledocholithiasis (koh-leh-DOH-koh-lih-THIGH-ah-sis) Presence of a gallstone in the common bile duct.

cholelithiasis (KOH-leh-lih-THIGH-ah-sis) Condition of having bile stones (gallstones).

cholelithotomy (KOH-leh-lih-THOT-oh-me) Surgical removal of a gallstone(s).

cholera (KOL-er-ah) Acute endemic infectious disease.

cholestatic (koh-les-TAT-ik) Stopping the flow of bile.

cholesteatoma (koh-less-tee-ah-TOE-mah) Yellow, waxy tumor arising in the middle ear.

cholesterol (koh-LESS-ter-ol) Steroid formed in liver cells; the most abundant steroid in tissues and circulates in the plasma attached to proteins of different densities.

choline (**KOH**-leen) An amine found in most tissues; a precursor for acetylcholine.

chondromalacia (**KON**-dro-mah-**LAY**-she-ah) Softening and degeneration of cartilage.

chondrosarcoma (**KON**-dro-sar-**KOH**-mah) Cancer arising from cartilage cells.

chordae tendineae (**KOR**-dee ten-**DIN**-ee) Tendinous cords attaching the bicuspid and tricuspid valves to the heart wall.

chorea (kor-**EE**-ah) Involuntary, irregular spasms of limb and facial muscles.

choriocarcinoma (**KOH**-ree-oh-kar-sih-**NOH**-mah) Highly malignant cancer in a testis or ovary.

chorion (**KOH**-ree-on) The fetal membrane that forms the placenta.

chorionic (koh-ree-**ON**-ick) Pertaining to the chorion.

chorionic villus (koh-ree-**ON**-ik **VILL**-us) Vascular process of the embryonic chorion to form the placenta.

choroid (**KOR**-oid) Region of the retina and uvea.

chromatid (**KROH**-ma-tid) One of the two strands of a chromosome.

chromatin (**KROH**-ma-tin) Substance composed of DNA that forms chromosomes during cell division.

chromosome (**KROH**-moh-sohm) Body in the nucleus that contains DNA and genes.

chronic (**KRON**-ik) Describes a persistent, long-term disease.

chronotropic (**KRONE**-oh-**TROH**-pic) Affecting the heart rate.

chyle (**KYLE**) A milky fluid that results from the digestion and absorption of fats in the small intestine.

chyme (**KYME**) Semifluid, partially digested food passed from the stomach into the duodenum.

chymotrypsin (kye-moh-**TRIP**-sin) Trypsin found in chyme.

ciliary body (**SILL**-ee-ary **BOD**-ee) Muscles that make the eye lens thicker and thinner.

cilium (**SILL**-ee-um) Hairlike motile projection from the surface of a cell. Plural *cilia*.

circulation (**SER**-kyu-**LAY**-shun) Continuous movement of blood through the heart and blood vessels.

circumcision (ser-kum-**SIZH**-un) To remove part or all of the prepuce.

circumduction (ser-kum-**DUCK**-shun) Movement of an extremity in a circular motion.

cirrhosis (sir-**ROE**-sis) Extensive fibrotic liver disease.

claudication (klaw-dih-**KAY**-shun) Intermittent leg pain and limping.

claustrophobia (klaw-stroh-**FOH**-be-ah) Pathologic fear of being trapped in a confined space.

clavicle (**KLAV**-ih-kul) Curved bone that forms the anterior part of the pectoral girdle.

clean (**KLENE**) Free from visible contamination.

cleft lip (**KLEFT LIP**) Congenital defect of the upper lip.

cleft palate (**KLEFT PAL**-ate) Congenital defect of the upper palate.

clitoris (**KLIT**-oh-ris) Erectile organ of the vulva.

clonic (**KLON**-ik) State of rapid successions of muscular contractions and relaxations.

closed fracture (**KLOSD FRAK**-chur) A bone is broken but the skin over it is intact.

Clostridium botulinum (klos-**TRID**-ee-um bot-you-**LIE**-num) Bacterium that causes food poisoning.

Clostridium difficile (klos-**TRID**-ee-um dif-ih-**SEE**-il) Gram-positive rod producing powerful exotoxins that cause colitis.

clot (**KLOT**) The mass of fibrin and cells that is produced in a wound.

coagulant (koh-ag-you-**LANT**) Substance that induces clotting.

coagulate (koh-**AG**-you-late) Form a clot.

coagulation (koh-ag-you-**LAY**-shun) The process of blood clotting.

coagulopathy (koh-ag-you-**LOP**-ah-thee) Disorder of blood clotting. Plural *coagulopathies*.

coarctation (koh-ark-**TAY**-shun) Constriction, stenosis, particularly of the aorta.

coccus (**KOK**-us) Round, spheroid bacterium. Plural *cocci*.

coccyx (**KOK**-sicks) Small tailbone at the lower end of the vertebral column.

cochlea (**KOK**-lee-ah) An intricate combination of passages; used to describe the part of the inner ear used in hearing.

cochlear (**KOK**-lee-ar) Pertaining to the cochlea.

coenzyme (koh-**EN**-zime) Substance required for an enzyme to function.

cognition (kog-**NIH**-shun) Process of acquiring knowledge through thinking, learning, and memory.

cognitive (**KOG**-nih-tiv) Pertaining to the mental activities of thinking and learning.

cognitive behavioral therapy (CBT) (**KOG**-nih-tiv be-**HAYV**-yur-al **THAIR**-ah-pee) Psychotherapy that emphasizes thoughts and attitudes in one's behavior.

cognitive processing therapy (**KOG**-nih-tiv **PROS**-es-ing **THAIR**-ah-pee) Psychotherapy to build skills to deal with effects of the trauma in other areas of life.

coitus (**KOH**-it-us) Sexual intercourse.

colic (**KOL**-ik) Spasmodic, crampy pains in the abdomen; in young infants, persistent crying and irritability thought to be arising from pain in the intestines.

colitis (koh-**LIE**-tis) Inflammation of the colon.

collagen (**KOL**-ah-jen) Major protein of connective tissue, cartilage, and bone.

collateral (koh-**LAT**-er-al) Situated at the side, often to bypass an obstruction.

Colles fracture (**KOL**-ez **FRAK**-chur) Fracture of the distal radius at the wrist.

colloid (**COLL**-oyd) Liquid containing suspended particles.

colon (**KOH**-lon) The large intestine, extending from the cecum to the rectum.

colonization (KOL-on-ih-ZAY-shun) Formation of a population of microorganisms.

colonoscopy (koh-lon-OSS-koh-pee) Examination of the inside of the colon by endoscopy.

color Doppler ultrasonography (DOP-ler UL-trah-soh-NOG-rah-fee) Computer-generated color image to show directions of blood flow.

colostomy (ko-LOSS-toe-me) Artificial opening from the colon to the outside of the body.

colostrum (koh-LOSS-trum) The first breast secretion at the end of pregnancy.

colpopexy (KOL-poh-peck-see) Surgical fixation of the vagina.

coma (KOH-mah) State of deep unconsciousness.

comatose (KOH-mah-toes) Being in a coma.

comedo (KOM-ee-doh) A whitehead or blackhead caused by too much sebum and too many keratin cells blocking the hair follicle. Plural *comedones.*

comminuted fracture (KOM-ih-nyu-ted FRAK-chur) A fracture in which the bone is broken into pieces.

comorbidity (koh-mor-BID-ih-tee) Presence of two or more diseases at the same time.

competent (KOM-peh-tent) Capable of performing a task or function.

complement (KOM-pleh-ment) Group of proteins in serum destroy bacteria and other cells.

complete (kom-PLEET) Whole, entire, total.

complete fracture (kom-PLEET FRAK-chur) A bone is fractured into two separate pieces.

compliance (kom-PLY-ance) Measure of the capacity of a chamber or hollow viscus to expand; for example, compliance of the lungs.

compression (kom-PRESH-un) A squeezing together so as to increase density and/or decrease a dimension of a structure.

compression fracture (kom-PRESH-un FRAK-chur) Fracture of a vertebra causing loss of height of the vertebra.

compulsion (kom-PULL-shun) Uncontrollable impulses to perform an act repetitively.

compulsive (kom-PULL-siv) Possessing uncontrollable impulses to perform an act repetitively.

conception (kon-SEP-shun) Fertilization of the egg by sperm to form a zygote.

concha (KON-kah) Shell-shaped bone on the medial wall of the nasal cavity. Plural *conchae.*

concussion (kon-KUSH-un) Mild head injury.

condom (KON-dom) A sheath or cover for the penis or vagina to prevent conception and infection.

conduction (kon-DUCK-shun) Process of transmitting energy.

conductive hearing loss (kon-DUK-tiv) Hearing loss caused by lesions in the outer ear or middle ear.

condyle (KON-dile) Large, smooth rounded expansion of the end of a bone that forms a joint with another bone.

condyloma (kon-dih-LOW-ma) Warty growth on external genitalia. Plural *condylomata.*

confusion (kon-FEW-zhun) Mental state in which environmental stimuli are not processed appropriately.

congenital (kon-JEN-ih-tal) Present at birth, either inherited or due to an event during gestation up to the moment of birth.

congruent (KON-gru-ent) Coinciding or agreeing with.

conization (koh-nih-ZAY-shun) Surgical excision of a cone-shaped piece of tissue.

conjunctiva (kon-junk-TIE-vah) Inner lining of the eyelids.

conjunctivitis (kon-junk-tih-VI-tis) Inflammation of the conjunctiva.

Conn syndrome (KON SIN-drom) Condition caused by excessive secretion of aldosterone. Also called *aldosteronism.*

conscious (KON-shus) Having present knowledge of oneself and one's surroundings.

consciousness (KON-shus-ness) The state of being aware of and responsive to the environment.

constipation (kon-stih-PAY-shun) Hard, infrequent bowel movements.

contagiosum (kon-TAY-jee-oh-sum) Infection spread from one person to another by direct contact.

contagious (kon-TAY-jus) Able to be transmitted, as infections transmitted from person to person or from person to air or surface to person.

contaminate (kon-TAM-in-ate) To cause the presence of an infectious agent to be on any surface.

contamination (KON-tam-ih-NAY-shun) Presence of an infectious agent on a surface or in a substance.

contraception (kon-trah-SEP-shun) Prevention of conception.

contraceptive (kon-trah-SEP-tiv) An agent that prevents conception.

contract (kon-TRAKT) Draw together or shorten.

contracture (kon-TRAK-chur) Muscle shortening due to spasm or fibrosis.

contrecoup (KON-treh-koo) Injury to the brain at a point directly opposite the point of original contact.

contusion (kon-TOO-zhun) Bruising of a tissue, including the brain.

conversion disorder (kon-VER-shun dis-OR-der) An unconscious emotional conflict is expressed as physical symptoms with no organic basis.

convulsion (kon-VUL-shun) Alternative name for seizure.

coordinate (ko-OR-din-ate) To bring together different structures into a harmonious function.

cor pulmonale (KOR pul-moh-NAH-lee) Right-sided heart failure arising from chronic lung disease.

coreceptor (koh-ree-SEP-tor) Cell surface protein that enhances the sensitivity of an antigen receptor.

cornea (KOR-nee-ah) The central, transparent part of the outer coat of the eye covering the iris and pupil.

coronal (KOR-oh-nal) Pertaining to the vertical plane dividing the body into anterior and posterior portions.

coronal plane (KOR-oh-nal PLAIN) Vertical plane dividing the body into anterior and posterior portions.

coronary circulation (KOR-oh-nair-ee SER-kyu-LAY-shun) Blood flow through the vessels supplying the heart.

corpus (KOR-pus) Major part of a structure. Plural *corpora*.

corpus albicans (KOR-pus AL-bih-kanz) An atrophied corpus luteum.

corpus callosum (KOR-pus kah-LOW-sum) Bridge of nerve fibers connecting the two cerebral hemispheres.

corpus luteum (KOR-pus LOO-teh-um) Yellow structure formed at the site of a ruptured ovarian follicle.

corpuscle (KOR-pus-ul) A blood cell.

cortex (KOR-teks) Outer portion of an organ, such as bone; *or* gray covering of cerebral hemispheres. Plural *cortices*.

corticoid (KOR-tih-koyd) One of the steroid hormones produced by the adrenal cortex. Also called *corticosteroid*.

corticosteroid (KOR-tih-koh-STEHR-oyd) A hormone produced by the adrenal cortex.

corticotropin (KOR-tih-koh-TROH-pin) Pituitary hormone that stimulates the cortex of the adrenal gland to secrete corticosteroids.

cortisol (KOR-tih-sol) One of the glucocorticoids produced by the adrenal cortex; has anti-inflammatory effects. Also called *hydrocortisone*.

coryza (ko-RYE-zah) Viral inflammation of the mucous membrane of the nose. Also called *rhinitis*.

counseling (KOWN-sel-ing) Professional relationship to transmit advice to direct the judgment of another.

coup (KOO) Injury to the brain occurring directly under the skull at the point of impact.

coxa (COCK-sah) Hip bone. Plural *coxae*.

cranial (KRAY-nee-al) Pertaining to the skull.

craniofacial (KRAY-nee-oh-FAY-shal) Pertaining to both the face and the cranium.

craniosacral (KRAY-nee-oh-SAY-kral) Referring to the cranium and sacrum.

cranium (KRAY-nee-um) The upper part of the skull that encloses and protects the brain.

craving (KRAY-ving) Deep longing or desire.

creatine kinase (KREE-ah-teen KI-naze) Enzyme elevated in plasma following heart muscle damage in myocardial infarction.

creatinine (kree-AT-ih-neen) Breakdown product of the skeletal muscle protein creatine.

cretin (KREH-tin) A person with severe congenital hypothyroidism.

cretinism (KREH-tin-izm) Condition of severe congenital hypothyroidism.

Creutzfeldt-Jakob disease (KROITS-felt-YAK-op DIZ-eez) Progressive incurable neurologic disease caused by infectious prions.

cricoid (CRY-koyd) Ring-shaped cartilage in the larynx.

crista ampullaris (KRIS-tah am-PULL-air-is) Mound of hair cells and gelatinous material in the ampulla of a semicircular canal.

criterion (kri-TEER-ee-on) Standard or rule for judging. Plural *criteria*.

Crohn disease (KRONE DIZ-eez) Inflammatory bowel disease with narrowing and thickening of the terminal small bowel. Also called *regional enteritis*.

croup (KROOP) Infection of the upper airways in children; characterized by a barking cough. Also called *laryngotracheobronchitis*.

crown (KROWN) Part of tooth above the gum.

crowning (KROWN-ing) During childbirth, when the maximum diameter of the baby's head comes through the vulvar ring.

cruciate (KRU-she-ate) Shaped like a cross.

cryokinetics (CRY-oh-kih-NET-iks) Combination of cold therapy with exercise.

cryoneurolysis (cry-oh-NYUR-oh-lie-sis) Temporary deactivation of nerve tissue using extreme cold.

cryopexy (cry-oh-PEX-ee) Repair of a detached retina by freezing it to surrounding tissue.

cryosurgery (cry-oh-SUR-jer-ee) Use of liquid nitrogen or argon gas in a probe to freeze and kill abnormal tissue.

cryotherapy (CRY-oh-THAIR-ah-pee) The use of cold in the treatment of injury.

cryptorchism (krip-TOR-kizm) Failure of one or both testes to descend into the scrotum.

curative (KYUR-ah-tiv) That which heals or cures.

curettage (kyu-reh-TAHZH) Scraping of the interior of a cavity.

curette (kyu-RET) Scoop-shaped instrument for scraping the interior of a cavity or removing new growths.

Cushing syndrome (KUSH-ing SIN-drom) Hypersecretion of cortisol (hydrocortisone) by the adrenal cortex.

cuspid (KUSS-pid) Tooth with one point.

cutaneous (kyu-TAY-nee-us) Pertaining to the skin.

cuticle (KEW-tih-cul) Nonliving epidermis at the base of the fingernails and toenails.

cyanocobalamin (SIGH-an-oh-koh-BAL-ah-min) Vitamin B_{12}.

cyanosis (sigh-ah-NO-sis) Blue discoloration of the skin, lips, and nail beds due to low levels of oxygen in the blood.

cyanotic (sigh-ah-NOT-ik) Marked by cyanosis.

cyst (SIST) An abnormal, fluid-containing sac.

cystic (SIS-tik) Relating to a cyst.

cystic fibrosis (CF) (SIS-tik fie-BRO-sis) Genetic disease in which excessive viscid mucus obstructs passages, including bronchi.

cystitis (sis-TIE-tis) Inflammation of the urinary bladder.

cystocele (SIS-toh-seal) Hernia of the bladder into the vagina.

cystopexy (SIS-toh-pek-see) Surgical procedure to support the urinary bladder.

cystoscope (SIS-toh-skope) An endoscope inserted to view the inside of the bladder.

cystoscopy (sis-TOS-koh-pee) The process of using a cystoscope.

cystourethrogram (sis-toh-you-REETH-roe-gram) X-ray image during voiding to show the structure and function of the bladder and urethra.

cytokine (**SIGH**-toh-kine) Proteins produced by different cells that communicate with other cells in the immune system.

cytosine (**SIGH**-toh-seen) One of the chemical bases found in, and comprising the sequence of, both DNA and RNA.

cytology (**SIGH**-tol-oh-gee) Study of the cell.

cytomegalovirus (sigh-toh-**MEG**-ah-loh-**VIE**-rus) A group of herpesviruses that can cause congenital infections.

cytoplasm (**SIGH**-toh-plazm) Clear, gelatinous substance that forms the substance of a cell except for the nucleus.

cytosine (**SIGH**-toh-seen) One of the chemicals found in both DNA and RNA.

cytotoxic (sigh-toh-**TOX**-ik) Destructive to cells.

D

dacryocystitis (**DAK**-re-oh-sis-**TIE**-tis) Inflammation of the lacrimal sac.

dacryostenosis (**DAK**-re-oh-ste-**NO**-sis) Narrowing of the nasolacrimal duct.

dandruff (**DAN**-druff) Seborrheic scales from the scalp.

death (DETH) Total and permanent cessation of all vital functions.

debridement (day-**BREED**-mon) The removal of injured or necrotic tissue.

decongestant (dee-con-**JESS**-tant) Agent that reduces the swelling and fluid in the nose and sinuses.

decubitus ulcer (de-**KYU**-bit-us **UL**-ser) Sore caused by lying down for long periods of time.

decussate (**DEE**-kuss-ate) Cross over like the arms of an "X."

defecation (def-eh-**KAY**-shun) Evacuation of feces from the rectum and anus.

defect (**DEE**-fect) An absence, malformation, or imperfection.

defective (dee-**FEK**-tiv) Imperfect.

defibrillation (dee-fib-rih-**LAY**-shun) Restoration of uncontrolled twitching of cardiac muscle fibers to normal rhythm.

defibrillator (dee-fib-rih-**LAY**-tor) Instrument for defibrillation.

deformity (de-**FOR**-mih-tee) A permanent structural deviation from the normal.

degenerative (dee-**JEN**-er-a-tiv) Relating to the deterioration of a structure.

deglutition (dee-glue-**TISH**-un) The act of swallowing.

dehydration (dee-high-**DRAY**-shun) Process of losing body water.

dehydroepiandrosterone (DHEA) (de-**HIGH**-droh-epee-an-**DROS**-ter-own) Precursor to testosterone; produced in the adrenal cortex.

delirium (de-**LIR**-ee-um) Acute altered state of consciousness with agitation and disorientation; condition is reversible.

deltoid (**DEL**-toyd) Large, fan-shaped muscle connecting the scapula and clavicle to the humerus.

delusion (de-**LOO**-shun) Fixed, unyielding, false belief or judgment held despite strong evidence to the contrary.

dementia (dee-**MEN**-she-ah) Chronic, progressive, irreversible loss of the mind's cognitive and intellectual functions.

demyelination (dee-**MY**-eh-lin-**A**-shun) Process of losing the myelin sheath of a nerve fiber.

dendrite (**DEN**-dright) Branched extension of the nerve cell body that receives nervous stimuli.

dental (**DEN**-tal) Pertaining to the teeth.

dentin (**DEN**-tin) Dense, ivorylike substance located under the enamel in a tooth.

dentist (**DEN**-tist) Legally qualified specialist in dentistry.

dentistry (**DEN**-tis-tree) Evaluation, diagnosis, prevention, and treatment of conditions of the oral cavity and associated structures.

deoxyribonucleic acid (DNA) (dee-**OCK**-see-**RYE**-boh-noo-**KLEE**-ik **ASS**-id) Source of hereditary characteristics found in chromosomes.

dependence (de-**PEN**-dense) State of needing someone or something.

dependent (de-**PEN**-dent) Having to rely on someone else.

depressant (de-**PRESS**-ant) Substance that diminishes activity, sensation, or tone.

depression (de-**PRESH**-un) Mental disorder with feelings of deep sadness and despair.

dermatitis (der-mah-**TYE**-tis) Inflammation of the skin.

dermatologist (der-mah-**TOL**-oh-jist) Medical specialist in diseases of the skin.

dermatology (der-mah-**TOL**-oh-jee) Medical specialty concerned with disorders of the skin.

dermatome (**DER**-mah-tome) The area of skin supplied by a single spinal nerve; alternatively, an instrument used for cutting thin slices.

dermatomyositis (**DER**-mah-toe-**MY**-oh-site-is) Inflammation of the skin and muscles.

dermis (**DER**-miss) Connective tissue layer of the skin beneath the epidermis.

detoxification (de-**TOKS**-ih-fi-**KAY**-shun) Removal of poison from a tissue or substance.

deviation (de-ve-**A**-shun) A turning aside from a normal course.

diabetes insipidus (dye-ah-**BEE**-teez in-**SIP**-ih-dus) Excretion of large amounts of dilute urine as a result of inadequate ADH production.

diabetes mellitus (dye-ah-**BEE**-teez **MEL**-ih-tus) Metabolic syndrome caused by absolute or relative insulin deficiency and/or insulin ineffectiveness.

diabetic (dye-ah-**BET**-ik) Pertaining to or suffering from diabetes.

diagnose (die-ag-**NOSE**) To make a diagnosis.

diagnosis (die-ag-**NO**-sis) The determination of the cause of a disease. Plural *diagnoses.*

diagnostic (die-ag-**NOS**-tik) Pertaining to or establishing a diagnosis.

dialectic (die-ah-**LEK**-tik) Logical argumentation.

dialysis (die-**AL**-ih-sis) An artificial method of filtration to remove excess waste materials and water from the body.

dialyzer (**DIE**-ah-lie-zer) Machine for dialysis.

diaphoresis (DIE-ah-foh-REE-sis) Sweat or perspiration.

diaphoretic (DIE-ah-foh-RET-ic) Pertaining to sweat or perspiration.

diaphragm (DIE-ah-fram) A ring and dome-shaped material inserted in the vagina to prevent pregnancy; *or* the musculomembranous partition separating the abdominal and thoracic cavities.

diaphragmatic (DIE-ah-frag-MAT-ic) Pertaining to the diaphragm.

diaphysis (die-AF-ih-sis) The shaft of a long bone.

diarrhea (die-ah-REE-ah) Abnormally frequent and loose stools.

diastasis (die-ASS-tah-sis) Separation of normally joined parts.

diastole (die-AS-toe-lee) Dilation of heart cavities, during which they fill with blood.

diet (DIE-et) Specific course of eating and drinking.

dietary (DIE-et-ary) Pertaining to a diet.

dietetics (die-eh-TET-iks) Application of diet to prevention and treatment of disease.

dietician (die-eh-TISH-un) Licensed professional in dietetics. Alternative spelling *dietitian*.

differential (dif-er-EN-shal) A differential white blood cell count lists percentages of the different leukocytes in a blood sample.

diffuse (dih-FUSE) To disseminate or spread out.

diffusion (dih-FYU-zhun) The means by which small particles move between tissues.

DiGeorge syndrome (dee-JORJ SIN-drome) Congenital absence of the thymus gland.

digestion (die-JEST-shun) Breakdown of food into elements suitable for cell metabolism.

digestive (die-JEST-iv) Relating to digestion.

digital (DIJ-ih-tal) Pertaining to a finger or toe.

diglyceride (die-GLISS-eh-ride) Substance with two fatty acids.

dilation (die-LAY-shun) Stretching or enlarging of an opening.

diode (DIE-ode) Allows electrical current to flow in one direction only.

dioxin (die-OK-sin) Carcinogenic contaminant in pesticides.

diphtheria (dif-THEER-ee-ah) Disease with a thick, membranous (leathery) coating of the pharynx.

diplegia (die-PLEE-jee-ah) Paralysis of all four limbs, with the two legs affected most severely.

disability (dis-ah-BILL-ih-tee) Diminished capacity to perform certain activities or functions.

disaccharide (die-SACK-ah-ride) A combination of two monosaccharides; for example, table sugar.

discipline (DIS-ih-plin) Training for proper conduct or action.

discrimination (DIS-krim-ih-NAY-shun) Ability to distinguish between different things.

disinfectant (dis-in-FEK-tant) Agent that disinfects.

disinfection (dis-in-FEK-shun) Process of destruction of microorganisms by chemical agents.

dislocation (dis-low-KAY-shun) The state of being completely out of joint.

displaced fracture (dis-PLAYSD FRAK-chur) A fracture in which the fragments are separated and are not in alignment.

disseminate (dih-SEM-in-ate) Widely scattered throughout the body or an organ.

dissociative identity disorder (di-SO-see-ah-tiv eye-DEN-tih-tee dis-OR-der) Mental disorder in which of an individual's personality is separated from the rest, leading to multiple personalities.

distal (DISS-tal) Situated away from the center of the body.

diuresis (die-you-REE-sis) Excretion of large volumes of urine.

diuretic (die-you-RET-ik) Agent that increases urine output.

diverticulitis (DIE-ver-tick-you-LIE-tis) Inflammation of the diverticula.

diverticulosis (DIE-ver-tick-you-LOW-sis) Presence of a number of small pouches in the wall of the large intestine.

diverticulum (die-ver-TICK-you-lum) A pouchlike opening or sac from a tubular structure (e.g., gut). Plural *diverticula*.

dizygotic (die-zye-GOT-ik) Twins from two separate zygotes.

dominant gene (DOM-ih-nant JEEN) Single allele that is expressed as a trait or characteristic.

dopamine (DOH-pah-meen) Neurotransmitter in some specific small areas of the brain.

Doppler (DOP-ler) Diagnostic instrument that sends an ultrasonic beam into the body.

Doppler ultrasonography (DOP-ler UL-trah-soh-NOG-rah-fee) Imaging that detects direction, velocity, and turbulence of blood flow; used in workup of stroke patients.

dormant (DOR-mant) Inactive.

dorsal (DOR-sal) Pertaining to the back or situated behind.

dorsum (DOR-sum) Upper, posterior, or back surface.

dosha (DOH-sha) Psychophysical constitution of the body in Ayurvedic medicine.

Down syndrome (DOWN SIN-drome) A syndrome with variable abnormalities associated with three chromosomes 21.

droplet (DROP-let) Globule of liquid; for example, that which is ejected from the mouth during speaking, coughing, sneezing.

Duchenne muscular dystrophy (DOO-shen MUSS-kyu-lar DISS-troh-fee) A condition with symmetrical weakness and wasting of pelvic, shoulder, and proximal limb muscles.

ductus arteriosus (DUK-tus ar-TEER-ih-OH-sus) Fetal vessel that connects the descending aorta with the left pulmonary artery.

ductus deferens (DUK-tus DEH-fuh-renz) Tube that receives sperm from the epididymis. Also known as *vas deferens*.

duodenal (du-oh-DEE-nal) Pertaining to the duodenum.

duodenum (du-oh-DEE-num) The first part of the small intestine; approximately 12 finger-breadths (9 to 10 inches) in length.

Dupuytren (du-pwe-TRAHN) Dupuytren contracture is thickening and shortening of fibrous bands in the palm of the hand.

dura mater (DYU-rah MAY-ter) Hard, fibrous outer layer of the meninges.

dwarfism (DWORF-izm) Short stature due to underproduction of growth hormone.

dysentery (DIS-en-tare-ee) Disease with diarrhea, bowel spasms, fever, and dehydration.

dysfunctional (dis-**FUNK**-shun-al) Having difficulty in performing.

dyslexia (dis-**LEK**-see-ah) Impaired reading and writing ability below the person's level of intelligence.

dyslexic (dis-**LEK**-sik) Pertaining to or suffering from dyslexia.

dyslipidemia (**DIS**-li-pi-**DEE**-me-ah) Abnormal (and "bad") levels of blood lipids.

dysmenorrhea (dis-men-oh-**REE**-ah) Painful and difficult menstruation.

dyspareunia (dis-pah-**RUE**-nee-ah) Pain during sexual intercourse.

dyspepsia (dis-**PEP**-see-ah) "Upset stomach," epigastric pain, nausea, and gas.

dysphagia (dis-**FAY**-jee-ah) Difficulty in swallowing.

dysplasia (dis-**PLAY**-zee-ah) Abnormal tissue formation.

dyspnea (disp-**NEE**-ah) Difficulty breathing.

dysrhythmia (dis-**RITH**-me-ah) An abnormal heart rhythm.

dysuria (dis-**YOU**-ree-ah) Difficulty or pain with urination.

E

eccrine (**EK**-rin) Coiled sweat gland that occurs in skin all over the body.

echinacea (ek-ih-**NAY**-sha) Spiky North American herb.

echocardiography (**EK**-oh-kar-dee-**OG**-rah-fee) Ultrasound recording of heart function.

echoencephalography (**EK**-oh-en-sef-ah-**LOG**-rah-fee) Use of ultrasound in the diagnosis of intracranial lesions.

eclampsia (ek-**LAMP**-see-uh) Convulsions in a patient with preeclampsia.

ecologic (ee-koh-**LOJ**-ik) Pertaining to the study of the environment.

ecology (ee-**KOL**-oh-jee) Interrelationship between living organisms with each other and the environment.

ectopic (ek-**TOP**-ik) Out of place, not in a normal position.

eczema (**EK**-zeh-mah) Inflammatory skin disease often with a serous discharge.

edema (ee-**DEE**-mah) Excessive accumulation of fluid in cells and tissues.

edematous (ee-**DEM**-ah-tus) Pertaining to or marked by edema.

effacement (ee-**FACE**-ment) Thinning of the cervix in relation to labor.

efferent (**EF**-eh-rent) Conducting impulses outward away from the brain or spinal cord.

effusion (eh-**FYU**-shun) Collection of fluid that has escaped from blood vessels into a cavity or tissues.

ejaculate (ee-**JACK**-you-late) To expel suddenly; *or* the semen expelled in ejaculation.

ejaculation (ee-**JACK**-you-**LAY**-shun) Process of expelling semen suddenly.

elective (e-**LEK**-tiv) Surgery that is not urgent or vital.

electrocardiogram (**ECG** or **EKG**) (ee-lek-troh-**KAR**-dee-oh-gram) Record of the electrical signals of the heart.

electrocardiograph (ee-lek-troh-**KAR**-dee-oh-graf) Machine that makes the electrocardiogram.

electrocardiography (ee-**LEK**-troh-kar-dee-**OG**-rah-fee) Interpretation of electrocardiograms.

electroconvulsive therapy (ee-**LEK**-troh-kon-**VUL**-siv **THAIR**-ah-pee) Passage of electric current through the brain to produce convulsions and treat persistent depression mania, and other disorders.

electrode (ee-**LEK**-trode) A device for conducting electricity.

electroencephalogram (**EEG**) (ee-**LEK**-troh-en-**SEF**-ah-low-gram) Record of the electrical activity of the brain.

electroencephalograph (ee-**LEK**-troh-en-**SEF**-ah-low-graf) Device used to record the electrical activity of the brain.

electroencephalography (ee-**LEK**-troh-en-**SEF**-ah-**LOG**-rah-fee) The process of recording the electrical activity of the brain.

electrolyte (ee-**LEK**-troh-lite) Substance that, when dissolved in a suitable medium, forms electrically charged particles.

electromagnetic (ee-**LEK**-troh-mag-**NET**-ik) Pertaining to energy propagated through matter and space.

electromyogram (ee-lek-troh-**MY**-oh-gram) Recording of electric currents associated with muscle action.

electromyography (ee-**LEK**-troh-my-**OG**-rah-fee) Recording of electrical activity in muscle.

electroneurodiagnostic (ee-**LEK**-troh-**NYUR**-oh-die-ag-**NOS**-tik) Pertaining to the use of electricity in the diagnosis of a neurologic disorder.

elimination (e-lim-ih-**NAY**-shun) Removal of waste material from the digestive tract.

emaciation (ee-may-see-**AY**-shun) Abnormal thinness.

embolus (**EM**-boh-lus) Detached piece of thrombus, mass of bacteria, quantity of air, or foreign body that blocks a vessel.

embryo (**EM**-bree-oh) Developing organism from conception until the end of the second month.

embryology (em-bree-**OL**-oh-jee) Science of the origin and early development of an organism.

embryonic (em-bree-**ON**-ic) Pertaining to the embryo.

emesis (**EM**-eh-sis) Vomit.

eminence (**EM**-ih-nens) A higher place or part.

emmetropia (emm-eh-**TROH**-pee-ah) Normal refractive condition of the eye.

empathy (**EM**-pah-thee) Ability to place yourself into the feelings, emotions, and reactions of another person.

emphysema (em-fih-**SEE**-mah) Dilation of respiratory bronchioles and alveoli.

empyema (**EM**-pie-**EE**-mah) Pus in a body cavity, particularly in the pleural cavity.

emulsify (eh-**MUL**-sih-fye) Break up into very small droplets to suspend in a solution (emulsion).

enamel (ee-**NAM**-el) Hard substance covering a tooth.

encephalitis (en-**SEF**-ah-**LIE**-tis) Inflammation of brain cells and tissues.

encephalocele (en-**SEF**-ah-loh-seal) Congenital defect of the cranium with herniation of brain tissue.

encephalomyelitis (en-**SEF**-ah-loh-**MY**-eh-lie-tis) Inflammation of the brain and spinal cord.

encode (en-**KODE**) Convert information.

encopresis (en-koh-**PREE**-sis) Repeated soiling with feces.

endarterectomy (**END**-ar-ter-**EK**-toe-me) Surgical removal of plaque from an artery.

endemic (en-**DEM**-ik) Disease always present in a community.

endocarditis (**EN**-doh-kar-**DIE**-tis) Inflammation of the lining of the heart.

endocardium (**EN**-doh-**KAR**-dee-um) The inside lining of the heart.

endocrine (**EN**-doh-krin) Pertaining to a gland that produces an internal or hormonal secretion and secretes it into the bloodstream.

endocrine gland (**EN**-doh-krin GLAND) A gland that produces an internal or hormonal secretion and secretes it into the bloodstream.

endocrinologist (**EN**-doh-krih-**NOL**-oh-jist) A medical specialist in endocrinology.

endocrinology (**EN**-doh-krih-**NOL**-oh-jee) Medical specialty concerned with the production and effects of hormones.

endogenous (en-**DOJ**-en-us) Produced within the organism.

endometrial (en-doh-**ME**-tree-al) Pertaining to the inner lining of the uterus.

endometriosis (**EN**-doh-me-tree-**OH**-sis) Endometrial tissue in the abdomen outside the uterus.

endometrium (en-doh-**ME**-tree-um) Inner lining of the uterus.

endoplasmic reticulum (**EN**-doh-**PLAZ**-mik reh-**TIC**-you-lum) Structure inside a cell that synthesizes steroids, detoxifies drugs, and manufactures cell membranes.

endorphin (en-**DOR**-fin) Natural substance in the brain that has the same effect as opium.

endoscope (**EN**-doh-skope) Instrument for examining the inside of a tubular or hollow organ.

endoscopy (en-**DOS**-koh-pee) The use of an endoscope.

endospore (**EN**-doh-spor) Spore produced inside a cell and capable of resisting heat, freezing, radiation, and chemicals.

endosteum (en-**DOSS**-tee-um) A membrane of tissue lining the inner (medullary) cavity of a long bone.

endotracheal (en-doh-**TRAY**-kee-al) Pertaining to being inside the trachea.

enema (**EN**-eh-mah) An injection of fluid into the rectum.

enteric (en-**TEHR**-ik) Pertaining to the intestine.

enteroscope (**EN**-ter-oh-**SKOPE**) Slender, tubular instrument with light source and camera to visualize the digestive tract.

enteroscopy (en-ter-**OSS**-koh-pee) The examination of the lining of the digestive tract.

enuresis (en-you-**REE**-sis) Bed-wetting; urinary incontinence.

environment (en-**VI**-ron-ment) All the external conditions affecting the life of an organism.

environmental (en-**VI**-ron-ment-al) Pertaining to the environment.

enzyme (**EN**-zime) Protein that induces changes in other substances.

eosinophil (ee-oh-**SIN**-oh-fill) An eosinophil's granules attract a rosy-red color on staining.

ependyma (ep-**EN**-dih-mah) Membrane lining the central canal of the spinal cord and the ventricles of the brain.

ependymoma (eh-pen-dih-**MOH**-mah) Benign tumor arising from cells lining the ventricles.

epicardium (**EP**-ih-kar-**DEE**-um) The outer layer of the heart wall.

epicondyle (ep-ih-**KON**-dile) Projection above the condyle for attachment of a ligament or tendon.

epidemic (ep-ih-**DEM**-ik) Outbreak in a community of a disease or a health-related behavior.

epidermis (ep-ih-**DER**-miss) Top layer of the skin.

epididymis (**EP**-ih-**DID**-ih-miss) Coiled tube attached to the testis.

epididymitis (**EP**-ih-did-ih-**MY**-tis) Inflammation of the epididymis.

epididymoorchitis (ep-ih-**DID**-ih-moh-or-**KIE**-tis) Inflammation of the epididymis and testicle. Also called *orchitis.*

epidural (ep-ih-**DYU**-ral) Above the dura.

epidural space (ep-ih-**DYU**-ral SPASE) Space between the dura mater and the wall of the vertebral canal or skull.

epigastric (ep-ih-**GAS**-trik) Abdominal region above the stomach.

epiglottis (ep-ih-**GLOT**-is) Leaf-shaped plate of cartilage that shuts off the larynx during swallowing.

epiglottitis (ep-ih-**GLOT**-eye-tis) Inflammation of the epiglottis.

epilepsy (**EP**-ih-**LEP**-see) Chronic brain disorder due to paroxysmal excessive neuronal discharges.

epinephrine (ep-ih-**NEF**-rin) Main catecholamine produced by the adrenal medulla. Also called *adrenaline.*

epiphyseal plate (eh-**PIF**-ih-see-al PLATE) Layer of cartilage between the epiphysis and metaphysis where bone growth occurs.

epiphysis (eh-**PIF**-ih-sis) Expanded area at the proximal and distal ends of a long bone that provides increased surface area for attachment of ligaments and tendons.

episiotomy (eh-piz-ee-**OT**-oh-me) Surgical incision of the vulva.

epispadias (ep-ih-**SPAY**-dee-as) Condition in which the urethral opening is on the dorsum of the penis.

epistaxis (ep-ih-**STAK**-sis) Nosebleed.

epithelium (ep-ih-**THEE**-lee-um) Tissue that covers surfaces or lines cavities.

equilibrium (ee-kwi-**LIB**-ree-um) Being evenly balanced.

erectile (ee-**REK**-tile) Capable of erection or being distended with blood.

erection (ee-**REK**-shun) Distended and rigid state of an organ.

ergonomic (err-go-**NOM**-ick) Term applied to a workplace tool or equipment designed to prevent worker injury and discomfort.

erosion (ee-**ROE**-shun) A shallow ulcer in the lining of a structure.

erythema infectiosum (er-ih-**THEE**-mah in-fek-she-**OH**-sum) Mild infectious disease of childhood with a flushed-cheek appearance. Also called *fifth disease.*

erythroblast (eh-RITH-ro-blast) Precursor to a red blood cell.

erythroblastosis fetalis (eh-RITH-ro-blast-oh-sis fee-TAH-lis) Hemolytic disease of the newborn due to Rh incompatibility.

erythrocyte (eh-RITH-roh-site) Another name for a red blood cell.

erythropoiesis (eh-RITH-ro-poy-EE-sis) The formation of red blood cells.

erythropoietin (eh-RITH-ro-POY-ee-tin) Protein secreted by the kidney that stimulates red blood cell production.

eschar (ESS-kar) The burned, dead tissue lying on top of third-degree burns.

Escherichia coli (esh-eh-RIK-ee-ah KOH-lie) Organism in the intestine; releases an exotoxin that causes diarrhea.

esophagitis (ee-SOF-ah-JI-tis) Inflammation of the lining of the esophagus.

esophagus (ee-SOF-ah-gus) Tube linking the pharynx and the stomach.

esotropia (es-oh-TROH-pee-ah) A turning of the eye inward toward the nose.

essential (eh-SEN-shal) Amino acids that cannot be synthesized by the body.

estrogen (ES-troh-jen) Generic term for hormones that stimulate female secondary sex characteristics.

ethmoid (ETH-moyd) Bone that forms the back of the nose and encloses numerous air cells.

eumelanin (YOU-mel-ah-nin) The dark form of the pigment melanin.

euphoria (yoo-FOR-ee-ah) Exaggerated feeling of well-being.

eupnea (yoop-NEE-ah) Normal breathing.

eustachian tube (you-STAY-shun TYUB) Tube that connects the middle ear to the nasopharynx. Also called *auditory tube.*

euthyroid (you-THIGH-royd) Normal thyroid function.

eversion (ee-VER-shun) A turning outward.

evolve (ee-VOLV) To develop gradually.

exacerbation (ek-zas-er-BAY-shun) Period in which there is an increase in the severity of a disease.

exanthem (ek-ZAN-them) Skin eruption or rash occurring as the outward sign of a viral or bacterial disease.

excoriate (eks-KOR-ee-ate) To scratch.

excoriation (eks-KOR-ee-AY-shun) Scratch marks.

excrement (EKS-kreh-ment) Waste matter such as feces.

excrete (eks-KREET) To pass out of the body waste products of metabolism.

excretion (eks-KREE-shun) Removal of waste products of metabolism out of the body.

exhale (EKS-hail) Breathe out.

exocrine gland (EK-soh-krin GLAND) A gland that secretes outwardly through excretory ducts.

exogenous (ex-OJ-en-us) Originating outside the organism.

exophthalmos (ek-sof-THAL-mos) Protrusion of the eyeball.

exotropia (ek-soh-TROH-pee-ah) A turning of the eye outward away from the nose.

expectorate (ek-SPEC-toh-rate) Cough up and spit out mucus from the respiratory tract.

expiration (EKS-pih-RAY-shun) Breathe out.

extension (eks-TEN-shun) Straighten a joint to increase its angle.

extracorporeal (EKS-trah-kor-POH-ree-al) Outside the body.

extravasate (eks-TRAV-ah-sate) To ooze out from a vessel into the tissues.

extrinsic (eks-TRIN-sik) Extrinsic eye muscles are located on the outside of the eye, as opposed to intrinsic muscles, which are located inside the eye.

F

facet (FAS-et) Small smooth area around a pain-producing nerve.

facial (FAY-shal) Seventh (VII) cranial nerve; supplying the forehead, nose, eyes, mouth, and jaws.

facies (FASH-eez) Facial expression and features characteristic of a specific disease.

fallopian tubes (fah-LOW-pee-an) Uterine tubes connected to the fundus of the uterus.

Fallot (fah-LOW) Person who first described the tetralogy of congenital heart defects.

fascia (FASH-ee-ah) Sheet of fibrous connective tissue.

fascicle (FAS-ih-kull) Bundle of muscle fibers.

fasciectomy (fash-ee-EK-toe-me) Surgical removal of fascia.

fasciitis (fash-ee-I-tis) Inflammation of the fascia.

fasciotomy (fash-ee-OT-oh-me) An incision through a band of fascia, usually to relieve pressure on underlying structures.

fat (FAT) Lipid that is solid at room temperature.

fatty acid (FAT-ee ASS-id) An acid obtained from the hydrolysis of fats.

febrile (FEB-ril or FEB-rile) Pertaining to or suffering from a fever.

fecal (FEE-kal) Pertaining to feces.

feces (FEE-sees) Undigested, waste material discharged from the bowel.

Feldenkrais method (FEL-den-kries METH-od) Series of exercises to discover new ways of pain-free movement.

femoral (FEM-oh-ral) Pertaining to the femur.

femur (FEE-mur) The thigh bone.

ferritin (FER-ih-tin) Iron-protein complex that regulates iron storage and transport.

fertilization (FER-til-eye-ZAY-shun) Union of a male sperm and a female egg.

fertilize (FER-til-ize) To penetrate an oocyte with a sperm so as to impregnate.

fertilizer (FER-tih-lie-zer) Substance used to increase the yield of crops.

festinant (FES-tih-nant) Shuffling, falling-forward gait.

fetal (FEE-tal) Pertaining to the fetus.

fetus (FEE-tus) Human organism from the end of the eighth week after conception to birth.

fever (FEE-ver) Increased body temperature that is a physiologic response to disease.

fiber (FIE-ber) Carbohydrate not digested by intestinal enzymes; *or* a strand or filament.

fibrillation (fi-brih-LAY-shun) Uncontrolled quivering or twitching of the heart muscle.

fibrin (FIE-brin) Stringy protein fiber that is a component of a blood clot.

fibrinogen (fie-BRIN-oh-jen) Precursor of fibrin in blood-clotting process.

fibroadenoma (FIE-broh-ad-en-OH-mah) Benign tumor containing much fibrous tissue.

fibroblast (FIE-bro-blast) Cell that forms collagen fibers.

fibrocartilage (fie-bro-KAR-til-age) Cartilage containing collagen fibers.

fibrocystic disease (fie-broh-SIS-tik DIZ-eez) Benign breast disease with multiple tiny lumps and cysts.

fibroid (FIE-broyd) Uterine tumor resembling fibrous tissue.

fibromyalgia (fie-bro-my-AL-jee-ah) Pain in the muscle fibers.

fibromyoma (FIE-bro-my-OH-mah) Benign neoplasm derived from smooth muscle containing fibrous tissue.

fibrosis (fie-BROH-sis) Repair of dead tissue cells by formation of fibrous tissue.

fibrous (FIE-brus) Tissue containing fibroblasts and fibers.

fibula (FIB-you-lah) The smaller of the two bones of the lower leg.

filter (FIL-ter) A porous substance through which a liquid or gas is passed to separate out contained particles; or to use a filter.

filtrate (FIL-trate) That which has passed through a filter.

filtration (fil-TRAY-shun) Process of passing liquid through a filter.

fimbria (FIM-bree-ah) A fringelike structure on the surface of a cell or microorganism. Plural *fimbriae.*

fissure (FISH-ur) Deep furrow or cleft. Plural *fissures.*

fistula (FIS-tyu-lah) Abnormal passage.

flagellum (fla-JELL-um) Tail of a sperm. Plural *flagella.*

flatulence (FLAT-you-lents) Excessive amount of gas in the stomach and intestines.

flatus (FLAY-tus) Gas or air expelled through the anus.

flavonoid (FLAY-vih-noid) A pigment found in fruit, wine, and tea. Also spelled *flavinoid.*

flex (FLEKS) To bend a joint so that the two parts come together.

flexion (FLEK-shun) Bend a joint to decrease its angle.

flexor (FLEK-sor) Muscle or tendon that flexes a joint.

flexure (FLEK-shur) A bend in a structure.

flora (FLO-rah) Microorganisms covering the exterior and interior of a healthy animal.

fluidized therapy (FLU-id-ized THAIR-ah-pee) Use of suspended particles in a hot air stream to apply heat.

fluidotherapy (FLU-id-oh-THAIR-ah-pee) A form of heat therapy.

fluorescein (flor-ESS-ee-in) Dye that produces a vivid green color under a blue light to diagnose corneal abrasions and foreign bodies.

fluoride (FLOR-ide) Chemical found in bones and teeth.

fluoroscopy (flor-OS-koh-pee) Examination of the structures of the body by x-rays.

folate (FO-late) Natural B_9 vitamin.

folic acid (FO-lik ASS-id) Synthetic B_9 vitamin.

follicle (FOLL-ih-kull) Spherical mass of cells containing a cavity or a small cul-de-sac, such as a hair follicle.

follicular (fo-LIK-you-lar) Pertaining to a follicle.

fomites (FO-my-teez) Bedding, clothing, towels, etc., that can harbor and transmit a disease agent.

foramen (fo-RAY-men) An opening through a structure. Plural *foramina.*

forceps extraction (FOR-seps ek-STRAK-shun) Assisted delivery of the baby by an instrument that grasps the head of the baby.

foreskin (FOR-skin) Skin that covers the glans penis.

fornix (FOR-niks) Arch-shaped, blind-ended part of the vagina behind and around the cervix. Plural *fornices.*

fovea centralis (FOH-vee-ah sen-TRAH-lis) Small pit in the center of the macula that has the highest visual acuity.

free radical (FREE RAD-ih-kal) Short-lived product of oxidation in a cell that can be damaging to the cell.

frenulum (FREN-you-lum) Fold of mucous membrane between the glans and the prepuce.

frequency (FREE-kwen-see) The number of times something happens in a given time (e.g., passing urine).

frontal (FRON-tal) Pertaining to the vertical plane dividing the body into anterior and posterior portions.

frontal lobe (FRON-tal LOBE) Area of brain behind the frontal bone.

fructosamine (FRUK-toe-sah-meen) Organic compound with fructose as its base.

fructose (FRUK-toes) Sugar found in fruits and honey.

function (FUNK-shun) The ability of an organ or tissue to perform its special work.

fundoscopy (fun-DOS-koh-pee) Examination of the fundus (retina) of the eye.

fundus (FUN-dus) Part farthest from the opening of a hollow organ.

fungicide (FUN-jee-side) Agent for destroying fungi.

fungus (FUN-gus) General term used to describe yeasts and molds. Plural *fungi.*

furuncle (FU-rung-kel) An infected hair follicle that spreads into the tissues around the follicle.

G

galactorrhea (gah-**LAK**-toe-**REE**-ah) Abnormal flow of milk from the breasts.

gallbladder (**GAWL**-blad-er) Receptacle on the inferior surface of the liver for storing bile.

gallstone (**GAWL**-stone) Hard mass of cholesterol, calcium, and bilirubin that can be formed in the gallbladder and bile duct.

galvanic (gal-**VAN**-ik) Pertaining to electric current.

ganglion (**GANG**-lee-on) Collection of nerve cell bodies outside the CNS; *or* a fluid-containing swelling attached to the synovial sheath of a tendon. Plural *ganglia*.

gastric (**GAS**-trik) Pertaining to the stomach.

gastrin (**GAS**-trin) Hormone secreted in the stomach that stimulates secretion of HCl and increases gastric motility.

gastritis (gas-**TRY**-tis) Inflammation of the lining of the stomach.

gastrocnemius (gas-trok-**NEE**-me-us) Major muscle in back of the lower leg (the calf).

gastrocolic reflex (gas-troh-**KOL**-ik **RE**-fleks) Taking food into the stomach leads to mass movement of feces in the colon and the desire to defecate.

gastroenteritis (**GAS**-troh-en-ter-**I**-tis) Inflammation of the stomach and intestines.

gastroenterologist (**GAS**-troh-en-ter-**OL**-oh-jist) Medical specialist in gastroenterology.

gastroenterology (**GAS**-troh-en-ter-**OL**-oh-gee) Medical specialty of the stomach and intestines.

gastroesophageal (**GAS**-troh-ee-sof-ah-**JEE**-al) Pertaining to the stomach and esophagus.

gastrointestinal (GI) (**GAS**-troh-in-**TESS**-tin-al) Relating to the stomach and intestines.

gastroscope (**GAS**-troh-skope) Endoscope for examining the inside of the stomach.

gastroscopy (gas-**TROS**-koh-pee) Endoscopic examination of the stomach.

Gaucher disease (go-**SHAY DIZ**-eez) Congenital disorder of fat metabolism.

gavage (guh-**VAHZH**) Forced feeding by stomach tube.

gene (**JEEN**) Functional segment of the DNA molecule.

genetic (jeh-**NET**-ik) Pertaining to a gene.

geneticist (jeh-**NET**-ih-sist) A specialist in genetics.

genetics (jeh-**NET**-iks) Science of the inheritance of characteristics.

genistein (**JEN**-is-tine) Flavonoid found in soy.

genital (**JEN**-ih-tal) Relating to reproduction or to the male or female sex organs.

genitalia (**JEN**-ih-**TAY**-lee-ah) External and internal organs of reproduction.

genome (**JEE**-nome) Complete set of genes.

genomics (jee-**NOME**-iks) Study of the structure, function, and information content of the genome.

genotype (jee-**NOH**-type) Specific genetic constitution of an individual.

geriatrician (jer-ee-ah-**TRISH**-an) Medical specialist in geriatrics.

geriatrics (jer-ee-**AT**-riks) Medical specialty that deals with the problems of old age.

gerontologist (jer-on-**TOL**-oh-jist) Medical specialist in gerontology.

gerontology (jer-on-**TOL**-oh-jee) Study of the process and problems of aging.

gestation (jes-**TAY**-shun) Period from conception to birth.

Giardia (jee-**AR**-dee-ah) Parasite in the small intestine.

giardiasis (jee-ar-**DIE**-ah-sis) Infection with *Giardia*, causing diarrhea.

gigantism (**JI**-gan-tizm) Abnormal height and size of the entire body.

gingiva (**JIN**-jih-vah) Tissue surrounding teeth and covering the jaw.

gingival (**JIN**-jih-vul) Pertaining to the gums.

gingivectomy (jin-jih-**VEC**-toe-me) Surgical removal of diseased gum tissue.

gingivitis (jin-jih-**VI**-tis) Inflammation of the gums.

Ginkgo **biloba** (**GING**-koh **BIL**-oh-bah) Extract of leaves used as a vasodilator.

ginseng (**JIN**-seng) Extract made from the root of a Chinese plant.

glans (**GLANZ**) Head of the penis or clitoris.

glaucoma (glau-**KOH**-mah) Increased intraocular pressure.

glia (**GLEE**-ah) Connective tissue that holds a structure together.

glioblastoma multiforme (**GLIE**-oh-blas-**TOE**-mah) A malignant form of brain cancer.

glioma (gli-**OH**-mah) Tumor arising in a glial cell.

globulin (**GLOB**-you-lin) Family of blood proteins.

glomerulonephritis (glo-**MER**-you-low-nef-**RYE**-tis) Infection of the glomeruli of the kidney.

glomerulus (glo-**MER**-you-lus) Plexus of capillaries; part of a nephron. Plural *glomeruli*.

glossodynia (gloss-oh-**DIN**-ee-ah) Painful, burning tongue.

glossopharyngeal (**GLOSS**-oh-fah-**RIN**-jee-al) Ninth (IX) cranial nerve; supplying the tongue and pharynx.

glottis (**GLOT**-is) Vocal apparatus of the larynx.

glucagon (**GLU**-kah-gon) Pancreatic hormone that supports blood glucose levels.

glucocorticoid (glu-co-**KOR**-tih-koyd) Hormone of the adrenal cortex that helps regulate glucose metabolism.

gluconeogenesis (**GLU**-ko-nee-oh-**JEN**-eh-sis) Formation of glucose from noncarbohydrate sources.

glucose (**GLU**-kose) The final product of carbohydrate digestion and the main sugar in the blood.

gluteal (**GLU**-tee-al) Pertaining to the buttocks.

gluten (**GLU**-ten) Insoluble protein found in wheat, barley, and oats.

gluteus (**GLU**-tee-us) Term that refers to a muscle in the buttocks.

glycemic index (glye-**SEE**-mic **IN**-deks) Measure of the rapidity in the rise of blood glucose after ingestion of carbohydrates.

glycemic load (glye-**SEE**-mic LOHD) Takes into account the amount of sugar available in the food to cause the rise in blood sugar.

glycogen (**GLYE**-koh-gen) The body's principal carbohydrate reserve, stored in the liver and skeletal muscle.

glycogenolysis (**GLYE**-koh-jen-oh-**LYE**-sis) Conversion of glycogen to glucose.

glycoprotein (**GLYE**-koh-**PRO**-teen) Combination of carbohydrate and protein.

glycosuria (**GLYE**-koh-**SYU**-ree-ah) Presence of glucose in urine.

glycosylated hemoglobin (Hb A1c) (**GLYE**-koh-sih-lay-ted **HE**-moh-**GLOW**-bin) Hemoglobin A fraction linked to glucose; used as an index of glucose control.

goiter (**GOY**-ter) Enlargement of the thyroid gland.

Golgi complex (**GOAL**-jee **KOM**-pleks) Organelle involved in synthesis of carbohydrates and glycoproteins.

gomphosis (gom-**FOE**-sis) Joint formed by a peg and socket. Plural *gomphoses.*

gonad (**GO**-nad) Testis or ovary. Plural *gonads.*

gonadotropin (**GO**-nad-oh-**TROH**-pin) Hormone capable of promoting gonad function.

gonorrhea (gon-oh-**REE**-ah) Specific contagious sexually transmitted infection.

gout (**GOWT**) Painful arthritis of the big toe and other joints.

grade (**GRAYD**) In cancer pathology, a classification of the rate of growth of cancer cells.

graft (**GRAFT**) Transplantation of living tissue.

Gram stain (**GRAM STAYN**) A method for differential staining of bacteria.

grand mal (**GRAHN MAL**) Old name for a generalized tonic-clonic seizure.

granulation (gran-you-**LAY**-shun) New fibrous tissue formed during wound healing.

granulocyte (**GRAN**-you-loh-site) A white blood cell that contains multiple small granules in its cytoplasm.

granulosa cell (gran-you-**LOH**-sah SELL) Cell lining the ovarian follicle.

Graves disease (**GRAVZ DIZ**-eez) Hyperthyroidism with toxic goiter.

gravid (**GRAV**-id) Pregnant.

gravida (**GRAV**-ih-dah) A pregnant woman.

gravidarum (gra-vih-**DAR**-um) Relating to pregnant women.

gray matter (**GRAY MATT**-er) Regions of the brain and spinal cord occupied by cell bodies and dendrites.

greenstick fracture (**GREEN**-stik **FRAK**-chur) A fracture in which one side of the bone is partially broken and the other side is bent; occurs mostly in children.

guanine (**GWAH**-neen) One of the chemical bases found in, and comprising the sequence of, both DNA and RNA.

Guillain-Barré syndrome (**GEE**-yan-bah-**RAY SIN**-drom) Disorder in which the body makes antibodies against myelin, disrupting nerve conduction.

gynecologist (guy-nih-**KOL**-oh-jist) Specialist in gynecology.

gynecology (guy-nih-**KOL**-oh-jee) Medical specialty for the care of the female reproductive system.

gynecomastia (**GUY**-nih-koh-**MAS**-tee-ah) Enlargement of the breast.

gyrus (**JI**-rus) Rounded elevation on the surface of the cerebral hemispheres. Plural *gyri.*

H

hairline fracture (**HAIR**-line **FRAK**-chur) A fracture without separation of the fragments.

halitosis (hal-ih-**TOE**-sis) Bad odor of the breath.

hallucination (hah-loo-sih-**NAY**-shun) Perception of an object or event when there is no such thing present.

hallux valgus (**HAL**-uks **VAL**-gus) Deviation of the big toe toward the lateral side of the foot.

handicap (**HAND**-ee-cap) Condition that interferes with a person's ability to function normally.

hapten (**HAP**-ten) Small molecule that has to bind to a larger molecule to form an antigen.

Hashimoto disease (hah-shee-**MOH**-toe **DIZ**-eez) Autoimmune disease of the thyroid gland. Also called *Hashimoto thyroiditis.*

haversian canals (hah-**VER**-shan ka-**NALS**) Vascular canals in bone. Also called *central canals.*

head (**HED**) The rounded extremity of a bone.

Heberden node (**HEH**-ber-den **NOHD**) Bony lump on the terminal phalanx of the fingers in osteoarthritis.

helix (**HE**-liks) A line in the shape of a coil.

helminth (**HELL**-minth) Any intestinal wormlike parasite.

hemangioma (he-**MAN**-jee-oh-mah) Abnormal mass of proliferating blood vessels.

hematemesis (he-mah-**TEM**-eh-sis) Vomiting of red blood.

hematochezia (he-mat-oh-**KEY**-zee-ah) The passage of red, bloody stools.

hematocrit (Hct) (**HE**-mat-oh-krit) Percentage of red blood cells in blood.

hematologist (he-mah-**TOL**-oh-jist) Specialist in hematology.

hematology (he-mah-**TOL**-oh-jee) Medical specialty of disorders of blood.

hematoma (he-mah-**TOH**-mah) Collection of blood that has escaped from the blood vessels into tissue. Also called *bruise.*

hematopoietic (**HE**-mah-toh-poy-**ET**-ick) Pertaining to the making of red blood cells.

hematuria (he-mah-**TYU**-ree-ah) Blood in the urine.

heme (**HEEM**) The iron-based component of hemoglobin that carries oxygen.

hemifacial (hem-ee-**FAY**-shal) Pertaining to one side of the face.

hemiparesis (**HEM**-ee-pah-**REE**-sis) Weakness of one side of the body.

hemiplegia (hem-ee-**PLEE**-jee-ah) Paralysis of one side of the body.

Hemoccult test (**HEEM**-oh-kult TEST) *Hemoccult* (trade name for a fecal occult blood test).

hemochromatosis (HE-mah-krom-ah-**TOE**-sis) Dangerously high levels of iron in the body with deposition of iron pigments in tissues.

hemodialysis (HE-moh-die-**AL**-ih-sis) An artificial method of filtration to remove excess waste materials and water directly from the blood.

hemodynamics (HE-moh-die-**NAM**-iks) The science of the blood flow through the circulation.

hemoglobin (HE-moh-**GLOW**-bin) Red-pigmented protein that is the main component of red blood cells.

hemoglobinopathy (HE-moh-**GLOW**-bih-**NOP**-ah-thee) Disease caused by the presence of an abnormal hemoglobin in the red blood cells.

hemolysis (he-**MOL**-ih-sis) Destruction of red blood cells so that hemoglobin is liberated.

hemolytic (he-moh-**LIT**-ik) Pertaining to the process of destruction of red blood cells.

hemophilia (he-moh-**FILL**-ee-ah) An inherited disease from a deficiency of clotting factor VIII.

hemoptysis (he-**MOP**-tih-sis) Bloody sputum.

hemorrhage (**HEM**-oh-raj) To bleed profusely.

hemorrhoid (**HEM**-oh-royd) Dilated rectal vein producing painful anal swelling. Plural *hemorrhoids*.

hemorrhoidectomy (**HEM**-oh-roy-**DEK**-toh-me) Surgical removal of hemorrhoids.

hemostasis (he-moh-**STAY**-sis) Controlling or stopping bleeding.

hemothorax (he-moh-**THOR**-ax) Blood in the pleural cavity.

heparin (**HEP**-ah-rin) An anticoagulant secreted particularly by liver cells.

hepatic (hep-**AT**-ik) Pertaining to the liver.

hepatitis (hep-ah-**TIE**-tis) Inflammation of the liver.

hepatocellular (**HEP**-ah-toe-**SELL**-you-lar) Pertaining to liver cells.

herbicide (**ER**-bih-side) Agent for destroying plants.

heredity (heh-**RED**-ih-tee) Transmission of characteristics from parents to offspring through genes.

hernia (**HER**-nee-ah) Protrusion of a structure through the tissue that normally contains it.

herniate (**HER**-nee-ate) To protrude.

herniation (**HER**-nee-ay-shun) Protrusion of an anatomical structure from its normal location.

herniorrhaphy (**HER**-nee-**OR**-ah-fee) Repair of a hernia.

herpangina (her-**PAN**-ji-nah) Ulcerative disease of the throat.

herpes simplex virus (HSV) (**HER**-peez **SIM**-pleks **VIE**-rus) Disease that manifests with painful, watery blisters on the skin and mucous membranes.

herpes zoster (**HER**-pees **ZOS**-ter) Painful eruption of vesicles that follows a dermatome or nerve root on one side of the body. Also called *shingles*.

heterograft (**HET**-er-oh-graft) A graft using tissue taken from another species. Also known as *xenograft*.

heterophile (**HET**-er-oh-file) Pertaining to antibodies present during a disease but not directed against the causative agent.

heterozygous (**HET**-er-oh-**ZIE**-gus) Carries a different version (allele) of a specific gene on each of the two corresponding chromosomes.

hiatus (high-**AY**-tus) An opening through a structure.

hilum (**HIGH**-lum) The site where the nerves and blood vessels enter and leave an organ. Plural *hila*.

hirsutism (**HER**-sue-tizm) Excessive body and facial hair.

histamine (**HISS**-tah-mean) Compound liberated in tissues as a result of injury or an allergic response.

histology (his-**TOL**-oh-jee) Structure and function of cells, tissues, and organs.

Hodgkin lymphoma (**HOJ**-kin lim-**FO**-muh) Disease marked by chronic enlargement of lymph nodes spreading to other nodes in an orderly way.

holistic (ho-**LIS**-tik) Pertaining to the care of the whole person in physical, mental, emotional, and spiritual dimensions.

homeopath (**HO**-mee-oh-path) Practitioner of homeopathy.

homeopathy (ho-mee-**OP**-ah-thee) Treatment of disease with minute doses of substances.

homeostasis (ho-mee-oh-**STAY**-sis) Stability or equilibrium of a system or the body's internal environment.

homicidal (hom-ih-**SIDE**-al) Having a tendency to commit homicide.

homicide (**HOM**-ih-side) Killing of one human by another.

homocysteine (ho-moh-**SIS**-teen) An amino acid similar to cysteine.

homograft (**HOH**-moh-graft) Skin graft from another person or a cadaver.

homozygous (hoh-moh-**ZIE**-gus) Having two identical copies of a specific gene on the two homologous chromosomes.

hordeolum (hor-**DEE**-oh-lum) Abscess in an eyelash follicle. Also called *stye*.

hormone (**HOR**-mohn) Chemical formed in one tissue or organ and carried by the blood to stimulate or inhibit a function of another tissue or organ.

Horner syndrome (**HOR**-ner **SIN**-drome) Disorder of the sympathetic nerves to the face and eye.

hospice (**HOS**-pis) Facility or program that provides care to the dying and their families.

host (HOST) Organism on which organisms live.

human immunodeficiency virus (HIV) (**HYU**-man **IM**-you-noh-dee-**FISH**-en-see **VIE**-rus) Etiologic agent of acquired immunodeficiency syndrome (AIDS).

human papilloma virus (HPV) (**HYU**-man pap-ih-**LOW**-mah **VIE**-rus) Causes warts on the skin and genitalia and can increase the risk for cervical cancer.

humerus (**HYU**-mer-us) Single bone of the upper arm.

humoral immunity (**HYU**-mor-al im-**YOU**-nih-tee) Defense mechanism arising from antibodies in the blood.

Huntington disease (HUN-ting-ton DIZ-eez) Progressive inherited, degenerative, incurable neurologic disease. Also called *Huntington chorea.*

hyaline (HIGH-ah-line) Cartilage that looks like frosted glass and contains fine collagen fibers.

hyaline membrane disease (HIGH-ah-line MEM-brain DIZ-eez) Respiratory distress syndrome of the newborn.

hydrocele (HIGH-droh-seal) Collection of fluid in the space of the tunica vaginalis.

hydrocephalus (high-droh-SEF-ah-lus) Enlarged head due to excess CSF in the cerebral ventricles.

hydrochloric acid (HCl) (high-droh-KLOR-ic ASS-id) The acid of gastric juice.

Hydrocollator (high-droh-KOLL-ay-tor) Synthetic hot or cold gel used to stimulate a rise or fall in tissue temperature.

hydrocortisone (high-droh-KOR-tih-sohn) Potent glucocorticoid with anti-inflammatory properties. Also called *cortisol.*

hydrogenated (HIGH-droh-jeh-NAY-ted) Addition of hydrogen to unsaturated oils to solidify them and produce trans fats.

hydronephrosis (HIGH-droh-neh-FRO-sis) Dilation of the pelvis and calyces of a kidney.

hydronephrotic (HIGH-droh-neh-FROT-ik) Pertaining to or suffering from the dilation of the pelvis and calyces of the kidney.

hymen (HIGH-men) Thin membrane partly occluding the vaginal orifice.

hyperactivity (HIGH-per-ac-TIV-ih-tee) Excessive restlessness and movement.

hyperbaric (high-per-BAR-ik) Pressure greater than atmospheric pressure.

hypercalcemia (HIGH-per-cal-SEE-me-ah) Excessive level of calcium in the blood.

hypercapnia (HIGH-per-KAP-nee-ah) Abnormal increase of carbon dioxide in the arterial bloodstream.

hypercarotenemia (HIGH-per-KAR-o-teh-NEE-me-ah) Excessive level of the yellow-red pigment carotene in the blood.

hyperemesis (high-per-EM-ee-sis) Excessive vomiting.

hyperflexion (high-per-FLEK-shun) Flexion of a limb or part beyond the normal limits.

hyperfractionated (high-per-FRAK-shun-ay-ted) Given in smaller amounts and more frequently.

hyperglycemia (HIGH-per-gly-SEE-me-ah) High level of glucose (sugar) in blood.

hyperglycemic (HIGH-per-gly-SEE-mik) Pertaining to high blood sugar.

hyperimmune globulin (HIGH-per-im-YUNE GLOB-you-lin) Immunoglobulin prepared from serum of people with a high antibody titer to a specific virus.

hyperinflation (HIGH-per-in-FLAY-shun) Overdistension of pulmonary alveoli with air resulting from airway obstruction.

hyperkalemia (HIGH-per-kah-LEE-me-ah) High level of potassium in the blood.

hypernatremia (HIGH-per-nah-TREE-me-ah) High level of sodium in the blood.

hyperopia (high-per-OH-pee-ah) Able to see distant objects but unable to see close objects.

hyperosmolar (HIGH-per-os-MOH-lar) Marked hyperglycemia without ketoacidosis.

hyperparathyroidism (HIGH-per-para-THIGH-royd-ism) Excessive levels of parathyroid hormone.

hyperplasia (high-per-PLAY-zee-ah) Increase in the *number* of the cells in a tissue or organ.

hyperpnea (high-perp-NEE-ah) Deeper and more rapid breathing than normal.

hypersecretion (HIGH-per-seh-KREE-shun) Excessive secretion of mucus (or enzymes or waste products).

hypersensitivity (HIGH-per-sen-sih-TIV-ih-tee) Exaggerated abnormal reaction to an allergen.

hypersplenism (high-per-SPLEN-izm) Condition in which the spleen removes blood components at an excessive rate.

hypertension (HIGH-per-TEN-shun) Persistent high arterial blood pressure.

hypertensive (HIGH-per-TEN-siv) Suffering from hypertension.

hyperthyroidism (high-per-THIGH-royd-ism) Excessive production of thyroid hormones.

hypertrophy (high-PER-troh-fee) Increase in size, but not in number, of an individual tissue element.

hypha (HIGH-fah) Branching tubular fungal cell. Plural *hyphae.*

hypnosis (hip-NOH-sis) Changed state of consciousness.

hypnotherapy (hip-noh-THAIR-ah-pee) Use of hypnosis in treatment of disorders.

hypochondriac (high-poh-KON-dree-ack) A person who exaggerates the significance of symptoms.

hypochondriasis (HIGH-poh-kon-DRY-ah-sis) Belief that a minor symptom indicates a severe disease.

hypochromic (high-poh-CROW-mik) Pale in color, as in RBCs when hemoglobin is deficient.

hypodermis (high-poh-DER-miss) Tissue layer below the dermis.

hypogastric (high-poh-GAS-trik) Abdominal region below the stomach.

hypoglossal (high-poh-GLOSS-al) Twelfth (XII) cranial nerve; supplying muscles of the tongue.

hypoglycemia (HIGH-poh-glie-SEE-me-ah) Low level of glucose (sugar) in the blood.

hypoglycemic (HIGH-poh-glie-SEE-mik) Pertaining to or suffering from hypoglycemia.

hypogonadism (HIGH-poh-GOH-nad-izm) Deficient gonad production of sperm or eggs or hormones.

hypokalemia (HIGH-poh-kah-LEE-me-ah) Low level of potassium in the blood.

hyponatremia (HIGH-poh-nah-TREE-me-ah) Low level of sodium in the blood.

hypoparathyroidism (HIGH-poh-para-THIGH-royd-ism) Deficient levels of parathyroid hormone.

hypophysis (high-POF-ih-sis) Another name for the pituitary gland.

hypopituitarism (HIGH-poh-pih-**TYU**-ih-tah-rizm) Condition of one or more deficient pituitary hormones.

hypospadias (high-poh-**SPAY**-dee-as) Urethral opening more proximal than normal on the ventral surface of the penis.

hypotension (HIGH-poh-**TEN**-shun) Persistent low arterial blood pressure.

hypothalamic (high-poh-tha-**LAM**-ik) Pertaining to the hypothalamus.

hypothalamus (high-poh-**THAL**-ah-muss) Area of gray matter forming part of the walls and floor of the third ventricle.

hypothenar (high-poh-**THAY**-nar) Fleshy eminence at the base of the little finger.

hypothermia (high-poh-**THER**-me-ah) Very low core body temperature.

hypothyroidism (high-poh-**THIGH**-royd-ism) Deficient production of thyroid hormones.

hypotonia (high-poh-**TOE**-nee-ah) Diminished muscle tone.

hypotonic (high-poh-**TON**-ik) Pertaining to or suffering from hypotonia.

hypovolemic (HIGH-poh-vo-**LEE**-mick) Having decreased blood volume in the body.

hypoxia (high-**POCK**-see-ah) Decrease below normal levels of oxygen in tissues, gases, or blood.

hypoxic (high-**POCK**-sik) Deficient in oxygen.

hysterectomy (his-ter-**EK**-toe-me) Surgical removal of the uterus.

hysterosalpingogram (HIS-ter-oh-sal-**PING**-oh-gram) Radiograph of the uterus and uterine tubes after injection of contrast material.

hysteroscopy (his-ter-**OS**-koh-pee) Visual inspection of the uterine cavity using an endoscope.

I

ictal (ICK-tal) Pertaining to, or condition caused by, a stroke or epilepsy.

idiopathic (ID-ih-oh-**PATH**-ik) Pertaining to a disease of unknown etiology.

ileocecal (ILL-ee-oh-**SEE**-cal) Pertaining to the junction of the ileum and cecum.

ileocecal sphincter (ILL-ee-oh-**SEE**-cal **SFINK**-ter) Band of muscle that encircles the junction of the ileum and cecum.

ileoscopy (ill-ee-**OS**-koh-pee) Endoscopic examination of the ileum.

ileostomy (ill-ee-**OS**-toe-me) Artificial opening from the ileum to the outside of the body.

ileum (ILL-ee-um) Third portion of the small intestine.

iliac (ILL-ee-ack) Pertaining to or near the ilium (pelvic bone).

ilium (ILL-ee-um) Large wing-shaped bone at the upper and posterior part of the pelvis. Plural *ilia*.

imagery (IM-aj-ree) Visualization of pleasant fantasies.

immune (im-**YUNE**) Protected from an infectious disease.

immune serum (im-**YUNE SEER**-um) Serum taken from another human or animal that has antibodies to a disease. Also called *antiserum*.

immunity (im-**YOU**-nih-tee) State of being protected.

immunization (im-you-nih-**ZAY**-shun) Administration of an agent to provide immunity.

immunize (IM-you-nize) To make resistant to an infectious disease.

immunoassay (IM-you-noh-**ASS**-ay) Biochemical test to measure the amount of a substance in a liquid, using the reaction of an antibody to its antigen.

immunodeficiency (IM-you-noh-dee-**FISH**-en-see) Failure of the immune system.

immunoglobulin (IM-you-noh-**GLOB**-you-lin) Specific protein evoked by an antigen. All antibodies are immunoglobulins.

immunologist (im-you-**NOL**-oh-jist) Medical specialist in immunology.

immunology (im-you-**NOL**-oh-jee) The science and practice of immunity and allergy.

immunosuppression (IM-you-noh-suh-**PRESH**-un) Suppression of the immune response by an outside agent, such as a drug.

impacted (im-**PAK**-ted) Immovably wedged, as with earwax blocking the external canal.

impacted fracture (im-**PAK**-ted **FRAK**-chur) A fracture in which one bone fragment is driven into the other.

impairment (im-**PAIR**-ment) Diminishing of normal function.

impedance (im-**PEE**-dahns) Resistance to the flow of an electric current.

impermeable (im-**PER**-me-ah-bull) Does not allow passage of anything.

impetigo (im-peh-**TIE**-go) Infection of the skin producing thick, yellow crusts.

implant (im-**PLANT**) To insert material into tissues; *or* the material inserted into tissues.

implantable (im-**PLAN**-tah-bul) Able to be inserted into tissues.

implantation (im-plan-**TAY**-shun) Attachment of a fertilized egg to the endometrium.

impotence (IM-poh-tence) Unable to achieve an erection.

impulsive (im-**PUL**-siv) Inability to resist performing inappropriate actions.

in situ (IN **SIGH**-tyu) In the correct place.

in utero (IN **YOU**-ter-oh) Within the womb; not yet born.

in vitro fertilization (IVF) (IN **VEE**-troh **FER**-til-eye-**ZAY**-shun) Process of combining a sperm and egg in a laboratory dish and placing the resulting embryos inside a uterus.

inattention (IN-ah-**TEN**-shun) Lack of concentration and direction.

incision (in-**SIZH**-un) A cut or surgical wound.

incisor (in-**SIGH**-zor) Chisel-shaped tooth.

incompatible (in-kom-**PAT**-ih-bul) Substances that interfere with each other physiologically.

incompetence (in-KOM-peh-tense) Failure of valves to close completely.

incomplete (in-kom-PLEET) Lacking some part.

incomplete fracture (in-kom-PLEET FRAK-chur) A fracture that does not extend across the bone, as in a hairline fracture.

incontinence (in-KON-tin-ence) Inability to prevent discharge of urine or feces.

incubation (in-kyu-BAY-shun) Process of developing an infection.

incus (IN-cuss) Middle one of the three ossicles in the middle ear; shaped like an anvil.

independence (in-de-PEN-denz) State of being independent.

independent (in-de-PEN-dent) Able to fend for oneself.

index (IN-deks) A standard indicator of measurement. Plural *indices.*

indole (IN-dole) A phytochemical that makes estrogen less effective.

infancy (IN-fan-see) The first year of life.

infant (IN-fant) Child in the first year of life.

infant formula (IN-fant FOR-myu-lah) Commercial product for infants manufactured from cows' milk or soy milk.

infarct (in-FARKT) Area of cell death resulting from an infarction.

infarction (in-FARK-shun) Sudden blockage of an artery.

infect (in-FEKT) To invade an organism with disease-producing microorganisms.

infection (in-FEK-shun) Invasion of the body by disease-producing microorganisms.

infectious (in-FEK-shus) Capable of being transmitted; *or* caused by infection by a microorganism.

inferior (in-FEE-ree-or) Situated below.

infertility (in-fer-TIL-ih-tee) Inability to conceive over a long period of time.

infestation (in-fes-TAY-shun) Act of being invaded on the skin by a troublesome other species, such as a parasite.

infiltrate (IN-fil-trate) To penetrate and invade into a tissue or cell.

infiltration (in-fil-TRAY-shun) The invasion into a tissue or cell.

inflate (in-FLAYT) Expand with air.

inflation (in-FLAY-shun) Process of expanding with air.

infundibulum (IN-fun-DIB-you-lum) Funnel-shaped structure. Plural *infundibula.*

infusion (in-FYU-zhun) Introduction intravenously of a substance other than blood.

ingestion (in-JEST-shun) Intake of food, either by mouth or through a nasogastric tube.

inguinal (IN-gwin-al) Pertaining to the groin.

inhale (IN-hail) Breathe in.

inherent (in-HAIR-ent) Occurring as a natural part of something.

inherited (in-HAIR-it-ed) Acquired through the genetic code.

innate (ih-NATE) Present at birth; arising from the intellect.

inotropic (IN-oh-TROH-pic) Affecting the contractility of cardiac muscle.

insanity (in-SAN-ih-tee) Nonmedical term for a person unable to be responsible for his or her actions.

insecticide (in-SEK-tih-side) Agent for destroying insects.

insemination (in-sem-ih-NAY-shun) Introduction of semen into the vagina.

insertion (in-SIR-shun) The insertion of a muscle is the attachment of a muscle to a more movable part of the skeleton, as distinct from the origin.

insomnia (in-SOM-nee-ah) Inability to sleep.

inspiration (in-spih-RAY-shun) Breathe in.

instability (in-stah-BIL-ih-tee) Abnormal tendency of a joint to partially or fully dislocate.

insufficiency (in-suh-FISH-en-see) Lack of completeness of function; in the heart, failure of a valve to close properly.

insulin (IN-syu-lin) A hormone secreted by the pancreas.

integrate (IN-teh-grate) To bring together into a complete and harmonious whole.

integument (in-TEG-you-ment) Organ system that covers the body, the skin being the main organ within the system.

integumentary (in-TEG-you-MEN-tah-ree) Pertaining to the covering of the body.

intellectual (in-teh-LEK-chu-al) Pertaining to the capacity for thinking and acquiring knowledge.

interatrial (IN-ter-AY-tree-al) Between the atria of the heart.

intercostal (IN-ter-KOS-tal) The space between two ribs.

intermittent (IN-ter-MIT-ent) Alternately ceasing and beginning again.

interosseous (in-ter-OSS-ee-us) A structure between bones, such as the muscles between the metacarpals.

interphalangeal (IN-ter-fay-LAN-jee-al) Pertaining to the joints between two phalanges.

interstitial (in-ter-STISH-al) Pertaining to spaces between cells in a tissue or organ.

interventricular (IN-ter-ven-TRIK-you-lar) Between the ventricles of the heart.

intervertebral (IN-ter-VER-teh-bral) The space between two vertebrae.

intestine (in-TES-tin) The digestive tube from stomach to anus.

intima (IN-tih-ma) Inner layer of a structure, particularly a blood vessel.

intolerance (in-TOL-er-ance) Inability of the small intestine to digest and dispose of a particular dietary constituent.

intracellular (in-trah-SELL-you-lar) Within the cell.

intracranial (in-trah-KRAY-nee-al) Within the cranium (skull).

intradermal (in-trah-DER-mal) Within the dermis.

intramuscular (in-trah-MUSS-kew-lar) Within the muscle.

intraocular (in-trah-OCK-you-lar) Pertaining to the inside of the eye.

intrathecal (**IN**-trah-**THEE**-kal) Within the subarachnoid or subdural space.

intrauterine (**IN**-trah-**YOU**-ter-ine) Inside the uterine cavity.

intravenous (**IN**-trah-**VEE**-nuss) Inside a vein.

intrinsic (in-**TRIN**-sik) Any muscle whose origin and insertion are entirely within the structure under consideration; for example, muscles inside the vocal cords or the eye.

intrinsic factor (in-**TRIN**-sik **FAK**-tor) Substance that makes the absorption of vitamin B_{12} happen.

intubation (**IN**-tyu-**BAY**-shun) Insertion of a tube into the trachea.

intussusception (**IN**-tuss-sus-**SEP**-shun) The slipping of one part of the bowel inside another to cause obstruction.

inversion (in-**VER**-shun) A turning inward.

involuntary (in-**VOL**-un-tah-ree) Not under control of the will.

involute (in-voh-**LUTE**) To return to a former condition; *or* decline associated with advanced age.

involution (in-voh-**LOO**-shun) A decrease in size or vigor.

iodine (**EYE**-oh-dine or **EYE**-oh-deen) Chemical element, the lack of which causes thyroid disease.

iris (**EYE**-ris) Colored portion of the eye with the pupil in its center.

irrigation (ih-rih-**GAY**-shun) Use of water to clean wax out of the external ear canal.

ischemia (is-**KEE**-me-ah) Lack of blood supply to a tissue.

ischium (**ISS**-kee-um) Lower and posterior part of the hip bone. Plural *ischia*.

Ishihara color system (ish-ee-**HAR**-ah) Test for color vision defects.

islet cells (**I**-let **SELLS**) Hormone-secreting cells of the pancreas.

islets of Langerhans (**EYE**-lets of **LAHNG**-er-hahnz) Areas of pancreatic cells that produce insulin and glucagon.

isoflavone (**I**-zo-**FLAY**-vone) Phytochemical that imitates estrogen.

isolate (**I**-so-late) To separate from others.

isotope (**I**-so-tope) Radioactive element used in diagnostic procedures.

isthmus (**IS**-mus) Part connecting two larger parts; for example, the uterus to the uterine tube.

J

Jaeger reading cards (**YA**-ger) Type in different sizes of print for testing near vision.

jaundice (**JAWN**-dis) Yellow staining of tissues with bile pigments, including bilirubin.

jejunum (je-**JEW**-num) Segment of small intestine between the duodenum and the ileum where most of the nutrients are absorbed.

jugular (**JUG**-you-lar) Pertaining to the throat.

juvenile (**JU**-ven-ile) Between the ages of 2 and 17 years.

K

Kaposi sarcoma (ka-**POH**-see sar-**KOH**-mah) A malignancy often seen in AIDS patients.

karyotype (**KAIR**-ee-oh-type) Map of chromosomes of an individual cell.

Kegel exercises (**KEG**-al **EKS**-er-size-ez) Contraction and relaxation of the pelvic floor muscles to improve urethral and rectal sphincter function.

keloid (**KEY**-loyd) Raised, irregular, lumpy, shiny scar due to excess collagen fiber production during healing of a wound.

keratin (**KER**-ah-tin) Protein found in the dead outer layer of skin and in nails and hair.

keratinocyte (ke-**RAT**-in-oh-site) Cell producing a tough, horny protein (keratin) in the process of differentiating into the dead cells of the stratum corneum.

keratomileusis (ker-ah-**TOE**-mill-oo-sis) A surgical procedure that involves cutting and shaping the cornea.

keratotomy (ker-ah-**TOT**-oh-mee) Incision in the cornea.

kernicterus (ker-**NICK**-ter-us) Bilirubin staining of the basal nuclei of the brain.

ketoacidosis (**KEY**-toe-as-ih-**DOE**-sis) Excessive production of ketones, making the blood acid.

ketone (**KEY**-tone) Chemical formed in uncontrolled diabetes or in starvation.

ketosis (key-**TOE**-sis) Excess production of ketones.

ki (**KEY**) Universal energy of life.

kidney (**KID**-nee) Organ of excretion.

kinesiology (ki-**NEE**-see-**OL**-oh-jee) Study of muscles and body parts involved in movement.

kleptomania (klep-toe-**MAY**-nee-ah) Uncontrollable need to steal

Klinefelter syndrome (**KLINE**-fel-ter **SIN**-drome) Genetic anomaly in males with XXY chromosomes.

Koplik spots (**KOP**-lik **SPOTZ**) Small red spots with a white center on the buccal mucosa early in measles.

kyphosis (ki-**FOH**-sis) A normal posterior curve of the thoracic spine that can be exaggerated in disease.

L

labium (**LAY**-bee-um) Fold of the vulva. Plural *labia*.

labor (**LAY**-bore) Process of expulsion of the fetus.

labrum (**LAY**-brum) Cartilage that forms a rim around the socket of the hip joint.

labyrinth (**LAB**-ih-rinth) The inner ear.

labyrinthitis (**LAB**-ih-rin-**THI**-tis) Inflammation of the inner ear.

laceration (lass-eh-**RAY**-shun) A tear of the skin.

lacrimal (**LAK**-rim-al) Pertaining to tears.

lactase (**LAK**-tase) Enzyme that breaks down lactose to glucose and galactose.

lactation (lak-**TAY**-shun) Production of milk.

lacteal (**LAK**-tee-al) A lymphatic vessel carrying chyle away from the intestine.

lactiferous (lak-**TIF**-er-us) Pertaining to or yielding milk.

lactose (**LAK**-toes) The disaccharide found in cow's milk.

lactovegetarian (**LAK**-toe-**VEJ**-eh-**TAR**-ee-an) Person whose diet consists of only plants and dairy products.

lacuna (la-**KOO**-nah) Small space or cavity within the matrix of bone. Plural *lacunae*.

lanugo (la-**NYU**-go) Fine, soft hair on the fetal body.

laparoscope (**LAP**-ah-roh-skope) Instrument (endoscope) used for viewing the abdominal contents.

laparoscopic (**LAP**-ah-rah-**SKOP**-ik) Pertaining to laparoscopy.

laparoscopy (lap-ah-**ROS**-koh-pee) Examination of the contents of the abdomen using an endoscope.

larva (**LAR**-vah) Stage in the development of an insect or intestinal parasite. Plural *larvae*.

laryngitis (lar-in-**JEYE**-tis) Inflammation of the larynx.

laryngopharynx (lah-**RING**-oh-**FAIR**-inks) Region of the pharynx below the epiglottis that includes the larynx.

laryngoscope (lah-**RING**-oh-skope) Hollow tube with a light and camera used to visualize or operate on the larynx.

laryngotracheobronchitis (lah-**RING**-oh-**TRAY**-kee-oh-brong-**KI**-tis) Inflammation of the larynx, trachea, and bronchi. Also called *croup*.

larynx (**LAIR**-inks) Organ of voice production.

laser (**LAY**-zer) Intense, narrow beam of monochromatic light.

laser surgery (**LAY**-zer **SUR**-jer-ee) Use of a concentrated, intense narrow beam of electromagnetic radiation for surgery.

latent (**LAY**-tent) Dormant, not discernible.

lateral (**LAT**-er-al) Situated at the side of a structure.

latex (**LAY**-tecks) Manufactured from the milky liquid in rubber plants; used for gloves in patient care.

latissimus dorsi (lah-**TISS**-ih-muss **DOOR**-sigh) The widest (broadest) muscle in the back.

lavage (lah-**VAHZH**) Washing out of a hollow cavity, tube, or organ.

legume (**LEG**-yoom) Family of plants including peas, beans, and lentils.

leiomyoma (**LIE**-oh-my-**OH**-mah) Benign neoplasm derived from smooth muscle.

lens (**LENZ**) Transparent refractive structure behind the iris.

lentigo (len-**TIE**-go) Age spot; small, flat, brown-black spot in the skin of older people. Plural *lentigines*.

leptin (**LEP**-tin) Hormone secreted by adipose tissue.

lesion (**LEE**-zhun) Pathologic change or injury in a tissue.

leukemia (loo-**KEE**-mee-ah) Disease in which the blood is taken over by white blood cells and their precursors.

leukocoria (loo-koh-**KOH**-ree-ah) Reflection in the pupil of a white mass in the eye.

leukocyte (**LOO**-koh-site) Another term for *white blood cell*. Alternative spelling *leucocyte*.

leukocytosis (**LOO**-koh-sigh-**TOE**-sis) An excessive number of white blood cells.

leukoencephalopathy (**LOO**-koh-en-sef-ah-**LOP**-ah-thee) Disease-producing destruction of white matter of the brain.

leukopenia (loo-koh-**PEE**-nee-ah) A deficient number of white blood cells.

leukoplakia (loo-koh-**PLAY**-kee-ah) White patch on the oral mucous membrane, often precancerous.

libido (li-**BEE**-doh) Sexual desire.

life expectancy (LIFE eck-**SPEK**-tan-see) Statistical determination of the number of years an individual is expected to live.

life span (LIFE SPAN) The age that a person reaches.

ligament (**LIG**-ah-ment) Band of fibrous tissue connecting two structures.

ligate (**LIE**-gate) Tie off a structure, such as a bleeding blood vessel.

ligation (lie-**GAY**-shun) Use of a tie to close a tube.

ligature (**LIG**-ah-chur) Thread or wire tied around a tubal structure to close it.

limbic (**LIM**-bic) Pertaining to the limbic system, an array of nerve fibers surrounding the thalamus.

linear fracture (**LIN**-ee-ar **FRAK**-chur) A fracture running parallel to the length of the bone.

lipase (**LIE**-paze) Enzyme that breaks down fat.

lipectomy (lip-**ECK**-toe-me) Surgical removal of adipose tissue.

lipid (**LIP**-id) General term for all types of fatty compounds; for example, cholesterol, triglycerides, and fatty acids.

lipoprotein (**LIE**-poh-pro-teen) Molecules made of combinations of fat and protein.

lithotripsy (**LITH**-oh-trip-see) Crushing stones by sound waves.

lithotripter (**LITH**-oh-trip-ter) Instrument that generates sound waves.

liver (**LIV**-er) Body's largest internal organ, located in the right upper quadrant of the abdomen.

lobe (**LOBE**) Subdivision of an organ or some other part.

lobectomy (low-**BECK**-toe-me) Surgical removal of a lobe of the lungs.

lochia (**LOW**-kee-uh) Vaginal discharge following childbirth.

locus (**LOW**-kus) A specific site; for example, the position a gene occupies on a chromosome.

longevity (lon-**JEV**-ih-tee) Duration of life beyond the normal expectation.

loop of Henle (LOOP of **HEN**-lee) Part of the renal tubule where reabsorption occurs.

lordosis (lore-**DOH**-sis) An exaggerated forward curvature of the lumbar spine.

louse (LOWSE) Parasitic insect. Plural *lice*.

lubricant (**LOO**-bri-cant) Substance for reducing friction.

lumbar (**LUM**-bar) Pertaining to the region in the back and sides between the ribs and pelvis.

lumen (**LOO**-men) The interior space of a tubelike structure.

lumpectomy (lump-**ECK**-toe-me) Removal of a lesion with preservation of surrounding tissue.

luteal (LOO-tee-al) Pertaining to a corpus luteum.

lutein (LOO-tee-in) Yellow pigment.

luteum (LOO-tee-um) Corpus luteum is the yellow (lutein) body formed after an ovarian follicle ruptures.

lycopene (LIE-koh-peen) Carotenoid that gives tomatoes their red color.

Lyme disease (LIME DIZ-eez) Disease transmitted by the bite of an infected deer tick.

lymph (LIMF) A clear fluid collected from tissues and transported by lymph vessels to the venous circulation.

lymphadenectomy (lim-FAD-eh-NECK-toe-me) Surgical excision of a lymph node.

lymphadenitis (lim-FAD-eh-neye-tis) Inflammation of a lymph node.

lymphadenopathy (lim-FAD-eh-NOP-ah-thee) Any disease process affecting a lymph node.

lymphangiogram (lim-FAN-jee-oh-gram) Radiographic images of lymph vessels and nodes following injection of contrast material.

lymphatic (lim-FAT-ik) Pertaining to lymph or the lymphatic system.

lymphedema (LIMF-e-dee-mah) Tissue swelling due to lymphatic obstruction.

lymphocyte (LIM-foh-site) Small white blood cell with a large nucleus.

lymphoid (LIM-foyd) Resembling lymphatic tissue.

lymphoma (lim-FO-muh) Any neoplasm of lymphatic tissue.

lysis (LIE-sis) Destruction of a cell; gradual decline of a disease (as opposed to a crisis).

lysosome (LIE-soh-sohm) Enzyme that digests foreign material and worn-out cell components.

lysozyme (LIE-soh-zime) Enzyme that dissolves the cell walls of bacteria.

M

macrocyte (MAK-roh-site) Large red blood cell.

macrocytic (mak-roh-SIT-ik) Pertaining to macrocytes.

macrophage (MAK-roh-fayj) Large white blood cell that removes bacteria, foreign particles, and dead cells.

macula (MAK-you-lah) Small area of special function; in the ear, a sensory receptor. Plural *maculae*.

macula lutea (MAK-you-lah LOO-tee-ah) Yellowish spot on the back of the retina; contains the fovea centralis.

macule (MAK-yul) Small, flat spot or patch on the skin.

majus (MAY-jus) Bigger or greater; for example, labia majora. Plural *majora*.

malabsorption (mal-ab-SORP-shun) Inadequate gastrointestinal absorption of nutrients.

malaria (mah-LAIR-ee-ah) Disease transmitted by the bite of a female *Anopheles* mosquito.

malformation (MAL-for-MAY-shun) Failure of proper or normal development.

malfunction (mal-FUNK-shun) Inadequate or abnormal function.

malignancy (mah-LIG-nan-see) Tumor that invades surrounding tissues and metastasizes to distant organs.

malignant (mah-LIG-nant) Capable of invading surrounding tissues and metastasizing to distant organs.

malleus (MAL-ee-us) Outer (lateral) one of the three ossicles in the middle ear; shaped like a hammer.

malnutrition (mal-nyu-TRISH-un) Inadequate nutrition from poor diet or inadequate absorption of nutrients.

malunion (mal-YOU-nee-un) Condition in which the two bony ends of a fracture fail to heal together correctly.

mammary (MAM-ah-ree) Relating to the lactating breast.

mammogram (MAM-oh-gram) The record produced by x-ray imaging of the breast.

mammography (mah-MOG-rah-fee) Process of x-ray examination of the breast.

mandible (MAN-di-bel) Lower jawbone.

mandibular (man-DIB-you-lar) Pertaining to the mandible.

mania (MAY-nee-ah) Mood disorder with hyperactivity, irritability, and rapid speech.

manic-depressive disorder (MAN-ik de-PRESS-iv dis-OR-der) An outdated name for bipolar disorder.

manipulation (mah-NIP-you-lay-shun) Hands-on adjustment of joints, particularly of the spine.

manipulative (mah-NIP-you-lay-tiv) Pertaining to manipulation.

Marfan syndrome (mahr-FAN SIN-drome) Genetic condition with malformation of elastic connective tissue.

marijuana (mar-ih-HWAN-ah) Dried, flowering leaves of the plant *Cannabis sativa*.

marrow (MAH-roe) Fatty, blood-forming tissue in the cavities of long bones.

massage (mah-SAHZH) Application of pressure or vibration to soft body tissues.

masseter (MASS-eh-ter) Muscle that closes the mouth.

mastalgia (mass-TAL-jee-uh) Pain in the breast.

mastectomy (mass-TECK-toe-me) Surgical excision of the breast.

masticate (MAS-tih-kate) To chew.

mastitis (mass-TIE-tis) Inflammation of the breast.

mastoid (MASS-toyd) Small bony protrusion immediately behind the ear.

maternal (mah-TER-nal) Pertaining to or derived from the mother.

matrix (MAY-triks) Substance that surrounds cells, is manufactured by the cells, and holds them together.

maturation (mat-you-RAY-shun) Process of achieving full development.

maxilla (mak-SILL-ah) Upper jawbone, containing right and left maxillary sinuses.

maximus (MAKS-ih-mus) The gluteus maximus muscle is the largest muscle in the body, covering a large part of each buttock.

McBurney point (mack-**BUR**-nee POYNT) One-third the distance from the anterior superior iliac spine to the umbilicus.

measles (**ME**-zelz) Acute, contagious disease of childhood. Also known as *rubeola.*

meatus (me-**AY**-tus) Passage or channel; also used to denote the external opening of a passage.

meconium (meh-**KOH**-nee-um) The first bowel movement of the newborn.

media (**ME**-dee-ah) Middle layer of a structure, particularly a blood vessel.

medial (**ME**-dee-al) Nearer to the middle of the body.

mediastinoscopy (**ME**-dee-ass-tih-**NOS**-koh-pee) Examination of the mediastinum using an endoscope.

mediastinum (**ME**-dee-ass-**TIE**-num) Area between the lungs containing the heart, aorta, venae cavae, esophagus, and trachea.

mediate (**ME**-dee-ate) Effect by means of an intermediary substance or person.

meditation (med-ih-**TAY**-shun) The focusing of attention or freeing the mind of thoughts as part of a formalized spiritual practice.

medius (**ME**-dee-us) The gluteus medius muscle is partly covered by the gluteus maximus; it originates on the ilium and is inserted into the femur.

medulla (meh-**DULL**-ah) Central portion of a structure surrounded by cortex.

medulla oblongata (meh-**DULL**-ah ob-lon-**GAH**-tah) Most posterior subdivision of the brainstem; continuation of the spinal cord.

megakaryocyte (**MEG**-ah-kair-ee-oh-site) Large cell with a large nucleus. Parts of the cytoplasm break off to form platelets.

megavitamin (meg-ah-**VIE**-tah-min) Large dose of a vitamin.

meiosis (my-**OH**-sis) Two rapid cell divisions, resulting in half the number of chromosomes.

melanin (**MEL**-ah-nin) Black pigment found in the skin, hair, and retina.

melanocyte (**MEL**-ann-oh-cyte) Cell that synthesizes (produces) melanin.

melanoma (**MEL**-ah-**NO**-mah) Malignant neoplasm formed from cells that produce melanin.

melatonin (mel-ah-**TONE**-in) Hormone formed by the pineal gland.

melena (mel-**EN**-ah) The passage of black, tarry stools.

membrane (**MEM**-brain) Thin layer of tissue covering a structure or cavity.

menarche (meh-**NAR**-key) First menstrual period.

Mendelian (men-**DEE**-lee-an) Described by Gregor Mendel.

Ménière disease (men-**YEAR DIZ**-eez) Disorder of the inner ear with a cluster of symptoms of acute attacks of tinnitus, vertigo, and hearing loss.

meninges (meh-**NIN**-jeez) Three-layered covering of the brain and spinal cord.

meningioma (meh-**NIN**-jee-**OH**-mah) Tumor arising from the arachnoid layer of the meninges.

meningitis (men-in-**JIE**-tis) Acute infectious disease of children and young adults.

meningocele (meh-**NING**-oh-seal) Protrusion of the meninges from the spinal cord or brain through a defect in the vertebral column or cranium.

meningococcal (meh-nin-goh-**KOK**-al) Pertaining to the *meningococcus* bacterium.

meningomyelocele (meh-**NIN**-goh-**MY**-el-oh-seal) Protrusion of the spinal cord and meninges through a defect in the vertebral arch of one or more vertebrae.

meniscectomy (men-ih-**SEK**-toh-me) Excision (cutting out) of all or part of a meniscus.

meniscus (meh-**NISS**-kuss) Disc of connective tissue cartilage between the bones of a joint; for example, in the knee joint. Plural *menisci.*

menopausal (**MEN**-oh-paws-al) Pertaining to menopause.

menopause (**MEN**-oh-paws) Permanent ending of menstrual periods.

menorrhagia (men-oh-**RAY**-jee-ah) Excessive menstrual bleeding.

menses (**MEN**-seez) Monthly uterine bleeding.

menstruate (**MEN**-stru-ate) The act of menstruation.

menstruation (men-stru-**AY**-shun) Synonym of *menses.*

meridian (meh-**RID**-ee-an) Energy line connecting different anatomical sites.

merocrine (**MARE**-oh-krin) Another name for *eccrine.*

mesentery (**MESS**-en-ter-ree) A double layer of peritoneum enclosing the abdominal viscera.

mesothelioma (**MEEZ**-oh-thee-lee-**OH**-mah) Cancer arising from the cells lining the pleura or peritoneum.

metabolic acidosis (met-ah-**BOL**-ik ass-ih-**DOE**-sis) Decreased pH in the blood and body tissues as a result of an upset in metabolism.

metabolism (meh-**TAB**-oh-lizm) The constantly changing physical and chemical processes occurring in the cell.

metacarpal (**MET**-ah-**KAR**-pal) The five bones between the carpus and the fingers.

metacarpophalangeal (**MET**-ah-**KAR**-poh-fay-**LAN**-jee-al) Pertaining to the joints between the metacarpal bones and the phalanges.

metaphysis (meh-**TAF**-ih-sis) Region between the diaphysis and the epiphysis where bone growth occurs.

metastasis (meh-**TAS**-tah-sis) Spread of a disease from one part of the body to another. Plural *metastases.*

metastasize (meh-**TAS**-tah-size) To spread to distant parts.

metastatic (meh-tah-**STAT**-ik) Pertaining to the character of cells that can metastasize.

metatarsus (**MET**-ah-**TAR**-sus) A collective term referring to the five parallel bones of the foot between the tarsus and the phalanges.

metrorrhagia (**MEH**-troh-**RAY**-jee-ah) Irregular uterine bleeding between menses.

microalbuminuria (**MY**-kroh-al-byu-min-**YOU**-ree-ah) Presence of very small quantities of albumin in urine that cannot be detected by conventional urine testing.

microaneurysm (my-kroh-**AN**-yu-rizm) Focal dilation of retinal capillaries.

microangiopathy (**MY**-kroh-an-jee-**OP**-ah-thee) Disease of the very small blood vessels (capillaries).

microarray (**MY**-kroh-ah-**RAY**) Technique for studying one gene in one experiment. Also called *gene chips.*

microbe (**MY**-krohb) Short for *microorganism.*

microcephaly (**MY**-kroh-**SEF**-ah-lee) An abnormally small head.

microcytic (my-kroh-**SIT**-ik) Pertaining to a small cell.

microglia (my-**KROH**-glee-ah) Small nervous tissue cells that are phagocytes.

microorganism (**MY**-kroh-**OR**-gan-izm) Any organism too small to be seen by the naked eye.

microscope (**MY**-kroh-skope) Instrument for viewing something small that cannot be seen in detail by the naked eye.

microscopic (**MY**-kroh-**SKOP**-ik) Visible only with the aid of a microscope.

micturate (**MIK**-choo-rate) Pass urine.

micturition (mik-choo-**RISH**-un) Act of passing urine.

migraine (**MY**-grain) Paroxysmal severe headache confined to one side of the head.

mineral (**MIN**-er-al) Inorganic compound usually found in earth's crust.

mineralocorticoid (**MIN**-er-al-oh-**KOR**-tih-koyd) Hormone of the adrenal cortex that influences sodium and potassium metabolism.

minimus (**MIN**-ih-mus) The gluteus minimus is the smallest of the gluteal muscles and lies under the gluteus medius.

minus (**MY**-nus) Smaller or lesser; for example, labia minora. Plural *minora.*

mitochondrion (my-toe-**KON**-dree-on) Organelle that generates, stores, and releases energy for cell activities. Plural *mitochondria.*

mitosis (my-**TOE**-sis) Cell division to create two identical cells, each with 46 chromosomes.

mitral (**MY**-tral) Shaped like the headdress of a Catholic bishop.

modality (moh-**DAL**-ih-tee) A form of therapeutic agent or regimen.

modify (**MOD**-ih-fie) Change the form or qualities of something.

molar (**MO**-lar) One of six teeth in each jaw that grind food.

molasses (mo-**LASS**-iz) Dark-colored syrup produced during the refining of sugar.

mold (MOLD) Filamentous fungus.

mole (MOLE) Benign localized area of melanin-producing cells.

molecule (**MOLL**-eh-kyul) Very small particle consisting of two or more atoms held tightly together.

molluscum (moh-**LUS**-kum) Soft, round tumor of the skin caused by a virus.

molluscum contagiosum (moh-**LUS**-kum kon-**TAY**-jee-oh-sum) An STD caused by a virus.

monoclonal (**MON**-oh-**KLO**-nal) Derived from a protein from a single clone of cells, all molecules of which are the same.

monocyte (**MON**-oh-site) Large white blood cell with a single nucleus.

monoglyceride (mon-oh-**GLISS**-eh-ride) A fatty substance with a single fatty acid.

mononeuropathy (**MON**-oh-nyu-**ROP**-ah-thee) Disorder affecting a single nerve.

mononucleosis (**MON**-oh-nyu-klee-**OH**-sis) Presence of large numbers of mononuclear leukocytes.

monoplegia (**MON**-oh-**PLEE**-jee-ah) Paralysis of one limb.

monosaccharide (**MON**-oh-**SACK**-ah-ride) Simplest form of sugar; for example, glucose.

Monospot test (**MON**-oh-spot TEST) Detects heterophile antibodies in infectious mononucleosis.

monozygotic (**MON**-oh-zye-**GOT**-ik) Twins from a single zygote.

mons pubis (MONZ **PYU**-bis) Fleshy pad with pubic hair, overlying the pubic bone.

Moro reflex (**MOR**-oh RE-fleks) Neonatal brainstem reflex. Also called *startle reflex.*

morphine (**MOR**-feen) Derivative of opium used as an analgesic or sedative.

mortality (mor-**TAL**-ih-tee) Fatal outcome or death rate.

morula (**MOR**-you-lah) Ball of cells formed from divisions of a zygote.

mosquito (mos-**KEY**-toe) Blood-sucking insect. Plural *mosquitoes.*

motile (**MOH**-til) Capable of spontaneous movement.

motility (moh-**TILL**-ih-tee) The ability for spontaneous movement.

motivation (moh-tih-**VAY**-shun) Force that enables a person to meet a need or achieve a goal.

motor (**MOH**-tor) Pertaining to nerves that send impulses out to cause muscles to contract or glands to secrete.

mouth (MOWTH) External opening of a cavity or canal.

mucin (**MYU**-sin) Protein element of mucus.

mucociliary (**MYU**-koh-**SIL**-ih-ah-ree) Pertaining to the ciliated epithelium lining the bronchial tree.

mucolytic (**MYU**-koh-**LIT**-ik) Agent capable of dissolving or liquefying mucus.

mucopurulent (myu-koh-**PYUR**-you-lent) Mixture of pus and mucus.

mucosa (myu-**KOH**-sah) Lining of a tubular structure. Another name for *mucous membrane.*

mucous (**MYU**-kus) Relating to mucus or the mucosa.

mucus (**MYU**-kus) Sticky secretion of cells in mucous membranes.

multidisciplinary (mul-tee-**DIS**-ih-plih-**NAR**-ee) Involving health care providers from more than one profession

multifocal (mul-tee-**FOH**-kal) Arising from many centers.

multimodal (mul-tee-**MOH**-dal) Using many methods.

multipara (mul-**TIP**-ah-ruh) Woman who has given birth to two or more children.

murmur (**MUR**-mur) Abnormal sound heard on auscultation of the heart or blood vessels.

Murphy sign (**MUR**-fee SINE) Tenderness in the right subcostal area on inspiration, associated with acute cholecystitis.

muscle (**MUSS**-el) Tissue consisting of contractile cells.

muscularis (muss-kyu-**LAR**-is) The muscular layer of a hollow organ or tube.

musculoskeletal (**MUSS**-kyu-loh-**SKEL**-eh-tal) Pertaining to the muscles and the bony skeleton.

mutagen (**MYU**-tah-jen) Agent that produces a mutation in a gene.

mutation (myu-**TAY**-shun) Change in the chemistry of a gene.

mute (**MYUT**) Unable or unwilling to speak.

mutism (**MYU**-tizm) Absence of speech.

myasthenia gravis (my-as-**THEE**-nee-ah **GRA**-vis) Disorder of fluctuating muscle weakness.

mycelium (my-**SEE**-lee-um) Mass of hyphae forming a colony of fungi.

mycologist (my-**KOL**-oh-jist) Specialist in mycology.

mycology (my-**KOL**-oh-jee) Study of fungi.

myelin (**MY**-eh-lin) Material of the sheath around the axon of a nerve.

myelitis (**MY**-eh-**LIE**-tis) Inflammation of the spinal cord.

myelocele (**MY**-eh-low-seal) Protrusion of the spinal cord through a defect in the vertebral arch.

myelography (my-eh-**LOG**-rah-fee) Radiography of the spinal cord and nerve roots after injection of a contrast medium into the subarachnoid space.

myeloid (**MY**-eh-loyd) Resembling cells derived from bone marrow.

myelomeningocele (**MY**-eh-low-meh-**NING**-oh-seal) Protrusion of the spinal cord and meninges through a defect in the vertebral arch of one or more vertebrae.

myocarditis (**MY**-oh-kar-**DIE**-tis) Inflammation of the heart muscle.

myocardium (**MY**-oh-**KAR**-dee-um) All the heart muscle.

myofascial (**MY**-oh-**FASH**-ee-al) Relating to the fascia surrounding and separating muscle tissue.

myoglobin (**MY**-oh-**GLOW**-bin) Protein of muscle that stores and transports oxygen.

myoma (my-**OH**-mah) Benign tumor of muscle.

myomectomy (my-oh-**MEK**-toe-me) Surgical removal of a myoma (fibroid).

myometrium (my-oh-**ME**-tree-um) Muscle wall of the uterus.

myopia (my-**OH**-pee-ah) Able to see close objects but unable to see distant objects.

myotherapy (**MY**-oh-**THAIR**-ah-pee) Treatment of muscles by massage.

myringotomy (mir-in-**GOT**-oh-me) Incision in the tympanic membrane.

myxedema (miks-eh-**DEE**-muh) Severe hypothyroidism.

N

narcissism (**NAR**-sih-sizm) Self-love; person interprets everything purely in relation to himself or herself.

narcissistic (**NAR**-sih-**SIS**-tik) Relating everything to oneself.

narcolepsy (**NAR**-coh-lep-see) Condition with frequent incidents of sudden, involuntary deep sleep.

narcotic (nar-**KOT**-ik) Drug derived from opium or a synthetic drug with similar effects.

naris (**NAH**-ris) Nostril. Plural *nares*.

nasal (**NAY**-zal) Pertaining to the nose.

nasogastric (**NAY**-zoh-**GAS**-trik) Pertaining to the nose and stomach.

nasolacrimal duct (**NAY**-zoh-**LAK**-rim-al DUKT) Passage from the lacrimal sac to the nose.

nasopharynx (**NAY**-zoh-**FAIR**-inks) Region of the pharynx at the back of the nose and above the soft palate.

natriuretic peptide (**NAH**-tree-you-**RET**-ik **PEP**-tide) Protein that increases the excretion of sodium.

naturopath (**NAH**-chur-oh-path) Practitioner of naturopathy.

naturopathic medicine (**NAH**-chur-oh-**PATH**-ik **MED**-ih-sin) A system of healing based on the healing power of nature.

naturopathy (nah-chur-**OP**-ah-thee) Holistic system of medicine with a natural approach to healing.

nebulizer (**NEB**-you-liz-er) Device used to deliver liquid medicine in a fine mist.

necrosis (neh-**KROH**-sis) Pathologic death of cells or tissue.

necrotic (neh-**KROT**-ik) Affected by necrosis.

necrotizing fasciitis (neh-kroh-**TIZE**-ing fash-eh-**EYE**-tis) Inflammation of fascia, producing death of the tissue.

Neisseria gonorrhoeae (ni-**SEE**-ree-ah gon-oh-**REE**-ee) Bacterium that causes gonorrhea.

neonatal (**NEE**-oh-**NAY**-tal) Pertaining to the newborn infant or the newborn period.

neonate (**NEE**-oh-nate) A newborn infant.

neoplasia (**NEE**-oh-**PLAY**-zee-ah) Process that results in formation of a tumor.

neoplasm (**NEE**-oh-plazm) A new growth, either a benign or malignant tumor.

neoplastic (**NEE**-oh-**PLAS**-tic) Pertaining to a neoplasm.

nephrectomy (neh-**FREK**-toe-me) Surgical removal of a kidney.

nephritis (neh-**FRY**-tis) Inflammation of the kidney.

nephrolithiasis (**NEF**-roe-lih-**THIGH**-ah-sis) Presence of a kidney stone.

nephrolithotomy (**NEF**-roe-lih-**THOT**-oh-me) Incision for removal of a stone.

nephrologist (neh-**FROL**-oh-jist) Medical specialist in disorders of the kidney.

nephrology (neh-**FROL**-oh-jee) Medical specialty of diseases of the kidney.

nephron (**NEF**-ron) Filtration unit of the kidney; glomerulus + renal tubule.

nephropathy (neh-**FROP**-ah-thee) Any disease of the kidney.

nephroscope (**NEF**-roe-skope) Endoscope used to view the inside of the kidney.

nephroscopy (neh-**FROS**-koh-pee) Examination of the kidney.

nephrotic syndrome (neh-**FROT**-ik **SIN**-drome) Glomerular disease with marked loss of protein. Also known as *nephrosis.*

nerve (NERV) A cord of fibers in connective tissue conduct impulses.

nerve conduction study (NERV kon-**DUK**-shun **STUD**-ee) Procedure for measuring the speed at which an electrical impulse travels along a nerve.

neural (**NYU**-ral) Pertaining to nervous tissue.

neural tube (**NYU**-ral TYUB) Embryologic tubelike structure that forms the brain and spinal cord.

neuralgia (nyu-**RAL**-jee-ah) Pain in the distribution of a nerve.

neurilemma (nyu-ri-**LEM**-ah) Covering of a nerve around the myelin sheath.

neuroglia (nyu-roh-**GLEE**-ah) Connective tissue holding nervous tissue together.

neurohypophysis (**NYUR**-oh-high-**POF**-ih-sis) Posterior lobe of the pituitary gland.

neurologist (nyu-**ROL**-oh-jist) Medical specialist in disorders of the nervous system.

neurology (nyu-**ROL**-oh-jee) Medical specialty of disorders of the nervous system.

neuromuscular (**NYUR**-oh-**MUSS**-kyu-lar) Pertaining to both nerves and muscles.

neuron (**NYUR**-on) Technical term for a nerve cell; consists of the cell body with its dendrites and axons.

neuropathy (nyu-**ROP**-ah-thee) Any disease of the nervous system.

neurosurgeon (**NYU**-roh-**SUR**-jun) Specialist in operating on the nervous system.

neurosurgery (**NYU**-roh-**SUR**-jer-ee) Medical specialty in surgery of the nervous system.

neurotoxin (**NYUR**-oh-tock-sin) Agent that poisons the nervous system.

neurotransmitter (**NYUR**-oh-trans-**MIT**-er) Chemical agent that relays messages from one nerve cell to the next.

neutropenia (**NEW**-troh-**PEE**-nee-uh) A deficiency of neutrophils.

neutrophil (**NEW**-troh-fill) A neutrophil's granules take up (purple) stain equally, whether the stain is acid or alkaline.

neutrophilia (**NEW**-troh-**FILL**-ee-ah) An increase in neutrophils.

nevus (**NEE**-vus) Congenital or acquired lesion of the skin. Plural *nevi.*

niacin (**NI**-ah-sin) Vitamin B$_3$.

nipple (**NIP**-el) Projection from the breast into which the lactiferous ducts open.

nitrite (**NI**-trite) Chemical formed in urine by *E. coli* and other microorganisms.

nitrogenous (ni-**TROJ**-en-us) Containing or generating nitrogen.

nocturia (nok-**TYU**-ree-ah) Excessive urination at night.

node (NOHD) A circumscribed mass of tissue.

nodule (**NOD**-yule) Small node or knotlike swelling.

nonessential (**NON**-ee-**SEN**-shal) Can be synthesized by the body.

nonunion (non-**YOU**-nee-un) Total failure of healing of a fracture.

norepinephrine (**NOR**-ep-ih-**NEFF**-rin) Parasympathetic neurotransmitter that is a catecholamine hormone of the adrenal gland. Also called *noradrenaline.*

nosocomial (noh-soh-**KOH**-mee-al) Acquired while in the hospital.

nuchal cord (**NYU**-kul KORD) Loop of umbilical cord around the fetal neck.

nucleolus (nyu-**KLEE**-oh-lus) Small mass within the nucleus.

nucleus (**NYU**-klee-us) Functional center of a cell or structure.

null cells (NULL SELLS) Lymphocytes with no surface markers, unlike T cells or B cells.

nutrient (**NYU**-tree-ent) A substance in food required for normal physiologic function.

nutrition (nyu-**TRISH**-un) The study of food and liquid requirements for normal function of the human body.

nutritionist (nyu-**TRISH**-un-ist) Certified professional in nutrition science.

nutritive (**NYU**-trih-tiv) Providing nourishment.

O

obesity (oh-**BEE**-sih-tee) Excessive amount of fat in the body.

oblique fracture (ob-**LEEK** **FRAK**-chur) A diagonal fracture across the long axis of the bone.

obsession (ob-**SESH**-un) Persistent, recurrent, uncontrollable thoughts or impulses.

obsessive (ob-**SES**-iv) Possessing persistent, recurrent, uncontrollable thoughts or impulses.

obstetrician (ob-steh-**TRISH**-un) Medical specialist in obstetrics.

obstetrics (OB) (ob-**STET**-ricks) Medical specialty for the care of women during pregnancy and the postpartum period.

occipital (ock-**SIP**-it-al) The back of the skull.

occipital lobe (ock-**SIP**-it-al LOBE) Posterior area of the cerebral hemispheres.

occlude (o-**KLUDE**) To close, plug, or completely obstruct.

occlusion (o-**KLU**-zhun) A complete obstruction.

occult (oh-**KULT**) Not visible on the surface.

occupational therapy (**OCK**-you-**PAY**-shun-al **THAIR**-ah-pee) Use of work and recreational activities to increase independent function.

ocular (**OCK**-you-lar) Pertaining to the eye.

oculomotor (**OCK**-you-loh-**MOH**-tor) Third (III) cranial nerve; moves the eye.

olfaction (ol-**FAK**-shun) Sense of smell.

olfactory (ol-**FAK**-toh-ree) First (I) cranial nerve; carries information related to the sense of smell.

oligodendrocyte (**OL**-ih-goh-**DEN**-droh-site) Connective tissue cell of the central nervous system that forms a myelin sheath.

oligodendroglioma (**OL**-ih-goh-**DEN**-droh-gly-**OH**-mah) A slow-growing tumor in the cerebral hemisphere of an adult.

oligohydramnios (**OL**-ih-goh-high-**DRAM**-nee-os) Too little amniotic fluid.

oliguria (ol-ih-**GYUR**-ee-ah) Scanty production of urine.

omentum (oh-**MEN**-tum) Membrane that encloses the bowels.

oncogene (**ONG**-koh-jeen) One of a family of genes involved in cell growth that work in concert to cause cancer.

oncogenic (**ONG**-koh-**JEN**-ik) Capable of producing a neoplasm.

oncologist (on-**KOL**-oh-jist) Medical specialist in oncology.

oncology (on-**KOL**-oh-jee) The science dealing with cancer.

onychomycosis (oh-ni-koh-my-**KOH**-sis) Condition of a fungus infection in a nail.

oocyte (**OH**-oh-site) Female egg cell.

oogenesis (oh-oh-**JEN**-eh-sis) Development of a female egg cell.

open fracture (**OH**-pen **FRAK**-chur) The skin over the fracture is broken.

ophthalmia neonatorum (off-**THAL**-me-ah ne-oh-nay-**TOR**-um) Conjunctivitis of the newborn.

ophthalmologist (off-thal-**MALL**-oh-jist) Medical specialist in ophthalmology.

ophthalmology (off-thal-**MALL**-oh-jee) Medical specialty that diagnoses and treats diseases of the eye.

ophthalmoscope (off-**THAL**-moh-skope) Instrument for viewing the retina.

ophthalmoscopic (**OFF**-thal-**MOS**-koh-pik) Pertaining to the use of an ophthalmoscope.

ophthalmoscopy (**OFF**-thal-**MOS**-koh-pee) The process of viewing the retina.

opiate (**OH**-pee-ate) A drug derived from opium.

opportunistic (**OP**-or-tyu-**NIS**-tik) An organism or a disease in a host with lowered resistance.

opportunistic infection (**OP**-or-tyu-**NIS**-tik in-**FEK**-shun) An infection that causes disease when the immune system is compromised for other reasons.

opposition (op-oh-**SIH**-shun) The movement of the thumb across the palm of the hand to touch the tips of the other fingers.

optic (**OP**-tick) Pertaining to the eye; *or* second (II) cranial nerve, which carries visual information.

optometrist (op-**TOM**-eh-trist) Someone who is skilled in the measurement of vision but cannot treat eye diseases or prescribe medication.

oral (**OR**-al) Pertaining to the mouth.

orbit (**OR**-bit) The bony socket that holds the eyeball.

orchiectomy (or-key-**ECK**-toe-me) Removal of one or both testes.

orchiopexy (**OR**-kee-oh-**PEK**-see) Surgical fixation of a testis in the scrotum.

orchitis (or-**KIE**-tis) Inflammation of the testis. Also called *epididymoorchitis*.

organ (**OR**-gan) Structure with specific functions in a body system.

organelle (**OR**-gah-nell) Part of a cell having a specialized function(s).

organic (or-**GAN**-ik) Compound with carbon atoms; *or* food produced without using chemicals.

organism (**OR**-gan-izm) Any whole, living individual whether animal or plant.

organophosphate (**OR**-ga-no-**FOS**-fate) Organic phosphorus compound used as an insecticide.

orifice (**OR**-ih-fis) Any opening or aperture.

origin (**OR**-ih-gin) Fixed source of a muscle at its attachment to bone.

oropharynx (**OR**-oh-**FAIR**-inks) Region at the back of the mouth between the soft palate and the tip of the epiglottis.

orthopedic (or-tho-**PEE**-dik) Pertaining to the correction and cure of deformities and diseases of the musculoskeletal system; originally, most of the deformities treated were in children. Also spelled *orthopaedic*.

orthopedist (or-tho-**PEE**-dist) Specialist in orthopedics.

orthopnea (or-**THOP**-nee-ah) Difficulty in breathing when lying flat.

orthopneic (or-**THOP**-nee-ik) Pertaining to or affected by orthopnea.

orthotic (or-**THOT**-ik) Orthopedic appliance used to correct an abnormality.

orthotist (or-**THOT**-ist) Maker and fitter of orthopedic appliances.

os (OS) Opening into a canal; for example, the cervix.

osmosis (oz-**MO**-sis) The passage of water across a cell membrane.

ossicle (**OS**-ih-kel) A small bone, particularly relating to the three bones in the middle ear.

osteoarthritis (**OS**-tee-oh-ar-**THRI**-tis) Chronic inflammatory disease of the joints with pain and loss of function.

osteoblast (**OS**-tee-oh-blast) Bone-forming cell.

osteoclast (**OS**-tee-oh-klast) Bone-removing cell.

osteocyte (**OS**-tee-oh-site) Bone-maintaining cell.

osteogenesis (**OS**-tee-oh-**JEN**-eh-sis) Creation of new bone.

osteogenesis imperfecta (**OS**-tee-oh-**JEN**-eh-sis im-per-**FEK**-tah) Inherited condition in which bone formation is incomplete, leading to fragile, easily broken bones.

osteogenic sarcoma (**OS**-tee-oh-**JEN**-ik sar-**KOH**-mah) Malignant tumor originating in bone-producing cells.

osteomalacia (**OS**-tee-oh-mah-**LAY**-she-ah) Soft, flexible bones lacking in calcium (rickets).

osteomyelitis (**OS**-tee-oh-my-eh-**LIE**-tis) Inflammation of bone tissue.

osteopath (**OS**-tee-oh-path) Practitioner of osteopathy.

osteopathy (**OS**-tee-**OP**-ah-thee) Medical practice based on maintaining the structural integrity of the musculoskeletal system.

osteopenia (OS-tee-oh-**PEE**-nee-ah) Decreased calcification of bone.

osteoporosis (OS-tee-oh-poh-**ROE**-sis) Condition in which the bones become more porous, brittle, and fragile and are more likely to fracture.

osteosarcoma (OS-tee-oh-sar-**KOH**-mah) Cancer arising in bone-forming cells.

ostomy (OS-toe-me) Surgery to create an artificial opening into a tubular structure.

otitis media (oh-**TIE**-tis **ME**-dee-ah) Inflammation of the middle ear.

otolith (OH-toe-lith) A calcium particle in the vestibule of the inner ear.

otologist (oh-**TOL**-oh-jist) Medical specialist in diseases of the ear.

otology (oh-**TOL**-oh-jee) Study of the function and diseases of the ear.

otomycosis (OH-toe-my-**KOH**-sis) Fungal infection of the external ear.

otorhinolaryngologist (oh-toe-rhino-lah-rin-**GOL**-oh-jist) Ear, nose, and throat medical specialist.

otosclerosis (oh-toe-sklair-**OH**-sis) Hardening at the junction of the stapes and oval window that causes loss of hearing.

otoscope (OH-toe-skope) Instrument for examining the ear.

otoscopic (oh-toe-**SKOP**-ik) Pertaining to examination with an otoscope.

otoscopy (oh-**TOS**-koh-pee) Examination of the ear.

ovarian (oh-**VAIR**-ee-an) Pertaining to the ovary.

ovary (OH-va-ree) One of the paired female egg-producing glands.

ovulation (OV-you-**LAY**-shun) Release of an oocyte from a follicle.

ovum (OH-vum) Egg. Also called *oocyte*. Plural *ova*.

oxygen (OCK-see-jen) The gas essential for life.

oxyhemoglobin (OCK-see-he-moh-**GLOW**-bin) Hemoglobin in combination with oxygen.

oxytocin (OCK-see-toe-sin) Pituitary hormone that stimulates the uterus to contract.

P

pacemaker (PACE-may-ker) Device that regulates cardiac electrical activity.

pain threshold (PANE **THRESH**-old) The point at which pain is first noticed.

palate (PAL-uht) Roof of the mouth.

palatine (PAL-ah-tine) Bone that forms the hard palate and parts of the nose and orbits.

palliative care (PAL-ee-ah-tiv KAIR) Care that relieves symptoms and pain without curing.

pallor (PAL-or) Paleness of the skin.

palm (PAHLM) The flat anterior surface of the hand.

palpate (PAL-pate) To examine with the fingers and hands.

palpation (pal-**PAY**-shun) An examination with the fingers and hands.

palpitation (pal-pih-**TAY**-shun) Forcible, rapid beat of the heart felt by the patient.

palsy (PAWL-zee) Paralysis or paresis from brain damage.

pancreas (PAN-kree-as) Lobulated gland, the head of which is tucked into the curve of the duodenum.

pancreatic (pan-kree-**AT**-ik) Pertaining to the pancreas.

pancreatitis (PAN-kree-ah-**TIE**-tis) Inflammation of the pancreas.

pancytopenia (PAN-site-oh-**PEE**-nee-ah) Deficiency of all types of blood cells.

pandemic (pan-**DEM**-ik) Disease attacking the population of a very large area.

panendoscopy (pan-en-**DOS**-koh-pee) Examination of the inside of the esophagus, stomach, and upper duodenum using a flexible fiber-optic endoscope.

panhypopituitarism (pan-**HIGH**-poh-pih-**TYU**-ih-tah-rizm) Deficiency of all the pituitary hormones.

pantothenic acid (PAN-toh-**THEN**-ik **ASS**-id) Coenzyme essential for cell function; vitamin B_5.

Pap test (PAP TEST) Examination of cells taken from the cervix.

papilla (pah-**PILL**-ah) Any small projection. Plural *papillae*.

papilledema (pah-pill-eh-**DEE**-mah) Swelling of the optic disc in the retina.

papilloma (pap-ih-**LOH**-mah) Benign projection of epithelial cells.

papule (PAP-yul) Small, circumscribed elevation on the skin.

para (PAH-rah) Abbreviation for number of deliveries.

paralysis (pah-**RAL**-ih-sis) Loss of voluntary movement.

paralytic (par-ah-**LYT**-ik) Pertaining to or suffering from paralysis.

paralyze (PAR-ah-lyze) To make incapable of movement.

parameter (pah-**RAM**-eh-ter) Evaluation or way of measuring.

paranasal (PAR-ah **NAY**-zal) Adjacent to the nose.

paranoia (par-ah-**NOY**-ah) Mental disorder with persecutory delusions.

paranoid (PAR-ah-noyd) Having delusions of persecution.

paraphimosis (PAR-ah-fi-**MOH**-sis) Condition in which a retracted prepuce cannot be pulled forward to cover the glans.

paraplegia (par-ah-**PLEE**-jee-ah) Paralysis of both lower extremities.

parasite (PAR-ah-site) An organism that attaches itself to, lives on or in, and derives its nutrition from another species.

parasitic (par-ah-**SIT**-ik) Pertaining to a parasite.

parasympathetic (par-ah-sim-pah-**THET**-ik) Pertaining to division of the autonomic nervous system; has opposite effects of the sympathetic division.

parathyroid (par-ah-**THIGH**-royd) Endocrine glands embedded in the back of the thyroid gland.

paraurethral (PAR-ah-you-REE-thral) Situated around the urethra.

parenchyma (pah-RENG-kih-mah) Characteristic functional cells of a gland or organ that are supported by the connective tissue framework.

parenteral (pah-REN-ter-al) Giving medication by any means other than the gastrointestinal tract.

paresis (par-EE-sis) Partial paralysis.

paresthesia (par-es-THEE-ze-ah) An abnormal sensation; for example, tingling, burning, pricking. Plural *paresthesias*.

parietal (pah-RYE-eh-tal) Pertaining to the outer layer of the pericardium and other body cavities; *or* the two bones forming the sidewalls and roof of the cranium.

parietal lobe (pah-RYE-eh-tal LOBE) Area of the brain under the parietal bone.

parity (PAIR-ih-tee) Number of deliveries.

Parkinson disease (PAR-kin-son DIZ-eez) Disease of muscular rigidity, tremors, and a masklike facial expression.

paronychia (par-oh-NICK-ee-ah) Infection alongside the nail.

parotid (pah-ROT-id) Parotid gland is the salivary gland beside the ear.

paroxysmal (par-ock-SIZ-mal) Occurring in sharp, spasmodic episodes.

particle (PAR-tih-kul) A small piece of matter.

particulate (par-TIK-you-late) Relating to a fine particle.

pasteurization (PAS-tyur-ih-ZAY-shun) The heating of fluids to moderate temperatures to destroy microorganisms.

patella (pah-TELL-ah) Thin, circular bone in front of the knee joint and embedded in the patellar tendon. Also called the *kneecap*.

patent (PAY-tent) Open.

patent ductus arteriosus (PAY-tent DUK-tus ar-TER-ee-oh-sus) An open, direct channel between the aorta and the pulmonary artery.

pathogen (PATH-oh-jen) A disease-causing microorganism.

pathologic fracture (path-oh-LOJ-ik FRAK-chur) Fracture occurring at a site already weakened by a disease process, such as cancer.

pathologic gambling (path-oh-LOJ-ik GAM-bling) Morbid, constant, uncontrollable, destructive gambling.

pathologist (pa-THOL-oh-jist) A specialist in pathology. (study of disease or characteristics of a particular disease).

pathology (pa-THOL-oh-jee) Medical specialty dealing with the structural and functional changes of a disease process; *or* the cause, development, and structural changes in disease.

pectin (PEK-tin) Plant fiber with the ability to thicken and solidify to a gel.

pectoral (PEK-tor-al) Pertaining to the chest.

pectoral girdle (PEK-tor-al GIR-del) Incomplete bony ring that attaches the upper limb to the axial skeleton.

pedal (PEED-al) Pertaining to the foot.

pediatrician (PEE-dee-ah-TRISH-an) Medical specialist in pediatrics.

pediatrics (pee-dee-AT-riks) Medical specialty of treating children during development from birth through adolescence.

pediculosis (peh-dick-you-LOH-sis) An infestation with lice.

peer (PEER) A person at the same level or standing.

pellagra (peh-LAG-rah) Disease due to dietary deficiency of niacin.

pelvic (PEL-vic) Pertaining to the pubic bone.

pelvis (PEL-vis) A cup-shaped cavity, as in the pelvis of the kidney; *or* a cup-shaped ring of bone.

penile (PEE-nile) Pertaining to the penis.

penis (PEE-nis) Conveys urine and semen to the outside.

pepsin (PEP-sin) Enzyme produced by the stomach that breaks down protein.

pepsinogen (pep-SIN-oh-jen) Converted by HCl in stomach to pepsin.

peptic (PEP-tik) Relating to the stomach and duodenum.

percentile (per-SEN-tile) One of a hundred groups in a distribution of variables.

perforated (PER-foh-ray-ted) Punctured with one or more holes.

perforation (per-foh-RAY-shun) Erosion that progresses to become a hole through the wall of a structure.

perfuse (per-FYUSE) To force blood to flow through a lumen or a vascular bed.

perfusion (per-FYU-shun) The act of perfusing.

pericarditis (PER-ih-kar-DIE-tis) Inflammation of the pericardium, the covering of the heart.

pericardium (per-ih-KAR-dee-um) Structure around the heart.

perimeter (peh-RIM-eh-ter) An edge or border.

perimetrium (per-ih-ME-tree-um) The covering of the uterus; part of the peritoneum.

perinatal (per-ih-NAY-tal) Around the time of birth.

perineal (PER-ih-NEE-al) Pertaining to the perineum.

perineum (PER-ih-NEE-um) Area between the thighs, extending from the coccyx to the pubis.

periodontal (PER-ee-oh-DON-tal) Around a tooth.

periodontics (PER-ee-oh-DON-tiks) Branch of dentistry specializing in disorders of tissues around the teeth.

periodontist (PER-ee-oh-DON-tist) Specialist in periodontics.

periodontitis (PER-ee-oh-don-TIE-tis) Inflammation of tissues around a tooth.

periorbital (per-ee-OR-bit-al) Pertaining to tissues around the orbit.

periosteum (PER-ee-OSS-tee-um) Fibrous membrane covering a bone.

peripheral (peh-RIF-er-al) Pertaining to the periphery or external boundary.

peripheral vision (peh-RIF-er-al VIZH-un) Ability to see objects as they come into the outer edges of the visual field.

periphery (peh-RIF-eh-ree) Outer part of a structure away from the center.

peristalsis (per-ih-**STAL**-sis) Waves of alternate contraction and relaxation of the intestinal wall to move food along the digestive tract.

peritoneal (**PER**-ih-toe-**NEE**-al) Pertaining to the peritoneum.

peritoneum (per-ih-toe-**NEE**-um) Membrane that lines the abdominal cavity.

peritonitis (**PER**-ih-toe-**NIE**-tis) Inflammation of the peritoneum.

peritubular (**PER**-ih-too-**BYU**-lar) Surrounding the small renal tubules.

permeable (**PER**-me-ah-bull) Allows passage of substances through a membrane.

pernicious anemia (per-**NISH**-us ah-**NEE**-me-ah) Chronic anemia due to lack of vitamin B$_{12}$.

pertussis (per-**TUSS**-is) Infectious disease with a spasmodic, intense cough ending on a whoop (stridor). Also known as *whooping cough.*

pes planus (PES **PLAY**-nuss) A flat foot with no plantar arch.

pessary (**PES**-ah-ree) Appliance inserted into the vagina to support the uterus.

pesticide (**PES**-tih-side) Agent for destroying flies, mosquitoes, and other pests.

petechia (peh-**TEE**-kee-ah) Pinpoint capillary hemorrhagic spot in the skin. Plural *petechiae.*

petit mal (peh-**TEE** MAL) Old name for an absence seizure.

Peyronie disease (pay-**ROH**-nee **DIZ**-eez) Penile bending and pain on erection.

phacoemulsification (fake-oh-ee-**MUL**-sih-fih-**KAY**-shun) Technique used to fragment the center of the lens into very tiny pieces and suck them out of the eye.

phagocyte (**FAG**-oh-site) Blood cell that ingests and destroys foreign particles and cells.

phagocytic (fag-oh-**SIT**-ik) Pertaining to phagocytes or phagocytosis.

phagocytize (**FAG**-oh-site-ize) Ingest foreign particles and cells.

phagocytosis (**FAG**-oh-sigh-**TOE**-sis) Process of ingestion and destruction.

phalanx (**FAY**-lanks) A bone of a finger or toe. Plural *phalanges.*

pharmacist (**FAR**-mah-sist) Person licensed by the state to prepare and dispense drugs.

pharmacology (far-mah-**KOLL**-oh-jee) Science of the preparation, uses, and effects of drugs.

pharmacy (**FAR**-mah-see) Facility licensed to prepare and dispense drugs.

pharyngitis (fair-in-**JIE**-tis) Inflammation of the pharynx.

pharynx (**FAIR**-inks) Air tube from the back of the nose to the larynx.

phenotype (**FEE**-noh-type) A visible trait.

phenylalanine (fen-il-**AL**-ah-neen) An amino acid.

phenylketonuria (**FEN**-il-**KEE**-toe-**NYU**-ree-ah) Hereditary disease with accumulation of phenylalanine and urinary excretion of its metabolites; leads to mental retardation if not controlled.

pheochromocytoma (fee-oh-**KRO**-moh-sigh-**TOE**-muh) Adenoma of the adrenal medulla secreting excessive catecholamines.

pheomelanin (**FEE**-oh-mel-ah-nin) The lighter form of melanin.

pheromone (**FER**-oh-moan) Substance that carries and generates a physical attraction for other people.

phimosis (fi-**MOH**-sis) Condition in which the prepuce cannot be retracted.

phlebitis (fleh-**BIE**-tis) Inflammation of a vein.

phlebotomist (fleh-**BOT**-oh-mist) Person skilled in taking blood from veins.

phlebotomy (fleh-**BOT**-oh-me) Taking blood from a vein.

phlegm (FLEM) Abnormal amounts of mucus expectorated from the respiratory tract.

phobia (**FOH**-be-ah) Pathologic fear or dread.

phonophoresis (foh-noh-for-**EE**-sis) Transport of one substance across the skin through the use of ultrasound.

phosphatase (**FOS**-fah-tase) Enzyme that liberates phosphorus.

photocoagulation (foh-toe-koh-ag-you-**LAY**-shun) The use of light (laser beam) to form a clot.

photodynamic (foh-toe-die-**NAM**-ik) Use of a light-sensitive drug with a laser beam to destroy cells.

photophobia (foh-toe-**FOH**-bee-ah) Fear of the light because it hurts the eyes.

photoreceptor (foh-toe-ree-**SEP**-tor) A photoreceptor cell receives light and converts it into electrical impulses.

photosensitivity (foh-toe-**SEN**-sih-tiv-ih-tee) Condition in which light produces pain in the eye.

phototherapy (foh-toe-**THAIR**-ah-pee) Treatment using light rays.

physiatrist (fih-**ZIE**-ah-trist) Specialist in physical medicine.

physiatry (fih-**ZIE**-ah-tree) Physical medicine.

physical medicine (**FIZ**-ih-cal **MED**-ih-sin) Diagnosis and treatment by means of remedial agents, such as exercises, manipulation, and heat.

physical therapy (**FIZ**-ih-cal **THAIR**-ah-pee) Use of remedial processes to overcome a physical defect. Also known as *physiotherapy.*

physiotherapy (**FIZ**-ee-oh-**THAIR**-ah-pee) Another term for *physical therapy.*

phytic acid (**FIE**-tik **ASS**-id) Component of fiber that can limit absorption of some minerals.

phytochemical (fie-toe-**KEM**-ih-kal) Biologically active, nonnutrient plant chemical.

pia mater (**PEE**-ah **MAY**-ter) Delicate inner layer of the meninges.

pica (**PIE**-kah) Eating substances not considered to be food.

pineal (**PIN**-ee-al) Pertaining to the pineal gland.

pink eye (PINK EYE) Conjunctivitis.

pinna (**PIN**-ah) Another name for *auricle.* Plural *pinnae.*

pinworm (**PIN**-worm) Intestinal parasite.

pitting edema (ee-**DEE**-mah) Edema that maintains for a time indentations made by applying pressure to the area.

pituitary (pih-**TOO**-ih-tary) Pertaining to the pituitary gland.

placebo (plah-**SEE**-boh) An inert compound with no innate therapeutic value.

placenta (plah-**SEN**-tah) Organ that allows metabolic interchange between the mother and the fetus.

plague (PLAYG) Infectious disease causing excessive mortality.

plantar reflex (**PLAN**-tar re-**FLEKS**) Neurologic response to stimulation of the sole of the foot.

plaque (PLAK) Patch of abnormal tissue.

plasma (**PLAZ**-mah) Fluid, noncellular component of blood.

plasma cell (**PLAZ**-mah SELL) Cell derived from B lymphocytes and active in formation of antibodies.

Plasmodium (plaz-**MOH**-dee-um) Causal agent for malaria.

platelet (**PLAYT**-let) Cell fragment involved in the clotting process. Also called *thrombocyte*.

pleura (**PLUR**-ah) Membrane covering the lungs and lining the ribs in the thoracic cavity. Plural *pleurae*.

pleurisy (**PLUR**-ih-see) Inflammation of the pleura.

plexus (**PLEK**-sus) A weblike network of joined nerves. Plural *plexuses*.

plica (**PLEE**-cah) Fold in a mucous membrane. Plural *plicae*.

pneumatic (new-**MAT**-ik) Pertaining to a structure filled with air.

pneumococcal (new-moh-**KOK**-al) Pertaining to the *Pneumococcus*.

pneumococcus (new-moh-**KOK**-us) Gram-positive cocci associated with respiratory infection. Plural *pneumococci*.

pneumoconiosis (new-moh-koh-nee-**OH**-sis) Fibrotic lung disease caused by the inhalation of different dusts.

pneumonectomy (**NEW**-moh-**NEK**-toe-me) Surgical removal of a whole lung.

pneumonia (new-**MOH**-nee-ah) Inflammation of the lung parenchyma.

pneumonic (new-**MON**-ik) Relating to pneumonia.

pneumothorax (new-moh-**THOR**-ax) Air in the pleural cavity.

podiatrist (po-**DIE**-ah-trist) Practitioner of podiatry.

podiatry (po-**DIE**-ah-tree) Specialty concerned with the diagnosis and treatment of disorders and injuries of the foot.

poikilocytic (**POY**-key-low-**SIT**-ik) Pertaining to an irregular-shaped RBC.

polarity (po-**LAR**-ih-tee) Possession of opposite characteristics.

poliomyelitis (**POE**-lee-oh-**MY**-eh-lie-tis) Inflammation of the gray matter of the spinal cord, leading to paralysis of the limbs and muscles of respiration.

pollutant (poh-**LOO**-tant) Substance that makes an environment unclean or impure.

pollution (poh-**LOO**-shun) Condition that is unclean, impure, and a danger to health.

polycystic (pol-ee-**SIS**-tik) Composed of many cysts.

polycythemia vera (**POL**-ee-sigh-**THEE**-me-ah) Chronic disease with bone marrow hyperplasia and an increase in the number of RBCs and blood volume.

polydipsia (pol-ee-**DIP**-see-ah) Excessive thirst.

polyhydramnios (**POL**-ee-high-**DRAM**-nee-os) Too much amniotic fluid.

polymenorrhea (**POL**-ee-men-oh-**REE**-ah) More than normal frequency of menses.

polymorphonuclear (**POL**-ee-more-foh-**NEW**-klee-ar) White blood cell with a multi-lobed nucleus.

polymyalgia rheumatica (poll-ee-my-**AL**-jee-ah rue-**MAT**-ick-ah) Pain in several muscle groups with systemic symptoms.

polyneuropathy (**POL**-ee-nyu-**ROP**-ah-thee) Disorder affecting many nerves.

polyp (**POL**-ip) Mass of tissue that projects into the lumen of the bowel.

polypectomy (pol-ip-**ECK**-toh-mee) Excision or removal of a polyp.

polyphagia (pol-ee-**FAY**-jee-ah) Excessive eating.

polyphenol (pol-ee-**FEE**-nol) Antioxidant found in grapes and tea.

polyposis (pol-ih-**POH**-sis) Presence of several polyps.

polysaccharide (pol-ee-**SACK**-ah-ride) A combination of many saccharides; for example, starch.

polysomnography (pol-ee-som-**NOG**-rah-fee) Test to monitor brain waves, muscle tension, eye movement, and oxygen levels in the blood as the patient sleeps.

polyuria (pol-ee-**YOU**-ree-ah) Excessive production of urine.

pons (PONZ) Part of the brainstem.

popliteal (pop-**LIT**-ee-al) Pertaining to the back of the knee.

popliteal fossa (pop-**LIT**-ee-al **FOSS**-ah) The hollow at the back of the knee.

portal; portal vein (**POR**-tal VANE) The vein that carries blood from the intestines to the liver.

postcoital (post-**KOH**-ih-tal) After sexual intercourse.

posterior (pos-**TER**-ee-or) Pertaining to the back surface of the body; situated behind.

postictal (post-**IK**-tal) Occurring after a seizure.

postmature (post-mah-**TYUR**) Infant born after 42 weeks of gestation.

postmaturity (post-mah-**TYUR**-ih-tee) Condition of being postmature.

postpartum (post-**PAR**-tum) After childbirth.

postpolio syndrome (PPS) (post-**POE**-lee-oh SIN-drome) Progressive muscle weakness in a person previously affected by polio.

postprandial (post-**PRAN**-dee-al) Following a meal.

postpubescent (post-pyu-**BESS**-ent) After the period of puberty.

posttraumatic (post-traw-**MAT**-ik) Occurring after and caused by trauma.

posture (**POSS**-chur) The carriage of the body as a whole and the position of the limbs.

Pott fracture (POT **FRAK**-chur) Fracture of the lower end of the fibula, often with fracture of the tibial malleolus.

prana (PRAH-nah) Vital power.

precancerous (pree-KAN-sir-us) Lesion from which a cancer can develop.

precipitate (pree-SIP-ih-tate) Very rapid and sudden, as labor and delivery.

precision (pree-SIH-zhun) Quality of being clearly defined or stated.

precursor (pree-KUR-sir) Cell or substance formed earlier in the development of the cell or substance.

prednisone (PRED-nih-zohn) A synthetic corticosteroid.

preeclampsia (pree-eh-KLAMP-see-uh) Hypertension, edema, and proteinuria during pregnancy.

preemie (PREE-me) Slang for *premature baby*.

pregnancy (PREG-nan-see) State of being pregnant.

pregnant (PREG-nant) Having conceived.

prehypertension (pree-HIGH-per-TEN-shun) Precursor to hypertension.

premature (pree-mah-TYUR) Occurring before the expected time; for example, an infant born before 37 weeks of gestation.

prematurity (pree-mah-TYUR-ih-tee) Condition of being premature.

premenstrual (pree-MEN-stru-al) Pertaining to the time immediately before the menses.

prenatal (pree-NAY-tal) Before birth.

prepatellar (pree-pah-TELL-ar) In front of the patella.

prepuce (PREE-puce) Fold of skin that covers the glans penis.

presbyopia (prez-bee-OH-pee-ah) Difficulty in nearsighted vision occurring in middle and old age.

preterm (PREE-term) Baby delivered before 37 weeks of gestation. Also called *premature*.

prevention (pree-VEN-shun) Process undertaken to prevent occurrence of a disease or health problem.

previa (PREE-vee-ah) Anything blocking the fetus during its birth; for example, an abnormally situated placenta, *placenta previa*.

priapism (PRY-ah-pizm) Persistent erection of the penis.

primary care (PRY-mah-ree KAIR) Comprehensive and preventive health care services that are the first point of care for a patient.

primigravida (pree-mih-GRAV-ih-dah) First pregnancy.

primipara (pree-MIP-ah-ruh) Woman who has given birth for the first time.

prion (PREE-on) Small infectious protein particle.

proctitis (prok-TIE-tis) Inflammation of the lining of the rectum.

proctoscopy (prok-TOSS-koh-pee) Examination of the inside of the anus by endoscopy.

prodromal (pro-DRO-mal) Beginning of disease, before the signs become overt.

progenitor (pro-JEN-it-or) Founder; beginning of an ancestry.

progesterone (pro-JESS-ter-own) Hormone that prepares the uterus for pregnancy.

progestin (pro-JESS-tin) A synthetic form of progesterone.

prognathism (PROG-nah-thizm) Condition of a forward-projecting jaw.

prognosis (prog-NO-sis) Forecasting of the probable course of a disease.

prolactin (pro-LAK-tin) Pituitary hormone that stimulates the production of milk.

prolactinoma (pro-lak-tih-NO-muh) Prolactin-producing tumor.

prolapse (pro-LAPS) The falling or slipping of a body part from its normal position.

proliferate (pro-LIF-eh-rate) To increase in number through reproduction.

pronate (PRO-nate) Rotate the forearm so that the surface of the palm faces posteriorly in the anatomical position.

pronation (pro-NAY-shun) Process of lying face-down or of turning a hand or foot with the volar (palm or sole) surface down.

prone (PRONE) Lying face-down, flat on your belly.

prophylactic (pro-fih-LAK-tik) The act or the agent that prevents a disease.

prophylaxis (pro-fih-LAX-is) Prevention of disease.

prostaglandin (PROS-tah-GLAN-din) Hormone present in many tissues, but first isolated from the prostate gland.

prostate (PROS-tate) Organ surrounding the beginning of the urethra.

prostatectomy (pross-tah-TEK-toe-me) Surgical removal of the prostate.

prostatic (pros-TAT-ik) Pertaining to the prostate.

prostatitis (pross-tah-TIE-tis) Inflammation of the prostate.

prosthesis (PROS-thee-sis) A manufactured substitute for a missing or diseased part of the body.

protease (PRO-tee-aze) Group of enzymes that break down protein.

protection (pro-TEK-shun) Defense against attack or invasion.

protein (PRO-teen) Class of food substances based on amino acids.

proteinuria (pro-tee-NYU-ree-ah) Presence of protein in urine.

prothrombin (pro-THROM-bin) Protein formed by the liver and converted to thrombin in the blood-clotting mechanism.

protocol (PRO-toe-kol) Detailed plan; for example, protocol for a regimen of therapy.

proton pump inhibitor (PPI) (PRO-ton PUMP in-HIB-ih-tor) Agent that blocks production of gastric acid.

protooncogene (pro-toe-ON-koh-jeen) A normal gene involved in normal cell growth.

provisional diagnosis (pro-VISH-un-al die-ag-NO-sis) A temporary diagnosis pending further examination or testing. Also called *preliminary diagnosis*.

proximal (PROK-sih-mal) Situated nearest to the center of the body.

pruritic (proo-RIT-ik) Itchy.

pruritus (proo-**RYE**-tus) Itching.

Pseudomonas (soo-doh-**MOH**-nas) Gram-negative aerobic rods.

psoriasis (so-**RYE**-ah-sis) Rash characterized by reddish, silver-scaled patches.

psychedelic (sigh-keh-**DEL**-ik) Agent that intensifies sensory perception.

psychiatric (sigh-kee-**AH**-trik) Pertaining to psychiatry.

psychiatrist (sigh-**KIGH**-ah-trist) Licensed medical specialist in psychiatry.

psychiatry (sigh-**KIGH**-ah-tree) Diagnosis and treatment of mental disorders.

psychoactive (sigh-koh-**AK**-tiv) Able to alter mood, behavior, and/or cognition.

psychoanalysis (sigh-koh-ah-**NAL**-ih-sis) Method of psychotherapy.

psychoanalyst (sigh-koh-**AN**-ah-list) Practitioner of psychoanalysis.

psychologic (sigh-koh-**LOJ**-ik) Pertaining to psychology.

psychological (sigh-koh-**LOJ**-ik-al) Pertaining to psychology.

psychologist (sigh-**KOL**-oh-jist) Licensed specialist in psychology.

psychology (sigh-**KOL**-oh-jee) Scientific study of the human mind and behavior.

psychopath (**SIGH**-koh-path) Person with antisocial personality disorder.

psychopharmacotherapy (**SIGH**-koh-**FAR**-mah-koh-**THAIR**-ah-pee) Drug treatment of mental disorders.

psychosis (sigh-**KOH**-sis) Disorder causing mental disruption and loss of contact with reality.

psychosocial (sigh-koh-**SOH**-shal) Involving both the mind and various social and community aspects of life.

psychosomatic (sigh-koh-soh-**MAT**-ik) Pertaining to disorders of the body usually resulting from disturbances of the mind.

psychotherapist (sigh-koh-**THAIR**-ah-pist) Practitioner of psychotherapy.

psychotherapy (sigh-koh-**THAIR**-ah-pee) Treatment of mental disorders through communication.

psychotic (sigh-**KOT**-ik) Pertaining to or affected by psychosis.

pterygoid (**TER**-ih-goyd) Pterygoid muscles are two wing-shaped muscles that open and close the mouth.

ptosis (**TOE**-sis) Sinking down of an eyelid or an organ.

pubarche (pyu-**BAR**-key) Development of pubic and axillary hair.

puberty (**PYU**-ber-tee) Process of maturing from child to young adult capable of reproducing.

pubic (**PYU**-bik) Pertaining to the pubis.

pubis (**PYU**-bis) Bony front arch of the pelvis of the hip. Also called *pubic bone.*

puerperium (pyu-er-**PEE**-ree-um) Six-week period after birth in which the uterus involutes.

pulmonary (**PULL**-moh-**NAR**-ee) Pertaining to the lungs and their blood supply.

pulmonologist (**PULL**-moh-**NOL**-oh-jist) Medical specialist in pulmonary disorders.

pulmonology (**PULL**-moh-**NOL**-oh-gee) Study of the lungs; *or* the medical specialty of disorders of the respiratory tract.

pulp (**PULP**) Dental pulp is the connective tissue in the cavity in the center of the tooth.

pupil (**PYU**-pill) The opening in the center of the iris that allows light to reach the lens. Plural *pupillae.*

purge (**PURJ**) Consciously throw up or cause bowel evacuation.

purging (**PURJ**-ing) The act of throwing up or evacuating the bowel.

purification (**PYUR**-if-ih-kay-shun) Make free from pathogens.

Purkinje fibers (per-**KIN**-jee fi-**BERS**) Network of nerve fibers in the myocardium.

purpura (**PUR**-pyu-rah) Skin hemorrhages that are red initially and then turn purple.

purulent (**PURE**-you-lent) Showing or containing a lot of pus.

pustule (**PUS**-tyul) Small protuberance on the skin that contains pus.

pyelitis (pie-eh-**LYE**-tis) Inflammation of the renal pelvis.

pyelogram (**PIE**-el-oh gram) X-ray image of the renal pelvis and ureters.

pyelonephritis (**PIE**-eh-loh-neh-**FRY**-tis) Inflammation of the kidney and renal pelvis.

pyloric (pie-**LOR**-ik) Pertaining to the pylorus.

pylorus (pie-**LOR**-us) Exit area of the stomach.

pyogenic (**PIE**-o-**JEN**-ik) Pus-producing.

pyorrhea (pie-oh-**REE**-ah) Purulent discharge.

pyrexia (pie-**REK**-see-ah) An abnormally high body temperature or fever.

pyridoxine (pir-ih-**DOK**-seen) Vitamin B_6.

pyromania (pie-roh-**MAY**-nee-ah) Morbid impulse to set fires

Q

Qigong (**CHEE**-gong) Exercises and breathing routines performed daily.

quadrant (**KWAD**-rant) One-quarter of a circle.

quadrantectomy (kwad-ran-**TEK**-toe-me) Surgical excision of a quadrant of the breast.

quadriceps femoris (**KWAD**-rih-seps **FEM**-or-is) An anterior thigh muscle with four heads.

quadriplegia (kwad-rih-**PLEE**-jee-ah) Paralysis of all four limbs.

quantum physics (**KWAHN**-tum **FIZ**-iks) The study of subatomic particles.

quiescent (kwi-**ESS**-ent) Latent, dormant.

quinoa (kee-**NO**-ah) Plant with edible seeds high in protein.

R

rabid (**RAB**-id) Suffering from rabies.

rabies (**RAY**-beez) Highly fatal infectious disease transmitted by the bite of infected animals.

radial (**RAY**-dee-al) Pertaining to the forearm.

radiation (ray-dee-AY-shun) A spreading out, as of anatomical parts.

radical (RAD-ih-cal) Extensive, as in complete removal of a diseased part.

radioactive (RAY-dee-oh-AK-tiv) Spontaneously emitting alpha, beta, or gamma rays.

radioactive iodine (RAY-dee-oh-AK-tiv EYE-oh-dine) Any of the various tracers that emit alpha, beta, or gamma rays.

radiologist (ray-dee-OL-oh-jist) Medical specialist in the use of x-rays and other imaging techniques.

radiology (ray-dee-OL-oh-jee) The study of medical imaging.

radionuclide (RAY-dee-oh-NYU-klide) Radioactive agent used in diagnostic imaging.

radiotherapy (RAY-dee-oh-THAIR-ah-pee) Treatment using radiation.

radius (RAY-dee-us) The forearm bone on the thumb side.

rale (RAHL) Crackle heard through a stethoscope when air bubbles through liquid in the lungs. Plural *rales*.

raphe (RAY-fee) Line separating two symmetrical structures.

rash (RASH) Cutaneous eruption.

reabsorption (ree-ab-SORP-shun) The taking back into the blood of substances that had previously been filtered out from it.

recessive gene (ree-SESS-iv JEEN) Allele that does not manifest as a trait or characteristic.

recombinant DNA (ree-KOM-bin-ant dee-en-a) DNA (deoxyribonucleic acid) altered by inserting a new sequence of DNA into the chain.

rectocele (REK-toe-seal) Hernia of the rectum into the vagina.

rectum (RECK-tum) Terminal part of the colon from the sigmoid to the anal canal.

recurrent (ree-KUR-ent) Symptoms or lesions returning after an intermission.

reduction (ree-DUCK-shun) The restoration of a structure to its normal position.

reflex (REE-fleks) An involuntary response to a stimulus.

reflexology (ree-flek-SOL-oh-jee) Stimulation of reflexes in the feet and hands, which correspond to other parts of the body.

reflux (REE-fluks) Backward flow.

refract (ree-FRACT) Make a change in the direction of, or bend, a ray of light.

regenerate (ree-JEN-eh-rate) Reconstitution of a lost part.

regimen (REJ-ih-men) Program of treatment.

regulate (REG-you-late) To control the way in which a process progresses.

regulation (reg-you-LAY-shun) Control of the way in which a process progresses.

regurgitate (ree-GUR-jih-tate) To flow backward; for example, through a heart valve.

regurgitation (ree-gur-jih-TAY-shun) Expel contents of the stomach into the mouth, short of vomiting.

rehabilitation (REE-hah-bill-ih-TAY-shun) Therapeutic restoration of an ability to function as before.

Reiki (RAY-kee) A healing method using the transfer of energy by placing hands on or near a patient.

remission (ree-MISH-un) Period in which there is a lessening or absence of the symptoms of a disease.

remit (ree-MIT) To diminish in intensity.

renal (REE-nal) Pertaining to the kidney.

renin (REE-nin) Enzyme secreted by the kidney that causes vasoconstriction.

replication (rep-lih-KAY-shun) Reproduction to produce an exact copy.

reproductive (ree-pro-DUC-tiv) Relating to the process by which organisms produce offspring.

resection (ree-SEK-shun) Removal of a specific part of an organ or structure.

resectoscope (ree-SEK-toe-skope) Endoscope for transurethral removal of lesions.

residual (re-ZID-you-al) Pertaining to anything left over.

resistance (ree-ZIS-tants) Ability of an organism to withstand the effects of an antagonistic agent.

resistant (ree-ZIS-tant) Able to resist.

resorption (ree-SORP-shun) Loss of substance, such as bone.

respiration (RES-pih-RAY-shun) Fundamental process of life used to exchange oxygen and carbon dioxide.

respirator (RES-pir-AY-tor) Another name for *ventilator*.

restorative rehabilitation (ree-STOR-ah-tiv REE-hah-bill-ih-TAY-shun) Promote renewal of health and strength.

rete testis (REE-teh TES-tis) Network of tubules between the seminiferous tubules and the epididymis.

retention (ree-TEN-shun) Holding back in the body what should normally be discharged (e.g., urine).

reticulum (reh-TIK-you-lum) Fine network of cells in the medulla oblongata.

retina (RET-ih-nah) Light-sensitive innermost layer of the eyeball.

retinaculum (ret-ih-NACK-you-lum) Fibrous ligament that keeps the tendons in place on the wrist so that they do not "bowstring" when the forearm muscles contract.

retinoblastoma (RET-in-oh-blas-TOE-mah) Malignant neoplasm of primitive retinal cells.

retinoid (RET-ih-noyd) A class of keratolytic agents.

retinopathy (ret-ih-NOP-ah-thee) Degenerative disease of the retina.

retraction (ree-TRAK-shun) A pulling back, as a pulling back of the intercostal spaces and the neck above the clavicle.

retrograde (RET-roh-grade) Reversal of a normal flow; for example, back from the bladder into the ureters.

retroversion (reh-troh-VER-shun) The tipping backward of the uterus.

retroverted (REH-troh-vert-ed) Tilted backward.

retrovirus (REH-troh-vie-rus) Virus that replicates in a host cell by converting its RNA core into DNA.

Reye syndrome (RAY SIN-drome) Encephalopathy and liver damage in children following an acute viral illness; linked to aspirin use.

rhabdomyolysis (RAB-doh-my-oh-LIE-sis) Destruction of muscle to produce myoglobin.

rhabdomyosarcoma (RAB-doh-MY-oh-sar-KOH-mah) Cancer derived from skeletal muscle.

rheumatism (RU-mat-izm) Pain in various parts of the musculoskeletal system.

rheumatoid arthritis (RA) (RHU-mah-toyd ar-THRI-tis) Disease of connective tissue, with arthritis as a major manifestation.

rhinitis (rye-NI-tis) Inflammation of the nasal mucosa. Also called *coryza*.

rhinoplasty (RYE-no-plas-tee) Surgical procedure to change the size or shape of the nose.

rhonchus (RONG-kuss) Wheezing sound heard on auscultation of the lungs; made by air passing through a constricted lumen. Plural *rhonchi*.

riboflavin (RYE-boh-flay-vin) Vitamin B$_2$.

ribonucleic acid (RNA) (RYE-boh-nyu-KLEE-ik ASS-id) Information carrier from DNA in the nucleus to the ribosome to produce protein molecules.

ribosome (RYE-bo-sohm) Structure in the cell that assembles amino acids into protein.

rickets (RICK-ets) Disease due to vitamin D deficiency, producing soft, flexible bones.

rigidity (ri-JID-ih-tee) Increased muscle tone at rest.

Rinne test (RIN-eh TEST) Test for conductive hearing loss.

ritual (RITCH-you-al) An activity or set of activities established and repeated.

Rolfing (ROLF-ing) Manipulation of connective tissue to realign and balance the whole body.

root (ROOT) Fundamental or beginning part of a structure.

rooting (rue-TING) A neonatal reflex to turn toward the nipple and open the mouth when a nipple is placed on the cheek.

rosacea (roh-ZAY-she-ah) Persistent erythematous rash of the central face.

roseola infantum (roh-ZEE-oh-lah in-FAN-tum) Skin rash in infants and young children caused by a herpesvirus.

rotator cuff (roh-TAY-tor CUFF) Part of the capsule of the shoulder joint.

Roux-en-Y (ROO-on-Y) Surgical procedure to reduce the size of the stomach.

ruga (ROO-ga) A fold, ridge, or crease. Plural *rugae*.

rumination (ROO-min-ay-shun) To bring back food into the mouth to chew over and over.

rupture (RUP-tyur) Break or tear of any organ or body part.

S

sacral (SAY-kral) In the neighborhood of the sacrum.

sacroiliac joint (say-kroh-ILL-ih-ak JOINT) The joint between the sacrum and the ilium.

sacrum (SAY-crum) Segment of the vertebral column that forms part of the pelvis.

sagittal (SAJ-ih-tal) Pertaining to the vertical plane through the body, dividing it into right and left portions.

saliva (sa-LIE-vah) Secretion in the mouth from salivary glands.

Salmonella (sal-moh-NELL-ah) Pathogenic Gram-negative rods causing dysentery.

salpingectomy (sal-pin-JECT-oh-me) Surgical removal of fallopian tube(s).

salpingitis (sal-pin-JIE-tis) Inflammation of the uterine tube.

sanitization (SAN-ih-tih-ZAY-shun) Process of using chemicals to remove pathogens from surfaces.

saphenous (SAPH-ih-nus) Relating to the saphenous vein in the thigh.

saponins (SAP-oh-nins) Phytochemicals that can prevent cancer cell replication.

sarcoidosis (sar-koy-DOH-sis) Granulomatous lesions of the lungs and other organs; cause is unknown.

sarcoma (sar-KOH-mah) A malignant tumor originating in connective tissue.

sarcopenia (sar-koh-PEE-nee-ah) Progressive loss of muscle mass and strength in aging.

saturated fatty acid (satch-you-RAY-ted FAT-ee ASS-id) Incapable of absorbing any more hydrogen, and is solid at room temperature.

scab (SKAB) Crust that forms over a wound or sore during healing.

scabies (SKAY-bees) Skin disease produced by mites.

scapula (SKAP-you-lah) Shoulder blade. Plural *scapulae*.

scapular (SKAP-you-lar) Pertaining to the shoulder blade.

scar (SKAR) Fibrotic seam that forms when a wound heals.

schizoid (SKITZ-oyd) Withdrawn, socially isolated.

schizophrenia (skitz-oh-FREE-nee-ah) Disorder of perception, thought, emotion, and behavior.

Schwann cell (SHWANN SELL) Connective tissue cell of the peripheral nervous system that forms a myelin sheath.

sciatic (sigh-AT-ik) Pertaining to the sciatic nerve or sciatica.

sciatica (sigh-AT-ih-kah) Pain from compression of L5 or S1 nerve roots.

scintigraphy (sin-TIG-rah-fee) Recording of radioactivity with a special camera.

sclera (SKLAIR-ah) Fibrous outer covering of the eyeball and the white of the eye.

scleritis (sklair-RI-tis) Inflammation of the sclera.

scleroderma (sklair-oh-DERM-ah) Thickening and hardening of the skin due to new collagen formation.

sclerose (skleh-ROZE) To harden or thicken.

sclerosis (skleh-ROH-sis) Thickening or hardening of a tissue.

sclerotherapy (SKLAIR-oh-THAIR-ah-pee) To collapse a vein by injecting a solution into it to harden it.

scoliosis (skoh-lee-OH-sis) An abnormal lateral curvature of the vertebral column.

scrotal (SKRO-tal) Pertaining to the scrotum.

scrotum (SKRO-tum) Sac containing the testes.

scurvy (SKUR-vee) Deficiency of vitamin C.

seasonal affective disorder (see-ZON-al af-FEK-tiv dis-OR-der) Depression that occurs at the same time every year, often in winter.

sebaceous glands (se-BAY-shus GLANZ) Glands in the dermis that open into hair follicles and secrete an oily fluid called sebum.

seborrhea (seb-oh-REE-ah) Excessive amount of sebum.

sebum (SEE-bum) Waxy secretion of the sebaceous glands.

secrete (se-KREET) To release or give off, as substances produced by cells.

secretin (se-KREE-tin) Hormone produced by the duodenum to stimulate pancreatic juice.

sedation (seh-DAY-shun) State of being calmed.

sedative (SED-ah-tiv) Agent that calms nervous excitement.

sedentary (sed-en-TER-ee) Accustomed to little exercise or movement.

sediment (SED-ih-ment) Insoluble material that settles to the bottom of a liquid.

sedimentation (SED-ih-men-TAY-shun) Formation of a sediment.

segment (SEG-ment) A section of an organ or structure.

segmentectomy (seg-men-TEK-toe-me) Surgical excision of a segment of a tissue or organ.

seizure (SEE-zhur) Event due to excessive electrical activity in the brain.

self-examination (self-ek-zam-ih-NAY-shun) The examination of part of one's own body.

self-mutilation (self-myu-tih-LAY-shun) Injury or disfigurement made to one's own body.

semen (SEE-men) Penile ejaculate containing sperm and seminal fluid.

semilunar (sem-ee-LOO-nar) Appears like a half moon.

seminal vesicle (SEM-in-al VES-ih-kull) Sac of the ductus deferens that produces seminal fluid.

seminiferous (sem-ih-NIF-er-us) Pertaining to carrying semen.

seminiferous tubule (sem-ih-NIF-er-us TU-byul) Coiled tubes in the testes that produce sperm.

seminoma (sem-ih-NO-mah) Neoplasm of germ cells of a testis.

semipermeable (sem-ee-PER-me-ah-bull) Freely permeable to water but not to solutes.

semipermeable membrane (sem-ee-PER-me-ah-bull MEM-brain) A membrane that allows only certain substances to pass through it.

senescence (seh-NES-ens) The state of being old.

senile (SEE-nile) Characteristic of old age.

senility (seh-NIL-ih-tee) Old age.

sensation (sen-SAY-shun) The conscious feeling of the effects of a stimulation.

sensorineural hearing loss (SEN-sor-ih-NYUR-al) Hearing loss caused by lesions of the inner ear or the auditory nerve.

sensory (SEN-soh-ree) Having the function of sensation; relating to structures of the nervous system that carry impulses to the brain.

sepsis (SEP-sis) Presence of pathogenic organisms or their toxins in blood or tissues.

septicemia (sep-tih-SEE-mee-ah) Microorganisms circulating in, and infecting, the blood (blood poisoning).

septum (SEP-tum) A wall dividing two cavities. Plural *septa*.

sequence (SEE-kwens) The succession of one event after another.

sequential (see-KWEN-shal) One event following after another.

serosa (seh-ROH-sa) Outermost covering of the alimentary tract.

serotonin (ser-oh-TOE-nin) A neurotransmitter in the central and peripheral nervous systems.

serous (SEER-us) Thicker and less transparent than water.

serum (SEER-um) Fluid remaining after removal of cells and fibrin clot.

sewage (SOO-aje) Waste matter from populated areas.

sharps (SHARPS) Any medical instrument capable of puncturing skin.

sharps container (SHARPS kon-TAY-ner) Puncture-resistant container for disposal of sharps.

Shigella (she-GEL-ah) Genus of Gram-negative rods.

shigellosis (shig-eh-LOH-sis) Dysentery caused by *Shigella*.

shock (SHOCK) Sudden physical or mental collapse or circulatory collapse.

shunt (SHUNT) A bypass or diversion of fluid, such as blood.

sibling (SIB-ling) Brother or sister.

sigmoid (SIG-moyd) Sigmoid colon is shaped like an "S."

sigmoidoscopy (sig-moi-DOS-koh-pee) Endoscopic examination of the sigmoid colon.

sign (SINE) Physical evidence of a disease process.

silicosis (sil-ih-KOH-sis) Fibrotic lung disease from inhaling silica particles.

simian crease (sih-ME-an KREES) Single crease across the palm of the hand; found in monkeys.

simulate (SIM-you-late) To imitate a disease process.

sinoatrial (SA) node (sigh-noh-AY-tree-al NODE) The center of modified cardiac muscle fibers in the wall of the right atrium that acts as the pacemaker for the heart rhythm.

sinus (SIGH-nus) Cavity or hollow space in a bone or other tissue.

sinus rhythm (SIGH-nus RITH-um) The normal (optimal) heart rhythm arising from the sinoatrial node.

sinusitis (sigh-nyu-SIGH-tis) Inflammation of the lining of a sinus.

Sjögren syndrome (SHOW-gren SIN-drome) Autoimmune disease that attacks the glands that produce saliva and tears.

Skene glands (SKEEN GLANZ) Paraurethral glands in the anterior wall of the vagina. Also called *paraurethral glands*.

smegma (SMEG-mah) Oily material produced by the glans and prepuce.

Snellen letter chart (SNEL-en) Test for acuity of distant vision.

snore (SNOR) Noise produced by vibrations in the structures of the nasopharynx.

sociopath (SO-see-oh-path) Person with antisocial personality disorder.

soleus (SO-lee-us) Large muscle of the calf.

somatic (soh-MAT-ik) Relating to the body in general; *or* pertaining to a division of the peripheral nervous system serving the skeletal muscles.

somatoform (soh-MAT-oh-form) Physical symptoms occurring without identifiable physical cause.

somatostatin (SO-mah-toh-STAT-in) Hormone that inhibits release of growth hormone and insulin.

somatotropin (SO-mah-toh-TROH-pin) Hormone of the anterior pituitary that stimulates growth of body tissues. Also called *growth hormone.*

sonogram (SON-oh-gram) Image obtained by using a sonograph.

sonograph (SON-oh-graf) Instrument that uses sound waves to create images of structures.

sonographer (so-NOG-rah-fer) The technician who performs a sonogram.

sorbitol (SOR-bih-tol) Alcohol derivative of glucose.

spasm (SPASM) Sudden involuntary contraction of a muscle group.

spasmodic (spaz-MOD-ik) Having intermittent spasms or contractions.

spastic (SPAZ-tik) Increased muscle tone on movement.

species (SPEE-sheez) A group of organisms with certain common characteristics.

specific (speh-SIF-ik) Relating to a particular entity.

specificity (spes-ih-FIS-ih-tee) State of having a fixed relation to a particular entity.

sperm (SPERM) Mature male sex cell. Also called *spermatozoon.*

spermatic (SPER-mat-ik) Pertaining to sperm.

spermatid (SPER-mah-tid) A cell late in the development process of sperm.

spermatocele (SPER-mat-oh-seal) Cyst of the epididymis that contains sperm.

spermatogenesis (SPER-mat-oh-JEN-eh-sis) The process by which male germ cells differentiate into sperm.

spermatozoa (SPER-mat-oh-ZOH-ah) Sperm (plural of *spermatozoon*).

spermicidal (SPER-mih-side-al) Pertaining to sperm.

spermicide (SPER-mih-side) Agent that destroys sperm.

sphenoid (SFEE-noyd) Wedge-shaped bone at the base of the skull.

spherocyte (SFEAR-oh-site) A spherical cell.

spherocytosis (SFEAR-oh-site-oh-sis) Presence of spherocytes in the blood.

sphincter (SFINK-ter) Band of muscle that encircles an opening; when it contracts, the opening squeezes closed.

sphygmomanometer (SFIG-moh-mah-NOM-ih-ter) Instrument for measuring arterial blood pressure.

spina bifida (SPY-nah BIH-fih-dah) Failure of one or more vertebral arches to close during fetal development.

spina bifida cystica (SIS-tik-ah) Meninges and spinal cord protruding through the absent vertebral arch and having the appearance of a cyst.

spina bifida occulta (OH-kul-tah) The deformity of the vertebral arch is not apparent from the skin surface.

spinal tap (SPY-nal TAP) Placement of a needle through an intervertebral space into the subarachnoid space to withdraw CSF.

spine (SPINE) Vertebral column; *or* a short projection from a bone.

spiral fracture (SPY-ral FRAK-chur) A fracture in the shape of a coil.

spirituality (SPEAR-ih-choo-AL-ity) Meaning to life that comes from the spirit or soul rather than the physical body.

spirochete (SPY-roh-keet) Spiral-shaped bacterium causing a sexually transmitted disease (syphilis).

spirometer (spy-ROM-eh-ter) An instrument used to measure respiratory volumes.

spirometry (spy-ROM-eh-tree) Use of a spirometer.

spirulina (spy-roo-LEE-nah) Commercial product of blue-green algae containing 60% to 70% protein.

spleen (SPLEEN) Vascular, lymphatic organ in the left upper quadrant of the abdomen.

splenectomy (sple-NECK-toe-me) Surgical removal of the spleen.

splenomegaly (sple-noh-MEG-ah-lee) Enlarged spleen.

spondylosis (spon-dih-LOH-sis) Degenerative osteoarthritis of the spine.

spongiform (SPON-jih-form) Looking like a sponge.

spongiosum (spun-jee-OH-sum) Spongelike tissue.

spore (SPOR) Generic term for any tiny compact cell produced during reproduction by bacteria.

sprain (SPRAIN) A wrench or tear in a ligament.

sputum (SPYU-tum) Matter coughed up and spat out by individuals with respiratory disorders.

squamous cell (SKWAY-mus SELL) Flat, scalelike epithelial cell.

stage (STAYJ) Definition of the extent and dissemination of a malignant neoplasm.

staging (STAY-jing) Process of determination of the extent of the distribution of a neoplasm.

stapes (STAY-peas) Inner (medial) one of the three ossicles of the middle ear; shaped like a stirrup.

Staphylococcus (STAF-ih-loh-KOK-us) Genus of Gram-positive bacteria that divide in more than one plane to form clusters. Plural *staphylococci.*

starch (STARCH) Complex carbohydrate made of multiple units of glucose attached together.

status (STAT-us) A state or condition

status epilepticus (STAT-us ep-ih-LEP-tik-us) A recurrent state of seizure activity lasting longer than a specific time frame (usually 30 minutes).

stem cell (STEM SELL) Undifferentiated cell found in a differentiated tissue that can divide to yield the specialized cells in that tissue.

stenosis (steh-NOH-sis) Narrowing of a canal or passage, as in the narrowing of a heart valve.

stent (STENT) Wire mesh tube used to keep arteries open.

stereopsis (ster-ee-OP-sis) Three-dimensional vision.

stereotactic (STER-ee-oh-TAK-tic) Pertaining to a precise three-dimensional method to locate a lesion.

stereotype (STER-ee-oh-tipe) An image held in common by members of a group.

sterile (STER-isle) Free from all living organisms and their spores; *or* unable to fertilize or reproduce.

sterility (steh-RIL-ih-tee) Inability to reproduce.

sterilization (STER-ih-lih-ZAY-shun) Process of making sterile.

sterilize (STER-ih-lize) To make sterile.

sternum (STIR-num) Long, flat bone forming the center of the anterior wall of the chest.

steroid (STER-oyd) Large family of chemical substances found in many drugs, hormones, and body components.

stethoscope (STETH-oh-skope) Instrument for listening to cardiac and respiratory sounds.

stimulant (STIM-you-lant) Agent that excites or strengthens functional activity.

stimulation (stim-you-LAY-shun) Arousal to increased functional activity.

stoma (STOW-mah) Artificial opening.

strabismus (strah-BIZ-mus) A turning of an eye away from its normal position.

strain (STRAIN) Overstretch or tear in a muscle or tendon.

stratum basale (STRAH-tum ba-SAL-eh) Deepest layer of the epidermis, from which the other cells originate and migrate.

streptococcal (strep-toe-KOK-al) Pertaining to the *Streptococcus*.

Streptococcus (strep-toe-KOK-us) Genus of Gram-positive bacteria that grow in chains. Plural *streptococci*.

streptokinase (strep-toe-KI-nase) An enzyme that dissolves clots.

striated muscle (STRI-ay-ted MUSS-el) Another term for *skeletal muscle.*

striation (stri-AY-shun) Stripes.

stricture (STRICK-shur) Narrowing of a tube.

stridor (STRY-door) High-pitched noise made when there is a respiratory obstruction in the larynx or trachea.

stroke (STROHK) Acute clinical event caused by an impaired cerebral circulation.

stroma (STROH-mah) Connective tissue framework that supports the parenchyma of an organ or gland.

subarachnoid space (sub-ah-RACK-noyd SPASE) Space between the pia mater and the arachnoid membrane.

subclavian (sub-CLAY-vee-an) Underneath the clavicle.

subcutaneous (sub-kew-TAY-nee-us) Below the skin. Also known as *hypodermic*.

subdural (sub-DUR-al) Located in the space between the dura mater and the arachnoid membrane.

sublingual (sub-LING-wal) Underneath the tongue.

subluxation (sub-luck-SAY-shun) An incomplete dislocation in which some contact between the joint surfaces remains.

submandibular (sub-man-DIB-you-lar) Underneath the mandible.

submucosa (sub-mew-KOH-sa) Tissue layer underneath the mucosa.

substernal (sub-STER-nal) Under the sternum or breastbone.

sucrose (SUE-krose) Table sugar.

suction (SUK-shun) Use of a catheter to clear the upper airway or other tubes.

sugar (SHUH-gar) Basic carbohydrate; term sometimes used for glucose or sucrose.

suicidal (SOO-ih-SIGH-dal) Wanting to kill oneself.

suicide (SOO-ih-side) The act of killing oneself.

sulcus (SUL-cuss) Groove on the surface of the cerebral hemispheres that separates gyri. Plural *sulci*.

superior (soo-PEE-ree-or) Situated above.

supinate (SOO-pih-nate) Rotate the forearm so that the surface of the palm faces anteriorly in the anatomical position.

supination (soo-pih-NAY-shun) Process of lying face-upward or turning an arm or foot so that the palm or sole is facing up.

supine (soo-PINE) Lying face-up, flat on your spine.

supplement (SUH-pleh-ment) Substance taken to remedy or prevent a deficiency.

suprapubic (SOO-prah-pyu-bik) Above the symphysis pubis.

surfactant (ser-FAK-tant) A protein and fat compound that creates surface tension to hold lung alveolar walls apart.

susceptible (suh-SEP-tih-bill) Capable of being affected by.

suture (SOO-chur) Place where two bones are joined together by a fibrous band continuous with their periosteum, as in the skull; *or* a stitch to hold the edges of a wound together. Plural *sutures*.

swab (SWOB) Wad of cotton used to remove or apply something from or to a surface.

sympathetic (sim-pah-THET-ik) Pertaining to the part of the autonomic nervous system operating at the unconscious level.

sympathy (SIM-pa-thee) Appreciation and concern for another person's mental and emotional state.

symphysis (SIM-feh-sis) Two bones joined by fibrocartilage. Plural *symphyses*.

symptom (SIMP-tum) Departure from normal health experienced by the patient.

symptomatic (simp-toe-MAT-ik) Pertaining to the symptoms of a disease.

synapse (SIN-aps) Junction between two nerve cells, or a nerve fiber and its target cell, where electrical impulses are transmitted between the cells.

synchondrosis (sin-kon-**DROH**-sis) A rigid articulation (joint) formed by cartilage. Plural *synchondroses.*

syncope (**SIN**-koh-peh) Temporary loss of consciousness and postural tone due to diminished cerebral blood flow.

syncytial (sin-**SISH**-ee-al) Pertaining to the syncytium.

syncytium (sin-**SISH**-ee-um) A multinucleated mass not separated into cells.

syndesmosis (sin-dez-**MOH**-sis) A rigid articulation (joint) formed by ligaments. Plural *syndesmoses.*

syndrome (**SIN**-drohm) Combination of signs and symptoms associated with a particular disease process.

synergist (**SIN**-er-jist) Agent or process that aids the action of another.

synovial (si-**NOH**-vee-al) Pertaining to synovial fluid and synovial membrane.

synthesis (**SIN**-the-sis) The process of building a compound from different elements.

synthetic (sin-**THET**-ik) Built up or put together from simpler compounds.

syphilis (**SIF**-ih-lis) Sexually transmitted disease caused by a spirochete.

syringomyelia (sih-**RING**-oh-my-**EE**-lee-ah) Abnormal longitudinal cavities in the spinal cord that cause paresthesias and muscle weakness.

systemic (sis-**TEM**-ik) Relating to the entire organism.

systemic lupus erythematosus (sis-**TEM**-ik **LOO**-pus er-ih-**THEE**-mah-toe-sus) Inflammatory connective tissue disease affecting the whole body.

systole (**SIS**-toe-lee) Contraction of the heart muscle.

T

tachycardia (tak-ih-**KAR**-dee-ah) Rapid heart rate (above 100 beats per minute).

tachypnea (tak-ip-**NEE**-ah) Rapid breathing.

tactile (**TAK**-tile) Relating to touch.

tai chi (tie-**CHEE**) Defined series of postures performed in fluid movement.

talipes (**TAL**-ip-eze) Deformity of the foot involving the talus.

talus (**TAY**-luss) The tarsal bone that articulates with the tibia to form the ankle joint.

tampon (**TAM**-pon) Plug or pack in a cavity to absorb or stop bleeding.

tamponade (tam-po-**NAID**) Pathologic compression of an organ such as the heart.

tangent (**TAN**-jent) Sudden change of course.

tangentiality (tan-jen-she-**AL**-ih-tee) Disturbance in thought processes, which move rapidly from one topic to another.

tapeworm (**TAPEWORM**) Intestinal parasitic worm.

tarsus (**TAR**-sus) The collection of seven bones in the foot that form the ankle and instep; *or* the flat fibrous plate that gives shape to the outer edges of the eyelids.

tartar (**TAR**-tar) Calcified deposit at the gingival margin of the teeth. Also called *dental calculus.*

taste (**TAYST**) Sensation from chemicals on the taste buds.

Tay-Sachs disease (**TAY**-**SAKS** **DIZ**-eez) Congenital fatal disorder of fat metabolism.

temperament (**TEM**-per-ah-ment) Predisposition to character or personality.

temporal (**TEM**-por-al) Bone that forms part of the base and sides of the skull.

temporal lobe (**TEM**-por-al LOBE) Posterior two-thirds of the cerebral hemispheres.

temporalis muscle (tem-poh-**RAHL**-is **MUSS**-el) Muscle attached to the temporal bone that opens and closes the jaw.

temporomandibular joint (TMJ) (**TEM**-por-oh-man-**DIB**-you-lar JOYNT) The joint between the temporal bone and the mandible.

tendinitis (ten-dih-**NYE**-tis) Inflammation of a tendon. Also spelled *tendonitis.*

tendon (**TEN**-dun) Fibrous band that connects muscle to bone.

tenosynovitis (**TEN**-oh-sine-oh-**VIE**-tis) Inflammation of a tendon and its surrounding synovial sheath.

teratogen (**TER**-ah-toe-jen) Agent that produces fetal deformities.

teratogenesis (**TER**-ah-toe-**JEN**-eh-sis) Process involved in producing fetal deformities.

teratogenic (**TER**-ah-toe-**JEN**-ik) Capable of producing fetal deformities.

teratoma (ter-ah-**TOE**-mah) Neoplasm of a testis or ovary containing multiple tissues from other sites in the body.

testicle (**TES**-tih-kul) One of the male reproductive glands. Also called *testis.*

testicular (tes-**TICK**-you-lar) Pertaining to the testicle.

testis (**TES**-tis) A synonym for testicle. Plural *testes.*

testosterone (tes-**TOSS**-ter-own) Powerful androgen produced by the testes.

tetanus (**TET**-ah-nuss) A disease with painful, tonic, muscular contractions caused by the toxin produced by *Clostridium tetani.*

tetany (**TET**-ah-nee) Severe muscle twitches, cramps, and spasms.

tetralogy (teh-**TRAL**-oh-jee) A set of four congenital heart defects.

tetralogy of Fallot (TOF) (teh-**TRAL**-oh-jee OF fah-**LOW**) Set of four congenital heart defects occurring together.

thalamus (**THAL**-ah-mus) Mass of gray matter underneath the ventricle in each cerebral hemisphere.

thalassemia (thal-ah-**SEE**-mee-ah) Group of inherited blood disorders that produce a hemolytic anemia.

thelarche (thee-**LAR**-key) Onset of breast development.

thenar (**THAY**-nar) The thenar eminence is the fleshy mass at the base of the thumb.

therapeutic (**THAIR**-ah-**PYU**-tik) Relating to the treatment of a disease or disorder.

therapist (THAIR-ah-pist) Professional trained in the practice of a particular therapy.

therapy (THAIR-ah-pee) Systematic treatment of a disease, dysfunction, or disorder.

thermotherapy (THER-moh-THAIR-ah-pee) The use of heat in treatment.

thiamine (THIGH-ah-min) Vitamin B$_1$.

thoracentesis (THOR-ah-sen-TEE-sis) Insertion of a needle into the pleural cavity to withdraw fluid or air. Also called *pleural tap*.

thoracic (THOR-ass-ik) Pertaining to the chest (thorax).

thoracoscopy (thor-ah-KOS-koh-pee) Examination of the pleural cavity with an endoscope.

thoracotomy (thor-ah-KOT-oh-me) Incision through the chest wall.

thorax (THO-racks) The part of the trunk between the abdomen and the neck.

thrombin (THROM-bin) Enzyme that forms fibrin.

thrombocyte (THROM-boh-site) Another name for *platelet.*

thrombocytopenia (THROM-boh-site-oh-PEE-nee-ah) Deficiency of platelets in circulating blood.

thromboembolism (THROM-boh-EM-boh-lizm) A piece of detached blood clot (embolus) blocking a distant blood vessel.

thrombolysis (throm-BOL-ih-sis) Dissolving a thrombus (clot).

thrombophlebitis (THROM-boh-fleh-BY-tis) Inflammation of a vein with clot formation.

thrombosis (throm-BOH-sis) Formation of a thrombus.

thrombus (THROM-bus) A clot attached to a diseased blood vessel or heart lining.

thrush (THRUSH) Infection with *Candida albicans.*

thymectomy (thigh-MEK-toe-me) Surgical removal of the thymus gland.

thymine (THIGH-meen) Chemical base found in, and comprising the sequence of, DNA but not RNA.

thymoma (thigh-MOH-mah) Benign tumor of the thymus.

thymus (THIGH-mus) Endocrine gland located in the mediastinum.

thyroid (THIGH-royd) Endocrine gland in the neck; *or* a cartilage of the larynx.

thyroid hormone (THIGH-royd HOR-mohn) Collective term for the two thyroid hormones, T3 and T4.

thyroid storm (THIGH-royd STORM) Medical crisis and emergency due to excess thyroid hormones.

thyroidectomy (thigh-roy-DEK-toe-me) Surgical removal of the thyroid gland.

thyroiditis (thigh-roy-DIE-tis) Inflammation of the thyroid gland.

thyrotoxicosis (THIGH-roe-toks-ih-KOH-sis) Disorder produced by excessive thyroid hormone production.

thyrotropin (thigh-roe-TROH-pin) Hormone from the anterior pituitary gland that stimulates function of the thyroid gland.

thyroxine (thigh-ROCK-sin) Thyroid hormone, T4, tetraiodothyronine.

tibia (TIB-ee-ah) The larger bone of the lower leg.

tic (TIK) Sudden, involuntary, repeated contraction of muscles.

tic douloureux (TIK duh-luh-RUE) Painful, sudden, spasmodic involuntary contractions of the facial muscles supplied by the trigeminal nerve. Also called *trigeminal neuralgia.*

tinea (TIN-ee-ah) General term for a group of related skin infections caused by different species of fungi.

tinnitus (TIN-ih-tus) Persistent ringing, whistling, clicking, or booming noise in the ears.

tissue (TISH-you) Collection of similar cells.

titer (TIE-ter) The strength of a substance in a solution as compared to a standard.

tolerance (TOL-er-ants) The capacity to become accustomed to a stimulus or drug.

tomography (toe-MOG-rah-fee) Radiographic image of a selected slice of tissue.

tone (TONE) Tension present in resting muscles.

tongue (TUNG) Mobile muscle mass in the mouth; bears the taste buds.

tonic (TON-ik) In a state of muscular contraction.

tonic-clonic (TON-ik-KLON-ik) The body alternates between excessive muscular rigidity (tonic) and jerking muscular contractions (clonic).

tonic-clonic seizure (TON-ik-KLON-ik SEE-zhur) Generalized seizure due to epileptic activity in all or most of the brain.

tonometer (toe-NOM-eh-ter) Instrument for determining intraocular pressure.

tonometry (toe-NOM-eh-tree) The measurement of intraocular pressure.

tonsil (TON-sill) Mass of lymphoid tissue on either side of the throat at the back of the tongue.

tonsillectomy (ton-sih-LEC-toh-me) Surgical removal of the tonsils.

tonsillitis (ton-sih-LIE-tis) Inflammation of the tonsils.

topical (TOP-ih-kal) Medication applied to the skin to obtain a local effect.

torsion (TOR-shun) The act or result of twisting.

Tourette syndrome (tur-ET SIN-drome) Disorder of multiple motor and vocal tics.

toxic (TOK-sick) Pertaining to a toxin.

toxicity (toks-ISS-ih-tee) The state of being poisonous.

toxin (TOK-sin) Poisonous substance formed by a cell or organism.

toxoid (TOK-soyd) Toxin treated to destroy its toxic capability but retain its antigenic capability.

toxoplasmosis (TOK-soh-plaz-MOH-sis) Parasitic infection acquired from undercooked meat from infected animals.

trachea (TRAY-kee-ah) Air tube from the larynx to the bronchi.

trachealis (tray-kee-AY-lis) Pertaining to the trachea.

tracheostomy (tray-kee-OST-oh-me) Incision into the windpipe, usually so that a tube can be inserted to assist breathing.

tracheotomy (tray-kee-OT-oh-me) Incision made into the trachea to create a tracheostomy.

tract (TRAKT) Bundle of nerve fibers with a common origin and destination.

traction (TRAK-shun) A pulling or dragging force.

trait (TRAYT) A discrete characteristic that has a known quality.

tranquilizer (TRANG-kwih-lie-zer) Agent that calms without sedating or depressing.

trans fatty acid (TRANZ FAT-ee ASS-id) Solid or semisolid product of hydrogenation of unsaturated plant oils.

transcatheter (trans-KATH-eh-ter) Catheter with a self-expanding mushroom device that is placed and left inside a PDA.

transcript (TRAN-skript) An exact copy or reproduction.

transcription (tran-SCRIP-shun) The action of making a copy of dictated material.

transcriptionist (tran-SCRIP-shun-ist) One who makes the copy of dictated material.

transdermal (trans-DER-mal) Going across or through the skin.

transducer (trans-DYU-sir) Device that converts energy from one form to another.

transfusion (trans-FYU-zhun) Transfer of blood or a blood component from donor to recipient.

transient (TRANZ-ee-ent) Lasting only a short time.

transplant (TRANZ-plant) The tissue or organ used; *or* the act of transferring tissue from one person to another.

transplantation (TRANZ-plan-TAY-shun) The moving of tissue or an organ from one person or place to another.

transverse (trans-VERS) Pertaining to the horizontal plane dividing the body into upper and lower portions.

transverse fracture (trans-VERS FRAK-chur) A fracture perpendicular to the long axis of the bone.

tremor (TREM-or) Small, shaking, involuntary, repetitive movements of hands, extremities, neck, or jaw.

triceps brachii (TRY-sepz BRAY-key-eye) Muscle of the arm that has three heads or points of origin.

trichinosis (trik-ih-NOH-sis) Disease from ingestion of undercooked pork containing a roundworm.

Trichomonas (trik-oh-MOH-nas) A parasite causing a sexually transmitted disease.

trichomoniasis (TRIK-oh-moh-NIE-ah-sis) Infection with *Trichomonas vaginalis*.

tricuspid (try-KUSS-pid) Having three points; a tricuspid heart valve has three flaps.

trigeminal (try-GEM-in-al) Fifth (V) cranial nerve, with its three different branches supplying the face.

triglyceride (tri-GLISS-eh-ride) Any of a group of fats containing three fatty acids.

triiodothyronine (tri-EYE-oh-doh-THY-roh-neen) Thyroid hormone T3.

trimester (TRY-mes-ter) One-third of the length of a full-term pregnancy.

triplegia (tri-PLEE-jee-ah) Paralysis of three limbs.

trisomy (TRI-so-me) Presence of an extra chromosome.

trochanter (troh-KAN-ter) One of two bony prominences near the head of the femur.

trochlear (TROHK-lee-are) Fourth (IV) cranial nerve; supplies one muscle of the eye.

tropic (TROH-pik) Tropic hormones stimulate other endocrine glands to produce hormones.

trypsin (TRIP-sin) Enzyme that breaks down protein.

tuberculosis (too-BER-kyu-LOW-sis) Infectious disease that can infect any organ or tissue.

tumor (TOO-mor) Any abnormal swelling.

tunica (TYU-nih-kah) A layer in the wall of a blood vessel or other tubular structure.

tunica vaginalis (TYU-nih-kah vaj-ih-NAHL-iss) Covering, particularly of a tubular structure. The tunica vaginalis is the sheath of the testis and epididymis.

turbinate (TUR-bin-ate) Another name for the nasal conchae on the lateral walls of the nasal cavity.

turmeric (ter-MER-ik) Spice used in Ayurvedic medicine.

Turner syndrome (TER-ner SIN-drome) Syndrome associated with a chromosome count of 45 and only one X chromosome.

tympanic (tim-PAN-ik) Pertaining to the tympanic membrane or tympanic cavity.

tympanostomy (tim-pan-OS-toe-me) Surgically created new opening in the tympanic membrane to allow fluid to drain from the middle ear.

typhoid (TIE-foyd) Acute infectious disease caused by *Salmonella typhi*.

U

ulcer (ULL-cer) Erosion of an area of skin or mucosa.

ulceration (ull-cer-A-shun) Formation of an ulcer.

ulcerative (UL-sir-ah-tiv) Marked by an ulcer or ulcers.

ulna (UL-na) The medial and larger bone of the forearm.

ulnar (UL-nar) Pertaining to the ulna or any of the structures (artery, vein, nerve) named after it.

ultrasonography (UL-trah-soh-NOG-rah-fee) Delineation of deep structures using sound waves.

ultrasound (UL-trah-sownd) Use of very high frequency sound waves.

ultraviolet (ul-trah-VIE-oh-let) Electromagnetic rays at higher frequency than the violet end of the spectrum.

umbilical (um-BIL-ih-kal) Pertaining to the umbilicus or the center of the abdomen.

umbilicus (um-BIL-ih-kus) Pit in the abdomen where the umbilical cord entered the fetus.

unconscious (un-KON-shus) Not conscious, lacking awareness.

unessential (un-ee-SEN-shal) Not of importance.

unipolar disorder (you-nih-POLE-ar dis-OR-der) Depression.

unsaturated fatty acid (un-SATCH-you-ray-ted FAT-ee ASS-id) Other atoms can be added to it.

uracil (**YUR**-ah-sil) Chemical found in RNA.

uranium (you-**RAY**-nee-um) Radioactive metallic element.

urea (you-**REE**-ah) End product of nitrogen metabolism.

uremia (you-**REE**-me-ah) The complex of symptoms arising from renal failure.

ureter (you-**RET**-er) Tube that connects the kidney to the urinary bladder.

ureteroscope (you-**REE**-ter-oh-scope) Endoscope to view the inside of the ureter.

ureteroscopy (you-**REE**-ter-os-koh-pee) Examination of the ureter.

urethra (you-**REE**-thra) Canal leading from the bladder to outside.

urethritis (you-ree-**THRI**-tis) Inflammation of the urethra.

urethrotomy (you-ree-**THROT**-oh-me) Incision of a stricture of the urethra.

urinalysis (you-rih-**NAL**-ih-sis) Examination of urine to separate it into its elements and define their kind and/or quantity.

urinary (**YUR**-in-ary) Pertaining to urine.

urinate (**YUR**-in-ate) To pass urine.

urination (yur-ih-**NAY**-shun) The act of passing urine.

urine (**YUR**-in) Fluid and dissolved substances excreted by the kidney.

urological (yur-oh-**LOJ**-ih-kal) Pertaining to urology.

urologist (you-**ROL**-oh-jist) Medical specialist in disorders of the urinary system.

urology (you-**ROL**-oh-jee) Medical specialty of disorders of the urinary system.

urticaria (ur-tee-**KARE**-ee-ah) Rash of itchy wheals (hives).

uterus (**YOU**-ter-us) Organ in which an egg develops into a fetus.

uvea (**YOU**-vee-ah) Middle coat of the eyeball—includes the iris, ciliary body, and choroid.

uveitis (you-vee-**I**-tis) Inflammation of the uvea.

uvula (**YOU**-vyu-lah) Fleshy projection of the soft palate.

V

vaccinate (**VAK**-sin-ate) To administer a vaccine.

vaccination (vak-sih-**NAY**-shun) Administration of a vaccine.

vaccine (**VAK**-seen) Preparation to generate active immunity.

vagina (vah-**JIE**-nah) Female genital canal extending from the uterus to the vulva.

vaginal (**VAJ**-in-al) Pertaining to the vagina.

vaginitis (vah-jih-**NIE**-tis) Inflammation of the vagina.

vaginosis (vah-jih-**NOH**-sis) Any disease of the vagina.

vagus (**VAY**-gus) Tenth (X) cranial nerve; supplies many different organs throughout the body.

varicocele (**VAIR**-ih-koh-seal) Varicose veins of the spermatic cord.

varicose (**VAIR**-ih-kos) Characterized by or affected with varices.

varicosities (vair-ih-**KOS**-ih-tees) Collection of varicose veins.

varix (**VAIR**-iks) Dilated, tortuous vein. Plural *varices.*

vasectomy (vah-**SEK**-toe-me) Excision of a segment of the ductus deferens.

vasoconstriction (**VAY**-soh-con-**STRIK**-shun) Reduction in diameter of a blood vessel.

vasodilation (**VAY**-soh-di-**LAY**-shun) Increase in diameter of a blood vessel.

vasopressin (vay-soh-**PRESS**-in) Pituitary hormone that constricts blood vessels and decreases urine output. Also called *antidiuretic hormone (ADH).*

vasovasostomy (**VAY**-soh-vay-**SOS**-toe-me) Reanastomosis of the ductus deferens to restore the flow of sperm. Also called *vasectomy reversal.*

vector (**VEK**-tor) A virus or other molecule used to carry a gene to target cells; *or* an animal or insect capable of transmitting an infection.

vegan (**VEE**-gan) One who eats plants and no animal or dairy products.

vegetative (**VEJ**-eh-tay-tiv) Functioning unconsciously as plant life is assumed to do.

vein (**VANE**) Blood vessel carrying blood toward the heart.

vena cava (**VEE**-nah **KAY**-vah) One of the two largest veins in the body. Plural *venae cavae.*

venogram (**VEE**-noh-gram) Radiograph of veins after injection of radiopaque contrast material.

venous (**VEE**-nuss) Pertaining to venous blood or the venous circulation.

ventilation (ven-tih-**LAY**-shun) Movement of gases into and out of the lungs.

ventilator (**VEN**-tih-**LAY**-tor) Device that breathes for the patient.

ventral (**VEN**-tral) Pertaining to the belly or situated nearer to the surface of the belly.

ventricle (**VEN**-trih-kel) A cavity of the heart or brain.

ventricular (ven-**TRIK**-you-lar) Pertaining to a ventricle.

venule (**VEN**-yule) Small vein leading from the capillary network.

vermiform (**VER**-mih-form) Worm shaped; used as a descriptor for the appendix.

vernix caseosa (**VER**-nicks kay-see-**OH**-sah) Cheesy substance covering the skin of the fetus.

verruca (ver-**ROO**-cah) Wart caused by a virus.

vertebra (**VER**-teh-brah) One of the bones of the spinal column. Plural *vertebrae.*

vertex (**VER**-teks) Topmost point of the vault of the skull.

vertigo (**VER**-tih-go) Sensation of spinning or whirling.

vesicle (**VES**-ih-kull) Small sac containing liquid; for example, a blister or semen.

vestibule (**VES**-tih-byul) Space at the entrance to a canal.

vestibulectomy (ves-tib-you-**LEK**-toe-me) Surgical excision of the vulva.

vestibulocochlear (ves-**TIB**-you-loh-**KOK**-lee-ar) Eighth (VIII) cranial nerve; carrying information for the senses of hearing and balance.

villus (**VILL**-us) Thin, hairlike projection, particularly of a mucous membrane lining a cavity. Plural *villi*.

viral (**VIE**-ral) Pertaining to a virus.

virilism (**VIR**-ih-lizm) Development of masculine characteristics by a woman or girl.

virulence (**VIR**-you-lence) The power of a toxin or pathogen.

virulent (**VIR**-you-lent) Extremely toxic or pathogenic.

virus (**VIE**-rus) Group of infectious agents that require living cells for growth and reproduction.

viscera (**VISS**-er-ah) Internal organs, particularly in the abdomen.

visceral (**VISS**-er-al) Pertaining to the internal organs.

viscosity (vis-**KOS**-ih-tee) The resistance of a fluid to flowing.

viscous (**VISS**-kus) Sticky; resistant to flow.

viscus (**VISS**-kus) Hollow, walled, internal organ.

visual acuity (**VIH**-zhoo-wal ah-**KYU**-ih-tee) Sharpness and clearness of vision.

visualization (**VIH**-zhoo-wah-lih-**ZAY**-shun) The forming of mental images or pictures.

vital signs (**VI**-tal SIGNS) A procedure during a physical examination in which temperature (T), pulse (P), respirations (R), and blood pressure (BP) are measured to assess general health and cardiorespiratory function.

vitamin (**VYE**-tah-min) Essential organic substance necessary in small amounts for normal cell function.

vitiligo (vit-ill-**EYE**-go) Nonpigmented white patches on otherwise normal skin.

vitreous humor (**VIT**-ree-us **HEW**-mor) A gelatinous liquid in the posterior cavity of the eyeball with the appearance of glass.

vocal (**VOH**-kal) Pertaining to the voice.

void (VOYD) To evacuate urine or feces.

voluntary muscle (**VOL**-un-tare-ee **MUSS**-el) Muscle that is under the control of the will.

vomer (**VOH**-mer) Lower nasal septum.

vulva (**VUL**-vah) Female external genitalia.

vulvodynia (vul-voh-**DIN**-ee-uh) Chronic vulvar pain.

vulvovaginal (**VUL**-voh-**VAJ**-ih-nal) Pertaining to the vulva and vagina.

vulvovaginitis (**VUL**-voh-vaj-ih-**NIE**-tis) Inflammation of the vagina and vulva.

W

warfarin (**WAR**-fuh-rin) Anticoagulant; also used as rat poison, trade name Coumadin.

Weber test (**VA**-ber TEST) Test for sensorineural hearing loss.

wheal (WHEEL) Small, itchy swelling of the skin. Wheals raised by an injection do not itch. Also called *hives*.

whiplash (**WHIP**-lash) Symptoms caused by sudden, uncontrolled extension and flexion of the neck, often in an automobile accident.

white matter (WITE **MATT**-er) Regions of the brain and spinal cord occupied by bundles of axons.

whooping cough (**WHO**-ping KAWF) Infectious disease with spasmodic, intense cough ending on a whoop (stridor). Also called *pertussis*.

Wilms tumor (WILMZ **TOO**-mor) Cancerous kidney tumor of childhood. Also known as *nephroblastoma*.

wound (WOOND) Any injury that interrupts the continuity of skin or a mucous membrane.

X

xenograft (**ZEN**-oh-graft) A graft from another species. Also known as *heterograft*.

Y

yeast (YEEST) Microscopic fungus.

yoga (**YOH**-gah) A system of lifestyle measures.

yolk sac (YOKE SACK) Source of blood cells and future sex cells for the fetus.

Z

zeaxanthin (**ZEE**-ah-**ZAN**-thin) Carotenoid found in pepper, corn, and spinach.

zygoma (zye-**GOH**-mah) Bone that forms the prominence of the cheek.

zygote (**ZYE**-goat) Cell resulting from the union of the sperm and egg.

PHOTO CREDITS

WELCOME CHAPTER

Opener, W.1-W.7, W.9, W.11: © The McGraw-Hill Companies, Inc./Rick Brady, photographer; **W.11:** Corbis RF; **W.12:** © The McGraw-Hill Companies, Inc./Rick Brady, photographer; **Page W-9:** © Vol. 115 PhotoDisc/Getty; **W.13:** © Vol. 66 PhotoDisc/Getty; **W.14:** © The McGraw-Hill Companies, Inc./Rick Brady, photographer; **W.15:** © Dynamicgraphics/Jupiter RF; **W.16:** © Vol. 15 PhotoDisc/Getty.

CHAPTER 1

Opener: © The McGraw-Hill Companies, Inc./Rick Brady, photographer.

CHAPTER 2

Opener: © Corbis RF; **2.2:** © Francis Leroy, Biocosmos/Photo Researchers Inc.; **2.7:** © The McGraw-Hill Companies, Inc./Dr. Alvin Telser; **2.10:** © The McGraw-Hill Companies/Joe DeGrandis, photographer; **2.11:** © The McGraw-Hill Companies, Inc./Eric Wise, photographer; **2.12, 2.14a-b:** © The McGraw-Hill Companies, Inc./Joe DeGrandis, photographer.

CHAPTER 3

Opener: © The McGraw-Hill Companies, Inc./Rick Brady, photographer; **3.4, 3.5:** © BioPhoto Associates/Photo Researchers Inc.; **3.6:** © James Stevenson/Photo Researchers, Inc.; **3.8:** © The McGraw-Hill Companies, Inc./Dennis Strete, photographer; **3.11:** © Medical-on-line/Alamy; **3.12:** © Dr. P. Marazzi/SPL/Photo Researchers, Inc.; **3.13:** © Kenneth Greer/Visuals Unlimited; **3.14:** © Logical Images; **3.15:** © SPL/Photo Researchers, Inc.; **3.16:** © Dr. P. Marazzi/SPL/Photo Researchers, Inc.; **3.17:** © Meckes/Ottawa/Photo Researchers, Inc.; **3.18:** © Dr P. Marazzi/SPL/Photo Researchers, Inc.; **3.19:** Courtesy Dr. Maureen Mayes; **3.20:** © Mediscan/Visuals Unlimited; **3.21:** © Medical-on-line/Alamy; **3.23:** © Kenneth Greer/Visuals Unlimited; **3.25 (all):** © The McGraw-Hill Companies, Inc./Joe DeGrandis, photographer; **3.28:** Reprinted from J. Walter Wilson, *Fungous Diseases of Man*, Plate 42 (middle right), © 1965, The Regents of the University of California; **3.29:** © Logical Images; **3.30a:** © Sheila Terry/Photo Researchers, Inc.; **3.30b:** © Dr. P. Marazzi/SPL/Photo Researchers, Inc.; **3.30c:** © John Radcliffe Hospital/Photo Researchers, Inc.; **3.34:** © Kenneth Greer/Visuals Unlimited.

CHAPTER 4

Opener: © The McGraw-Hill Companies, Inc./Rick Brady, photographer; **4.1:** © The McGraw-Hill Companies, Inc./Joe DeGrandis, photographer; **4.3:** © Phototake Inc./Alamy; **4.4:** © Western Opthamolic Hospital/Photo Researchers Inc.; **4.5:** © SPL/Photo Researchers, Inc.; **4.6** © Mediscan; **4.7:** © ISM/Phototake; **4.9:** © BioPhoto Associates/Photo Researchers Inc.; **4.10:** © Matt Harris Photography/Alamy; **4.18:** © Phototake Inc./Alamy; **4.19:** © National Eye Institute, National Institutes of Health; **4.20:** © Dr. P. Marazzi/SPL/Photo Researchers, Inc.; **4.21** © National Eye Institute, National Institutes of Health; **4.22:** © Paul Parker/Photo Researchers Inc.; **4.23:** © Volume 58/PhotoDisc/Getty; **4.24:** © Chris Barry/Phototake; **4.25:** © National Eye Institute, National Institutes of Health; **4.26:** © Lisa Klancher; **4.29a:** © The McGraw-Hill Companies, Inc./Rick Brady, photographer; **4.29b:** Courtesy Richmond Products, Inc.; **4.30:** © St. Bartholomew's Hospital/Photo Researchers, Inc.; **Page 118:** © The McGraw-Hill Companies, Inc./Rick Brady, photographer; **4.35:** © ISM/Phototake; **4.37:** © Lester V. Bergman/Corbis; **4.38:** © ISM/Phototake; **4.39:** © Collection CNRI/Phototake; **4.40:** © ISM/Phototake.

CHAPTER 5

Opener: © The McGraw-Hill Companies, Inc./Rick Brady, photographer; **5.2:** © The McGraw-Hill Companies, Inc./Christine Eckel, photographer; **5.4:** © Dr. Michael Klein/Peter Arnold, Inc.; **5.5:** © The McGraw-Hill Companies, Inc./Joe DeGrandis, photographer; **5.7:** © SPL/Photo Researchers Inc.; **5.8:** © SIU/Visuals Unlimited; **5.13 (all):** © The McGraw-Hill Companies, Inc./Tim Vacula, photographer; **5.14 (all):** © The McGraw-Hill Companies, Inc./Eric Wise, photographer; **5.15a:** © Du Cane Medical Imaging Ltd./Photo Researchers, Inc.; **5.15b:** © Logical Images; **5.18:** © The McGraw-Hill Companies, Inc./Rick Brady, photographer; **5.30:** © Zephyr/Photo Researchers, Inc.; **5.31:** © The McGraw-Hill Companies, Inc./Christine Eckel, photographer; **5.32:** The McGraw-Hill Companies, Inc./Eric Wise, photographer; **5.33:** © Dr. P. Marazzi/SPL/Photo Researchers Inc.; **5.34:** © Ralph Hutchings/Visuals Unlimited; **5.35:** © Dr. P. Marazzi/SPL/Photo Researchers, Inc.; **5.39:** © Mediscan/Visuals Unlimited; **5.40:** © AJPhoto/Photo Researchers Inc.; **5.43:** © Charles McRae, M.D./Visuals Unlimited; **5.46:** © Sovereign/Phototake Inc.

CHAPTER 6

Opener: © The McGraw-Hill Companies, Inc./Rick Brady, photographer; **6.8:** © Photo Network Stock/Grant Heilman Photography Inc.; **6.9:** © ISM/Phototake; **6.10:** © Medical-on-line/Alamy; **6.11:** © Mediscan/VisualsUnlimited; **6.19:** © CNRI/SPL/Photo Researchers Inc.; **6.24:** © Dr. Joseph William/Phototake; **6.26:** © SIU Biomedical/Photo Researchers, Inc.; **6.31:** © Phototake Inc./Alamy; **6.32:** © CNRI/Photo Researchers, Inc.; **6.34:** © Susan Leavine/Photo Researchers Inc.; **6.35:** © SPL/Photo Researchers Inc.; **6.36:** © Dr. P. Marazzi/SPL/Photo Researchers, Inc.

CHAPTER 7

Opener: © Vol. 40/PhotoDisc/Getty; **7.1:** © The McGraw-Hill Companies, Inc./Eric Wise, photographer; **7.2b:** © Bill Longcore/Photo Researchers, Inc.; **7.5a-b:** © Ed Reschke; **7.6:** © Dr. E. Walker/Photo Researchers, Inc.; **7.7:** © Meckes/Ottawa/Photo Researchers, Inc.; **7.8–7.12:** © Ed Reschke; **7.13:** © Andrew Syred/SPL/Photo Researchers, Inc.; **7.15:** © Oliver Meckes/Photo Researchers, Inc.; **7.16a:** Medical-on-line/Alamy; **7.16b:** © Dr. P. Marazzi/SPL, Photo Researchers, Inc.; **7.16c:** © Paul Cox/Alamy.

CHAPTER 8

Opener, 8.11: © The McGraw-Hill Companies, Inc./Rick Brady, photographer; **8.13 a-b:** © Ed Reschke; **8.14:** © Pasieka/SPL/Photo Researchers, Inc.; **8.16:** © Wellcome Photo Library; **8.22:** © Carolina Biological/Visuals Unlimited; **8.24:** © Dr. P. Marazzi/Photo Researchers, Inc.

CHAPTER 9

Opener: © The McGraw-Hill Companies, Inc./Rick Brady, photographer; **9.7:** © Phototake; **9.12:** © Ralph Hutchings/Visuals Unlimited; **9.13:** © SIU/Visuals Unlimited; **9.16a-b:** © Ralph Hutchings/Visuals Unlimited;

9.18: © Collection CNRI/Phototake; **9.19:** © Wellcome Photo Library; **9.20:** © Garo/Photo Researchers, Inc.

CHAPTER 10

Opener: © The McGraw-Hill Companies, Inc./Rick Brady, photographer; **10.18a-b:** © Phototake Inc./Alamy; **10.19a:** © Wellcome Photo Library; **10.19b:** © R. Spencer Phippen/Phototake Inc.; **10.20:** © Rachel Epstein/The Image Works; **10.21:** © Simon Fraser/Photo Researchers, Inc.; **10.24a:** © ISM/Phototake Inc.; **10.24b:** © Scott Camazine/Alamy; **10.25:** © NIH/Phototake Inc.; **10.26:** © Medicscan; **10.27:** © James Cavallini/Photo Researchers Inc.; **10.28a:** © Wellcome Photo Library; **10.28b:** © Simon Fraser/Newcastle Hospitals NHS/SPL/Photo Researchers, Inc.; **10.29:** © Bart's Medical Library/Phototake Inc.; **10.30:** © O.J. Staats/Custom Medical Stock Photo; **10.31:** © Dr. M.A. Ansary/Custom Medical Stock Photography; **10.33b:** © NMSB/Custom Medical Stock Photo; **10.35a-b:** © Phototake Inc./Alamy; **10.36:** © Marcus E. Raichle.

CHAPTER 11

Opener: © The McGraw-Hill Companies, Inc./Rick Brady, photographer; **11.1b:** © CNRI/SPL/Photo Researchers, Inc.; **11.4:** © Per H. Kjeldsen; **11.7:** © Medical-on-Line/Alamy; **11.11:** © Saturn Stills/SPL/Photo Researchers, Inc.; **11.12:** © SPL/Photo Researchers, Inc.

CHAPTER 12

Opener: © The McGraw-Hill Companies, Inc./Rick Brady, photographer; **12.6:** © Brian Evans/Photo Researchers Inc.; **12.8a:** © Phototake; **12.8b:** © The McGraw-Hill Companies, Inc./Photo by Alvin Telser; **12.11:** © Wellcome Photo Library; **12.12:** © English/Custom Medical Stock Photo.

CHAPTER 13

Opener: © The McGraw-Hill Companies, Inc./Rick Brady, photographer; **13.3:** © CNRI/Photo Researchers, Inc.; **13.4, 13.5:** © Biophoto Associates/Photo Researchers, Inc.; **13.6, 13.7:** © Kenneth Greer/Visuals Unlimited; **13.10:** © SPL/Photo Researchers, Inc.; **13.14:** © Dr. Landrum Shettles; **13.16:** © The William Boyd Museum, Dept. of Pathology and Laboratory Medicine, The University of British Columbia; **13.17:** © Wellcome Photo Library; **13.18:** © The William Boyd Museum, Dept. of Pathology and Laboratory Medicine, The University of British Columbia; **13.19:** © Parviz M. Pour/Photo Researchers Inc.; **13.21:** © Corbis RF; **13.23:** © Getty RF; **13.28:** © BrandX Pictures/Punchstock; **13.30:** © Photo Researchers, Inc.; **13.34:** © Visuals Unlimited; **13.36:** © EP Vol. 90/Getty Images; **13.37:** © Wellcome Photo Library; **13.38:** © ALIX/Phanie/Photo Researchers, Inc.; **13.39:** © TSI/Getty Images; **13.40, 13.41:** © Biophoto Associates/Photo Researchers, Inc.

CHAPTER 14

Opener: © The McGraw-Hill Companies, Inc./Rick Brady, photographer; **14.5:** © Robert Eric/Corbis; **14.6:** Reprinted by permission of publisher from Albert Mendeloff, "Acromegaly, diabetes, hypermetabolism, proteinuria, and heart failure." *American Journal of Medicine*, 20:1, 01-56, p. 135; **14.7:** © Frank Trapper/Corbis; **14.9:** © Biophoto Associates/Photo Researchers, Inc.; **14.10:** © Lester V. Bergman/Corbis; **14.11:** © Dr. P. Marazzi/SPL/Photo Researchers, Inc.; **14.12:** © Mediscan, London; **14.15:** © Bettmann/Corbis; **14.17a-b:** Reprinted from *Atlas of Pediatric Physical Diagnosis*, 3/e by Zitelli and Davis, fig. 19.17, 1997. Mosby-Wolfe Europe Limited, London, UK; **14.18a:** © AP/Wide World Photos; **14.18b:** © Bettmann/Corbis.

CHAPTER 15

Opener: © The McGraw-Hill Companies, Inc./Rick Brady, photographer; **15.4:** © The McGraw-Hill Companies, Inc./Dennis Strete, photographer; **15.6:** © NYU Franklin New Fund/Phototake; **15.7:** © Science VU/Visuals Unlimited; **15.8:** © SPL/Photo Researchers, Inc.

CHAPTER 16

Opener: © The McGraw-Hill Companies, Inc./Rick Brady, photographer; **16.3:** © St. Bartholomew's Hospital, London/Photo Researchers, Inc.; **16.4:** © Sally and Richard Greenhill/Alamy; **16.5:** © Scott Camazine/Alamy; **16.6:** © Medical-on-Line/Alamy; **16.7:** © NMSB/Custom Medical Stock Photo; **16.8:** © Susan Leavines/Photo Researchers, Inc.; **16.9:** © Wellcome Medical Trust Library; **16.10:** © David Parker/Photo Researchers, Inc.; **16.11:** © Barry Slaven, MD, PhD/Phototake; **16.12:** © Wong Adam/Redlink/Corbis; **16.13:** © Pasieka/SPL/Photo Researchers, Inc.

CHAPTER 17

Opener: © The McGraw-Hill Companies, Inc./Rick Brady, photographer; **17.1:** © Vol. 12/PhotoLink/Getty Images; **17.2:** © The McGraw-Hill Companies, Inc./Elite Images; **17.3:** © Vol. 83/Corbis; **17.4:** © OS49 PhotoDisc/Getty; **17.5:** © Biophoto Associates/Photo Researchers, Inc.; **17.6:** © Wellcome Photo Library; **17.7:** © Vol. 20/PhotoDisc/Getty; **17.8a-b:** © Vol. OS49/PhotoDisc/Getty; **17.9:** © Photo Network Stock/Grant Heilman Photography Inc.; **17.11:** © Gary D. McMichael/Photo Researchers, Inc.

CHAPTER 18

Opener: © The McGraw-Hill Companies, Inc./Rick Brady, photographer; **18.1a-b:** © Courtesy of North Coast Medical; **18.2a:** © Mediscan/Visuals Unlimited; **18.2b:** © AJPhoto/Photo Researchers Inc. **18.3:** © The McGraw-Hill Companies, Inc./Rick Brady, photographer; **18.4:** © Roger Ressmeyer/Corbis; **18.5:** © Mona Reeder/Dallas Morning News/Corbis; **18.6–18.10:** © The McGraw-Hill Companies, Inc./Rick Brady, photographer.

CHAPTER 19

Opener: © The McGraw-Hill Companies, Inc./Rick Brady, photographer; **19.1:** © Vol. 15 PhotoDisc/Getty; **19.2:** © Will & Deni McIntyre/Photo Researchers Inc.; **19.3:** © Paul Almasy/Corbis; **19.4:** © Dr. P. Marazzi/SPL/Photo Researchers Inc.; **19.5:** © Royalty-Free/Corbis; **19.6:** © Masterfile.

CHAPTER 20

Opener: © Mark Pearson/Alamy; **20.4:** © Kathy Park Talaro; **20.5, 20.6:** Centers for Disease Control and Prevention; **20.7:** © Custom Medical Stock Photo; **20.9:** © Dr. Jack M. Bostrack/Visuals Unlimited; **20.10:** © Kathy Park Talaro; **20.11:** © CNRI/SPL/Photo Researchers, Inc.; **20.12:** © Dennis Kunkel Microscopy, Inc./Phototake Inc./Alamy; **20.13:** Credit: Dr. S. Knutton from D.R. Lloyd and S. Knurron, *Infection and Immunity*, January 1987, p. 86–92. © ASM; **20.14, 20.15:** Centers for Disease Control and Prevention; **20.16:** © Vol. 18 PhotoDisc/Getty; **20.17a-b:** Dr. Judy A. Murphy, San Joaquin Delta College, Department of Microscopy, Stockton, CA; **20.18:** © Dr. P. Marazzi/SPL/Photo Researchers, Inc.; **20.19:** National Genome New Institute/NIH; **20.20:** © Eric Grave/Photo Researchers, Inc.; **20.21:** © Henry Westheim Photography/Alamy; **20.22:** © Taylor Jorjorian/Alamy; **20.23:** © The McGraw-Hill Companies, Inc./Rick Brady, photographer.

CHAPTER 21

Opener: © Lauren Shear/Photo Researchers Inc.; **21.2:** © CNRI/Photo Researchers, Inc.; **21.7:** © Hattie Young/Photo Researchers, Inc.

CHAPTER 22

Opener: © The McGraw-Hill Companies, Inc./Rick Brady, photographer; **22.2:** © Steve Gschmeissner/SPL/Photo Researchers, Inc.; **22.3:** © Ed Reschke; **22.4:** © The McGraw-Hill Companies, Inc./Jill Braaten, photographer; **22.5:** © Getty RF; **22.6:** © Garry D. McMichael/Photo Researchers, Inc.; **22.7:** © Medical Elements PhotoDisc/Getty Images; **22.8:** © Dynamic Graphics/RF/Jupiter; **22.9:** © Tomas del Amo/Alamy; **22.10:** © Vol. 40 PhotoDisc/GettyImages; **22.11:** © ISM/Phototake, Inc.; **22.12:** © Wellcome Photo Library; **22.14:** Courtesy Varian Medical Systems.

CHAPTER 23

Opener: © Corbis RF; **23.1:** © garythephotographer; **23.2:** © Vol. 189 Corbis RF; **23.3:** © Vol. 67 PhotoDisc/Getty Images; **23.4:** © Image Source/Alamy; **23.5:** © Vol.189 Corbis RF; **23.6:** © The McGraw-Hill Companies, Inc./Rick Brady, photographer; **23.7:** © Will & Deni McIntyre/Photo Researchers, Inc.; **23.8:** © Scott Camazine/Photo-Researchers, Inc.; **23.9:** © Dag Sundberg/Alamy.

ILLUSTRATION CREDITS

WELCOME CHAPTER

W.10: Adapted from *Integrated Basic Sciences: PreTest Self-Assessment and Review,* by Earl Brown. Copyright © 1998 The McGraw-Hill Companies, Inc. Reprinted with permission.

CHAPTER 1

Table 1.5: Adapted from *Anatomy and Physiology* 3e, by Kenneth S. Saladin. Copyright © 2004 The McGraw-Hill Companies, Inc. Reprinted with permission.

CHAPTER 2

Table 2.1: Adapted from *Hole's Human Anatomy and Physiology,* 10, by Shier, Butler, and Lewis. Copyright © 2004 The McGraw-Hill Companies, Inc. Reprinted with permission.; **Table 2.2:** Adapted from *Hole's Human Anatomy and Physiology,* 10, by Shier, Butler, and Lewis. Copyright © 2004 The McGraw-Hill Companies, Inc. Reprinted with permission.

CHAPTER 4

Figure 4.28: The images were reproduced, with permission, from Ishihara's Tests for Colour Deficiency published by KANEHARA TRADING INC., located at Tokyo in Japan. But tests for color deficiency cannot be conducted with this material. For accurate testing, the original plates should be used.; **Figure 4.29b:** Courtesy of Richmond Products.

CHAPTER 9

TA 8.2: Courtesy of Bibbero Systems, Inc, Petaluma, CA.

CHAPTER 12

Case Report 13.3: Courtesy of Bibbero Systems, Inc, Petaluma, CA.

CHAPTER 17

Table 17.1: Based on U.S. Department of Agriculture (USDA), www.mypyramid.gov, 2005.; **Figure 17.10:** NIH Publication.;

Figure 17.12: Copyright © 2000 Oldways Preservation & Exchange Trust.; **Figure 17.13:** From *JAMA,* 2001; 285(3), pp. 2486–97. Reprinted with permission from the American Medical Association. **Figure 17.14:** U.S. Department of Agriculture (USDA).

CHAPTER 22

Table 22.1: From National Vital Statistic Report, October 2004.

From *Anatomy & Physiology: The Unity and Form of Function,* (3rd edition), by K. S. Saladin, 2004, Dubuque, IA: The McGraw-Hill Companies, Inc.: Unnumbered figure page 26; Figures 2.1, 2.3, 2.4, 2.5, 2.6, 2.8, 2.9, 2.13, unnumbered figure page 44, 3.1, 3.7, 3.22, 3.24, 3.25, 3.27, 3.30, 3.31, 3.32, 3.33, 4.27, 4.31, 4.36, 4.41, 4.43, 4.44, 5.1, 5.6, 5.10, 5.11, 5.12, 5.26, 5.27, 5.28, 6.12, 6.13, 6.14, 6.15, 6.16, 6.22, 6.23, 6.25, 6.27, 6.29, 6.30, 6.33, 7.4, 7.18, 8.1, 8.2, 8.4, 8.5, 8.6, 8.7, 8.12, 8.18, 8.19, 8.20, 8.21, 8.23, unnumbered figure page 334, 9.1, 9.2, 9.3, 9.4, 9.5, 9.6, 9.8, 9.10, 9.14, 10.1, 10.2, 10.3, 10.4, 10.12, 10.13, 10.14, 10.15, 10.16, 10.17, 10.23, 10.34, 11.1a, 11.2b, 11.6, 11.8, 11.10, 12.1, 12.2, 12.3, 12.7, 13.1, 13.2, 13.8, 13.11, 13.12, 13.13, 13.15, 13.24, 13.26, 13.27, 13.29, 13.31, 13.33, 13.35, 14.1, 14.2, 14.3, 14.4, 14.8, 14.13, 14.14, 14.16, 14.19, 15.1, 15.3, 15.5, 16.1, 16.2, 20.3, 21.1, 21.3.

From *Human Anatomy,* by K. S. Saladin, 2005, Dubuque, IA: The McGraw-Hill Companies, Inc.: Figures 3.3, unnumbered figure page 86, 4.1, 4.2, 4.14, 5.9, 5.17, 5.20, 5.21, 5.22, 5.23, 5.25, 5.29, 5.31, 5.36, 5.37, 5.41, 5.42, 5.44, 5.45, 6.2, 6.3, 6.4, 6.7, 6.20, 6.21, 10.7, 10.8, unnumbered figure page 477, 13.25, 15.2.

From *Human Anatomy,* by M. McKinley and V. D. O'Loughlin, 2006, Dubuque, IA: The McGraw-Hill Companies, Inc.: Figures 3.26, 4.11, 4.12, 4.13, 4.15, 4.16, 4.17, 4.42, unnumbered figure page 142, 5.2, 5.3, 5.16, 6.6, 6.18, 8.15, 9.9, 9.15, 9.17, 9.21, 10.5, 10.6, 10.10, 10.33, 11.5, 11.9, 12.8, 12.9, 12.10, 13.22.

From *Hole's Human Anatomy & Physiology,* (10th edition), by D. Shier, J. Butler, and R. Lewis, 2004, Dubuque, IA: The McGraw-Hill Companies, Inc.: Figures 2.6, 3.2, 4.8, 4.32, 4.34, 5.24, 5.36, 5.38, 6.1, 6.5, 6.17, 7.2, 7.3, 7.17, 8.8, 8.9, 8.17, 9.6, 10.9, 10.11, 10.30, 11.2a, 12.4, 12.5, 13.9.

From *Microbiology: A Systems Approach,* by M. K. Cowan and K. P. Talaro, 2006, Dubuque, IA: The McGraw-Hill Companies, Inc.: Figures 15.9, 20.1, 20.8, 20.19.

From *Medical Assisting: Administrative and Clinical Competencies,* (2nd edition), by B. Ramutkowski, K. A. Booth, D. J. Pugh, S. Thomson, and L. Whicker, 2005, Dubuque, IA: The McGraw-Hill Companies, Inc.: Figures 3-9, 3-10, 11.14.

From *Anatomy & Physiology,* (7th edition), by R. R. Seeley, T. D. Stephens, and P. Tate, 2006, Dubuque, IA: The McGraw-Hill Companies, Inc.: Figures 5.9, 5.19, unnumbered figure page 200, 6.28, 6.32, 7.1, 8.3, 8.10, 9.11, 11.3.

From *Pathophysiology: Concepts and Applications for Health Care Professionals* (3rd edition), by T. J. Nowak and A. G. Handford, 2004, Dubuque, IA: The McGraw-Hill Companies, Inc.: Figures 20.2, 22.1.

From *Identification, Evaluation, and Treatment of Overweight and Obesity in Adults: The Practical Guide.* Bethesda, MD: National Institutes of Health 2000; NIH publication 00-4064: Figure 17.10.

From Executive Summary of the Third Report of the National Cholesterol Education Program (NCEP) Expert Panel on Detection, Evaluation, and Treatment of High Blood Cholesterol in Adults (Adult Treatment Panel III). JAMA 2001; 285(3): 2486–97: Figure 17.13.

From United States Department of Agriculture: Figure 17.14.

From *Genetics: Analysis and Principles* (3rd edition), by R. J. Brooker, 2009, Dubuque, IA: The McGraw-Hill Companies, Inc.: Figure 21.4.

From *Medical Genetics,* by G. H. Sack, Jr., 1998, New York: The McGraw-Hill Companies, Inc.: Figure 21.5.

A